Ackley & Ladwig's

# Guide to
# NURSING
# DIAGNOSIS

SEVENTH EDITION

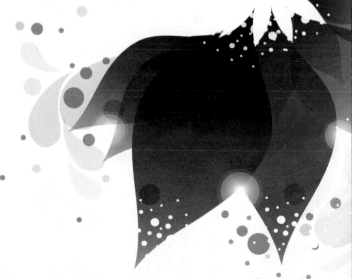

Ackley & Ladwig's

# Guide to
# NURSING
# DIAGNOSIS

SEVENTH EDITION

**Marina Reyna Martinez-Kratz,**
MS, RN, CNE

Professor
Department of Nursing
Jackson College
Jackson, Michigan

**Mary Beth Flynn Makic,**
PhD, RN, CCNS, CCRN-K, FAAN, FNAP, FCNS

Professor
Program Director, Adult-Gerontology Clinical Nurse Specialist
    Program
College of Nursing
University of Colorado
Aurora, Colorado

ELSEVIER

3251 Riverport Lane
St. Louis, Missouri 63043

ACKLEY AND LADWIG'S GUIDE TO NURSING      ISBN: 978-0-323-81271-9
DIAGNOSIS, SEVENTH EDITION
**Copyright © 2023 by Elsevier Inc. All rights reserved.**

No part of this publication may be reproduced or transmitted in any form or by any
means, electronic or mechanical, including photocopying, recording, or any information
storage and retrieval system, without permission in writing from the publisher. Details on
how to seek permission, further information about the Publisher's permissions policies,
and our arrangements with organizations such as the Copyright Clearance Center and the
Copyright Licensing Agency can be found at our website: www.elsevier.com/permissions.

This book and the individual contributions contained in it are protected under copyright
by the Publisher (other than as may be noted herein).

T. Heather Herdman/Shigemi Kamitsuru/Camila Takáo Lopes (Eds.), NANDA
International, Inc. *Nursing Diagnoses: Definitions and Classification 2021-2023*, twelfth
edition. © 2021 NANDA International, ISBN 978-1-68420-454-0. Used by arrangement
with the Thieme Group, Stuttgart/New York. In order to make safe and effective
judgments using NANDA-I diagnoses, it is essential that nurses refer to the definitions
and defining characteristics of the diagnoses listed in this work.

---

**Notice**

Practitioners and researchers must always rely on their own experience and knowledge in evaluating and using any information, methods, compounds or experiments
described herein. Because of rapid advances in the medical sciences, in particular,
independent verification of diagnoses and drug dosages should be made. To the
fullest extent of the law, no responsibility is assumed by Elsevier, authors, editors
or contributors for any injury and/or damage to persons or property as a matter of
products liability, negligence or otherwise, or from any use or operation of any methods, products, instructions, or ideas contained in the material herein.

---

Previous editions copyrighted 2020, 2017, 2014, 2011, 2008, and 2006.

*Senior Content Strategist:* Sandra Clark
*Senior Content Development Specialist:* Rae L. Robertson
*Publishing Services Manager:* Julie Eddy
*Book Production Specialist:* Clay S. Broeker
*Design Direction:* Patrick Ferguson

Printed in Canada

Last digit is the print number:   9  8  7  6  5  4  3  2  1

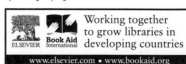

Working together
to grow libraries in
developing countries

www.elsevier.com • www.bookaid.org

# DEDICATION

*To all the nurses who are working on the front lines. To my best friend and the love of my life, Kent Martinez-Kratz. To my children, Maxwell, Jesse, and Sierra, whose love, inspiration, and wit make my life complete. To my first fans, my parents Angel and Eva and siblings Debra and Jason. To Gail Ladwig, for being the absolute best nursing professor, mentor, colleague, and comadre. Finally, to Betty Ackley's memory, for inspiring excellence in nursing education and practice.*

**Marina Reyna Martinez-Kratz**

*To nursing colleagues throughout the world who continue to demonstrate our un-wavering commitment to providing exceptional physical, emotional, and spiritual care. Special thanks to my family. To my husband and children, whose unconditional love and support are ever present in my life. To my parents and sisters for always encouraging me to follow my passion. Finally, to Betty Ackley and Gail Ladwig for their steadfast commitment to the profession of nursing as expert teachers and prolific authors. Your leadership and spirit continue to inform nursing practice excellence.*

**Mary Beth Flynn Makic**

# ACKNOWLEDGMENTS

The authors would like to thank the following individuals for their contributions to *Ackley and Ladwig's Nursing Diagnosis Handbook: An Evidence-Based Guide to Planning Care,* thirteenth edition, by Mary Beth Flynn Makic and Marina Reyna Martinez-Kratz, from which this book has been developed:

**Keith A. Anderson, PhD, MSW**

**Amanda Andrews, BSc (Hons), MA**

**Carla Aresco, MSL, CRNP**

**Suzanne C. Ashworth, MSN, APRN, CCRN, CCNS**

**Kathaleen C. Bloom, PhD, CNM**

**Susan Bonini, EdD, MSN, RN**

**Monica Brock, MSN, RN, CCRN, CNEcl**

**Elyse Bueno, MS, ACCNS-AG, CCRN, NE-BC**

**Stacey M. Carroll, PhD, APRN-BC**

**Nadia Ali Muhammad Ali Charania, PhD, RN**

**Nichol Chesser, RN, CNM, DNP**

**Lorraine Chiappetta, MSN, RN, CNE**

**JoAnn Coar, MSN, RN-BC, A-GNP-C, CWOCN**

**Maureen F. Cooney, DNP, FNP-BC, ACHPN, AP-PMN**

**Mary Rose Day, DN, MA, PGDip PHN, BSc, RPHN, RM, RGN**

**Helen I. de Graaf-Waar, MSc, RN**

**Mary E. Desmond, PhD, RN, MA, MSN, AHN-BC**

**Julianne E. Doubet, BSN, RN, EMT-B**

**Margaret M. Egan-Touw, DNP, RN, CNE**

**Dawn Fairlie, PhD, NP**

**Arlene T. Farren, PhD, RN, AOCN, CTN-A**

**Judith Ann Floyd, PhD, RN, FNAP, FAAN**

**Meredith Ford, MSN, RN, CNE**

**Katherine Foss, MSN, RN**

**Maria Galletto, MSN, RN, CNL, CPHQ**

**Tracy P. George, DNP, APRN-BC, CNE**

Susanne W. Gibbons, PhD, C-ANP/GNP

Barbara A. Given, PhD, RN, FAAN

Pauline McKinney Green, PhD, RN, CNE

Sherry A. Greenberg, PhD, RN, GNP-BC, FGSA, FAANP, FAAN

Linda J. Hassler, DNP, RN, GCNS-BC, FGNLA

Dianne F. Hayward, RN, MSN, WHNP

Kelly Henrichs, DNP, RN, GNP-BC

Dina M. Hewett, PhD, RN, NEA-BC

Patricia Hindin, PhD, CNM

Paula D. Hopper, MSN, RN, CNE

Wendie A. Howland, MN, RN-BC, CRRN, CCM, CNLCP, LNCC

Teri Hulett, RN, BSN, CIC, FAPIC

Nicole Huntley, MS, RN, APN, ACCNS-AG

Olga F. Jarrín, PhD, RN

Laura King, DNP, RN, MSN, CNE

Rachel Klompmaker, BScN, NP-PHC, MScN

Gail B. Ladwig, MSN, RN

Patrick Luna, MSN, RN, CEN, NRP

Mary Beth Flynn Makic, PhD, RN, CCNS, CCRN-K, FAAN, FNAP, FCNS

Mary Patricia Mancuso, MA

Marina Reyna Martinez-Kratz, MS, RN, CNE

Lauren McAlister, MSN, FNP-BC, DNP

Kimberly S. Meyer, PhD, ACNP-BC, CNRN

Daniela Moscarella, DNP, APN, CPNP-PC, CCRN-K

Morgan Nestingen, MSN, APRN, AGCNS-BC, OCN, ONN-CG

Katherina A. Nikzad-Terhune, PhD, MSW

Darcy O'Banion, RN, MS, ACCNS-AG

Kenneth J. Oja, PhD, RN

Kristen A. Oster, DNP, APRN, ACNS-BC, CNOR, CNS-CP

Kathleen L. Patusky, PhD, MA, RN, CNS

Kim L. Paxton, DNP, APRN, ANP-BC, LHIT-C

Nishat S. Poppy, BSN, RN

Ann Will Poteet, MS, RN, CNS, AGNP-C

Margaret Quinn, DNP, CPNP, CNE

Friso Raemaekers, B Health, RN, CEN

Barbara A. Reyna, PhD, RN, NNP-BC

Mamilda Robinson, DNP, APN, PMHNP-BC

Kimberly Anne Rumsey, MSN, RN, CNE

Debra Siela, PhD, RN, ACNS-BC, CCRN-K, CNE, RRT

Tammy Spencer, DNP, RN, CNE, AGCNS-BC, CCNS

Bernie St. Aubyn, BSc (Hons), MSc

Denise Sullivan, MSN, ANP-BC, ACHPN, AP-PMN

Jacquelyn Svoboda, DNP, RN, WHNP-C

Philemon Tedros, BSN, RN

Krystal Chamberlain Tenure, MSN, RN, CCRN, SCRN

Rosemary Timmerman, DNP, APRN, CCNS, CCRN-CSC-CMC

Janelle M. Tipton, DNP, APRN-CNS, AOCN

Mary Velahos, BSN

Barbara Baele Vincensi, PhD, RN, FNP-BC

Jody L. Vogelzang, PhD, RDN, CHES, FAND

Suzanne White, MSN, RN, PHCNS-BC

David M. Wikstrom, BSN, RN, CMSRN

Ruth A. Wittmann-Price, PhD, RN, CNS, CNE, CNEcl. CHSE, ANEF, FAAN

Wendy Worden, MS, APRN, CNS, CRRN, CWCN

## Assess

Assess the client using the format provided by the clinical setting. Collect data including client's symptoms, clinical state, and known medical or psychiatric diagnoses.

## Diagnose

Use Section I, Guide to Nursing Diagnoses, and locate the client's symptoms, clinical state, medical or psychiatric diagnoses, and anticipated or prescribed diagnostic studies or surgical interventions (listed in alphabetical order). Note suggestions for appropriate nursing diagnoses.

Then use Section II, Guide to Planning Care, to evaluate each suggested nursing diagnosis and "related to" etiology statement. Section II is a listing of care plans according to NANDA-I, arranged alphabetically by diagnostic concept, for each nursing diagnosis referred to in Section I. Determine the appropriateness of each nursing diagnosis by comparing the Defining Characteristics and/or Risk Factors to the client data collected.

## Determine Outcomes

Use Section II, Guide to Planning Care, to find appropriate outcomes for the client.

## Plan Interventions

Use Section II, Guide to Planning Care, to find appropriate interventions for the client.

## Give Nursing Care

Administer nursing care following the plan of care based on the interventions.

## Evaluate Nursing Care

Evaluate nursing care administered using the Client Outcomes. If the outcomes were not met and the nursing interventions were not effective, reassess the client and determine if the appropriate nursing diagnoses were made.

## Document

Document all of the previous steps using the format provided in the clinical setting.

# CONTENTS

## SECTION I Guide to Nursing Diagnosis, 1

An alphabetized list of medical, surgical, and psychiatric diagnoses; diagnostic procedures, clinical states, symptoms, and problems, with suggested nursing diagnoses.

## SECTION II Guide to Planning Care, 157

The definition, defining characteristics, risk factors, related factors, client outcomes, interventions, geriatric interventions, pediatric interventions, critical care interventions, home care interventions, culturally competent nursing interventions (when appropriate), and client/family teaching and discharge planning for each alphabetized nursing diagnosis.

## APPENDIX

Nursing Care Plans for Hearing Loss and Vision Loss, 841

## BIBLIOGRAPHY, 851

## INDEX, 881

# CONTENTS

**SECTION I** Guide to Nursing Practice

**SECTION II**

# GUIDE TO NURSING DIAGNOSIS

Section I is an alphabetical listing of client symptoms, client problems, medical diagnoses, psychosocial diagnoses, and clinical states. Each of these will have a list of possible nursing diagnoses. You may use this section to find suggestions for nursing diagnoses for your client.

• Assess the client using the format provided by the clinical setting.

• Locate the client's symptoms, problems, clinical state, diagnoses, surgeries, and diagnostic testing in the alphabetical listing contained in this section.

• Note suggestions given for appropriate nursing diagnoses.

• Evaluate the suggested nursing diagnoses to determine whether they are appropriate for the client and are supported by the information that was found in the assessment.

• Use Section II (which contains an alphabetized list of all NANDA-I approved nursing diagnoses) to validate this information and check the definition, defining characteristics (if appropriate), risk factors, related factors, at risk populations, and associated conditions. Determine whether the nursing diagnosis you have selected is appropriate for the client.

SECTION

1

# A

## ABDOMINAL DISTENTION

**Chronic Functional Constipation** r/t habitually suppresses urge to defecate, impaired physical mobility, inadequate dietary intake, insufficient fiber intake, insufficient fluid intake

**Constipation** r/t decreased activity, decreased fluid intake, decreased fiber intake, pathological process

**Dysfunctional Gastrointestinal Motility** r/t decreased perfusion of intestines, medication effect

**Nausea** r/t irritation of gastrointestinal tract

**Imbalanced Nutrition: Less Than Body Requirements** r/t nausea, vomiting

**Acute Pain** r/t retention of air, gastrointestinal secretions

**Delayed Surgical Recovery** r/t retention of gas, secretions

## ABDOMINAL HYSTERECTOMY

*See Hysterectomy*

## ABDOMINAL PAIN

**Dysfunctional Gastrointestinal Motility** r/t decreased perfusion, medication effect

**Acute Pain** r/t injury, pathological process

## ABDOMINAL SURGERY

**Constipation** r/t decreased activity, decreased fluid intake, anesthesia, opioids

**Dysfunctional Gastrointestinal Motility** r/t medication or anesthesia effect, trauma from surgery

**Imbalanced Nutrition: Less Than Body Requirements** r/t high metabolic needs, decreased ability to ingest or digest food

**Acute Pain** r/t surgical procedure

**Ineffective Peripheral Tissue Perfusion** r/t immobility, abdominal surgery

**Risk for Delayed Surgical Recovery:** Risk factor: extensive surgical procedure

**Risk for Surgical Site Infection:** Risk factor: invasive procedure

**Risk for Thrombosis:** Risk factor: impaired physical mobility, smoking

**Readiness for Enhanced Knowledge:** expresses an interest in learning

*See Surgery, Perioperative Care; Surgery, Postoperative Care; Surgery, Preoperative Care*

## ABDOMINAL TRAUMA

**Disturbed Body Image** r/t scarring, change in body function, need for temporary colostomy

**Ineffective Breathing Pattern** r/t abdominal distention, pain

**Deficient Fluid Volume** r/t hemorrhage, active fluid volume loss

**Dysfunctional Gastrointestinal Motility** r/t decreased perfusion

**Acute Pain** r/t abdominal trauma

**Risk for Bleeding:** Risk factor: trauma and possible contusion/rupture of abdominal organs

**Risk for Infection:** Risk factor: possible perforation of abdominal structures

## ABLATION, RADIOFREQUENCY CATHETER

**Fear** r/t invasive procedure

**Risk for Decreased Cardiac Tissue Perfusion:** Risk factor: catheterization of heart

## ABORTION, INDUCED

**Compromised Family Coping** r/t unresolved feelings about decision

**Acute Pain** r/t surgical intervention

**Chronic Low Self-Esteem** r/t feelings of guilt

**Chronic Sorrow** r/t loss of potential child

**Risk for Bleeding:** Risk factor: trauma from abortion

**Risk for Infection:** Risk factors: open uterine blood vessels, dilated cervix

**Risk for Post-Trauma Syndrome:** Risk factor: psychological trauma of abortion

**Risk for Spiritual Distress:** Risk factor: perceived moral implications of decision

**Readiness for Enhanced Health Literacy:** expresses desire to enhance personal health care decisions

**Readiness for Enhanced Knowledge:** expresses an interest in learning

**A**

## ABORTION, SPONTANEOUS

**Disturbed Body Image** r/t perceived inability to carry pregnancy, produce child

**Disabled Family Coping** r/t unresolved feelings about loss

**Ineffective Coping** r/t personal vulnerability

**Interrupted Family Processes** r/t unmet expectations for pregnancy and childbirth

**Fear** r/t implications for future pregnancies

**Risk for Maladaptive Grieving** r/t loss of fetus

**Acute Pain** r/t uterine contractions, surgical intervention

**Situational Low Self-Esteem** r/t feelings about loss of fetus

**Chronic Sorrow** r/t loss of potential child

**Risk for Bleeding:** Risk factor: trauma from abortion

**Risk for Infection:** Risk factors: septic or incomplete abortion of products of conception, open uterine blood vessels, dilated cervix

**Risk for Post-Trauma Syndrome:** Risk factor: psychological trauma of abortion

**Risk for Spiritual Distress:** Risk factor: loss of fetus

**Readiness for Enhanced Knowledge:** expresses an interest in learning

## ABRUPTIO PLACENTAE <36 WEEKS

**Anxiety** r/t unknown outcome, change in birth plans

**Death Anxiety** r/t unknown outcome, hemorrhage, or pain

**Interrupted Family Processes** r/t unmet expectations for pregnancy and childbirth

**Fear** r/t threat to well-being of self and fetus

**Impaired Gas Exchange: Placental** r/t decreased uteroplacental area

**Acute Pain** r/t irritable uterus, hypertonic uterus

**Impaired Tissue Integrity: Maternal** r/t possible uterine rupture

**Risk for Bleeding:** Risk factor: separation of placenta from uterus causing bleeding

**Risk for Infection:** Risk factor: partial separation of placenta

**Risk for Disturbed Maternal–Fetal Dyad:** Risk factors: trauma of process, lack of energy of mother

**Risk for Shock:** Risk factor: separation of placenta from uterus

**Readiness for Enhanced Knowledge:** expresses an interest in learning

## ABSCESS FORMATION

**Acute Pain** r/t inflammation

**Ineffective Protection** r/t inadequate nutrition, abnormal blood profile, drug therapy, depressed immune function

**Impaired Tissue Integrity** r/t altered circulation, nutritional deficit or excess

**Readiness for Enhanced Knowledge:** expresses an interest in learning

## ABUSE, CHILD

*See Child Abuse*

## ABUSE, SPOUSE, PARENT, OR SIGNIFICANT OTHER

**Anxiety** r/t threat to self-concept, situational crisis of abuse

**Caregiver Role Strain** r/t chronic illness, self-care deficits, lack of respite care, extent of caregiving required

**Impaired Verbal Communication** r/t psychological barriers of fear

**Compromised Family Coping** r/t abusive patterns

**Defensive Coping** r/t low self-esteem

**Disturbed Family Identity Syndrome** r/t unaddressed domestic violence

**Dysfunctional Family Processes** r/t inadequate coping skills

**Insomnia** r/t psychological stress

**Post-Trauma Syndrome** r/t history of abuse

**Powerlessness** r/t lifestyle of helplessness

**Chronic Low Self-Esteem** r/t negative family interactions

**Risk for Impaired Emancipated Decision-Making:** Risk factor: inability to verbalize needs and wants

**Risk for Female Genital Mutilation:** Risk factor: lack of family knowledge about impact of practice on physical health

**Risk for Self-Directed Violence:** Risk factor: history of abuse

## ACCESSORY MUSCLE USE (TO BREATHE)

**Ineffective Breathing Pattern** (See **Breathing Pattern, Ineffective,** Section II)

*See Asthma; Bronchitis; COPD (Chronic Obstructive Pulmonary Disease); Respiratory Infections, Acute Childhood (Croup, Epiglottis, Pertussis, Pneumonia, Respiratory Syncytial Virus)*

## ACCIDENT PRONE

**Frail Elderly Syndrome** r/t history of falls

**Acute Confusion** r/t altered level of consciousness

**Ineffective Coping** r/t personal vulnerability, situational crises

**Ineffective Impulse Control** (See **Impulse Control, Ineffective,** Section II)

**Risk for Injury:** Risk factor: history of accidents

**Wandering** r/t overstimulating environment

## ACHALASIA

**Ineffective Coping** r/t chronic disease

**Acute Pain** r/t stasis of food in esophagus

**Impaired Swallowing** r/t neuromuscular impairment

**Risk for Aspiration:** Risk factor: nocturnal regurgitation

## ACID-BASE IMBALANCES

**Risk for Electrolyte Imbalance:** Risk factors: renal dysfunction, diarrhea, treatment-related side effects (e.g., medications, drains)

## ACIDOSIS, METABOLIC

**Acute Confusion** r/t acid-base imbalance, associated electrolyte imbalance

**Impaired Memory** r/t effect of metabolic acidosis on brain function

**Imbalanced Nutrition: Less Than Body Requirements** r/t inability to ingest, absorb nutrients

**Risk for Electrolyte Imbalance:** Risk factor: effect of metabolic acidosis on renal function

**Risk for Injury:** Risk factors: disorientation, weakness, stupor

**Risk for Decreased Cardiac Tissue Perfusion:** Risk factor: dysrhythmias from hyperkalemia

**Risk for Shock:** Risk factors: abnormal metabolic state, presence of acid state impairing function, decreased tissue perfusion

## ACIDOSIS, RESPIRATORY

**Decreased Activity Tolerance** r/t imbalance between oxygen supply and demand

**Impaired Gas Exchange** r/t ventilation-perfusion imbalance

**Impaired Memory** r/t hypoxia

**Risk for Decreased Cardiac Tissue Perfusion:** Risk factor: dysrhythmias associated with respiratory acidosis

## ACNE

**Disturbed Body Image** r/t biophysical changes associated with skin disorder

**Ineffective Health Self-Management** r/t insufficient knowledge of therapeutic regimen

**Impaired Skin Integrity** r/t hormonal changes (adolescence, menstrual cycle)

## ACROMEGALY

**Decreased Activity Tolerance**

**Ineffective Airway Clearance** r/t airway obstruction by enlarged tongue

**Disturbed Body Image** r/t changes in body function and appearance

**Impaired Physical Mobility** r/t joint pain

**Risk for Decreased Cardiac Tissue Perfusion:** Risk factor: increased atherosclerosis from abnormal health status

**Risk for Unstable Blood Glucose Level:** Risk factor: abnormal physical health status

**Sexual Dysfunction** r/t changes in hormonal secretions

**Risk for Overweight:** Risk factor: energy expenditure less than energy intake

**A**

## ACTIVITY INTOLERANCE, POTENTIAL TO DEVELOP

**Decreased Activity Tolerance** r/t sedentary behavior, deconditioning

## ACUTE ABDOMINAL PAIN

**Deficient Fluid Volume** r/t air and fluids trapped in bowel, inability to drink

**Acute Pain** r/t pathological process

**Risk for Dysfunctional Gastrointestinal Motility:** Risk factor: ineffective gastrointestinal tissue perfusion

*See Abdominal Pain*

## ACUTE ALCOHOL INTOXICATION

**Ineffective Breathing Pattern** r/t depression of the respiratory center from excessive alcohol intake

**Acute Confusion** r/t central nervous system depression

**Dysfunctional Family Processes** r/t abuse of alcohol

**Risk for Aspiration:** Risk factor: depressed reflexes with acute vomiting

**Risk for Infection:** Risk factor: impaired immune system from malnutrition associated with chronic excessive alcohol intake

**Risk for Injury:** Risk factor: chemical (alcohol)

## ACUTE BACK PAIN

**Anxiety** r/t situational crisis, back injury

**Constipation** r/t decreased activity, effect of pain medication

**Ineffective Coping** r/t situational crisis, back injury

**Impaired Physical Mobility** r/t pain

**Acute Pain** r/t back injury

**Readiness for Enhanced Knowledge:** expresses an interest in learning

## ACUTE CONFUSION

*See Confusion, Acute*

## ACUTE CORONARY SYNDROME

**Decreased Cardiac Output** r/t cardiac disorder

**Risk for Decreased Cardiac Tissue Perfusion** (See **Cardiac Tissue Perfusion, Risk for Decreased,** Section II)

*See Angina; Myocardial Infarction (MI)*

## ACUTE LYMPHOCYTIC LEUKEMIA (ALL)

*See Cancer; Chemotherapy; Child with Chronic Condition; Leukemia*

## ACUTE RENAL FAILURE

*See Renal Failure*

## ACUTE RESPIRATORY DISTRESS SYNDROME

*See ARDS (Acute Respiratory Distress Syndrome)*

## ACUTE SUBSTANCE WITHDRAWAL

**Acute Substance Withdrawal Syndrome:** Risk factor: developed dependence to alcohol or other addictive substances

**Anxiety** r/t unknown outcome of withdrawal sequence, physiological effects

**Imbalanced Energy Field** r/t hyperactivity of energy flow

**Impaired Comfort** r/t restlessness and agitation

**Acute Confusion** r/t effects of substance withdrawal

**Ineffective Coping** r/t situational crisis, withdrawal

**Labile Emotional Control** r/t lack of control over the progression of withdrawal process

**Fear** r/t threat to well-being of self

**Insomnia** r/t physical and psychological effects of substance withdrawal

**Imbalanced Nutrition: Less than Body Requirements** r/t nausea, anxiety

**Powerlessness** r/t loss of ability to control withdrawal process

**Risk for Acute Confusion:** Risk factor: possible alteration in level of consciousness

**Risk for Injury:** Risk factor: alteration in sensory perceptual functioning

**Risk for Suicidal Behavior:** Risk factor: psychic pain

**Risk for Other-Directed Violence:** Risk factors: poor impulse control, hallucinations

**Risk for Self-Directed Violence:** Risk factors: poor impulse control, hallucinations

## ADAMS–STOKES SYNDROME

*See Dysrhythmia*

## ADDICTION

*See Alcoholism; Substance Abuse*

## ADDISON'S DISEASE

**Decreased Activity Tolerance** r/t weakness, fatigue

**Disturbed Body Image** r/t increased skin pigmentation

**Deficient Fluid Volume** r/t failure of regulatory mechanisms

**Imbalanced Nutrition: Less than Body Requirements** r/t chronic illness

**Risk for Injury:** Risk factor: weakness

**Readiness for Enhanced Knowledge:** expresses an interest in learning

## ADENOIDECTOMY

**Acute Pain** r/t surgical incision

**Ineffective Airway Clearance** r/t hesitation or reluctance to cough as a result of pain, fear

**Nausea** r/t anesthesia effects, drainage from surgery

**Risk for Aspiration:** Risk factors: postoperative drainage, impaired swallowing

**Risk for Bleeding:** Risk factor: surgical incision

**Risk for Deficient Fluid Volume:** Risk factors: decreased intake as a result of painful swallowing, effects of anesthesia

**Risk for Dry Mouth:** Risk factor: mouth breathing due to nasal congestion

**Risk for Imbalanced Nutrition: Less than Body Requirements:** Risk factor: reluctance to swallow

**Readiness for Enhanced Knowledge:** expresses an interest in learning

## ADHESIONS, LYSIS OF

*See Abdominal Surgery*

## ADJUSTMENT DISORDER

**Anxiety** r/t inability to cope with psychosocial stressor

**Ineffective Coping** r/t stressors

**Impaired Mood Regulation** r/t emotional instability

**Labile Emotional Control** r/t emotional disturbance

**Risk-Prone Health Behavior** r/t assault to self-esteem

**Disturbed Personal Identity** r/t psychosocial stressor (specific to individual)

**Situational Low Self-Esteem** r/t change in role function

**Impaired Social Interaction** r/t absence of significant others or peers

## ADJUSTMENT IMPAIRMENT

**Risk-Prone Health Behavior** (See **Health Behavior, Risk-Prone,** Section II)

## ADOLESCENT, PREGNANT

**Anxiety** r/t situational and maturational crisis, pregnancy

**Disturbed Body Image** r/t pregnancy superimposed on developing body

**Decisional Conflict: Keeping Child Versus Giving up Child Versus Abortion** r/t lack of experience with decision-making, interference with decision-making, multiple or divergent sources of information, lack of support system

**Disabled Family Coping** r/t highly ambivalent family relationships, chronically unresolved feelings of guilt, anger, despair

**Ineffective Coping** r/t situational and maturational crisis, personal vulnerability

**Ineffective Denial** r/t fear of consequences of pregnancy becoming known

**Ineffective Adolescent Eating Dynamics** r/t lack of knowledge of nutritional needs during pregnancy

**Interrupted Family Processes** r/t unmet expectations for adolescent, situational crisis

**Fear** r/t labor and delivery

**Deficient Knowledge** r/t pregnancy, infant growth and development, parenting

A

**Imbalanced Nutrition: Less than Body Requirements** r/t lack of knowledge of nutritional needs during pregnancy and as growing adolescent

**Ineffective Role Performance** r/t pregnancy

**Situational Low Self-Esteem** r/t feelings of shame and guilt about becoming or being pregnant

**Impaired Social Interaction** r/t self-concept disturbance

**Social Isolation** r/t absence of supportive significant others

**Risk for Impaired Attachment:** Risk factor: anxiety associated with the parent role

**Risk for Disturbed Family Identity Syndrome**: Risk Factor: excessive stress

**Risk for Urge Urinary Incontinence:** Risk factor: pressure on bladder by growing uterus

**Risk for Disturbed Maternal–Fetal Dyad:** Risk factors: immaturity, substance use

**Risk for Impaired Parenting:** Risk factors: adolescent parent, unplanned or unwanted pregnancy, single parent

**Readiness for Enhanced Childbearing Process:** reports appropriate prenatal lifestyle

**Readiness for Enhanced Health Literacy:** expresses desire to enhance social support for health

**Readiness for Enhanced Knowledge:** expresses an interest in learning

## ADOPTION, GIVING CHILD UP FOR

**Decisional Conflict** r/t unclear personal values or beliefs, perceived threat to value system, support system deficit

**Ineffective Coping** r/t stress of loss of child

**Interrupted Family Processes** r/t conflict within family regarding relinquishment of child

**Maladaptive Grieving** r/t loss of child, loss of role of parent

**Insomnia** r/t depression or trauma of relinquishment of child

**Social Isolation** r/t making choice that goes against values of significant others

**Chronic Sorrow** r/t loss of relationship with child

**Risk for Spiritual Distress:** Risk factor: perceived moral implications of decision

**Readiness for Enhanced Spiritual Well-Being:** harmony with self-regarding final decision

## ADRENOCORTICAL INSUFFICIENCY

**Deficient Fluid Volume** r/t insufficient ability to reabsorb water

**Ineffective Protection** r/t inability to tolerate stress

**Delayed Surgical Recovery** r/t inability to respond to stress

**Risk for Shock:** Risk factors: deficient fluid volume, decreased cortisol to initiate stress response to insult to body

*See Addison's Disease; Shock, Hypovolemic*

## ADVANCE DIRECTIVES

**Death Anxiety** r/t planning for end-of-life health decisions

**Decisional Conflict** r/t unclear personal values or beliefs, perceived threat to value system, support system deficit

**Maladaptive Grieving** r/t possible loss of self, significant other

**Readiness for Enhanced Spiritual Well-Being:** harmonious interconnectedness with self, others, higher power, God

## AFFECTIVE DISORDERS

*See Depression (Major Depressive Disorder); Dysthymic Disorder; Manic Disorder, Bipolar I; SAD (Seasonal Affective Disorder)*

## AGE-RELATED MACULAR DEGENERATION

*See Macular Degeneration*

## AGGRESSIVE BEHAVIOR

**Fear** r/t real or imagined threat to own well-being

**Risk for Other-Directed Violence** (See Violence, Other-Directed, Risk for, Section II)

## AGING

**Death Anxiety** r/t fear of unknown, loss of self, impact on significant others

**Impaired Dentition** r/t ineffective oral hygiene

**Risk for Frail Elderly Syndrome:** Risk factors: >70 years, activity intolerance, impaired vision

**Maladaptive Grieving** r/t multiple losses, impending death

**Ineffective Health Maintenance Behaviors** r/t powerlessness

**Hearing Loss** r/t exposure to loud noises, aging

**Impaired Urinary Elimination** r/t impaired vision, impaired cognition, neuromuscular limitations, altered environmental factors

**Impaired Resilience** r/t aging, multiple losses

**Sleep Deprivation** r/t aging-related sleep-stage shifts

**Risk for Caregiver Role Strain:** Risk factor: inability to handle increasing needs of significant other

**Risk for Impaired Emancipated Decision-Making:** Risk factor: inability to process information regarding health care decisions

**Risk for Injury:** Risk factors: vision loss, hearing loss, decreased balance, decreased sensation in feet

**Risk for Loneliness:** Risk factors: inadequate support system, role transition, health alterations, depression, fatigue

**Risk for Ineffective Thermoregulation:** Risk factor: aging

**Readiness for Enhanced Community Coping:** providing social support and other resources identified as needed for elderly client

**Readiness for Enhanced Family Coping:** ability to gratify needs, address adaptive tasks

**Readiness for Enhanced Health Self-Management:** knowledge about medication, nutrition, exercise, coping strategies

**Readiness for Enhanced Knowledge:** specify need to improve health

**Readiness for Enhanced Nutrition:** need to improve health

**Readiness for Enhanced Relationship:** demonstrates understanding of partner's insufficient function

**Readiness for Enhanced Sleep:** need to improve sleep

**Readiness for Enhanced Spiritual Well-Being:** one's experience of life's meaning, harmony with self, others, higher power, God, environment

## AGITATION

**Acute Confusion** r/t side effects of medication, hypoxia, decreased cerebral perfusion, alcohol abuse or withdrawal, substance abuse or withdrawal, sensory deprivation or overload

**Sleep Deprivation** r/t sustained inadequate sleep hygiene, sundown syndrome

## AGORAPHOBIA

**Anxiety** r/t real or perceived threat to physical integrity

**Ineffective Coping** r/t inadequate support systems

**Fear** r/t leaving home, going out in public places

**Impaired Social Interaction** r/t disturbance in self-concept

**Social Isolation** r/t altered thought process

## AGRANULOCYTOSIS

**Delayed Surgical Recovery** r/t abnormal blood profile

**Risk for Infection:** Risk factor: abnormal blood profile

**Readiness for Enhanced Knowledge:** expresses an interest in learning

## AIDS (ACQUIRED IMMUNODEFICIENCY SYNDROME)

**Death Anxiety** r/t fear of premature death

**Disturbed Body Image** r/t chronic contagious illness, cachexia

**Caregiver Role Strain** r/t unpredictable illness course, presence of situation stressors

**Diarrhea** r/t inflammatory bowel changes

**A**

**Interrupted Family Processes** r/t distress about diagnosis of human immunodeficiency virus (HIV) infection

**Fatigue** r/t disease process, stress, decreased nutritional intake

**Fear** r/t powerlessness, threat to well-being

**Maladaptive Grieving: Family/Parental** r/t potential or impending death of loved one

**Maladaptive Grieving: Individual** r/t loss of physical and psychosocial well-being

**Hopelessness** r/t deteriorating physical condition

**Imbalanced Nutrition: Less than Body Requirements** r/t decreased ability to eat and absorb nutrients as a result of anorexia, nausea, diarrhea; oral candidiasis

**Chronic Pain** r/t tissue inflammation and destruction

**Impaired Resilience** r/t chronic illness

**Situational Low Self-Esteem** r/t crisis of chronic contagious illness

**Ineffective Sexuality Pattern** r/t possible transmission of disease

**Social Isolation** r/t self-concept disturbance, therapeutic isolation

**Chronic Sorrow** r/t chronic illness

**Spiritual Distress** r/t challenged beliefs or moral system

**Risk for Deficient Fluid Volume:** Risk factors: diarrhea, vomiting, fever, bleeding

**Risk for Infection:** Risk factor: inadequate immune system

**Risk for Loneliness:** Risk factor: social isolation

**Risk for Impaired Oral Mucous Membrane Integrity:** Risk factor: immunological deficit

**Risk for Impaired Skin Integrity:** Risk factors: immunological deficit, diarrhea

**Risk for Spiritual Distress:** Risk factor: physical illness

**Readiness for Enhanced Health Literacy:** expresses desire to enhance understanding of health information to make health care choices

**Readiness for Enhanced Knowledge:** expresses an interest in learning

*See AIDS, Child; Cancer; Pneumonia*

## AIDS, CHILD

**Impaired Parenting** r/t congenital acquisition of infection secondary to intravenous (IV) drug use, multiple sexual partners, history of contaminated blood transfusion

**Risk for Disturbed Family Identity Syndrome:** Risk factor: excessive stress

*See AIDS (Acquired Immunodeficiency Syndrome); Child with Chronic Condition; Hospitalized Child; Terminally Ill Child, Adolescent; Terminally Ill Child, Infant/Toddler; Terminally Ill Child, Preschool Child; Terminally Ill Child, School-Age Child/Preadolescent; Terminally Ill Child/Death of Child, Parent*

## AIDS DEMENTIA

**Chronic Confusion** r/t viral invasion of nervous system

*See Dementia*

## AIRWAY OBSTRUCTION/ SECRETIONS

**Ineffective Airway Clearance** (See **Airway Clearance, Ineffective,** Section II)

## ALCOHOL WITHDRAWAL

**Anxiety** r/t situational crisis, withdrawal

**Acute Confusion** r/t effects of alcohol withdrawal

**Ineffective Coping** r/t personal vulnerability

**Dysfunctional Family Processes** r/t abuse of alcohol

**Insomnia** r/t effect of alcohol withdrawal, anxiety

**Imbalanced Nutrition: Less than Body Requirements** r/t poor dietary habits

**Chronic Low Self-Esteem** r/t repeated unmet expectations

**Acute Substance Withdrawal Syndrome:** Risk factor: developed dependence to alcohol

**Risk for Deficient Fluid Volume:** Risk factors: excessive diaphoresis, agitation, decreased fluid intake

**Risk for Other-Directed Violence:** Risk factor: substance withdrawal

**Risk for Self-Directed Violence:** Risk factor: substance withdrawal

**Readiness for Enhanced Knowledge:** expresses an interest in learning

## ALCOHOLISM

**Anxiety** r/t loss of control

**Risk-Prone Health Behavior** r/t lack of motivation to change behaviors, addiction

**Acute Confusion** r/t alcohol abuse

**Chronic Confusion** r/t neurological effects of chronic alcohol intake

**Defensive Coping** r/t denial of reality of addiction

**Disabled Family Coping** r/t codependency issues due to alcoholism

**Ineffective Coping** r/t use of alcohol to cope with life events

**Labile Emotional Control** r/t substance abuse

**Ineffective Denial** r/t refusal to acknowledge addiction

**Dysfunctional Family Processes** r/t alcohol abuse

**Ineffective Home Maintenance Behaviors** r/t memory deficits, fatigue

**Insomnia** r/t irritability, nightmares, tremors

**Impaired Memory** r/t alcohol abuse

**Self-Neglect** r/t effects of alcohol abuse

**Imbalanced Nutrition: Less than Body Requirements** r/t anorexia, inappropriate diet with increased carbohydrates

**Powerlessness** r/t alcohol addiction

**Ineffective Protection** r/t malnutrition, sleep deprivation

**Chronic Low Self-Esteem** r/t failure at life events

**Social Isolation** r/t unacceptable social behavior, values

**Acute Substance Withdrawal Syndrome:** Risk factor: developed dependence to alcohol

**Risk for Injury:** Risk factor: alteration in sensory or perceptual function

**Risk for Loneliness:** Risk factor: unacceptable social behavior

**Risk for Acute Substance Withdrawal Syndrome:** Risk factor: developed dependence to alcohol

**Risk for Other-Directed Violence:** Risk factors: reactions to substances used, impulsive behavior, disorientation, impaired judgment

**Risk for Self-Directed Violence:** Risk factors: reactions to substances used, impulsive behavior, disorientation, impaired judgment

## ALCOHOLISM, DYSFUNCTIONAL FAMILY PROCESSES

**Dysfunctional Family Processes** (See **Family Processes, Dysfunctional,** Section II)

**Disturbed Family Identity Syndrome:** Risk factor: excessive stress

## ALKALOSIS

*See Metabolic Alkalosis*

## ALL (ACUTE LYMPHOCYTIC LEUKEMIA)

*See Cancer; Chemotherapy; Child with Chronic Condition; Leukemia*

## ALLERGIES

**Risk for Allergy Reaction:** Risk factors: chemical factors, dander, environmental substances, foods, insect stings, medications

**Risk for Latex Allergy Reaction:** Risk factor: repeated exposure to products containing latex

**Readiness for Enhanced Knowledge:** expresses an interest in learning

## ALOPECIA

**Disturbed Body Image** r/t loss of hair, change in appearance

**Readiness for Enhanced Knowledge:** expresses an interest in learning

## ALS (AMYOTROPHIC LATERAL SCLEROSIS)

*See Amyotrophic Lateral Sclerosis (ALS)*

## ALTERED MENTAL STATUS

*See Confusion, Acute; Confusion, Chronic; Memory Deficit*

## ALZHEIMER'S DISEASE

**Caregiver Role Strain** r/t duration and extent of caregiving required

**A**

**Chronic Confusion** r/t loss of cognitive function

**Compromised Family Coping** r/t interrupted family processes

**Frail Elderly Syndrome** r/t alteration in cognitive functioning

**Ineffective Home Maintenance Behaviors** r/t impaired cognitive function, inadequate support systems

**Hopelessness** r/t deteriorating condition

**Insomnia** r/t neurological impairment, daytime naps

**Impaired Memory** r/t neurological disturbance

**Impaired Physical Mobility** r/t severe neurological dysfunction

**Self-Neglect** r/t loss of cognitive function

**Powerlessness** r/t deteriorating condition

**Self-Care Deficit: Specify** r/t loss of cognitive function, psychological impairment

**Social Isolation** r/t fear of disclosure of memory loss

**Wandering** r/t cognitive impairment, frustration, physiological state

**Risk for Chronic Functional Constipation:** Risk factor: impaired cognitive functioning

**Risk for Injury:** Risk factor: confusion

**Risk for Loneliness:** Risk factor: potential social isolation

**Risk for Relocation Stress Syndrome:** Risk factors: impaired psychosocial health, decreased health status

**Risk for Other-Directed Violence:** Risk factors: frustration, fear, anger, loss of cognitive function

**Readiness for Enhanced Knowledge:** Caregiver: expresses an interest in learning
*See Dementia*

## AMD (AGE-RELATED MACULAR DEGENERATION)
*See Macular Degeneration*

## AMENORRHEA
**Imbalanced Nutrition: Less than Body Requirements** r/t inadequate food intake
*See Sexuality, Adolescent*

## AMI (ACUTE MYOCARDIAL INFARCTION)
*See MI (Myocardial Infarction)*

## AMNESIA
**Acute Confusion** r/t alcohol abuse, delirium, dementia, drug abuse

**Dysfunctional Family Processes** r/t alcohol abuse, inadequate coping skills

**Impaired Memory** r/t excessive environmental disturbance, neurological disturbance

**Post-Trauma Syndrome** r/t history of abuse, catastrophic illness, disaster, accident

## AMNIOCENTESIS
**Anxiety** r/t threat to self and fetus, unknown future

**Decisional Conflict** r/t choice of treatment pending results of test

**Risk for Infection:** Risk factor: invasive procedure

## AMNIONITIS
*See Chorioamnionitis*

## AMNIOTIC MEMBRANE RUPTURE
*See Premature Rupture of Membranes*

## AMPUTATION
**Disturbed Body Image** r/t negative effects of amputation, response from others

**Maladaptive Grieving** r/t loss of body part, future lifestyle changes

**Impaired Physical Mobility** r/t musculoskeletal impairment, limited movement

**Acute Pain** r/t surgery, phantom limb sensation

**Chronic Pain** r/t surgery, phantom limb sensation

**Ineffective Peripheral Tissue Perfusion** r/t impaired arterial circulation

**Impaired Skin Integrity** r/t poor healing, prosthesis rubbing

**Risk for Bleeding:** Risk factor: vulnerable surgical site

**Risk for Impaired Tissue Integrity:** Risk factor: mechanical factors impacting site

**Readiness for Enhanced Knowledge:** expresses an interest in learning

## AMYOTROPHIC LATERAL SCLEROSIS (ALS)

**Death Anxiety** r/t impending progressive loss of function leading to death

**Ineffective Breathing Pattern** r/t compromised muscles of respiration

**Impaired Verbal Communication** r/t weakness of muscles of speech, deficient knowledge of ways to compensate and alternative communication devices

**Decisional Conflict: Ventilator Therapy** r/t unclear personal values or beliefs, lack of relevant information

**Impaired Resilience** r/t perceived vulnerability

**Chronic Sorrow** r/t chronic illness

**Impaired Swallowing** r/t weakness of muscles involved in swallowing

**Impaired Spontaneous Ventilation** r/t weakness of muscles of respiration

**Risk for Aspiration:** Risk factor: impaired swallowing

**Risk for Spiritual Distress:** Risk factor: chronic debilitating condition

*See Neurological Disorders*

## ANAL FISTULA

*See Hemorrhoidectomy*

## ANAPHYLACTIC SHOCK

**Deficient Fluid Volume** r/t compromised regulatory mechanism

**Ineffective Airway Clearance** r/t laryngeal edema, bronchospasm

**Risk for Latex Allergy Reaction** r/t abnormal immune mechanism response

**Impaired Spontaneous Ventilation** r/t acute airway obstruction from anaphylaxis process

## ANAPHYLAXIS PREVENTION

**Risk for Allergy Reaction** (See **Allergy Reaction, Risk for,** Section II)

## ANASARCA

**Excess Fluid Volume** r/t excessive fluid intake, cardiac/renal dysfunction, loss of plasma proteins

**Risk for Decreased Cardiac Output:** Risk factor: imbalanced fluid volume

**Risk for Impaired Skin Integrity:** Risk factor: impaired circulation to skin from edema

## ANEMIA

**Anxiety** r/t cause of disease

**Impaired Comfort** r/t feelings of always being cold from decreased hemoglobin and decreased metabolism

**Fatigue** r/t decreased oxygen supply to the body, increased cardiac workload

**Impaired Memory** r/t change in cognition from decreased oxygen supply to the body

**Delayed Surgical Recovery** r/t decreased oxygen supply to body, increased cardiac workload

**Risk for Bleeding** (See **Bleeding, Risk for,** Section II)

**Risk for Injury:** Risk factor: alteration in peripheral sensory perception

**Readiness for Enhanced Knowledge:** expresses an interest in learning

## ANEMIA, IN PREGNANCY

**Anxiety** r/t concerns about health of self and fetus

**Fatigue** r/t decreased oxygen supply to the body, increased cardiac workload

**Risk for Infection:** Risk factor: reduction in oxygen-carrying capacity of blood

**Risk for Disturbed Maternal–Fetal Dyad:** Risk factor: compromised oxygen transport

**Readiness for Enhanced Knowledge:** expresses an interest in learning

## ANEMIA, SICKLE CELL

*See Anemia; Sickle Cell Anemia/Crisis*

## ANENCEPHALY

*See Neural Tube Defects (Meningocele, Myelomeningocele, Spina Bifida, Anencephaly)*

## ANEURYSM, ABDOMINAL AORTIC REPAIR SURGERY

**Risk for Deficient Fluid Volume:** Risk factor: hemorrhage r/t potential abnormal blood loss

**Risk for Surgical Site Infection:** Risk factor: invasive procedure

*See Abdominal Surgery*

## ANEURYSM, CEREBRAL

*See Craniectomy/Craniotomy; Subarachnoid Hemorrhage*

## ANGER

**Anxiety** r/t situational crisis

**Defensive Coping** r/t inability to acknowledge responsibility for actions and results of actions

**Labile Emotional Control** r/t stressors

**Fear** r/t environmental stressor, hospitalization

**Maladaptive Grieving** r/t significant loss

**Risk-Prone Health Behavior** r/t assault to self-esteem, disability requiring change in lifestyle, inadequate support system

**Powerlessness** r/t health care environment

**Risk for Compromised Human Dignity:** Risk factors: inadequate participation in decision-making, perceived dehumanizing treatment, perceived humiliation, exposure of the body, cultural incongruity

**Risk for Post-Trauma Syndrome:** Risk factor: inadequate social support

**Risk for Other-Directed Violence:** Risk factors: history of violence, rage reaction

**Risk for Self-Directed Violence:** Risk factors: history of violence, history of abuse, rage reaction

## ANGINA

**Decreased Activity Tolerance** r/t acute pain, dysrhythmias

**Anxiety** r/t situational crisis

**Decreased Cardiac Output** r/t myocardial ischemia, medication effect, dysrhythmia

**Ineffective Coping** r/t personal vulnerability to situational crisis of new diagnosis, deteriorating health

**Ineffective Denial** r/t deficient knowledge of need to seek help with symptoms

**Maladaptive Grieving** r/t pain, loss of health

**Acute Pain** r/t myocardial ischemia

**Ineffective Sexuality Pattern** r/t disease process, medications, loss of libido

**Readiness for Enhanced Knowledge:** expresses an interest in learning

*See MI (Myocardial Infarction)*

## ANGIOCARDIOGRAPHY (CARDIAC CATHETERIZATION)

*See Cardiac Catheterization*

## ANGIOPLASTY, CORONARY

**Fear** r/t possible outcome of interventional procedure

**Ineffective Peripheral Tissue Perfusion** r/t vasospasm, hematoma formation

**Risk for Bleeding:** Risk factors: possible damage to coronary artery, hematoma formation

**Risk for Decreased Cardiac Tissue Perfusion:** Risk factors: ventricular ischemia, dysrhythmias

**Readiness for Enhanced Knowledge:** expresses an interest in learning

## ANOMALY, FETAL/NEWBORN (PARENT DEALING WITH)

**Anxiety** r/t threat to role functioning, situational crisis

**Decisional Conflict: Interventions for Fetus or Newborn** r/t lack of relevant information, spiritual distress, threat to value system

**Disabled Family Coping** r/t chronically unresolved feelings about loss of perfect baby

**Ineffective Coping** r/t personal vulnerability in situational crisis

**Interrupted Family Processes** r/t unmet expectations for perfect baby, lack of adequate support systems

**Fear** r/t real or imagined threat to baby, implications for future pregnancies, powerlessness

**Maladaptive Grieving** r/t loss of ideal child

**Hopelessness** r/t long-term stress, deteriorating physical condition of child, lost spiritual belief

**Deficient Knowledge** r/t limited exposure to situation

**Impaired Parenting** r/t interruption of bonding process

**Powerlessness** r/t complication threatening fetus or newborn

**Parental Role Conflict** r/t separation from newborn, intimidation with invasive or restrictive modalities, specialized care center policies

**Situational Low Self-Esteem** r/t perceived inability to produce a perfect child

**Social Isolation** r/t alterations in child's physical appearance, altered state of wellness

**Chronic Sorrow** r/t loss of ideal child, inadequate bereavement support

**Spiritual Distress** r/t test of spiritual beliefs

**Risk for Impaired Attachment:** Risk factor: ill infant unable to effectively initiate parental contact as result of altered behavioral organization

**Risk for Disorganized Infant Behavior:** Risk factor: congenital disorder

**Risk for Impaired Parenting:** Risk factors: interruption of bonding process; unrealistic expectations for self, infant, or partner; perceived threat to own emotional survival; severe stress; lack of knowledge

**Risk for Spiritual Distress:** Risk factor: lack of normal child to raise and carry on family name

### ANORECTAL ABSCESS

**Disturbed Body Image** r/t odor and drainage from rectal area

**Acute Pain** r/t inflammation of perirectal area

**Risk for Constipation:** Risk factor: fear of painful elimination

**Readiness for Enhanced Knowledge:** expresses an interest in learning

### ANOREXIA

**Deficient Fluid Volume** r/t inability to drink

**Imbalanced Nutrition: Less than Body Requirements** r/t loss of appetite, nausea, vomiting, laxative abuse

**Delayed Surgical Recovery** r/t inadequate nutritional intake

**Risk for Delayed Surgical Recovery:** Risk factor: inadequate nutritional intake

### ANOREXIA NERVOSA

**Decreased Activity Tolerance** r/t fatigue, weakness

**Disturbed Body Image** r/t misconception of actual body appearance

**Constipation** r/t lack of adequate food, fiber, and fluid intake

**Defensive Coping** r/t psychological impairment, eating disorder

**Disabled Family Coping** r/t highly ambivalent family relationships

**Ineffective Denial** r/t fear of consequences of therapy, possible weight gain

**Diarrhea** r/t laxative abuse

**Interrupted Family Processes** r/t situational crisis

**Ineffective Adolescent Eating Dynamics** r/t food refusal

**Ineffective Family Health Self-Management** r/t family conflict, excessive demands on family associated with complexity of condition and treatment

**Imbalanced Nutrition: Less than Body Requirements** r/t inadequate food intake, excessive exercise

**Chronic Low Self-Esteem** r/t repeated unmet expectations

**Ineffective Sexuality Pattern** r/t loss of libido from malnutrition

**Risk for Infection:** Risk factor: malnutrition resulting in depressed immune system

**Risk for Spiritual Distress:** Risk factor: low self-esteem

*See Maturational Issues, Adolescent*

### ANOSMIA (SMELL, LOSS OF ABILITY TO)

**Imbalanced Nutrition: Less than Body Requirements** r/t loss of appetite associated with loss of smell

### ANTEPARTUM PERIOD

*See Pregnancy, Normal; Prenatal Care, Normal*

**A**

## ANTERIOR REPAIR, ANTERIOR COLPORRHAPHY

**Urinary Retention** r/t edema of urinary structures

**Risk for Urge Urinary Incontinence:** Risk factor: trauma to bladder

**Readiness for Enhanced Knowledge:** expresses an interest in learning

*See Vaginal Hysterectomy*

## ANTICOAGULANT THERAPY

**Risk for Bleeding:** Risk factor: altered clotting function from anticoagulant

**Risk for Deficient Fluid Volume: Hemorrhage:** Risk factor: altered clotting mechanism

**Readiness for Enhanced Knowledge:** expresses an interest in learning

## ANTISOCIAL PERSONALITY DISORDER

**Defensive Coping** r/t excessive use of projection

**Ineffective Coping** r/t frequently violating the norms and rules of society

**Labile Emotional Control** r/t psychiatric disorder

**Hopelessness** r/t abandonment

**Impaired Social Interaction** r/t sociocultural conflict, chemical dependence, inability to form relationships

**Spiritual Distress** r/t separation from religious or cultural ties

**Ineffective Health Self-Management** r/t excessive demands on family

**Risk for Loneliness:** Risk factor: inability to interact appropriately with others

**Risk for Impaired Parenting:** Risk factors: inability to function as parent or guardian, emotional instability

**Risk for Self-Mutilation:** Risk factors: self-hatred, depersonalization

**Risk for Other-Directed Violence:** Risk factor: history of violence, altered thought patterns

## ANURIA

*See Renal Failure*

## ANXIETY

(See **Anxiety,** Section II)

## ANXIETY DISORDER

**Ineffective Activity Planning** r/t unrealistic perception of events

**Anxiety** r/t unmet security and safety needs

**Death Anxiety** r/t fears of unknown, powerlessness

**Decisional Conflict** r/t low self-esteem, fear of making a mistake

**Defensive Coping** r/t overwhelming feelings of dread

**Disabled Family Coping** r/t ritualistic behavior, actions

**Imbalanced Energy Field** r/t feelings of restlessness and apprehension

**Impaired Mood Regulation** r/t functional impairment, impaired social functioning, alteration in sleep pattern

**Ineffective Coping** r/t inability to express feelings appropriately

**Ineffective Denial** r/t overwhelming feelings of hopelessness, fear, threat to self

**Insomnia** r/t psychological impairment, emotional instability

**Labile Emotional Control** r/t emotional instability

**Powerlessness** r/t lifestyle of helplessness

**Self-Care Deficit** r/t ritualistic behavior, activities

**Sleep Deprivation** r/t prolonged psychological discomfort

**Risk for Spiritual Distress:** Risk factor: psychological distress

**Readiness for Enhanced Knowledge:** expresses an interest in learning

## AORTIC VALVULAR STENOSIS

*See Congenital Heart Disease/Cardiac Anomalies*

## APHASIA

**Anxiety** r/t situational crisis of aphasia

**Impaired Verbal Communication** r/t decrease in circulation to brain

**Ineffective Coping** r/t loss of speech

**Ineffective Health Maintenance Behaviors** r/t deficient knowledge regarding information on aphasia and alternative communication techniques

## APLASTIC ANEMIA

**Decreased Activity Tolerance** r/t imbalance between oxygen supply and demand

**Fear** r/t ability to live with serious disease

**Risk for Bleeding:** Risk factor: inadequate clotting factors

**Risk for Infection:** Risk factor: inadequate immune function

**Readiness for Enhanced Knowledge:** expresses an interest in learning

## APNEA IN INFANCY

*See Premature Infant (Child); Premature Infant (Parent); SIDS (Sudden Infant Death Syndrome)*

## APNEUSTIC RESPIRATIONS

**Ineffective Breathing Pattern** r/t perception or cognitive impairment, neurological impairment

## APPENDECTOMY

**Deficient Fluid Volume** r/t fluid restriction, hypermetabolic state, nausea, vomiting

**Acute Pain** r/t surgical incision

**Delayed Surgical Recovery** r/t rupture of appendix

**Risk for Infection:** Risk factors: perforation or rupture of appendix, peritonitis

**Risk for Surgical Site Infection:** Risk factor: surgical incision

**Readiness for Enhanced Knowledge:** expresses an interest in learning

*See Hospitalized Child; Surgery, Postoperative Care*

## APPENDICITIS

**Deficient Fluid Volume** r/t anorexia, nausea, vomiting

**Acute Pain** r/t inflammation

**Risk for Infection:** Risk factor: possible perforation of appendix

**Readiness for Enhanced Knowledge:** expresses an interest in learning

## APPREHENSION

**Anxiety** r/t threat to self-concept, threat to health status, situational crisis

**Death Anxiety** r/t apprehension over loss of self, consequences to significant others

## ARDS (ACUTE RESPIRATORY DISTRESS SYNDROME)

**Ineffective Airway Clearance** r/t excessive tracheobronchial secretions

**Death Anxiety** r/t seriousness of physical disease

**Impaired Gas Exchange** r/t damage to alveolar-capillary membrane, change in lung compliance

**Impaired Spontaneous Ventilation** r/t damage to alveolar-capillary membrane

*See Ventilated Client, Mechanically*

## ARRHYTHMIA

*See Dysrhythmia*

## ARTERIAL INSUFFICIENCY

**Ineffective Peripheral Tissue Perfusion** r/t interruption of arterial flow

**Delayed Surgical Recovery** r/t ineffective tissue perfusion

## ARTHRITIS

**Decreased Activity Tolerance** r/t chronic pain, fatigue, weakness

**Disturbed Body Image** r/t ineffective coping with joint abnormalities

**Impaired Physical Mobility** r/t joint impairment

**Chronic Pain** r/t progression of joint deterioration

**Self-Care Deficit: Specify** r/t pain with movement, damage to joints

**Readiness for Enhanced Knowledge:** expresses an interest in learning

*See JRA (Juvenile Rheumatoid Arthritis)*

## ARTHROCENTESIS

**Acute Pain** r/t invasive procedure

## ARTHROPLASTY (TOTAL HIP REPLACEMENT)

*See Total Joint Replacement (Total Hip/Total Knee/Shoulder); Surgery,*

*Perioperative Care; Surgery, Postoperative Care; Surgery, Preoperative Care*

## ARTHROSCOPY

**Impaired Physical Mobility** r/t surgical trauma of knee

**Readiness for Enhanced Knowledge:** expresses an interest in learning

## ASCITES

**Ineffective Breathing Pattern** r/t increased abdominal girth

**Imbalanced Nutrition: Less than Body Requirements** r/t loss of appetite

**Chronic Pain** r/t altered body function

**Readiness for Enhanced Knowledge:** expresses an interest in learning

*See Ascites; Cancer; Cirrhosis*

## ASPERGER'S SYNDROME

**Ineffective Relationship** r/t poor communication skills, lack of empathy

*See Autism*

## ASPHYXIA, BIRTH

**Ineffective Breathing Pattern** r/t depression of breathing reflex secondary to anoxia

**Ineffective Coping** r/t uncertainty of child outcome

**Fear (Parental)** r/t concern over safety of infant

**Impaired Gas Exchange** r/t poor placental perfusion, lack of initiation of breathing by newborn

**Maladaptive Grieving** r/t loss of perfect child, concern of loss of future abilities

**Impaired Spontaneous Ventilation** r/t brain injury

**Risk for Impaired Attachment:** Risk factors: ill infant who is unable to initiate parental contact, hospitalization in critical care environment

**Risk for Delayed Child Development**: Risk factors: lack of oxygen to brain

**Risk for Disorganized Infant Behavior:** Risk factor: lack of oxygen to brain

**Risk for Injury:** Risk factor: lack of oxygen to brain

**Risk for Ineffective Cerebral Tissue Perfusion:** Risk factor: poor placental perfusion or cord compression resulting in lack of oxygen to brain

## ASPIRATION, DANGER OF

**Risk for Aspiration** (See **Aspiration, Risk for,** Section II)

## ASSAULT VICTIM

**Post-Trauma Syndrome** r/t assault

**Rape-Trauma Syndrome** r/t rape

**Impaired Resilience** r/t frightening experience, post-trauma stress response

**Risk for Post-Trauma Syndrome:** Risk factors: perception of event, inadequate social support, unsupportive environment, diminished ego strength, duration of event

**Risk for Spiritual Distress:** Risk factors: physical, psychological stress

## ASSAULTIVE CLIENT

**Risk for Injury:** Risk factors: confused thought process, impaired judgment

**Risk for Other-Directed Violence:** Risk factors: paranoid ideation, anger

## ASTHMA

**Decreased Activity Tolerance** r/t fatigue, energy shift to meet muscle needs for breathing to overcome airway obstruction

**Ineffective Airway Clearance** r/t tracheobronchial narrowing, excessive secretions

**Anxiety** r/t inability to breathe effectively, fear of suffocation

**Disturbed Body Image** r/t decreased participation in physical activities

**Ineffective Breathing Pattern** r/t anxiety

**Ineffective Coping** r/t personal vulnerability to situational crisis

**Ineffective Health Self-Management** (See **Health Management, Ineffective,** Section II)

**Ineffective Home Maintenance Behaviors** r/t deficient knowledge regarding control of environmental triggers

**Sleep Deprivation** r/t ineffective breathing pattern, cough

**Readiness for Enhanced Health Self-Management** (See **Health Self-Management, Readiness for Enhanced,** Section II)

**Readiness for Enhanced Knowledge:** expresses an interest in learning

*See Child with Chronic Condition; Hospitalized Child*

## ATAXIA

**Anxiety** r/t change in health status

**Disturbed Body Image** r/t staggering gait

**Impaired Physical Mobility** r/t neuromuscular impairment

**Risk for Falls:** Risk factors: gait alteration, instability

## ATELECTASIS

**Ineffective Breathing Pattern** r/t loss of functional lung tissue, depression of respiratory function or hypoventilation because of pain

**Impaired Gas Exchange** r/t decreased alveolar-capillary surface

**Anxiety** r/t alteration in respiratory pattern

*See Atelectasis*

## ATHEROSCLEROSIS

*See MI (Myocardial Infarction); CVA (Cerebrovascular Accident); Peripheral Vascular Disease (PVD)*

## ATHLETE'S FOOT

**Impaired Skin Integrity** r/t effects of fungal agent

**Readiness for Enhanced Knowledge:** expresses an interest in learning

*See Pruritus*

## ATN (ACUTE TUBULAR NECROSIS)

*See Renal Failure*

## ATRIAL FIBRILLATION

*See Dysrhythmia*

## ATRIAL SEPTAL DEFECT

*See Congenital Heart Disease/Cardiac Anomalies*

## ATTENTION DEFICIT DISORDER

**Risk-Prone Health Behavior** r/t intense emotional state

**Disabled Family Coping** r/t significant person with chronically unexpressed feelings of guilt, anxiety, hostility, and despair

**Ineffective Impulse Control** (See **Impulse Control, Ineffective,** Section II)

**Chronic Low Self-Esteem** r/t difficulty in participating in expected activities, poor school performance

**Social Isolation** r/t unacceptable social behavior

**Risk for Delayed Child Development:** Risk factor: behavior disorders

**Risk for Falls:** Risk factor: rapid non-thinking behavior

**Risk for Loneliness:** Risk factor: social isolation

**Risk for Impaired Parenting:** Risk factor: lack of knowledge of factors contributing to child's behavior

**Risk for Spiritual Distress:** Risk factor: poor relationships

## AUTISM

**Impaired Verbal Communication** r/t speech and language delays

**Compromised Family Coping** r/t parental guilt over etiology of disease, inability to accept or adapt to child's condition, inability to help child and other family members seek treatment

**Disturbed Personal Identity** r/t inability to distinguish between self and environment, inability to identify own body as separate from those of other people, inability to integrate concept of self

**Self-Neglect** r/t impaired socialization

**Impaired Social Interaction** r/t communication barriers, inability to relate to others, failure to develop peer relationships

**Risk for Delayed Child Development:** Risk factor: autism

**Risk for Disturbed Family Identity Syndrome**: Risk factor: excessive stress

**Risk for Loneliness:** Risk factor: difficulty developing relationships with other people

**B**

**Risk for Self-Mutilation:** Risk factor: autistic state

**Risk for Other-Directed Violence:** Risk factors: frequent destructive rages toward others secondary to extreme response to changes in routine, fear of harmless things

**Risk for Self-Directed Violence:** Risk factors: frequent destructive rages toward self, secondary to extreme response to changes in routine, fear of harmless things

*See Child with Chronic Condition*

## AUTONOMIC DYSREFLEXIA

**Autonomic Dysreflexia** r/t bladder distention, bowel distention, noxious stimuli

**Risk for Autonomic Dysreflexia:** Risk factors: bladder distention, bowel distention, noxious stimuli

## AUTONOMIC HYPERREFLEXIA

*See Autonomic Dysreflexia*

# B

## BABY CARE

**Readiness for Enhanced Childbearing Process:** demonstrates appropriate feeding and baby care techniques, along with attachment to infant and providing a safe environment

**Anxiety** r/t situational crisis, back injury

**Ineffective Coping** r/t situational crisis, back injury

**Impaired Physical Mobility** r/t pain

**Acute Pain** r/t back injury

**Chronic Pain** r/t back injury

**Risk for Constipation:** Risk factors: decreased activity, side effect of pain medication

**Risk for Disuse Syndrome:** Risk factor: severe pain

**Readiness for Enhanced Knowledge:** expresses an interest in learning

## BACTEREMIA

**Risk for Infection:** Risk factor: compromised immune system

**Risk for Shock:** Risk factor: development of systemic inflammatory response from presence of bacteria in bloodstream

## BALANCED ENERGY FIELD

**Imbalanced Energy Field** (See **Energy Field, Imbalanced,** Section II)

## BARREL CHEST

*See Aging (if appropriate); COPD (Chronic Obstructive Pulmonary Disease)*

## BATHING/HYGIENE PROBLEMS

**Impaired Mobility** r/t chronic physically limiting condition

**Self-Neglect** (See **Self-Neglect,** Section II)

**Bathing Self-Care Deficit** (See **Self-Care Deficit, bathing,** Section II)

## BATTERED CHILD SYNDROME

**Dysfunctional Family Processes** r/t inadequate coping skills

**Sleep Deprivation** r/t prolonged psychological discomfort

**Chronic Sorrow** r/t situational crises

**Risk for Post-Trauma Syndrome:** Risk factors: physical abuse, incest, rape, molestation

**Risk for Self-Mutilation:** Risk factors: feelings of rejection, dysfunctional family

**Risk for Suicidal Behaviors:** Risk factor: childhood abuse

*See Child Abuse*

## BATTERED PERSON

*See Abuse, Spouse, Parent, or Significant Other*

## BEDBUGS, INFESTATION

**Ineffective Home Maintenance Behaviors** r/t deficient knowledge regarding prevention of bedbug infestation

**Impaired Skin Integrity** r/t bites of bedbugs

*See Pruritus*

## BED MOBILITY, IMPAIRED

**Impaired Bed Mobility** (See **Mobility, Bed, Impaired,** Section II)

## BED REST, PROLONGED

**Decreased Diversional Activity Engagement** r/t prolonged bed rest

**Impaired Bed Mobility** r/t neuromuscular impairment

**Social Isolation** r/t prolonged bed rest

**Risk for Chronic Functional Constipation:** Risk factor: insufficient physical activity

**Risk for Disuse Syndrome:** Risk factor: prolonged immobility

**Risk for Frail Elderly Syndrome:** Risk factor: prolonged immobility

**Risk for Loneliness:** Risk factor: prolonged bed rest

**Risk for Overweight:** Risk factor: energy expenditure below energy intake

**Risk for Pressure Ulcer:** Risk factor: prolonged immobility

**Risk for Thrombosis:** Risk factor: prolonged immobility

### BEDSORES

*See Pressure Ulcer*

### BEDWETTING

**Ineffective Health Maintenance Behaviors** r/t unachieved developmental level, neuromuscular immaturity, diseases of the urinary system

### BELL'S PALSY

**Disturbed Body Image** r/t loss of motor control on one side of face

**Imbalanced Nutrition: Less than Body Requirements** r/t difficulty with chewing

**Acute Pain** r/t inflammation of facial nerve

**Risk for Injury (Eye):** Risk factors: decreased tears, decreased blinking of eye

**Readiness for Enhanced Knowledge:** expresses an interest in learning

### BENIGN PROSTATIC HYPERTROPHY

*See BPH (Benign Prostatic Hypertrophy); Prostatic Hypertrophy*

### BEREAVEMENT

**Maladaptive Grieving** r/t loss of significant person

**Insomnia** r/t grief

**Risk for Maladaptive Grieving:** Risk factor: emotional instability, lack of social support

**Risk for Spiritual Distress:** Risk factor: death of a loved one

### BILIARY ATRESIA

**Anxiety** r/t surgical intervention, possible liver transplantation

**Impaired Comfort** r/t inflammation of skin, itching

**Imbalanced Nutrition: Less than Body Requirements** r/t decreased absorption of fat and fat-soluble vitamins, poor feeding

**Risk for Bleeding:** Risk factors: vitamin K deficiency, altered clotting mechanisms

**Ineffective Breathing Pattern** r/t enlarged liver, development of ascites

**Risk for Impaired Skin Integrity:** Risk factor: pruritus

*See Child with Chronic Condition; Cirrhosis; Hospitalized Child*

### BILIARY CALCULUS

*See Cholelithiasis*

### BILIARY OBSTRUCTION

*See Jaundice*

### BILIRUBIN ELEVATION IN NEONATE

*See Hyperbilirubinemia, Neonatal*

### BIOPSY

**Fear** r/t outcome of biopsy

**Readiness for Enhanced Knowledge:** expresses an interest in learning

### BIOTERRORISM

**Contamination** r/t exposure to bioterrorism

**Risk for Infection:** Risk factor: exposure to harmful biological agent

**Risk for Post-Trauma Syndrome:** Risk factor: perception of event of bioterrorism

### BIPOLAR DISORDER I (MOST RECENT EPISODE, DEPRESSED OR MANIC)

**Ineffective Activity Planning** r/t unrealistic perception of events

**Fatigue** r/t psychological demands

**Risk-Prone Health Behavior:** Risk factor: low state of optimism

**B**

**Ineffective Health Maintenance Behaviors** r/t lack of ability to make good judgments regarding ways to obtain help

**Self-Care Deficit: Specify** r/t depression, cognitive impairment

**Chronic Low Self-Esteem** r/t repeated unmet expectations

**Social Isolation** r/t ineffective coping

**Risk for Maladaptive Grieving:** Risk factor: lack of previous resolution of former grieving response

**Risk for Loneliness:** Risk factors: stress, conflict

**Risk for Spiritual Distress:** Risk factor: mental illness

**Risk for Suicidal Behavior:** Risk factors: psychiatric disorder, poor support system

*See Depression (Major Depressive Disorder); Manic Disorder, Bipolar I*

### BIRTH ASPHYXIA

*See Asphyxia, Birth*

### BIRTH CONTROL

*See Contraceptive Method*

### BLADDER CANCER

**Urinary Retention** r/t clots obstructing urethra

*See Cancer; TURP (Transurethral Resection of the Prostate)*

### BLADDER DISTENTION

**Urinary Retention** r/t high urethral pressure caused by weak detrusor, inhibition of reflex arc, blockage, strong sphincter

### BLADDER TRAINING

**Disturbed Body Image** r/t difficulty maintaining control of urinary elimination

**Disability-Associated Urinary Incontinence** r/t altered environment; sensory, cognitive, mobility deficit

**Stress Urinary Incontinence** r/t degenerative change in pelvic muscles and structural supports

**Urge Urinary Incontinence** r/t decreased bladder capacity, increased urine concentration, overdistention of bladder

**Readiness for Enhanced Knowledge:** expresses an interest in learning

### BLADDER TRAINING, CHILD

*See Toilet Training*

### BLEEDING TENDENCY

**Risk for Bleeding** (See **Bleeding, Risk for,** Section II)

**Risk for Delayed Surgical Recovery:** Risk factor: bleeding tendency

### BLEPHAROPLASTY

**Disturbed Body Image** r/t effects of surgery

**Readiness for Enhanced Knowledge:** expresses an interest in learning

### BLINDNESS

**Interrupted Family Processes** r/t shift in health status of family member (change in visual acuity)

**Ineffective Home Maintenance Behaviors** r/t decreased vision

**Ineffective Role Performance** r/t alteration in health status (change in visual acuity)

**Self-Care Deficit: Specify** r/t inability to see to be able to perform activities of daily living

**Risk for Injury:** Risk factor: sensory dysfunction

**Readiness for Enhanced Knowledge:** expresses an interest in learning

### BLOOD DISORDER

**Ineffective Protection** r/t abnormal blood profile

**Risk for Bleeding:** Risk factor: abnormal blood profile

*See ITP (Idiopathic Thrombocytopenic Purpura); Hemophilia; Lacerations; Shock, Hypovolemic*

### BLOOD GLUCOSE CONTROL

**Risk for Unstable Blood Glucose Level** (See **Glucose Level, Blood, Unstable, Risk for,** Section II)

### BLOOD PRESSURE ALTERATION

*See Hypotension; HTN (Hypertension)*

(See **Unstable Blood Pressure, Risk for,** Section II)

## BLOOD TRANSFUSION

**Anxiety** r/t possibility of harm from transfusion

*See Anemia*

## BODY DYSMORPHIC DISORDER

**Anxiety** r/t perceived defect of body

**Disturbed Body Image** r/t over-involvement in physical appearance

**Chronic Low Self-Esteem** r/t lack of self-valuing because of perceived body defects

**Social Isolation** r/t distancing self from others because of perceived self-body defects

**Risk for Suicidal Behavior:** Risk factor: perceived defects of body affecting self-valuing and hopes

## BODY IMAGE CHANGE

**Disturbed Body Image** (See **Body Image, Disturbed,** Section II)

## BODY TEMPERATURE, ALTERED

**Ineffective Thermoregulation** (See **Thermoregulation, Ineffective,** Section II)

## BONE MARROW BIOPSY

**Fear** r/t unknown outcome of results of biopsy

**Acute Pain** r/t bone marrow aspiration

**Readiness for Enhanced Knowledge:** expresses an interest in learning

*See Disease Necessitating Bone Marrow Biopsy (e.g., Leukemia)*

## BORDERLINE PERSONALITY DISORDER

**Ineffective Activity Planning** r/t unrealistic perception of events

**Anxiety** r/t perceived threat to self-concept

**Defensive Coping** r/t difficulty with relationships, inability to accept blame for own behavior

**Ineffective Coping** r/t use of maladjusted defense mechanisms (e.g., projection, denial)

**Powerlessness** r/t lifestyle of helplessness

**Social Isolation** r/t immature interests

**Ineffective Family Health Self-Management** r/t manipulative behavior of client

**Risk for Caregiver Role Strain:** Risk factors: inability of care receiver to accept criticism, care receiver taking advantage of others to meet own needs or having unreasonable expectations

**Risk for Self-Mutilation:** Risk factors: ineffective coping, feelings of self-hatred

**Risk for Spiritual Distress:** Risk factor: poor relationships associated with abnormal behaviors

**Risk for Self-Directed Violence:** Risk factors: feelings of need to punish self, manipulative behavior

## BOREDOM

**Decreased Diversional Activity Engagement** r/t environmental lack of diversional activity

**Impaired Mood Regulation** r/t emotional instability

**Social Isolation** r/t altered state of wellness

## BOTULISM

**Deficient Fluid Volume** r/t profuse diarrhea

**Readiness for Enhanced Knowledge:** expresses an interest in learning

## BOWEL INCONTINENCE

**Impaired Bowel Continence** r/t decreased awareness of need to defecate, loss of sphincter control, fecal impaction

**Readiness for Enhanced Knowledge:** expresses an interest in learning

## BOWEL OBSTRUCTION

**Constipation** r/t decreased motility, intestinal obstruction

**Deficient Fluid Volume** r/t inadequate fluid volume intake, fluid loss in bowel

**Imbalanced Nutrition: Less than Body Requirements** r/t nausea, vomiting

**Acute Pain** r/t pressure from distended abdomen

## BOWEL RESECTION

*See Abdominal Surgery*

**B**

## BOWEL SOUNDS, ABSENT OR DIMINISHED

**Constipation** r/t decreased or absent peristalsis

**Deficient Fluid Volume** r/t inability to ingest fluids, loss of fluids in bowel

**Delayed Surgical Recovery** r/t inability to obtain adequate nutritional status

**Risk for Dysfunctional Gastrointestinal Motility** (See **Gastrointestinal Motility, Dysfunctional, Risk for,** Section II)

## BOWEL SOUNDS, HYPERACTIVE

**Diarrhea** r/t increased gastrointestinal motility

## BOWEL TRAINING

**Impaired Bowel Continence** r/t loss of control of rectal sphincter

**Readiness for Enhanced Knowledge:** expresses an interest in learning

## BOWEL TRAINING, CHILD

*See Toilet Training*

## BPH (BENIGN PROSTATIC HYPERTROPHY)

**Ineffective Health Maintenance Behaviors** r/t deficient knowledge regarding self-care with prostatic hypertrophy

**Insomnia** r/t nocturia

**Urinary Retention** r/t obstruction of urethra

**Risk for Urge Urinary Incontinence:** Risk factors: detrusor muscle instability with impaired contractility, involuntary sphincter relaxation

**Risk for Infection:** Risk factors: urinary residual after voiding, bacterial invasion of bladder

**Readiness for Enhanced Knowledge:** expresses an interest in learning

*See Prostatic Hypertrophy*

## BRADYCARDIA

**Decreased Cardiac Output** r/t slow heart rate supplying inadequate amount of blood for body function

**Risk for Ineffective Cerebral Tissue Perfusion:** Risk factors: decreased cardiac output secondary to bradycardia, vagal response

**Readiness for Enhanced Knowledge:** expresses an interest in learning

## BRADYPNEA

**Ineffective Breathing Pattern** r/t neuromuscular impairment, pain, musculoskeletal impairment, perception or cognitive impairment, anxiety, fatigue or decreased energy, effects of drugs

*See Sleep Apnea* (See **Airway Clearance, Ineffective,** Section II)

## BRAIN INJURY

**Risk for Ineffective Thermoregulation:** Risk factor: posttraumatic inflammation or infection

*See Intracranial Pressure, Increased*

## BRAIN SURGERY

*See Craniectomy/Craniotomy*

## BRAIN TUMOR

**Acute Confusion** r/t pressure from tumor

**Fear** r/t threat to well-being

**Maladaptive Grieving** r/t potential loss of physiological-psychosocial well-being

**Acute Pain** r/t pressure from tumor

**Vision Loss** r/t tumor growth compressing optic nerve and/or brain tissue

**Risk for Injury:** Risk factors: sensory-perceptual alterations, weakness

**Risk for Ineffective Thermoregulation:** Risk factor: changes in metabolic activity of the brain

*See Cancer; Chemotherapy; Child with Chronic Condition; Craniectomy/ Craniotomy; Hospitalized Child; Radiation Therapy; Terminally Ill Child, Adolescent; Terminally Ill Child, Infant/ Toddler; Terminally Ill Child, Preschool Child; Terminally Ill Child, School-Age Child/Preadolescent; Terminally Ill Child/ Death of Child, Parent*

## BRAXTON HICKS CONTRACTIONS

**Decreased Activity Tolerance** r/t increased contractions with increased gestation

**Anxiety** r/t uncertainty about beginning labor

**Fatigue** r/t lack of sleep

**Stress Urinary Incontinence** r/t increased pressure on bladder with contractions

**Insomnia** r/t contractions when lying down

**Ineffective Sexuality Pattern** r/t fear of contractions associated with loss of infant

## BREAST BIOPSY

**Fear** r/t potential for diagnosis of cancer

**Risk for Spiritual Distress:** Risk factor: fear of diagnosis of cancer

**Readiness for Enhanced Knowledge:** expresses an interest in learning

## BREAST CANCER

**Death Anxiety** r/t diagnosis of cancer

**Ineffective Coping** r/t treatment, prognosis

**Fear** r/t diagnosis of cancer

**Sexual Dysfunction** r/t loss of body part, partner's reaction to loss

**Chronic Sorrow** r/t diagnosis of cancer, loss of body integrity

**Risk for Spiritual Distress:** Risk factor: fear of diagnosis of cancer

**Readiness for Enhanced Health Literacy:** expresses desire to enhance understanding of health information to make health care choices

**Readiness for Enhanced Knowledge:** expresses an interest in learning

*See Cancer; Chemotherapy; Mastectomy; Radiation Therapy*

## BREAST EXAMINATION, SELF

*See SBE (Self–Breast Examination)*

## BREAST LUMPS

**Fear** r/t potential for diagnosis of cancer

**Readiness for Enhanced Knowledge:** expresses an interest in learning

## BREAST PUMPING

**Risk for Infection:** Risk factors: possible contaminated breast pump, incomplete emptying of breast

**Risk for Impaired Skin Integrity:** Risk factor: high suction

**Readiness for Enhanced Knowledge:** expresses an interest in learning

## BREASTFEEDING, EFFECTIVE

**Readiness for Enhanced Breastfeeding** (See Breastfeeding, Readiness for Enhanced, Section II)

## BREASTFEEDING, INEFFECTIVE

**Ineffective Breastfeeding** (See Breastfeeding, Ineffective, Section II)

*See Ineffective Infant Suck-Swallow Response; Painful Breasts, Engorgement; Painful Breasts, Sore Nipples*

## BREASTFEEDING, INTERRUPTED

**Interrupted Breastfeeding** (See Breastfeeding, Interrupted, Section II)

## BREAST MILK PRODUCTION, INSUFFICIENT

**Insufficient Breast Milk Production** (See Breast Milk Production, Insufficient, Section II)

## BREATH SOUNDS, DECREASED OR ABSENT

*See Atelectasis; Pneumothorax*

## BREATHING PATTERN ALTERATION

**Ineffective Breathing Pattern** r/t neuromuscular impairment, pain, musculoskeletal impairment, perception or cognitive impairment, anxiety, decreased energy or fatigue

## BREECH BIRTH

**Fear: Maternal** r/t danger to infant, self

**Impaired Gas Exchange: Fetal** r/t compressed umbilical cord

**Risk for Aspiration: Fetal:** Risk factor: birth of body before head

**Risk for Impaired Tissue Integrity: Fetal:** Risk factor: difficult birth

**Risk for Impaired Tissue Integrity: Maternal:** Risk factor: difficult birth

## BRONCHITIS

**Ineffective Airway Clearance** r/t excessive thickened mucus secretion

**Readiness for Enhanced Health Self-Management:** wishes to stop smoking

**Readiness for Enhanced Knowledge:** expresses an interest in learning

## BRONCHOPULMONARY DYSPLASIA

**Decreased Activity Tolerance** r/t imbalance between oxygen supply and demand

**Excess Fluid volume** r/t sodium and water retention

**Imbalanced Nutrition: Less than Body Requirements** r/t poor feeding, increased caloric needs as a result of increased work of breathing

*See Child with Chronic Condition; Hospitalized Child; Respiratory Conditions of the Neonate*

## BRONCHOSCOPY

**Risk for Aspiration:** Risk factor: temporary loss of gag reflex

**Risk for Injury:** Risk factors: complication of pneumothorax, laryngeal edema, hemorrhage (if biopsy done)

## BRUITS, CAROTID

**Risk for Ineffective Cerebral Tissue Perfusion:** Risk factors: interruption of carotid blood flow to brain

## BRYANT'S TRACTION

*See Traction and Casts*

## BUCK'S TRACTION

*See Traction and Casts*

## BUERGER'S DISEASE

*See Peripheral Vascular Disease (PVD)*

## BULIMIA

**Disturbed Body Image** r/t misperception about actual appearance, body weight

**Compromised Family Coping** r/t chronically unresolved feelings of guilt, anger, hostility

**Defensive Coping** r/t eating disorder

**Diarrhea** r/t laxative abuse

**Fear** r/t food ingestion, weight gain

**Imbalanced Nutrition: Less than Body Requirements** r/t induced vomiting, excessive exercise, laxative abuse

**Ineffective Adolescent Eating Dynamics** r/t overeating, leading to purge

**Powerlessness** r/t urge to purge self after eating

**Chronic Low Self-Esteem** r/t lack of positive feedback

*See Maturational Issues, Adolescent*

## BULLYING

**Anxiety** r/t specific or nonspecific threat to self

**Impaired Social Interaction** r/t dysfunctional interactions with others

**Fear** r/t perceived threat to self

**Risk for Compromised Human Dignity:** Risk factors: dehumanizing treatment, humiliation

**Risk for Other-Directed Violence:** Risk factors: social isolation, unresolved interpersonal conflicts

**Risk for Powerlessness:** Risk factor: ineffective coping strategies

**Risk for Impaired Resilience:** Risk factor: insufficient familial and social support

**Risk for Self-Directed violence:** Risk factors: unresolved interpersonal conflicts, social isolation

**Risk for Chronic Low Self-Esteem:** Risk factors: ineffective coping strategies, absence of sense of belonging, inadequate respect from others

## BUNION

**Readiness for Enhanced Knowledge:** expresses an interest in learning

## BUNIONECTOMY

**Impaired physical Mobility** r/t sore foot

**Impaired Walking** r/t pain associated with surgery

**Risk for Surgical Site Infection:** Risk factors: surgical incision

**Readiness for Enhanced Knowledge:** expresses an interest in learning

## BURN RISK

**Risk for Thermal Injury** (See **Thermal Injury, Risk for,** Section II)

## BURNS

**Anxiety** r/t burn injury, treatments

**Disturbed Body Image** r/t altered physical appearance

**Decreased Diversional Activity Engagement** r/t long-term hospitalization

**Fear** r/t pain from treatments, possible permanent disfigurement

**Deficient Fluid Volume** r/t loss of protective skin

**Maladaptive Grieving** r/t loss of bodily function, loss of future hopes and plans

**Hypothermia** r/t impaired skin integrity

**Impaired Physical Mobility** r/t pain, musculoskeletal impairment, contracture formation

**Imbalanced Nutrition: Less than Body Requirements** r/t increased metabolic needs, anorexia, protein and fluid loss

**Acute Pain** r/t burn injury, treatments

**Chronic Pain** r/t burn injury, treatments

**Ineffective Peripheral Tissue Perfusion** r/t circumferential burns, impaired arterial/venous circulation

**Post-Trauma Syndrome** r/t life-threatening event

**Impaired Skin Integrity** r/t injury of skin

**Delayed Surgical Recovery** r/t ineffective tissue perfusion

**Risk for Ineffective Airway Clearance:** Risk factors: potential tracheobronchial obstruction, edema

**Risk for Deficient Fluid Volume:** Risk factors: loss from skin surface, fluid shift

**Risk for Infection:** Risk factors: loss of intact skin, trauma, invasive sites

**Risk for Peripheral Neurovascular Dysfunction:** Risk factor: eschar formation with circumferential burn

**Risk for Post-Trauma Syndrome:** Risk factors: perception, duration of event that caused burns

**Risk for Ineffective Thermoregulation:** Risk factor: disruption of skin integrity

**Readiness for Enhanced Knowledge:** expresses an interest in learning

*See Hospitalized Child; Safety, Childhood*

## BURSITIS

**Impaired Physical Mobility** r/t inflammation in joint

**Acute Pain** r/t inflammation in joint

## BYPASS GRAFT

*See Coronary Artery Bypass Grafting (CABG)*

## CABG (CORONARY ARTERY BYPASS GRAFTING)

*See Coronary Artery Bypass Grafting (CABG)*

## CACHEXIA

**Frail Elderly Syndrome** r/t fatigue, feeding self-care deficit

**Imbalanced Nutrition: Less than Body Requirements** r/t inability to ingest food because of physiological factors

**Risk for Infection:** Risk factor: inadequate nutrition

## CALCIUM ALTERATION

*See Hypercalcemia; Hypocalcemia*

## CANCER

**Decreased Activity Tolerance** r/t side effects of treatment, weakness from cancer

**Death Anxiety** r/t unresolved issues regarding dying

**Disturbed Body Image** r/t side effects of treatment, cachexia

**Decisional Conflict** r/t selection of treatment choices, continuation or discontinuation of treatment, "do not resuscitate" decision

**Constipation** r/t side effects of medication, altered nutrition, decreased activity

**Compromised Family Coping** r/t prolonged disease or disability progression that

**C**

exhausts supportive ability of significant others

**Ineffective Coping** r/t personal vulnerability in situational crisis, terminal illness

**Ineffective Denial** r/t complicated grieving process

**Fear** r/t serious threat to well-being

**Maladaptive Grieving** r/t potential loss of significant others, high risk for infertility

**Ineffective Health Maintenance Behaviors** r/t deficient knowledge regarding prescribed treatment

**Hopelessness** r/t loss of control, terminal illness

**Insomnia** r/t anxiety, pain

**Impaired Physical Mobility** r/t weakness, neuromusculoskeletal impairment, pain

**Imbalanced Nutrition: Less than Body Requirements** r/t loss of appetite, difficulty swallowing, side effects of chemotherapy, obstruction by tumor

**Impaired Oral Mucous Membrane Integrity** r/t chemotherapy, effects of radiation, oral pH changes, decreased oral secretions

**Chronic Pain** r/t metastatic cancer

**Powerlessness** r/t treatment, progression of disease

**Ineffective Protection** r/t cancer suppressing immune system

**Ineffective Role Performance** r/t change in physical capacity, inability to resume prior role

**Self-Care Deficit: Specify** r/t pain, intolerance to activity, decreased strength

**Impaired Skin Integrity** r/t immunological deficit, immobility

**Social Isolation** r/t hospitalization, lifestyle changes

**Chronic Sorrow** r/t chronic illness of cancer

**Spiritual Distress** r/t test of spiritual beliefs

**Risk for Bleeding:** Risk factor: bone marrow depression from chemotherapy

**Risk for Disuse Syndrome:** Risk factors: immobility, fatigue

**Risk for Ineffective Home Maintenance Behaviors:** Risk factor: lack of familiarity with community resources

**Risk for Infection:** Risk factor: inadequate immune system

**Risk for Impaired Resilience:** Risk factors: multiple stressors, pain, chronic illness

**Risk for Spiritual Distress:** Risk factor: physical illness of cancer

**Readiness for Enhanced Knowledge:** expresses an interest in learning

**Readiness for enhanced spiritual well-being:** desire for harmony with self, others, higher power, God, when faced with serious illness

*See Chemotherapy; Child with Chronic Condition; Hospitalized Child; Leukemia; Radiation Therapy; Terminally Ill Child, Adolescent; Terminally Ill Child, Infant/Toddler; Terminally Ill Child, Preschool Child; Terminally Ill Child, School-Age Child/Preadolescent; Terminally Ill Child/Death of Child, Parent*

## CANDIDIASIS, ORAL

**Readiness for Enhanced Knowledge:** expresses an interest in learning

**Impaired Oral Mucous Membrane Integrity** r/t overgrowth of infectious agent, depressed immune function

**Acute Pain** r/t oral condition

## CAPILLARY REFILL TIME, PROLONGED

**Impaired Gas Exchange** r/t ventilation perfusion imbalance

**Ineffective Peripheral Tissue Perfusion** r/t interruption of arterial flow

*See Shock, Hypovolemic*

## CARBON MONOXIDE POISONING

*See Smoke Inhalation*

## CARDIAC ARREST

**Post-Trauma Syndrome** r/t experiencing serious life event

*See Dysrhythmia; MI (Myocardial Infarction)*

## CARDIAC CATHETERIZATION

**Fear** r/t invasive procedure, uncertainty of outcome of procedure

**Risk for Injury: Hematoma:** Risk factor: invasive procedure

**Risk for Decreased Cardiac Tissue Perfusion:** Risk factors: ventricular ischemia, dysrhythmia

**Risk for Peripheral Neurovascular Dysfunction:** Risk factor: vascular obstruction

**Risk for Impaired Tissue Integrity:** Risk factor: invasive procedure

**Readiness for Enhanced Knowledge:** expresses an interest in learning postprocedure care, treatment, and prevention of coronary artery disease

## CARDIAC DISORDERS IN PREGNANCY

**Decreased Activity Tolerance** r/t cardiac pathophysiology, increased demand for cardiac output because of pregnancy, weakness, fatigue

**Death Anxiety** r/t potential danger of condition

**Compromised Family Coping** r/t prolonged hospitalization or maternal incapacitation that exhausts supportive capacity of significant others

**Ineffective Coping** r/t personal vulnerability

**Interrupted Family Processes** r/t hospitalization, maternal incapacitation, changes in roles

**Fatigue** r/t physiological, psychological, and emotional demands

**Fear** r/t potential maternal effects, potential poor fetal or maternal outcome

**Powerlessness** r/t illness-related regimen

**Ineffective Role Performance** r/t changes in lifestyle, expectations from disease process with superimposed pregnancy

**Situational Low Self-Esteem** r/t situational crisis, pregnancy

**Social Isolation** r/t limitations of activity, bed rest or hospitalization, separation from family and friends

**Risk for Decreased Cardiac Tissue Perfusion:** Risk factor: strain on compromised heart from work of pregnancy, delivery

**Risk for Imbalanced Fluid Volume:** Risk factor: sudden changes in circulation after delivery of placenta, compromised regulatory mechanism with increased afterload, preload, circulating blood volume

**Risk for Impaired Gas Exchange:** Risk factor: pulmonary edema

**Risk for Disturbed Maternal–Fetal Dyad:** Risk factor: compromised oxygen transport

**Risk for impaired Resilience:** Risk factors: multiple stressors, fear

**Risk for Spiritual Distress:** Risk factor: fear of diagnosis for self and infant

**Readiness for Enhanced Knowledge:** expresses an interest in learning

## CARDIAC DYSRHYTHMIA

*See Dysrhythmia*

## CARDIAC OUTPUT, DECREASED

**Decreased Cardiac Output** r/t cardiac dysfunction

**Decreased Cardiac Output** (See **Cardiac Output, Decreased,** Section II)

**Risk for Decreased Cardiac Output** (See **Cardiac Output, Risk for Decreased,** Section II)

## CARDIAC TAMPONADE

**Decreased Cardiac Output** r/t fluid in pericardial sac

*See Pericarditis*

## CARDIOGENIC SHOCK

*See Shock, Cardiogenic*

## CAREGIVER ROLE STRAIN

**Caregiver Role Strain** (See **Caregiver Role Strain,** Section II)

**Risk for Impaired Resilience:** Risk factor: stress of prolonged caregiving

## CARIOUS TEETH

*See Cavities in Teeth*

## CAROTID ENDARTERECTOMY

**Fear** r/t surgery in vital area

**Risk for Ineffective Airway Clearance:** Risk factor: hematoma compressing trachea

**Risk for Bleeding:** Risk factor: possible hematoma formation, trauma to region

**Risk for Ineffective Cerebral Tissue Perfusion:** Risk factors: hemorrhage, clot formation

**Readiness for Enhanced Knowledge:** expresses an interest in learning

## CARPAL TUNNEL SYNDROME

**Impaired Physical Mobility** r/t neuromuscular impairment

**Chronic Pain** r/t unrelieved pressure on median nerve

**Self-Care Deficit: Bathing, Dressing, Feeding** r/t pain

## CARPOPEDAL SPASM

*See Hypocalcemia*

## CASTS

**Decreased Diversional Activity Engagement** r/t physical limitations from cast

**Impaired Physical Mobility** r/t limb immobilization

**Self-Care Deficit: Bathing, Dressing, Feeding** r/t presence of cast(s) on upper extremities

**Self-Care Deficit: Toileting** r/t presence of cast(s) on lower extremities

**Impaired Walking** r/t cast(s) on lower extremities, fracture of bones

**Risk for Peripheral Neurovascular Dysfunction:** Risk factors: mechanical compression from cast, trauma from fracture

**Risk for Impaired Skin Integrity:** Risk factor: unrelieved pressure on skin from cast

**Readiness for Enhanced Knowledge:** expresses an interest in learning

*See Traction and Casts*

## CATARACT EXTRACTION

**Anxiety** r/t threat of permanent vision loss, surgical procedure

**Vision Loss** r/t edema from surgery (see Appendix E on Evolve)

**Risk for Injury:** Risk factors: increased intraocular pressure, accommodation to new visual field

**Readiness for Enhanced Knowledge:** expresses an interest in learning

## CATATONIC SCHIZOPHRENIA

**Impaired Verbal Communication** r/t cognitive impairment

**Impaired Memory** r/t cognitive impairment

**Impaired Physical Mobility** r/t cognitive impairment, maintenance of rigid posture, inappropriate or bizarre postures

**Imbalanced Nutrition: Less than Body Requirements** r/t decrease in outside stimulation, loss of perception of hunger, resistance to instructions to eat

**Social Isolation** r/t inability to communicate, immobility

*See Schizophrenia*

## CATHETERIZATION, URINARY

**Risk for Infection:** Risk factor: invasive procedure

**Readiness for Enhanced Knowledge:** expresses an interest in learning

## CAVITIES IN TEETH

**Impaired Dentition** r/t ineffective oral hygiene, barriers to self-care, economic barriers to professional care, nutritional deficits, dietary habits

## CELIAC DISEASE

**Diarrhea** r/t malabsorption of food, immune effects of gluten on gastrointestinal system

**Imbalanced Nutrition: Less than Body Requirements** r/t malabsorption caused by immune effects of gluten

**Readiness for Enhanced Knowledge:** expresses an interest in learning

## CELLULITIS

**Acute Pain** r/t inflammatory changes in tissues from infection

**Impaired Tissue Integrity** r/t inflammatory process damaging skin and underlying tissue

**Ineffective Peripheral Tissue Perfusion** r/t edema of extremities

**Risk for Vascular Trauma:** Risk factor: infusion of antibiotics

**Readiness for Enhanced Knowledge:** expresses an interest in learning

## CELLULITIS, PERIORBITAL

**Acute Pain** r/t edema and inflammation of skin/tissues

**Impaired Skin Integrity** r/t inflammation or infection of skin, tissues

**Vision Loss** r/t decreased visual field secondary to edema of eyelids (see Appendix E on Evolve)

**Readiness for Enhanced Knowledge:** expresses an interest in learning

*See Hospitalized Child*

## CENTRAL LINE INSERTION

**Risk for Infection:** Risk factor: invasive procedure

**Risk for Vascular Trauma** (See **Vascular Trauma, Risk for,** Section II)

**Readiness for Enhanced Knowledge:** expresses an interest in learning

## CEREBRAL ANEURYSM

*See Craniectomy/Craniotomy; Intracranial Pressure, Increased; Subarachnoid Hemorrhage*

## CEREBRAL PALSY

**Impaired Verbal Communication** r/t impaired ability to articulate or speak words because of facial muscle involvement

**Decreased Diversional Activity Engagement** r/t physical impairments, limitations on ability to participate in recreational activities

**Impaired Physical Mobility** r/t spasticity, neuromuscular impairment or weakness

**Imbalanced Nutrition: Less than Body Requirements** r/t spasticity, feeding or swallowing difficulties

**Self-Care Deficit: Specify** r/t neuromuscular impairments, sensory deficits

**Impaired Social Interaction** r/t impaired communication skills, limited physical activity, perceived differences from peers

**Chronic Sorrow** r/t presence of chronic disability

**Risk for Adult Falls:** Risk factor: impaired physical mobility

**Risk for Child Falls**: Risk factor: impaired physical mobility

**Risk for Injury:** Risk factors: muscle weakness, inability to control spasticity

**Risk for Impaired Parenting:** Risk factor: caring for child with overwhelming needs resulting from chronic change in health status

**Risk for Spiritual Distress:** Risk factor: psychological stress associated with chronic illness

*See Child with Chronic Condition*

## CEREBRAL PERFUSION

**Risk for Ineffective Cerebral Tissue Perfusion** (See **Cerebral Tissue Perfusion, Ineffective, Risk for,** Section II)

## CEREBROVASCULAR ACCIDENT (CVA)

*See CVA (Cerebrovascular Accident)*

## CERVICITIS

**Ineffective Health Maintenance Behaviors** r/t deficient knowledge regarding care and prevention of condition

**Ineffective Sexuality Pattern** r/t abstinence during acute stage

**Risk for Infection:** Risk factors: spread of infection, recurrence of infection

## CESAREAN DELIVERY

**Disturbed Body Image** r/t surgery, unmet expectations for childbirth

**Interrupted Family Processes** r/t unmet expectations for childbirth

**Fear** r/t perceived threat to own well-being, outcome of birth

**Impaired Physical Mobility** r/t pain

**Acute Pain** r/t surgical incision

**Ineffective Role Performance** r/t unmet expectations for childbirth

**Situational Low Self-Esteem** r/t inability to deliver child vaginally

**Risk for Bleeding:** Risk factor: surgery

**Risk for Imbalanced Fluid Volume:** Risk factors: loss of blood, fluid shifts

**Risk for Surgical Site Infection:** Risk factor: surgical incision

**Risk for Urinary Retention:** Risk factor: regional anesthesia

**Readiness for Enhanced Childbearing Process:** a pattern of preparing for, maintaining, and strengthening care of newborn

**Readiness for Enhanced Knowledge:** expresses an interest in learning

## CHEMICAL DEPENDENCE

*See Alcoholism; Substance Abuse*

## CHEMOTHERAPY

**Death Anxiety** r/t chemotherapy not accomplishing desired results

**Disturbed Body Image** r/t loss of weight, loss of hair

**Fatigue** r/t disease process, anemia, drug effects

**Nausea** r/t effects of chemotherapy

**Imbalanced Nutrition: Less than Body Requirements** r/t side effects of chemotherapy

**Impaired Oral Mucous Membrane Integrity** r/t effects of chemotherapy

**Ineffective Protection** r/t suppressed immune system, decreased platelets

**Risk for Bleeding:** Risk factors: tumor eroding blood vessel, stress effects on gastrointestinal system

**Risk for Infection:** Risk factor: immunosuppression

**Risk for Vascular Trauma:** Risk factor: infusion of irritating medications

**Readiness for Enhanced Knowledge:** expresses an interest in learning
*See Cancer*

## CHEST PAIN

**Fear** r/t potential threat of death

**Acute Pain** r/t myocardial injury, ischemia

**Risk for Decreased Cardiac Tissue Perfusion:** Risk factor: ventricular ischemia
*See Angina; MI (Myocardial Infarction)*

## CHEST TUBES

**Ineffective Breathing Pattern** r/t asymmetrical lung expansion secondary to pain

**Impaired Gas Exchange** r/t decreased functional lung tissue

**Acute Pain** r/t presence of chest tubes, injury

**Risk for Injury:** Risk factor: presence of invasive chest tube

## CHEYNE-STOKES RESPIRATION

**Ineffective Breathing pattern** r/t critical illness

## CHICKENPOX

*See Communicable Diseases, Childhood*

## CHILD ABUSE

**Interrupted Family Processes** r/t inadequate coping skills

**Fear** r/t threat of punishment for perceived wrongdoing

**Insomnia** r/t hypervigilance, fear

**Imbalanced Nutrition: Less than Body Requirements** r/t inadequate caretaking

**Acute Pain** r/t physical injuries

**Impaired Parenting** r/t psychological impairment, physical or emotional abuse of parent, substance abuse, unrealistic expectations of child

**Ineffective Child Eating Dynamics** r/t hostile parental relationship

**Post-Trauma Syndrome** r/t physical abuse, incest, rape, molestation

**Chronic Low Self-Esteem** r/t lack of positive feedback, excessive negative feedback

**Impaired Skin Integrity** r/t altered nutritional state, physical abuse

**Social Isolation: Family Imposed** r/t fear of disclosure of family dysfunction and abuse

**Risk for Poisoning:** Risk factors: inadequate safeguards, lack of proper safety precautions, accessibility of illicit substances because of impaired home maintenance

**Risk for Suffocation:** Risk factors: unattended child, unsafe environment

**Risk for Physical Trauma:** Risk factors: inadequate precautions, cognitive or emotional difficulties

## CHILDBEARING PROBLEMS

**Ineffective Childbearing Process** (See **Childbearing Process, Ineffective,** Section II)

**Risk for Ineffective Childbearing Process** (See **Childbearing Process, Risk for Ineffective,** Section II)

## CHILD NEGLECT

*See Child Abuse; Failure to Thrive*

## CHILD WITH CHRONIC CONDITION

**Decreased Activity Tolerance** r/t fatigue associated with chronic illness

**Compromised Family Coping** r/t prolonged overconcern for child; distortion of reality regarding child's health problem, including extreme denial about its existence or severity

**Disabled Family Coping** r/t prolonged disease or disability progression that exhausts supportive capacity of significant others

**Ineffective Coping: Child** r/t situational or maturational crises

**Decisional Conflict** r/t treatment options, conflicting values

**Decreased Diversional Activity Engagement** r/t immobility, monotonous environment, frequent or lengthy treatments, reluctance to participate, self-imposed social isolation

**Interrupted Family Processes** r/t intermittent situational crisis of illness, disease, hospitalization

**Ineffective Health Maintenance Behaviors** r/t exhausting family resources (finances, physical energy, support systems)

**Ineffective Home Maintenance Behaviors** r/t overtaxed family members (e.g., exhausted, anxious)

**Hopelessness: Child** r/t prolonged activity restriction, long-term stress, lack of involvement in or passively allowing care as a result of parental overprotection

**Insomnia: Child or Parent** r/t time-intensive treatments, exacerbation of condition, 24-hour care needs

**Deficient Knowledge** r/t knowledge or skill acquisition regarding health practices, acceptance of limitations, promotion of maximal potential of child, self-actualization of rest of family

**Imbalanced Nutrition: Less than Body Requirements** r/t anorexia, fatigue from physical exertion

**Risk for Overweight** r/t effects of steroid medications on appetite

**Chronic Pain** r/t physical, biological, chemical, or psychological factors

**Powerlessness: Child** r/t health care environment, illness-related regimen, lifestyle of learned helplessness

**Parental Role Conflict** r/t separation from child as a result of chronic illness, home care of child with special needs, interruptions of family life resulting from home care regimen

**Chronic Low Self-Esteem** r/t actual or perceived differences; peer acceptance; decreased ability to participate in physical, school, and social activities

**Ineffective Sexuality Pattern: Parental** r/t disrupted relationship with sexual partner

**Impaired Social Interaction** r/t developmental lag or delay, perceived differences

**Social Isolation: Family** r/t actual or perceived social stigmatization, complex care requirements

**Chronic Sorrow** r/t developmental stages and missed opportunities or milestones that bring comparisons with social or personal norms, unending caregiving as reminder of loss

**Risk for Delayed Child Development:** Risk factor: chronic illness

**Risk for Infection:** Risk factor: debilitating physical condition

**Risk for Impaired Parenting:** Risk factors: impaired or disrupted bonding, caring for child with perceived overwhelming care needs

**Readiness for Enhanced Family Coping:** impact of crisis on family values, priorities, goals, or relationships; changes in family choices to optimize wellness

## CHILDBIRTH

**Readiness for Enhanced Childbearing Process** (See **Childbearing Process, Readiness for Enhanced,** Section II)

*See Labor, Normal; Postpartum, Normal Care*

## CHILDHOOD OBESITY

**Obesity** r/t disordered eating behaviors

**Risk for Unstable Blood Glucose Level:** Risk factor: excessive weight gain

**Risk for Metabolic Syndrome:** Risk factors: obesity, sedentary lifestyle

**Readiness for Enhanced Exercise Engagement:** expresses desire to engage in regular exercise

**Readiness for Enhanced Knowledge:** expresses desire to make healthier nutrition choices

## CHILLS

**Hyperthermia** r/t infectious process

## CHLAMYDIA INFECTION

*See STD (Sexually Transmitted Disease)*

## CHLOASMA

**Disturbed Body Image** r/t change in skin color

## CHOKING OR COUGHING WITH EATING

**Impaired Swallowing** r/t neuromuscular impairment

**Risk for Aspiration:** Risk factors: depressed cough and gag reflexes

## CHOLECYSTECTOMY

**Imbalanced Nutrition: Less than Body Requirements** r/t high metabolic needs, decreased ability to digest fatty foods

**Acute Pain** r/t trauma from surgery

**Risk for Deficient Fluid Volume:** Risk factors: restricted intake, nausea, vomiting

**Risk for Surgical Site Infection:** Risk factor: invasive procedure

**Readiness for Enhanced Knowledge:** expresses an interest in learning

*See Abdominal Surgery*

## CHOLELITHIASIS

**Nausea** r/t obstruction of bile

**Imbalanced Nutrition: Less than Body Requirements** r/t anorexia, nausea, vomiting

**Acute Pain** r/t obstruction of bile flow, inflammation in gallbladder

**Readiness for Enhanced Knowledge:** expresses an interest in learning

## CHORIOAMNIONITIS

**Anxiety** r/t threat to self and infant

**Maladaptive Grieving** r/t guilt about potential loss of ideal pregnancy and birth

**Hyperthermia** r/t infectious process

**Situational Low Self-Esteem** r/t guilt about threat to infant's health

**Risk for Infection:** Risk factors: infection transmission from mother to fetus; infection in fetal environment

## CHRONIC CONFUSION

*See Confusion, Chronic*

## CHRONIC FUNCTIONAL CONSTIPATION

(See **Constipation, Chronic Functional,** Section II)

(See **Constipation, Chronic Functional, Risk for,** Section II)

## CHRONIC LYMPHOCYTIC LEUKEMIA

*See Cancer; Chemotherapy; Leukemia*

## CHRONIC OBSTRUCTIVE PULMONARY DISEASE (COPD)

*See COPD (Chronic Obstructive Pulmonary Disease)*

## CHRONIC PAIN

*See Pain Management, Chronic*

## CHRONIC RENAL FAILURE (CHRONIC RENAL DISEASE)

*See Renal Failure*

## CHVOSTEK'S SIGN

*See Hypocalcemia*

## CIRCUMCISION

**Acute Pain** r/t surgical intervention

**Risk for Bleeding:** Risk factor: surgical trauma

**Risk for Infection:** Risk factor: surgical wound

**Readiness for Enhanced Knowledge: Parent:** expresses an interest in learning

## CIRRHOSIS

**Chronic Confusion** r/t chronic organic disorder with increased ammonia levels, substance abuse

**Defensive Coping** r/t inability to accept responsibility to stop substance abuse

**Fatigue** r/t malnutrition

**Ineffective Health Maintenance Behaviors** r/t deficient knowledge regarding correlation between lifestyle habits and disease process

**Nausea** r/t irritation to gastrointestinal system

**Imbalanced Nutrition: Less than Body Requirements** r/t loss of appetite, nausea, vomiting

**Chronic Pain** r/t liver enlargement

**Chronic Low Self-Esteem** r/t chronic illness

**Chronic Sorrow** r/t presence of chronic illness

**Risk for Bleeding:** Risk factors: impaired blood coagulation, bleeding from portal hypertension

**Risk for Injury:** Risk factors: substance intoxication, potential delirium tremens

**Risk for Impaired Oral Mucous Membrane Integrity:** Risk factors: altered nutrition, inadequate oral care

**Risk for Impaired Skin Integrity:** Risk factors: altered nutritional state, altered metabolic state

## CLEFT LIP/CLEFT PALATE

**Ineffective Airway Clearance** r/t common feeding and breathing passage, postoperative laryngeal, incisional edema

**Ineffective Breastfeeding** r/t infant anomaly

**Impaired Verbal Communication** r/t inadequate palate function, possible hearing loss from infected eustachian tubes

**Fear: Parental** r/t special care needs, surgery

**Maladaptive Grieving** r/t loss of perfect child

**Ineffective Infant Feeding Dynamics** r/t fear resulting in inadequate feeding

**Ineffective Infant Suck-Swallow Response** r/t cleft lip, cleft palate

**Impaired Physical Mobility** r/t imposed restricted activity, use of elbow restraints

**Impaired Oral Mucous Membrane Integrity** r/t surgical correction

**Acute Pain** r/t surgical correction, elbow restraints

**Impaired Skin Integrity** r/t incomplete joining of lip, palate ridges

**Chronic Sorrow** r/t birth of child with congenital defect

**Risk for Aspiration:** Risk factor: common feeding and breathing passage

**Risk for Disturbed Body Image:** Risk factors: disfigurement, speech impediment

**Risk for Deficient Fluid Volume:** Risk factor: inability to take liquids in usual manner

**Risk for Infection:** Risk factors: invasive procedure, disruption of eustachian tube development, aspiration

**Readiness for Enhanced Knowledge: Parent:** expresses an interest in learning

## CLOTTING DISORDER

**Fear** r/t threat to well-being

**Risk for Bleeding:** Risk factor: impaired clotting

**Readiness for Enhanced Knowledge:** expresses an interest in learning

*See Anticoagulant Therapy; DIC (Disseminated Intravascular Coagulation); Hemophilia*

## COCAINE BABY

*See Neonatal Abstinence Syndrome*

## CODEPENDENCY

**Caregiver Role Strain** r/t codependency

**Impaired Verbal Communication** r/t psychological barriers

**Ineffective Coping** r/t inadequate support systems

**Decisional Conflict** r/t support system deficit

**Ineffective Denial** r/t unmet self-needs

**Powerlessness** r/t lifestyle of helplessness

## COLD, VIRAL

*See Infectious Processes*

## COLECTOMY

**Constipation** r/t decreased activity, decreased fluid intake

**Imbalanced Nutrition: Less than Body Requirements** r/t high metabolic needs, decreased ability to ingest or digest food

**Acute Pain** r/t recent surgery

**Risk for Surgical Site Infection:** Risk factor: invasive procedure

**Readiness for Enhanced Knowledge:** expresses an interest in learning

*See Abdominal Surgery*

## COLITIS

**Diarrhea** r/t inflammation in colon

**Deficient Fluid Volume** r/t frequent stools

**Acute Pain** r/t inflammation in colon

**Readiness for Enhanced Knowledge:** expresses an interest in learning

*See Crohn's Disease; Inflammatory Bowel Disease (Child and Adult)*

## COLLAGEN DISEASE

*See specific disease (e.g., Lupus Erythematosus; JRA [Juvenile Rheumatoid Arthritis]); Congenital Heart Disease/ Cardiac Anomalies*

## COLOSTOMY

**Disturbed Body Image** r/t presence of stoma, daily care of fecal material

**Ineffective Sexuality Pattern** r/t altered body image, self-concept

**Social Isolation** r/t anxiety about appearance of stoma and possible leakage of stool

**Risk for Constipation:** Risk factor: inappropriate diet

**Risk for Diarrhea:** Risk factor: inappropriate diet

**Risk for Impaired Skin Integrity:** Risk factor: irritation from bowel contents

**Readiness for Enhanced Knowledge:** expresses an interest in learning

## COLPORRHAPHY, ANTERIOR

*See Vaginal Hysterectomy*

## COMA

**Death Anxiety: Significant Others** r/t unknown outcome of coma state

**Interrupted Family Processes** r/t illness or disability of family member

**Disability-Associated Urinary Incontinence** r/t presence of comatose state

**Self-Care Deficit** r/t neuromuscular impairment

**Ineffective Family Health Self-Management** r/t complexity of therapeutic regimen

**Risk for Aspiration:** Risk factors: impaired swallowing, loss of cough or gag reflex

**Risk for Disuse Syndrome:** Risk factor: altered level of consciousness impairing mobility

**Risk for Dry Mouth:** Risk factor: inability to perform own oral care

**Risk for Hypothermia:** Risk factors: inactivity, possible pharmaceutical agents, possible hypothalamic injury

**Risk for Injury:** Risk factor: potential seizure activity

**Risk for Corneal Injury:** Risk factor: suppressed corneal reflex

**Risk for Urinary Tract Injury:** Risk factor: long-term use of urinary catheter

**Risk for Impaired Oral Mucous Membrane Integrity:** Risk factors: dry mouth, inability to do own mouth care

**Risk for Pressure Ulcer:** Risk factor: prolonged immobility

**Risk for Impaired Skin Integrity:** Risk factor: immobility

**Risk for Spiritual Distress: Significant Others:** Risk factors: loss of ability to relate to loved one, unknown outcome of coma

**Risk for Impaired Tissue Integrity:** Risk factor: impaired physical mobility

*See Head Injury; Subarachnoid Hemorrhage; Intracranial Pressure, Increased*

## COMFORT, LOSS OF

**Impaired Comfort** (See **Comfort, Impaired,** Section II)

**Readiness for Enhanced Comfort** (See **Comfort, Readiness for Enhanced,** Section II)

## COMMUNICABLE DISEASES, CHILDHOOD (E.G., MEASLES, MUMPS, RUBELLA, CHICKENPOX, SCABIES, LICE, IMPETIGO)

**Impaired Comfort** r/t pruritus, inflammation or infection of skin, subdermal organisms

**Decreased Diversional Activity Engagement** r/t imposed isolation from peers, disruption in usual play activities, fatigue, activity intolerance

**Ineffective Health Maintenance Behaviors** r/t nonadherence to appropriate immunization schedules, lack of prevention of transmission of infection

**Acute Pain** r/t impaired skin integrity, edema

**Risk for Infection: Transmission to Others:** Risk factor: contagious organisms

*See Meningitis/Encephalitis; Respiratory Infections, Acute Childhood*

## COMMUNICATION

**Readiness for Enhanced Communication** (See **Communication, Readiness for Enhanced,** Section II)

## COMMUNICATION PROBLEMS

**Impaired Verbal Communication** (See **Communication, Verbal, Impaired,** Section II)

## COMMUNITY COPING

**Ineffective Community Coping** (See **Coping, Community, Ineffective,** Section II)

**Readiness for Enhanced Community Coping:** community sense of power to manage stressors, social supports available, resources available for problem solving

## COMMUNITY HEALTH PROBLEMS

**Deficient community Health** (See **Health, Deficient, Community,** Section II)

## COMPANION ANIMAL

**Anxiety** r/t environmental and personal stressors

**Impaired Comfort** r/t insufficient environmental control

## COMPARTMENT SYNDROME

**Fear** r/t possible loss of limb, damage to limb

**Acute Pain** r/t pressure in compromised body part

**Ineffective Peripheral Tissue Perfusion** r/t increased pressure within compartment

## COMPULSION

*See OCD (Obsessive-Compulsive Disorder)*

## CONDUCTION DISORDERS (CARDIAC)

*See Dysrhythmia*

## CONFUSION, ACUTE

**Acute Confusion** r/t older than 70 years of age with hospitalization, alcohol abuse, delirium, dementia, substance abuse

**Frail Elderly Syndrome** r/t impaired memory

**Risk for Acute Confusion:** Risk factor: alteration in level of consciousness

## CONFUSION, CHRONIC

**Chronic Confusion** r/t dementia, Korsakoff's psychosis, multi-infarct dementia, cerebrovascular accident, head injury

**Frail Elderly Syndrome** r/t impaired memory

**Impaired Memory** r/t fluid and electrolyte imbalance, neurological disturbances, excessive environmental disturbances, anemia, acute or chronic hypoxia, decreased cardiac output

**Impaired Mood Regulation** r/t emotional instability

*See Alzheimer's Disease; Dementia*

**C**

## CONGENITAL HEART DISEASE/ CARDIAC ANOMALIES

**Decreased Activity Tolerance** r/t fatigue, generalized weakness, lack of adequate oxygenation

**Ineffective Breathing Pattern** r/t pulmonary vascular disease

**Decreased Cardiac Output** r/t cardiac dysfunction

**Excess Fluid Volume** r/t cardiac dysfunction, side effects of medication

**Impaired Gas Exchange** r/t cardiac dysfunction, pulmonary congestion

**Imbalanced Nutrition: Less than Body Requirements** r/t fatigue, generalized weakness, inability of infant to suck and feed, increased caloric requirements

**Risk for Deficient Fluid Volume:** Risk factor: side effects of diuretics

**Risk for Disorganized Infant Behavior:** Risk factor: invasive procedures

**Risk for Poisoning:** Risk factor: potential toxicity of cardiac medications

**Risk for Ineffective Thermoregulation:** Risk factor: neonatal age

*See Child with Chronic Condition; Hospitalized Child*

## CONGESTIVE HEART FAILURE (CHF)

*See Heart Failure*

## CONJUNCTIVITIS

**Acute Pain** r/t inflammatory process

**Vision Loss** r/t change in visual acuity resulting from inflammation

## CONSCIOUSNESS, ALTERED LEVEL OF

**Acute Confusion** r/t alcohol abuse, delirium, dementia, drug abuse, head injury

**Chronic Confusion** r/t multi-infarct dementia, Korsakoff's psychosis, head injury, cerebrovascular accident, neurological deficit

**Disability-Associated Urinary Incontinence** r/t neurological dysfunction

**Impaired Memory** r/t neurological disturbances

**Self-Care Deficit: Specify** r/t neuromuscular impairment

**Risk for Aspiration:** Risk factors: impaired swallowing, loss of cough or gag reflex

**Risk for Disuse Syndrome:** Risk factor: impaired mobility resulting from altered level of consciousness

**Risk for Dry Mouth:** Risk factor: inability to perform own oral care

**Risk for Falls:** Risk factor: diminished mental status

**Risk for Impaired Oral Mucous Membrane Integrity:** Risk factors: dry mouth, interrupted oral care

**Risk for Ineffective Cerebral Tissue Perfusion:** Risk factors: increased intracranial pressure, altered cerebral perfusion

**Risk for Impaired Skin Integrity:** Risk factor: immobility

*See Coma; Head Injury; Subarachnoid Hemorrhage; Intracranial Pressure, Increased*

## CONSTIPATION

**Constipation** (See **Constipation**, Section II)

## CONSTIPATION, CHRONIC FUNCTIONAL

**Constipation** (See **Constipation, Chronic Functional,** Section II)

## CONSTIPATION, PERCEIVED

**Perceived Constipation** (See **Perceived Constipation,** Section II)

## CONSTIPATION, RISK FOR

**Risk for Constipation** (See **Constipation, Risk for,** Section II)

**Risk for Chronic Functional Constipation** (See **Constipation, Chronic Functional, Risk for,** Section II)

## CONTAMINATION

**Contamination** (See **Contamination**, Section II)

**C**

**Risk for Contamination** (See **Contamination, Risk for,** Section II)

## CONTINENT ILEOSTOMY (KOCK POUCH)

**Ineffective Coping** r/t stress of disease, exacerbations caused by stress

**Imbalanced Nutrition: Less than Body Requirements** r/t malabsorption from disease process

**Risk for Injury:** Risk factors: failure of valve, stomal cyanosis, intestinal obstruction

**Readiness for Enhanced Knowledge:** expresses an interest in learning

*See Abdominal Surgery; Crohn's Disease*

## CONTRACEPTIVE METHOD

**Decisional Conflict: Method of Contraception** r/t unclear personal values or beliefs, lack of experience or interference with decision-making, lack of relevant information, support system deficit

**Ineffective Sexuality Pattern** r/t fear of pregnancy

**Readiness for Enhanced Health Self-Management:** requesting information about available and appropriate birth control methods

## CONVULSIONS

**Anxiety** r/t concern over controlling convulsions

**Impaired Memory** r/t neurological disturbance

**Risk for Aspiration:** Risk factor: impaired swallowing

**Risk for Injury:** Risk factor: seizure activity

**Readiness for Enhanced Knowledge:** expresses an interest in learning

*See Seizure Disorders, Adult; Seizure Disorders, Childhood*

## COPD (CHRONIC OBSTRUCTIVE PULMONARY DISEASE)

**Decreased Activity Tolerance** r/t imbalance between oxygen supply and demand

**Ineffective Airway Clearance** r/t bronchoconstriction, increased mucus, ineffective cough, infection

**Anxiety** r/t breathlessness, change in health status

**Death Anxiety** r/t seriousness of medical condition, difficulty being able to "catch breath," feeling of suffocation

**Interrupted Family Processes** r/t role changes

**Impaired Gas Exchange** r/t ventilation-perfusion inequality

**Ineffective Health Self-Management** (See **Health Management, Ineffective,** Section II)

**Imbalanced Nutrition: Less than Body Requirements** r/t decreased intake because of dyspnea, unpleasant taste in mouth left by medications, increased need for calories from work of breathing

**Powerlessness** r/t progressive nature of disease

**Self-Care Deficit** r/t fatigue from the increased work of breathing

**Chronic Low Self-Esteem** r/t chronic illness

**Sleep Deprivation** r/t breathing difficulties when lying down

**Impaired Social Interaction** r/t social isolation because of oxygen use, activity intolerance

**Chronic Sorrow** r/t presence of chronic illness

**Risk for Infection:** Risk factor: stasis of respiratory secretions

**Readiness for Enhanced Health Self-Management** (See **Health Management, Readiness for Enhanced,** Section II)

## COPING

**Readiness for Enhanced Coping** (See **Coping, Readiness for Enhanced,** Section II)

**Risk for Complicated Immigration Transition:** Risk factors: insufficient knowledge about the process to access resources in the host country, insufficient social support in the host country, overt discrimination

## COPING PROBLEMS

**Compromised Family Coping** (See **Coping, Compromised Family,** Section II)

**Defensive Coping** (See **Coping, Defensive,** Section II)

**Disabled Family Coping** (See **Coping, Disabled Family,** Section II)

**Ineffective Coping** (See **Coping, Ineffective,** Section II)

**Ineffective Community Coping** (See **Coping, Ineffective Community,** Section II)

### CORNEAL INJURY

**Risk for Corneal Injury** (See **Corneal Injury, Risk for,** Section II)

### CORNEAL REFLEX, ABSENT

**Risk for Injury:** Risk factors: accidental corneal abrasion, drying of cornea

### CORNEAL TRANSPLANT

**Risk for Surgical Site Infection:** Risk factors: invasive procedure, surgery

**Readiness for Enhanced Health Self-Management:** describes need to rest and avoid strenuous activities during healing phase

### CORONARY ARTERY BYPASS GRAFTING (CABG)

**Decreased Cardiac Output** r/t dysrhythmia, depressed cardiac function, change in preload, contractility or afterload

**Fear** r/t outcome of surgical procedure

**Deficient Fluid Volume** r/t intraoperative blood loss, use of diuretics in surgery

**Acute Pain** r/t traumatic surgery

**Risk for Perioperative Positioning Injury:** Risk factors: hypothermia, extended supine position

**Risk for Surgical Site Infection:** Risk factor: surgical incision

**Risk for Impaired Tissue Integrity:** Risk factor: surgical procedure

**Readiness for Enhanced Knowledge:** expresses an interest in learning

### COSTOVERTEBRAL ANGLE TENDERNESS

*See Kidney Stone; Pyelonephritis*

### COUGH, INEFFECTIVE

**Ineffective Airway Clearance** r/t decreased energy, fatigue, normal aging changes

*See Bronchitis; COPD (Chronic Obstructive Pulmonary Disease); Pulmonary Edema*

### CRACKLES IN LUNGS, COARSE

**Ineffective Airway Clearance** r/t excessive secretions in airways, ineffective cough

*See Heart Failure; Pneumonia; Pulmonary Edema*

### CRACKLES IN LUNGS, FINE

**Ineffective Breathing Pattern** r/t fatigue, surgery, decreased energy

*See Bronchitis or Pneumonia (if from pulmonary infection); Congestive Heart Failure (CHF) (if cardiac in origin); Infection, Potential for*

### CRANIECTOMY/CRANIOTOMY

**Frail Elderly Syndrome** r/t alteration in cognition

**Fear** r/t threat to well-being

**Impaired Memory** r/t neurological surgery

**Acute Pain** r/t recent brain surgery, increased intracranial pressure

**Risk for Ineffective Cerebral Tissue Perfusion:** Risk factors: cerebral edema, increased intracranial pressure

**Risk for Injury:** Risk factor: potential confusion

*See Coma (if relevant)*

### CREPITATION, SUBCUTANEOUS

*See Pneumothorax*

### CRISIS

**Anxiety** r/t threat to or change in environment, health status, interaction patterns, situation, self-concept, or role functioning; threat of death of self or significant other

**Death Anxiety** r/t feelings of hopelessness associated with crisis

**Compromised Family Coping** r/t situational or developmental crisis

**Ineffective Coping** r/t situational or maturational crisis

**Fear** r/t crisis situation

Maladaptive Grieving r/t potential significant loss

Impaired Resilience r/t onset of crisis

Situational Low Self-Esteem r/t perception of inability to handle crisis

Stress Overload (See Stress Overload, Section II)

Risk for Spiritual Distress: Risk factors: physical or psychological stress, natural disasters, situational losses, maturational losses

## CROHN'S DISEASE

Anxiety r/t change in health status

Ineffective Coping r/t repeated episodes of diarrhea

Diarrhea r/t inflammatory process

Ineffective Health Maintenance Behaviors r/t deficient knowledge regarding management of disease

Imbalanced Nutrition: Less than Body Requirements r/t diarrhea, altered ability to digest and absorb food

Acute Pain r/t increased peristalsis

Powerlessness r/t chronic disease

Risk for Deficient Fluid Volume: Risk factor: abnormal fluid loss with diarrhea

## CROUP

*See Respiratory Infections, Acute Childhood (Croup, Epiglottitis, Pertussis, Pneumonia, Respiratory)*

## CRYOSURGERY FOR RETINAL DETACHMENT

*See Retinal Detachment*

## CUSHING'S SYNDROME

Decreased Activity Tolerance r/t fatigue, weakness

Disturbed Body Image r/t change in appearance from disease process

Excess Fluid Volume r/t failure of regulatory mechanisms

Sexual Dysfunction r/t loss of libido

Impaired Skin Integrity r/t thin vulnerable skin from effects of increased cortisol

Risk for Infection: Risk factor: suppression of immune system caused by increased cortisol levels

Risk for Injury: Risk factors: decreased muscle strength, brittle bones

Readiness for Enhanced Knowledge: expresses an interest in learning

**C**

## CUTS (WOUNDS)

*See Lacerations*

## CVA (CEREBROVASCULAR ACCIDENT)

Anxiety r/t situational crisis, change in physical or emotional condition

Disturbed Body Image r/t chronic illness, paralysis

Caregiver Role Strain r/t cognitive problems of care receiver, need for significant home care

Impaired Verbal Communication r/t pressure damage, decreased circulation to brain in speech center informational sources

Chronic Confusion r/t neurological changes

Constipation r/t decreased activity

Ineffective Coping r/t disability

Interrupted Family Processes r/t illness, disability of family member

Frail Elderly Syndrome r/t alteration in cognitive functioning

Maladaptive Grieving r/t loss of health

Ineffective Home Maintenance Behaviors r/t neurological disease affecting ability to perform activities of daily living

Disability-Associated Urinary Incontinence r/t neurological dysfunction

Impaired Memory r/t neurological disturbances

Impaired Physical Mobility r/t loss of balance and coordination

Unilateral Neglect r/t disturbed perception from neurological damage

Self-Care Deficit: Specify r/t decreased strength and endurance, paralysis

Impaired Social interaction r/t limited physical mobility, limited ability to communicate

Impaired Swallowing r/t neuromuscular dysfunction

Impaired Transfer Ability r/t limited physical mobility

**Vision Loss** r/t pressure damage to visual centers in the brain (*see Appendix E on Evolve*)

**Impaired Walking** r/t loss of balance and coordination

**Risk for Aspiration:** Risk factors: impaired swallowing, loss of gag reflex

**Risk for Chronic Functional Constipation:** Risk factor: immobility

**Risk for Disuse Syndrome:** Risk factor: paralysis

**Risk for Adult Falls:** Risk factor: paralysis, decreased balance

**Risk for Injury:** Risk factors: vision loss, decreased tissue perfusion with loss of sensation

**Risk for Ineffective Cerebral Tissue Perfusion:** Risk factor: clot, emboli, or hemorrhage from cerebral vessel

**Risk for Impaired Skin Integrity:** Risk factor: immobility

**Readiness for Enhanced Knowledge:** expresses an interest in learning

## CYANOSIS, CENTRAL WITH CYANOSIS OF ORAL MUCOUS MEMBRANES

**Impaired Gas Exchange** r/t alveolar-capillary membrane changes

## CYANOSIS, PERIPHERAL WITH CYANOSIS OF NAIL BEDS

**Ineffective Peripheral Tissue Perfusion** r/t interruption of arterial flow, severe vasoconstriction, cold temperatures

## CYSTIC FIBROSIS

**Decreased Activity Tolerance** r/t imbalance between oxygen supply and demand

**Ineffective Airway Clearance** r/t increased production of thick mucus

**Anxiety** r/t dyspnea, oxygen deprivation

**Disturbed Body Image** r/t changes in physical appearance, treatment of chronic lung disease (clubbing, barrel chest, home oxygen therapy)

**Impaired Gas Exchange** r/t ventilation-perfusion imbalance

**Ineffective Home Maintenance Behaviors** r/t extensive daily treatment, medications necessary for health

**Imbalanced Nutrition: Less than Body Requirements** r/t anorexia; decreased absorption of nutrients, fat; increased work of breathing

**Chronic Sorrow** r/t presence of chronic disease

**Risk for Caregiver Role Strain:** Risk factors: illness severity of care receiver, unpredictable course of illness

**Risk for Deficient Fluid Volume:** Risk factors: decreased fluid intake, increased work of breathing

**Risk for Infection:** Risk factors: thick, tenacious mucus; harboring of bacterial organisms; immunocompromised state

**Risk for Spiritual Distress:** Risk factor: presence of chronic disease

*See Child with Chronic Condition; Hospitalized Child; Terminally Ill Child, Adolescent; Terminally Ill Child, Infant/ Toddler; Terminally Ill Child, Preschool Child; Terminally Ill Child, School-Age Child/Preadolescent; Terminally Ill Child/ Death of Child, Parent*

## CYSTITIS

**Acute Pain: Dysuria** r/t inflammatory process in bladder and urethra

**Impaired Urinary Elimination: Frequency** r/t urinary tract infection

**Urge Urinary Incontinence:** Risk factor: infection in bladder

**Readiness for Enhanced Knowledge:** expresses an interest in learning

## CYSTOCELE

**Stress Urinary Incontinence** r/t prolapsed bladder

**Readiness for Enhanced Knowledge:** expresses an interest in learning

## CYSTOSCOPY

**Urinary Retention** r/t edema in urethra obstructing flow of urine

**Risk for Infection:** Risk factor: invasive procedure

**Readiness for Enhanced Knowledge:** expresses an interest in learning

# D

## DEAFNESS

**Impaired Verbal Communication** r/t impaired hearing

**Hearing Loss** r/t alteration in sensory reception, transmission, integration

**Risk for Injury:** Risk factor: alteration in sensory perception

## DEATH

**Risk for Sudden Infant Death** (See **Sudden Infant Death, Risk for,** Section II)

## DEATH, ONCOMING

**Death Anxiety** r/t unresolved issues surrounding dying

**Compromised Family Coping** r/t client's inability to provide support to family

**Ineffective Coping** r/t personal vulnerability

**Fear** r/t threat of death

**Maladaptive Grieving** r/t loss of significant other

**Powerlessness** r/t effects of illness, oncoming death

**Social Isolation** r/t altered state of wellness

**Spiritual Distress** r/t intense suffering

**Readiness for Enhanced Spiritual Well-Being:** desire of client and family to be in harmony with each other, higher power, God

*See Terminally Ill Child, Adolescent; Terminally Ill Child, Infant/Toddler; Terminally Ill Child, Preschool Child; Terminally Ill Child, School-Age Child/ Preadolescent; Terminally Ill Child/Death of Child, Parent*

## DECISIONS, DIFFICULTY MAKING

**Decisional Conflict** r/t support system deficit, perceived threat to value system, multiple or divergent sources of information, lack of relevant information, unclear personal values or beliefs

**Risk for Impaired Emancipated Decision-Making:** Risk factor: insufficient self-confidence in decision-making

**Readiness for Enhanced Decision-Making** (See **Decision-Making, Readiness for Enhanced,** Section II)

## DECUBITUS ULCER

*See Pressure Ulcer; Pressure Injury*

## DEEP VEIN THROMBOSIS (DVT)

*See DVT (Deep Vein Thrombosis); Venous Thromboembolism*

## DEFENSIVE BEHAVIOR

**Defensive Coping** r/t nonacceptance of blame, denial of problems or weakness

**Ineffective Denial** r/t inability to face situation realistically

## DEHISCENCE, ABDOMINAL

**Fear** r/t threat of death, severe dysfunction

**Acute Pain** r/t stretching of abdominal wall

**Impaired Skin Integrity** r/t altered circulation, malnutrition, opening in incision

**Delayed Surgical Recovery** r/t altered circulation, malnutrition, opening in incision

**Impaired Tissue Integrity** r/t exposure of abdominal contents to external environment

**Risk for Deficient Fluid Volume:** Risk factor: altered circulation associated with opening of wound and exposure of abdominal contents

**Risk for Surgical Site Infection:** Risk factors: loss of skin integrity, open surgical wound

## DEHYDRATION

**Deficient Fluid Volume** r/t active fluid volume loss

**Impaired Oral Mucous Membrane Integrity** r/t decreased salivation, fluid deficit

**Risk for Chronic Functional Constipation:** Risk factor: decreased fluid volume

**Risk for Dry Mouth:** Risk factor: decreased fluid volume

**Risk for Ineffective Thermoregulation:** Risk factor: decreased fluid volume

**Risk for Unstable Blood Pressure:** Risk factor: hypotension caused by insufficient fluid volume

D

*See Burns; Heat Stroke; Vomiting; Diarrhea*

## DELIRIUM

**Acute Confusion** r/t effects of medication, response to hospitalization, alcohol abuse, substance abuse, sensory deprivation or overload, infection, polypharmacy

**Impaired Memory** r/t delirium

**Sleep Deprivation** r/t sustained inadequate sleep hygiene

**Risk for Injury:** Risk factor: altered level of consciousness

## DELIRIUM TREMENS (DT)

*See Alcohol Withdrawal*

## DELIVERY

*See Labor, Normal*

## DELUSIONS

**Impaired Verbal Communication** r/t psychological impairment, delusional thinking

**Acute Confusion** r/t alcohol abuse, delirium, dementia, substance abuse

**Ineffective Coping** r/t distortion and insecurity of life events

**Fear** r/t content of intrusive thoughts

**Risk for Other-Directed Violence:** Risk factor: delusional thinking

**Risk for Self-Directed Violence:** Risk factor: delusional thinking

## DEMENTIA

**Chronic Confusion** r/t neurological dysfunction

**Interrupted Family Processes** r/t disability of family member

**Frail Elderly Syndrome** r/t alteration in cognitive functioning

**Ineffective Home Maintenance Behaviors** r/t inadequate support system, neurological dysfunction

**Imbalanced Nutrition: Less than Body Requirements** r/t neurological impairment

**Disability-Associated Urinary Incontinence** r/t neurological dysfunction

**Insomnia** r/t neurological impairment, naps during the day

**Impaired Physical Mobility** r/t alteration in cognitive function

**Self-Neglect** r/t cognitive impairment

**Self-Care Deficit: Specify** r/t psychological or neuromuscular impairment

**Chronic Sorrow: Significant Other** r/t chronic long-standing disability, loss of mental function

**Impaired Swallowing** r/t neuromuscular changes associated with long-standing dementia

**Risk for Caregiver Role Strain:** Risk factors: number of caregiving tasks, duration of caregiving required

**Risk for Chronic Functional Constipation:** Risk factor: decreased fluid intake

**Risk for Adult Falls:** Risk factor: diminished mental status

**Risk for Frail Elderly Syndrome:** Risk factors: cognitive impairment

**Risk for Injury:** Risk factors: confusion, decreased muscle coordination

**Risk for Impaired Skin Integrity:** Risk factors: altered nutritional status, immobility

## DENIAL OF HEALTH STATUS

**Ineffective Denial** r/t lack of perception about the health status effects of illness

**Ineffective Health Self-Management** r/t denial of seriousness of health situation

## DENTAL CARIES

**Impaired Dentition** r/t ineffective oral hygiene, barriers to self-care, economic barriers to professional care, nutritional deficits, dietary habits

**Ineffective Health Maintenance Behaviors** r/t lack of knowledge regarding prevention of dental disease

## DEPRESSION (MAJOR DEPRESSIVE DISORDER)

**Death Anxiety** r/t feelings of lack of self-worth

**Constipation** r/t inactivity, decreased fluid intake

**Fatigue** r/t psychological demands

**Ineffective Health Maintenance Behaviors** r/t lack of ability to make good judgments regarding ways to obtain help

**Hopelessness** r/t feeling of abandonment, long-term stress

**Impaired Mood Regulation** r/t emotional instability

**Insomnia** r/t inactivity

**Self-Neglect** r/t depression, cognitive impairment

**Powerlessness** r/t pattern of helplessness

**Chronic Low Self-Esteem** r/t repeated unmet expectations

**Sexual Dysfunction** r/t loss of sexual desire

**Social Isolation** r/t ineffective coping

**Chronic Sorrow** r/t unresolved grief

**Risk for Maladaptive Grieving:** Risk factor: lack of previous resolution of former grieving response

**Risk for Suicidal Behaviors:** Risk factor: grieving, hopelessness

## DERMATITIS

**Anxiety** r/t situational crisis imposed by illness

**Impaired Comfort** r/t itching

**Impaired Skin Integrity** r/t side effect of medication, allergic reaction

**Readiness for Enhanced Knowledge:** expresses an interest in learning

*See Itching*

## DESPONDENCY

**Hopelessness** r/t long-term stress

*See Depression (Major Depressive Disorder)*

## DESTRUCTIVE BEHAVIOR TOWARD OTHERS

**Risk-Prone Health Behavior** r/t intense emotional state

**Ineffective Coping** r/t situational crises, maturational crises, disturbance in pattern of appraisal of threat

**Risk for Other-Directed Violence** (See Violence, Other-Directed, Risk for, Section II)

## DEVELOPMENTAL CONCERNS

**Risk for Delayed Child Development:** Risk factor: growth and development lag

**Risk for Delayed Infant Motor Development:** Risk factor: growth and development lag

## DIABETES IN PREGNANCY

*See Gestational Diabetes (Diabetes in Pregnancy)*

## DIABETES INSIPIDUS

**Deficient Fluid Volume** r/t inability to conserve fluid

**Ineffective Health Maintenance Behaviors** r/t deficient knowledge regarding care of disease, importance of medications

## DIABETES MELLITUS

**Ineffective Health Maintenance Behaviors** r/t complexity of therapeutic regimen

**Ineffective Health Self-Management** (See Health Management, Ineffective, Section II)

**Imbalanced Nutrition: Less than Body Requirements** r/t inability to use glucose (type 1 [insulin-dependent] diabetes)

**Risk for Overweight:** Risk factor: excessive intake of nutrients (type 2 diabetes)

**Ineffective Peripheral Tissue Perfusion** r/t impaired arterial circulation

**Powerlessness** r/t perceived lack of personal control

**Sexual Dysfunction** r/t neuropathy associated with disease

**Vision Loss** r/t ineffective tissue perfusion of retina

**Risk for Unstable Blood Glucose Level** (See Glucose Level, Blood, Unstable, Risk for, Section II)

**Risk for Infection:** Risk factors: hyperglycemia, impaired healing, circulatory changes

**Risk for Injury:** Risk factors: hypoglycemia or hyperglycemia from failure to consume adequate calories, failure to take insulin

**Risk for Dysfunctional Gastrointestinal Motility:** Risk factor: complication of diabetes

**Risk for Metabolic Syndrome:** Risk factor: complication of diabetes

**Risk for Impaired Skin Integrity:** Risk factor: loss of pain perception in extremities

**Risk for Delayed Surgical Recovery:** Risk factor: impaired healing due to circulatory changes

**Readiness for Enhanced Health Literacy:** expresses desire to enhance understanding of health information to make health care choices

**Readiness for Enhanced Health Self-Management** (See Health Self-Management, **Readiness for Enhanced,** Section II)

**Readiness for Enhanced Knowledge:** expresses an interest in learning

*See Hyperglycemia; Hypoglycemia*

## DIABETES MELLITUS, JUVENILE (INSULIN-DEPENDENT DIABETES MELLITUS TYPE 1)

**Risk-Prone Health Behavior** r/t inadequate comprehension, inadequate social support, low self-efficacy, impaired adjustment attributable to adolescent maturational crises

**Disturbed Body Image** r/t imposed deviations from biophysical and psychosocial norm, perceived differences from peers

**Impaired Comfort** r/t insulin injections, peripheral blood glucose testing

**Ineffective Health Maintenance Behaviors** r/t inadequate trust in health care professional, ineffective communication skills, ineffective coping strategies, ineffective family coping

**Imbalanced Nutrition: Less than Body Requirements** r/t inability of body to adequately metabolize and use glucose and nutrients, increased caloric needs of child to promote growth and physical activity participation with peers

**Risk for Metabolic Syndrome:** Risk factor: complication of diabetes

**Readiness for Enhanced Knowledge:** expresses an interest in learning

*See Diabetes Mellitus; Child with Chronic Condition; Hospitalized Child*

## DIABETIC COMA

**Acute Confusion** r/t hyperglycemia, presence of excessive metabolic acids

**Deficient Fluid Volume** r/t hyperglycemia resulting in polyuria

**Ineffective Health Self-Management** r/t lack of understanding of preventive measures, adequate blood glucose control

**Risk for Unstable Blood Glucose Level** (See **Glucose Level, Blood, Unstable, Risk for,** Section II)

**Risk for Infection:** Risk factors: hyperglycemia, changes in vascular system

*See Diabetes Mellitus*

## DIABETIC KETOACIDOSIS

*See Ketoacidosis, Diabetic*

## DIABETIC NEUROPATHY

*See Neuropathy, Peripheral*

## DIABETIC RETINOPATHY

**Maladaptive Grieving** r/t loss of vision

**Ineffective Health Maintenance Behaviors** r/t deficient knowledge regarding preserving vision with treatment if possible, use of low-vision aids

*See Vision Impairment; Blindness*

## DIALYSIS

*See Hemodialysis; Peritoneal Dialysis*

## DIAPHRAGMATIC HERNIA

*See Hiatal Hernia*

## DIARRHEA

**Diarrhea** r/t infection, change in diet, gastrointestinal disorders, stress, medication effect, impaction

**Deficient Fluid Volume** r/t excessive loss of fluids in liquid stools

**Risk for Electrolyte Imbalance:** Risk factor: effect of loss of electrolytes from frequent stools

## DIC (DISSEMINATED INTRAVASCULAR COAGULATION)

**Fear** r/t threat to well-being

**Deficient Fluid Volume: Hemorrhage** r/t depletion of clotting factors

**Risk for Bleeding:** Risk factors: microclotting within vascular system, depleted clotting factors

## DIGITALIS TOXICITY

**Decreased Cardiac Output** r/t drug toxicity affecting cardiac rhythm, rate

**Ineffective Health Self-Management** r/t deficient knowledge regarding action, appropriate method of administration of digitalis

## DIGNITY, LOSS OF

**Risk for Compromised Human Dignity** (See **Human Dignity, Compromised, Risk for,** Section II)

## DILATION AND CURETTAGE (D&C)

**Acute Pain** r/t uterine contractions

**Risk for Bleeding:** Risk factor: surgical procedure

**Risk for Surgical Site Infection:** Risk factor: surgical procedure

**Ineffective Sexuality Pattern** r/t painful coitus, fear associated with surgery on genital area

**Readiness for Enhanced Knowledge:** expresses an interest in learning

## DIRTY BODY (FOR PROLONGED PERIOD)

**Self-Neglect** r/t mental illness, substance abuse, cognitive impairment

## DISCHARGE PLANNING

**Ineffective Home Maintenance Behaviors** r/t family member's disease or injury interfering with home maintenance

**Deficient Knowledge** r/t lack of exposure to information for home care

**Relocation Stress Syndrome:** Risk factors: insufficient predeparture counseling, insufficient support system, unpredictability of experience

**Readiness for Enhanced Health Literacy:** expresses desire to enhance understanding of health information to make health care choices

**Readiness for Enhanced Knowledge:** expresses an interest in learning

## DISCOMFORTS OF PREGNANCY

**Disturbed Body Image** r/t pregnancy-induced body changes

**Impaired Comfort** r/t enlarged abdomen, swollen feet

**Fatigue** r/t hormonal, metabolic, body changes

**Stress Urinary Incontinence** r/t enlarged uterus, fetal movement

**Insomnia** r/t psychological stress, fetal movement, muscular cramping, urinary frequency, shortness of breath

**Nausea** r/t hormone effect

**Acute Pain: Headache** r/t hormonal changes of pregnancy

**Acute Pain: Leg Cramps** r/t nerve compression, calcium/phosphorus/potassium imbalance

**Risk for Constipation:** Risk factors: decreased intestinal motility, inadequate fiber in diet

**Risk for Injury:** Risk factors: faintness and/or syncope caused by vasomotor lability or postural hypotension, venous stasis in lower extremities

## DISLOCATION OF JOINT

**Acute Pain** r/t dislocation of a joint

**Self-Care Deficit** r/t inability to use a joint

**Risk for Injury:** Risk factor: unstable joint

## DISSECTING ANEURYSM

**Fear** r/t threat to well-being

*See Abdominal Surgery; Aneurysm, Abdominal Aortic Repair*

## DISSEMINATED INTRAVASCULAR COAGULATION (DIC)

*See DIC (Disseminated Intravascular Coagulation)*

## DISSOCIATIVE IDENTITY DISORDER (NOT OTHERWISE SPECIFIED)

**Anxiety** r/t psychosocial stress

**Ineffective Coping** r/t personal vulnerability in crisis of accurate self-perception

**Disturbed Personal Identity** r/t inability to distinguish self-caused by multiple personality disorder, depersonalization, disturbance in memory

**Impaired Memory** r/t altered state of consciousness

*See Multiple Personality Disorder (Dissociative Identity Disorder)*

## DISTRESS

**Anxiety** r/t situational crises, maturational crises

**Death Anxiety** r/t denial of one's own mortality or impending death

## DISUSE SYNDROME, POTENTIAL TO DEVELOP

**Risk for Disuse Syndrome:** Risk factors: paralysis, mechanical immobilization, prescribed immobilization, severe pain, altered level of consciousness

## DIVERSIONAL ACTIVITY ENGAGEMENT, LACK OF

**Decreased Diversional Activity Engagement** r/t environmental lack of diversional activity as in frequent hospitalizations, lengthy treatments

## DIVERTICULITIS

**Constipation** r/t dietary deficiency of fiber and roughage

**Diarrhea** r/t increased intestinal motility caused by inflammation

**Deficient Knowledge** r/t diet needed to control disease, medication regimen

**Imbalanced Nutrition: Less than Body Requirements** r/t loss of appetite

**Acute Pain** r/t inflammation of bowel

**Risk for Deficient Fluid Volume:** Risk factor: diarrhea

## DIZZINESS

**Decreased Cardiac Output** r/t alteration in heart rate and rhythm, altered stroke volume

**Deficient Knowledge** r/t actions to take to prevent or modify dizziness and prevent falls

**Impaired Physical Mobility** r/t dizziness

**Risk for Adult Falls:** Risk factor: difficulty maintaining balance

**Risk for Ineffective Cerebral Tissue Perfusion:** Risk factor: interruption of cerebral arterial blood flow

## DOMESTIC VIOLENCE

**Impaired Verbal Communication** r/t psychological barriers of fear

**Compromised Family Coping** r/t abusive patterns

**Defensive Coping** r/t low self-esteem

**Disturbed Family Identity Syndrome** r/t domestic violence

**Dysfunctional Family Processes** r/t inadequate coping skills

**Fear** r/t threat to self-concept, situational crisis of abuse

**Insomnia** r/t psychological stress

**Post-Trauma Syndrome** r/t history of abuse

**Powerlessness** r/t lifestyle of helplessness

**Situational Low Self-Esteem** r/t negative family interactions

**Risk for Compromised Resilience:** Risk factor: effects of abuse

**Risk for Other-Directed Violence:** Risk factor: history of abuse

## DOWN SYNDROME

*See Child with Chronic Condition; Intellectual Disability*

## DRESS SELF (INABILITY TO)

**Dressing Self-Care Deficit** r/t intolerance to activity, decreased strength and endurance, pain, discomfort, perceptual or cognitive impairment, neuromuscular impairment, musculoskeletal impairment, depression, severe anxiety

## DRIBBLING OF URINE

**Urinary Retention** r/t degenerative changes in pelvic muscles and urinary structures

**Stress Urinary Incontinence** r/t degenerative changes in pelvic muscles and urinary structures

## DROOLING

**Impaired Swallowing** r/t neuromuscular impairment, mechanical obstruction

**Risk for Aspiration:** Risk factor: impaired swallowing

## DROPOUT FROM SCHOOL

**Impaired Resilience** (See **Resilience, Individual, Impaired,** Section II)

**Anxiety** r/t conflict about life goals

**Ineffective Coping** r/t inadequate resources

## DRUG ABUSE

*See Substance Abuse*

## DRUG WITHDRAWAL

*See Acute Substance Withdrawal Syndrome*

## DRY EYE

**Risk for Dry Eye:** Risk factors (See **Dry Eye, Risk for,** Section II)

**Risk for Corneal Injury:** Risk factor: suppressed corneal reflex

**Readiness for Enhanced Knowledge:** expresses an interest in learning

*See Conjunctivitis; Keratoconjunctivitis Sicca (Dry Eye Syndrome)*

## DRY MOUTH

**Risk for Dry Mouth:** Risk factors (See **Dry Mouth, Risk for,** Section II)

**Risk for Impaired Oral Mucous Membrane Integrity:** Risk factor: reduced quality or quantity of saliva caused by decreased fluid volume

## DT (DELIRIUM TREMENS)

*See Alcohol Withdrawal*

## DVT (DEEP VEIN THROMBOSIS)

**Constipation** r/t inactivity, bed rest

**Impaired Physical Mobility** r/t pain in extremity

**Acute Pain** r/t vascular inflammation, edema

**Ineffective Peripheral Tissue Perfusion** r/t deficient knowledge of aggravating factors

**Delayed Surgical Recovery** r/t impaired physical mobility

**Readiness for Enhanced Knowledge:** expresses an interest in learning

**Risk for Ineffective Thermoregulation:** Risk factor: inactivity

*See Anticoagulant Therapy; Venous Thromboembolism, Risk for* (See Section II)

## DYING CLIENT

*See Terminally Ill Adult; Terminally Ill Adolescent; Terminally Ill Child, Infant/ Toddler; Terminally Ill Child, Preschool Child; Terminally Ill Child, School-Age Child/Preadolescent; Terminally Ill Child/ Death of Child, Parent*

## DYSFUNCTIONAL EATING PATTERN

**Imbalanced Nutrition: Less than Body Requirements** r/t psychological factors

**Risk for Overweight:** Risk factor: psychological factors

*See Anorexia Nervosa; Bulimia; Maturational Issues, Adolescent; Obesity*

## DYSFUNCTIONAL FAMILY UNIT

*See Family Problems*

## DYSFUNCTIONAL VENTILATORY WEANING

**Dysfunctional Ventilatory Weaning Response** r/t physical, psychological, situational factors

## DYSMENORRHEA

**Nausea** r/t prostaglandin effect

**Acute Pain** r/t cramping from hormonal effects

**Readiness for Enhanced Knowledge:** expresses an interest in learning

## DYSPAREUNIA

**Sexual Dysfunction** r/t lack of lubrication during intercourse, alteration in reproductive organ function

## DYSPEPSIA

**Anxiety** r/t pressures of personal role

**Acute Pain** r/t gastrointestinal disease, consumption of irritating foods

**D**

**D**

**Readiness for Enhanced Knowledge:** expresses an interest in learning

## DYSPHAGIA

**Impaired Swallowing** r/t neuromuscular impairment

**Risk for Aspiration:** Risk factor: loss of gag or cough reflex

## DYSPHASIA

**Impaired Verbal Communication** r/t decrease in circulation to brain

**Impaired Social Interaction** r/t difficulty in communicating

## DYSPNEA

**Decreased Activity Tolerance** r/t imbalance between oxygen supply and demand

**Ineffective Breathing Pattern** r/t compromised cardiac or pulmonary function, decreased lung expansion, neurological impairment affecting respiratory center, extreme anxiety

**Fear** r/t threat to state of well-being, potential death

**Impaired Gas Exchange** r/t alveolar-capillary damage

**Insomnia** r/t difficulty breathing, positioning required for effective breathing

**Sleep Deprivation** r/t ineffective breathing pattern

## DYSRHYTHMIA

**Decreased Activity Tolerance** r/t decreased cardiac output

**Decreased Cardiac Output** r/t alteration in heart rate, rhythm

**Fear** r/t threat of death, change in health status

**Risk for Ineffective Cerebral Tissue Perfusion:** Risk factor: decreased blood supply to the brain from dysrhythmia

**Risk for Unstable Blood Pressure** r/t cardiac arrhythmia and electrolyte imbalance

**Readiness for Enhanced Knowledge:** expresses an interest in learning

## DYSTHYMIC DISORDER

**Ineffective Coping** r/t impaired social interaction

**Ineffective Health Maintenance Behaviors** r/t inability to make good judgments regarding ways to obtain help

**Insomnia** r/t anxious thoughts

**Chronic Low Self-Esteem** r/t repeated unmet expectations

**Ineffective Sexuality Pattern** r/t loss of sexual desire

**Social Isolation** r/t ineffective coping

*See Depression (Major Depressive Disorder)*

## DYSTOCIA

**Anxiety** r/t difficult labor, deficient knowledge regarding normal labor pattern

**Ineffective Coping** r/t situational crisis

**Fatigue** r/t prolonged labor

**Maladaptive Grieving** r/t loss of ideal labor experience

**Acute Pain** r/t difficult labor, medical interventions

**Powerlessness** r/t perceived inability to control outcome of labor

**Risk for Bleeding:** Risk factor: hemorrhage secondary to uterine atony

**Risk for Ineffective Cerebral Tissue Perfusion (Fetal):** Risk factor: difficult labor and birth

**Risk for Infection:** Risk factor: prolonged rupture of membranes

**Risk for Impaired Tissue Integrity (Maternal and Fetal):** Risk factor: difficult labor

## DYSURIA

**Impaired Urinary Elimination** r/t infection/inflammation of the urinary tract

**Risk for Urge Urinary Incontinence:** Risk factor: detrusor hyperreflexia from infection in the urinary tract

**Acute Pain** r/t infection/inflammation of the urinary tract

# E

## EAR SURGERY

**Acute Pain** r/t edema in ears from surgery

**Hearing Loss** r/t invasive surgery of ears, dressings

**Risk for Delayed Child Development:** Risk factor: hearing impairment

**Risk for Adult Falls:** Risk factor: dizziness from excessive stimuli to vestibular apparatus

**Readiness for Enhanced Knowledge:** expresses an interest in learning

*See Hospitalized Child*

## EARACHE

**Acute Pain** r/t trauma, edema, infection

**Hearing Loss** r/t altered sensory reception, transmission

## EATING DYNAMICS, ADOLESCENT

**Imbalanced Nutrition: Less than Body Requirements** r/t negative perception of one's body

**Ineffective Adolescent Eating Dynamics** r/t altered family dynamics, eating disorder, excessive stress

**Risk for Overweight:** Risk factor: media influence resulting in unhealthy choices, insufficient interest in physical activity

**Readiness for Enhanced Health Literacy:** expresses desire to learn to make healthy food choices

## EATING DYNAMICS, CHILD

**Imbalanced Nutrition: Less than Body Requirements** r/t excessive of parental control over quantity and choices of foods

**Ineffective Child Eating Dynamics** r/t bribing child to eat, forcing child to eat

**Risk for Delayed Child Development:** Risk factor: inadequate nutrition to meet metabolic needs for normal development

**Risk for Overweight:** Risk factors: unhealthy choices, frequent snacking, low physical activity

## EATING DYNAMICS, INFANT

*See Feeding Dynamics, Infant*

## ECLAMPSIA

**Interrupted Family Processes** r/t unmet expectations for pregnancy and childbirth

**Fear** r/t threat of well-being to self and fetus

**Risk for Aspiration:** Risk factor: seizure activity

**Risk for Ineffective Cerebral Tissue Perfusion: Fetal:** Risk factor: uteroplacental insufficiency

**Risk for Imbalanced Fluid Volume:** Risk factor: decreased urine output as a result of renal dysfunction

**Risk for unstable Blood Pressure:** Risk factor: hypertension caused by excess fluid volume

## ECMO (EXTRACORPOREAL MEMBRANE OXYGENATOR)

**Death Anxiety** r/t emergency condition, hemorrhage

**Decreased Cardiac Output** r/t altered contractility of the heart

**Impaired Gas Exchange** (See **Gas Exchange, Impaired,** Section II)

*See Respiratory Conditions of the Neonate*

## ECT (ELECTROCONVULSIVE THERAPY)

**Decisional Conflict** r/t lack of relevant information

**Fear** r/t real or imagined threat to well-being

**Impaired Memory** r/t effects of treatment

*See Depression (Major Depressive Disorder)*

## ECTOPIC PREGNANCY

**Death Anxiety** r/t emergency condition, hemorrhage

**Disturbed Body Image** r/t negative feelings about body and reproductive functioning

**Fear** r/t threat to self, surgery, implications for future pregnancy

**Acute Pain** r/t stretching or rupture of implantation site

**Ineffective Role Performance** r/t loss of pregnancy

**Situational Low Self-Esteem** r/t loss of pregnancy, inability to carry pregnancy to term

**E**

**Chronic Sorrow** r/t loss of pregnancy, potential loss of fertility

**Risk for Bleeding:** Risk factor: possible rupture of implantation site, surgical trauma

**Risk for Ineffective Coping:** Risk factor: loss of pregnancy

**Risk for Interrupted Family Processes:** Risk factor: situational crisis

**Risk for Infection:** Risk factors: traumatized tissue, surgical procedure

**Risk for Spiritual Distress:** Risk factor: grief process

### ECZEMA

**Disturbed Body Image** r/t change in appearance from inflamed skin

**Impaired Comfort: Pruritus** r/t inflammation of skin

**Impaired Skin Integrity** r/t side effect of medication, allergic reaction

**Readiness for Enhanced Knowledge:** expresses an interest in learning

### ED (ERECTILE DYSFUNCTION)

*See Erectile Dysfunction (ED); Impotence*

### EDEMA

**Excess Fluid Volume** r/t excessive fluid intake, cardiac dysfunction, renal dysfunction, loss of plasma proteins

**Ineffective Health Maintenance Behaviors** r/t deficient knowledge regarding treatment of edema

**Risk for Impaired Skin Integrity:** Risk factors: impaired circulation, fragility of skin

*See Heart Failure; Renal Failure*

### ELDER ABUSE

*See Abuse, Spouse, Parent, or Significant Other*

### ELDERLY

*See Aging; Frail Elderly Syndrome*

### ELECTROCONVULSIVE THERAPY

*See ECT (Electroconvulsive Therapy)*

### ELECTROLYTE IMBALANCE

**Risk for Electrolyte Imbalance** (See **Electrolyte Imbalance, Risk for,** Section II)

**Risk for Unstable Blood Pressure:** Risk factor: fluid volume changes

### EMACIATED PERSON

**Frail Elderly Syndrome** r/t living alone, malnutrition, alteration in cognitive functioning

**Imbalanced Nutrition: Less than Body Requirements** r/t inability to ingest food, digest food, absorb nutrients because of biological, psychological, economic factors

### EMANCIPATED DECISION-MAKING, IMPAIRED

**Risk for Impaired Emancipated Decision-Making:** Risk factor: inability or unwillingness to verbalize needs and wants

**Readiness for Enhanced Emancipated Decision-Making:** expresses desire to enhance decision-making process

### EMBOLECTOMY

**Fear** r/t threat of great bodily harm from embolus

**Ineffective Peripheral Tissue Perfusion** r/t presence of embolus

**Risk for Bleeding:** Risk factors: postoperative complication, surgical area

*See Surgery, Postoperative Care*

### EMBOLI

*See Pulmonary Embolism (PE)*

### EMBOLISM IN LEG OR ARM

**Ineffective Peripheral Tissue Perfusion** r/t arterial/venous obstruction from clot

*See DVT (Deep Vein Thrombosis); Risk for Thrombosis*

### EMESIS

**Nausea** (See **Nausea,** Section II)

*See Vomiting*

### EMOTIONAL PROBLEMS

*See Coping Problems*

### EMPATHY

**Readiness for Enhanced Community Coping:** social supports, being available for problem solving

**Readiness for Enhanced Family Coping:** basic needs met, desire to move to higher level of health

**Readiness for Enhanced Spiritual Well-Being:** desire to establish interconnectedness through spirituality

## EMPHYSEMA

*See COPD (Chronic Obstructive Pulmonary Disease)*

## EMPTINESS

**Social Isolation** r/t inability to engage in satisfying personal relationships

**Chronic Sorrow** r/t unresolved grief

**Spiritual Distress** r/t separation from religious or cultural ties

## ENCEPHALITIS

*See Meningitis/Encephalitis*

## ENDOCARDIAL CUSHION DEFECT

*See Congenital Heart Disease/Cardiac Anomalies*

## ENDOCARDITIS

**Decreased Activity Tolerance** r/t reduced cardiac reserve, prescribed bed rest

**Decreased Cardiac Output** r/t inflammation of lining of heart and change in structure of valve leaflets, increased myocardial workload

**Risk for Imbalanced Nutrition: Less than Body Requirements:** Risk factors: fever, hypermetabolic state associated with fever

**Risk for Ineffective Cerebral Tissue Perfusion:** Risk factor: possible presence of emboli in cerebral circulation

**Risk for Ineffective Peripheral Tissue Perfusion:** Risk factor: possible presence of emboli in peripheral circulation

**Readiness for Enhanced Knowledge:** expresses an interest in learning

## ENDOMETRIOSIS

**Maladaptive Grieving** r/t possible infertility

**Nausea** r/t prostaglandin effect

**Acute Pain** r/t onset of menses with distention of endometrial tissue

**Sexual Dysfunction** r/t painful intercourse

**Readiness for Enhanced Knowledge:** expresses an interest in learning

## ENDOMETRITIS

**Anxiety** r/t, fear of unknown

**Ineffective Thermoregulation** r/t infectious process

**Acute Pain** r/t infectious process in reproductive tract

**Readiness for Enhanced Knowledge:** expresses an interest in learning

## ENURESIS

**Ineffective Health Maintenance Behaviors** r/t unachieved developmental task, neuromuscular immaturity, diseases of urinary system

*See Toilet Training*

## ENVIRONMENTAL INTERPRETATION PROBLEMS

*See Chronic Confusion*

## EPIDIDYMITIS

**Anxiety** r/t situational crisis, pain, threat to future fertility

**Acute Pain** r/t inflammation in scrotal sac

**Ineffective Sexuality Pattern** r/t edema of epididymis and testes

**Readiness for Enhanced Knowledge:** expresses an interest in learning

## EPIGLOTTITIS

*See Respiratory Infections, Acute Childhood (Croup, Epiglottitis, Pertussis, Pneumonia, Respiratory Syncytial Virus)*

## EPILEPSY

**Anxiety** r/t threat to role functioning

**Ineffective Health Self-Management** r/t deficient knowledge regarding seizure control

**Impaired Memory** r/t seizure activity

**Risk for Aspiration:** Risk factors: impaired swallowing, excessive secretions

**Risk for Injury:** Risk factor: environmental factors during seizure

**E**

**Readiness for Enhanced Knowledge:** expresses an interest in learning

*See Seizure Disorders, Adult; Seizure Disorders, Childhood (Epilepsy, Febrile Seizures, Infantile Spasms)*

## EPISIOTOMY

**Anxiety** r/t fear of pain

**Disturbed Body Image** r/t fear of resuming sexual relations

**Impaired Physical Mobility** r/t pain, swelling, tissue trauma

**Acute Pain** r/t tissue trauma

**Sexual Dysfunction** r/t altered body structure, tissue trauma

**Impaired Skin Integrity** r/t perineal incision

**Risk for Infection:** Risk factor: tissue trauma

## EPISTAXIS

**Fear** r/t large amount of blood loss

**Risk for Deficient Fluid Volume:** Risk factor: excessive blood loss

## EPSTEIN-BARR VIRUS

*See Mononucleosis*

## ERECTILE DYSFUNCTION (ED)

**Situational Low Self-Esteem** r/t physiological crisis, inability to practice usual sexual activity

**Sexual Dysfunction** r/t altered body function

**Readiness for Enhanced Knowledge:** information regarding treatment for erectile dysfunction

*See Impotence*

## *ESCHERICHIA COLI* INFECTION

**Fear** r/t serious illness, unknown outcome

**Deficient Knowledge** r/t how to prevent disease; care of self with serious illness

*See Gastroenteritis; Gastroenteritis, Child; Hospitalized Child*

## ESOPHAGEAL VARICES

**Fear** r/t threat of death from hematemesis

**Risk for Bleeding:** Risk factors: portal hypertension, distended variceal vessels that can easily rupture

*See Cirrhosis*

## ESOPHAGITIS

**Acute Pain** r/t inflammation of esophagus

**Readiness for Enhanced Knowledge:** expresses an interest in learning

## EVISCERATION

*See Dehiscence, Abdominal*

## EXHAUSTION

**Impaired Resilience** (See **Resilience, Individual, Impaired,** Section II)

**Disturbed Sleep Pattern** (See **Sleep Pattern, Disturbed,** Section II)

## EXPOSURE TO HOT OR COLD ENVIRONMENT

**Hyperthermia** r/t exposure to hot environment, abnormal reaction to anesthetics

**Hypothermia** r/t exposure to cold environment

**Risk for Ineffective Thermoregulation:** Risk factors: extremes of environmental temperature, inappropriate clothing for environmental temperature

## EXTERNAL FIXATION

**Disturbed Body Image** r/t trauma, change to affected part

**Risk for Infection:** Risk factor: presence of pins inserted into bone

*See Fracture*

## EXTRACORPOREAL MEMBRANE OXYGENATOR (ECMO)

*See ECMO (Extracorporeal Membrane Oxygenator)*

## EYE DISCOMFORT

**Risk for Dry Eye** (See **Eye, Dry, Risk for,** Section II)

**Risk for Corneal Injury:** Risk factors: exposure of the eyeball, blinking less than five times per minute

## EYE SURGERY

**Anxiety** r/t possible loss of vision

**Self-Care Deficit: Specify** r/t impaired vision

**Vision Loss** r/t surgical procedure, eye pathology

**Risk for Injury:** Risk factor: impaired vision

**Readiness for Enhanced Knowledge:** expresses an interest in learning

*See Hospitalized Child*

# F

## FAILURE TO THRIVE, CHILD

**Disorganized Infant Behavior** (See **Infant Behavior, Disorganized,** Section II)

**Ineffective Child Eating Dynamics** r/t lack of knowledge or resources regarding nutritional needs of child

**Ineffective Infant Feeding Dynamics** r/t lack of knowledge regarding nutritional needs of infant

**Ineffective Infant Suck-Swallow Response** r/t unsatisfactory sucking behavior

**Insomnia** r/t inconsistency of caretaker; lack of quiet, consistent environment

**Imbalanced Nutrition: Less than Body Requirements** r/t inadequate type or amounts of food for infant or child, inappropriate feeding techniques

**Impaired Parenting** r/t lack of parenting skills, inadequate role modeling

**Chronic Low Self-Esteem: Parental** r/t feelings of inadequacy, support system deficiencies, inadequate role model

**Social Isolation** r/t limited support systems, self-imposed situation

**Risk for Impaired Attachment:** Risk factor: inability of parents to meet infant's needs

**Readiness for Enhanced Knowledge:** parent expresses willingness to learn how to meet infant/child nutritional needs

## FALLS, RISK FOR

**Risk for Adult Falls** (See **Adult Falls, Risk for,** Section II)

**Risk for Child Falls** (See **Child Falls, Risk for,** Section II)

## FAMILY PROBLEMS

**Compromised Family Coping** (See **Coping, Family, Compromised,** Section II)

**Disabled Family Coping** (See **Coping, Family, Disabled,** Section II)

**Interrupted Family Processes** r/t situation transition and/or crises, developmental transition and/or crises

**Ineffective Family Health Self-Management** (See **Family Health Management, Ineffective,** Section II)

**Readiness for Enhanced Family Coping:** needs sufficiently gratified, adaptive tasks effectively addressed to enable goals of self-actualization to surface

## FAMILY PROCESS

**Dysfunctional Family Processes** (See **Family Processes, Dysfunctional,** Section II)

**Interrupted Family Processes** (See **Family Processes, Interrupted,** Section II)

**Readiness for Enhanced Family Processes** (See **Family Processes, Readiness for Enhanced,** Section II)

**Readiness for Enhanced Relationship** (See **Relationship, Readiness for Enhanced,** Section II)

## FATIGUE

**Fatigue** (See **Fatigue,** Section II)

## FEAR

**Death Anxiety** r/t fear of death

**Fear** r/t identifiable physical or psychological threat to person

## FEBRILE SEIZURES

*See Seizure Disorders, Childhood (Epilepsy, Febrile Seizures, Infantile Spasms)*

## FECAL IMPACTION

*See Impaction of Stool*
(See **Constipation,** Section II)
(See **Constipation, Chronic Functional,** Section II)

## FECAL INCONTINENCE

**Impaired Bowel Continence** r/t neurological impairment, gastrointestinal disorders, anorectal trauma, weakened perineal muscles

**F**

## FEEDING DYNAMICS, INFANT

**Ineffective Infant Eating Dynamics** r/t inappropriate transition to sold foods

**Ineffective Infant Suck-Swallow Response** r/t unsatisfactory sucking behavior

**Risk for Caregiver Role Strain:** Risk factor: fatigue leading to ineffective or insufficient feeding

**Risk for Impaired Attachment:** Risk factor: inability physically or psychologically to meet nutritional needs of newborn

**Risk for Impaired Parenting:** Risk factors: stress, sleep deprivation, insufficient knowledge, and/or social isolation

**Readiness for Enhanced Health Literacy:** expresses a desire to enhance knowledge of appropriate feeding dynamics for each developmental stage (See **Ineffective Feeding Dynamics, Infant,** Section II)

## FEEDING PROBLEMS, NEWBORN

**Ineffective Breastfeeding** (See **Breastfeeding, Ineffective,** Section II)

**Ineffective Infant Feeding Dynamics** r/t attachment issues, lack of knowledge of appropriate methods of feeding infant for each stage of development

**Ineffective Infant Suck-Swallow Response** r/t unsatisfactory sucking behavior

**Insufficient Breast Milk Production** (See **Breast Milk Production, Insufficient,** Section II)

**Disorganized Infant Behavior** r/t prematurity, immature neurological system

**Ineffective Infant Feeding Dynamics** r/t parental lack of knowledge of appropriate feeding methods for each stage of development

**Ineffective Infant Feeding Pattern** r/t prematurity, neurological impairment or delay, oral hypersensitivity, prolonged nothing-by-mouth status

**Impaired Swallowing** r/t prematurity

**Neonatal Abstinence Syndrome:** At-risk population: in utero substance exposure secondary to maternal substance use

**Nipple-Areolar Complex Injury** r/t maternal impatience with breastfeeding process

**Risk for Deficient Fluid Volume:** Risk factor: inability to take in adequate amount of fluids

## FEMALE GENITAL MUTILATION

**Acute Pain** r/t traumatic surgical procedure

**Anxiety** r/t situational crisis

**Disturbed Body Image** r/t scarring, changes in body function

**Fear** r/t threat to well-being

**Powerlessness** r/t absence of control of decision-making

**Impaired Skin Integrity** r/t traumatic surgical procedure

**Impaired Tissue Integrity** r/t wound, potential for infection

**Risk for Compromised Human Dignity:** Risk factor: dehumanizing treatment

**Risk for Infection:** Risk factor: invasive procedure

**Risk for Post-Trauma Syndrome:** Risk factor: experiencing traumatic surgery

**Risk for Chronic Low Self-Esteem:** Risk factor: cultural incongruence (See **Female Genital Mutilation, Risk for,** Section II)

## FEMORAL POPLITEAL BYPASS

**Anxiety** r/t threat to or change in health status

**Acute Pain** r/t surgical trauma, edema in surgical area

**Ineffective Peripheral Tissue Perfusion** r/t impaired arterial circulation

**Risk for Bleeding:** Risk factor: surgery on arteries

**Risk for Surgical Site Infection:** Risk factor: invasive procedure

## FETAL ALCOHOL SYNDROME

*See Neonatal Abstinence Syndrome*

## FETAL DISTRESS/ NONREASSURING FETAL HEART RATE PATTERN

**Fear** r/t threat to fetus

**Ineffective Peripheral Tissue Perfusion: fetal** r/t interruption of umbilical cord blood flow

## FEVER

**Ineffective Thermoregulation** r/t infectious process

## FIBROCYSTIC BREAST DISEASE

*See Breast Lumps*

## FILTHY HOME ENVIRONMENT

**Ineffective Home Maintenance Behaviors** (See **Home Maintenance Behaviors, Ineffective,** Section II)

**Self-Neglect** r/t mental illness, substance abuse, cognitive impairment

## FINANCIAL CRISIS IN THE HOME ENVIRONMENT

**Ineffective Home Maintenance Behaviors** r/t insufficient finances

## FISTULECTOMY

*See Hemorrhoidectomy*

## FLAIL CHEST

**Ineffective Breathing Pattern** r/t chest trauma

**Fear** r/t difficulty breathing

**Impaired Gas Exchange** r/t loss of effective lung function

**Impaired Spontaneous Ventilation** r/t paradoxical respirations

## FLASHBACKS

**Post-Trauma Syndrome** r/t catastrophic event

## FLAT AFFECT

**Hopelessness** r/t prolonged activity restriction creating isolation, failing or deteriorating physiological condition, long-term stress, abandonment, lost belief in transcendent values or higher power or God

**Risk for Loneliness:** Risk factors: social isolation, lack of interest in surroundings

*See Depression (Major Depressive Disorder); Dysthymic Disorder*

## FLUID VOLUME DEFICIT

**Deficient Fluid Volume** r/t active fluid loss, vomiting, diarrhea, failure of regulatory mechanisms

**Risk for Shock:** Risk factors: hypovolemia, sepsis, systemic inflammatory response syndrome (SIRS)

**Risk for Unstable Blood Pressure:** Risk factor: hypotension, excessive loss or insufficient intake of fluid

## FLUID VOLUME EXCESS

**Excess Fluid Volume** r/t compromised regulatory mechanism, excess sodium intake

**Risk for Unstable Blood Pressure:** Risk factor: hypertension, excessive intake or retention of fluid

## FLUID VOLUME IMBALANCE, RISK FOR

**Risk for Imbalanced Fluid Volume:** Risk factor: major invasive surgeries

## FOOD ALLERGIES

**Diarrhea** r/t immune effects of offending food on gastrointestinal system

**Risk for Allergy Reaction:** Risk factor: specific foods

**Readiness for Enhanced Knowledge:** expresses an interest in learning

*See Anaphylactic Shock*

## FOODBORNE ILLNESS

**Diarrhea** r/t infectious material in gastrointestinal tract

**Deficient Fluid Volume** r/t active fluid loss from vomiting and diarrhea

**Deficient Knowledge** r/t care of self with serious illness, prevention of further incidences of foodborne illness

**Nausea** r/t contamination irritating stomach

**Risk for Dysfunctional Gastrointestinal Motility:** Risk factor: contaminated food

*See Gastroenteritis; Gastroenteritis, Child; Hospitalized Child;* Escherichia coli *Infection*

## FOOD INTOLERANCE

**Risk for Dysfunctional Gastrointestinal Motility:** Risk factor: food intolerance

**F**

## FOREIGN BODY ASPIRATION

**Ineffective Airway Clearance** r/t obstruction of airway

**Ineffective Health Maintenance Behaviors** r/t parental deficient knowledge regarding high-risk items

**Risk for Suffocation:** Risk factor: inhalation of small objects

*See Safety, Childhood*

## FORMULA FEEDING OF INFANT

**Maladaptive Grieving: Maternal** r/t loss of desired breastfeeding experience

**Ineffective Infant Feeding Dynamics** r/t lack of knowledge of appropriate methods of feeding infant for each stage of development

**Ineffective Infant Suck-Swallow Response** r/t unsatisfactory sucking behavior

**Risk for Constipation: Infant:** Risk factor: iron-fortified formula

**Risk for Infection: Infant:** Risk factors: lack of passive maternal immunity, supine feeding position, contamination of formula

**Readiness for Enhanced Knowledge:** expresses an interest in learning

## FRACTURE

**Decreased Diversional Activity Engagement** r/t immobility

**Impaired Physical Mobility** r/t limb immobilization

**Acute Pain** r/t muscle spasm, edema, trauma

**Post-Trauma Syndrome** r/t catastrophic event

**Impaired Walking** r/t limb immobility

**Risk for Ineffective Peripheral Tissue Perfusion:** Risk factors: immobility, presence of cast

**Risk for Peripheral Neurovascular Dysfunction:** Risk factors: mechanical compression, treatment of fracture

**Risk for Impaired Skin Integrity:** Risk factors: immobility, presence of cast

**Risk for Thrombosis:** Risk factors: trauma, immobility

**Readiness for Enhanced Knowledge:** expresses an interest in learning

## FRACTURED HIP

*See Hip Fracture*

## FRAIL ELDERLY SYNDROME

**Decreased Activity Tolerance** r/t sensory changes

**Risk for Frail Elderly Syndrome** (See **Frail Elderly Syndrome, Risk for,** Section II)

**Risk for Injury:** Risk factors: impaired vision, impaired gait

**Risk for Powerlessness:** Risk factor: inability to maintain independence

## FREQUENCY OF URINATION

**Stress Urinary Incontinence** r/t degenerative change in pelvic muscles and structural support

**Urge Urinary Incontinence** r/t decreased bladder capacity, irritation of bladder stretch receptors causing spasm, alcohol, caffeine, increased fluids, increased urine concentration, overdistended bladder

**Impaired Urinary Elimination** r/t urinary tract infection

**Urinary Retention** r/t high urethral pressure caused by weak detrusor, inhibition of reflex arc, strong sphincter, blockage

## FRIENDSHIP

**Readiness for Enhanced Relationship:** expresses desire to enhance communication between partners

## FROSTBITE

**Acute Pain** r/t decreased circulation from prolonged exposure to cold

**Ineffective Peripheral Tissue Perfusion** r/t damage to extremities from prolonged exposure to cold

**Impaired Tissue Integrity** r/t freezing of skin and tissues

**Risk for Ineffective Thermoregulation:** Risk factor: prolonged exposure to cold

*See Hypothermia*

## FROTHY SPUTUM

*See CHF (Congestive Heart Failure); Pulmonary Edema; Seizure Disorders, Adult; Seizure Disorders, Childhood*

*(Epilepsy, Febrile Seizures, Infantile Spasms)*

## FUSION, LUMBAR

**Anxiety** r/t fear of surgical procedure, possible recurring problems

**Impaired Physical Mobility** r/t limitations from surgical procedure, presence of brace

**Acute Pain** r/t discomfort at bone donor site, surgical operation

**Risk for Injury:** Risk factor: improper body mechanics

**Risk for Perioperative Positioning Injury:** Risk factor: immobilization during surgery

**Readiness for Enhanced Knowledge:** expresses an interest in learning

## G

## GAG REFLEX, DEPRESSED OR ABSENT

**Impaired Swallowing** r/t neuromuscular impairment

**Risk for Aspiration:** Risk factors: depressed cough or gag reflex

## GALLOP RHYTHM

**Decreased Cardiac Output** r/t decreased contractility of heart

## GALLSTONES

*See Cholelithiasis*

## GANG MEMBER

**Impaired Resilience** (See **Resilience, Individual, Impaired,** Section II)

## GANGRENE

**Fear** r/t possible loss of extremity

**Ineffective Peripheral Tissue Perfusion** r/t obstruction of arterial flow

*See Diabetes Mellitus; Peripheral Vascular Disease*

## GAS EXCHANGE, IMPAIRED

**Impaired Gas Exchange** r/t ventilation-perfusion imbalance

**Dysfunctional Ventilatory Weaning Response** r/t psychomotor agitation

## GASTRIC ULCER

*See GI Bleed (Gastrointestinal Bleeding); Ulcer, Peptic (Duodenal or Gastric)*

## GASTRITIS

**Imbalanced Nutrition: Less than Body Requirements** r/t vomiting, inadequate intestinal absorption of nutrients, restricted dietary regimen

**Acute Pain** r/t inflammation of gastric mucosa

**Risk for Deficient Fluid Volume:** Risk factors: excessive loss from gastrointestinal tract from vomiting, decreased intake

## GASTROENTERITIS

**Diarrhea** r/t infectious process involving intestinal tract

**Deficient Fluid Volume** r/t excessive loss from gastrointestinal tract from diarrhea, vomiting

**Nausea** r/t irritation to gastrointestinal system

**Imbalanced Nutrition: Less than Body Requirements** r/t vomiting, inadequate intestinal absorption of nutrients, restricted dietary intake

**Acute Pain** r/t increased peristalsis causing cramping

**Risk for Electrolyte Imbalance:** Risk factor: loss of gastrointestinal fluids high in electrolytes

**Readiness for Enhanced Knowledge:** expresses an interest in learning

*See Gastroenteritis, Child*

## GASTROENTERITIS, CHILD

**Impaired Skin Integrity: Diaper Rash** r/t acidic excretions on perineal tissues

**Readiness for Enhanced Knowledge:** expresses an interest in learning

**Acute Pain** r/t increased peristalsis causing cramping

*See Gastroenteritis; Hospitalized Child*

## GASTROESOPHAGEAL REFLUX DISEASE (GERD)

**Ineffective Airway Clearance** r/t reflux of gastric contents into esophagus and tracheal or bronchial tree

**Ineffective Health Maintenance Behaviors** r/t deficient knowledge regarding antireflux regimen (e.g., positioning, change in diet)

**Acute Pain** r/t irritation of esophagus from gastric acids

**Risk for Aspiration:** Risk factor: entry of gastric contents in tracheal or bronchial tree

## GASTROESOPHAGEAL REFLUX, CHILD

**Ineffective Airway Clearance** r/t reflux of gastric contents into esophagus and tracheal or bronchial tree

**Anxiety: Parental** r/t possible need for surgical intervention

**Deficient Fluid Volume** r/t persistent vomiting

**Imbalanced Nutrition: Less than Body Requirements** r/t poor feeding, vomiting

**Risk for Aspiration:** Risk factor: entry of gastric contents in tracheal or bronchial tree

**Risk for Impaired Parenting:** Risk factors: disruption in bonding as a result of irritable or inconsolable infant; lack of sleep for parents

**Readiness for Enhanced Knowledge:** expresses an interest in learning

*See Child with Chronic Condition; Hospitalized Child*

## GASTROINTESTINAL BLEEDING (GI BLEED)

*See GI Bleed (Gastrointestinal Bleeding)*

## GASTROINTESTINAL HEMORRHAGE

*See GI Bleed (Gastrointestinal Bleeding)*

## GASTROINTESTINAL SURGERY

**Risk for Injury:** Risk factor: inadvertent insertion of nasogastric tube through gastric incision line

*See Abdominal Surgery*

## GASTROSCHISIS/OMPHALOCELE

**Ineffective Airway Clearance** r/t complications of anesthetic effects

**Impaired Gas Exchange** r/t effects of anesthesia, subsequent atelectasis

**Maladaptive Grieving** r/t threatened loss of infant, loss of perfect birth or infant because of serious medical condition

**Risk for Deficient Fluid Volume:** Risk factors: inability to feed because of condition, subsequent electrolyte imbalance

**Risk for Infection:** Risk factor: disrupted skin integrity with exposure of abdominal contents

**Risk for Injury:** Risk factors: disrupted skin integrity, ineffective protection

## GASTROSTOMY

**Risk for Impaired Skin Integrity:** Risk factor: presence of gastric contents on skin

*See Tube Feeding*

## GENDER DYSPHORIA

**Anxiety** r/t conflict between physical (assigned) gender and gender they identify with

**Decisional Conflict** r/t uncertainty about choices regarding gender reassignment

**Disturbed Body Image** r/t alteration in self-perception, inability to identify with own body

**Ineffective Denial** r/t insufficient emotional support

**Fear** r/t victimization

**Disturbed Personal Identity** r/t gender confusion

**Ineffective Sexuality Pattern** r/t conflict surrounding gender identity

**Risk for Compromised Human Dignity:** Risk factor: cultural incongruence, humiliation

**Readiness for Enhanced Decision-Making:** expresses desire to enhance understanding of choices for decision-making

## GENITAL HERPES

*See Herpes Simplex II*

## GENITAL WARTS

*See STD (Sexually Transmitted Disease)*

## GERD

*See Gastroesophageal Reflux Disease (GERD)*

## GESTATIONAL DIABETES (DIABETES IN PREGNANCY)

**Anxiety** r/t threat to self and/or fetus

**Impaired Nutrition: Less than Body Requirements** r/t decreased insulin production and glucose uptake in cells

**Risk for Overweight: Fetal** r/t excessive glucose uptake

**Impaired Nutrition: More than Body Requirements: Fetal** r/t excessive glucose uptake

**Risk for Unstable Blood Glucose:** Risk factor: excessive intake of carbohydrates

**Risk for Disturbed Maternal–Fetal Dyad:** Risk factor: impaired glucose metabolism

**Risk for Impaired Tissue Integrity: Fetal:** Risk factors: large infant, congenital defects, birth injury

**Risk for Impaired Tissue Integrity: Maternal:** Risk factor: delivery of large infant

**Readiness for Enhanced Knowledge:** expresses an interest in learning

*See Diabetes Mellitus*

## GI BLEED (GASTROINTESTINAL BLEEDING)

**Fatigue** r/t loss of circulating blood volume, decreased ability to transport oxygen

**Fear** r/t threat to well-being, potential death

**Deficient Fluid Volume** r/t gastrointestinal bleeding, hemorrhage

**Imbalanced Nutrition: Less than Body Requirements** r/t nausea, vomiting

**Acute Pain** r/t irritated mucosa from acid secretion

**Risk for Ineffective Coping:** Risk factors: personal vulnerability in crisis, bleeding, hospitalization

**Readiness for Enhanced Knowledge:** expresses an interest in learning

## GINGIVITIS

**Impaired Oral Mucous Membrane Integrity** r/t ineffective oral hygiene

## GLAUCOMA

**Deficient Knowledge** r/t treatment and self-care for disease

*See Vision Impairment*

## GLOMERULONEPHRITIS

**Excess Fluid Volume** r/t renal impairment

**Imbalanced Nutrition: Less than Body Requirements** r/t anorexia, restrictive diet

**Acute Pain** r/t edema of kidney

**Readiness for Enhanced Knowledge:** expresses an interest in learning

## GLUTEN ALLERGY

*See Celiac Disease*

## GONORRHEA

**Acute Pain** r/t inflammation of reproductive organs

**Risk for Infection:** Risk factor: spread of organism throughout reproductive organs

**Readiness for Enhanced Knowledge:** expresses an interest in learning

*See STD (Sexually Transmitted Disease)*

## GOUT

**Impaired Physical Mobility** r/t musculoskeletal impairment

**Chronic Pain** r/t inflammation of affected joint

**Readiness for Enhanced Knowledge:** expresses an interest in learning

## GRANDIOSITY

**Defensive Coping** r/t inaccurate perception of self and abilities

## GRAND MAL SEIZURE

*See Seizure Disorders, Adult; Seizure Disorders, Childhood (Epilepsy, Febrile Seizures, Infantile Spasms)*

## GRANDPARENTS RAISING GRANDCHILDREN

**Anxiety** r/t change in role status

**Decisional Conflict** r/t support system deficit

**Parental Role Conflict** r/t change in parental role

**Compromised Family Coping** r/t family role changes

**Interrupted Family Processes** r/t family roles shift

**G**

**Ineffective Role Performance** r/t role transition, aging

**Ineffective Family Health Self-Management** r/t excessive demands on individual or family

**Risk for Impaired Parenting:** Risk factor: role strain

**Risk for Powerlessness:** Risk factors: role strain, situational crisis, aging

**Risk for Spiritual Distress:** Risk factor: life change

**Readiness for Enhanced Parenting:** physical and emotional needs of children are met

## GRAVES' DISEASE

*See Hyperthyroidism*

## GRIEVING, MALADAPTIVE

**Complicated Grieving** r/t expected or sudden death of a significant other with whom there was a volatile relationship, emotional instability, lack of social support

**Risk for Maladaptive Grieving:** Risk factors: death of a significant other with whom there was a volatile relationship, emotional instability, lack of social support

## GROOM SELF (INABILITY TO)

**Bathing Self-Care Deficit** (See **Self-Care Deficit, Bathing,** Section II)

**Dressing Self-Care Deficit** (See **Self-Care Deficit, Dressing,** Section II)

## GROWTH AND DEVELOPMENT LAG

*See Failure to Thrive, Child*

## GUILLAIN-BARRÉ SYNDROME

**Dysfunctional Ventilatory Weaning Response** r/t fatigue

**Impaired Spontaneous Ventilation** r/t weak respiratory muscles

**Risk for Aspiration:** Risk factors: ineffective cough; depressed gag reflex

*See Neurological Disorders*

## GUILT

**Maladaptive Grieving** r/t potential loss of significant person, animal, prized material possession, change in life role

**Impaired Resilience** (See **Resilience, Individual, Impaired,** Section II)

**Situational Low Self-Esteem** r/t unmet expectations of self

**Risk for Maladaptive Grieving:** Risk factors: actual loss of significant person, animal, prized material possession, change in life role

**Risk for Post-Trauma Syndrome:** Risk factor: exaggerated sense of responsibility for traumatic event

**Readiness for Enhanced Spiritual Well-Being:** desire to be in harmony with self, others, higher power or God

## HAIR LOSS

**Disturbed Body Image** r/t psychological reaction to loss of hair

**Imbalanced Nutrition: Less than Body Requirements** r/t inability to ingest food because of biological, psychological, economic factors

## HALITOSIS

**Impaired Dentition** r/t ineffective oral hygiene

**Impaired Oral Mucous Membrane Integrity** r/t ineffective oral hygiene

## HALLUCINATIONS

**Anxiety** r/t threat to self-concept

**Acute Confusion** r/t alcohol abuse, delirium, dementia, mental illness, substance abuse

**Ineffective Coping** r/t distortion and insecurity of life events

**Risk for Self-Mutilation:** Risk factor: command hallucinations

**Risk for Other-Directed Violence:** Risk factors: catatonic excitement, manic excitement, rage or panic reactions, response to violent internal stimuli

**Risk for Self-Directed Violence:** Risk factors: catatonic excitement, manic excitement, rage or panic reactions, response to violent internal stimuli

## HEADACHE

**Acute Pain** r/t lack of knowledge of pain control techniques or methods to prevent headaches

**Ineffective Health Self-Management** r/t lack of knowledge, identification, elimination of aggravating factors

## HEAD INJURY

**Ineffective Breathing Pattern** r/t pressure damage to breathing center in brainstem

**Acute Confusion** r/t increased intracranial pressure

**Risk for Ineffective Cerebral Tissue Perfusion:** Risk factors: effects of increased intracranial pressure, trauma to brain

*See Neurological Disorders*

## HEALTH BEHAVIOR, RISK-PRONE

**Risk-Prone Health Behavior:** Risk factors (See **Health Behavior, Risk-Prone,** Section II)

**Risk for Metabolic Syndrome** r/t obesity

## HEALTH MAINTENANCE PROBLEMS

**Ineffective Health Maintenance Behaviors** (See **Health Maintenance Behaviors, Ineffective,** Section II)

**Ineffective Health Self-Management** (See **Health Self-Management, Ineffective,** Section II)

## HEALTH-SEEKING PERSON

**Readiness for Enhanced Health literacy** (See **Health Literacy, Readiness for Enhanced,** Section II)

**Readiness for Enhanced Health Self-Management** (See **Health Self-Management, Readiness for Enhanced,** Section II)

## HEARING IMPAIRMENT

**Impaired Verbal Communication** r/t inability to hear own voice

**Hearing Loss** (see Appendix E on Evolve)

**Social Isolation** r/t difficulty with communication

## HEART ATTACK

*See MI (Myocardial Infarction)*

## HEARTBURN

**Nausea** r/t gastrointestinal irritation

**Acute Pain: Heartburn** r/t inflammation of stomach and esophagus

**Risk for Imbalanced Nutrition: Less than Body Requirements:** Risk factor: pain after eating

**Readiness for Enhanced Knowledge:** expresses an interest in learning

*See Gastroesophageal Reflux Disease (GERD)*

## HEART FAILURE

**Decreased Activity Tolerance** r/t weakness, fatigue, shortness of breath

**Decreased Cardiac Output** r/t impaired cardiac function, increased preload, decreased contractility, increased afterload

**Constipation** r/t activity intolerance

**Fatigue** r/t disease process with decreased cardiac output

**Fear** r/t threat to one's own well-being

**Excess Fluid Volume** r/t impaired excretion of sodium and water

**Impaired Gas Exchange** r/t excessive fluid in interstitial space of lungs

**Powerlessness** r/t illness-related regimen

**Risk for Shock (Cardiogenic):** Risk factors: decreased contractility of heart, increased afterload

**Readiness for Enhanced Health Management** (See **Health Management, Readiness for Enhanced,** Section II)

*See Child with Chronic Condition; Congenital Heart Disease/Cardiac Anomalies; Hospitalized Child*

## HEART SURGERY

*See Coronary Artery Bypass Grafting (CABG)*

## HEAT STROKE

**Deficient Fluid Volume** r/t profuse diaphoresis from high environmental temperature

**Hyperthermia** r/t vigorous activity, high environmental temperature, inappropriate clothing

**H**

**H**

## HEMATEMESIS

*See GI Bleed (Gastrointestinal Bleeding)*

## HEMATURIA

*See Kidney Stone; UTI (Urinary Tract Infection)*

## HEMIANOPIA

**Anxiety** r/t change in vision

**Unilateral Neglect** r/t effects of disturbed perceptual abilities

**Risk for Injury:** Risk factor: disturbed sensory perception

## HEMIPLEGIA

**Anxiety** r/t change in health status

**Disturbed Body Image** r/t functional loss of one side of body

**Impaired Physical Mobility** r/t loss of neurological control of involved extremities

**Self-Care Deficit: Specify** r/t neuromuscular impairment

**Impaired Sitting** r/t partial paralysis

**Impaired Standing** r/t partial paralysis

**Impaired Transfer Ability** r/t partial paralysis

**Unilateral Neglect** r/t effects of disturbed perceptual abilities

**Impaired Walking** r/t loss of neurological control of involved extremities

**Risk for Adult Falls:** Risk factor: impaired mobility

**Risk for Impaired Skin Integrity:** Risk factors: alteration in sensation, immobility; pressure over bony prominence

*See CVA (Cerebrovascular Accident)*

## HEMODIALYSIS

**Ineffective Coping** r/t situational crisis

**Interrupted Family Processes** r/t changes in role responsibilities as a result of therapy regimen

**Excess Fluid Volume** r/t renal disease with minimal urine output

**Powerlessness** r/t treatment regimen

**Risk for Caregiver Role Strain:** Risk factor: complexity of care receiver treatment

**Risk for Electrolyte Imbalance:** Risk factor: effect of metabolic state on renal function

**Risk for deficient Fluid Volume:** Risk factor: excessive removal of fluid during dialysis

**Risk for Infection:** Risk factors: exposure to blood products, risk for developing hepatitis B or C, impaired immune system

**Risk for Injury:** Risk factors: clotting of blood access, abnormal surface for blood flow

**Risk for Impaired Tissue Integrity:** Risk factor: mechanical factor associated with fistula formation

**Readiness for Enhanced Knowledge:** expresses an interest in learning

*See Renal Failure; Renal Failure, Child with Chronic Condition*

## HEMODYNAMIC MONITORING

**Risk for Infection:** Risk factor: invasive procedure

**Risk for Injury:** Risk factors: inadvertent wedging of catheter, dislodgment of catheter, disconnection of catheter

**Risk for Impaired Tissue Integrity:** Risk factor: invasive procedure

*See Shock, Cardiogenic; Shock, Hypovolemic; Shock, Septic*

## HEMOLYTIC UREMIC SYNDROME

**Fatigue** r/t decreased red blood cells

**Fear** r/t serious condition with unknown outcome

**Deficient Fluid Volume** r/t vomiting, diarrhea

**Nausea** r/t effects of uremia

**Risk for Injury:** Risk factors: decreased platelet count, seizure activity

**Risk for Impaired Skin Integrity:** Risk factor: diarrhea

*See Hospitalized Child; Renal Failure, Acute/Chronic, Child*

## HEMOPHILIA

**Fear** r/t high risk for AIDS infection from contaminated blood products

**Impaired Physical Mobility** r/t pain from acute bleeds, imposed activity restrictions, joint pain

**Acute Pain** r/t bleeding into body tissues

**Risk for Bleeding:** Risk factors: deficient clotting factors, child's developmental level, age-appropriate play, inappropriate use of toys or sports equipment

**Readiness for Enhanced Knowledge:** expresses an interest in learning

*See Child with Chronic Condition; Hospitalized Child; Maturational Issues, Adolescent*

## HEMOPTYSIS

**Fear** r/t serious threat to well-being

**Risk for Ineffective Airway Clearance:** Risk factor: obstruction of airway with blood and mucus

**Risk for Deficient Fluid Volume:** Risk factor: excessive loss of blood

## HEMORRHAGE

**Fear** r/t threat to well-being

**Deficient Fluid Volume** r/t massive blood loss

*See Hypovolemic Shock*

## HEMORRHOIDECTOMY

**Anxiety** r/t embarrassment, need for privacy

**Constipation** r/t fear of pain with defecation

**Acute Pain** r/t surgical procedure

**Urinary Retention** r/t pain, anesthetic effect

**Risk for Bleeding:** Risk factors: inadequate clotting, trauma from surgery

**Readiness for Enhanced Knowledge:** expresses an interest in learning

## HEMORRHOIDS

**Impaired Comfort** r/t itching in rectal area

**Constipation** r/t painful defecation, poor bowel habits

**Impaired Sitting** r/t pain and pressure

**Readiness for Enhanced Knowledge:** expresses an interest in learning

## HEMOTHORAX

**Deficient Fluid Volume** r/t blood in pleural space

*See Pneumothorax*

## HEPATITIS

**Decreased Activity Tolerance** r/t weakness or fatigue caused by infection

**Decreased Diversional Activity Engagement** r/t isolation

**Fatigue** r/t infectious process, altered body chemistry

**Imbalanced Nutrition: Less than Body Requirements** r/t anorexia, impaired use of proteins and carbohydrates

**Acute Pain** r/t edema of liver, bile irritating skin

**Social Isolation** r/t treatment-imposed isolation

**Risk for Imbalanced Fluid Volume:** Risk factor: excessive loss of fluids from vomiting and diarrhea

**Readiness for Enhanced Knowledge:** expresses an interest in learning

## HERNIA

*See Hiatal Hernia; Inguinal Hernia Repair*

## HERNIATED DISK

*See Low Back Pain*

## HERNIORRHAPHY

*See Inguinal Hernia Repair*

## HERPES IN PREGNANCY

**Fear** r/t threat to fetus, impending surgery

**Situational Low Self-Esteem** r/t threat to fetus as a result of disease process

**Risk for Infection: Infant:** Risk factors: transplacental transfer during primary herpes, exposure to active herpes during birth process

*See Herpes Simplex II*

## HERPES SIMPLEX I

**Impaired Oral Mucous Membrane Integrity** r/t inflammatory changes in mouth

## HERPES SIMPLEX II

**Ineffective Health Maintenance Behaviors** r/t deficient knowledge regarding treatment, prevention, spread of disease

**Acute Pain** r/t active herpes lesion

**H**

**Situational Low Self-Esteem** r/t expressions of shame or guilt

**Sexual Dysfunction** r/t disease process

**Impaired Tissue Integrity** r/t active herpes lesion

**Impaired Urinary Elimination** r/t pain with urination

## HERPES ZOSTER

*See Shingles*

## HHNS (HYPEROSMOLAR HYPERGLYCEMIC NONKETOTIC SYNDROME)

*See Hyperosmolar Hyperglycemic Nonketotic Syndrome (HHNS)*

## HIATAL HERNIA

**Ineffective Health Maintenance Behaviors** r/t deficient knowledge regarding care of disease

**Nausea** r/t effects of gastric contents in esophagus

**Imbalanced Nutrition: Less than Body Requirements** r/t pain after eating

**Acute Pain** r/t gastroesophageal reflux

## HIP FRACTURE

**Acute Confusion** r/t sensory overload, sensory deprivation, medication side effects, advanced age, pain

**Constipation** r/t immobility, opioids, anesthesia

**Fear** r/t outcome of treatment, future mobility, present helplessness

**Impaired Physical Mobility** r/t surgical incision, temporary absence of weight bearing, pain when walking

**Acute Pain** r/t injury, surgical procedure, movement

**Powerlessness** r/t health care environment

**Self-Care Deficit: Specify** r/t musculoskeletal impairment

**Impaired Transfer Ability** r/t immobilization of hip

**Impaired Walking** r/t temporary absence of weight bearing

**Risk for Bleeding:** Risk factors: postoperative complication, surgical blood loss

**Risk for Surgical Site Infection:** Risk factor: invasive procedure

**Risk for Injury:** Risk factors: activities such as greater than 90-degree flexion of hips that can result in dislodged prosthesis, unsteadiness when ambulating

**Risk for Perioperative Positioning Injury:** Risk factors: immobilization, muscle weakness, emaciation

**Risk for Peripheral Neurovascular Dysfunction:** Risk factors: trauma, vascular obstruction, fracture

**Risk for Impaired Skin Integrity:** Risk factor: immobility

**Risk for Thrombosis:** Risk factors: immobility, trauma

## HIP REPLACEMENT

*See Total Joint Replacement (Total Hip/ Total Knee/Shoulder)*

## HIRSCHSPRUNG'S DISEASE

**Constipation: Bowel Obstruction** r/t inhibited peristalsis as a result of congenital absence of parasympathetic ganglion cells in distal colon

**Maladaptive Grieving** r/t loss of perfect child, birth of child with congenital defect even though child expected to be normal within 2 years

**Imbalanced Nutrition: Less than Body Requirements** r/t anorexia, pain from distended colon

**Acute Pain** r/t distended colon, incisional postoperative pain

**Impaired Skin Integrity** r/t stoma, potential skin care problems associated with stoma

**Readiness for Enhanced Knowledge:** expresses an interest in learning

*See Hospitalized Child*

## HIRSUTISM

**Disturbed Body Image** r/t excessive hair

## HITTING BEHAVIOR

**Acute Confusion** r/t dementia, alcohol abuse, drug abuse, delirium

**Risk for Other-Directed Violence** (See **Violence, Other-Directed, Risk for,** Section II)

## HIV (HUMAN IMMUNODEFICIENCY VIRUS)

**Fear** r/t possible death

**Ineffective Protection** r/t depressed immune system

**Readiness for Enhanced Health Literacy:** expresses desire to enhance understanding of health information to make health care choices

*See AIDS (Acquired Immunodeficiency Syndrome)*

## HODGKIN'S DISEASE

*See Anemia; Cancer; Chemotherapy*

## HOMELESSNESS

**Ineffective Home Maintenance Behaviors** r/t impaired cognitive or emotional functioning, inadequate support system, insufficient finances

## HOME MAINTENANCE PROBLEMS

**Ineffective Home Maintenance Behaviors** (See **Home Maintenance, Impaired,** Section II)

**Self-Neglect** r/t mental illness, substance abuse, cognitive impairment

**Powerlessness** r/t interpersonal interactions

**Risk for Physical Trauma:** Risk factor: being in high-crime neighborhood

## HOPE

**Readiness for Enhanced Hope** (See **Hope, Readiness for Enhanced,** Section II)

## HOPELESSNESS

**Hopelessness** (See **Hopelessness,** Section II)

## HOSPITALIZED CHILD

**Decreased Activity Tolerance** r/t fatigue associated with acute illness

**Anxiety: Separation: Child** r/t familiar surroundings and separation from family and friends

**Compromised Family Coping** r/t possible prolonged hospitalization that exhausts supportive capacity of significant people

**Ineffective Coping: Parent** r/t possible guilt regarding hospitalization of child, parental inadequacies

**Decreased Diversional Activity Engagement** r/t immobility, monotonous environment, frequent or lengthy treatments, reluctance to participate, therapeutic isolation, separation from peers

**Interrupted Family Processes** r/t situational crisis of illness, disease, hospitalization

**Fear** r/t deficient knowledge or maturational level with fear of unknown, mutilation, painful procedures, surgery

**Hopelessness: Child** r/t prolonged activity restriction, uncertain prognosis

**Insomnia: Child or Parent** r/t 24-hour care needs of hospitalization

**Acute Pain** r/t treatments, diagnostic or therapeutic procedures, disease process

**Powerlessness: Child** r/t health care environment, illness-related regimen

**Risk for Impaired Attachment:** Risk factor: separation

**Risk for Injury:** Risk factors: unfamiliar environment, developmental age, lack of parental knowledge regarding safety (e.g., side rails, IV site/pole)

**Risk for Imbalanced Nutrition: Less than Body Requirements:** Risk factors: anorexia, absence of familiar foods, cultural preferences

**Readiness for Enhanced Family Coping:** impact of crisis on family values, priorities, goals, relationships in family

*See Child with Chronic Condition*

## HOSTILE BEHAVIOR

**Risk for Other-Directed Violence:** Risk factor: antisocial personality disorder

## HTN (HYPERTENSION)

**Ineffective Health Self-Management** (See **Health Management, Ineffective,** Section II)

**Readiness for Enhanced Health Self-Management** (See **Health Management, Readiness for Enhanced,** Section II)

**Risk for Overweight:** Risk factor: lack of knowledge of relationship between diet and disease process

## HUMAN ENERGY FIELD

**Energy Field, Imbalanced** (See **Imbalanced Energy Field,** Section II)

## HUMILIATING EXPERIENCE

**Risk for Compromised Human Dignity** (See **Human Dignity, Compromised, Risk for,** Section II)

## HUNTINGTON'S DISEASE

**Decisional Conflict** r/t whether to have children

*See Neurological Disorders*

## HYDROCELE

**Acute Pain** r/t severely enlarged hydrocele

**Ineffective Sexuality Pattern** r/t recent surgery on area of scrotum

## HYDROCEPHALUS

**Decisional Conflict** r/t unclear or conflicting values regarding selection of treatment modality

**Interrupted Family processes** r/t situational crisis

**Imbalanced Nutrition: Less than Body Requirements** r/t inadequate intake as a result of anorexia, nausea, vomiting, feeding difficulties

**Risk for Infection:** Risk factor: sequelae of invasive procedure (shunt placement)

**Risk for Ineffective Cerebral Tissue Perfusion:** Risk factors: interrupted flow, hypervolemia of cerebral ventricles

**Risk for Adult Falls:** Risk factors: acute illness, alteration in cognitive functioning

*See Normal Pressure Hydrocephalus (NPH); Child with Chronic Condition; Hospitalized Child; Premature Infant (Child); Premature Infant (Parent)*

## HYGIENE, INABILITY TO PROVIDE OWN

**Frail Elderly Syndrome** r/t living alone

**Self-Neglect** (See **Self-Neglect,** Section II)

**Bathing Self-Care Deficit** (See **Self-Care Deficit, Bathing,** Section II)

## HYPERACTIVE SYNDROME

**Decisional Conflict** r/t multiple or divergent sources of information regarding education, nutrition, medication regimens; willingness to change own food habits; limited resources

**Parental Role Conflict: When Siblings Present** r/t increased attention toward hyperactive child

**Compromised Family Coping** r/t unsuccessful strategies to control excessive activity, behaviors, frustration, anger

**Ineffective Impulse Control** r/t disorder of development, environment that might cause frustration or irritation

**Ineffective Role Performance: Parent** r/t stressors associated with dealing with hyperactive child, perceived or projected blame for causes of child's behavior, unmet needs for support or care, lack of energy to provide for those needs

**Chronic Low Self-Esteem** r/t inability to achieve socially acceptable behaviors; frustration; frequent reprimands, punishment, or scolding for uncontrolled activity and behaviors; mood fluctuations and restlessness; inability to succeed academically; lack of peer support

**Impaired Social Interaction** r/t impulsive and overactive behaviors, concomitant emotional difficulties, distractibility and excitability

**Risk for Impaired Parenting:** Risk factor: disruptive or uncontrollable behaviors of child

**Risk for Other-Directed Violence: Parent or Child:** Risk factors: frustration with disruptive behavior, anger, unsuccessful relationships

## HYPERBILIRUBINEMIA, NEONATAL

**Anxiety: Parent** r/t threat to infant, unknown future

**Parental Role Conflict** r/t interruption of family life because of care regimen

**Neonatal Hyperbilirubinemia** r/t abnormal breakdown of red blood cells following birth

**Imbalanced Nutrition: Less than Body Requirements: Infant** r/t disinterest in feeding because of jaundice-related lethargy

**Risk for Injury: Infant:** Risk factors: kernicterus, phototherapy lights

**Risk for Ineffective Thermoregulation:** Risk factor: phototherapy

**Readiness for Enhanced Health Self-Management: Parents:** expresses desire to manage treatment: assessment of jaundice when infant is discharged from the hospital, when to call the physician, and possible preventive measures such as frequent breastfeeding (See **Neonatal Hyperbilirubinemia, Risk for,** Section II)

## HYPERCALCEMIA

**Decreased Cardiac Output** r/t bradydysrhythmia

**Impaired Physical Mobility** r/t decreased muscle tone

**Imbalanced Nutrition: Less than Body Requirements** r/t gastrointestinal manifestations of hypercalcemia (nausea, anorexia, ileus)

**Risk for Disuse Syndrome:** Risk factor: comatose state impairing mobility

## HYPERCAPNIA

**Fear** r/t difficulty breathing

**Impaired Gas Exchange** r/t ventilation-perfusion imbalance, retention of carbon dioxide

*See ARDS (Adult Respiratory Distress Syndrome); COPD (Chronic Obstructive Pulmonary Disorder); Sleep Apnea*

## HYPEREMESIS GRAVIDARUM

**Anxiety** r/t threat to self and infant, hospitalization

**Deficient Fluid Volume** r/t excessive vomiting

**Ineffective Home Maintenance Behaviors** r/t chronic nausea, inability to function

**Nausea** r/t hormonal changes of pregnancy

**Imbalanced Nutrition: Less than Body Requirements** r/t excessive vomiting

**Powerlessness** r/t health care regimen

**Social Isolation** r/t hospitalization

**Risk for Electrolyte Imbalance:** Risk factor: vomiting

## HYPERGLYCEMIA

**Ineffective Health Self-Management** r/t complexity of therapeutic regimen, decisional conflicts, economic difficulties, unsupportive family, insufficient cues to action, deficient knowledge, mistrust, lack of acknowledgment of seriousness of condition

**Risk for Unstable Blood Glucose Level** (See **Glucose Level, Blood, Unstable, Risk for,** Section II)

*See Diabetes Mellitus*

## HYPERKALEMIA

**Risk for Decreased Activity Tolerance:** Risk factor: muscle weakness

**Risk for Decreased Cardiac Tissue Perfusion:** Risk factor: abnormal electrolyte level affecting heart rate and rhythm

**Risk for Excess Fluid Volume:** Risk factor: untreated renal failure

## HYPERNATREMIA

**Risk for Imbalanced Fluid Volume:** Risk factors: abnormal water loss, inadequate water intake

## HYPEROSMOLAR HYPERGLYCEMIC NONKETOTIC SYNDROME (HHNS)

**Acute Confusion** r/t dehydration, electrolyte imbalance

**Deficient Fluid Volume** r/t polyuria, hyperglycemia, inadequate fluid intake

**Risk for Electrolyte Imbalance:** Risk factor: effect of metabolic state on kidney function

**Risk for Injury: Seizures:** Risk factors: hyperosmolar state, electrolyte imbalance

**H**

*See Diabetes Mellitus; Diabetes Mellitus, Juvenile (Insulin-Dependent Diabetes Mellitus Type 1)*

## HYPERPHOSPHATEMIA

**Deficient Knowledge** r/t dietary changes needed to control phosphate levels

*See Renal Failure*

## HYPERSENSITIVITY TO SLIGHT CRITICISM

**Defensive Coping** r/t situational crisis, psychological impairment, substance abuse

## HYPERTENSION (HTN)

*See HTN (Hypertension)*

**Risk for Decreased Cardiac Output:** Risk factors: decreased contractility and altered conductivity associated with myocardial damage

**Risk for Unstable Blood Pressure** (See **Unstable Blood Pressure, Risk for,** Section II)

## HYPERTHERMIA

**Hyperthermia** (See **Hyperthermia,** Section II)

## HYPERTHYROIDISM

**Anxiety** r/t increased stimulation, loss of control

**Diarrhea** r/t increased gastric motility

**Insomnia** r/t anxiety, excessive sympathetic discharge

**Imbalanced Nutrition: Less than Body Requirements** r/t increased metabolic rate, increased gastrointestinal activity

**Risk for Injury: Eye Damage:** Risk factor: protruding eyes without sufficient lubrication

**Risk for Unstable Blood Pressure** r/t hyperthyroidism

**Readiness for Enhanced Knowledge:** expresses an interest in learning

## HYPERVENTILATION

**Ineffective Breathing Pattern** r/t anxiety, acid-base imbalance

*See Anxiety Disorder; Dyspnea; Heart Failure*

## HYPOCALCEMIA

**Decreased Activity Tolerance** r/t neuromuscular irritability

**Ineffective Breathing Pattern** r/t laryngospasm

**Imbalanced Nutrition: Less than Body Requirements** r/t effects of vitamin D deficiency, renal failure, malabsorption, laxative use

## HYPOGLYCEMIA

**Acute Confusion** r/t insufficient blood glucose to brain

**Ineffective Health Self-Management** r/t deficient knowledge regarding disease process, self-care

**Imbalanced Nutrition: Less than Body Requirements** r/t imbalance of glucose and insulin level

**Risk for Unstable Blood Glucose Level** (See **Glucose Level, Blood, Unstable, Risk for,** Section II)

*See Diabetes Mellitus; Diabetes Mellitus, Juvenile (IDDM Type 1)*

## HYPOKALEMIA

**Decreased Activity Tolerance** r/t muscle weakness

**Risk for Decreased Cardiac Tissue Perfusion:** Risk factor: possible dysrhythmia from electrolyte imbalance

## HYPOMAGNESEMIA

**Imbalanced Nutrition: Less than Body Requirements** r/t deficient knowledge of nutrition, alcoholism

*See Alcoholism*

## HYPOMANIA

**Insomnia** r/t psychological stimulus

*See Manic Disorder, Bipolar I*

## HYPONATREMIA

**Acute Confusion** r/t electrolyte imbalance

**Excess Fluid Volume** r/t excessive intake of hypotonic fluids

**H**

**Risk for Injury:** Risk factors: seizures, new onset of confusion

## HYPOPLASTIC LEFT LUNG

*See Congenital Heart Disease/Cardiac Anomalies*

## HYPOTENSION

**Decreased Cardiac Output** r/t decreased preload, decreased contractility

**Risk for Deficient Fluid Volume:** Risk factor: excessive fluid loss

**Risk for Ineffective Cerebral Tissue Perfusion:** Risk factors: hypovolemia, decreased contractility, decreased afterload

**Risk for Shock** (See **Shock, Risk for,** Section II)

**Risk for Unstable Blood Pressure** (See **Unstable Blood Pressure, Risk for,** Section II)

*See Dehydration; Heart Failure; MI (Myocardial Infarction)*

## HYPOTHERMIA

**Hypothermia** (See **Hypothermia,** Section II)

**Risk for Hypothermia** (See **Hypothermia, Risk for,** Section II)

## HYPOTHYROIDISM

**Decreased Activity Tolerance** r/t muscular stiffness, shortness of breath on exertion

**Constipation** r/t decreased gastric motility

**Impaired Gas Exchange** r/t respiratory depression

**Impaired Skin Integrity** r/t edema, dry or scaly skin

**Risk for Overweight:** Risk factor: decreased metabolic process

## HYPOVOLEMIC SHOCK

*See Shock, Hypovolemic*

## HYPOXIA

**Acute Confusion** r/t decreased oxygen supply to brain

**Fear** r/t breathlessness

**Impaired Gas Exchange** r/t altered oxygen supply, inability to transport oxygen

**Risk for Shock** (See **Shock, Risk for,** Section II)

## HYSTERECTOMY

**Constipation** r/t opioids, anesthesia, bowel manipulation during surgery

**Ineffective Coping** r/t situational crisis of surgery

**Maladaptive Grieving** r/t change in body image, loss of reproductive status

**Acute Pain** r/t surgical injury

**Sexual Dysfunction** r/t disturbance in self-concept

**Urinary Retention** r/t edema in area, anesthesia, opioids, pain

**Risk for Bleeding:** Risk factor: surgical procedure

**Risk for Constipation:** Risk factors: opioids, anesthesia, bowel manipulation during surgery

**Risk for Ineffective Peripheral Tissue Perfusion:** Risk factor: deficient knowledge of aggravating factors

**Risk for Surgical Site Infection:** Risk factor: invasive procedure

**Readiness for Enhanced Knowledge:** Expresses an interest in learning

*See Surgery, Perioperative Care; Surgery, Preoperative Care; Surgery, Postoperative Care*

# I

## IBS (IRRITABLE BOWEL SYNDROME)

**Constipation** r/t low-residue diet, stress

**Diarrhea** r/t increased motility of intestines associated with disease process, stress

**Ineffective Health Self-Management** r/t deficient knowledge, powerlessness

**Chronic Pain** r/t spasms, increased motility of bowel

**Risk for Electrolyte Imbalance:** Risk factor: diarrhea

**Readiness for Enhanced Health Self-Management:** expresses desire to manage illness and prevent onset of symptoms

## ICD (IMPLANTABLE CARDIOVERTER/DEFIBRILLATOR)

**Anxiety** r/t possible dysrhythmia, threat of death

**Decreased Cardiac Output** r/t possible dysrhythmia

**Readiness for Enhanced Knowledge:** expresses an interest in learning

## IDDM (INSULIN-DEPENDENT DIABETES MELLITUS)

*See Diabetes Mellitus*

## IDENTITY DISTURBANCE/ PROBLEMS

**Disturbed Personal Identity** r/t situational crisis, psychological impairment, chronic illness, pain

**Risk for Disturbed Personal Identity** (See **Identity, Personal, Risk for Disturbed,** Section II)

## IDIOPATHIC THROMBOCYTOPENIC PURPURA (ITP)

*See ITP (Idiopathic Thrombocytopenic Purpura)*

## ILEAL CONDUIT

**Disturbed Body Image** r/t presence of stoma

**Ineffective Health Self-Management** r/t new skills required to care for appliance and self

**Ineffective Sexuality Pattern** r/t altered body function and structure

**Social Isolation** r/t alteration in physical appearance, fear of accidental spill of urine

**Risk for Latex Allergy Reaction:** Risk factor: repeated exposures to latex associated with treatment and management of disease

**Risk for Impaired Skin Integrity:** Risk factor: difficulty obtaining tight seal of appliance

**Readiness for Enhanced Knowledge:** expresses an interest in learning

## ILEOSTOMY

**Disturbed Body Image** r/t presence of stoma

**Diarrhea** r/t dietary changes, alteration in intestinal motility

**Deficient Knowledge** r/t limited practice of stoma care, dietary modifications

**Ineffective Sexuality Pattern** r/t altered body function and structure

**Social Isolation** r/t alteration in physical appearance, fear of accidental spill of ostomy contents

**Risk for Impaired Skin Integrity:** Risk factors: difficulty obtaining tight seal of appliance, caustic drainage

**Readiness for Enhanced Knowledge:** expresses an interest in learning

## ILEUS

**Deficient Fluid Volume** r/t loss of fluids from vomiting, fluids trapped in bowel

**Dysfunctional Gastrointestinal Motility** r/t effects of surgery, decreased perfusion of intestines, medication effect, immobility

**Nausea** r/t gastrointestinal irritation

**Acute Pain** r/t pressure, abdominal distention

**Readiness for Enhanced Knowledge:** expresses an interest in learning

## IMMIGRATION TRANSITION, RISK FOR COMPLICATED

**Anxiety** r/t changes in safety and security needs

**Fear** r/t unfamiliar environment, separation from support system, possible language barrier

**Impaired Social Interaction** r/t possible communication or sociocultural barriers

**Risk for Loneliness:** Risk factor: separation from support system

**Risk for Powerlessness:** Risk factor: insufficient social support

**Risk for Relocation Stress Syndrome:** Risk factors: insufficient support system, social isolation, and potential communication barriers

**Risk for Impaired Resilience:** Risk factor: decreased ability to adapt to adverse or changing situations

**Readiness for Enhanced Coping:** expresses desire to enhance social support

**Readiness for Enhanced Knowledge:** expresses a desire to become familiar with resources within their environment

## IMMOBILITY

**Ineffective Breathing Pattern** r/t inability to deep breathe in supine position

**Acute Confusion: Elderly** r/t sensory deprivation from immobility

**Constipation** r/t immobility

**Risk for Frail Elderly Syndrome:** Risk factors: low physical activity, bed rest

**Impaired Physical Mobility** r/t medically imposed bed rest

**Ineffective Peripheral Tissue Perfusion** r/t interruption of venous flow

**Powerlessness** r/t forced immobility from health care environment

**Impaired Walking** r/t limited physical mobility, deconditioning of body

**Risk for Disuse Syndrome:** Risk factor: immobilization

**Risk for Impaired Skin Integrity:** Risk factors: pressure over bony prominences, shearing forces when moved; pressure from devices

**Risk for Impaired Tissue Integrity:** Risk factors: mechanical factors from pressure over bony prominences, shearing forces when moved; pressure from devices

**Risk for Overweight:** Risk factor: energy expenditure less than energy intake

**Risk for Thrombosis:** Risk factor: lack of physical activity

**Readiness for Enhanced Knowledge:** expresses an interest in learning

## IMMUNIZATION

(See **Readiness for Enhanced Health Literacy,** Section II)

(See **Readiness for Enhanced Health Self-Management,** Section II)

## IMMUNOSUPPRESSION

**Risk for Infection:** Risk factors: immunosuppression; exposure to disease outbreak

**Impaired Social Interaction** r/t therapeutic isolation

## IMPACTION OF STOOL

**Constipation** r/t decreased fluid intake, less than adequate amounts of fiber and bulk-forming foods in diet, medication effect, or immobility

## IMPAIRED SITTING

**Impaired Physical Mobility** r/t musculoskeletal, cognitive, or neuromuscular disorder

## IMPAIRED STANDING

**Decreased Activity Tolerance** r/t insufficient physiological or psychological energy

**Powerlessness** r/t loss of function

## IMPERFORATE ANUS

**Anxiety** r/t ability to care for newborn

**Deficient Knowledge** r/t home care for newborn

**Impaired Skin Integrity** r/t pruritus

## IMPETIGO

**Impaired Skin Integrity** r/t infectious disease

**Readiness for Enhanced Knowledge:** expresses an interest in learning

*See Communicable Diseases, Childhood (e.g., Measles, Mumps, Rubella, Chickenpox, Scabies, Lice)*

## IMPLANTABLE CARDIOVERTER/ DEFIBRILLATOR (ICD)

*See ICD (Implantable Cardioverter/ Defibrillator)*

## IMPOTENCE

**Situational Low Self-Esteem** r/t physiological crisis, inability to practice usual sexual activity

**Sexual Dysfunction** r/t altered body function

**Readiness for Enhanced Knowledge:** treatment information for erectile dysfunction

*See Erectile Dysfunction (ED)*

## IMPULSIVENESS

**Ineffective Impulse Control** (See **Impulse Control, Ineffective,** Section II)

## INACTIVITY

**Decreased Activity Tolerance** r/t imbalance between oxygen supply and demand, sedentary lifestyle, weakness, immobility

**Hopelessness** r/t deteriorating physiological condition, long-term stress, social isolation

**Impaired Physical Mobility** r/t intolerance to activity, decreased strength and endurance, depression, severe anxiety, musculoskeletal impairment, perceptual or cognitive impairment, neuromuscular impairment, pain, discomfort

**Risk for Constipation:** Risk factor: insufficient physical activity

## INCOMPETENT CERVIX

*See Premature Dilation of the Cervix (Incompetent Cervix)*

## INCONTINENCE OF STOOL

**Disturbed Body Image** r/t inability to control elimination of stool

**Impaired Bowel Continence** r/t decreased awareness of need to defecate, loss of sphincter control

**Toileting Self-Care Deficit** r/t cognitive impairment, neuromuscular impairment, perceptual impairment, weakness

**Situational Low Self-Esteem** r/t inability to control elimination of stool

**Risk for Impaired Skin Integrity:** Risk factor: presence of stool

## INCONTINENCE OF URINE

**Disability-Associated Urinary Incontinence** r/t altered environment; sensory, cognitive, or mobility deficits

**Stress Urinary Incontinence** (See **Incontinence, Urinary, Stress,** Section II)

**Urge Urinary Incontinence** (See **Incontinence, Urinary, Urge,** Section II)

**Toileting Self-Care Deficit** r/t cognitive impairment

**Situational Low Self-Esteem** r/t inability to control passage of urine

**Risk for Impaired Skin Integrity:** Risk factor: presence of urine on perineal skin

## INDIGESTION

**Nausea** r/t gastrointestinal irritation

**Imbalanced Nutrition: Less than Body Requirements** r/t discomfort when eating

## INDUCTION OF LABOR

**Anxiety** r/t medical interventions, powerlessness

**Decisional Conflict** r/t perceived threat to idealized birth

**Ineffective Coping** r/t situational crisis of medical intervention in birthing process

**Acute Pain** r/t contractions

**Situational Low Self-Esteem** r/t inability to carry out normal labor

**Risk for Injury: Maternal and Fetal:** Risk factors: hypertonic uterus, potential prematurity of newborn

**Readiness for Enhanced Family Processes:** family support during induction of labor

## INFANT APNEA

*See Premature Infant (Child); Respiratory Conditions of the Neonate; Sudden Infant Death Syndrome (SIDS)*

## INFANT BEHAVIOR

**Disorganized Infant Behavior** r/t pain, oral/motor problems, feeding intolerance, environmental overstimulation, lack of containment or boundaries, prematurity, invasive or painful procedures

**Risk for Disorganized Infant Behavior:** Risk factors: pain, oral/motor problems, environmental overstimulation, lack of containment or boundaries

**Readiness for Enhanced Organized Infant behavior:** stable physiologic measures, use of some self-regulatory measures

## INFANT CARE

**Readiness for Enhanced Childbearing Process:** a pattern of preparing for, maintaining, and strengthening care of newborn infant

## INFANT FEEDING DYNAMIC, INEFFECTIVE

**Ineffective Infant Feeding Dynamic** r/t prematurity, neurological impairment or delay, oral hypersensitivity, prolonged nothing-by-mouth order

## INFANT OF DIABETIC MOTHER

**Decreased Cardiac Output** r/t cardiomegaly

**Deficient Fluid Volume** r/t increased urinary excretion and osmotic diuresis

**Imbalanced Nutrition: Less than Body Requirements** r/t hypotonia, lethargy, poor sucking, postnatal metabolic changes from hyperglycemia to hypoglycemia and hyperinsulinism

**Risk for Impaired Gas Exchange:** Risk factors: increased incidence of cardiomegaly, prematurity

**Risk for Unstable Blood Glucose Level:** Risk factor: metabolic change from hyperglycemia to hypoglycemia and hyperinsulinism

**Risk for Disturbed Maternal–Fetal Dyad:** Risk factor: impaired glucose metabolism

*See Premature Infant (Child); Respiratory Conditions of the Neonate*

## INFANT OF SUBSTANCE-ABUSING MOTHER

*See Neonatal Abstinence Syndrome*

## INFANTILE POLYARTERITIS

*See Kawasaki Disease*

## INFECTION, POTENTIAL FOR

**Risk for Infection** (See **Infection, Risk for,** Section II)

## INFECTIOUS PROCESSES

**Impaired Comfort** r/t distressing symptoms

**Diarrhea** r/t gastrointestinal inflammation

**Ineffective Health Maintenance Behaviors** r/t knowledge deficit regarding transmission, symptoms, and treatment

**Ineffective Health Self-Management** r/t lack of knowledge regarding preventive immunizations

**Ineffective Protection** r/t inadequate nutrition, abnormal blood profiles, drug therapies, treatments

**Impaired Social Interaction** r/t therapeutic isolation

**Risk for Electrolyte Imbalance:** Risk factors: vomiting, diarrhea

**Risk for Deficient Fluid Volume:** Risk factors: vomiting, diarrhea, inadequate fluid intake

**Risk for Infection:** Risk factor: increased environmental exposure when in close proximity to infected persons

**Risk for Surgical Site Infection** r/t immunosuppression

**Risk for Ineffective Thermoregulation:** Risk factor: infectious process

**Readiness for Enhanced Knowledge:** expresses desire for information regarding prevention and treatment

## INFERTILITY

**Ineffective Health Self-Management** r/t deficient knowledge about infertility

**Powerlessness** r/t infertility

**Chronic Sorrow** r/t inability to conceive a child

**Spiritual Distress** r/t inability to conceive a child

## INFLAMMATORY BOWEL DISEASE (CHILD AND ADULT)

**Ineffective Coping** r/t repeated episodes of diarrhea

**Diarrhea** r/t effects of inflammatory changes of the bowel

**Deficient Fluid Volume** r/t frequent and loose stools

**Imbalanced Nutrition: Less than Body Requirements** r/t anorexia, decreased absorption of nutrients from gastrointestinal tract

**Acute Pain** r/t abdominal cramping and anal irritation

**Impaired Skin Integrity** r/t frequent stools, development of anal fissures

**Social Isolation** r/t diarrhea

*See Child with Chronic Condition; Crohn's Disease; Hospitalized Child; Maturational Issues, Adolescent*

## INFLUENZA

*See Infectious Processes*

## INGUINAL HERNIA REPAIR

**Impaired Physical Mobility** r/t pain at surgical site and fear of causing hernia to rupture

**Acute Pain** r/t surgical procedure

**Urinary Retention** r/t possible edema at surgical site

**Risk for Surgical Site Infection:** Risk factor: surgical procedure

## INJURY

**Risk for Adult Falls:** Risk factors: orthostatic hypotension, impaired physical mobility, diminished mental status

**Risk for Child Falls:** Risk factors: impaired physical mobility, diminished mental status

**Risk for Injury:** Risk factor: environmental conditions interacting with client's adaptive and defensive resources

**Risk for Corneal Injury:** Risk factors: blinking less than five times per minute, mechanical ventilation, pharmaceutical agent, prolonged hospitalization

**Risk for Thermal Injury:** Risk factors: cognitive impairment, inadequate supervision, developmental level

**Risk for Urinary Tract Injury:** Risk factor: inflammation and/or infection from long-term use of urinary catheter

## INSOMNIA

(See **Insomnia,** Section II)

## INSULIN SHOCK

*See Hypoglycemia*

## INTELLECTUAL DISABILITY

**Impaired Verbal Communication** r/t developmental delay

**Interrupted Family Processes** r/t crisis of diagnosis and situational transition

**Maladaptive Grieving** r/t loss of perfect child, birth of child with congenital defect or subsequent head injury

**Deficient Community Health** r/t lack of programs to address developmental deficiencies

**Ineffective Home Maintenance Behaviors** r/t insufficient support systems

**Self-Neglect** r/t learning disability

**Self-Care Deficit: Bathing, Dressing, Feeding, Toileting** r/t perceptual or cognitive impairment

**Self-Mutilation** r/t inability to express tension verbally

**Social Isolation** r/t delay in accomplishing developmental tasks

**Spiritual Distress** r/t chronic condition of child with special needs

**Stress Overload** r/t intense, repeated stressor (chronic condition)

**Impaired Swallowing** r/t neuromuscular impairment

**Risk for Ineffective Activity Planning** r/t inability to process information

**Risk for Impaired Religiosity:** Risk factor: social isolation

**Risk for Self-Mutilation:** Risk factors: separation anxiety, depersonalization

**Readiness for Enhanced Family Coping:** adaptation and acceptance of child's condition and needs

*See Child with Chronic Condition; Safety, Childhood*

## INTERMITTENT CLAUDICATION

**Deficient Knowledge** r/t lack of knowledge of cause and treatment of peripheral vascular diseases

**Acute Pain** r/t decreased circulation to extremities with activity

**Ineffective Peripheral Tissue Perfusion** r/t interruption of arterial flow

**Risk for Injury:** Risk factor: tissue hypoxia

**Readiness for Enhanced Knowledge:** prevention of pain and impaired circulation

*See Peripheral Vascular Disease (PVD)*

## INTERNAL CARDIOVERTER/ DEFIBRILLATOR (ICD)

*See ICD (Implantable Cardioverter/ Defibrillator)*

## INTERNAL FIXATION

**Impaired Walking** r/t repair of fracture

**Risk for Infection:** Risk factors: traumatized tissue, broken skin

*See Fracture*

## INTERSTITIAL CYSTITIS

**Acute Pain** r/t inflammatory process

**Impaired Urinary Elimination** r/t inflammation of bladder

**Risk for Infection:** Risk factor: suppressed inflammatory response

**Readiness for Enhanced Knowledge:** expresses an interest in learning

## INTERVERTEBRAL DISK EXCISION

*See Laminectomy*

## INTESTINAL OBSTRUCTION

*See Ileus; Bowel Obstruction*

## INTESTINAL PERFORATION

*See Peritonitis*

## INTOXICATION

**Anxiety** r/t loss of control of actions

**Acute Confusion** r/t alcohol abuse

**Ineffective Coping** r/t use of mind-altering substances as a means of coping

**Impaired Memory** r/t effects of alcohol on mind

**Risk for Aspiration:** Risk factors: diminished mental status, vomiting

**Risk for Adult Falls:** Risk factor: diminished mental status

**Risk for Other-Directed Violence:** Risk factor: inability to control thoughts and actions

## INTRAAORTIC BALLOON COUNTERPULSATION

**Anxiety** r/t device providing cardiovascular assistance

**Decreased Cardiac Output** r/t heart dysfunction needing counterpulsation

**Compromised Family Coping** r/t seriousness of significant other's medical condition

**Impaired Physical Mobility** r/t restriction of movement because of mechanical device

**Risk for Peripheral Neurovascular Dysfunction:** Risk factors: vascular obstruction of balloon catheter, thrombus formation, emboli, edema

**Risk for Infection:** Risk factor: invasive procedure

**Risk for Impaired Tissue Integrity:** Risk factor: invasive procedure

## INTRACRANIAL PRESSURE, INCREASED

**Ineffective Breathing Pattern** r/t pressure damage to breathing center in brainstem

**Acute Confusion** r/t increased intracranial pressure

**Impaired Memory** r/t neurological disturbance

**Vision Loss** r/t pressure damage to sensory centers in brain

**Risk for Ineffective Cerebral Tissue Perfusion:** Risk factors: body position, cerebral vessel circulation deficits

*See Head Injury; Subarachnoid Hemorrhage*

## INTRAUTERINE GROWTH RETARDATION

**Anxiety: Maternal** r/t threat to fetus

**Ineffective Coping: Maternal** r/t situational crisis, threat to fetus

**Impaired Gas Exchange** r/t insufficient placental perfusion

**Imbalanced Nutrition: Less than Body Requirements** r/t insufficient placenta

**Situational Low Self-Esteem: Maternal** r/t guilt about threat to fetus

**Spiritual Distress** r/t unknown outcome of fetus

**Risk for Powerlessness:** Risk factor: unknown outcome of fetus

## INTRAVENOUS THERAPY

**Risk for Vascular Trauma:** Risk factor: infusion of irritating chemicals

## INTUBATION, ENDOTRACHEAL OR NASOGASTRIC

**Disturbed Body Image** r/t altered appearance with mechanical devices

**Impaired Verbal Communication** r/t endotracheal tube

**Imbalanced Nutrition: Less than Body Requirements** r/t inability to ingest food because of the presence of tubes

**Impaired Oral Mucous Membrane** r/t presence of tubes

**Acute Pain** r/t presence of tube

## IODINE REACTION WITH DIAGNOSTIC TESTING

**Risk for Adverse Reaction to Iodinated Contrast Media** (See **Reaction to Iodinated Contrast Media, Risk for Adverse,** Section II)

## IRREGULAR PULSE

*See Dysrhythmia*

## IRRITABLE BOWEL SYNDROME (IBS)

*See IBS (Irritable Bowel Syndrome)*

## ISOLATION

**Impaired Resilience** (See **Resilience, Individual, Impaired,** Section II)

**Social Isolation** (See **Social Isolation,** Section II)

## ITCHING

*See Pruritus*

## ITP (IDIOPATHIC THROMBOCYTOPENIC PURPURA)

**Decreased Diversional Activity Engagement** r/t activity restrictions, safety precautions

**Ineffective Protection** r/t decreased platelet count

**Risk for Bleeding:** Risk factors: decreased platelet count, developmental level, age-appropriate play

*See Hospitalized Child*

# J

## JAUNDICE

**Imbalanced Nutrition: Less than Body Requirements** r/t decreased appetite with liver disorder

**Risk for Bleeding:** Risk factor: impaired liver function

**Risk for Impaired Liver Function:** Risk factors: possible viral infection, medication effect

**Risk for Impaired Skin Integrity:** Risk factors: pruritus, itching

*See Cirrhosis; Hepatitis*

## JAUNDICE, NEONATAL

*See Hyperbilirubinemia, Neonatal*

## JAW PAIN AND HEART ATTACKS

*See Angina; Chest Pain; MI (Myocardial Infarction)*

## JAW SURGERY

**Deficient Knowledge** r/t emergency care for wired jaws (e.g., cutting bands and wires), oral care

**Imbalanced Nutrition: Less than Body Requirements** r/t jaws wired closed, difficulty eating

**Acute Pain** r/t surgical procedure

**Impaired Swallowing** r/t edema from surgery

**Risk for Aspiration:** Risk factor: wired jaws

## JITTERY

**Anxiety** r/t unconscious conflict about essential values and goals, threat to or change in health status

**Death Anxiety** r/t unresolved issues relating to end of life

**Risk for Post-Trauma Syndrome:** Risk factors: occupation, survivor's role in event, inadequate social support

## JOCK ITCH

**Ineffective Health Self-Management** r/t prevention and treatment of disorder

**Impaired Skin Integrity** r/t moisture and irritating or tight-fitting clothing

*See Pruritus*

## JOINT DISLOCATION

*See Dislocation of Joint*

## JOINT PAIN

*See Arthritis; Bursitis; JRA (Juvenile Rheumatoid Arthritis); Osteoarthritis; Rheumatoid Arthritis (RA)*

## JOINT REPLACEMENT

**Risk for Peripheral Neurovascular Dysfunction:** Risk factor: orthopedic surgery

**Risk for Impaired Tissue Integrity:** Risk factor: invasive procedure

*See Total Joint Replacement (Total Hip/ Total Knee/Shoulder)*

## JRA (JUVENILE RHEUMATOID ARTHRITIS)

**Impaired Comfort** r/t altered health status

**Fatigue** r/t chronic inflammatory disease

**Impaired Physical Mobility** r/t pain, restricted joint movement

**Acute Pain** r/t swollen or inflamed joints, restricted movement, physical therapy

**Self-Care Deficit:** feeding, bathing, dressing, toileting r/t restricted joint movement, pain

**Risk for Compromised Human Dignity:** Risk factors: perceived intrusion by clinicians, invasion of privacy

**Risk for Injury:** Risk factors: impaired physical mobility, splints, adaptive devices, increased bleeding potential from antiinflammatory medications

**Risk for Impaired Resilience:** Risk factor: chronic condition

**Risk for Situational Low Self-Esteem:** Risk factor: disturbed body image

**Risk for Impaired Skin Integrity:** Risk factors: splints, adaptive devices

*See Child with Chronic Condition; Hospitalized Child*

## KAPOSI'S SARCOMA

**Risk for Maladaptive Grieving:** Risk factor: loss of social support

**Risk for Impaired Religiosity:** Risk factors: illness/hospitalization, ineffective coping

**Risk for Impaired Resilience:** Risk factor: serious illness

*See AIDS (Acquired Immunodeficiency Syndrome)*

## KAWASAKI DISEASE

**Anxiety: Parental** r/t progression of disease, complications of arthritis, and cardiac involvement

**Impaired Comfort** r/t altered health status

**Hyperthermia** r/t inflammatory disease process

**Imbalanced Nutrition: Less than Body Requirements** r/t impaired oral mucous membrane integrity

**Impaired Oral Mucous Membrane Integrity** r/t inflamed mouth and pharynx; swollen lips that become dry, cracked, fissured

**Acute Pain** r/t enlarged lymph nodes; erythematous skin rash that progresses to desquamation, peeling, denuding of skin

**Impaired Skin integrity** r/t inflammatory skin changes

**Risk for Imbalanced Fluid Volume:** Risk factor: hypovolemia

**Risk for Decreased Cardiac Tissue Perfusion:** Risk factor: cardiac involvement

**Risk for Dry Mouth:** Risk factor: decreased fluid intake

*See Hospitalized Child*

## KELOIDS

**Disturbed Body Image** r/t presence of scar tissue at site of a healed skin injury

**Readiness for Enhanced Health Self-Management:** desire to have information to manage condition

## KERATOCONJUNCTIVITIS SICCA (DRY EYE SYNDROME)

**Risk for Dry Eye:** Risk factors: aging, staring at a computer screen for long intervals

**Risk for Infection:** Risk factor: dry eyes that are more vulnerable to infection

**Risk for Corneal Injury:** Risk factors: dry eye, exposure of the eyeball

*See Conjunctivitis*

## KERATOPLASTY

*See Corneal Transplant*

## KETOACIDOSIS, ALCOHOLIC

*See Alcohol Withdrawal; Alcoholism*

## KETOACIDOSIS, DIABETIC

**Deficient Fluid Volume** r/t excess excretion of urine, nausea, vomiting, increased respiration

**Impaired Memory** r/t fluid and electrolyte imbalance

**Imbalanced Nutrition: Less than Body Requirements** r/t body's inability to use nutrients

**Risk for Unstable Blood Glucose Level:** Risk factor: deficient knowledge of diabetes management (e.g., action plan)

**Risk for Powerlessness:** Risk factor: illness-related regimen

**Risk for Impaired Resilience:** Risk factor: complications of disease

*See Diabetes Mellitus*

## KEYHOLE HEART SURGERY

*See MIDCAB (Minimally Invasive Direct Coronary Artery Bypass)*

## KIDNEY DISEASE SCREENING

**Readiness for Enhanced Health Self-Management:** seeks information for screening

**Risk for Electrolyte Imbalance** r/t renal dysfunction

## KIDNEY FAILURE

*See Renal Failure*

## KIDNEY FAILURE ACUTE/CHRONIC, CHILD

*See Renal Failure, Acute/Chronic, Child*

## KIDNEY FAILURE, NONOLIGURIC

*See Renal Failure, Nonoliguric*

## KIDNEY STONE

**Acute Pain** r/t obstruction from kidney calculi

**Impaired Urinary Elimination: Urgency and Frequency** r/t anatomical obstruction, irritation caused by stone

**Risk for Infection:** Risk factor: obstruction of urinary tract with stasis of urine

**Readiness for Enhanced Knowledge:** expresses an interest in learning about prevention of stones

## KIDNEY TRANSPLANT

**Ineffective Protection** r/t immunosuppressive therapy

**Readiness for Enhanced Decision-Making:** expresses desire to enhance understanding of choices

**Readiness for Enhanced Family Processes:** adapting to life without dialysis

**Readiness for Enhanced Health Self-Management:** desire to manage the treatment and prevention of complications after transplantation

**Readiness for Enhanced Spiritual Well-Being:** heightened coping, living without dialysis

*See Renal Failure, Kidney Transplantation, Donor; Kidney Transplantation, Recipient; Nephrectomy; Surgery, Perioperative Care; Surgery, Postoperative Care; Surgery, Preoperative Care*

## KIDNEY TRANSPLANTATION, DONOR

**Impaired Emancipated Decision-Making** r/t harvesting of kidney from traumatized donor

**Moral Distress** r/t conflict among decision makers, end-of-life decisions, time constraints for decision-making

**Spiritual Distress** r/t grieving from loss of significant person

**Risk for Surgical Site Infection:** Risk factor: surgical procedure

**Readiness for Enhanced Communication:** expressing thoughts and feelings about situation

**Readiness for Enhanced Family Coping:** decision to allow organ donation

**Readiness for Enhanced Emancipated Decision-Making:** expresses desire to enhance understanding and meaning of choices

**Readiness for Enhanced Resilience:** decision to donate organs

**Readiness for Enhanced Spirituality:** inner peace resulting from allowance of organ donation

*See Nephrectomy*

## KIDNEY TRANSPLANTATION, RECIPIENT

**Anxiety** r/t possible rejection, procedure

**Ineffective Health Maintenance Behaviors** r/t long-term home treatment after transplantation, diet, signs of rejection, use of medications

**Deficient Knowledge** r/t specific nutritional needs, possible paralytic ileus, fluid or sodium restrictions

**Impaired Urinary Elimination** r/t possible impaired renal function

**Risk for Bleeding:** Risk factor: surgical procedure

**Risk for Infection:** Risk factor: use of immunosuppressive therapy to control rejection

**Risk for Surgical Site Infection:** Risk factor: surgical procedure

**Risk for Shock:** Risk factor: possible hypovolemia

**Risk for Spiritual Distress:** Risk factor: obtaining transplanted kidney from someone's traumatic loss

**Readiness for Enhanced Spiritual Well-Being:** acceptance of situation

## KIDNEY TUMOR

*See Wilms' Tumor*

## KISSING DISEASE

*See Mononucleosis*

## KNEE REPLACEMENT

*See Total Joint Replacement (Total Hip/Total Knee/Shoulder)*

## KNOWLEDGE

**Readiness for Enhanced Knowledge** (See Knowledge, Readiness for Enhanced, Section II)

## KNOWLEDGE, DEFICIENT

**Ineffective Health maintenance behaviors** r/t lack of or significant alteration in communication skills (written, verbal, and/or gestural)

**Deficient Knowledge** (See Knowledge, Deficient, Section II)

**Readiness for Enhanced Knowledge** (See Knowledge, Readiness for Enhanced, Section II)

## KOCK POUCH

*See Continent Ileostomy (Kock Pouch)*

## KORSAKOFF'S SYNDROME

**Acute Confusion** r/t alcohol abuse

**Dysfunctional Family Processes** r/t alcoholism as possible cause of syndrome

**Impaired Memory** r/t neurological changes associated with excessive alcohol intake

**Self-Neglect** r/t cognitive impairment from chronic alcohol abuse

**Risk for Adult Falls:** Risk factor: cognitive impairment from chronic alcohol abuse

**Risk for Injury:** Risk factors: sensory dysfunction, lack of coordinaltion when ambulating from chronic alcohol abuse

**Risk for Impaired Liver function:** Risk factor: substance abuse (alcohol)

**Risk for Imbalanced Nutrition: Less than Body Requirements:** Risk factor: lack of adequate balanced intake from chronic alcohol abuse

# L

## LABOR, INDUCTION OF

*See Induction of Labor*

## LABOR, NORMAL

**Anxiety** r/t fear of the unknown, situational crisis

**Impaired Comfort** r/t labor

**Fatigue** r/t childbirth

**Deficient Knowledge** r/t lack of preparation for labor

**Labor Pain** r/t uterine contractions, stretching of cervix and birth canal

**Impaired Tissue Integrity** r/t passage of infant through birth canal, episiotomy

**Risk for Ineffective Childbearing Process** (See Childbearing Process, Section II)

**Risk for Adult Falls:** Risk factors: excessive loss or shift in intravascular fluid volume, orthostatic hypotension

**Risk for Deficient Fluid Volume:** Risk factor: excessive loss of blood

**Risk for Infection:** Risk factors: multiple vaginal examinations, tissue trauma, prolonged rupture of membranes

**Risk for Injury: Fetal:** Risk factor: hypoxia

**Risk for Post-Trauma Syndrome:** Risk factors: trauma or violence associated with labor pains, medical or surgical interventions, history of sexual abuse

**Readiness for Enhanced Childbearing Process:** responds appropriately, is proactive, bonds with infant, uses support systems

**Risk for Nipple-Areolar Complex Injury:** breast engorgement; inappropriate positioning of the mother during breastfeeding

**Readiness for Enhanced Family Coping:** significant other provides support during labor

**Readiness for Enhanced Health Management:** prenatal care and childbirth education birth process

**Readiness for Enhanced Power:** expresses readiness to enhance participation in choices regarding treatment during labor

## LABOR PAIN

**Labor Pain** r/t uterine contractions, stretching of cervix and birth canal

## LABYRINTHITIS

**Ineffective Health Self-Management** r/t delay in seeking treatment for respiratory and ear infections

**Risk for Injury** r/t dizziness

**Readiness for Enhanced Health Management:** management of episodes

*See Ménière's Disease*

## LACERATIONS

**Readiness for Enhanced Health Management:** appropriate care of injury

**Risk for Infection:** Risk factor: broken skin

**Risk for Physical Trauma:** Risk factor: children playing with dangerous objects

## LACTATION

*See Breastfeeding, Ineffective; Breastfeeding, Interrupted*

## LACTIC ACIDOSIS

**Decreased Cardiac Output** r/t altered heart rate/rhythm, preload, and contractility

**Risk for Electrolyte Imbalance:** Risk factor: impaired regulatory mechanism

**Risk for Decreased Cardiac Tissue Perfusion:** Risk factor: hypoxia

**Impaired Gas Exchange** r/t ineffective breathing pattern, pain, ineffective airway clearance

*See Ketoacidosis, Diabetic*

## LACTOSE INTOLERANCE

**Readiness for Enhanced Knowledge:** interest in identifying lactose intolerance, treatment, and substitutes for milk products

*See Abdominal Distention; Diarrhea*

## LAMINECTOMY

**Anxiety** r/t change in health status, surgical procedure

**Impaired Comfort** r/t surgical procedure

**Deficient Knowledge** r/t appropriate postoperative and postdischarge activities

**Impaired Physical Mobility** r/t neuromuscular impairment

**Acute Pain** r/t localized inflammation and edema

**Urinary Retention** r/t competing sensory impulses, effects of opioids or anesthesia

**Risk for Bleeding:** Risk factor: surgery

**Risk for Surgical Site Infection:** Risk factor: invasive procedure, surgery

**Risk for Perioperative Positioning Injury:** Risk factor: prone position

*See Surgery, Perioperative Care; Surgery, Postoperative Care; Surgery, Preoperative Care*

## LANGUAGE IMPAIRMENT

*See Speech Disorders*

## LAPAROSCOPIC LASER CHOLECYSTECTOMY

*See Cholecystectomy; Laser Surgery*

## LAPAROSCOPY

**Urge Urinary Incontinence** r/t pressure on the bladder from gas

**Acute Pain: Shoulder** r/t gas irritating the diaphragm

## LAPAROTOMY

*See Abdominal Surgery*

## LARGE BOWEL RESECTION

*See Abdominal Surgery*

## LARYNGECTOMY

**Ineffective Airway Clearance** r/t surgical removal of glottis, decreased humidification

**Death Anxiety** r/t unknown results of surgery

**Disturbed Body Image** r/t change in body structure and function

**Impaired Comfort** r/t surgery

**Impaired Verbal Communication** r/t removal of larynx

**Interrupted Family Processes** r/t surgery, serious condition of family member, difficulty communicating

**Grieving** r/t loss of voice, fear of death

**Ineffective Health Self-Management** r/t deficient knowledge regarding self-care with laryngectomy

**Imbalanced Nutrition: Less than Body Requirements** r/t absence of oral feeding, difficulty swallowing, increased need for fluids

**Impaired Oral Mucous Membrane** r/t absence of oral feeding

**Chronic Sorrow** r/t change in body image

**Impaired Swallowing** r/t edema, laryngectomy tube

**Risk for Electrolyte Imbalance:** Risk factor: fluid imbalance

**Risk for Maladaptive Grieving:** Risk factors: loss, major life event

**Risk for Compromised Human Dignity:** Risk factor: inability to communicate

**Risk for Surgical Site Infection:** Risk factors: invasive procedure, surgery

**Risk for Powerlessness:** Risk factors: chronic illness, change in communication

**Risk for Impaired Resilience:** Risk factor: change in health status

**Risk for Situational Low Self-Esteem:** Risk factor: disturbed body image

## LASER SURGERY

**Impaired Comfort** r/t surgery

**Constipation** r/t laser intervention in vulval and perianal areas

**Deficient Knowledge** r/t preoperative and postoperative care associated with laser procedure

**Acute Pain** r/t heat from laser

**Risk for Bleeding:** Risk factor: surgery

**Risk for Infection:** Risk factor: delayed heating reaction of tissue exposed to laser

**Risk for Injury:** Risk factor: accidental exposure to laser beam

## LASIK EYE SURGERY (LASER-ASSISTED IN SITU KERATOMILEUSIS)

**Impaired Comfort** r/t surgery

**Decisional Conflict** r/t decision to have surgery

**Risk for Infection:** Risk factor: invasive procedure/surgery

**Readiness for Enhanced Health Management:** surgical procedure preoperative and postoperative teaching and expectations

## LATEX ALLERGY REACTION

**Risk for Latex Allergy Reaction** (See **Latex Allergy Reaction, Risk for,** Section II)

**Readiness for Enhanced Knowledge:** prevention and treatment of exposure to latex products

## LAXATIVE ABUSE

**Perceived Constipation** r/t health belief, faulty appraisal, impaired thought processes

## LEAD POISONING

**Contamination** r/t flaking, peeling paint in presence of young children

**Ineffective Home Maintenance Behaviors** r/t presence of lead paint

**Risk for Delayed Child Development:** Risk factor: lead poisoning

## LEFT HEART CATHETERIZATION

*See Cardiac Catheterization*

## LEGIONNAIRES' DISEASE

**Contamination** r/t contaminated water in air-conditioning systems

*See Pneumonia*

## LENS IMPLANT

*See Cataract Extraction; Vision Impairment*

## LETHARGY/LISTLESSNESS

**Frail Elderly Syndrome** r/t alteration in cognitive function

**Fatigue** r/t decreased metabolic energy production

**Insomnia** r/t internal or external stressors

**Risk for Ineffective Cerebral Tissue Perfusion:** Risk factor: carbon dioxide retention and/or lack of oxygen supply to brain

## LEUKEMIA

**Ineffective Protection** r/t abnormal blood profile

**Fatigue** r/t abnormal blood profile and/or side effects of chemotherapy treatment

**Risk for Imbalanced Fluid Volume:** Risk factors: nausea, vomiting, bleeding, side effects of treatment

**Risk for Infection:** Risk factor: ineffective immune system

**Risk for Impaired Resilience:** Risk factor: serious illness

*See Cancer; Chemotherapy*

## LEUKOPENIA

**Ineffective Protection** r/t leukopenia

**Risk for Infection:** Risk factor: low white blood cell count

## LEVEL OF CONSCIOUSNESS, DECREASED

*See Confusion, Acute; Confusion, Chronic*

## LICE

**Impaired Comfort** r/t inflammation, pruritus

**Readiness for Enhanced Health Management:** preventing and treating infestation

**Ineffective Home Maintenance Behaviors** r/t close unsanitary, overcrowded conditions

**Self-Neglect** r/t lifestyle

*See Communicable Diseases, Childhood (e.g., Measles, Mumps, Rubella, Chickenpox, Scabies, Lice)*

## LIFESTYLE, SEDENTARY

**Sedentary Lifestyle** (See **Sedentary Lifestyle,** Section II)

**Risk for Ineffective Peripheral Tissue Perfusion:** Risk factor: lack of movement

**Decreased Activity Tolerance:** Related factor: impaired physical mobility

## LIGHTHEADEDNESS

*See Dizziness; Vertigo; Falls*

## LIMB REATTACHMENT PROCEDURES

**Anxiety** r/t unknown outcome of reattachment procedure, use and appearance of limb

**Disturbed Body Image** r/t unpredictability of function and appearance of reattached body part

**Grieving** r/t unknown outcome of reattachment procedure

**Spiritual Distress** r/t anxiety about condition

**Stress Overload** r/t multiple coexisting stressors, physical demands

**Risk for Bleeding:** Risk factor: severed vessels

**Risk for Perioperative Positioning Injury:** Risk factor: immobilization

**Risk for Peripheral Neurovascular Dysfunction:** Risk factors: trauma, orthopedic and neurovascular surgery, compression of nerves and blood vessels

**Risk for Powerlessness:** Risk factor: unknown outcome of procedure

**Risk for Impaired Religiosity:** Risk factors: suffering, hospitalization

*See Surgery, Postoperative Care*

## LIPOSUCTION

**Disturbed Body Image** r/t dissatisfaction with unwanted fat deposits in body

**Risk for Impaired Resilience:** Risk factor: body image disturbance

**Readiness for Enhanced Decision-Making:** expresses desire to make decision regarding liposuction

**Readiness for Enhanced Self-Concept:** satisfaction with new body image

*See Surgery, Perioperative Care; Surgery, Postoperative Care; Surgery, Preoperative Care*

## LITHOTRIPSY

**Readiness for Enhanced Health Management:** expresses desire for information related to procedure and aftercare and prevention of stones

*See Kidney Stone*

## LIVER BIOPSY

**Anxiety** r/t procedure and results

**Risk for Deficient Fluid Volume:** Risk factor: hemorrhage from biopsy site

**Risk for Infection:** Risk factor: invasive procedure

**Risk for Powerlessness:** Risk factor: inability to control outcome of procedure

## LIVER CANCER

**Risk for Bleeding:** Risk factor: liver dysfunction

**Risk for Adult Falls:** Risk factor: confusion associated with liver dysfunction

**Risk for Impaired Liver Function:** Risk factor: disease process

**Risk for Impaired Resilience:** Risk factor: serious illness

*See Cancer; Chemotherapy; Radiation Therapy*

## LIVER DISEASE

*See Cirrhosis; Hepatitis*

## LIVER FUNCTION

**Risk for Impaired Liver Function** (See **Liver Function, Impaired, Risk for,** Section II)

## LIVER TRANSPLANT

**Impaired Comfort** r/t surgical pain

**Decisional Conflict** r/t acceptance of donor liver

**Ineffective Protection** r/t immunosuppressive therapy

**Risk for Impaired Liver Function:** Risk factors: possible rejection, infection

**Readiness for Enhanced Family Processes:** change in physical needs of family member

**Readiness for Enhanced Health Management:** desire to manage the treatment and prevention of complications after transplantation

**Readiness for Enhanced Spiritual Well-Being:** heightened coping

*See Surgery, Perioperative Care; Surgery, Postoperative Care; Surgery, Preoperative Care*

## LIVING WILL

**Moral Distress** r/t end-of-life decisions

**Readiness for Enhanced Decision-Making:** expresses desire to enhance understanding of choices for decision-making

**Readiness for Enhanced Relationship:** shares information with others

**Readiness for Enhanced Religiosity:** request to meet with religious leaders or facilitators

**Readiness for Enhanced Resilience:** uses effective communication

**Readiness for Enhanced Spiritual Well-Being:** acceptance of and preparation for end of life

*See Advance Directives*

## LOBECTOMY

*See Thoracotomy*

**L**

## LONELINESS

**Spiritual Distress** r/t loneliness, social alienation

**Risk for Loneliness** (See **Loneliness, Risk for,** Section II)

**Risk for Impaired Religiosity:** Risk factor: lack of social interaction

**Readiness for Enhanced Hope:** expresses desire to enhance interconnectedness with others

**Readiness for Enhanced Relationship:** expresses satisfaction with complementary relationship between partners

## LOOSE STOOLS (BOWEL MOVEMENTS)

**Diarrhea** r/t increased gastric motility

**Risk for Dysfunctional Gastrointestinal Motility** (See **Gastrointestinal Motility, Dysfunctional, Risk for,** Section II)

*See Diarrhea*

## LOSS OF BLADDER CONTROL

*See Incontinence of Urine*

## LOSS OF BOWEL CONTROL

*See Incontinence of Stool*

## LOU GEHRIG'S DISEASE

*See Amyotrophic Lateral Sclerosis (ALS)*

## LOW BACK PAIN

**Impaired Comfort** r/t back pain

**Ineffective Health Maintenance Behaviors** r/t deficient knowledge regarding self-care with back pain

**Impaired Physical Mobility** r/t back pain

**Chronic Pain** r/t degenerative processes, musculotendinous strain, injury, inflammation, congenital deformities

**Urinary Retention** r/t possible spinal cord compression

**Risk for Powerlessness:** Risk factor: living with chronic pain

**Readiness for Enhanced Health Management:** expresses desire for information to manage pain

## LOW BLOOD GLUCOSE

*See Hypoglycemia*

## LOW BLOOD PRESSURE

*See Hypotension*

## LOWER GI BLEEDING

*See GI Bleed (Gastrointestinal Bleeding)*

## LUMBAR PUNCTURE

**Anxiety** r/t invasive procedure and unknown results

**Deficient Knowledge** r/t information about procedure

**Acute Pain** r/t possible loss of cerebrospinal fluid

**Risk for Ineffective Cerebral Tissue Perfusion:** Risk factor: treatment-related side effects

**Risk for Infection:** Risk factor: invasive procedure

## LUMPECTOMY

**Decisional Conflict** r/t treatment choices

**Readiness for Enhanced Knowledge:** preoperative and postoperative care

**Readiness for Enhanced Spiritual Well-Being:** hope of benign diagnosis

*See Cancer*

## LUNG CANCER

*See Cancer; Chemotherapy; Radiation Therapy; Thoracotomy*

## LUNG SURGERY

*See Thoracotomy*

## LUPUS ERYTHEMATOSUS

**Disturbed Body Image** r/t change in skin, rash, lesions, ulcers, mottled erythema

**Fatigue** r/t increased metabolic requirements

**Ineffective Health Maintenance Behaviors** r/t deficient knowledge regarding medication, diet, activity

**Acute Pain** r/t inflammatory process

**Powerlessness** r/t unpredictability of course of disease

**Impaired Religiosity** r/t ineffective coping with disease

**Chronic Sorrow** r/t presence of chronic illness

**Spiritual Distress** r/t chronicity of disease, unknown etiology

**Risk for Decreased Cardiac Tissue Perfusion:** Risk factor: altered circulation

**Risk for Impaired Resilience:** Risk factor: chronic disease

**Risk for Impaired Skin Integrity:** Risk factors: chronic inflammation, edema, altered circulation

## LYME DISEASE

**Impaired Comfort** r/t inflammation

**Fatigue** r/t increased energy requirements

**Deficient Knowledge** r/t lack of information concerning disease, prevention, treatment

**Acute Pain** r/t inflammation of joints, urticaria, rash

**Chronic Pain** r/t chronic inflammation

**Risk for Decreased Cardiac Output:** Risk factor: dysrhythmia

**Risk for Powerlessness:** Risk factor: possible chronic condition

## LYMPHEDEMA

**Disturbed Body Image** r/t change in appearance of body part with edema

**Excess Fluid Volume** r/t compromised regulatory system; inflammation, obstruction, or removal of lymph glands

**Deficient Knowledge** r/t management of condition

**Risk for Infection:** Risk factors: abnormal lymphatic system allowing stasis of fluids with decreased resistance to infection

**Risk for Situational Low Self-Esteem:** Risk factor: disturbed body image

**Ineffective Lymphedema Self-Management** r/t difficulty managing complex treatment regimen

**Risk for Ineffective Lymphedema Self-Management:** Risk factors: decreased perceived quality of life; inadequate commitment to a plan of action; unrealistic perception of susceptibility to sequelae

## LYMPHOMA

*See Cancer*

# M

## MACULAR DEGENERATION

**Anxiety** r/t expressed insecurity with visual loss

**Ineffective Coping** r/t visual loss

**Compromised Family Coping** r/t deteriorating vision of family member

**Risk-Prone Health Behavior** r/t deteriorating vision while trying to maintain usual lifestyle

**Hopelessness** r/t deteriorating vision

**Sedentary Lifestyle** r/t visual loss

**Self-Neglect** r/t change in vision

**Social Isolation** r/t inability to drive because of visual changes

**Risk for Falls:** Risk factor: visual difficulties

**Risk for Injury:** Risk factor: inability to distinguish traffic lights and safety signs

**Risk for Powerlessness:** Risk factor: deteriorating vision

**Risk for Impaired Religiosity:** Risk factor: possible lack of transportation to church

**Risk for Impaired Resilience:** Risk factor: changing vision

**Readiness for Enhanced Health Management:** appropriate choices of daily activities for meeting the goals of a treatment program

## MAGNETIC RESONANCE IMAGING (MRI)

*See MRI (Magnetic Resonance Imaging)*

## MAJOR DEPRESSIVE DISORDER

*See Depression (Major Depressive Disorder)*

## MALABSORPTION SYNDROME

**Diarrhea** r/t lactose intolerance, gluten sensitivity, resection of small bowel

**Dysfunctional Gastrointestinal Motility** r/t disease state

**Deficient Knowledge** r/t lack of information about diet and nutrition

**Imbalanced Nutrition: Less than Body Requirements** r/t inability of body to absorb nutrients because of physiological factors

**Risk for Electrolyte Imbalance:** Risk factors: hypovolemia, hyponatremia, hypokalemia

**Risk for Imbalanced Fluid Volume:** Risk factors: diarrhea, hypovolemia

*See Abdominal Distention*

## MALADAPTIVE BEHAVIOR

*See Crisis; Post-Trauma Syndrome; Suicide Attempt*

## MALAISE

*See Fatigue*

## MALARIA

**Contamination** r/t geographic area

**Risk for Contamination:** Risk factors: increased environmental exposure (not wearing protective clothing, not using insecticide or repellant on skin, clothing, and in room in areas in which infected mosquitoes are present); inadequate defense mechanisms (inappropriate use of prophylactic regimen)

**Risk for Impaired Liver Function:** Risk factor: complications of disease

**Readiness for Enhanced Community Coping:** uses resources available for problem-solving

**Readiness for Enhanced Health Management:** expresses desire to enhance immunization status/vaccination status

**Readiness for Enhanced Resilience:** immunization status

*See Anemia*

## MALE INFERTILITY

*See Erectile Dysfunction (ED); Infertility*

## MALIGNANCY

*See Cancer*

## MALIGNANT HYPERTENSION (ARTERIOLAR NEPHROSCLEROSIS)

**Decreased Cardiac Output** r/t altered afterload, altered contractility

**Fatigue** r/t disease state, increased blood pressure

**Excess Fluid Volume** r/t decreased kidney function

**Risk for Ineffective Cerebral Tissue Perfusion:** Risk factor: elevated blood pressure damaging cerebral vessels

**Risk for Acute Confusion:** Risk factors: increased blood urea nitrogen or creatinine levels

**Risk for Imbalanced Fluid Volume:** Risk factors: hypertension, altered kidney function

**Risk for Unstable Blood Pressure:** Risk factor: damaged vessels due to disease process

**Readiness for Enhanced Health Management:** expresses desire to manage the illness, high blood pressure

## MALIGNANT HYPERTHERMIA

**Hyperthermia** r/t anesthesia reaction associated with inherited condition

**Readiness for Enhanced Health Management:** knowledge of risk factors

**Risk for Shock** r/t deficient fluid volume

## MALNUTRITION

**Insufficient Breast Milk Production** (See **Breast Milk, Insufficient Production,** Section II)

**Frail Elderly Syndrome** r/t undetected malnutrition

**Deficient Knowledge** r/t misinformation about normal nutrition, social isolation, lack of food preparation facilities

**Imbalanced Nutrition: Less than Body Requirements** r/t inability to ingest food, digest food, or absorb nutrients because of biological, psychological, or economic factors; institutionalization (i.e., lack of menu choices)

**Ineffective Protection** r/t inadequate nutrition

**Ineffective Health Management** r/t inadequate nutrition

**Self-Neglect** r/t inadequate nutrition

**Risk for Powerlessness:** Risk factor: possible inability to provide adequate nutrition

## MAMMOGRAPHY

**Readiness for Enhanced Health Management:** follows guidelines for screening

**Readiness for Enhanced Resilience:** responsibility for self-care

## MANIC DISORDER, BIPOLAR I

**Anxiety** r/t change in role function

**Ineffective Coping** r/t situational crisis

**Ineffective Denial** r/t fear of inability to control behavior

**Interrupted Family Processes** r/t family member's illness

**Risk-Prone Health Behavior** r/t low self-efficacy

**Ineffective Health Management** r/t unpredictability of client, excessive demands on family, chronic illness, social support deficit

**Ineffective Home Maintenance Behaviors** r/t altered psychological state, inability to concentrate

**Disturbed Personal Identity** r/t manic state

**Insomnia** r/t constant anxious thoughts

**Imbalanced Nutrition: Less than Body Requirements** r/t lack of time and motivation to eat, constant movement

**Impaired individual Resilience** r/t psychological disorder

**Ineffective Role Performance** r/t impaired social interactions

**Self-Neglect** r/t manic state

**Sleep Deprivation** r/t hyperagitated state

**Risk for Ineffective Activity Planning** r/t inability to process information

**Risk for Caregiver Role Strain:** Risk factor: unpredictability of condition

**Risk for Imbalanced Fluid Volume:** Risk factor: hypovolemia

**Risk for Powerlessness:** Risk factor: inability to control changes in mood

**Risk for Spiritual Distress:** Risk factor: depression

**Risk for Suicidal Behavior:** Risk factor: bipolar disorder

**Risk for Self-Directed Violence:** Risk factors: hallucinations, delusions

**Risk for Other-Directed Violence:** Risk factor: pathologic intoxication

**Readiness for Enhanced Hope:** expresses desire to enhance problem-solving goals

## MANIPULATIVE BEHAVIOR

**Defensive Coping** r/t superior attitude toward others

**Ineffective Coping** r/t inappropriate use of defense mechanisms

**Self-Mutilation** r/t use of manipulation to obtain nurturing relationship with others

**Self-Neglect** r/t maintaining control

**Impaired Social Interaction** r/t self-concept disturbance

**Risk for Loneliness:** Risk factor: inability to interact appropriately with others

**Risk for Situational Low Self-Esteem:** Risk factor: history of learned helplessness

**Risk for Self-Mutilation:** Risk factor: inability to cope with increased psychological or physiological tension in healthy manner

## MARFAN SYNDROME

**Decreased Cardiac Output** r/t dilation of the aortic root, dissection or rupture of the aorta

**Risk for Decreased Cardiac Tissue Perfusion:** Risk factor: heart-related complications from Marfan syndrome

**Risk for Impaired Cardiovascular Function:** Risk factor: heart-related valve disorders form Marfan syndrome

**Readiness for Enhanced Health Management:** describes reduction of risk factors

*See Mitral Valve Prolapse; Scoliosis*

## MASTECTOMY

**Disturbed Body Image** r/t loss of sexually significant body part

M

**Impaired Comfort** r/t altered body image; difficult diagnosis

**Death Anxiety** r/t threat of mortality associated with breast cancer

**Fatigue** r/t increased metabolic requirements

**Fear** r/t change in body image, prognosis

**Deficient Knowledge** r/t self-care activities

**Insomnia** r/t impaired health status

**Nausea** r/t chemotherapy

**Acute Pain** r/t surgical procedure

**Sexual Dysfunction** r/t change in body image, fear of loss of femininity

**Chronic Sorrow** r/t disturbed body image, unknown long-term health status

**Spiritual Distress** r/t change in body image

**Risk for Surgical Site Infection:** Risk factors: surgical procedure, broken skin

**Risk for Impaired Physical Mobility:** Risk factors: nerve or muscle damage, pain

**Risk for Post-Trauma Syndrome:** Risk factors: loss of body part, surgical wounds

**Risk for Powerlessness:** Risk factor: fear of unknown outcome of procedure

**Risk for Impaired Resilience:** Risk factor: altered body image

*See Cancer; Modified Radical Mastectomy; Surgery, Perioperative Care; Surgery, Postoperative Care; Surgery, Preoperative Care*

## MASTITIS

**Anxiety** r/t threat to self, concern over safety of milk for infant

**Ineffective Breastfeeding** r/t breast pain, conflicting advice from health care providers

**Deficient Knowledge** r/t antibiotic regimen, comfort measures

**Acute Pain** r/t infectious disease process, swelling of breast tissue

**Ineffective Role Performance** r/t change in capacity to function in expected role

## MATERNAL INFECTION

**Ineffective Protection** r/t invasive procedures, traumatized tissue

*See Postpartum, Normal Care*

## MATURATIONAL ISSUES, ADOLESCENT

**Ineffective Coping** r/t maturational crises

**Risk-Prone Health Behavior** r/t inadequate comprehension, negative attitude toward health care

**Interrupted Family Processes** r/t developmental crises of adolescence resulting from challenge of parental authority and values, situational crises from change in parental marital status

**Deficient Knowledge: Potential for Enhanced Health Maintenance** r/t information misinterpretation, lack of education regarding age-related factors

**Impaired Social Interaction** r/t ineffective, unsuccessful, or dysfunctional interaction with peers

**Social Isolation** r/t perceived alteration in physical appearance, social values not accepted by dominant peer group

**Risk for Ineffective Activity Planning:** Risk factor: unrealistic perception of personal competencies

**Risk for Disturbed Personal Identity:** Risk factor: maturational issues

**Risk for Injury:** Risk factor: thrill-seeking behaviors

**Risk for Chronic Low Self-Esteem:** Risk factor: lack of sense of belonging in peer group

**Risk for Situational Low Self-Esteem:** Risk factor: developmental changes

**Readiness for Enhanced Communication:** expressing willingness to communicate with parental figures

**Readiness for Enhanced Relationship:** expresses desire to enhance communication with parental figures

*See Sexuality, Adolescent; Substance Misuse (if relevant)*

## MAZE III PROCEDURE

*See Dysrhythmia; Open Heart Surgery*

## MD (MUSCULAR DYSTROPHY)

*See Muscular Dystrophy (MD)*

## MEASLES (RUBEOLA)

*See Communicable Diseases, Childhood (e.g., Measles, Mumps, Rubella, Chickenpox, Scabies, Lice)*

## MECONIUM ASPIRATION

*See Respiratory Conditions of the Neonate*

## MECONIUM DELAYED

**Risk for Neonatal Hyperbilirubinemia:** Risk factor: delayed meconium

## MEDICAL MARIJUANA

**Imbalanced Nutrition: Less than Body Requirements** r/t eating disorder, appetite loss, effects of chemotherapy

**Chronic Pain Syndrome** r/t persistence of pain as a result of physical injury or condition

**Nausea** r/t effects of chemotherapy

## MELANOMA

**Disturbed Body Image** r/t altered pigmentation, surgical incision

**Death Anxiety** r/t threat of mortality associated with cancer

**Fear** r/t threat to well-being

**Ineffective Health Maintenance Behaviors** r/t deficient knowledge regarding self-care and treatment of melanoma

**Acute Pain** r/t surgical incision

**Chronic Sorrow** r/t disturbed body image, unknown long-term health status

**Readiness for Enhanced Health Management:** describes reduction of risk factors; protection from sunlight's ultraviolet rays

*See Cancer*

## MELENA

**Fear** r/t presence of blood in feces

**Risk for Imbalanced Fluid volume:** Risk factor: hemorrhage

*See GI Bleed (Gastrointestinal Bleeding)*

## MEMORY DEFICIT

**Impaired Memory** (See **Memory, Impaired,** Section II)

## MÉNIÈRE'S DISEASE

**Risk for Injury:** Risk factor: symptoms of disease

**Readiness for Enhanced Health Management:** expresses desire to manage illness

*See Dizziness; Nausea; Vertigo*

## MENINGITIS/ENCEPHALITIS

**Ineffective Airway Clearance** r/t seizure activity

**Impaired Comfort** r/t altered health status

**Excess Fluid Volume** r/t increased intracranial pressure, syndrome of inappropriate secretion of antidiuretic hormone

**Impaired Mobility** r/t neuromuscular or central nervous system insult

**Acute Pain** r/t biological injury

**Risk for Aspiration:** Risk factor: seizure activity

**Risk for Acute Confusion:** Risk factor: infection of brain

**Risk for Falls:** Risk factors: neuromuscular dysfunction and confusion

**Risk for Injury:** Risk factor: seizure activity

**Risk for Impaired Resilience:** Risk factor: illness

**Risk for Shock:** Risk factor: infectious process

**Risk for Ineffective Cerebral Tissue Perfusion:** Risk factors: cerebral tissue edema and inflammation of meninges, increased intracranial pressure; infection

**Risk for Ineffective Thermoregulation:** Risk factor: infectious process

**Risk for Unstable Blood Pressure** r/t fluid shifts

*See Hospitalized Child*

## MENINGOCELE

*See Neural Tube Defects*

## MENOPAUSE

**Impaired Comfort** r/t symptoms associated with menopause

**Insomnia** r/t hormonal shifts

**M**

**Impaired Memory** r/t change in hormonal levels

**Sexual Dysfunction** r/t menopausal changes

**Ineffective Sexuality Pattern** r/t altered body structure, lack of lubrication, lack of knowledge of artificial lubrication

**Ineffective Thermoregulation** r/t changes in hormonal levels

**Risk for Urge Urinary Incontinence:** Risk factor: changes in hormonal levels affecting bladder function

**Risk for Overweight:** Risk factor: change in metabolic rate caused by fluctuating hormone levels

**Risk for Powerlessness:** Risk factor: changes associated with menopause

**Risk for Impaired Resilience:** Risk factor: menopause

**Risk for Situational Low Self-Esteem:** Risk factors: developmental changes, menopause

**Readiness for Enhanced Health Management:** verbalized desire to manage menopause

**Readiness for Enhanced Self-Care:** expresses satisfaction with body image

**Readiness for Enhanced Spiritual Well-Being:** desire for harmony of mind, body, and spirit

## MENORRHAGIA

**Fear** r/t loss of large amounts of blood

**Risk for Deficient Fluid Volume:** Risk factor: excessive loss of menstrual blood

## MENTAL ILLNESS

**Defensive Coping** r/t psychological impairment, substance misuse

**Ineffective Coping** r/t situational crisis, coping with mental illness

**Compromised Family Coping** r/t lack of available support from client

**Disabled Family Coping** r/t chronically unexpressed feelings of guilt, anxiety, hostility, or despair

**Ineffective Denial** r/t refusal to acknowledge abuse problem, fear of the social stigma of disease

**Risk-Prone Health Behavior** r/t low self-efficacy

**Disturbed Personal Identity** r/t psychoses

**Ineffective Relationship** r/t effects of mental illness in partner relationship

**Chronic Sorrow** r/t presence of mental illness

**Stress Overload** r/t multiple coexisting stressors

**Ineffective Family Health Self-Management** r/t chronicity of condition, unpredictability of client, unknown prognosis

**Risk for Loneliness:** Risk factor: social isolation

**Risk for Powerlessness:** Risk factor: lifestyle of helplessness

**Risk for Impaired Resilience:** Risk factor: chronic illness

**Risk for Chronic Low Self-Esteem:** Risk factor: presence of mental illness/repeated negative reinforcement

## METABOLIC ACIDOSIS

*See Ketoacidosis, Alcoholic; Ketoacidosis, Diabetic*

## METABOLIC ALKALOSIS

**Deficient Fluid Volume** r/t fluid volume loss, vomiting, gastric suctioning, failure of regulatory mechanisms

## METABOLIC IMBALANCE SYNDROME

**Ineffective Health Maintenance Behaviors** r/t deficient knowledge regarding basic health practice

**Obesity** r/t energy expenditure below energy intake

**Risk for Unstable Blood Glucose Level:** Risk factor: variations in serum glucose levels

## METASTASIS

*See Cancer*

## METHICILLIN-RESISTANT *STAPHYLOCOCCUS AUREUS* (MRSA)

*See MRSA (Methicillin-Resistant* Staphylococcus aureus*)*

## MI (MYOCARDIAL INFARCTION)

**Decreased Activity Tolerance** r/t imbalance between oxygen supply and demand

**Anxiety** r/t threat of death, possible change in role status

**Death Anxiety** r/t seriousness of medical condition

**Constipation** r/t decreased peristalsis from decreased physical activity, medication effect, change in diet

**Ineffective Family Coping** r/t spouse or significant other's fear of partner loss

**Ineffective Denial** r/t fear, deficient knowledge about heart disease

**Interrupted Family Processes** r/t crisis, role change

**Fear** r/t threat to well-being

**Ineffective Health Maintenance Behaviors** r/t deficient knowledge regarding self-care and treatment

**Acute Pain** r/t myocardial tissue damage from inadequate blood supply

**Situational Low Self-Esteem** r/t crisis of MI

**Ineffective Sexuality Pattern** r/t fear of chest pain, possibility of heart damage

**Risk for Powerlessness:** Risk factor: acute illness

**Risk for Shock:** Risk factors: hypotension, myocardial dysfunction, hypoxia

**Risk for Spiritual Distress:** Risk factor: physical illness

**Risk for Decreased Cardiac Output:** Risk factors: alteration in heart rate, rhythm, and contractility

**Risk for Decreased Cardiac Tissue Perfusion:** Risk factors: coronary artery spasm, hypertension, hypotension, hypoxia

**Risk for Unstable Blood Pressure** r/t cardiac dysrhythmia

**Readiness for Enhanced Knowledge:** expresses an interest in learning about condition

*See Angioplasty, Coronary; Coronary Artery Bypass Grafting (CABG)*

## MIDCAB (MINIMALLY INVASIVE DIRECT CORONARY ARTERY BYPASS)

**Risk for Bleeding:** Risk factor: surgery

**Readiness for Enhanced Health Management:** preoperative and postoperative care associated with surgery

**Risk for Surgical Site Infection:** Risk factor: surgical procedure

*See Angioplasty, Coronary; Coronary Artery Bypass Grafting (CABG)*

## MIDLIFE CRISIS

**Ineffective Coping** r/t inability to deal with changes associated with aging

**Powerlessness** r/t lack of control over life situation

**Spiritual Distress** r/t questioning beliefs or value system

**Risk for Disturbed Personal Identity:** Risk factor: alteration in social roles

**Risk for Chronic Low Self-Esteem:** Risk factor: ineffective coping with loss

**Readiness for Enhanced Relationship:** meets goals for lifestyle change

**Readiness for Enhanced Spiritual Well-Being:** desire to find purpose and meaning to life

## MIGRAINE HEADACHE

**Ineffective Health Maintenance Behaviors** r/t deficient knowledge regarding prevention and treatment of headaches

**Readiness for Enhanced Health Management:** expresses desire to manage illness

**Acute Pain: Headache** r/t vasodilation of cerebral and extracerebral vessels

**Risk for Impaired Resilience:** Risk factors: chronic illness, disabling pain

## MILITARY FAMILIES, PERSONNEL

**Anxiety** r/t apprehension and helplessness caused by uncertainty of family members' situation

**Interrupted Family Processes** r/t possible change in family roles, decrease in available emotional support

**M**

**Relocation Stress Syndrome** r/t unpredictability of experience, powerlessness, significant environmental change

## MILK INTOLERANCE
*See Lactose Intolerance*

## MINIMALLY INVASIVE DIRECT CORONARY ARTERY BYPASS (MIDCAB)
*See MIDCAB (Minimally Invasive Direct Coronary Artery Bypass)*

## MISCARRIAGE
*See Pregnancy Loss*

## MITRAL STENOSIS
**Decreased Activity Tolerance** r/t imbalance between oxygen supply and demand

**Anxiety** r/t possible worsening of symptoms, activity intolerance, fatigue

**Decreased Cardiac Output** r/t incompetent heart valves, abnormal forward or backward blood flow, flow into a dilated chamber, flow through an abnormal passage between chambers

**Fatigue** r/t reduced cardiac output

**Ineffective Health Maintenance Behaviors** r/t deficient knowledge regarding self-care with disorder

**Risk for Decreased Cardiac Tissue Perfusion:** Risk factor: incompetent heart valve

**Risk for Infection:** Risk factors: invasive procedure, risk for endocarditis

## MITRAL VALVE PROLAPSE
**Anxiety** r/t symptoms of condition: palpitations, chest pain

**Fatigue** r/t abnormal catecholamine regulation, decreased intravascular volume

**Fear** r/t lack of knowledge about mitral valve prolapse, feelings of having heart attack

**Ineffective Health Maintenance Behaviors** r/t deficient knowledge regarding methods to relieve pain and treat dysrhythmia and shortness of breath, need for prophylactic antibiotics before invasive procedures

**Acute Pain** r/t mitral valve regurgitation

**Risk for Ineffective Cerebral Tissue Perfusion:** Risk factor: postural hypotension

**Risk for Infection:** Risk factor: invasive procedures

**Risk for Powerlessness:** Risk factor: unpredictability of onset of symptoms

**Readiness for Enhanced Knowledge:** expresses interest in learning about condition

## MOBILITY, IMPAIRED BED
**Impaired Bed Mobility** (See **Mobility, Bed, Impaired,** Section II)

## MOBILITY, IMPAIRED PHYSICAL
**Impaired Physical Mobility** (See **Mobility, Physical, Impaired,** Section II)

**Risk for Falls:** Risk factor: impaired physical mobility

## MOBILITY, IMPAIRED WHEELCHAIR
**Impaired Wheelchair Mobility** (See **Mobility, Wheelchair, Impaired,** Section II)

## MODIFIED RADICAL MASTECTOMY
**Readiness for Enhanced Communication:** willingness to enhance communication
*See Mastectomy*

## MONONUCLEOSIS
**Decreased Activity Tolerance** r/t generalized weakness

**Impaired Comfort** r/t sore throat, muscle aches

**Fatigue** r/t disease state, stress

**Ineffective Health Maintenance Behaviors** r/t deficient knowledge concerning transmission and treatment of disease

**Acute Pain** r/t enlargement of lymph nodes, oropharyngeal edema

**Impaired Swallowing** r/t enlargement of lymph nodes, oropharyngeal edema

**Risk for Injury:** Risk factor: possible rupture of spleen

**Risk for Loneliness:** Risk factor: social isolation

## MOOD DISORDERS

**Caregiver Role Strain** r/t overwhelming needs of care receiver, unpredictability of mood alterations

**Labile Emotional Control** (See **Labile Emotional Control,** Section II)

**Risk-Prone Health Behavior** r/t hopelessness, altered locus of control

**Impaired Mood Regulation** (See **Mood Regulation, Impaired,** Section II)

**Self-Neglect** r/t inability to care for self

**Social Isolation** r/t alterations in mental status

**Risk for Situational Low Self-Esteem:** Risk factor: unpredictable changes in mood

**Readiness for Enhanced Communication:** expresses feelings

*See specific disorder: Depression (Major Depressive Disorder); Dysthymic Disorder; Hypomania; Manic Disorder, Bipolar I*

## MOON FACE

**Disturbed Body Image** r/t change in appearance from disease and medication(s)

**Risk for Situational Low Self-Esteem:** Risk factor: change in body image

*See Cushing's Syndrome*

## MORAL/ETHICAL DILEMMAS

**Impaired Emancipated Decision-Making** r/t questioning personal values and belief, which alter decision

**Moral Distress** r/t conflicting information guiding moral or ethical decision-making

**Risk for Powerlessness:** Risk factor: lack of knowledge to make a decision

**Risk for Spiritual Distress:** Risk factor: moral or ethical crisis

**Readiness for Enhanced Emancipated Decision-Making:** expresses desire to enhance congruency of decisions with personal values and goals

**Readiness for Enhanced Religiosity:** requests assistance in expanding religious options

**Readiness for Enhanced Resilience:** vulnerable state

**Readiness for Enhanced Spiritual Well-Being:** request for interaction with others regarding difficult decisions

## MORNING SICKNESS

*See Hyperemesis Gravidarum; Pregnancy, Normal*

## MOTION SICKNESS

*See Labyrinthitis*

## MOTTLING OF PERIPHERAL SKIN

**Ineffective Peripheral Tissue Perfusion** r/t interruption of arterial flow, decreased circulating blood volume

**Risk for Shock:** Risk factor: inadequate circulation to perfuse body

## MOURNING

*See Grieving*

## MOUTH LESIONS

*See Mucous Membrane Integrity, Impaired Oral*

## MRI (MAGNETIC RESONANCE IMAGING)

**Anxiety** r/t fear of being in closed spaces

**Readiness for Enhanced Health Management:** describes reduction of risk factors associated with exam

**Deficient Knowledge** r/t unfamiliarity with information resources; exam information

**Readiness for Enhanced Knowledge:** expresses interest in learning about exam

## MRSA (METHICILLIN-RESISTANT *STAPHYLOCOCCUS AUREUS*)

**Impaired Skin Integrity** r/t infection

**Delayed Surgical Recovery** r/t infection

**Ineffective Thermoregulation** r/t severe infection stimulating immune system

**Impaired Tissue Integrity** r/t wound, infection

**Risk for Loneliness:** Risk factor: physical isolation

**Risk for Impaired Resilience:** Risk factor: illness

**Risk for Shock:** Risk factor: sepsis

**M**

## MS (MULTIPLE SCLEROSIS)

*See Multiple Sclerosis*

## MUCOCUTANEOUS LYMPH NODE SYNDROME

*See Kawasaki Disease*

## MUCOUS MEMBRANE INTEGRITY, IMPAIRED ORAL

**Impaired Oral Mucous Membrane Integrity** (See **Oral Mucous Membrane Integrity, Impaired,** Section II)

## MULTI-INFARCT DEMENTIA

*See Dementia*

## MULTIPLE GESTATIONS

**Anxiety** r/t uncertain outcome of pregnancy

**Death Anxiety** r/t maternal complications associated with multiple gestations

**Insufficient Breast Milk Production** r/t multiple births

**Ineffective Childbearing Process** r/t unavailable support system

**Fatigue** r/t physiological demands of a multifetal pregnancy and/or care of more than one infant

**Ineffective Home Maintenance Behaviors** r/t fatigue

**Stress Urinary Incontinence** r/t increased pelvic pressure

**Insomnia** r/t impairment of normal sleep pattern; parental responsibilities

**Deficient Knowledge** r/t caring for more than one infant

**Neonatal Hyperbilirubinemia** r/t feeding pattern not well established

**Deficient Knowledge** r/t caring for more than one infant

**Imbalanced Nutrition: Less than Body Requirements** r/t physiological demands of a multifetal pregnancy

**Stress Overload** r/t multiple coexisting stressors, family demands

**Impaired Walking** r/t increased uterine size

**Risk for Ineffective Breastfeeding:** Risk factors: lack of support, physical demands of feeding more than one infant

**Risk for Delayed Child Development: Fetus:** Risk factor: multiple gestations

**Risk for Neonatal Hyperbilirubinemia:** Risk factors: abnormal weight loss, prematurity, feeding pattern not well established

**Readiness for Enhanced Childbearing Process:** demonstrates appropriate care for infants and mother

**Readiness for Enhanced Family Processes:** family adapting to change with more than one infant

## MULTIPLE PERSONALITY DISORDER (DISSOCIATIVE IDENTITY DISORDER)

**Anxiety** r/t loss of control of behavior and feelings

**Disturbed Body Image** r/t psychosocial changes

**Defensive Coping** r/t unresolved past traumatic events, severe anxiety

**Ineffective Coping** r/t history of abuse

**Hopelessness** r/t long-term stress

**Disturbed Personal Identity** r/t severe child abuse

**Chronic Low Self-Esteem** r/t rejection, failure

**Risk for Self-Mutilation:** Risk factor: need to act out to relieve stress

**Readiness for Enhanced Communication:** willingness to discuss problems associated with condition

*See Dissociative Identity Disorder (Not Otherwise Specified)*

## MULTIPLE SCLEROSIS (MS)

**Ineffective Activity Planning** r/t unrealistic perception of personal competence

**Ineffective Airway Clearance** r/t decreased energy or fatigue

**Impaired Physical Mobility** r/t neuromuscular impairment

**Self-Neglect** r/t functional impairment

**Powerlessness** r/t progressive nature of disease

**Self-Care Deficit: Specify** r/t neuromuscular impairment

**Sexual Dysfunction** r/t biopsychosocial alteration of sexuality

**Chronic Sorrow** r/t loss of physical ability

**Spiritual Distress** r/t perceived hopelessness of diagnosis

**Urinary Retention** r/t inhibition of the reflex arc

**Risk for Disuse Syndrome:** Risk factor: physical immobility

**Risk for Injury:** Risk factors: altered mobility, sensory dysfunction

**Risk for Imbalanced Nutrition: Less than Body Requirements:** Risk factors: impaired swallowing, depression

**Risk for Powerlessness:** Risk factor: chronic illness

**Risk for Impaired Religiosity:** Risk factor: illness

**Risk for Thermal Injury:** Risk factor: neuromuscular impairment

**Readiness for Enhanced Health Management:** expresses a desire to manage condition

**Readiness for Enhanced Self-Care:** expresses desire to enhance knowledge of strategies and responsibility for self-care

**Readiness for Enhanced Spiritual Well-Being:** struggling with chronic debilitating condition

*See Neurological Disorders*

## MUMPS

*See Communicable Diseases, Childhood (e.g., Measles, Mumps, Rubella, Chickenpox, Scabies, Lice)*

## MURMURS

**Decreased Cardiac Output** r/t altered preload/afterload

**Risk for Decreased Cardiac Tissue Perfusion:** Risk factor: incompetent valve

**Risk for Fatigue:** Risk factor: decreased cardiac output

## MUSCULAR ATROPHY/WEAKNESS

**Risk for Disuse Syndrome:** Risk factor: impaired physical mobility

**Risk for Adult Falls:** Risk factor: impaired physical mobility

**Risk for Child Falls:** Risk factor: impaired physical mobility

## MUSCULAR DYSTROPHY (MD)

**Decreased Activity Tolerance** r/t fatigue, muscle weakness

**Ineffective Activity Planning** r/t unrealistic perception of personal competence

**Ineffective Airway Clearance** r/t muscle weakness and decreased ability to cough

**Constipation** r/t immobility

**Fatigue** r/t increased energy requirements to perform activities of daily living

**Impaired Physical Mobility** r/t muscle weakness and development of contractures

**Imbalanced Nutrition: Less than Body Requirements** r/t impaired swallowing or chewing

**Self-Care Deficit: Feeding, Bathing, Dressing, Toileting** r/t muscle weakness and fatigue

**Self-Neglect** r/t functional impairment

**Impaired Transfer Ability** r/t muscle weakness

**Impaired Swallowing** r/t neuromuscular impairment

**Impaired Walking** r/t muscle weakness

**Risk for Aspiration:** Risk factor: impaired swallowing

**Risk for Decreased Cardiac Tissue Perfusion:** Risk factor: hypoxia associated with cardiomyopathy

**Risk for Disuse Syndrome:** Risk factor: complications of immobility

**Risk for Falls:** Risk factor: muscle weakness

**Risk for Infection:** Risk factor: pooling of pulmonary secretions as a result of immobility and muscle weakness

**Risk for Injury:** Risk factors: muscle weakness and unsteady gait

**Risk for Overweight:** Risk factor: inactivity

**Risk for Powerlessness:** Risk factor: chronic condition

**Risk for Impaired Religiosity:** Risk factor: illness

**Risk for Impaired Resilience:** Risk factor: chronic illness

**Risk for Situational Low Self-Esteem:** Risk factor: presence of chronic condition

**Risk for Impaired Skin Integrity:** Risk factors: immobility, braces, or adaptive devices

**Readiness for Enhanced Self-Concept:** acceptance of strength and abilities

*See Child with Chronic Condition; Hospitalized Child*

## MVC (MOTOR VEHICLE CRASH)

*See Fracture; Head Injury; Injury; Pneumothorax*

## MYASTHENIA GRAVIS

**Ineffective Airway Clearance** r/t decreased ability to cough and swallow

**Interrupted Family Processes** r/t crisis of dealing with diagnosis

**Fatigue** r/t paresthesia, aching muscles, weakness of muscles

**Impaired Physical Mobility** r/t defective transmission of nerve impulses at the neuromuscular junction

**Imbalanced Nutrition: Less than Body Requirements** r/t difficulty eating and swallowing

**Impaired Swallowing** r/t neuromuscular impairment

**Risk for Caregiver Role Strain:** Risk factors: severity of illness of client, overwhelming needs of client

**Risk for Impaired Religiosity:** Risk factor: illness

**Risk for Impaired Resilience:** Risk factor: new diagnosis of chronic, serious illness

**Readiness for Enhanced Spiritual Well-Being:** heightened coping with serious illness

*See Neurological Disorders*

## MYCOPLASMA PNEUMONIA

*See Pneumonia*

## MYELOCELE

*See Neural Tube Defects*

## MYELOMENINGOCELE

*See Neural Tube Defects*

## MYOCARDIAL INFARCTION (MI)

*See MI (Myocardial Infarction)*

## MYOCARDITIS

**Decreased Activity Tolerance** r/t reduced cardiac reserve and prescribed bed rest

**Decreased Cardiac Output** r/t altered preload/afterload

**Fear** r/t dyspnea and reduced cardiac reserve

**Deficient Knowledge** r/t treatment of disease

**Risk for Decreased Cardiac Tissue Perfusion:** Risk factors: hypoxia, hypovolemia, cardiac tamponade

**Readiness for Enhanced Knowledge:** treatment of disease

*See Heart Failure, if appropriate*

## MYRINGOTOMY

**Fear** r/t hospitalization, surgical procedure

**Ineffective Health Maintenance** r/t deficient knowledge regarding care after surgery

**Acute Pain** r/t surgical procedure

**Risk for Surgical Site Infection:** Risk factor: invasive procedure

*See Ear Surgery*

## MYXEDEMA

*See Hypothyroidism*

# N

## NARCISSISTIC PERSONALITY DISORDER

**Defensive Coping** r/t grandiose sense of self

**Impaired Emancipated Decision-Making** r/t lack of realistic problem-solving skills

**Interrupted Family Processes** r/t taking advantage of others to achieve own goals

**Risk-Prone Health Behavior** r/t low self-efficacy

**Disturbed Personal Identity** r/t psychological impairment

**Ineffective Relationship** r/t lack of mutual support/respect between partners

**Impaired Individual Resilience** r/t psychological disorders

**Impaired Social Interaction** r/t self-concept disturbance

**Risk for Loneliness:** Risk factors: emotional deprivation, social isolation

## NARCOLEPSY

**Anxiety** r/t fear of lack of control over falling asleep

**Disturbed Sleep Pattern** r/t uncontrollable desire to sleep

**Risk for Physical Trauma:** Risk factor: falling asleep during potentially dangerous activity

**Readiness for Enhanced Sleep:** expresses willingness to enhance sleep

## NARCOTIC USE

*See Opioid Use (preferred terminology)*

## NASOGASTRIC SUCTION

**Impaired Oral Mucous Membrane Integrity** r/t presence of nasogastric tube

**Risk for Electrolyte Imbalance:** Risk factor: loss of gastrointestinal fluids that contain electrolytes

**Risk for Imbalanced Fluid Volume:** Risk factor: loss of gastrointestinal fluids without adequate replacement

**Risk for Dysfunctional Gastrointestinal Motility:** Risk factor: decreased intestinal motility

## NAUSEA

**Nausea** (See **Nausea,** Section II)

## NEAR-DROWNING

**Ineffective Airway Clearance** r/t aspiration of fluid

**Aspiration** r/t aspiration of fluid into lungs

**Fear: Parental** r/t possible death of child, possible permanent and debilitating sequelae

**Impaired Gas Exchange** r/t laryngospasm, holding breath, aspiration, inflammation

**Maladaptive Grieving** r/t potential death of child, unknown sequelae, guilt about accident

**Ineffective Health Maintenance Behaviors** r/t parental deficient knowledge regarding safety measures appropriate for age

**Hypothermia** r/t central nervous system injury, prolonged submersion in cold water

**Risk for Delayed Child Development:** Risk factors: hypoxemia, cerebral anoxia

**Risk for Maladaptive Grieving:** Risk factors: potential death of child, unknown sequelae, guilt about accident

**Risk for Infection:** Risk factors: aspiration, invasive monitoring

**Risk for Ineffective Cerebral Tissue Perfusion:** Risk factor: hypoxia

**Readiness for Enhanced Spiritual Well-Being:** struggle with survival of life-threatening situation

*See Child with Chronic Condition; Hospitalized Child; Safety, Childhood; Terminally Ill Child/Death of Child, Parent*

## NEARSIGHTEDNESS

**Readiness for Enhanced Health Management:** need for correction of myopia

## NEARSIGHTEDNESS; CORNEAL SURGERY

*See LASIK Eye Surgery (Laser-Assisted in Situ Keratomileusis)*

## NECK VEIN DISTENTION

**Decreased Cardiac Output** r/t decreased contractility of heart resulting in increased preload

**Excess Fluid Volume** r/t excess fluid intake, compromised regulatory mechanisms

**Risk for Thrombosis** r/t blood coagulation disorders

*See Congestive Heart Failure (CHF); Heart Failure*

## NECROSIS, KIDNEY TUBULAR; NECROSIS, ACUTE TUBULAR

*See Renal Failure*

## NECROTIZING ENTEROCOLITIS

**Ineffective Breathing Pattern** r/t abdominal distention, hypoxia

**Diarrhea** r/t infection

**Impaired Bowel Continence** r/t infection

**Deficient Fluid Volume** r/t vomiting, gastrointestinal bleeding

**Neonatal Hyperbilirubinemia** r/t feeding pattern not well established

**Imbalanced Nutrition: Less than Body Requirements** r/t decreased ability to absorb nutrients, decreased perfusion to gastrointestinal tract

**Risk for Dysfunctional Gastrointestinal Motility:** Risk factor: infection

**Risk for Infection:** Risk factors: bacterial invasion of gastrointestinal tract, invasive procedures

*See Hospitalized Child; Premature Infant (Child)*

## NEGATIVE FEELINGS ABOUT SELF

**Chronic Low Self-Esteem** r/t long-standing negative self-evaluation

**Self-Neglect** r/t negative feelings

**Readiness for Enhanced Self-Concept:** expresses willingness to enhance self-concept

## NEGLECT, UNILATERAL

**Unilateral Neglect** (See **Unilateral Neglect,** Section II)

## NEGLECTFUL CARE OF FAMILY MEMBER

**Caregiver Role Strain** r/t overwhelming care demands of family member, lack of social or financial support

**Disabled Family Coping** r/t highly ambivalent family relationships, lack of respite care

**Interrupted Family Processes** r/t situational transition or crisis

**Deficient Knowledge** r/t care needs

**Impaired Individual Resilience** r/t vulnerability from neglect

**Risk for Compromised Human Dignity:** Risk factor: inadequate participation in decision-making

## NEONATAL ABSTINENCE SYNDROME

**Ineffective Airway Clearance** r/t pooling of secretions from lack of adequate cough reflex, effects of viral or bacterial lower airway infection as a result of altered protective state

**Interrupted Breastfeeding** r/t use of drugs or alcohol by mother

**Ineffective Childbearing Process** r/t inconsistent prenatal health visits, suboptimal maternal nutrition, substance abuse

**Impaired Comfort** r/t irritability and inability to relax

**Diarrhea** r/t effects of withdrawal, increased peristalsis from hyperirritability

**Disorganized Infant Behavior** r/t exposure and/or withdrawal from toxic substances (alcohol or drugs), lack of attachment

**Imbalanced Nutrition: Less than Body Requirements** r/t feeding problems; uncoordinated or ineffective suck and swallow; effects of diarrhea, vomiting, or colic associated with maternal substance abuse

**Impaired Parenting** r/t impaired or absent attachment behaviors, inadequate support systems

**Ineffective Infant Suck-Swallow Response** r/t uncoordinated or ineffective sucking reflex, neurological delay

**Disturbed Sleep Pattern** r/t hyperirritability or hypersensitivity to environmental stimuli

**Risk for Impaired Attachment:** Risk factor: (parent) substance misuse, inability to meet infant's needs

**Risk for Delayed Child Development:** Risk factor: effects of prenatal substance abuse

**Risk for Infection:** Risk factor: stress effects of withdrawal

**Risk for Disturbed Maternal–Fetal Dyad:** Risk factor: substance abuse

**Risk for Sudden Infant Death:** Risk factor: prenatal illicit drug exposure

**Risk for Ineffective Thermoregulation:** Risk factor: immature nervous system

*See Anomaly, Fetal/Newborn (Parent Dealing with); Cerebral Palsy; Child with Chronic Condition; Failure to Thrive; Hospitalized Child; Hyperactive Syndrome; Premature Infant/Child; Sudden Infant Death, Risk for*

## NEONATAL HYPERBILIRUBINEMIA

Neonatal Hyperbilirubinemia (See **Neonatal Hyperbilirubinemia,** Section II)

## NEONATE

**Readiness for Enhanced Childbearing Process:** appropriate care of newborn

*See Newborn, Normal; Newborn, Postmature; Newborn, Small for Gestational Age (SGA)*

## NEOPLASM

**Fear** r/t possible malignancy

*See Cancer*

## NEPHRECTOMY

**Anxiety** r/t surgical recovery, prognosis

**Ineffective Breathing Pattern** r/t location of surgical incision

**Constipation** r/t lack of return of peristalsis

**Acute Pain** r/t incisional discomfort

**Spiritual Distress** r/t chronic illness

**Risk for Bleeding:** Risk factor: surgery

**Risk for Imbalanced Fluid Volume:** Risk factors: vascular losses, decreased intake

**Risk for Surgical Site Infection:** Risk factor: surgical procedure

## NEPHROSTOMY, PERCUTANEOUS

**Acute Pain** r/t invasive procedure

**Impaired Urinary Elimination** r/t nephrostomy tube

**Risk for Infection:** Risk factor: invasive procedure

## NEPHROTIC SYNDROME

**Decreased Activity Tolerance** r/t generalized edema

**Disturbed Body Image** r/t edematous appearance and side effects of steroid therapy

**Excess Fluid Volume** r/t edema resulting from oncotic fluid shift caused by serum protein loss and kidney retention of salt and water

**Imbalanced Nutrition: Less than Body Requirements** r/t anorexia, protein loss

**Imbalanced Nutrition: More than Body Requirements** r/t increased appetite attributable to steroid therapy

**Social Isolation** r/t edematous appearance

**Risk for Infection:** Risk factor: altered immune mechanisms caused by disease and effects of steroids

**Risk for Impaired Skin Integrity:** Risk factor: edema

*See Child with Chronic Condition; Hospitalized Child*

## NEURAL TUBE DEFECTS (MENINGOCELE, MYELOMENINGOCELE, SPINA BIFIDA, ANENCEPHALY)

**Chronic Functional Constipation** r/t immobility or less than adequate mobility

**Maladaptive Grieving** r/t loss of perfect child, birth of child with congenital defect

**Mixed Urinary Incontinence** r/t neurogenic impairment

**Urge Urinary Incontinence** r/t neurogenic impairment

**Impaired Mobility** r/t neuromuscular impairment

**Chronic Low Self-Esteem** r/t perceived differences, decreased ability to participate in physical and social activities at school

**Impaired Skin Integrity** r/t incontinence

**Risk for Delayed Child Development:** Risk factor: inadequate nutrition

**Risk for Latex Allergy Reaction:** Risk factor: multiple exposures to latex products

**Risk for Imbalanced Nutrition: More than Body Requirements:** Risk factors: diminished, limited, or impaired physical activity

**Risk for Powerlessness:** Risk factor: debilitating disease

**Risk for Impaired Skin Integrity: Lower Extremities:** Risk factor: decreased sensory perception

**Readiness for Enhanced Family Coping:** effective adaptive response by family members

**Readiness for Enhanced Family Processes:** family supports each other

**N**

*See Child with Chronic Condition; Premature Infant (Child)*

## NEURALGIA

*See Trigeminal Neuralgia*

## NEURITIS (PERIPHERAL NEUROPATHY)

**Decreased Activity Tolerance** r/t pain with movement

**Ineffective Health Maintenance Behaviors** r/t deficient knowledge regarding self-care with neuritis

**Acute Pain** r/t stimulation of affected nerve endings, inflammation of sensory nerves

*See Neuropathy, Peripheral*

## NEUROGENIC BLADDER

**Mixed Urinary Incontinence** r/t neurological impairment

**Urinary Retention** r/t interruption in the lateral spinal tracts

## NEUROLOGICAL DISORDERS

**Ineffective Airway Clearance** r/t perceptual or cognitive impairment, decreased energy, fatigue

**Acute Confusion** r/t dementia, alcohol abuse, drug abuse, delirium

**Ineffective Coping** r/t disability requiring change in lifestyle

**Interrupted Family Processes** r/t situational crisis, illness, or disability of family member

**Maladaptive Grieving** r/t loss of usual body functioning

**Ineffective Home Maintenance Behaviors** r/t client's or family member's disease

**Risk for Corneal Injury:** Risk factor: lack of spontaneous blink reflex

**Impaired Memory** r/t neurological disturbance

**Impaired Physical Mobility** r/t neuromuscular impairment

**Imbalanced Nutrition: Less than Body Requirements** r/t impaired swallowing, depression, difficulty feeding self

**Powerlessness** r/t progressive nature of disease

**Self-Care Deficit: Specify** r/t neuromuscular dysfunction

**Sexual Dysfunction** r/t biopsychosocial alteration of sexuality

**Social Isolation** r/t altered state of wellness

**Impaired Swallowing** r/t neuromuscular dysfunction

**Risk for Disuse Syndrome:** Risk factors: physical immobility, neuromuscular dysfunction

**Risk for Injury:** Risk factors: altered mobility, sensory dysfunction, cognitive impairment

**Risk for Ineffective Cerebral Tissue Perfusion:** Risk factor: cerebral disease/injury

**Risk for Impaired Religiosity:** Risk factor: life transition

**Risk for Impaired Skin Integrity:** Risk factors: altered sensation, altered mental status, paralysis

*See specific condition: Alcohol Withdrawal; Amyotrophic Lateral Sclerosis (ALS); CVA (Cerebrovascular Accident); Delirium; Dementia; Guillain-Barré Syndrome; Head Injury; Huntington's Disease; Spinal Cord Injury; Myasthenia Gravis; Muscular Dystrophy (MD); Parkinson's Disease*

## NEUROPATHY, PERIPHERAL

**Chronic Pain** r/t damage to nerves in the peripheral nervous system as a result of medication side effects, vitamin deficiency, or diabetes

**Ineffective Thermoregulation** r/t decreased ability to regulate body temperature

**Risk for Injury:** Risk factors: lack of muscle control, decreased sensation

**Risk for Impaired Skin Integrity:** Risk factor: poor perfusion

**Risk for Thermal Injury:** Risk factor: nerve damage

*See Peripheral Vascular Disease (PVD)*

## NEUROSURGERY

*See Craniectomy/Craniotomy*

N

## NEWBORN, NORMAL

**Breastfeeding** r/t normal oral structure and gestational age greater than 34 weeks

**Ineffective Thermoregulation** r/t immaturity of neuroendocrine system

**Risk for Sudden Infant Death:** Risk factors: lack of knowledge regarding infant sleeping in prone or side-lying position, prenatal or postnatal infant smoke exposure, infant overheating or overwrapping, loose articles in the sleep environment

**Risk for Infection:** Risk factors: open umbilical stump, immature immune system

**Risk for Injury:** Risk factors: immaturity, need for caretaking

**Readiness for Enhanced Childbearing Process:** appropriate care of newborn

**Readiness for Enhanced Organized Infant Behavior:** demonstrates adaptive response to pain

**Readiness for Enhanced Parenting:** providing emotional and physical needs of infant

## NEWBORN, POSTMATURE

**Hypothermia** r/t depleted stores of subcutaneous fat

**Impaired Skin Integrity** r/t cracked and peeling skin as a result of decreased vernix

**Risk for Ineffective Airway Clearance:** Risk factor: meconium aspiration

**Risk for Unstable Blood Glucose Level:** Risk factor: depleted glycogen stores

## NEWBORN, SMALL FOR GESTATIONAL AGE (SGA)

**Neonatal Hyperbilirubinemia** r/t neonate age and difficulty feeding

**Imbalanced Nutrition: Less than Body Requirements** r/t history of placental insufficiency

**Ineffective Thermoregulation** r/t decreased brown fat, subcutaneous fat

**Risk for Delayed Child Development:** Risk factor: history of placental insufficiency

**Risk for Injury:** Risk factors: hypoglycemia, perinatal asphyxia, meconium aspiration

**Risk for Sudden Infant Death:** Risk factor: low birth weight

## NICOTINE ADDICTION

**Risk-Prone Health Behavior** r/t smoking

**Ineffective Health Maintenance Behaviors** r/t lack of ability to make a judgment about smoking cessation

**Risk for Impaired Skin Integrity:** Risk factor: poor tissue perfusion associated with nicotine

**Powerlessness** r/t perceived lack of control over ability to give up nicotine

**Readiness for Enhanced Emancipated Decision-Making:** expresses desire to enhance understanding and meaning of choices

**Readiness for Enhanced Health Literacy:** expresses desire to enhance understanding of health information to make health care choices

**Readiness for Enhanced Health Management:** expresses desire to learn measures to stop smoking

## NIDDM (NON–INSULIN-DEPENDENT DIABETES MELLITUS)

**Readiness for Enhanced Health Management:** expresses desire for information on exercise and diet to manage diabetes

*See Diabetes Mellitus*

## NIGHTMARES

**Post-Trauma Syndrome** r/t disaster, war, epidemic, rape, assault, torture, catastrophic illness, or accident

## NIPPLE SORENESS

**Impaired Comfort** r/t physical condition

*See Painful Breasts, Sore Nipples; Sore Nipples, Breastfeeding*

## NOCTURIA

**Urge Urinary Incontinence** r/t decreased bladder capacity, irritation of bladder stretch receptors causing spasm, alcohol, caffeine, increased fluids, increased urine concentration, overdistention of bladder

**N**

**Impaired Urinary Elimination** r/t sensory motor impairment, urinary tract infection

**Risk for Powerlessness:** Risk factor: inability to control nighttime voiding

## NOCTURNAL MYOCLONUS

*See Restless Leg Syndrome; Stress*

## NOCTURNAL PAROXYSMAL DYSPNEA

*See PND (Paroxysmal Nocturnal Dyspnea)*

## NON–INSULIN-DEPENDENT DIABETES MELLITUS (NIDDM)

*See Diabetes Mellitus*

## NORMAL PRESSURE HYDROCEPHALUS (NPH)

**Impaired Verbal Communication** r/t obstruction of flow of cerebrospinal fluid affecting speech

**Acute Confusion** r/t increased intracranial pressure caused by obstruction to flow of cerebrospinal fluid

**Impaired Memory** r/t neurological disturbance

**Risk for Ineffective Cerebral Tissue Perfusion:** Risk factor: fluid pressing on the brain

**Risk for Adult Falls:** Risk factor: unsteady gait as a result of obstruction of cerebrospinal fluid

**Risk for Child Falls:** Risk factor: unsteady gait as a result of obstruction of cerebrospinal fluid

## NSTEMI (NON–ST-ELEVATION MYOCARDIAL INFARCTION)

*See MI (Myocardial Infarction)*

## NURSING

*See Breastfeeding, Effective; Breastfeeding, Ineffective; Breastfeeding, Interrupted; Nipple-Areolar Complex Injury*

## NUTRITION

**Readiness for Enhanced Nutrition** (See **Nutrition, Readiness for Enhanced,** Section II)

## NUTRITION, IMBALANCED

**Imbalanced Nutrition: Less than Body Requirements** (See **Nutrition: Less than Body Requirements, Imbalanced,** Section II)

**Obesity** (See **Obesity,** Section II)

**Overweight** (See **Overweight,** Section II)

**Risk for Dry Mouth** r/t depression

**Risk for Overweight** (See **Overweight, Risk for,** Section II)

**Risk for Metabolic Syndrome** r/t inadequate dietary habits

## OBESITY

**Disturbed Body Image** r/t eating disorder, excess weight

**Risk-Prone Health Behavior** r/t negative attitude toward health care

**Obesity** (See **Obesity,** Section II)

**Chronic Low Self-Esteem** r/t ineffective coping, overeating

**Risk for Metabolic Syndrome:** Risk factor: obesity

**Risk for Ineffective Peripheral Tissue Perfusion:** Risk factor: sedentary lifestyle

**Readiness for Enhanced Nutrition:** expresses willingness to enhance nutrition

## OBS (ORGANIC BRAIN SYNDROME)

*See Organic Mental Disorders; Dementia*

## OBSESSIVE-COMPULSIVE DISORDER (OCD)

*See OCD (Obsessive-Compulsive Disorder)*

## OBSTRUCTION, BOWEL

*See Bowel Obstruction*

## OBSTRUCTIVE SLEEP APNEA

**Insomnia** r/t blocked airway

**Obesity** r/t excessive intake related to metabolic need

*See PND (Paroxysmal Nocturnal Dyspnea)*

## OCD (OBSESSIVE-COMPULSIVE DISORDER)

**Ineffective Activity Planning** r/t unrealistic perception of events

**Anxiety** r/t threat to self-concept, unmet needs

**Impaired Emancipated Decision-Making** r/t inability to make a decision for fear of reprisal

**Disabled Family Coping** r/t family process being disrupted by client's ritualistic activities

**Ineffective Coping** r/t expression of feelings in an unacceptable way, ritualistic behavior

**Risk-Prone Health Behavior** r/t inadequate comprehension associated with repetitive thoughts

**Powerlessness** r/t unrelenting repetitive thoughts to perform irrational activities

**Impaired Individual Resilience** r/t psychological disorder

**Risk for Situational Low Self-Esteem:** Risk factor: inability to control repetitive thoughts and actions

## OCCUPATIONAL INJURY

**Fatigue** r/t lack of sleep

**Deficient Knowledge** r/t inadequate training, improper use of equipment

**Stress Overload** r/t feelings of pressure

**Risk for Occupational Injury** (See **Risk for Occupational Injury,** Section II)

## ODD (OPPOSITIONAL DEFIANT DISORDER)

**Anxiety** r/t feelings of anger and hostility toward authority figures

**Ineffective Coping** r/t lack of self-control or perceived lack of self-control

**Disabled Family Coping** r/t feelings of anger, hostility; defiant behavior toward authority figures

**Risk-Prone Health Behavior** r/t multiple stressors associated with condition

**Ineffective Impulse Control** r/t anger/compunction to engage in disruptive behaviors

**Chronic or Situational Low Self-Esteem** r/t poor self-control and disruptive behaviors

**Impaired Social Interaction** r/t being touchy or easily annoyed, blaming others for own mistakes, constant trouble in school

**Social Isolation** r/t unaccepted social behavior

**Ineffective Family Health Self-Management** r/t difficulty in limit setting and managing oppositional behaviors

**Risk for Ineffective Activity Planning:** Risk factors: unrealistic perception of events, hedonism, insufficient social support

**Risk for Impaired Parenting:** Risk factors: children's difficult behaviors and inability to set limits

**Risk for Powerlessness:** Risk factor: inability to deal with difficult behaviors

**Risk for Spiritual Distress:** Risk factors: anxiety and stress in dealing with difficult behaviors

**Risk for Other-Directed Violence:** Risk factors: history of violence, threats of violence against others, history of antisocial behavior, history of indirect violence

## OLDER ADULT

*See Aging*

## OLIGURIA

**Deficient Fluid Volume** r/t active fluid loss, failure of regulatory mechanism, inadequate intake

**Risk for Electrolyte Imbalance** r/t inadequate knowledge of modifiable factors

*See Cardiac Output, Decreased; Renal Failure; Shock, Hypovolemic*

## OMPHALOCELE

*See Gastroschisis/Omphalocele*

## OOPHORECTOMY

**Risk for Ineffective Sexuality Pattern:** Risk factor: altered body function

*See Surgery, Perioperative Care; Surgery, Postoperative Care; Surgery, Preoperative Care*

## OPCAB (OFF-PUMP CORONARY ARTERY BYPASS)

*See Angioplasty, Coronary; Coronary Artery Bypass Grafting (CABG)*

**O**

## OPEN HEART SURGERY

**Risk for Decreased Cardiac Tissue Perfusion:** Risk factor: cardiac surgery

*See Coronary Artery Bypass Grafting (CABG); Dysrhythmia*

## OPEN REDUCTION OF FRACTURE WITH INTERNAL FIXATION (FEMUR)

**Anxiety** r/t outcome of corrective procedure

**Impaired Physical Mobility** r/t postoperative position, abduction of leg, avoidance of acute flexion

**Powerlessness** r/t loss of control, unanticipated change in lifestyle

**Risk for Surgical Site Infection:** Risk factor: surgical procedure

**Risk for Perioperative Positioning injury:** Risk factor: immobilization

**Risk for Peripheral Neurovascular Dysfunction:** Risk factors: mechanical compression, orthopedic surgery, immobilization

**Risk for Thrombosis:** Risk factor: impaired mobility

*See Surgery, Postoperative Care*

## OPIOID ADDICTION

*See Substance Abuse*

## OPIOID USE

**Acute Pain** r/t physical injury or surgical procedure

**Chronic Pain Syndrome** r/t prolonged use of opioids

**Risk for Constipation:** Risk factor: effects of opioids on peristalsis

*See Substance Abuse; Substance Withdrawal; Pain Management, Acute; Pain Management, Chronic*

## OPPORTUNISTIC INFECTION

**Delayed Surgical Recovery** r/t abnormal blood profiles, impaired healing

**Risk for Infection:** Risk factor: abnormal blood profiles

*See AIDS (Acquired Immunodeficiency Syndrome); HIV (Human Immunodeficiency Virus)*

## OPPOSITIONAL DEFIANT DISORDER (ODD)

*See ODD (Oppositional Defiant Disorder)*

## ORAL MUCOUS MEMBRANE INTEGRITY, IMPAIRED

**Impaired Oral Mucous Membrane Integrity** (See **Oral Mucous Membrane Integrity, Impaired,** Section II)

## ORAL THRUSH

**Impaired Oral Mucous Membrane Integrity:** Risk factors: effects of chemotherapy, radiotherapy, oral trauma, immune system disease

*See Candidiasis, Oral*

## ORCHITIS

**Readiness for Enhanced Health Self-Management:** follows recommendations for mumps vaccination

*See Epididymitis*

## ORGANIC MENTAL DISORDERS

**Chronic Confusion** r/t progressive impairment in cognitive functioning

**Frail Elderly Syndrome** r/t alteration in cognitive function

**Impaired Social Interaction** r/t disturbed thought processes

**Risk for Disturbed Personal Identity:** Risk factor: delusions/fluctuating perceptions of stimuli

*See Dementia*

## ORTHOPEDIC TRACTION

**Ineffective Role Performance** r/t limited physical mobility

**Impaired Social Interaction** r/t limited physical mobility

**Impaired Transfer Ability** r/t limited physical mobility

**Risk for Impaired Religiosity:** Risk factor: immobility

*See Traction and Casts*

## ORTHOPNEA

**Ineffective Breathing Pattern** r/t inability to breathe with head of bed flat

**Decreased Cardiac Output** r/t inability of heart to meet demands of body

## ORTHOSTATIC HYPOTENSION

*See Dizziness*

## OSTEOARTHRITIS

**Acute Pain** r/t movement

**Impaired Walking** r/t inflammation and damage to joints

*See Arthritis*

## OSTEOMYELITIS

**Decreased Diversional Activity Engagement** r/t prolonged immobilization, hospitalization

**Fear: Parental** r/t concern regarding possible growth plate damage caused by infection, concern that infection may become chronic

**Ineffective Health Maintenance Behaviors** r/t continued immobility at home, possible extensive casts, continued antibiotics

**Impaired Physical Mobility** r/t imposed immobility as a result of infected area

**Acute Pain** r/t inflammation in affected extremity

**Ineffective Thermoregulation** r/t infectious process

**Risk for Constipation:** Risk factor: immobility

**Risk for Infection:** Risk factor: inadequate primary and secondary defenses

**Risk for Impaired Skin Integrity:** Risk factor: irritation from splint or cast

*See Hospitalized Child*

## OSTEOPOROSIS

**Deficient Knowledge** r/t diet, exercise, need to abstain from alcohol and nicotine

**Impaired Physical Mobility** r/t pain, skeletal changes

**Imbalanced Nutrition: Less than Body Requirements** r/t inadequate intake of calcium and vitamin D

**Acute Pain** r/t fracture, muscle spasms

**Risk for Injury: Fracture:** Risk factors: lack of activity, risk of falling resulting from environmental hazards, neuromuscular disorders, diminished senses, cardiovascular responses to drugs

**Risk for Adult Falls** r/t decreased lower extremity strength

**Risk for Powerlessness:** Risk factor: debilitating disease

**Readiness for Enhanced Health Self-Management:** expresses desire to manage the treatment of illness and prevent complications

## OSTOMY

*See Child with Chronic Condition; Colostomy; Ileal Conduit; Ileostomy*

## OTITIS MEDIA

**Acute Pain** r/t inflammation, infectious process

**Risk for Delayed Child Development: Speech and Language:** Risk factor: frequent otitis media

**Anxiety** r/t pain

**Risk for Infection:** Risk factors: eustachian tube obstruction, traumatic eardrum perforation, infectious process

**Readiness for Enhanced Knowledge:** information on treatment and prevention of disease

## OVARIAN CARCINOMA

**Death Anxiety** r/t unknown outcome, possible poor prognosis

**Fear** r/t unknown outcome, possible poor prognosis

**Ineffective Health Maintenance Behaviors** r/t deficient knowledge regarding self-care, treatment of condition

**Readiness for Enhanced Family Processes:** family functioning meets needs of client

**Readiness for Enhanced Resilience:** participates in support groups

**O**

*See Chemotherapy; Hysterectomy;
Radiation Therapy*

# P

## PACEMAKER

**Anxiety** r/t change in health status, presence of pacemaker

**Death Anxiety** r/t worry over possible malfunction of pacemaker

**Deficient Knowledge** r/t self-care program, when to seek medical attention

**Acute Pain** r/t surgical procedure

**Risk for Bleeding:** Risk factor: surgery

**Risk for Decreased Cardiac Tissue Perfusion:** Risk factor: pacemaker malfunction

**Risk for Impaired Cardiovascular Function:** Risk factor: cardiac dysrhythmias

**Risk for Infection:** Risk factors: invasive procedure, presence of foreign body (catheter and generator)

**Risk for Powerlessness:** Risk factor: presence of electronic device to stimulate heart

**Readiness for Enhanced Health Management:** appropriate health care management of pacemaker

## PAGET'S DISEASE

**Disturbed Body Image** r/t possible enlarged head, bowed tibias, kyphosis

**Deficient Knowledge** r/t appropriate diet high in protein and calcium, mild exercise

**Chronic Sorrow** r/t chronic condition with altered body image

**Risk for Physical Trauma: Fracture:** Risk factor: excessive bone destruction

## PAIN MANAGEMENT, ACUTE

**Acute Pain** r/t injury or surgical procedure

**Imbalanced Energy Field** r/t unpleasant sensory and emotional feelings

## PAIN MANAGEMENT, CHRONIC

**Chronic Pain** (See **Pain, Chronic,** Section II)

**Chronic Pain Syndrome** r/t persistent pain affecting daily living

**Risk for Constipation:** Risk factor: effects of medications on peristalsis

**Readiness for Enhanced Knowledge:** expresses a desire to learn alternative methods of nonpharmaceutical pain control

*See Substance Misuse*

## PAINFUL BREASTS, ENGORGEMENT

**Acute Pain** r/t distention of breast tissue

**Ineffective Role Performance** r/t change in physical capacity to assume role of breastfeeding mother

**Impaired Tissue Integrity** r/t excessive fluid in breast tissues

**Risk for Ineffective Breastfeeding:** Risk factors: pain, infant's inability to latch on to engorged breast

**Risk for Infection:** Risk factor: milk stasis

**Risk for Nipple-Areolar Complex Injury** r/t breast engorgement

## PAINFUL BREASTS, SORE NIPPLES

**Insufficient Breast Milk Production** r/t long breastfeeding time/pain response

**Ineffective Breastfeeding** r/t pain

**Acute Pain** r/t cracked nipples

**Ineffective Role Performance** r/t change in physical capacity to assume role of breastfeeding mother

**Impaired Skin Integrity** r/t mechanical factors involved in suckling, breastfeeding management

**Nipple-Areolar Complex Injury** r/t maternal impatience with the breastfeeding process

**Risk for Infection:** Risk factor: break in skin

## PALLOR OF EXTREMITIES

**Ineffective Peripheral Tissue Perfusion** r/t interruption of vascular flow

*See Shock; Peripheral Vascular disease (PVD)*

## PALPITATIONS (HEART PALPITATIONS)

*See Dysrhythmia*

## PANCREATIC CANCER

**Death Anxiety** r/t possible poor prognosis of disease process

**Ineffective Family Coping** r/t poor prognosis

**Fear** r/t poor prognosis of the disease

**Maladaptive Grieving** r/t shortened lifespan

**Deficient Knowledge** r/t disease-induced diabetes, home management

**Spiritual Distress** r/t poor prognosis

**Risk for impaired Liver Function:** Risk factor: complications from underlying disease

*See Cancer; Chemotherapy; Radiation Therapy; Surgery, Perioperative Care; Surgery, Postoperative Care; Surgery, Preoperative Care*

## PANCREATITIS

**Ineffective Breathing Pattern** r/t splinting from severe pain, disease process, and inflammation

**Ineffective Denial** r/t ineffective coping, alcohol use

**Diarrhea** r/t decrease in pancreatic secretions resulting in steatorrhea

**Deficient Fluid Volume** r/t vomiting, decreased fluid intake, fever, diaphoresis, fluid shifts

**Ineffective Health Maintenance Behaviors** r/t deficient knowledge concerning diet, alcohol use, medication

**Nausea** r/t irritation of gastrointestinal system

**Imbalanced Nutrition: Less than Body Requirements** r/t inadequate dietary intake, increased nutritional needs as a result of acute illness, increased metabolic needs caused by increased body temperature, disease process

**Acute Pain** r/t irritation and edema of the inflamed pancreas

**Chronic Sorrow** r/t chronic illness

**Readiness for Enhanced Comfort:** expresses desire to enhance comfort

## PANIC DISORDER (PANIC ATTACKS)

**Ineffective Activity Planning** r/t unrealistic perception of events

**Anxiety** r/t situational crisis

**Ineffective Coping** r/t personal vulnerability

**Risk-Prone Health Behavior** r/t low self-efficacy

**Disturbed Personal Identity** r/t situational crisis

**Post-Trauma Syndrome** r/t previous catastrophic event

**Social Isolation** r/t fear of lack of control

**Risk for Loneliness:** Risk factor: inability to socially interact because of fear of losing control

**Risk for Post-Trauma Syndrome:** Risk factors: perception of the event, diminished ego strength

**Risk for Powerlessness:** Risk factor: ineffective coping skills

**Readiness for Enhanced Coping:** seeks problem-oriented and emotion-oriented strategies to manage condition

*See Anxiety; Anxiety Disorder*

## PARALYSIS

**Disturbed Body Image** r/t biophysical changes, loss of movement, immobility

**Impaired Comfort** r/t prolonged immobility

**Constipation** r/t effects of spinal cord disruption, inadequate fiber in diet

**Ineffective Health Maintenance Behaviors** r/t deficient knowledge regarding self-care with paralysis

**Ineffective Home Maintenance Behaviors** r/t physical disability

**Mixed Urinary Incontinence** r/t neurological impairment

**Impaired Physical Mobility** r/t neuromuscular impairment

**Impaired Wheelchair Mobility** r/t neuromuscular impairment

**Self-Neglect** r/t functional impairment

**Powerlessness** r/t illness-related regimen

**Self-Care Deficit: Specify** r/t neuromuscular impairment

**Sexual Dysfunction** r/t loss of sensation, biopsychosocial alteration

**Chronic Sorrow** r/t loss of physical mobility

**Impaired Transfer Ability** r/t paralysis

**P**

**Risk for Autonomic Dysreflexia:** Risk factor: cause of paralysis

**Risk for Disuse Syndrome:** Risk factor: paralysis

**Risk for Adult Falls:** Risk factor: paralysis

**Risk for Injury:** Risk factors: altered mobility, sensory dysfunction

**Risk for Post-Trauma Syndrome:** Risk factor: event causing paralysis

**Risk for Impaired Religiosity:** Risk factors: immobility, possible lack of transportation

**Risk for Impaired Resilience:** Risk factor: chronic disability

**Risk for Situational Low Self-Esteem:** Risk factor: change in body image and function

**Risk for Impaired Skin integrity:** Risk factors: altered circulation, altered sensation, immobility

**Risk for Thrombosis:** Risk factor: prolonged immobility

**Readiness for Enhanced Self-Care:** expresses desire to enhance knowledge and responsibility for strategies for self-care

*See Child with Chronic Condition; Hemiplegia; Hospitalized Child; Neural Tube Defects (Meningocele, Myelomeningocele, Spina Bifida, Anencephaly); Spinal Cord Injury*

## PARALYTIC ILEUS

**Constipation** r/t decreased gastrointestinal motility

**Deficient Fluid Volume** r/t loss of fluids from vomiting, retention of fluid in bowel

**Dysfunctional Gastrointestinal Motility** r/t recent abdominal surgery, electrolyte imbalance

**Nausea** r/t gastrointestinal irritation

**Acute Pain** r/t pressure, abdominal distention, presence of nasogastric tube

*See Bowel Obstruction*

## PARANOID PERSONALITY DISORDER

**Ineffective Activity Planning** r/t unrealistic perception of events

**Anxiety** r/t uncontrollable intrusive, suspicious thoughts

**Risk-Prone Health Behavior** r/t intense emotional state

**Disturbed Personal Identity** r/t difficulty with reality testing

**Impaired Individual Resilience** r/t psychological disorder

**Chronic Low Self-Esteem** r/t inability to trust others

**Social Isolation** r/t inappropriate social skills

**Risk for Loneliness:** Risk factor: social isolation

**Risk for Other-Directed Violence:** Risk factor: being suspicious of others and their actions

## PARAPLEGIA

*See Spinal Cord Injury*

## PARATHYROIDECTOMY

**Anxiety** r/t surgery

**Risk for Ineffective Airway Clearance:** Risk factors: edema or hematoma formation, airway obstruction

**Risk for Bleeding:** Risk factor: surgery

**Risk for Impaired Verbal Communication:** Risk factors: possible laryngeal damage, edema

**Risk for Infection:** Risk factor: surgical procedure

*See Hypocalcemia*

## PARENT ATTACHMENT

**Risk for Impaired Attachment** (See **Attachment, Impaired, Risk for,** Section II)

**Readiness for Enhanced Childbearing Process:** demonstrates appropriate care of newborn

*See Parental Role Conflict*

## PARENTAL ROLE CONFLICT

**Parental Role Conflict** (See **Role Conflict, Parental,** Section II)

**Ineffective Relationship** r/t unrealistic expectations

**Chronic Sorrow** r/t difficult parent–child relationship

**Risk for Spiritual Distress:** Risk factor: altered relationships

**Readiness for Enhanced Parenting:**
willingness to enhance parenting

### PARENTING

**Readiness for Enhanced Parenting** (See
**Parenting, Readiness for Enhanced,** Section II)

### PARENTING, IMPAIRED

**Impaired Parenting** (See **Parenting,
Impaired,** Section II)

**Chronic Sorrow** r/t difficult parent–child
relationship

**Risk for Spiritual Distress:** Risk factor:
altered relationships

### PARENTING, RISK FOR IMPAIRED

**Risk for Impaired Parenting** (See **Parenting,
Impaired, Risk for,** Section II)

*See Parenting, Impaired*

### PARESTHESIA

**Risk for Injury:** Risk factors: inability to feel
temperature changes, pain

**Risk for Impaired Skin Integrity:** Risk factor:
impaired sensation

**Risk for Thermal Injury:** Risk factor:
neuromuscular impairment

### PARKINSON'S DISEASE

**Impaired Verbal Communication** r/t
decreased speech volume, slowness of
speech, impaired facial muscles

**Constipation** r/t weakness of muscles,
lack of exercise, inadequate fluid intake,
decreased autonomic nervous system activity

**Frail Elderly Syndrome** r/t chronic illness

**Imbalanced Nutrition: Less than Body
Requirements** r/t tremor, slowness in eating,
difficulty in chewing and swallowing

**Chronic Sorrow** r/t loss of physical capacity

**Risk for Injury:** Risk factors: tremors, slow
reactions, altered gait

*See Neurologic Disorders*

### PAROXYSMAL NOCTURNAL DYSPNEA (PND)

*See PND (Paroxysmal Nocturnal Dyspnea)*

### PATENT DUCTUS ARTERIOSUS (PDA)

*See Congenital Heart Disease/Cardiac
Anomalies*

### PATIENT-CONTROLLED ANALGESIA (PCA)

*See PCA (Patient-Controlled Analgesia)*

### PATIENT EDUCATION

**Deficient Knowledge** r/t lack of exposure to
information misinterpretation, unfamiliarity
with information resources to manage
illness

**Readiness for Enhanced Emancipated
Decision-Making:** expresses desire to
enhance understanding of choices for
decision-making

**Readiness for Enhanced Knowledge
(Specify):** interest in learning

**Readiness for Enhanced Health
Management:** expresses desire for
information to manage the illness

### PCA (PATIENT-CONTROLLED ANALGESIA)

**Deficient Knowledge** r/t self-care of pain
control

**Nausea** r/t side effects of medication

**Risk for Injury:** Risk factors: possible
complications associated with PCA

**Risk for Vascular Trauma:** Risk factors:
insertion site and length of insertion
time

**Readiness for Enhanced Knowledge:**
appropriate management of PCA

**Acute Pain:** guarding behaviors

### PECTUS EXCAVATUM

*See Marfan Syndrome*

### PEDICULOSIS

*See Lice*

### PEG (PERCUTANEOUS ENDOSCOPIC GASTROSTOMY)

*See Tube Feeding*

## PELVIC INFLAMMATORY DISEASE (PID)

*See PID (Pelvic Inflammatory Disease)*

## PENILE PROSTHESIS

**Ineffective Sexuality Pattern** r/t use of penile prosthesis

**Risk for Surgical Site Infection:** Risk factor: invasive surgical procedure

**Risk for Situational Low Self-Esteem:** Risk factor: ineffective sexuality pattern

**Readiness for Enhanced Health Management:** seeks information regarding care and use of prosthesis

*See Erectile Dysfunction (ED); Impotence*

## PEPTIC ULCER

*See Ulcer, Peptic (Duodenal or Gastric)*

## PERCUTANEOUS TRANSLUMINAL CORONARY ANGIOPLASTY (PTCA)

*See Angioplasty, Coronary*

## PERICARDIAL FRICTION RUB

**Decreased Cardiac Output** r/t inflammation

**Acute Pain** r/t inflammation, effusion

**Risk for Decreased Cardiac Tissue Perfusion:** Risk factors: inflammation in pericardial sac, fluid accumulation compressing heart

## PERICARDITIS

**Decreased Activity Tolerance** r/t reduced cardiac reserve, prescribed bed rest

**Decreased Cardiac Output** r/t impaired cardiac function from inflammation of pericardial sac

**Risk for Decreased Cardiac Tissue Perfusion:** Risk factor: inflammation in pericardial sac

**Deficient Knowledge** r/t unfamiliarity with information sources

**Risk for Imbalanced Nutrition: Less than Body Requirements:** Risk factors: fever, hypermetabolic state associated with fever

**Acute Pain** r/t biological injury, inflammation

## PERIODONTAL DISEASE

**Risk for Impaired Oral Mucous Membrane Integrity** (See **Oral Mucous Membrane Integrity, Impaired, Risk for,** Section II)

## PERIOPERATIVE HYPOTHERMIA

**Risk for Perioperative Hypothermia** (See **Perioperative Hypothermia, Risk for,** Section II)

## PERIOPERATIVE POSITIONING

**Risk for Perioperative Positioning Injury** (See **Perioperative Positioning injury, Risk for,** Section II)

## PERIPHERAL NEUROPATHY

*See Neuropathy, Peripheral*

## PERIPHERAL NEUROVASCULAR DYSFUNCTION

**Risk for Peripheral Neurovascular Dysfunction** (See **Peripheral Neurovascular Dysfunction, Risk for,** Section II)

*See Neuropathy, Peripheral; Peripheral Vascular Disease (PVD)*

## PERIPHERAL VASCULAR DISEASE (PVD)

**Ineffective Health Maintenance Behaviors** r/t deficient knowledge regarding self-care and treatment of disease

**Chronic Pain: Intermittent Claudication** r/t ischemia

**Ineffective Peripheral Tissue Perfusion** r/t disease process

**Risk for Adult Falls:** Risk factor: altered mobility

**Risk for Injury:** Risk factors: tissue hypoxia, altered mobility, altered sensation

**Risk for Peripheral Neurovascular Dysfunction:** Risk factor: possible vascular obstruction

**Risk for Impaired Tissue Integrity:** Risk factor: altered circulation or sensation

**Readiness for Enhanced Health Management:** self-care and treatment of disease

*See Neuropathy, Peripheral; Peripheral Neurovascular Dysfunction*

## PERITONEAL DIALYSIS

**Ineffective Breathing Pattern** r/t pressure from dialysate

**Impaired Comfort** r/t instillation of dialysate, temperature of dialysate

**Ineffective Home Maintenance Behaviors** r/t complex home treatment of client

**Deficient Knowledge** r/t treatment procedure, self-care with peritoneal dialysis

**Chronic Sorrow** r/t chronic disability

**Risk for Ineffective Coping:** Risk factor: disability requiring change in lifestyle

**Risk for Unstable Blood Glucose Level:** Risk factors: increased concentrations of glucose in dialysate, ineffective medication management

**Risk for Imbalanced Fluid Volume:** Risk factor: medical procedure

**Risk for Infection: Peritoneal:** Risk factors: invasive procedure, presence of catheter, dialysate

**Risk for Powerlessness:** Risk factors: chronic condition and care involved

*See Child with Chronic Condition; Hemodialysis; Hospitalized Child; Renal Failure; Renal Failure, Acute/Chronic, Child*

## PERITONITIS

**Ineffective Breathing Pattern** r/t pain, increased abdominal pressure

**Constipation** r/t decreased oral intake, decrease of peristalsis

**Deficient Fluid Volume** r/t retention of fluid in bowel with loss of circulating blood volume

**Nausea** r/t gastrointestinal irritation

**Imbalanced Nutrition: Less than Body Requirements** r/t nausea, vomiting

**Acute Pain** r/t inflammation and infection of gastrointestinal system

**Risk for Dysfunctional Gastrointestinal Motility:** Risk factor: gastrointestinal disease

**Risk for Infection** r/t inadequate knowledge to avoid exposure to pathogens

## PERNICIOUS ANEMIA

**Diarrhea** r/t malabsorption of nutrients

**Fatigue** r/t imbalanced nutrition: less than body requirements

**Impaired Memory** r/t lack of adequate red blood cells

**Nausea** r/t altered oral mucous membrane; sore tongue, bleeding gums

**Imbalanced Nutrition: Less than Body Requirements** r/t lack of appetite associated with nausea and altered oral mucous membrane

**Impaired Oral Mucous Membrane Integrity** r/t vitamin deficiency; inability to absorb vitamin $B_{12}$ associated with lack of intrinsic factor

**Risk for Adult Falls:** Risk factors: dizziness, lightheadedness

**Risk for Peripheral Neurovascular Dysfunction:** Risk factor: anemia

## PERSISTENT FETAL CIRCULATION

*See Congenital Heart Disease/Cardiac Anomalies*

## PERSONAL IDENTITY PROBLEMS

**Disturbed Personal Identity** (See **Identity, Personal, Disturbed,** Section II)

**Risk for Disturbed Personal Identity** (See **Disturbed Personal Identity, Risk for,** Section II)

## PERSONALITY DISORDER

**Ineffective Activity Planning** r/t unrealistic perception of events

**Impaired Individual Resilience** r/t psychological disorder

*See specific disorder: Antisocial Personality Disorder; Borderline Personality Disorder; OCD (Obsessive-Compulsive Disorder); Paranoid Personality Disorder*

## PERTUSSIS (WHOOPING COUGH)

**Risk for Impaired Emancipated Decision-Making:** Risk factor: indecision regarding administration of usual childhood vaccinations

*See Respiratory Infections, Acute Childhood*

## PESTICIDE CONTAMINATION

**Contamination** r/t use of environmental contaminants; pesticides

**Risk for Allergy Reaction:** Risk factor: repeated exposure to pesticides

## PETECHIAE

*See Anticoagulant Therapy; Clotting Disorder; DIC (Disseminated Intravascular Coagulation); Hemophilia*

## PETIT MAL SEIZURE

**Readiness for Enhanced Health Management:** wears medical alert bracelet; limits hazardous activities such as driving, swimming, working at heights, operating equipment

*See Epilepsy*

## PHARYNGITIS

*See Sore Throat*

## PHENYLKETONURIA (PKU)

*See PKU (Phenylketonuria)*

## PHEOCHROMOCYTOMA

**Anxiety** r/t symptoms from increased catecholamines—headache, palpitations, sweating, nervousness, nausea, vomiting, syncope

**Ineffective Health Maintenance Behaviors** r/t deficient knowledge regarding treatment and self-care

**Insomnia** r/t high levels of catecholamines

**Nausea** r/t increased catecholamines

**Risk for Decreased Cardiac Tissue Perfusion:** Risk factor: hypertension

*See Surgery, Perioperative Care; Surgery, Postoperative Care; Surgery, Preoperative Care*

## PHLEBITIS

*See Thrombophlebitis*

## PHOBIA (SPECIFIC)

**Fear** r/t presence or anticipation of specific object or situation

**Powerlessness** r/t anxiety about encountering unknown or known entity

**Impaired Individual Resilience** r/t psychological disorder

**Readiness for Enhanced Power:** expresses readiness to enhance identification of choices that can be made for change

*See Anxiety; Anxiety Disorder; Panic Disorder (Panic Attacks)*

## PHOTOSENSITIVITY

**Ineffective Health Maintenance Behaviors** r/t deficient knowledge regarding medications inducing photosensitivity

**Risk for Dry Eye:** Risk factors: pharmaceutical agents, sunlight exposure

**Risk for Impaired Skin Integrity:** Risk factor: exposure to sun

## PHYSICAL ABUSE

*See Abuse, Child; Abuse, Spouse, Parent, or Significant Other*

## PICA

**Anxiety** r/t stress

**Imbalanced Nutrition: Less than Body Requirements** r/t eating nonnutritive substances

**Impaired Parenting** r/t lack of supervision, food deprivation

**Risk for Constipation:** Risk factor: presence of undigestible materials in gastrointestinal tract

**Risk for Dysfunctional Gastrointestinal Motility:** Risk factor: abnormal eating behavior

**Risk for Infection:** Risk factor: ingestion of infectious agents via contaminated substances

**Risk for Poisoning:** Risk factor: ingestion of substances containing lead

*See Anemia*

## PID (PELVIC INFLAMMATORY DISEASE)

**Ineffective Health Maintenance Behaviors** r/t deficient knowledge regarding self-care, treatment of disease

**Acute Pain** r/t biological injury; inflammation, edema, congestion of pelvic tissues

**Ineffective Sexuality Pattern** r/t medically imposed abstinence from sexual activities until acute infection subsides, change in reproductive potential

**Risk for Infection:** Risk factors: insufficient knowledge to avoid exposure to pathogens; proper hygiene, nutrition, other health habits

*See Maturational Issues, Adolescent; STD (Sexually Transmitted Disease)*

## PIH (PREGNANCY-INDUCED HYPERTENSION/PREECLAMPSIA)

**Anxiety** r/t fear of the unknown, threat to self and infant, change in role functioning

**Death Anxiety** r/t threat of preeclampsia

**Decreased Diversional Activity Engagement** r/t bed rest

**Interrupted Family Processes** r/t situational crisis

**Ineffective Home Maintenance Behaviors** r/t bed rest

**Deficient Knowledge** r/t lack of experience with situation

**Impaired Physical Mobility** r/t medically prescribed limitations

**Impaired Parenting** r/t prescribed bed rest

**Powerlessness** r/t complication threatening pregnancy, medically prescribed limitations

**Ineffective Role Performance** r/t change in physical capacity to assume role of pregnant woman or resume other roles

**Situational Low Self-Esteem** r/t loss of idealized pregnancy

**Impaired Social Interaction** r/t imposed bed rest

**Risk for Imbalanced Fluid Volume:** Risk factors: hypertension, altered kidney function

**Risk for Injury: Fetal:** Risk factors: decreased uteroplacental perfusion, seizures

**Risk for Injury: Maternal:** Risk factors: vasospasm, high blood pressure

**Risk for Unstable Blood Pressure:** Risk factor: hypertension, imbalanced fluid volume

**Readiness for Enhanced Knowledge:** exhibits desire for information on managing condition

## PILOERECTION

**Hypothermia** r/t exposure to cold environment

## PINK EYE

*See Conjunctivitis*

## PINWORMS

**Impaired Comfort** r/t itching

**Ineffective Home Maintenance Behaviors** r/t inadequate cleaning of bed linen and toilet seats

**Insomnia** r/t discomfort

**Readiness for Enhanced Health Management:** proper handwashing; short, clean fingernails; avoiding hand, mouth, nose contact with unwashed hands; appropriate cleaning of bed linen and toilet seats

## PITUITARY TUMOR, BENIGN

*See Cushing's Disease*

## PKU (PHENYLKETONURIA)

**Risk for Delayed Child Development:** Risk factors: not following strict dietary program; eating foods extremely low in phenylalanine; avoiding eggs, milk, any foods containing aspartame (e.g., NutraSweet)

**Readiness for Enhanced Health Management:** testing for PKU and following prescribed dietary regimen

## PLACENTA ABRUPTIO

**Death Anxiety** r/t threat of mortality associated with bleeding

**Fear** r/t threat to self and fetus

**Ineffective Health Maintenance Behaviors** r/t deficient knowledge regarding treatment and control of hypertension associated with placenta abruptio

**Acute Pain: Abdominal/Back** r/t premature separation of placenta before delivery

**Risk for Bleeding:** Risk factor: placenta abruptio

P

**Risk for Deficient Fluid Volume:** Risk factor: maternal blood loss

**Risk for Powerlessness:** Risk factors: complications of pregnancy and unknown outcome

**Risk for Shock:** Risk factor: hypovolemia

**Risk for Spiritual Distress:** Risk factor: fear from unknown outcome of pregnancy

## PLACENTA PREVIA

**Death Anxiety** r/t threat of mortality associated with bleeding

**Disturbed Body Image** r/t negative feelings about body and reproductive ability, feelings of helplessness

**Ineffective Coping** r/t threat to self and fetus

**Decreased Diversional Activity Engagement** r/t long-term hospitalization

**Interrupted Family Processes** r/t maternal bed rest, hospitalization

**Fear** r/t threat to self and fetus, unknown future

**Ineffective Home Maintenance Behaviors** r/t maternal bed rest, hospitalization

**Impaired Physical Mobility** r/t medical protocol, maternal bed rest

**Ineffective Role Performance** r/t maternal bed rest, hospitalization

**Situational Low Self-Esteem** r/t situational crisis

**Spiritual Distress** r/t inability to participate in usual religious rituals, situational crisis

**Risk for Bleeding:** Risk factor: placenta previa

**Risk for Constipation:** Risk factors: bed rest, pregnancy

**Risk for Deficient Fluid Volume:** Risk factor: maternal blood loss

**Risk for Imbalanced Fluid Volume:** Risk factor: maternal blood loss

**Risk for Injury: Fetal and Maternal:** Risk factors: threat to uteroplacental perfusion, hemorrhage

**Risk for Disturbed Maternal–Fetal Dyad:** Risk factor: complication of pregnancy

**Risk for Impaired Parenting:** Risk factors: maternal bed rest, hospitalization

**Risk for Ineffective Peripheral Tissue Perfusion: Placental:** Risk factors: dilation of cervix, loss of placental implantation site

**Risk for Powerlessness:** Risk factors: complications of pregnancy, unknown outcome

**Risk for Shock:** Risk factor: hypovolemia

## PLANTAR FASCIITIS

**Impaired Comfort** r/t inflamed structures of feet

**Impaired Physical Mobility** r/t discomfort

**Acute Pain** r/t inflammation

**Chronic Pain** r/t inflammation

## PLEURAL EFFUSION

**Ineffective Breathing Pattern** r/t pain

**Excess Fluid Volume** r/t compromised regulatory mechanisms; heart, liver, or kidney failure

**Acute Pain** r/t inflammation, fluid accumulation

## PLEURAL FRICTION RUB

**Ineffective Breathing Pattern** r/t pain

**Acute Pain** r/t inflammation, fluid accumulation

## PLEURAL TAP

*See Pleural Effusion*

## PLEURISY

**Ineffective Breathing Pattern** r/t pain

**Impaired Gas Exchange** r/t ventilation perfusion imbalance

**Acute Pain** r/t pressure on pleural nerve endings associated with fluid accumulation or inflammation

**Impaired Walking** r/t activity intolerance, inability to "catch breath"

**Risk for Ineffective Airway Clearance:** Risk factors: increased secretions, ineffective cough because of pain

**Risk for Infection:** Risk factor: exposure to pathogens

## PMS (PREMENSTRUAL SYNDROME)

**Fatigue** r/t hormonal changes

**Excess Fluid Volume** r/t alterations of hormonal levels inducing fluid retention

**Deficient Knowledge** r/t methods to deal with and prevent syndrome

**Acute Pain** r/t hormonal stimulation of gastrointestinal structures

**Risk for Powerlessness:** Risk factors: lack of knowledge and ability to deal with symptoms

**Risk for Impaired Resilience:** Risk factor: PMS symptoms

**Readiness for Enhanced Communication:** willingness to express thoughts and feelings about PMS

**Readiness for Enhanced Health Management:** desire for information to manage and prevent symptoms

## PND (PAROXYSMAL NOCTURNAL DYSPNEA)

**Anxiety** r/t inability to breathe during sleep

**Ineffective Breathing Pattern** r/t increase in carbon dioxide levels, decrease in oxygen levels

**Insomnia** r/t suffocating feeling from fluid in lungs on awakening from sleep

**Sleep Deprivation** r/t inability to breathe during sleep

**Risk for Decreased Cardiac Tissue Perfusion:** Risk factor: hypoxia

**Risk for Powerlessness:** Risk factor: inability to control nocturnal dyspnea

**Readiness for Enhanced Sleep:** expresses willingness to learn measures to enhance sleep

## PNEUMONECTOMY

*See Thoracotomy*

## PNEUMONIA

**Decreased Activity Tolerance** r/t imbalance between oxygen supply and demand

**Ineffective Airway Clearance** r/t inflammation and presence of secretions

**Impaired Gas Exchange** r/t decreased functional lung tissue

**Dysfunctional Adult Ventilatory Weaning Response** r/t fatigue

**Ineffective Health Management** r/t deficient knowledge regarding self-care and treatment of disease

**Imbalanced Nutrition: Less than Body Requirements** r/t loss of appetite

**Impaired Oral Mucous Membrane Integrity** r/t dry mouth from mouth breathing, decreased fluid intake

**Ineffective Thermoregulation** r/t infectious process

**Risk for Acute Confusion:** Risk factors: underlying illness, hypoxia

**Risk for Deficient Fluid Volume:** Risk factor: inadequate intake of fluids

**Risk for Vascular Trauma:** Risk factor: irritation from intravenous antibiotics

*See Respiratory Infections, Acute Childhood*

## PNEUMOTHORAX

**Fear** r/t threat to own well-being, difficulty breathing

**Impaired Gas Exchange** r/t ventilation-perfusion imbalance, decreased functional lung tissue

**Impaired Spontaneous Ventilation** r/t respiratory muscle fatigue with difficulty breathing

**Acute Pain** r/t recent injury, coughing, deep breathing

**Risk for Injury:** Risk factor: possible complications associated with closed chest drainage system

*See Chest Tubes*

## POISONING, RISK FOR

**Risk for Poisoning** (See **Poisoning, Risk for,** Section II)

## POLIOMYELITIS

*See Paralysis*

## POLYDIPSIA

*See Diabetes Mellitus*

## POLYPHAGIA

**Readiness for Enhanced Nutrition:** knowledge of appropriate diet for diabetes

*See Diabetes Mellitus*

P

## POLYURIA

*See Diabetes Mellitus*

## POSTOPERATIVE CARE

*See Surgery, Postoperative Care*

## POSTPARTUM DEPRESSION

**Anxiety** r/t new responsibilities of parenting

**Disturbed Body Image** r/t normal postpartum recovery

**Ineffective Childbearing Process** r/t depression/lack of support system

**Ineffective Coping** r/t hormonal changes

**Fatigue** r/t childbirth, postpartum state, crying child

**Risk-Prone Health Behavior** r/t lack of support systems

**Ineffective Home Maintenance Behaviors** r/t fatigue, care of newborn

**Hopelessness** r/t stress, exhaustion

**Deficient Knowledge** r/t lifestyle changes

**Impaired Parenting** r/t hormone-induced depression

**Ineffective Role Performance** r/t new responsibilities of parenting

**Sexual Dysfunction** r/t fear of another pregnancy, postpartum pain, lochia flow

**Sleep Deprivation** r/t environmental stimulation of newborn

**Impaired Social Interaction** r/t change in role functioning

**Risk for Disturbed Personal Identity:** Risk factor: role change/depression/inability to cope

**Risk for Situational Low Self-Esteem:** Risk factor: decreased power over feelings of sadness

**Risk for Spiritual Distress:** Risk factors: altered relationships, social isolation

**Readiness for Enhanced Hope:** expresses desire to enhance hope and interconnectedness with others

*See Depression (Major Depressive Disorder)*

## POSTPARTUM HEMORRHAGE

**Decreased Activity Tolerance** r/t anemia from loss of blood

**Death Anxiety** r/t threat of mortality associated with bleeding

**Disturbed Body Image** r/t loss of ideal childbirth

**Insufficient Breast Milk Production** r/t fluid volume depletion

**Interrupted Breastfeeding** r/t separation from infant for medical treatment

**Decreased Cardiac Output** r/t hypovolemia

**Fear** r/t threat to self, unknown future

**Deficient Fluid Volume** r/t uterine atony, loss of blood

**Ineffective Home Maintenance Behaviors** r/t lack of stamina

**Deficient Knowledge** r/t lack of exposure to situation

**Acute Pain** r/t nursing and medical interventions to control bleeding

**Ineffective Peripheral Tissue Perfusion** r/t hypovolemia

**Risk for Bleeding:** Risk factor: postpartum complications

**Risk for Impaired Childbearing:** Risk factor: postpartum complication

**Risk for Imbalanced Fluid Volume:** Risk factor: maternal blood loss

**Risk for Infection:** Risk factors: loss of blood, depressed immunity

**Risk for Impaired Parenting:** Risk factor: weakened maternal condition

**Risk for Powerlessness:** Risk factor: acute illness

**Risk for Shock:** Risk factor: hypovolemia

## POSTPARTUM, NORMAL CARE

**Anxiety** r/t change in role functioning, parenting

**Effective Breastfeeding** r/t basic breastfeeding knowledge, support of partner and health care provider

**Fatigue** r/t childbirth, new responsibilities of parenting, body changes

**Acute Pain** r/t episiotomy, lacerations, bruising, breast engorgement, headache, sore nipples, epidural or intravenous site, hemorrhoids

**Sexual Dysfunction** r/t recent childbirth

**Impaired Tissue Integrity** r/t episiotomy, lacerations

**Sleep Deprivation** r/t care of infant

**Impaired Urinary Elimination** r/t effects of anesthesia, tissue trauma

**Risk for Constipation:** Risk factors: hormonal effects on smooth muscles, fear of straining with defecation, effects of anesthesia

**Risk for Infection:** Risk factors: tissue trauma, blood loss

**Readiness for Enhanced Family Coping:** adaptation to new family member

**Readiness for Enhanced Hope:** desire to increase hope

**Readiness for Enhanced Parenting:** expresses willingness to enhance parenting skills

## POST-TRAUMA SYNDROME

**Post-Trauma Syndrome** (See **Post-Trauma Syndrome,** Section II)

## POST-TRAUMA SYNDROME, RISK FOR

**Risk for Post-Trauma Syndrome** (See **Post-Trauma Syndrome, Risk for,** Section II)

## POSTTRAUMATIC STRESS DISORDER (PTSD)

*See PTSD (Post-Traumatic Stress Disorder)*

## POTASSIUM, INCREASE/DECREASE

*See Hyperkalemia; Hypokalemia*

## POWER/POWERLESSNESS

**Powerlessness** (See **Powerlessness,** Section II)

**Risk for Powerlessness** (See **Powerlessness, Risk for,** Section II)

**Readiness for Enhanced Power** (See **Power, Readiness for Enhanced,** Section II)

## PREECLAMPSIA

*See PIH (Pregnancy-Induced Hypertension/Preeclampsia)*

## PREGNANCY, CARDIAC DISORDERS

*See Cardiac Disorders in Pregnancy*

## PREGNANCY-INDUCED HYPERTENSION/PREECLAMPSIA (PIH)

*See PIH (Pregnancy-Induced Hypertension/Preeclampsia)*

## PREGNANCY LOSS

**Anxiety** r/t threat to role functioning, health status, situational crisis

**Compromised Family Coping** r/t lack of support by significant other because of personal suffering

**Ineffective Coping** r/t situational crisis

**Maladaptive Grieving** r/t loss of pregnancy, fetus, or child

**Acute Pain** r/t surgical intervention

**Ineffective Role Performance** r/t inability to assume parenting role

**Ineffective Sexuality Pattern** r/t self-esteem disturbance resulting from pregnancy loss and anxiety about future pregnancies

**Chronic Sorrow** r/t loss of a fetus or child

**Spiritual Distress** r/t intense suffering from loss of child

**Risk for Deficient Fluid Volume:** Risk factor: blood loss

**Risk for Maladaptive Grieving:** Risk factor: loss of pregnancy

**Risk for Infection:** Risk factor: retained products of conception

**Risk for Powerlessness:** Risk factor: situational crisis

**Risk for Ineffective Relationship:** Risk factor: poor communication skills in dealing with the loss

**Risk for Spiritual Distress:** Risk factor: intense suffering

**Readiness for Enhanced Communication:** willingness to express feelings and thoughts about loss

P

**Readiness for Enhanced Hope:** expresses desire to enhance hope

**Readiness for Enhanced Spiritual Well-Being:** desire for acceptance of loss

## PREGNANCY, NORMAL

**Anxiety** r/t unknown future, threat to self secondary to pain of labor

**Disturbed Body Image** r/t altered body function and appearance

**Interrupted Family Processes** r/t developmental transition of pregnancy

**Fatigue** r/t increased energy demands

**Fear** r/t labor and delivery

**Deficient Knowledge** r/t primiparity

**Nausea** r/t hormonal changes of pregnancy

**Imbalanced Nutrition: Less than Body Requirements** r/t growing fetus, nausea

**Imbalanced Nutrition: More than Body Requirements** r/t deficient knowledge regarding nutritional needs of pregnancy

**Sleep Deprivation** r/t uncomfortable pregnancy state

**Impaired Urinary Elimination** r/t frequency caused by increased pelvic pressure and hormonal stimulation

**Risk for Constipation:** Risk factor: pregnancy

**Risk for Sexual Dysfunction:** Risk factors: altered body function, self-concept, body image with pregnancy

**Readiness for Enhanced Childbearing Process:** appropriate prenatal care

**Readiness for Enhanced Family Coping:** satisfying partner relationship, attention to gratification of needs, effective adaptation to developmental tasks of pregnancy

**Readiness for Enhanced Family Processes:** family adapts to change

**Readiness for Enhanced Health Management:** seeks information for prenatal self-care

**Readiness for Enhanced Nutrition:** desire for knowledge of appropriate nutrition during pregnancy

**Readiness for Enhanced Parenting:** expresses willingness to enhance parenting skills

**Readiness for Enhanced Relationship:** meeting developmental goals associated with pregnancy

**Readiness for Enhanced Spiritual Well-Being:** new role as parent

*See Discomforts of Pregnancy*

## PREMATURE DILATION OF THE CERVIX (INCOMPETENT CERVIX)

**Ineffective Activity Planning** r/t unrealistic perception of events

**Ineffective Coping** r/t bed rest, threat to fetus

**Decreased Diversional Activity Engagement** r/t bed rest

**Fear** r/t potential loss of infant

**Maladaptive Grieving** r/t potential loss of infant

**Deficient Knowledge** r/t treatment regimen, prognosis for pregnancy

**Impaired Physical Mobility** r/t imposed bed rest to prevent preterm birth

**Powerlessness** r/t inability to control outcome of pregnancy

**Ineffective Role Performance** r/t inability to continue usual patterns of responsibility

**Situational Low Self-Esteem** r/t inability to complete normal pregnancy

**Sexual Dysfunction** r/t fear of harm to fetus

**Impaired Social Interaction** r/t bed rest

**Risk for Infection:** Risk factor: invasive procedures to prevent preterm birth

**Risk for Injury: Fetal:** Risk factors: preterm birth, use of anesthetics

**Risk for Injury: Maternal:** Risk factor: surgical procedures to prevent preterm birth (e.g., cerclage)

**Risk for Impaired Resilience:** Risk factor: complication of pregnancy

**Risk for Spiritual Distress:** Risk factors: physical/psychological stress

## PREMATURE INFANT (CHILD)

**Insufficient Breast Milk Production** r/t ineffective sucking, latching on of the infant

**Impaired Gas Exchange** r/t effects of cardiopulmonary insufficiency

**Disorganized Infant Behavior** r/t prematurity

**Insomnia** r/t noisy and noxious intensive care environment

**Neonatal Hyperbilirubinemia** r/t infant experiences difficulty making transition to extrauterine life

**Imbalanced Nutrition: Less than Body Requirements** r/t delayed or understimulated rooting reflex, easy fatigue during feeding, diminished endurance

**Impaired Swallowing** r/t decreased or absent gag reflex, fatigue

**Ineffective Thermoregulation** r/t large body surface/weight ratio, immaturity of thermal regulation, state of prematurity

**Risk for Delayed Child Development:** Risk factor: prematurity

**Risk for Infection:** Risk factors: inadequate, immature, or undeveloped acquired immune response

**Risk for Injury:** Risk factor: prolonged mechanical ventilation, retinopathy of prematurity (ROP) secondary to 100% oxygen environment

**Risk for Neonatal Hyperbilirubinemia:** Risk factor: late preterm birth

**Readiness for Enhanced Organized Infant Behavior:** use of some self-regulatory measures

## PREMATURE INFANT (PARENT)

**Ineffective Breastfeeding** r/t disrupted establishment of effective pattern secondary to prematurity or insufficient opportunities

**Decisional Conflict** r/t support system deficit, multiple sources of information

**Compromised Family Coping** r/t disrupted family roles and disorganization, prolonged condition exhausting supportive capacity of significant persons

**Ineffective Infant Feeding Dynamics** r/t insufficient knowledge of nutritional needs

**Maladaptive Grieving** r/t loss of perfect child possibly leading to complicated grieving

**Risk for Maladaptive Grieving (Prolonged)** r/t unresolved conflicts

**Parental Role Conflict** r/t expressed concerns, expressed inability to care

for child's physical, emotional, or developmental needs

**Chronic Sorrow** r/t threat of loss of a child, prolonged hospitalization

**Spiritual Distress** r/t challenged belief or value systems regarding moral or ethical implications of treatment plans

**Risk for Impaired Attachment:** Risk factors: separation, physical barriers, lack of privacy

**Risk for Disturbed Maternal–Fetal Dyad:** Risk factor: complication of pregnancy

**Risk for Powerlessness:** Risk factor: inability to control situation

**Risk for Impaired Resilience:** Risk factor: premature infant

**Risk for Spiritual Distress:** Risk factor: challenged belief or value systems regarding moral or ethical implications of treatment plans

**Readiness for Enhanced Family Process:** adaptation to change associated with premature infant

*See Child with Chronic Condition; Hospitalized Child*

## PREMATURE RUPTURE OF MEMBRANES

**Anxiety** r/t threat to infant's health status

**Disturbed Body Image** r/t inability to carry pregnancy to term

**Ineffective Coping** r/t situational crisis

**Maladaptive Grieving** r/t potential loss of infant

**Situational Low Self-Esteem** r/t inability to carry pregnancy to term

**Risk for Ineffective Childbearing Process:** Risk factor: complication of pregnancy

**Risk for Infection:** Risk factor: rupture of membranes

**Risk for Injury: Fetal:** Risk factor: risk of premature birth

## PREMENSTRUAL TENSION SYNDROME (PMS)

*See PMS (Premenstrual Tension Syndrome)*

## PRENATAL CARE, NORMAL

**Readiness for Enhanced Childbearing Process:** appropriate prenatal lifestyle

**Readiness for Enhanced Knowledge:** appropriate prenatal care

**Readiness for Enhanced Spiritual Well-Being:** new role as parent

*See Pregnancy, Normal*

## PRENATAL TESTING

**Anxiety** r/t unknown outcome, delayed test results

**Acute Pain** r/t invasive procedures

**Risk for Infection:** Risk factor: invasive procedures during amniocentesis or chorionic villus sampling

**Risk for Injury:** Risk factor: invasive procedures

## PREOPERATIVE TEACHING

*See Surgery, Preoperative Care*

## PRESSURE INJURY

**Impaired Bed Mobility** r/t intolerance to activity, pain, cognitive impairment, depression, severe anxiety, severity of illness

**Imbalanced Nutrition: Less than Body Requirements** r/t limited access to food, inability to absorb nutrients because of biological factors, anorexia

**Acute Pain** r/t tissue destruction, exposure of nerves

**Impaired Skin Integrity: Stage I or II Pressure Injury** r/t physical immobility, mechanical factors, altered circulation, skin irritants, excessive moisture

**Impaired Tissue Integrity: Stage III or IV Pressure Injury** r/t altered circulation, impaired physical mobility, excessive moisture

**Risk for Infection:** Risk factors: physical immobility, mechanical factors (shearing forces, pressure, restraint, altered circulation, skin irritants, excessive moisture, open wound)

**Risk for Adult Pressure Injury** (See **Adult Pressure Injury,** Section II)

**Risk for Child Pressure Injury** (See **Child Pressure Injury,** Section II)

**Risk for Neonate Pressure Injury** (See **Neonate Pressure Injury,** Section II)

## PRETERM LABOR

**Anxiety** r/t threat to fetus, change in role functioning, change in environment and interaction patterns, use of tocolytic drugs

**Ineffective Coping** r/t situational crisis, preterm labor

**Decreased Diversional Activity Engagement** r/t long-term hospitalization

**Risk for Maladaptive Grieving** r/t loss of idealized pregnancy, potential loss of fetus

**Ineffective Home Maintenance Behaviors** r/t medical restrictions

**Impaired Physical Mobility** r/t medically imposed restrictions

**Ineffective Role Performance** r/t inability to carry out normal roles secondary to bed rest or hospitalization, change in expected course of pregnancy

**Situational Low Self-Esteem** r/t threatened ability to carry pregnancy to term

**Sexual Dysfunction** r/t actual or perceived limitation imposed by preterm labor and/or prescribed treatment, separation from partner because of hospitalization

**Sleep Deprivation** r/t change in usual pattern secondary to contractions, hospitalization, treatment regimen

**Impaired Social Interaction** r/t prolonged bed rest or hospitalization

**Risk for Injury: Fetal:** Risk factors: premature birth, immature body systems

**Risk for Injury: Maternal:** Risk factor: use of tocolytic drugs

**Risk for Powerlessness:** Risk factor: lack of control over preterm labor

**Risk for Vascular Trauma:** Risk factor: intravenous medication

**Readiness for Enhanced Childbearing Process:** appropriate prenatal lifestyle

**Readiness for Enhanced Comfort:** expresses desire to enhance relaxation

**P**

Readiness for Enhanced Communication: willingness to discuss thoughts and feelings about situation

## PROBLEM-SOLVING DYSFUNCTION

Defensive Coping r/t situational crisis

Impaired Emancipated Decision-Making r/t problem-solving dysfunction

Risk for Chronic Low Self-Esteem: Risk factor: repeated failures

Readiness for Enhanced Communication: willing to share ideas with others

Readiness for Enhanced Relationship: shares information and ideas between partners

Readiness for Enhanced Resilience: identifies available resources

Readiness for Enhanced Spiritual Well-Being: desires to draw on inner strength and find meaning and purpose to life

## PROJECTION

Anxiety r/t threat to self-concept

Defensive Coping r/t inability to acknowledge that own behavior may be a problem, blaming others

Chronic Low Self-Esteem r/t failure

Impaired Social Interaction r/t self-concept disturbance, confrontational communication style

Risk for Loneliness: Risk factor: blaming others for problems

See Paranoid Personality Disorder

## PROLAPSED UMBILICAL CORD

Fear r/t threat to fetus, impending surgery

Ineffective Peripheral Tissue Perfusion: Fetal r/t interruption in umbilical blood flow

Risk for Ineffective Cerebral Tissue Perfusion: Fetal: Risk factor: cord compression

Risk for Injury: Risk factor (maternal): emergency surgery

See TURP (Transurethral Resection of the Prostate)

## PROSTATIC HYPERTROPHY

Ineffective Health Maintenance Behaviors r/t deficient knowledge regarding self-care and prevention of complications

Sleep Deprivation r/t nocturia

Urinary Retention r/t obstruction

Risk for Infection: Risk factors: urinary residual after voiding, bacterial invasion of bladder

See BPH (Benign Prostatic Hypertrophy)

## PROSTATITIS

Impaired Comfort r/t inflammation

Ineffective Health Maintenance Behaviors r/t deficient knowledge regarding treatment

Urge Urinary Incontinence r/t irritation of bladder

Ineffective Protection r/t depressed immune system

## PRURITUS

Impaired Comfort r/t inflammation of skin causing itching

Deficient Knowledge r/t methods to treat and prevent itching

Risk for Impaired Skin Integrity: Risk factors: scratching, dry skin

## PSORIASIS

Disturbed Body Image r/t lesions on body

Impaired Comfort r/t irritated skin

Ineffective Health Maintenance Behaviors r/t deficient knowledge regarding treatment modalities

Powerlessness r/t lack of control over condition with frequent exacerbations and remissions

Impaired Skin Integrity r/t lesions on body

## PSYCHOSIS

Ineffective Activity Planning r/t compromised ability to process information

Ineffective Health Maintenance Behaviors r/t cognitive impairment, ineffective individual and family coping

Self-Neglect r/t mental disorder

Impaired Individual Resilience r/t psychological disorder

**Situational Low Self-Esteem** r/t excessive use of defense mechanisms (e.g., projection, denial, rationalization)

**Risk for Disturbed Personal Identity:** Risk factor: psychosis

**Impaired Mood Regulation** r/t psychosis

**Risk for Post-Trauma Syndrome:** Risk factor: diminished ego strength

*See Schizophrenia*

## PTCA (PERCUTANEOUS TRANSLUMINAL CORONARY ANGIOPLASTY)

*See Angioplasty, Coronary*

## PTSD (POSTTRAUMATIC STRESS DISORDER)

**Anxiety** r/t exposure to internal or external cues that symbolize or resemble an aspect of the traumatic event

**Chronic Sorrow** r/t chronic disability (e.g., physical, mental)

**Death Anxiety** r/t psychological stress associated with traumatic event

**Ineffective Breathing Pattern** r/t hyperventilation associated with anxiety

**Ineffective Coping** r/t extreme anxiety

**Ineffective Impulse Control** r/t thinking of initial trauma experience

**Ineffective Relationship** r/t stressors

**Insomnia** r/t recurring nightmares

**Post-Trauma Syndrome** r/t exposure to a traumatic event

**Sleep Deprivation** r/t nightmares interrupting sleep associated with traumatic event

**Spiritual Distress** r/t feelings of detachment or estrangement from others

**Risk for Impaired Resilience:** Risk factor: chronicity of existing crisis

**Risk for Powerlessness:** Risk factors: flashbacks, reliving event

**Risk for Ineffective Relationship:** Risk factor: stressful life events

**Risk for Self- or Other-Directed Violence:** Risk factors: fear of self or others

**Readiness for Enhanced Comfort:** expresses desire to enhance relaxation

**Readiness for Enhanced Communication:** willingness to express feelings and thoughts

**Readiness for Enhanced Spiritual Well-Being:** desire for harmony after stressful event

## PULMONARY EDEMA

**Anxiety** r/t fear of suffocation

**Ineffective Airway Clearance** r/t presence of tracheobronchial secretions

**Decreased Cardiac Output** r/t increased preload, infective forward perfusion

**Impaired Gas Exchange** r/t extravasation of extravascular fluid in lung tissues and alveoli

**Ineffective Health Maintenance Behaviors** r/t deficient knowledge regarding treatment regimen

**Sleep Deprivation** r/t inability to breathe

**Risk for Acute Confusion:** Risk factor: hypoxia

*See Heart Failure*

## PULMONARY EMBOLISM (PE)

**Anxiety** r/t fear of suffocation

**Decreased Cardiac Output** r/t right ventricular failure secondary to obstructed pulmonary artery

**Fear** r/t severe pain, possible death

**Impaired Gas Exchange** r/t altered blood flow to alveoli secondary to embolus

**Deficient Knowledge** r/t activities to prevent embolism, self-care after diagnosis of embolism

**Acute Pain** r/t biological injury, lack of oxygen to cells

**Ineffective Peripheral Tissue Perfusion** r/t deep vein thrombus formation

**Risk for Thrombosis** r/t sedentary lifestyle

*See Anticoagulant Therapy*

## PULMONARY STENOSIS

*See Congenital Heart Disease/Cardiac Anomalies*

## PULSE DEFICIT

**Risk for Decreased Cardiac Output** r/t dysrhythmia

*See Dysrhythmia*

## PULSE OXIMETRY

**Readiness for Enhanced Knowledge:** information about treatment regimen

*See Hypoxia*

## PULSE PRESSURE, INCREASED

*See Intracranial Pressure, Increased*

## PULSE PRESSURE, NARROWED

*See Shock, Hypovolemic*

## PULSES, ABSENT OR DIMINISHED PERIPHERAL

**Ineffective Peripheral Tissue Perfusion** r/t interruption of arterial flow

**Risk for Peripheral Neurovascular Dysfunction:** Risk factors: fractures, mechanical compression, orthopedic surgery trauma, immobilization, burns, vascular obstruction

## PURPURA

*See Clotting Disorder*

## PYELONEPHRITIS

**Ineffective Health Maintenance Behaviors** r/t deficient knowledge regarding self-care, treatment of disease, prevention of further urinary tract infections

**Acute Pain** r/t inflammation and irritation of urinary tract

**Disturbed Sleep Pattern** r/t urinary frequency

**Impaired Urinary Elimination** r/t irritation of urinary tract

## PYLORIC STENOSIS

**Imbalanced Nutrition: Less than Body Requirements** r/t vomiting secondary to pyloric sphincter obstruction

**Acute Pain** r/t abdominal fullness

**Risk for Decreased Fluid Volume:** Risk factors: vomiting, dehydration

*See Hospitalized Child*

## PYLOROMYOTOMY (PYLORIC STENOSIS REPAIR)

*See Surgery Preoperative Care, Perioperative Care, Postoperative Care*

# R

## RA (RHEUMATOID ARTHRITIS)

*See Rheumatoid Arthritis (RA)*

## RABIES

**Ineffective Health Maintenance Behaviors** r/t deficient knowledge regarding care of wound, isolation, and observation of infected animal

**Acute Pain** r/t multiple immunization injections

**Risk for Ineffective Cerebral Tissue Perfusion:** Risk factor: rabies virus

## RADIAL NERVE DYSFUNCTION

**Acute Pain** r/t trauma to hand or arm

**Chronic Pain** r/t trauma hand or arm

*See Neuropathy, Peripheral*

## RADIATION THERAPY (RADIOTHERAPY)

**Decreased Activity Tolerance** r/t fatigue from possible anemia

**Disturbed Body Image** r/t change in appearance, hair loss

**Diarrhea** r/t irradiation effects

**Fatigue** r/t malnutrition from lack of appetite, nausea, and vomiting; side effect of radiation

**Deficient Knowledge** r/t what to expect with radiation therapy, how to do self-care

**Nausea** r/t side effects of radiation

**Imbalanced Nutrition: Less than Body Requirements** r/t anorexia, nausea, vomiting, irradiation of areas of pharynx and esophagus

**Impaired Oral Mucous Membrane Integrity** r/t irradiation effects

**Ineffective Protection** r/t suppression of bone marrow

**Risk for Dry Mouth:** Risk factor: possible side effect of radiation treatments

**Risk for Impaired Oral Mucous Membrane Integrity:** Risk factor: radiation treatments

**Risk for Powerlessness:** Risk factors: medical treatment and possible side effects

**R**

**Risk for Impaired Resilience:** Risk factor: radiation treatment

**Risk for Impaired Skin Integrity:** Risk factor: irradiation effects

**Risk for Spiritual Distress:** Risk factors: radiation treatment, prognosis

**Ineffective Dry Eye Self-Management** inattentive to dry eye symptoms from radiotherapy treatment regimen

## RADICAL NECK DISSECTION

*See Laryngectomy*

## RAGE

**Risk-Prone Health Behavior** r/t multiple stressors

**Labile Emotional Control** r/t psychiatric disorders and mood disorders

**Impaired Individual Resilience** r/t poor impulse control

**Stress Overload** r/t multiple coexisting stressors

**Risk for Self-Mutilation:** Risk factor: command hallucinations

**Risk for Suicidal Behavior:** Risk factor: desire to kill self

**Risk for Other-Directed Violence:** Risk factors: panic state, manic excitement, organic brain syndrome

## RAPE-TRAUMA SYNDROME

**Rape-Trauma Syndrome** (See **Rape-Trauma Syndrome,** Section II)

**Chronic Sorrow** r/t forced loss of virginity

**Risk for Ineffective Childbearing Process** r/t to trauma and violence

**Risk for Post-Trauma Syndrome:** Risk factor: trauma or violence associated with rape

**Risk for Powerlessness:** Risk factor: inability to control thoughts about incident

**Risk for Ineffective Relationship:** Risk factor: trauma and violence

**Risk for Chronic Low Self-Esteem:** Risk factors: perceived lack of respect from others, feeling violated

**Risk for Spiritual Distress:** Risk factor: forced loss of virginity

## RASH

**Impaired Comfort** r/t pruritus

**Impaired Skin Integrity** r/t mechanical trauma

**Risk for Infection:** Risk factors: traumatized tissue, broken skin

## RATIONALIZATION

**Defensive Coping** r/t situational crisis, inability to accept blame for consequences of own behavior

**Ineffective Denial** r/t fear of consequences, actual or perceived loss

**Impaired Individual Resilience** r/t psychological disturbance

**Risk for Post-Trauma Syndrome:** Risk factor: survivor's role in event

**Readiness for Enhanced Communication:** expresses desire to share thoughts and feelings

**Readiness for Enhanced Spiritual Well-Being:** possibility of seeking harmony with self, others, higher power, God

## RATS, RODENTS IN HOME

**Ineffective Home Maintenance Behaviors** r/t lack of knowledge, insufficient finances

**Risk for Allergy Reaction:** Risk factor: repeated exposure to environmental contamination

*See Filthy Home Environment*

## RAYNAUD'S DISEASE

**Deficient Knowledge** r/t lack of information about disease process, possible complications, self-care needs regarding disease process and medication

**Ineffective Peripheral Tissue Perfusion** r/t transient reduction of blood flow

**Acute Pain** r/t transient reduction in blood flow

## RDS (RESPIRATORY DISTRESS SYNDROME)

*See Respiratory Conditions of the Neonate*

## RECTAL FULLNESS

**Chronic Functional Constipation** r/t decreased activity level, decreased fluid intake, inadequate fiber in diet, decreased peristalsis, side effects of antidepressant or antipsychotic therapy

**Risk for Chronic Functional Constipation:** Risk factor: habitual denial of or ignoring urge to defecate

## RECTAL LUMP

*See Hemorrhoids*

## RECTAL PAIN/BLEEDING

**Chronic Functional Constipation** r/t pain on defecation

**Deficient Knowledge** r/t possible causes of rectal bleeding, pain, treatment modalities

**Acute Pain** r/t pressure of defecation

**Risk for Bleeding:** Risk factor: rectal disease

## RECTAL SURGERY

*See Hemorrhoidectomy*

## RECTOCELE REPAIR

**Chronic Functional Constipation** r/t painful defecation

**Ineffective Health Maintenance Behaviors** r/t deficient knowledge of postoperative care of surgical site, dietary measures, exercise to prevent constipation

**Acute Pain** r/t surgical procedure

**Urinary Retention** r/t edema from surgery

**Risk for Bleeding:** Risk factor: surgery

**Risk for Surgical Site Infection:** Risk factors: surgical procedure, possible contamination of area with feces

## REFLEX INCONTINENCE

**Mixed Urinary Incontinence** (See **Incontinence, Urinary, Mixed,** Section II)

## REGRESSION

**Anxiety** r/t threat to or change in health status

**Defensive Coping** r/t denial of obvious problems, weaknesses

**Self-Neglect** r/t functional impairment

**Powerlessness** r/t health care environment

**Impaired Individual Resilience** r/t psychological disturbance

**Ineffective Role Performance** r/t powerlessness over health status

*See Hospitalized Child; Separation Anxiety*

## REGRETFUL

**Anxiety** r/t situational or maturational crises

**Death Anxiety** r/t feelings of not having accomplished goals in life

**Risk for Spiritual Distress:** Risk factor: inability to forgive

## REHABILITATION

**Ineffective Coping** r/t loss of normal function

**Impaired Physical Mobility** r/t injury, surgery, psychosocial condition warranting rehabilitation

**Self-Care Deficit: Specify** r/t impaired physical mobility

**Risk for Adult Falls:** Risk factor: physical deconditioning

**Risk for Child Falls:** Risk factor: Decreased lower extremity strength

**Readiness for Enhanced Comfort:** expresses desire to enhance feeling of comfort

**Readiness for Enhanced Self-Concept:** accepts strengths and limitations

**Readiness for Enhanced Health Self-Management:** expresses desire to manage rehabilitation

## RELATIONSHIP

**Ineffective Relationship** (See **Ineffective Relationship,** Section II)

**Readiness for Enhanced Relationship** (See **Risk for Enhanced Relationship,** Section II)

## RELAXATION TECHNIQUES

**Anxiety** r/t situational crisis

**Readiness for Enhanced Comfort:** expresses desire to enhance relaxation

**Readiness for Enhanced Health Self-Management:** desire to manage illness

**Readiness for Enhanced Religiosity:** requests religious materials or experiences

**Readiness for Enhanced Resilience:** desire to enhance resilience

**R**

**Readiness for Enhanced Self-Concept:** willingness to enhance self-concept

**Readiness for Enhanced Spiritual Well-Being:** seeking comfort from higher power

## RELIGIOSITY

**Impaired Religiosity** (See **Religiosity, Impaired,** Section II)

**Risk for Impaired Religiosity** (See **Religiosity, Impaired, Risk for,** Section II)

**Readiness for Enhanced Religiosity** (See **Religiosity, Readiness for Enhanced,** Section II)

## RELIGIOUS CONCERNS

**Spiritual Distress** r/t separation from religious or cultural ties

**Risk for Impaired Religiosity:** Risk factors: ineffective support, coping, caregiving

**Risk for Spiritual Distress:** Risk factors: physical or psychological stress

**Readiness for Enhanced Spiritual Well-Being:** desire for increased spirituality

## RELOCATION STRESS SYNDROME

**Relocation Stress Syndrome** (See **Relocation Stress Syndrome,** Section II)

**Risk for Relocation Stress Syndrome** (See **Relocation Stress Syndrome, Risk for,** Section II)

## RENAL FAILURE

**Decreased Activity Tolerance** r/t effects of anemia, heart failure

**Death Anxiety** r/t unknown outcome of disease

**Decreased Cardiac Output** r/t effects of heart failure, elevated potassium levels interfering with conduction system

**Impaired Comfort** r/t pruritus

**Ineffective Coping** r/t depression resulting from chronic disease

**Fatigue** r/t effects of chronic uremia and anemia

**Excessive Fluid Volume** r/t decreased urine output, sodium retention, inappropriate fluid intake

**Ineffective Health Self-Management** r/t complexity of health care regimen,

inadequate number of cues to action, perceived barriers, powerlessness

**Imbalanced Nutrition: Less than Body Requirements** r/t anorexia, nausea, vomiting, altered taste sensation, dietary restrictions

**Impaired Oral Mucous Membrane Integrity** r/t irritation from nitrogenous waste products

**Chronic Sorrow** r/t chronic illness

**Spiritual Distress** r/t dealing with chronic illness

**Impaired Urinary Elimination** r/t effects of disease, need for dialysis

**Risk for Electrolyte Imbalance:** Risk factor: renal dysfunction

**Risk for Infection:** Risk factor: altered immune functioning

**Risk for Injury:** Risk factors: bone changes, neuropathy, muscle weakness

**Risk for Impaired Oral Mucous Membrane Integrity:** Risk factors: dehydration, effects of uremia

**Risk for Powerlessness:** Risk factor: chronic illness

**Risk for Sepsis:** Risk factor: infection

## RENAL FAILURE ACUTE/CHRONIC, CHILD

**Disturbed Body Image** r/t growth retardation, bone changes, visibility of dialysis access devices (shunt, fistula), edema

**Decreased Diversional Activity Engagement** r/t immobility during dialysis

*See Child with Chronic Condition; Hospitalized Child*

## RENAL FAILURE, NONOLIGURIC

**Anxiety** r/t change in health status

**Risk for Deficient Fluid Volume:** Risk factor: loss of large volumes of urine

*See Renal Failure*

## RESPIRATORY ACIDOSIS

*See Acidosis, Respiratory*

## RESPIRATORY CONDITIONS OF THE NEONATE (RESPIRATORY DISTRESS SYNDROME [RDS], MECONIUM ASPIRATION, DIAPHRAGMATIC HERNIA)

**Ineffective Airway Clearance** r/t sequelae of attempts to breathe in utero resulting in meconium aspiration

**Fatigue** r/t increased energy requirements and metabolic demands

**Impaired Gas Exchange** r/t decreased surfactant, immature lung tissue

**Dysfunctional Ventilator Weaning Response** r/t immature respiratory system

**Risk for Infection:** Risk factors: tissue destruction or irritation as a result of aspiration of meconium fluid

*See Bronchopulmonary Dysplasia; Hospitalized Child; Premature Infant, Child*

## RESPIRATORY DISTRESS

*See Dyspnea*

## RESPIRATORY DISTRESS SYNDROME (RDS)

*See Respiratory Conditions of the Neonate*

## RESPIRATORY INFECTIONS, ACUTE CHILDHOOD (CROUP, EPIGLOTTITIS, PERTUSSIS, PNEUMONIA, RESPIRATORY SYNCYTIAL VIRUS)

**Decreased Activity Tolerance** r/t generalized weakness, dyspnea, fatigue, poor oxygenation

**Ineffective Airway Clearance** r/t excess tracheobronchial secretions

**Ineffective Breathing Pattern** r/t inflamed bronchial passages, coughing

**Fear** r/t oxygen deprivation, difficulty breathing

**Deficient Fluid Volume** r/t insensible losses (fever, diaphoresis), inadequate oral fluid intake

**Impaired Gas Exchange** r/t insufficient oxygenation as a result of inflammation or edema of epiglottis, larynx, bronchial passages

**Imbalanced Nutrition: Less than Body Requirements** r/t anorexia, fatigue, generalized weakness, poor sucking and breathing coordination, dyspnea

**Ineffective Thermoregulation** r/t infectious process

**Risk for Aspiration:** Risk factors: inability to coordinate breathing, coughing, sucking

**Risk for Infection: Transmission to Others:** Risk factor: virulent infectious organisms

**Risk for Injury (to Pregnant Others):** Risk factors: exposure to aerosolized medications (e.g., ribavirin, pentamidine), resultant potential fetal toxicity

**Risk for Suffocation:** Risk factors: inflammation of larynx, epiglottis

*See Hospitalized Child*

## RESPIRATORY SYNCYTIAL VIRUS

*See Respiratory Infections, Acute Childhood*

## RESTLESS LEG SYNDROME

**Disturbed Sleep Pattern** r/t leg discomfort during sleep relieved by frequent leg movement

**Chronic Pain** r/t leg discomfort

*See Stress*

## RETINAL DETACHMENT

**Anxiety** r/t change in vision, threat of loss of vision

**Deficient Knowledge** r/t symptoms, need for early intervention to prevent permanent damage

**Vision Loss** r/t impaired visual acuity

**Risk for Ineffective Home Maintenance Behaviors:** Risk factors: postoperative care, activity limitations, care of affected eye

**Risk for Impaired Resilience:** Risk factor: possible loss of vision

*See Vision Impairment*

## RETINOPATHY, DIABETIC

*See Diabetic Retinopathy*

**R**

## RETINOPATHY OF PREMATURITY (ROP)

**Risk for Injury:** Risk factors: prolonged mechanical ventilation, ROP secondary to 100% oxygen environment

*See Retinal Detachment*

## RH FACTOR INCOMPATIBILITY

**Anxiety** r/t unknown outcome of pregnancy

**Neonatal Hyperbilirubinemia** r/t Rh factor incompatibility

**Deficient Knowledge** r/t treatment regimen from lack of experience with situation

**Powerlessness** r/t perceived lack of control over outcome of pregnancy

**Risk for Injury: Fetal:** Risk factors: intrauterine destruction of red blood cells, transfusions

**Risk for Neonatal Hyperbilirubinemia:** Risk factor: Rh factor incompatibility

**Readiness for Enhanced Health Management:** prenatal care, compliance with diagnostic and treatment regimen

## RHABDOMYOLYSIS

**Ineffective Coping** r/t seriousness of condition

**Impaired Physical Mobility** r/t myalgia and muscle weakness

**Risk for Deficient Fluid Volume:** Risk factor: reduced blood flow to kidneys

**Risk for Shock:** Risk factor: hypovolemia

**Readiness for Enhanced Health Management:** seeks information to avoid condition

*See Kidney Failure*

## RHEUMATIC FEVER

*See Endocarditis*

## RHEUMATOID ARTHRITIS (RA)

**Imbalanced Nutrition: Less than Body Requirements** r/t loss of appetite

**Chronic Pain** r/t joint inflammation

**Disturbed Body Image** r/t joint deformity and muscle atrophy

**Impaired Physical Mobility** r/t pain, impaired joints

**Risk for Impaired Resilience:** Risk factor: chronic, painful, progressive disease

*See Arthritis; JRA (Juvenile Rheumatoid Arthritis)*

## RIB FRACTURE

**Ineffective Breathing Pattern** r/t fractured ribs

**Acute Pain** r/t movement, deep breathing

**Impaired Gas Exchange** r/t ventilation-perfusion imbalance, decreased depth of ventilation

## RIDICULE OF OTHERS

**Defensive Coping** r/t situational crisis, psychological impairment, substance abuse

**Risk for Post-Trauma Syndrome:** Risk factor: perception of event

## RINGWORM OF BODY

**Impaired Comfort** r/t pruritus

**Impaired Skin Integrity** r/t presence of macules associated with fungus

*See Itching; Pruritus*

## RINGWORM OF NAILS

**Disturbed Body Image** r/t appearance of nails, removed nails

## RINGWORM OF SCALP

**Disturbed Body Image** r/t possible hair loss (alopecia)

*See Itching; Pruritus*

## ROACHES, INVASION OF HOME WITH

**Ineffective Home Maintenance Behaviors** r/t lack of knowledge, insufficient finances

*See Filthy Home Environment*

## ROLE PERFORMANCE, ALTERED

**Ineffective Role Performance** (See **Role Performance, Ineffective,** Section II)

## ROP (RETINOPATHY OF PREMATURITY)

*See Retinopathy of Prematurity (ROP)*

**R**

## RSV (RESPIRATORY SYNCYTIAL VIRUS)

*See Respiratory Infection, Acute Childhood*

## RUBELLA

*See Communicable Diseases, Childhood (e.g., Measles, Mumps, Rubella, Chickenpox, Scabies, Lice, Impetigo)*

## RUBOR OF EXTREMITIES

**Ineffective Peripheral Tissue Perfusion** r/t interruption of arterial flow

*See Peripheral Vascular Disease (PVD)*

## RUPTURED DISK

*See Low Back Pain*

# S

## SAD (SEASONAL AFFECTIVE DISORDER)

**Readiness for Enhanced Resilience:** uses SAD lights during winter months

*See Depression (Major Depressive Disorder)*

## SADNESS

**Risk for Maladaptive Grieving** r/t actual or perceived loss

**Impaired Mood Regulation** r/t chronic illness (See **Mood Regulation, Impaired,** Section II)

**Spiritual Distress** r/t intense suffering

**Risk for Powerlessness:** Risk factor: actual or perceived loss

**Risk for Spiritual Distress:** Risk factor: loss of loved one

**Readiness for Enhanced Communication:** willingness to share feelings and thoughts

**Readiness for Enhanced Spiritual Well-Being:** desire for harmony after actual or perceived loss

*See Depression (Major Depressive Disorder); Major Depressive Disorder*

## SAFE SEX

**Readiness for Enhanced Health Self-Management:** takes appropriate precautions during sexual activity to keep from contracting sexually transmitted disease

*See Sexuality, Adolescent; STD (Sexually Transmitted Disease)*

## SAFETY, CHILDHOOD

**Deficient Knowledge: Potential for Enhanced Health Self-Maintenance** r/t parental knowledge and skill acquisition regarding appropriate safety measures

**Risk for Aspiration** (See **Aspiration, Risk for,** Section II)

**Risk for Injury:** Risk factors: developmental age, altered home maintenance

**Risk for Impaired Parenting:** Risk factors: lack of available and effective role model, lack of knowledge, misinformation from other family members (old wives' tales)

**Risk for Poisoning:** Risk factors: use of lead-based paint; presence of asbestos or radon gas; drugs not locked in cabinet; household products left in accessible area (bleach, detergent, drain cleaners, household cleaners); alcohol and perfume within reach of child; presence of poisonous plants; atmospheric pollutants

**Risk for Thermal injury:** Risk factor: inadequate supervision

**Readiness for Enhanced Childbearing Process:** expresses appropriate knowledge for care of child

## SALMONELLA

**Impaired Home Maintenance** r/t improper preparation or storage of food, lack of safety measures when caring for pet reptile

**Risk for Shock:** Risk factors: hypovolemia, diarrhea, sepsis

**Readiness for Enhanced Health Self-Management:** avoiding improperly prepared or stored food, wearing gloves when handling pet reptiles or their feces

*See Gastroenteritis; Gastroenteritis, Child*

## SALPINGECTOMY

**Decisional Conflict** r/t sterilization procedure

**Maladaptive Grieving** r/t possible loss from tubal pregnancy

**S**

**Risk for Impaired Urinary Elimination:** Risk factor: trauma to ureter during surgery

*See Hysterectomy; Surgery, Perioperative Care; Surgery, Postoperative Care; Surgery, Preoperative Care*

## SARCOIDOSIS

**Anxiety** r/t change in health status

**Impaired Gas Exchange** r/t ventilation-perfusion imbalance

**Ineffective Health Maintenance Behaviors** r/t deficient knowledge regarding home care and medication regimen

**Acute Pain** r/t possible disease affecting joints

**Ineffective Protection** r/t immune disorder

**Risk for Decreased Cardiac Tissue Perfusion:** Risk factor: dysrhythmias

**Risk for Impaired Skin integrity:** Risk factor: immunological disorder

## SBE (SELF–BREAST EXAMINATION)

**Readiness for Enhanced Health Self-Management:** desires to have information about SBE

**Readiness for Enhanced Knowledge:** SBE

## SCABIES

*See Communicable Diseases, Childhood (e.g., Measles, Mumps, Rubella, Chickenpox, Scabies, Lice, Impetigo)*

## SCARED

**Anxiety** r/t threat of death, threat to or change in health status

**Death Anxiety** r/t unresolved issues surrounding end-of-life decisions

**Fear** r/t hospitalization, real or imagined threat to own well-being

**Impaired Individual Resilience** r/t violence

**Readiness for Enhanced Communication:** willingness to share thoughts and feelings

## SCHIZOPHRENIA

**Ineffective Activity Planning** r/t compromised ability to process information

**Anxiety** r/t unconscious conflict with reality

**Impaired Verbal Communication** r/t psychosis, disorientation, inaccurate perception, hallucinations, delusions

**Ineffective Coping** r/t inadequate support systems, unrealistic perceptions, inadequate coping skills, disturbed thought processes, impaired communication

**Decreased Diversional Activity Engagement** r/t social isolation, possible regression

**Interrupted Family Processes** r/t inability to express feelings, impaired communication

**Fear** r/t altered contact with reality

**Ineffective Health Maintenance Behaviors** r/t cognitive impairment, ineffective individual and family coping, lack of material resources

**Ineffective Family Health Self-Management** r/t chronicity and unpredictability of condition

**Ineffective Home Maintenance Behaviors** r/t impaired cognitive or emotional functioning, insufficient finances, inadequate support systems

**Hopelessness** r/t long-term stress from chronic mental illness

**Disturbed Personal Identity** r/t psychiatric disorder

**Impaired Memory** r/t psychosocial condition

**Imbalanced Nutrition: Less than Body Requirements** r/t fear of eating, lack of awareness of hunger, disinterest toward food

**Impaired Individual Resilience** r/t psychological disorder

**Self-Care Deficit: Specify** r/t loss of contact with reality, impairment of perception

**Self-Neglect** r/t psychosis

**Sleep Deprivation** r/t intrusive thoughts, nightmares

**Impaired Social Interaction** r/t impaired communication patterns, self-concept disturbance, disturbed thought processes

**Social Isolation** r/t lack of trust, regression, delusional thinking, repressed fears

**Chronic Sorrow** r/t chronic mental illness

**Spiritual Distress** r/t loneliness, social alienation

**Risk for Caregiver Role Strain:** Risk factors: bizarre behavior of client, chronicity of condition

**Risk for Compromised Human Dignity:** Risk factor: stigmatizing label

**Risk for Loneliness:** Risk factor: inability to interact socially

**Risk for Post-Trauma Syndrome:** Risk factor: diminished ego strength

**Risk for Powerlessness:** Risk factor: intrusive, distorted thinking

**Risk for Impaired Religiosity:** Risk factors: ineffective coping, lack of security

**Risk for Suicidal Behavior:** Risk factor: psychiatric illness

**Risk for Self-Directed Violence:** Risk factors: lack of trust, panic, hallucinations, delusional thinking

**Risk for Other-Directed Violence:** Risk factor: psychotic disorder

**Readiness for Enhanced Hope:** expresses desire to enhance interconnectedness with others and problem-solve to meet goals

**Readiness for Enhanced Power:** expresses willingness to enhance participation in choices for daily living and health and enhance knowledge for participation in change

## SCIATICA

*See Neuropathy, Peripheral*

## SCOLIOSIS

**Risk-Prone Health Behavior** r/t lack of developmental maturity to comprehend long-term consequences of noncompliance with treatment procedures

**Disturbed Body Image** r/t use of therapeutic braces, postsurgery scars, restricted physical activity

**Impaired Comfort** r/t altered health status and body image

**Impaired Gas Exchange** r/t restricted lung expansion as a result of severe presurgery curvature of spine, immobilization

**Ineffective Health Maintenance Behaviors** r/t deficient knowledge regarding treatment modalities, restrictions, home care, postoperative activities

**Impaired Physical Mobility** r/t restricted movement, dyspnea caused by severe curvature of spine

**Acute Pain** r/t musculoskeletal restrictions, surgery, reambulation with cast or spinal rod

**Impaired Skin Integrity** r/t braces, casts, surgical correction

**Chronic Sorrow** r/t chronic disability

**Risk for Perioperative Positioning Injury:** Risk factor: prone position

**Risk for Impaired Resilience:** Risk factor: chronic condition

**Readiness for Enhanced Health Self-Management:** desires knowledge regarding treatment for condition

*See Hospitalized Child; Maturational Issues, Adolescent*

## SEDENTARY LIFESTYLE

**Decreased Activity Tolerance** r/t sedentary lifestyle

**Sedentary Lifestyle** (See **Sedentary Lifestyle,** Section II)

**Obesity** (See **Obesity,** Section II)

**Overweight** (See **Overweight,** Section II)

**Risk for Overweight** (See **Overweight,** Section II)

**Risk for Ineffective Peripheral Tissue Perfusion:** Risk factor: insufficient knowledge of aggravating factors (e.g., immobility, obesity)

**Readiness for Enhanced Coping:** seeking knowledge of new strategies to adjust to sedentary lifestyle

## SEIZURE DISORDERS, ADULT

**Acute Confusion** r/t postseizure state

**Social Isolation** r/t unpredictability of seizures, community-imposed stigma

**Risk for Ineffective Airway Clearance:** Risk factor: accumulation of secretions during seizure

**Risk for Child Falls:** Risk factor: uncontrolled seizure activity

**Risk for Powerlessness:** Risk factor: possible seizure

**Risk for Impaired Resilience:** Risk factor: chronic illness

**Readiness for Enhanced Knowledge:** anticonvulsive therapy

**Readiness for Enhanced Self-Care:** expresses desire to enhance knowledge and responsibility for self-care

*See Epilepsy*

## SEIZURE DISORDERS, CHILDHOOD (EPILEPSY, FEBRILE SEIZURES, INFANTILE SPASMS)

**Ineffective Health Maintenance Behaviors** r/t lack of knowledge regarding anticonvulsive therapy, fever reduction (febrile seizures)

**Social Isolation** r/t unpredictability of seizures, community-imposed stigma

**Risk for Ineffective Airway Clearance:** Risk factor: accumulation of secretions during seizure

**Risk for Delayed Child Development:** Risk factors: effects of seizure disorder, parental overprotection

**Risk for Child Falls:** Risk factor: possible seizure

**Risk for Injury:** Risk factors: uncontrolled movements during seizure, falls, drowsiness caused by anticonvulsants

*See Epilepsy*

## SELF–BREAST EXAMINATION (SBE)

*See SBE (Self–Breast Examination)*

## SELF-CARE

**Readiness for Enhanced Self-Care** (See **Self-Care, Readiness for Enhanced,** Section II)

## SELF-CARE DEFICIT, BATHING

**Bathing Self-Care Deficit** (See **Self-Care Deficit, Bathing,** Section II)

## SELF-CARE DEFICIT, DRESSING

**Dressing Self-Care Deficit** (See **Self-Care Deficit, Dressing,** Section II)

## SELF-CARE DEFICIT, FEEDING

**Feeding Self-Care Deficit** (See **Self-Care Deficit, Feeding,** Section II)

## SELF-CARE DEFICIT, TOILETING

**Toileting Self-Care Deficit** (See **Self-Care Deficit, Toileting,** Section II)

## SELF-CONCEPT

**Readiness for Enhanced Self-Concept** (See **Self-Concept, Readiness for Enhanced,** Section II)

## SELF-DESTRUCTIVE BEHAVIOR

**Post-Trauma Syndrome** r/t unresolved feelings from traumatic event

**Risk for Self-Mutilation:** Risk factors: feelings of depression, rejection, self-hatred, depersonalization; command hallucinations

**Risk for Suicidal Behavior:** Risk factor: history of self-destructive behavior

**Risk for Self-Directed Violence:** Risk factors: panic state, history of child abuse, toxic reaction to medication

## SELF-ESTEEM, CHRONIC LOW

**Chronic Low Self-Esteem** (See **Self-Esteem, Low, Chronic,** Section II)

**Risk for Disturbed Personal Identity:** Risk factor: chronic low self-esteem

## SELF-ESTEEM, SITUATIONAL LOW

**Situational Low Self-Esteem** (See **Self-Esteem, Low, Situational,** Section II)

**Risk for Situational Low Self-Esteem** (See **Self-Esteem, Low, Situational, Risk For,** Section II)

## SELF-MUTILATION

**Ineffective Impulse Control** r/t ineffective management of anxiety

**Self-Mutilation** (See **Self-Mutilation,** Section II)

**Risk for Self-Mutilation** (See **Self-Mutilation, Risk for,** Section II)

## SENILE DEMENTIA

**Ineffective Relationship** r/t cognitive changes in one partner

**S**

**Sedentary Lifestyle** r/t lack of interest in movement

*See Dementia*

## SEPARATION ANXIETY

**Ineffective Coping** r/t maturational and situational crises, vulnerability related to developmental age, hospitalization, separation from family and familiar surroundings, multiple caregivers

**Insomnia** r/t separation for significant others

**Risk for Impaired Attachment:** Risk factor: separation

*See Hospitalized Child*

## SEPSIS, CHILD

**Impaired Gas Exchange** r/t pulmonary inflammation associated with disease process

**Imbalanced Nutrition: Less than Body Requirements** r/t anorexia, generalized weakness, poor sucking reflex

**Delayed Surgical Recovery** r/t presence of infection

**Ineffective Thermoregulation** r/t infectious process, septic shock

**Ineffective Peripheral Tissue Perfusion** r/t arterial or venous blood flow exchange problems, septic shock

**Risk for Deficient Fluid Volume:** Risk factor: inflammation leading to decreased systemic vascular resistance

**Risk for Impaired Skin Integrity:** Risk factor: desquamation caused by disseminated intravascular coagulation

*See Hospitalized Child; Premature Infant, Child*

## SEPTICEMIA

**Imbalanced Nutrition: Less than Body Requirements** r/t anorexia, generalized weakness

**Ineffective Peripheral Tissue Perfusion** r/t decreased systemic vascular resistance

**Risk for Deficient Fluid Volume:** Risk factors: vasodilation of peripheral vessels, leaking of capillaries

**Risk for Shock:** Risk factors: hypotension, hypovolemia

**Risk for Unstable Blood Pressure:** Risk factor: hypovolemia

*See Sepsis, Child; Shock, Septic*

## SERVICE ANIMAL

**Readiness for Enhanced Power:** expresses desire to enhance independence with actions for change

**Readiness for Enhanced Resilience:** expresses desire to enhance involvement in activities, desire to enhance environmental safety

## SEVERE ACUTE RESPIRATORY SYNDROME (SARS)

*See Pneumonia*

## SEXUAL DYSFUNCTION

**Sexual Dysfunction** r/t insufficient knowledge about sexual function

**Ineffective Relationship** r/t reported sexual dissatisfaction between partners

**Chronic Sorrow** r/t loss of ideal sexual experience, altered relationships

**Risk for Situational Low Self-Esteem:** Risk factor: alteration in body function

*See Erectile Dysfunction (ED)*

## SEXUAL HARASSMENT VICTIM

**Anxiety** r/t situational crisis

**Risk for Compromised Human Dignity:** Risk factors: humiliation, dehumanizing treatment

**Risk for Post-Trauma Syndrome:** Risk factors: perceived traumatic event, insufficient social support

**Risk for Spiritual Distress:** Risk factors: physical, psychological stress

*See Assault Victim*

## SEXUALITY, ADOLESCENT

**Disturbed Body Image** r/t anxiety caused by unachieved developmental milestone (puberty) or deficient knowledge regarding reproductive maturation with expressed concerns regarding lack of growth of secondary sex characteristics

S

**Impaired Emancipated Decision-Making: Sexual Activity** r/t undefined personal values or beliefs, multiple or divergent sources of information, lack of relevant information

**Ineffective Impulse control** r/t denial of consequences of actions

**Deficient Knowledge: Potential for Enhanced Health Self-Maintenance** r/t multiple or divergent sources of information or lack of relevant information regarding sexual transmission of disease, contraception, prevention of toxic shock syndrome

*See Maturational Issues, Adolescent*

## SEXUALITY PATTERN, INEFFECTIVE

**Ineffective Sexuality Pattern** (See **Sexuality Pattern, Ineffective,** Section II)

## SEXUALLY TRANSMITTED DISEASE (STD)

*See STD (Sexually Transmitted Disease)*

## SHAKEN BABY SYNDROME

**Impaired Parenting** r/t stress, history of being abusive

**Impaired Individual Resilience** r/t poor impulse control

**Stress Overload** r/t intense repeated family stressors, family violence

**Risk for Other-Directed Violence:** Risk factors: history of violence against others, perinatal complications

*See Child Abuse; Suspected Child Abuse and Neglect (SCAN), Child; Suspected Child Abuse and Neglect (SCAN), Parent*

## SHAKINESS

**Anxiety** r/t situational or maturational crisis, threat of death

## SHAME

**Situational Low Self-Esteem** r/t inability to deal with past traumatic events, blaming of self for events not in one's control

## SHINGLES

**Acute Pain** r/t vesicular eruption along the nerves

**Ineffective Protection** r/t abnormal blood profiles

**Social Isolation** r/t altered state of wellness, contagiousness of disease

**Risk for Infection:** Risk factor: tissue destruction

*See Itching*

## SHIVERING

**Impaired Comfort** r/t altered health status

**Fear** r/t serious threat to health status

**Hypothermia** r/t exposure to cool environment

**Ineffective Thermoregulation** r/t serious infectious process resulting in immune response of fever

*See Shock, Septic*

## SHOCK, CARDIOGENIC

**Decreased Cardiac Output** r/t decreased myocardial contractility, dysrhythmia

## SHOCK, HYPOVOLEMIC

**Deficient Fluid Volume** r/t abnormal loss of fluid, trauma, third spacing

## SHOCK, SEPTIC

**Deficient Fluid Volume** r/t abnormal loss of intravascular fluid, pooling of blood in peripheral circulation, overwhelming inflammatory response

**Ineffective Protection** r/t inadequately functioning immune system

*See Sepsis, Child; Septicemia*

## SHOULDER REPAIR

**Self-Care Deficit: Bathing, Dressing, Feeding** r/t immobilization of affected shoulder

**Risk for Perioperative Positioning Injury:** Risk factor: immobility

*See Surgery, Preoperative Care; Surgery, Perioperative Care; Surgery, Postoperative Care; Total Joint Replacement (Total Hip/Total Knee/Shoulder)*

## SICKLE CELL ANEMIA/CRISIS

**Decreased Activity Tolerance** r/t fatigue, effects of chronic anemia

**S**

**Deficient Fluid Volume** r/t decreased intake, increased fluid requirements during sickle cell crisis, decreased ability of kidneys to concentrate urine

**Impaired Physical Mobility** r/t pain, fatigue

**Acute Pain** r/t viscous blood, tissue hypoxia

**Ineffective Peripheral Tissue Perfusion** r/t effects of red cell sickling, infarction of tissues

**Risk for Decreased Cardiac Tissue Perfusion:** Risk factors: effects of red cell sickling, infarction of tissues

**Risk for Infection:** Risk factor: alterations in splenic function

**Risk for Impaired Resilience:** Risk factor: chronic illness

**Risk for Ineffective Cerebral Tissue Perfusion:** Risk factors: effects of red cell sickling, infarction of tissues

*See Child with Chronic Condition; Hospitalized Child*

## SIDS (SUDDEN INFANT DEATH SYNDROME)

**Anxiety: Parental Worry** r/t life-threatening event

**Interrupted Family Processes** r/t stress as a result of special care needs of infant with apnea

**Maladaptive Grieving** r/t potential loss of infant

**Insomnia: Parental/Infant** r/t home apnea monitoring

**Deficient Knowledge: Potential For Enhanced Health Self-Maintenance** r/t knowledge or skill acquisition of cardiopulmonary resuscitation and home apnea monitoring

**Impaired Resilience** r/t sudden loss

**Risk for Sudden Infant Death** (See **Sudden Infant Death, Risk for,** Section II)

**Risk for Powerlessness:** Risk factor: unanticipated life-threatening event

*See Terminally Ill Child/Death of Child, Parent*

## SITTING PROBLEMS

**Impaired Sitting** (See **Sitting, Impaired,** Section II)

## SITUATIONAL CRISIS

**Imbalanced Energy Field** r/t hyperactivity of the energy flow

**Ineffective Coping** r/t situational crisis

**Interrupted Family Processes** r/t situational crisis

**Risk for Ineffective Activity Planning:** Risk factor: inability to process information

**Risk for Disturbed Personal Identity:** Risk factor: situational crisis

**Readiness for Enhanced Communication:** willingness to share feelings and thoughts

**Readiness for Enhanced Religiosity:** requests religious material and/or experiences

**Readiness for Enhanced Resilience:** desire to enhance resilience

**Readiness for Enhanced Spiritual Well-Being:** desire for harmony following crisis

## SJS (STEVENS-JOHNSON SYNDROME)

*See Stevens-Johnson Syndrome (SJS)*

## SKIN CANCER

**Ineffective Health Maintenance Behaviors** r/t deficient knowledge regarding self-care with skin cancer

**Ineffective Protection** r/t weakened immune system

**Impaired Tissue Integrity** r/t abnormal cell growth in skin, treatment of skin cancer

**Readiness for Enhanced Health Self-Management:** follows preventive measures

**Readiness for Enhanced Knowledge:** self-care to prevent and treat skin cancer

## SKIN DISORDERS

**Impaired Skin Integrity** (See **Skin Integrity, Impaired,** Section II)

## SKIN TURGOR, CHANGE IN ELASTICITY

**Deficient Fluid Volume** r/t active fluid loss

## SLEEP

**Readiness for Enhanced Sleep** (See **Sleep, Readiness for Enhanced,** Section II)

**S**

## SLEEP APNEA

**Ineffective Breathing Pattern** r/t obesity, substance misuse, enlarged tonsils, smoking, or neurological pathology such as a brain tumor

**Impaired Comfort** r/t use of bilevel positive airway pressure (BiPAP)/continuous positive airway pressure (CPAP) machine

## SLEEP DEPRIVATION

**Fatigue** r/t lack of sleep

**Sleep Deprivation** (See **Sleep Deprivation,** Section II)

**Insomnia** (See **Insomnia,** Section II)

## SLEEP PROBLEMS

**Insomnia** (See **Insomnia,** Section II)

## SLEEP PATTERN, DISTURBED, PARENT/CHILD

**Insomnia: Child** r/t anxiety or fear

**Insomnia: Parent** r/t parental responsibilities, stress

*See Suspected Child Abuse and Neglect (SCAN), Child; Suspected Child Abuse and Neglect (SCAN), Parent*

## SLURRING OF SPEECH

**Impaired Verbal Communication** r/t decrease in circulation to brain, brain tumor, anatomical defect, cleft palate

**Situational Low Self-Esteem** r/t speech impairment

*See Communication Problems*

## SMALL BOWEL RESECTION

*See Abdominal Surgery*

## SMELL, LOSS OF ABILITY TO

**Risk for Injury:** Risk factors: inability to detect gas fumes, smoke smells

*See Anosmia (Smell, Loss of Ability to)*

## SMOKE INHALATION

**Ineffective Airway Clearance** r/t smoke inhalation

**Impaired Gas Exchange** r/t ventilation-perfusion imbalance

**Risk for Acute Confusion:** Risk factor: decreased oxygen supply

**Risk for Infection:** Risk factors: inflammation, ineffective airway clearance, pneumonia

**Risk for Poisoning:** Risk factor: exposure to carbon monoxide

**Readiness for Enhanced Health Self-Management:** functioning smoke detectors and carbon monoxide detectors in home and work, escape route planned and reviewed

*See Atelectasis; Burns; Pneumonia*

## SMOKING BEHAVIOR

**Insufficient Breast Milk Production** r/t smoking

**Risk-Prone Health Behavior** Risk factor: smoking

**Ineffective Health Maintenance Behaviors** r/t denial of effects of smoking, lack of effective support for smoking withdrawal

**Readiness for Enhanced Knowledge:** expresses interest in smoking cessation

**Risk for Dry Eye:** Risk factor: smoking

**Risk for Ineffective Peripheral Tissue Perfusion:** Risk factor: effect of nicotine

**Risk for Thermal Injury:** Risk factor: unsafe smoking behavior

**Readiness for Enhanced Health Literacy:** verbalizes desire to enhance understanding of health information to make health care choices

## SOCIAL INTERACTION, IMPAIRED

**Impaired Social Interaction** (See **Social Interaction, Impaired,** Section II)

## SOCIAL ISOLATION

**Social Isolation** (See **Social Isolation,** Section II)

## SOCIOPATHIC PERSONALITY

*See Antisocial Personality Disorder*

## SODIUM, DECREASE/INCREASE

*See Hyponatremia; Hypernatremia*

S

## SOMATIZATION DISORDER

**Anxiety** r/t unresolved conflicts channeled into physical complaints or conditions

**Ineffective Coping** r/t lack of insight into underlying conflicts

**Ineffective Denial** r/t displaced psychological stress to physical symptoms

**Nausea** r/t anxiety

**Chronic Pain** r/t unexpressed anger, multiple physical disorders, depression

**Impaired Individual Resilience** r/t possible psychological disorders

## SORE NIPPLES, BREASTFEEDING

**Ineffective Breastfeeding** r/t deficient knowledge regarding correct feeding procedure

**Nipple-Areolar Complex Injury** r/t breast engorgement

*See Painful Breasts, Sore Nipples*

## SORE THROAT

**Impaired Comfort** r/t sore throat

**Deficient Knowledge** r/t treatment, relief of discomfort

**Impaired Oral Mucous Membrane Integrity** r/t inflammation or infection of oral cavity

**Impaired Swallowing** r/t irritation of oropharyngeal cavity

**Risk for Dry Mouth:** Risk factor: painful swallowing

## SORROW

**Maladaptive Grieving** r/t loss of significant person, object, or role

**Chronic Sorrow** (See **Sorrow, Chronic,** Section II)

**Readiness for Enhanced Communication:** expresses thoughts and feelings

**Readiness for Enhanced Spiritual Well-Being:** desire to find purpose and meaning of loss

## SPASTIC COLON

*See IBS (Irritable Bowel Syndrome)*

## SPEECH DISORDERS

**Anxiety** r/t difficulty with communication

**Impaired Verbal Communication** r/t anatomical defect, cleft palate, psychological barriers, decrease in circulation to brain

## SPINA BIFIDA

*See Neural Tube Defects (Meningocele, Myelomeningocele, Spina Bifida, Anencephaly)*

## SPINAL CORD INJURY

**Decreased Diversional Activity Engagement** r/t long-term hospitalization, frequent lengthy treatments

**Fear** r/t powerlessness over loss of body function

**Disturbed Body Image** r/t alteration in body function

**Chronic Functional Constipation** r/t inhibition of reflex arc

**Maladaptive Grieving** r/t loss of usual body function

**Ineffective Coping** r/t inability to meet basic needs and insufficient sense of control

**Sedentary Lifestyle** r/t lack of resources or interest

**Impaired Physical Mobility** r/t neuromuscular impairment

**Impaired Wheelchair Mobility** r/t neuromuscular impairment

**Impaired Standing** r/t spinal cord injury

**Urinary Retention** r/t inhibition of reflex arc

**Risk for Autonomic Dysreflexia:** Risk factors: bladder or bowel distention, skin irritation, deficient knowledge of client and caregiver

**Risk for Ineffective Breathing Pattern:** Risk factor: neuromuscular impairment

**Risk for Infection:** Risk factors: chronic disease, stasis of body fluids

**Risk for Loneliness:** Risk factor: physical immobility

**Risk for Powerlessness:** Risk factor: loss of function

**Risk for Adult Pressure Injury:** Risk factor: immobility and decreased sensation

**Risk for Child Pressure Injury:** Risk factor: immobility and decreased sensation

**S**

**Risk for Thermal Injury:** Risk factor: physical immobility

**Risk for Thrombosis:** Risk factor: physical immobility

*See Child with Chronic Condition; Hospitalized Child; Neural Tube Defects (Meningocele, Myelomeningocele, Spina Bifida, Anencephaly); Paralysis*

## SPINAL FUSION

**Impaired Bed Mobility** r/t impaired ability to turn side to side while keeping spine in proper alignment

**Impaired Physical Mobility** r/t musculoskeletal impairment associated with surgery, possible back brace

**Readiness for Enhanced Knowledge:** expresses interest in information associated with surgery

**Risk for Adult Pressure Injury:** Risk factor: immobility

**Risk for Child Pressure Injury:** Risk factor: immobility

*See Acute Back Pain; Scoliosis; Surgery, Preoperative Care; Surgery, Perioperative Care; Surgery, Postoperative Care*

## SPIRITUAL DISTRESS

**Spiritual Distress** (See **Spiritual Distress,** Section II)

**Risk for Chronic Low Self-Esteem:** Risk factor: unresolved spiritual issues

**Risk for Spiritual Distress** (See **Spiritual Distress, Risk for,** Section II)

## SPIRITUAL WELL-BEING

**Readiness for Enhanced Spiritual Well-Being** (See **Spiritual Well-Being, Readiness for Enhanced,** Section II)

## SPLENECTOMY

*See Abdominal Surgery*

## SPRAINS

**Acute Pain** r/t physical injury

**Impaired Physical Mobility** r/t injury

**Impaired Walking** r/t injury

## STABLE BLOOD PRESSURE, RISK FOR UNSTABLE

**Deficient Knowledge** r/t inconsistency with medication regiment (See **Unstable Blood Pressure, Risk for,** Section II)

## STANDING PROBLEMS

**Impaired Standing** (See **Impaired Standing,** Section II)

## STAPEDECTOMY

**Hearing Loss** r/t edema from surgery

**Acute Pain** r/t headache

**Risk for Adult Falls:** Risk factor: dizziness

**Risk for Infection:** Risk factor: invasive procedure

## STASIS ULCER

**Impaired Tissue Integrity** r/t chronic venous congestion

**Risk for Infection:** Risk factor: open wound

*See CHF (Congestive Heart Failure); Varicose Veins*

## STD (SEXUALLY TRANSMITTED DISEASE)

**Impaired Comfort** r/t infection

**Fear** r/t altered body function, risk for social isolation, fear of incurable illness

**Ineffective Health Maintenance Behaviors** r/t deficient knowledge regarding transmission, symptoms, treatment of STD

**Ineffective Sexuality Pattern** r/t illness, altered body function, need for abstinence to heal

**Social Isolation** r/t fear of contracting or spreading disease

**Risk for Infection: Spread of Infection:** Risk factor: lack of knowledge concerning transmission of disease

**Readiness for Enhanced Knowledge:** seeks information regarding prevention and treatment of STDs

*See Maturational Issues, Adolescent; PID (Pelvic Inflammatory Disease)*

## STEMI (ST-ELEVATION MYOCARDIAL INFARCTION)

*See MI (Myocardial Infarction)*

## STENT (CORONARY ARTERY STENT)

**Risk for Injury:** Risk factor: complications associated with stent placement

**Risk for Decreased Cardiac Tissue Perfusion:** Risk factor: possible restenosis

**Risk for Vascular Trauma:** Risk factors: insertion site, catheter width

**Readiness for Enhanced Decision-Making:** expresses desire to enhance risk-benefit analysis, understanding and meaning of choices, and decisions regarding treatment

*See Angioplasty, Coronary; Cardiac Catheterization*

## STERILIZATION SURGERY

**Decisional Conflict** r/t multiple or divergent sources of information, unclear personal values or beliefs

*See Surgery, Preoperative Care; Surgery, Perioperative Care; Surgery, Postoperative Care; Tubal Ligation; Vasectomy*

## STERTOROUS RESPIRATIONS

**Ineffective Airway Clearance** r/t pharyngeal obstruction

## STEVENS-JOHNSON SYNDROME (SJS)

**Impaired Oral Mucous Membrane Integrity** r/t immunocompromised condition associated with allergic medication reaction

**Acute Pain** r/t painful skin lesions and painful mucosa lesions

**Impaired Skin Integrity** r/t allergic medication reaction

**Risk for Deficient Fluid Volume:** Risk factors: factors affecting fluid needs (hypermetabolic state, fever), excessive losses through normal routes (vomiting and diarrhea)

**Risk for Infection:** Risk factor: sloughing skin

**Risk for Impaired Liver Function:** Risk factor: impaired immune response

## STILLBIRTH

*See Pregnancy Loss*

## STOMA

*See Colostomy; Ileostomy*

## STOMATITIS

**Impaired Oral Mucous Membrane Integrity** r/t pathological conditions of oral cavity; side effects of chemotherapy

**Risk for Impaired Oral Mucous Membrane Integrity** (See **Impaired Oral Mucous Membrane Integrity, Risk for,** Section II)

## STOOL, HARD/DRY

**Chronic Functional Constipation** r/t inadequate fluid intake, inadequate fiber intake, decreased activity level, decreased gastric motility

## STRAINING WITH DEFECATION

**Chronic Functional Constipation** r/t less than adequate fluid intake, less than adequate dietary intake

**Risk for Decreased Cardiac Output:** Risk factor: vagal stimulation with dysrhythmia resulting from Valsalva maneuver

## STREP THROAT

**Risk for Infection:** Risk factor: exposure to pathogen

*See Sore Throat*

## STRESS

**Anxiety** r/t feelings of helplessness, feelings of being threatened

**Ineffective Coping** r/t ineffective use of problem-solving process, feelings of apprehension or helplessness

**Fear** r/t powerlessness over feelings

**Stress Overload** r/t intense or multiple stressors

**Readiness for Enhanced Communication:** shows willingness to share thoughts and feelings

**Readiness for Enhanced Spiritual Well-Being:** expresses desire for harmony and peace in stressful situation

*See Anxiety*

**S**

## STRESS URINARY INCONTINENCE

**Stress Urinary Incontinence** r/t degenerative change in pelvic muscles

## STRIDOR

**Ineffective Airway Clearance** r/t obstruction, tracheobronchial infection, trauma

## STROKE

*See CVA (Cerebrovascular Accident)*

## STUTTERING

**Anxiety** r/t impaired verbal communication

**Impaired Verbal Communication** r/t anxiety, psychological problems

## SUBARACHNOID HEMORRHAGE

**Acute Pain: Headache** r/t irritation of meninges from blood, increased intracranial pressure

**Risk for Ineffective Cerebral Tissue Perfusion:** Risk factor: bleeding from cerebral vessel

*See Intracranial Pressure, Increased*

## SUBSTANCE MISUSE

**Acute Substance Withdrawal Syndrome:** Risk factor: developed dependence to alcohol or other addictive substances

**Anxiety** r/t threat to self-concept, lack of control of drug use

**Compromised Family Coping** r/t codependency issues

**Defensive Coping** r/t substance misuse

**Disabled Family Coping** r/t differing coping styles between support persons

**Ineffective Coping** r/t use of substances to cope with life events

**Ineffective Denial** r/t refusal to acknowledge substance misuse problem

**Dysfunctional Family Processes** r/t substance misuse

**Risk-Prone Health Behavior** r/t addiction

**Deficient Community Health** r/t prevention and control of illegal substances in community

**Ineffective Impulse Control** r/t addictive process

**Insomnia** r/t irritability, nightmares, tremors

**Imbalanced Nutrition: Less than Body Requirements** r/t poor eating habits

**Powerlessness** r/t feeling unable to change patterns of drug abuse

**Ineffective Relationship** r/t inability for well-balanced collaboration between partners

**Sexual Dysfunction** r/t actions and side effects of drugs

**Sleep Deprivation** r/t prolonged psychological discomfort

**Impaired Social Interaction** r/t disturbed thought processes from drug abuse

**Risk for Acute Substance Withdrawal Syndrome:** Risk factor: developed dependence to alcohol or other addictive substances

**Risk for Impaired Attachment:** Risk factor: substance misuse

**Risk for Injury:** Risk factors: hallucinations, drug effects

**Risk for Disturbed Personal Identity:** Risk factor: ingestion/inhalation of toxic chemicals

**Risk for Chronic Low Self-Esteem:** Risk factors: perceived lack of respect from others, repeated failures, repeated negative reinforcement

**Risk for Thermal Injury:** Risk factor: intoxication with drugs or alcohol

**Risk for Unstable Blood Pressure:** Risk factor: vasoconstriction of cardiac arteries

**Risk for Vascular Trauma:** Risk factor: chemical irritant self injected into veins

**Risk for Self-Directed Violence:** Risk factors: reactions to substances used, impulsive behavior, disorientation, impaired judgment

**Risk for Other-Directed Violence:** Risk factor: poor impulse control

**Readiness for Enhanced Coping:** seeking social support and knowledge of new strategies

**Readiness for Enhanced Self-Concept:** accepting strengths and limitations

*See Alcoholism*

## SUBSTANCE MISUSE, ADOLESCENT

*See Alcoholism; Maturational Issues, Adolescent; Substance Misuse*

## SUBSTANCE MISUSE IN PREGNANCY

**Ineffective Childbearing Process** r/t substance misuse

**Defensive Coping** r/t denial of situation, differing value system

**Ineffective Health Self-Management** r/t addiction

**Deficient Knowledge** r/t lack of exposure to information regarding effects of substance misuse in pregnancy

**Neonatal Abstinence Syndrome** r/t in utero substance exposure secondary to maternal substance use

**Risk for Impaired Attachment:** Risk factors: substance misuse, inability of parent to meet infant's or own personal needs

**Risk for Infection:** Risk factors: intravenous drug use, lifestyle

**Risk for Injury: Fetal:** Risk factor: effects of drugs on fetal growth and development

**Risk for Injury: Maternal:** Risk factor: drug or alcohol misuse

**Risk for Impaired Parenting:** Risk factor: lack of ability to meet infant's needs due to addiction with use of alcohol or drugs

*See Alcoholism; Substance Misuse*

## SUBSTANCE WITHDRAWAL

*See Acute Substance Withdrawal Syndrome*

## SUCKING REFLEX

**Effective Breastfeeding** r/t regular and sustained sucking and swallowing at breast

## SUDDEN INFANT DEATH SYNDROME (SIDS)

*See SIDS (Sudden Infant Death Syndrome)*

## SUFFOCATION, RISK FOR

**Risk for Suffocation** (See **Suffocation, Risk for,** Section II)

## SUICIDE ATTEMPT

**Risk-Prone Health Behavior** r/t low self-efficacy

**Ineffective Coping** r/t anger, complicated grieving

**Hopelessness** r/t perceived or actual loss, substance misuse, low self-concept, inadequate support systems

**Ineffective Impulse Control** r/t inability to modulate stress, anxiety

**Post-Trauma Syndrome** r/t history of traumatic events, abuse, rape, incest, war, torture

**Impaired Individual Resilience** r/t poor impulse control

**Situational Low Self-Esteem** r/t guilt, inability to trust, feelings of worthlessness or rejection

**Social Isolation** r/t inability to engage in satisfying personal relationships

**Spiritual Distress** r/t hopelessness, despair

**Risk for Post-Trauma Syndrome:** Risk factor: survivor's role in suicide attempt

**Risk for Suicidal Behavior** (See **Suicide, Risk for,** Section II)

**Readiness for Enhanced Communication:** willingness to share thoughts and feelings

**Readiness for Enhanced Spiritual Well-Being:** desire for harmony and inner strength to help redefine purpose for life

*See Violent Behavior*

## SUPPORT SYSTEM, INADEQUATE

**Readiness for Enhanced Family Coping:** ability to adapt to tasks associated with care, support of significant other during health crisis

**Readiness for Enhanced Family Processes:** activities support the growth of family members

**Readiness for Enhanced Parenting:** children or other dependent person(s) expressing satisfaction with home environment

## SUPPRESSION OF LABOR

*See Preterm Labor*

**S**

## SURGERY, PERIOPERATIVE CARE

**Risk for Imbalanced Fluid Volume:** Risk factor: surgery

**Risk for Perioperative Hypothermia:** Risk factors: inadequate covering of client, cold surgical room

**Risk for Perioperative Positioning Injury:** Risk factors: predisposing condition, prolonged surgery

## SURGERY, POSTOPERATIVE CARE

**Decreased Activity Tolerance** r/t pain, surgical procedure

**Anxiety** r/t change in health status, hospital environment

**Deficient Knowledge** r/t postoperative expectations, lifestyle changes

**Nausea** r/t manipulation of gastrointestinal tract, postsurgical anesthesia

**Imbalanced Nutrition: Less than Body Requirements** r/t anorexia, nausea, vomiting, decreased peristalsis

**Ineffective Peripheral Tissue Perfusion** r/t hypovolemia, circulatory stasis, obesity, prolonged immobility, decreased coughing, decreased deep breathing

**Acute Pain** r/t inflammation or injury in surgical area

**Delayed Surgical Recovery** r/t extensive surgical procedure, postoperative surgical infection

**Urinary Retention** r/t anesthesia, pain, fear, unfamiliar surroundings, client's position

**Risk for Bleeding:** Risk factor: surgical procedure

**Risk for Ineffective Breathing Pattern:** Risk factors: pain, location of incision, effects of anesthesia or opioids

**Risk for Constipation:** Risk factors: decreased activity, decreased food or fluid intake, anesthesia, pain medication

**Risk for Imbalanced Fluid Volume:** Risk factors: hypermetabolic state, fluid loss during surgery, presence of indwelling tubes, fluids used to distend organ structures being absorbed into body

**Risk for Surgical Site Infection:** Risk factors: invasive procedure, pain, anesthesia, location of incision, weakened cough as a result of aging

## SURGERY, PREOPERATIVE CARE

**Anxiety** r/t threat to or change in health status, situational crisis, fear of the unknown

**Insomnia** r/t anxiety about upcoming surgery

**Deficient Knowledge** r/t preoperative procedures, postoperative expectations

**Readiness for Enhanced Knowledge:** shows understanding of preoperative and postoperative expectations for self-care

## SURGICAL RECOVERY, DELAYED

**Delayed Surgical Recovery** (See **Surgical Recovery, Delayed,** Section II)

**Risk for Delayed Surgical Recovery** (See **Surgical Recovery, Delayed, Risk for,** Section II)

## SURGICAL SITE INFECTION

**Anxiety** r/t unforeseen result of surgery

**Impaired Comfort** r/t surgical site pain

**Risk for Ineffective Thermoregulation:** Risk factor: infectious process

**Risk for Delayed Surgical Recovery:** Risk factor: interrupted healing of surgical site

**Readiness for Enhanced Knowledge:** expresses desire for knowledge of prevention and symptoms of infection

## SUSPECTED CHILD ABUSE AND NEGLECT (SCAN), CHILD

**Ineffective Activity Planning** r/t lack of family support

**Anxiety: Child** r/t threat of punishment for perceived wrongdoing

**Deficient Community Health** r/t inadequate reporting and follow-up of SCAN

**Disturbed Personal Identity** r/t dysfunctional family processes

**Rape-Trauma Syndrome** r/t altered lifestyle because of abuse, changes in residence

**Risk for Impaired Resilience:** Risk factor: adverse situation

**Readiness for Enhanced Community Coping:** obtaining resources to prevent child abuse, neglect

*See Child Abuse; Hospitalized Child;
Maturational Issues, Adolescent*

## SUSPECTED CHILD ABUSE AND NEGLECT (SCAN), PARENT

**Disabled Family Coping** r/t dysfunctional family, underdeveloped nurturing parental role, lack of parental support systems or role models

**Dysfunctional Family Processes** r/t inadequate coping skills

**Ineffective Health Maintenance Behaviors** r/t deficient knowledge of parenting skills as result of unachieved developmental tasks

**Impaired Home Maintenance** r/t disorganization, parental dysfunction, neglect of safe and nurturing environment

**Ineffective Impulse Control** r/t projection of anger, frustration onto child

**Impaired Parenting** r/t unrealistic expectations of child; lack of effective role model; unmet social, emotional, or maturational needs of parents; interruption in bonding process

**Impaired Individual Resilience** r/t poor impulse control

**Chronic Low Self-Esteem** r/t lack of successful parenting experiences

**Risk for Other-Directed Violence: Parent to Child:** Risk factors: inadequate coping mechanisms, unresolved stressors, unachieved maturational level by parent

## SUSPICION

**Disturbed Personal Identity** r/t psychiatric disorder

**Powerlessness** r/t repetitive paranoid thinking

**Impaired Social Interaction** r/t disturbed thought processes, paranoid delusions, hallucinations

**Disturbed Thought Process** r/t psychiatric disorder

**Risk for Self-Directed Violence:** Risk factor: inability to trust

**Risk for Other-Directed Violence:** Risk factor: impulsiveness

## SWALLOWING DIFFICULTIES

**Impaired Swallowing** (See **Swallowing, Impaired,** Section II)

**Risk for Aspiration** r/t difficulty swallowing

## SYNCOPE

**Anxiety** r/t fear of falling

**Impaired Physical Mobility** r/t fear of falling

**Ineffective Health Management Behaviors** r/t lack of knowledge in how to prevent syncope

**Social Isolation** r/t fear of falling

**Risk for Decreased Cardiac Output:** Risk factor: dysrhythmia

**Risk for Adult Falls:** Risk factor: syncope

**Risk for Injury:** Risk factors: altered sensory perception, transient loss of consciousness, risk for falls

**Risk for Ineffective Cerebral Tissue Perfusion:** Risk factor: interruption of blood flow

## SYPHILIS

*See STD (Sexually Transmitted Disease)*

## SYSTEMIC LUPUS ERYTHEMATOSUS

*See Lupus Erythematosus*

# T

## T & A (TONSILLECTOMY AND ADENOIDECTOMY)

**Ineffective Airway Clearance** r/t hesitation or reluctance to cough because of pain

**Deficient Knowledge: Potential for Enhanced Health Maintenance Behaviors** r/t insufficient knowledge regarding postoperative nutritional and rest requirements, signs and symptoms of complications, positioning

**Nausea** r/t gastric irritation, pharmaceuticals, anesthesia

**Acute Pain** r/t surgical incision

**Risk for Aspiration:** Risk factors: postoperative drainage and impaired swallowing

**Risk for Deficient Fluid Volume:** Risk factors: decreased intake because of painful swallowing, effects of anesthesia (nausea, vomiting), hemorrhage

**Risk for Imbalanced Nutrition: Less than Body Requirements:** Risk factors: hesitation or reluctance to swallow

## TACHYCARDIA

*See Dysrhythmia*

## TACHYPNEA

**Ineffective Breathing Pattern** r/t pain, anxiety, hypoxia

*See cause of Tachypnea*

## TARDIVE DYSKINESIA

**Ineffective Health Self-Management** r/t complexity of therapeutic regimen or medication

**Deficient Knowledge** r/t cognitive limitation in assimilating information relating to side effects associated with neuroleptic medications

**Risk for Injury:** Risk factor: drug-induced abnormal body movements

## TASTE ABNORMALITY

**Frail Elderly Syndrome** r/t chronic illness

## TB (PULMONARY TUBERCULOSIS)

**Ineffective Airway Clearance** r/t increased secretions, excessive mucus

**Ineffective Breathing Pattern** r/t decreased energy, fatigue

**Fatigue** r/t disease state

**Impaired Gas Exchange** r/t disease process

**Ineffective Health Self-Management** r/t deficient knowledge of prevention and treatment regimen

**Ineffective Home Maintenance Behaviors** r/t client or family member with disease

**Ineffective Thermoregulation** r/t presence of infection

**Risk for Infection:** Risk factor: insufficient knowledge regarding avoidance of exposure to pathogens

**Readiness for Enhanced Health Self-Management:** takes medications according to prescribed protocol for prevention and treatment

## TBI (TRAUMATIC BRAIN INJURY)

**Interrupted Family Processes** r/t traumatic injury to family member

**Chronic Sorrow** r/t change in health status and functional ability

**Risk for Post-Trauma Syndrome:** Risk factor: perception of event causing TBI

**Risk for Impaired Religiosity:** Risk factor: impaired physical mobility

**Risk for Impaired Resilience:** Risk factor: crisis of injury

*See Head Injury; Neurologic Disorders*

## TD (TRAVELER'S DIARRHEA)

*See Traveler's Diarrhea (TD)*

## TECHNOLOGY ADDICTION

**Decreased Diversional Activity Engagement** r/t insufficient motivation to separate from electronic devices

**Impaired Social Interaction** r/t lack of desire to engage in personal face-to-face contact with others

**Risk for Impaired Attachment:** Risk factor: preoccupation with electronic devices

**Risk for Impaired Parenting:** Risk factor: insufficient uninterrupted meaningful interaction between parent and child as the result of preoccupation with electronic devices

**Risk for Ineffective Relationship:** Risk factor: ineffective face-to-face communication skills

## TEMPERATURE, DECREASED

**Hypothermia** r/t exposure to cold environment

## TEMPERATURE, HIGH

**Hyperthermia** r/t neurological damage, disease condition with high temperature, excessive heat, inflammatory response

## TEMPERATURE REGULATION, IMPAIRED

**Ineffective Thermoregulation** r/t trauma, illness, cerebral injury

## TEN (TOXIC EPIDERMAL NECROLYSIS)

*See Toxic Epidermal Necrolysis (TEN)*

## TENS UNIT (TRANSCUTANEOUS ELECTRICAL NERVE STIMULATION)

**Risk for Unstable Blood Pressure:** Risk factor: improper use of TENS unit (front of neck)

**Readiness for Enhanced Comfort:** expresses desire to enhance resolution of complaints

## TENSION

**Anxiety** r/t threat to or change in health status, situational crisis

**Readiness for Enhanced Communication:** expresses willingness to share feelings and thoughts

*See Stress*

## TERMINALLY ILL ADULT

**Death Anxiety** r/t unresolved issues relating to death and dying

**Imbalanced Energy Field** r/t weak energy field patterns

**Risk for Spiritual Distress:** Risk factor: impending death

**Readiness for Enhanced Religiosity.** requests religious material and/or experiences

**Readiness for Enhanced Spiritual Well-Being:** desire to achieve harmony of mind, body, spirit

*See Terminally Ill Child/Death of Child, Parent*

## TERMINALLY ILL CHILD, ADOLESCENT

**Disturbed Body Image** r/t effects of terminal disease, already critical feelings of group identity and self-image

**Ineffective Coping** r/t inability to establish personal and peer identity because of the threat of being different or not being healthy, inability to achieve maturational tasks

**Impaired Social Interaction** r/t forced separation from peers

*See Child with Chronic Condition; Hospitalized Child, Terminally Ill Child/Death of Child, Parent*

## TERMINALLY ILL CHILD, INFANT/TODDLER

**Ineffective Coping** r/t separation from parents and familiar environment from inability to understand dying process

*See Child with Chronic Condition, Terminally Ill Child/Death of Child, Parent*

## TERMINALLY ILL CHILD, PRESCHOOL CHILD

**Fear** r/t perceived punishment, bodily harm, feelings of guilt caused by magical thinking (i.e., believing that thoughts cause events)

*See Child with Chronic Condition, Terminally Ill Child/Death of Child, Parent*

## TERMINALLY ILL CHILD, SCHOOL-AGE CHILD/PREADOLESCENT

**Fear** r/t perceived punishment, body mutilation, feelings of guilt

**Maladaptive Grieving** r/t difficulty dealing with concurrent crises

*See Child with Chronic Condition, Terminally Ill Child/Death of Child, Parent*

## TERMINALLY ILL CHILD/DEATH OF CHILD, PARENT

**Compromised Family Coping** r/t inability or unwillingness to discuss impending death and feelings with child or support child through terminal stages of illness

**Decisional Conflict** r/t continuation or discontinuation of treatment, do-not-resuscitate decision, ethical issues regarding organ donation

**Ineffective Denial** r/t complicated grieving

**Interrupted Family Processes** r/t situational crisis

**Maladaptive Grieving** r/t death of child

**Hopelessness** r/t overwhelming stresses caused by terminal illness

**Insomnia** r/t grieving process

**Impaired Parenting** r/t risk for overprotection of surviving siblings

**Powerlessness** r/t inability to alter course of events

**Impaired Social Interaction** r/t complicated grieving

**Social Isolation: Imposed by Others** r/t feelings of inadequacy in providing support to grieving parents

**Social Isolation: Self-Imposed** r/t unresolved grief, perceived inadequate parenting skills

**Spiritual Distress** r/t sudden and unexpected death, prolonged suffering before death, questioning the death of youth, questioning the meaning of one's own existence

**Risk for Maladaptive Grieving:** Risk factors: prolonged, unresolved, obstructed progression through stages of grief and mourning

**Risk for Impaired Resilience:** Risk factor: impending death

**Readiness for Enhanced Family Coping:** impact of crisis on family values, priorities, goals, or relationships; expressed interest or desire to attach meaning to child's life and death

## TETRALOGY OF FALLOT

*See Congenital Heart Disease/Cardiac Anomalies*

## TETRAPLEGIA

**Autonomic Dysreflexia** r/t bladder or bowel distention, skin irritation, infection, deficient knowledge of client and caregiver

**Maladaptive Grieving** r/t loss of previous functioning

**Powerlessness** r/t inability to perform previous activities

**Impaired Sitting** r/t paralysis of extremities

**Impaired Spontaneous Ventilation** r/t loss of innervation of respiratory muscles, respiratory muscle fatigue

**Risk for Aspiration:** Risk factor: inadequate ability to protect airway from neurological damage

**Risk for Infection:** Risk factor: urinary stasis

**Risk for Impaired Skin Integrity:** Risk factor: physical immobilization and decreased sensation

**Risk for Adult Pressure Injury:** Risk factor: immobility and sensory loss

**Risk for Child Pressure Injury:** Risk factor: immobility and sensory loss

**Risk for Ineffective Thermoregulation:** Risk factors: inability to move to increase temperature, possible presence of infection to increase temperature

## THERMOREGULATION, INEFFECTIVE

**Ineffective Thermoregulation** (See **Thermoregulation, Ineffective,** Section II)

**Risk for Ineffective Thermoregulation** (See **Ineffective Thermoregulation, Risk for,** Section II)

## THORACENTESIS

*See Pleural Effusion*

## THORACOTOMY

**Decreased Activity Tolerance** r/t pain, imbalance between oxygen supply and demand, presence of chest tubes

**Ineffective Airway Clearance** r/t drowsiness, pain with breathing and coughing

**Ineffective Breathing Pattern** r/t decreased energy, fatigue, pain

**Deficient Knowledge** r/t self-care, effective breathing exercises, pain relief

**Acute Pain** r/t surgical procedure, coughing, deep breathing

**Risk for Bleeding:** Risk factor: surgery

**Risk for Surgical Site Infection:** Risk factor: invasive procedure

**Risk for Injury:** Risk factor: disruption of closed-chest drainage system

**Risk for Perioperative Positioning Injury:** Risk factors: lateral positioning, immobility

**Risk for Vascular Trauma:** Risk factors: chemical irritant; antibiotics

## THOUGHT DISORDERS

*See Schizophrenia*

## THROMBOCYTOPENIC PURPURA

*See ITP (Idiopathic Thrombocytopenic Purpura)*

## THROMBOPHLEBITIS

*See Deep Vein Thrombosis (DVT)*

## THYROIDECTOMY

**Risk for Ineffective Airway Clearance:** Risk factor: edema or hematoma formation, airway obstruction

**Risk for Impaired Verbal Communication:** Risk factors: edema, pain, vocal cord or laryngeal nerve damage

**Risk for Injury:** Risk factor: possible parathyroid damage or removal

*See Surgery, Preoperative Care; Surgery, Perioperative Care; Surgery, Postoperative Care*

## TIA (TRANSIENT ISCHEMIC ATTACK)

**Acute Confusion** r/t hypoxia

**Readiness for Enhanced Health Self-Management:** obtains knowledge regarding treatment prevention of inadequate oxygenation

*See Syncope*

## TIC DISORDER

*See Tourette's Syndrome (TS)*

## TINEA CAPITIS

**Impaired Comfort** r/t inflammation from skin irritation

*See Ringworm of Scalp*

## TINEA CORPORIS

*See Ringworm of Body*

## TINEA CRURIS

*See Jock Itch; Itching; Pruritus*

## TINEA PEDIS

*See Athlete's Foot; Itching; Pruritus*

## TINEA UNGUIUM (ONYCHOMYCOSIS)

*See Ringworm of Nails*

## TINNITUS

**Ineffective Health Maintenance Behaviors** r/t deficient knowledge regarding self-care with tinnitus

**Hearing Loss** r/t ringing in ears obscuring hearing

## TISSUE DAMAGE, INTEGUMENTARY

**Impaired Tissue Integrity** (See **Tissue Integrity, Impaired,** Section II)

**Risk for Impaired Tissue Integrity** (See **Tissue Integrity, Impaired, Risk for,** Section II)

## TISSUE PERFUSION, PERIPHERAL

**Ineffective Peripheral Tissue Perfusion** (See **Tissue Perfusion, Peripheral, Ineffective,** Section II)

**Risk for Ineffective Peripheral Tissue Perfusion** (See **Tissue Perfusion, Peripheral, Ineffective, Risk for,** Section II)

## TOILETING PROBLEMS

**Toileting Self-Care Deficit** r/t impaired transfer ability, impaired mobility status, intolerance of activity, neuromuscular impairment, cognitive impairment

**Impaired Transfer Ability** r/t neuromuscular deficits

## TOILET TRAINING

**Deficient Knowledge: Parent** r/t signs of child's readiness for training

**Risk for Constipation:** Risk factor: withholding stool

**Risk for Infection:** Risk factor: withholding urination

## TONSILLECTOMY AND ADENOIDECTOMY (T & A)

*See T & A (Tonsillectomy and Adenoidectomy)*

## TOOTHACHE

**Impaired Dentition** r/t ineffective oral hygiene, barriers to self-care, economic barriers to professional care, nutritional deficits, lack of knowledge regarding dental health

**Acute Pain** r/t inflammation, infection

## TOTAL ANOMALOUS PULMONARY VENOUS RETURN

*See Congenital Heart Disease/Cardiac Anomalies*

T

## TOTAL JOINT REPLACEMENT (TOTAL HIP/TOTAL KNEE/SHOULDER)

**Disturbed Body Image** r/t large scar, presence of prosthesis

**Impaired Physical Mobility** r/t musculoskeletal impairment, surgery, prosthesis

**Risk for Injury: Neurovascular:** Risk factors: altered peripheral tissue perfusion, impaired mobility, prosthesis

**Risk for Peripheral Neurovascular Dysfunction:** Risk factors: immobilization, surgical procedure

**Ineffective Peripheral Tissue Perfusion** r/t surgery

*See Surgery, Preoperative Care; Surgery, Perioperative Care; Surgery, Postoperative Care*

## TOTAL PARENTERAL NUTRITION (TPN)

*See TPN (Total Parenteral Nutrition)*

## TOURETTE'S SYNDROME (TS)

**Hopelessness** r/t inability to control behavior

**Impaired Individual Resilience** r/t uncontrollable behavior

**Risk for Situational Low Self-Esteem:** Risk factors: uncontrollable behavior, motor and phonic tics

*See Attention Deficit Disorder*

## TOXEMIA

*See PIH (Pregnancy-Induced Hypertension/Preeclampsia)*

## TOXIC EPIDERMAL NECROLYSIS (TEN) (ERYTHEMA MULTIFORME)

**Death Anxiety** r/t uncertainty of prognosis

**Risk for Shock** r/t deficient fluid volume

## TPN (TOTAL PARENTERAL NUTRITION)

**Imbalanced Nutrition: Less than Body Requirements** r/t inability to digest food or absorb nutrients as a result of biological or psychological factors

**Risk for Electrolyte Imbalance:** Risk factor: need for regulation of electrolytes in TPN fluids

**Risk for Excess Fluid Volume:** Risk factor: rapid administration of TPN

**Risk for Unstable Blood Glucose Level:** Risk factor: high glucose levels in TPN to be regulated according to blood glucose levels

**Risk for Infection:** Risk factors: concentrated glucose solution, invasive administration of fluids

**Risk for Vascular Trauma:** Risk factors: insertion site, length of treatment time

## TRACHEOESOPHAGEAL FISTULA

**Ineffective Airway Clearance** r/t aspiration of feeding because of inability to swallow

**Imbalanced Nutrition: Less than Body Requirements** r/t difficulties swallowing

**Risk for Aspiration:** Risk factor: common passage of air and food

**Risk for Vascular Trauma:** Risk factors: venous medications and site

*See Respiratory Conditions of the Neonate; Hospitalized Child*

## TRACHEOSTOMY

**Ineffective Airway Clearance** r/t increased secretions, mucous plugs

**Anxiety** r/t impaired verbal communication, ineffective airway clearance

**Disturbed Body Image** r/t abnormal opening in neck

**Impaired Verbal Communication** r/t presence of mechanical airway

**Deficient Knowledge** r/t self-care, home maintenance management

**Acute Pain** r/t edema, surgical procedure

**Risk for Aspiration:** Risk factor: presence of tracheostomy

**Risk for Bleeding:** Risk factor: surgical incision

**Risk for Surgical Site Infection:** Risk factors: invasive procedure, pooling of secretions

## TRACTION AND CASTS

**Constipation** r/t immobility

T

**Decreased Diversional Activity Engagement** r/t immobility

**Impaired Physical Mobility** r/t imposed restrictions on activity because of bone or joint disease injury

**Acute Pain** r/t immobility, injury, or disease

**Self-Care Deficit: Feeding, Dressing, Bathing, Toileting** r/t degree of impaired physical mobility, body area affected by traction or cast

**Impaired Transfer Ability** r/t presence of traction, casts

**Risk for Disuse Syndrome:** Risk factor: mechanical immobilization

**Risk for Child Pressure Injury:** Risk factor: immobility and pressure over bony prominence

*See Casts*

## TRANSFER ABILITY

**Impaired Transfer Ability** (See **Transfer Ability, Impaired,** Section II)

## TRANSIENT ISCHEMIC ATTACK (TIA)

*See TIA (Transient Ischemic Attack)*

## TRANSPOSITION OF GREAT VESSELS

*See Congenital Heart Disease/Cardiac Anomalies*

## TRANSURETHRAL RESECTION OF THE PROSTATE (TURP)

*See TURP (Transurethral Resection of the Prostate)*

## TRAUMA IN PREGNANCY

**Anxiety** r/t threat to self or fetus, unknown outcome

**Deficient Knowledge** r/t lack of exposure to situation

**Acute Pain** r/t trauma

**Impaired Skin Integrity** r/t trauma

**Risk for Bleeding:** Risk factor: trauma

**Risk for Deficient Fluid Volume:** Risk factor: fluid loss

**Risk for Infection:** Risk factor: traumatized tissue

**Risk for Injury: Fetal:** Risk factor: premature separation of placenta

**Risk for Disturbed Maternal–Fetal Dyad:** Risk factor: complication of pregnancy

## TRAUMA, PHYSICAL, RISK FOR

**Risk for Physical Trauma** (See **Physical Trauma, Risk for,** Section II)

## TRAUMATIC BRAIN INJURY (TBI)

*See TBI (Traumatic Brain Injury); Intracranial Pressure, Increased*

## TRAUMATIC EVENT

**Post-Trauma Syndrome** r/t previously experienced trauma

## TRAVELER'S DIARRHEA (TD)

**Diarrhea** r/t travel with exposure to different bacteria, viruses

**Risk for Deficient Fluid Volume:** Risk factor: excessive loss of fluids

**Risk for Infection:** Risk factors: insufficient knowledge regarding avoidance of exposure to pathogens (water supply, iced drinks, local cheese, ice cream, undercooked meat, fish and shellfish, uncooked vegetables, unclean eating utensils, improper handwashing)

## TREMBLING OF HANDS

**Fear** r/t threat to or change in health status, threat of death, situational crisis

## TRICUSPID ATRESIA

*See Congenital Heart Disease/Cardiac Anomalies*

## TRIGEMINAL NEURALGIA

**Ineffective Health Self-Management** r/t deficient knowledge regarding prevention of stimuli that trigger pain

**Imbalanced Nutrition: Less than Body Requirements** r/t pain when chewing

**Acute Pain** r/t irritation of trigeminal nerve

**Risk for Corneal Injury:** Risk factor: possible decreased corneal sensation

## TRUNCUS ARTERIOSUS

*See Congenital Heart Disease/Cardiac Anomalies*

## TS (TOURETTE'S SYNDROME)

*See Tourette's Syndrome (TS)*

## TSE (TESTICULAR SELF-EXAMINATION)

**Readiness for Enhanced Health Self-Management:** seeks information regarding self-examination

## TUBAL LIGATION

**Decisional Conflict** r/t tubal sterilization

*See Laparoscopy*

## TUBE FEEDING

**Risk for Aspiration:** Risk factors: improper placement of feeding tube, improper positioning of client during and after feeding, excessive residual feeding or lack of digestion, altered gag reflex

**Risk for Deficient Fluid Volume:** Risk factor: inadequate water administration with concentrated feeding

**Risk for Imbalanced Nutrition: Less than Body Requirements:** Risk factors: intolerance to tube feeding, inadequate calorie replacement to meet metabolic needs

**Impaired Bowel Continence:** Risk factor: tube feeding osmolality too high for proper nutrient absorption

## TUBERCULOSIS (TB)

*See TB (Pulmonary Tuberculosis)*

## TURP (TRANSURETHRAL RESECTION OF THE PROSTATE)

**Deficient Knowledge** r/t postoperative self-care, home maintenance management

**Acute Pain** r/t incision, irritation from catheter, bladder spasms, kidney infection

**Urinary Retention** r/t obstruction of urethra or catheter with clots

**Risk for Bleeding:** Risk factor: surgery

**Risk for Deficient Fluid Volume:** Risk factors: fluid loss, possible bleeding

**Risk for Urge Urinary Incontinence:** Risk factor: edema from surgical procedure

**Risk for Infection:** Risk factors: invasive procedure, route for bacteria entry

**Risk for Urinary Tract Injury:** Risk factor: invasive procedure

## ULCER, PEPTIC (DUODENAL OR GASTRIC)

**Fatigue** r/t loss of blood, chronic illness

**Ineffective Health Maintenance Behaviors** r/t lack of knowledge regarding health practices to prevent ulcer formation

**Nausea** r/t gastrointestinal irritation

**Acute Pain** r/t irritated mucosa from acid secretion

*See GI Bleed (Gastrointestinal Bleeding)*

## ULCERATIVE COLITIS

*See Inflammatory Bowel Disease (Child and Adult)*

## ULCERS, STASIS

*See Stasis Ulcer*

## UNILATERAL NEGLECT OF ONE SIDE OF BODY

**Unilateral Neglect** (See **Unilateral Neglect,** Section II)

## UNSANITARY LIVING CONDITIONS

**Impaired Home Maintenance** r/t impaired cognitive or emotional functioning, lack of knowledge, insufficient finances, addiction

**Risk for Allergy Reaction:** Risk factor: exposure to environmental contaminants

## UPPER RESPIRATORY INFECTION

*See Cold, Viral*

## URGENCY TO URINATE

**Urge Urinary Incontinence** (See **Incontinence, Urinary, Urge,** Section II)

**Risk for Urge Urinary Incontinence** (See **Incontinence, Urinary, Urge, Risk for,** Section II)

## URINARY CATHETER

**Risk for Urinary Tract Injury:** Risk factors: confused client, long-term use of catheter, large retention balloon or catheter, perirectal burn injured client

# Vascular Dementia (Formerly Called Multi-Infarct Dementia) 153

**Risk for Infection:** Risk factors: difficulty managing long-term invasive urinary catheter devices

## URINARY DIVERSION
*See Ileal Conduit*

## URINARY ELIMINATION, IMPAIRED
**Impaired Urinary Elimination** (See **Urinary Elimination, Impaired,** Section II)

## URINARY INCONTINENCE
*See Incontinence of Urine*

## URINARY RETENTION
**Urinary Retention** (See **Urinary Retention,** Section II)

## URINARY TRACT INFECTION (UTI)
*See UTI (Urinary Tract Infection)*

## UROLITHIASIS
*See Kidney Stone*

## UTERINE ATONY IN LABOR
*See Dystocia*

## UTERINE ATONY IN POSTPARTUM
*See Postpartum Hemorrhage*

## UTERINE BLEEDING
*See Hemorrhage; Postpartum Hemorrhage; Shock, Hypovolemic*

## UTI (URINARY TRACT INFECTION)
**Ineffective Health Maintenance Behaviors** r/t deficient knowledge regarding methods to treat and prevent UTIs, prolonged use of indwelling urinary catheter

**Acute Pain: Dysuria** r/t inflammatory process in bladder

**Impaired Urinary Elimination: Frequency** r/t urinary tract infection

**Risk for Acute Confusion:** Risk factor: infectious process

**Risk for Urge Urinary Incontinence:** Risk factor: hyperreflexia from cystitis

**Risk for Urinary Tract Injury:** Risk factors: confused client, long-term use of catheter, large retention balloon or catheter

# V

## VAD (VENTRICULAR ASSIST DEVICE)
*See Ventricular Assist Device (VAD)*

## VAGINAL HYSTERECTOMY
**Urinary Retention** r/t edema at surgical site

**Risk for Urge Urinary Incontinence:** Risk factors: edema, congestion of pelvic tissues

**Risk for Infection:** Risk factor: surgical site

**Risk for Perioperative Positioning Injury:** Risk factor: lithotomy position

## VAGINITIS
**Impaired Comfort** r/t pruritus, itching

**Ineffective Health Maintenance Behaviors** r/t deficient knowledge regarding self-care with vaginitis

**Ineffective Sexuality Pattern** r/t abstinence during acute stage, pain

## VAGOTOMY
*See Abdominal Surgery*

## VALUE SYSTEM CONFLICT
**Decisional Conflict** r/t unclear personal values or beliefs

**Spiritual Distress** r/t challenged value system

**Readiness for Enhanced Spiritual Well-Being:** desire for harmony with self, others, higher power, God

## VARICOSE VEINS
**Ineffective Health Maintenance Behaviors** r/t deficient knowledge regarding health care practices, prevention, treatment regimen

**Chronic Pain** r/t impaired circulation

**Ineffective Peripheral Tissue Perfusion** r/t venous stasis

**Risk for Impaired Tissue Integrity:** Risk factor: altered peripheral tissue perfusion

## VASCULAR DEMENTIA (FORMERLY CALLED MULTI-INFARCT DEMENTIA)
*See Dementia*

## VASECTOMY

**Decisional Conflict** r/t surgery as method of permanent sterilization

## VENEREAL DISEASE

*See STD (Sexually Transmitted Disease)*

## VENOUS THROMBOEMBOLISM (VTE)

**Anxiety** r/t lack of circulation to body part

**Acute Pain** r/t vascular obstruction

**Ineffective Peripheral Tissue Perfusion** r/t interruption of circulatory flow

**Risk for Peripheral Neurovascular Dysfunction:** Risk factor: vascular obstruction

## VENTILATED CLIENT, MECHANICALLY

**Ineffective Airway Clearance** r/t increased secretions, decreased cough and gag reflex

**Ineffective Breathing Pattern** r/t decreased energy and fatigue as a result of possible altered nutrition: less than body requirements, neurological disease or damage

**Impaired Verbal Communication** r/t presence of endotracheal tube, inability to phonate

**Fear** r/t inability to breathe on own, difficulty communicating

**Impaired Gas Exchange** r/t ventilation-perfusion imbalance

**Powerlessness** r/t health treatment regimen

**Social Isolation** r/t impaired mobility, ventilator dependence

**Impaired Spontaneous Ventilation** r/t metabolic factors, respiratory muscle fatigue

**Dysfunctional Ventilatory Weaning Response** r/t psychological, situational, physiological factors

**Risk for Adult Falls:** Risk factors: impaired mobility, decreased muscle strength

**Risk for Child Falls:** Risk factors: impaired mobility, decreased lower extremity strength

**Risk for Infection:** Risk factors: presence of endotracheal tube, pooled secretions

**Risk for Pressure Ulcer:** Risk factor: decreased mobility

**Risk for Impaired Resilience:** Risk factor: illness

*See Child With Chronic Condition; Hospitalized Child; Respiratory Conditions of the Neonate*

## VENTRICULAR ASSIST DEVICE (VAD)

**Anxiety** r/t possible failure of device

**Risk for Infection:** Risk factor: device insertion site

**Risk for Vascular Trauma:** Risk factor: insertion site

**Readiness for Enhanced Decision-Making:** expresses desire to enhance the understanding of the meaning of choices regarding implanting a VAD

*See Open Heart Surgery*

## VENTRICULAR FIBRILLATION

*See Dysrhythmia*

## VETERANS

**Anxiety** r/t possible unmet needs, both physical and psychological

**Risk for Post-Trauma Syndrome:** Risk factors: witnessing death, survivor role, guilt, environment not conducive to needs

**Risk for Suicide:** Risk factors: substance abuse, insufficient social support, physical injury, psychiatric disorder

## VERTIGO

*See Syncope*

## VIOLENT BEHAVIOR

**Risk for Other-Directed Violence** (See **Violence, Other-Directed, Risk for,** Section II)

**Risk for Self-Directed Violence** (See **Violence, Self-Directed, Risk for,** Section II)

## VIRAL GASTROENTERITIS

**Diarrhea** r/t infectious process, Norovirus

**Deficient Fluid Volume** r/t vomiting, diarrhea

**Ineffective Health Self-Management** r/t inadequate handwashing

*See Gastroenteritis, Child*

## VISION IMPAIRMENT

**Fear** r/t loss of sight

**Social Isolation** r/t altered state of wellness, inability to see

**Risk for Impaired Resilience:** Risk factor: presence of new crisis

*See Blindness; Cataracts; Glaucoma*

## VOMITING

**Nausea** r/t infectious processes, chemotherapy, postsurgical anesthesia, irritation to the gastrointestinal system, stimulation of neuropharmacological mechanisms

**Imbalanced Nutrition: Less than Body Requirements** r/t inability to ingest food

**Risk for Electrolyte Imbalance:** Risk factor: vomiting

## VTE (VENOUS THROMBOEMBOLISM)

**Risk for Thrombosis** r/t ineffective management of preventive measures, immobility, dehydration

(See **Venous Thromboembolism, Risk for,** Section II)

# W

## WALKING IMPAIRMENT

**Impaired Walking** (See **Walking, Impaired,** Section II)

## WANDERING

**Wandering** (See **Wandering,** Section II)

## WEAKNESS

**Fatigue** r/t decreased or increased metabolic energy production

**Risk for Adult Falls:** Risk factor: weakness

## WEIGHT GAIN

**Overweight** (See **Overweight,** Section II)

**Risk for Metabolic Syndrome** r/t absence of interest in improving health behaviors

## WEIGHT LOSS

**Imbalanced Nutrition: Less than Body Requirements** r/t inability to ingest food

because of biological, psychological, economic factors

## WELLNESS-SEEKING BEHAVIOR

**Readiness for Enhanced Health Self-Management:** Expresses desire for increased control of health practice

## WERNICKE-KORSAKOFF SYNDROME

*See Korsakoff's Syndrome*

## WEST NILE VIRUS

*See Meningitis/Encephalitis*

## WHEELCHAIR USE PROBLEMS

**Impaired Wheelchair Mobility** (See **Mobility, Wheelchair, Impaired,** Section II)

## WHEEZING

**Ineffective Airway Clearance** r/t tracheobronchial obstructions, secretions

**Ineffective Breathing Pattern** r/t tracheobronchial obstructions and fatigue

## WILMS' TUMOR

**Chronic Functional Constipation** r/t obstruction associated with presence of tumor

**Acute Pain** r/t pressure from tumor

*See Chemotherapy; Hospitalized Child; Radiation Therapy; Surgery, Preoperative Care; Surgery, Perioperative Care; Surgery, Postoperative Care*

## WITHDRAWAL FROM ALCOHOL

*See Alcohol Withdrawal*

## WITHDRAWAL FROM DRUGS

*See Acute Substance Withdrawal Syndrome; Substance Misuse*

## WOUND DEBRIDEMENT

**Acute Pain** r/t debridement of wound

**Impaired Tissue Integrity** r/t debridement, open wound

**Risk for Infection:** Risk factors: open wound, presence of bacteria

## WOUND DEHISCENCE, EVISCERATION

**Fear** r/t client fear of body parts "falling out," surgical procedure not going as planned

**Disturbed Body Image** r/t change in body structure and wound appearance

**Imbalanced Nutrition: Less than Body Requirements** r/t inability to digest nutrients, need for increased protein for healing

**Risk for Deficient Fluid Volume:** Risk factors: inability to ingest nutrients, obstruction, fluid loss

**Risk for Injury:** Risk factor: exposed abdominal contents

**Risk for Delayed Surgical Recovery:** Risk factors: separation of wound, exposure of abdominal contents

**Risk for Surgical Site Infection:** Risk factor: open wound after surgical procedure

## WOUND INFECTION

**Disturbed Body Image** r/t open wound

**Imbalanced Nutrition: Less than Body Requirements** r/t biological factors, infection, fever

**Ineffective Thermoregulation** r/t infection in wound resulting in fever

**Impaired Tissue Integrity** r/t wound, presence of infection

**Risk for Imbalanced Fluid Volume:** Risk factor: increased metabolic rate

**Risk for Infection: Spread of:** Risk factor: imbalanced nutrition: less than body requirements

**Risk for Delayed Surgical Recovery:** Risk factor: presence of infection

## WOUNDS, OPEN

*See Lacerations*

**W**

# II

# GUIDE TO PLANNING CARE

Section II is a collection of NANDA-I nursing diagnosis care plans. The care plans are arranged alphabetically by diagnostic concept. Each care plan includes the diagnosis label, domain and class, definition, defining characteristics, and (if appropriate) risk factors, related factors, at-risk populations, and associated conditions. Risk diagnoses, however, only contain definition and risk factors. Care plans include suggested outcomes and interventions for all nursing diagnoses.

*MAKING AN ACCURATE NURSING DIAGNOSIS*
Verify the accuracy of the previously suggested nursing diagnoses (from Section I) or from the alphabetized list (front/back of the book) for the client.
- Read the definition for the suggested nursing diagnosis and determine if it is appropriate.
- Compare the Defining Characteristics with the symptoms that were identified from the client data collected.

*or*
- Compare the Risk Factors with the factors that were identified from the client data collected.

*WRITING OUTCOMES STATEMENTS AND NURSING INTERVENTIONS*
After selecting the appropriate nursing diagnosis, use this section to identify appropriate client outcomes and interventions.
- Follow this care plan to administer evidence-based nursing care to the client.
- Document all steps and evaluate and update the care plan as needed.

# GUIDE TO

# Decreased Activity Tolerance   A

**Domain 4** Activity/rest    **Class 2** Activity/exercise

## NANDA-I Definition

Insufficient endurance to complete required or desired daily activities.

## Defining Characteristics

Abnormal blood pressure response to activity; abnormal heart rate response to activity; anxious when activity is required; electrocardiogram change; exertional discomfort; exertional dyspnea; expresses fatigue; generalized weakness

## Related Factors

Decreased muscle strength; depressive symptoms; fear of pain; imbalance between oxygen supply/demand; impaired physical mobility; inexperience with an activity; insufficient muscle mass; malnutrition; pain; physical deconditioning; sedentary lifestyle

## At-Risk Population

Individuals with history of decreased activity tolerance; older adults

## Associated Conditions

Neoplasms; neurodegenerative diseases; respiration disorders; traumatic brain injuries; vitamin D deficiency

## Client Outcomes

### Client Will (Specify Time Frame)

- Participate in prescribed physical activity with appropriate changes in heart rate, blood pressure, and breathing rate; maintain monitor patterns (rhythm and ST segment) within normal limits
- State symptoms of adverse effects of exercise and report onset of symptoms immediately
- Maintain normal skin color; skin is warm and dry with activity
- Verbalize an understanding of the need to gradually increase activity based on testing, tolerance, and symptoms
- Demonstrate increased tolerance to activity

## Nursing Interventions

- Determine cause of decreased activity tolerance (see Related Factors) and decide whether cause is physical, psychological, or motivational.
- If mainly on bed rest, minimize cardiovascular, neuromuscular, and skeletal deconditioning by positioning the client in an upright position several times daily as tolerated and perform simple range-of-motion (ROM) techniques (passive or active).
- Assess the client daily for appropriateness of activity and bed rest orders. Mobilize the client as soon as possible.

• = Independent     ▲ = Collaborative

- If the client is mostly immobile, consider use of a transfer chair or a chair that becomes a stretcher.
- When appropriate, gradually increase activity, allowing the client to assist with positioning, transferring, and self-care as able. Progress the client from sitting in bed to dangling, to standing, to ambulation. Always have the client dangle at the bedside before standing to evaluate for postural hypotension.
▲ When getting a client up, observe for symptoms of intolerance such as nausea, pallor, dizziness, visual dimming, and impaired consciousness, as well as changes in vital signs; manual blood pressure monitoring is more accurate than use of an automated blood pressure device.
- If the client has symptoms of postural hypotension, such as dizziness, lightheadedness, or pallor, take precautions, such as dangling the client and applying leg compression stockings, before the client stands.
- Perform ROM exercises if the client is unable to tolerate activity or is mostly immobile. See care plan for Risk for **Disuse** Syndrome.
- Monitor and record the client's ability to tolerate activity: changes in mentation, pulse rate, blood pressure, respiratory pattern, dyspnea, use of accessory muscles, and skin color before, during, and after the activity. If the following signs and symptoms of cardiac decompensation develop, activity should be stopped immediately:
  ○ Lightheadedness, confusion, ataxia, pallor, cyanosis, nausea, or any peripheral circulatory insufficiency
  ○ Onset of chest discomfort or pain
  ○ Changes in heart rate: increased, decreased, palpitations, dysrhythmia
  ○ Drop in blood pressure or hypotension
  ○ Rise in blood pressure or hypertension
  ○ Dyspnea
  ○ Decreased oxygen saturation
  ○ Excessive fatigue
▲ Instruct the client to stop the activity immediately and report to the health care provider if the client is experiencing the following symptoms: new or worsened intensity or increased frequency of discomfort; tightness or pressure in chest, back, neck, jaw, shoulders, and/or arms; palpitations; dizziness; weakness; unusual and extreme fatigue; or excessive air hunger.
- Observe and document skin integrity several times a day. Decreased **Activity** Tolerance, if resulting in immobility, may lead to pressure ulcers. Mechanical pressure, moisture, friction, and shearing forces

all predispose to their development. Refer to the care plan Risk for Impaired **Skin** Integrity.
- Assess for constipation. If present, refer to care plan for **Constipation.** Decreased **Activity** Tolerance is associated with increased risk of **Constipation.**
▲ Refer the client to physical therapy to help increase activity levels and strength.
▲ Consider a dietitian referral to assess nutritional needs related to decreased activity tolerance; provide nutrition as indicated. If the client is unable to eat food, use enteral or parenteral feedings as needed.
- Recognize that malnutrition causes significant morbidity because of the loss of lean body mass.
- Provide emotional support and encouragement to the client to gradually increase activity. Work with the client to set mutual goals that increase activity levels.
▲ Observe for pain before activity. If possible, treat pain before activity and ensure that the client is not heavily sedated.
▲ Obtain any necessary assistive devices or equipment needed before ambulating the client (e.g., walkers, canes, crutches, portable oxygen).
▲ Use a gait-walking belt when ambulating the client.

**Decreased Activity Tolerance Due to Respiratory Disease**
- If the client is able to walk and has chronic obstructive pulmonary disease (COPD), use the traditional 6-minute walk distance to evaluate activity tolerance with ambulation.
▲ Ensure that the client with pulmonary diseases has oxygen saturation testing with exercise. Use supplemental oxygen to keep oxygen saturation 90% or above or as prescribed with activity.
- Monitor a respiratory client's response to activity by observing for symptoms of respiratory intolerance, such as increased dyspnea, loss of ability to control breathing rhythmically, use of accessory muscles, nasal flaring, appearance of facial distress, and skin tone changes such as pallor and cyanosis, changes in mentation, or inability to talk during activity.
- Instruct and assist the client in using conscious, controlled breathing techniques during exercise, including pursed-lip breathing, and inspiratory muscle use.
▲ Evaluate the client's nutritional status. Use nutritional supplements to increase nutritional level if needed. Refer to a dietitian if indicated.
▲ For the client in the intensive care unit, consider mobilizing the client with passive exercise.

• = Independent        ▲ = Collaborative

▲ Refer the COPD client to a pulmonary rehabilitation program.

**Decreased Activity Tolerance Due to Cardiovascular Disease**

• If the client is able to walk and has heart failure, consider use of the 6-minute walk test to determine physical ability.

• Allow for periods of rest before and after planned exertion periods such as meals, baths, treatments, and physical activity.

▲ Refer to a heart failure program or cardiac rehabilitation program for education, evaluation, and guided support to increase activity and rebuild life.

▲ Refer to a community support program that includes support of significant others.

• See care plan for Decreased **Cardiac** Output for further interventions.

**Pediatric**

• Focus interview questions toward exercise tolerance, specifically including any history of asthma exacerbations.

**Geriatric**

• Slow the pace of care. Allow the client extra time to perform physical activities. Slow gait in older adults may be related to fear of falling, decreased strength in muscles, reduced balance or visual acuity, knee flexion contractures, and foot pain.

• Encourage families to help/allow an older client to be independent in whatever activities possible.

▲ Assess for swaying, poor balance, weakness, and fear of falling while older clients stand/walk. Refer to physical therapy if appropriate.

• Refer to the care plan for Risk for Adult **Falls** and Impaired **Walking.**

▲ Initiate ambulation by simply ambulating a client a few steps from bed to chair, once a health care provider's out-of-bed order is obtained.

▲ Evaluate medications the client is taking to see if they could be causing Decreased **Activity** Tolerance.

▲ Refer the disabled older client to physical therapy for functional training including gait training, stepping, and sit-to-stand exercises, or for strength training.

**Home Care**

▲ Begin discharge planning as soon as possible with the case manager or social worker to assess the need for home support systems and the need for community or home health services.

▲ Assess the home environment for factors that contribute to decreased activity tolerance such as stairs or distance to the bathroom. Refer the client for occupational therapy, if needed, and to assist the client in restructuring the home and ADL patterns.

• = Independent                    ▲ = Collaborative

▲ Refer the client for physical therapy for strength training and possible **A** weight training to regain strength, increase endurance, and improve balance. If the client is homebound, the physical therapist can also initiate cardiac rehabilitation.

• Encourage progress with positive feedback. The client's experience should be validated within expected norms. Recognition of progress enhances motivation.

• Teach the client/family the importance of and methods for setting priorities for activities, especially those having a high energy demand (e.g., home/family events). Instruct on realistic expectations.

• Encourage routine low-level exercise periods such as a daily short walk or chair exercises.

• Provide the client/family with resources such as senior centers, exercise classes, educational and recreational programs, and volunteer opportunities that can aid in promoting socialization and appropriate activity. Social isolation can be an outcome of and contribute to Decreased **Activity** Tolerance.

• Instruct the client and family on the importance of maintaining proper nutrition and use of dietary supplements as indicated. Illness may suppress appetite, leading to inadequate nutrition.

▲ Refer to medical social services as necessary to assist the family in adjusting to major changes in patterns of living because of Decreased **Activity** Tolerance.

▲ Assess the need for long-term supports for optimal activity tolerance of priority activities (e.g., assistive devices, oxygen, medication, catheters, massage), especially for a hospice client. Evaluate intermittently.

▲ Refer to home health aide services to support the client and family through changing levels of activity tolerance. Introduce aide support early. Instruct the aide to promote independence in activity as tolerated.

• Allow terminally ill clients and their families to guide care. Control by the client or family respects their autonomy and promotes effective coping.

• Provide increased attention to comfort and dignity of the terminally ill client in care planning.

▲ Institute case management of frail elderly to support continued independent living.

**Client/Family Teaching and Discharge Planning**

• Instruct the client on techniques for avoiding Decreased **Activity** Tolerance, such as controlled breathing techniques.

• = Independent          ▲ = Collaborative

**A**
- Teach the client techniques to decrease dizziness from postural hypotension when changing positions, especially when standing up.
- Help client with energy conservation and work simplification techniques in ADLs.
- Describe to the client the symptoms of Decreased **Activity** Tolerance, including which symptoms to report to the health care provider.
- Explain to the client how to use assistive devices, oxygen, or medications before or during activity.
- Help the client set up an activity log to record exercise and exercise tolerance.

# Risk for Decreased Activity Tolerance

**Domain 4** Activity/rest     **Class 2** Activity/exercise
## NANDA-I Definition
Susceptible to experiencing insufficient endurance to complete required or desired daily activities.
## Risk Factors
Decreased muscle strength; depressive symptoms; fear of pain; imbalance between oxygen supply/demand; impaired physical mobility; inexperience with an activity; insufficient muscle mass; malnutrition; pain; physical deconditioning; sedentary lifestyle
## At-Risk Population
Individuals with history of decreased activity tolerance; older adults
## Associated Conditions
Neoplasms; neurodegenerative diseases; respiration disorders; traumatic brain injuries; vitamin D deficiency
## Client Outcomes, Nursing Interventions, and Client/Family Teaching and Discharge Planning
Refer to care plan for Decreased **Activity** Tolerance.

# Ineffective Activity Planning

**Domain 9** Coping/stress tolerance     **Class 2** Coping responses
## NANDA-I Definition
Inability to prepare for a set of actions fixed in time and under certain conditions.

• = Independent            ▲ = Collaborative

## Defining Characteristics

Absence of plan; excessive anxiety about a task; inadequate health resources; inadequate organizational skills; pattern of failure; reports fear of performing a task; unmet goals for chosen activity

## Related Factors

Flight behavior when faced with proposed solution; hedonism; inadequate information processing ability; inadequate social support; unrealistic perception of event; unrealistic perception of personal abilities

## At-Risk Population

Individuals with history of procrastination

## Client Outcomes

### Client Will (Specify Time Frame)

- Verbalize need for self-directed activity
- Choose the health care option that fits his or her lifestyle within an appropriate amount of time that allows enactment of the choice
- Describe how the chosen option fits into current lifestyle before or after the decision has been made
- Verbalize the need for a behavioral change to improve physical activity
- Offer alternative options to those with barriers to participating in physical activity

## Nursing Interventions

- Identify the client's perception of the problem and how they envision their participation to improve goal setting.
- Identify the informational needs of the client such as client's understanding of health condition, treatment options, health system processes, diet, exercise, and access to important telephone numbers.
- Address the client's fears and anxieties and encourage him or her to modify their cognitive approach to planning.
- Client verbalizes need for behavioral change for improved physical activity.
- Encourage clients to verbalize the need for physical activity to help reduce role overload.
- ▲ Determine factors that will increase opportunities to successfully plan activities and increase the success of the project: financial resources; family situation; prior medical, psychiatric, and psychosocial conditions; material resources; and the ability to manage stress.
- ▲ Encourage physical actively. Collaborate with occupational and/or physical therapy to establish activity opportunities and limitations.

### Pediatric

- Begin activity planning in preschool-age children of working parents.
- Establish a contract.

• = Independent          ▲ = Collaborative

**A**

- Provide support to the schools for physical activities in all school venues.
- Support safe neighborhood activity programs.

**Geriatric**

- Plan activities for older clients.
- Plan activities for older clients with impaired mental function.
- Community-based activities for older adults.

**Multicultural**

- Provide literature and information in the appropriate language for the client who speaks little to no English.
- Preplanning educational programs for the culturally diverse population needs to be developed.
- ▲ Support and education by the physician and family on how exercise can help reduce and/or prevent falls of older adults improves adherence to physical activity.

**Home Care**

- Have a preplanned activity exercise for the home client with a debilitating musculoskeletal disease to help improve functional status.
- Assess the home environment for barriers that can impact the client's motivation to be a participant in the activity planned.
- Home care for the cardiac rehabilitation client.
- For additional interventions, refer to care plans for **Anxiety,** Readiness for Enhanced Family **Coping,** Readiness for Enhanced **Decision-Making, Fear,** Readiness for Enhanced **Hope,** Readiness for Enhanced **Power,** Readiness for Enhanced **Spiritual** Well-Being, and Readiness for Enhanced **Health** Self-Management.

# Risk for Ineffective Activity Planning

**Domain 9** Coping/stress tolerance     **Class 2** Coping responses

## NANDA-I Definition

Susceptible to an inability to prepare for a set of actions fixed in time and under certain conditions, which may compromise health.

## Risk Factors

Flight behavior when faced with proposed solution; hedonism; inadequate information processing ability; inadequate social support; unrealistic perception of event; unrealistic perception of personal abilities

## At-Risk Population

Individuals with history of procrastination

**Client Outcomes, Nursing Interventions, and Client/Family Teaching and Discharge Planning**

Refer to care plan for Ineffective **Activity** Planning.

# Ineffective Airway Clearance

**Domain 11** Safety/protection    **Class 2** Physical injury

## NANDA-I Definition

Reduced ability to clear secretions or obstructions from the respiratory tract to maintain a clear airway.

## Defining Characteristics

Absence of cough; adventitious breath sounds; altered respiratory rhythm; altered thoracic percussion; altered thoraco-vocal fremitus; bradypnea; cyanosis; difficulty verbalizing; diminished breath sounds; excessive sputum; hypoxemia; ineffective cough; ineffective sputum elimination; nasal flaring; orthopnea; psychomotor agitation; subcostal retraction; tachypnea; use of accessory muscles of respiration

## Related Factors

Dehydration; excessive mucus; exposure to harmful substance; fear of pain; foreign body in airway; inattentive to second-hand smoke; mucus plug; retained secretions; smoking

## At-Risk Population

Children; infants

## Associated Conditions

Airway spasm; allergic airway; asthma; chronic obstructive pulmonary disease; congenital heart disease; critical illness; exudate in the alveoli; general anesthesia; hyperplasia of the bronchial walls; neuromuscular diseases; respiratory tract infection

## Client Outcomes

**Client Will (Specify Time Frame)**

- Demonstrate effective coughing and clear breath sounds
- Maintain a patent airway at all times
- Explain methods useful to enhance secretion removal
- Explain the significance of changes in sputum to include color, character, amount, and odor
- Identify and avoid specific factors that inhibit effective airway clearance

## Nursing Interventions

- Auscultate breath sounds every 1 to 4 hours. The presence of crackles and wheezes may alert the nurse to airway obstruction, which may lead to or exacerbate existing hypoxia.

• = Independent          ▲ = Collaborative

- Monitor respiratory patterns, including rate, depth, and effort.
- Monitor blood gas values and pulse oxygen saturation levels as available. An oxygen saturation of less than 90% (normal: 95%–100%) or a partial pressure of oxygen of less than 80 mm Hg (normal: 80–100 mm Hg) indicates significant oxygenation problems (Bickley et al, 2020a).
▲ Administer oxygen as ordered. Oxygen administration has been shown to correct hypoxemia (Sauls, 2021).
- Position the client in a semirecumbent position with the head of the bed at a 30- to 45-degree angle to decrease the aspiration of gastric, oral, and nasal secretions (Siela, 2010; Vollman, Sole, & Quinn, 2017; Sauls, 2021).
- Help the client deep breathe and perform controlled coughing. Have the client inhale deeply, hold breath for several seconds, and cough two or three times with mouth open while tightening the upper abdominal muscles.
- If the client has obstructive lung disease, such as chronic obstructive pulmonary disease (COPD), cystic fibrosis, or bronchiectasis, consider helping the client use the forced expiratory technique, the "huff cough." The client does a series of coughs while saying the word "huff."
▲ Encourage the client to use an incentive spirometer. Recognize that controlled coughing and deep breathing may be just as effective as incentive spirometry (Chalmers, Aliberti, & Blasi, 2015).
- Encourage activity and ambulation as tolerated. If the client cannot be ambulated, turn the client from side to side at least every 2 hours.
- Encourage fluid intake of up to 2500 mL/day within cardiac or renal reserve.
▲ Administer medications such as bronchodilators or inhaled steroids as ordered. Watch for side effects such as tachycardia or anxiety with bronchodilators or inflamed pharynx with inhaled steroids.
▲ Provide percussion, vibration, and oscillation as appropriate for individual client needs.
- Use of positive expiratory pressure (PEP) with a mask for airway clearance shows a significant reduction in pulmonary exacerbations in people with cystic fibrosis (McIlwaine, Button, & Nevitt, 2019).
- Observe sputum, noting color, odor, and volume.

**Critical Care**

▲ In intubated clients, body positioning and mobilization may optimize airway secretion clearance. Lateral rotational movement provides continuous postural drainage and mobilization of secretions (St. Clair & MacDermott, 2017).

• = Independent          ▲ = Collaborative

A

- Reposition the client as needed. Use rotational or kinetic bed therapy in clients for whom side-to-side turning is contraindicated or difficult.
- If the client is intubated, consider use of kinetic therapy, using a kinetic bed that slowly moves the client with 40-degree turns.
- Assess for the presence or absence of a gag reflex.
▲ Early mobility and physical rehabilitation can reduce muscle weakness, mechanical ventilation duration, intensive care unit stay, delirium, and hospitalization.
- If the client is intubated and is stable, consider getting the client up to sit at the edge of the bed, transfer to a chair, or walk as appropriate, if an effective multiprofessional team is developed to keep the client safe (Dirkes & Kozlowski, 2019).
- When suctioning an endotracheal tube or tracheostomy tube for a client on a ventilator, do the following:
  ○ Explain the process of suctioning beforehand and ensure the client is not in pain or overly anxious. Suctioning can be a frightening experience; an explanation along with adequate pain relief or needed sedation can reduce stress, anxiety, and pain (Seckel, 2017).
  ○ Hyperoxygenate before and between endotracheal suction sessions. Studies have demonstrated that hyperoxygenation may help prevent oxygen desaturation in a suctioned client (Pedersen et al, 2009; Siela, 2010; Seckel, 2017; Vollman, Sole, & Quinn, 2017).
  ○ Suction for less than 15 seconds. Studies demonstrated that because of a drop in the partial pressure of oxygen with suctioning, preferably no more than 10 seconds should be used actually suctioning, with the entire procedure taking 15 seconds (Pedersen et al, 2009; Seckel, 2017).
  ○ Use a closed, in-line suction system. Closed in-line suctioning has minimal effects on heart rate, respiratory rate, tidal volume, and oxygen saturation and may reduce contamination (Seckel, 2017).
  ○ Avoid saline instillation during suctioning.
  ○ Use of a subglottic suctioning endotracheal tube reduces the incidence of VAP or ventilator-associated complications (Vollman, Sole, & Quinn, 2017; Pozuelo-Carrascosa et al, 2020). A decrease in mortality occurs with use of subglottic secretion drainage (Pozuelo-Carrascosa et al, 2020).
  ○ Document results of coughing and suctioning, particularly client tolerance and secretion characteristics such as color, odor, and volume (Seckel, 2017).

• = Independent          ▲ = Collaborative

**A**

**Pediatric**

- Educate parents about the risk factors for ineffective airway clearance such as foreign body ingestion and passive smoke exposure.
- Educate children and parents on the importance of adherence to peak expiratory flow monitoring for asthma self-management.
- Educate parents and other caregivers that cough and cold medications bought over the counter are not safe for a child younger than 2 unless specifically ordered by a health care provider.
- See the care plan for Risk for **Suffocation.**

**Geriatric**

- Encourage ambulation as tolerated without causing exhaustion.
- Actively encourage older adults to deep breathe and cough.
- Ensure adequate hydration within cardiac and renal reserves.

**Home Care**

- Some of the above interventions may be adapted for home care use.
- ▲ Begin discharge planning as soon as possible with case manager or social worker to assess need for home support systems, assistive devices, and community or home health services.
- Assess home environment for factors that exacerbate airway clearance problems (e.g., presence of allergens, lack of adequate humidity in air, poor air flow, stressful family relationships).
- Assess affective climate within family and family support system. Refer to care plan for **Caregiver** Role Strain.
- Refer to GOLD guidelines for management of home care and indications of hospital admission criteria. http://www.goldcopd.org/.
- When respiratory procedures are being implemented, explain equipment and procedures to family members and caregivers, and provide needed emotional support.
- When electrically based equipment for respiratory support is being implemented, evaluate home environment for electrical safety, proper grounding, and so on. Ensure that notification is sent to the local utility company, the emergency medical team, and police and fire departments.
- Provide family with support for care of a client with chronic or terminal illness.
- Witnessing breathing difficulties and facing concerns of dealing with chronic or terminal illness can create fear in caregiver. Fear inhibits effective coping. Refer to care plans for **Anxiety** and **Powerlessness.**
- Instruct the client to avoid exposure to persons with upper respiratory infections, avoid crowds of people, and wash hands after each exposure to groups of people or public places.

• = Independent          ▲ = Collaborative

▲ Determine client adherence to medical regimen. Instruct the client and family on importance of reporting effectiveness of current medications to health care provider.

• Teach the client when and how to use inhalant or nebulizer treatments at home.

• Teach the client/family importance of maintaining regimen and having "as-needed" drugs easily accessible at all times.

• Instruct the client and family on the importance of maintaining proper nutrition, adequate fluids, rest, and behavioral pacing for energy conservation and rehabilitation.

• Instruct in use of dietary supplements as indicated.

• Identify an emergency plan, including criteria for use.

▲ Refer for home health aide services for assistance with activities of daily living (ADLs). Clients with decreased oxygenation and copious respiratory secretions are often unable to maintain energy for ADLs.

▲ Assess family for role changes and coping skills. Refer to medical social services as necessary.

▲ For the client dying at home with a terminal illness, if the "death rattle" is present with gurgling, rattling, or crackling sounds in the airway with each breath, recognize that anticholinergic medications can often help control symptoms, if given early in the process.

▲ For the client with a death rattle, nursing care includes turning to mobilize secretions, keeping the head of the bed elevated for postural drainage of secretions, and avoiding suctioning.

**Client/Family Teaching and Discharge Planning**

▲ Teach the importance of not smoking. Refer to a smoking cessation program, and encourage clients who relapse to keep trying to quit. Ensure that the client receives appropriate medications to support smoking cessation from the primary health care provider.

▲ Teach the client how to use a flutter clearance device if ordered, which vibrates to loosen mucus and gives positive pressure to keep airways open.

▲ Teach the client how to use peak expiratory flow rate (PEFR) meter if ordered and when to seek medical attention if PEFR reading drops. Also teach how to use metered dose inhalers and self-administer inhaled corticosteroids as ordered following precautions to decrease side effects.

• Teach the client how to deep breathe and cough effectively. Controlled coughing uses the diaphragmatic muscles, making the cough more forceful and effective (Sommers et al, 2015).

• = Independent          ▲ = Collaborative

- Teach the client/family to identify and avoid specific factors that exacerbate ineffective airway clearance, including known allergens and especially smoking (if relevant) or exposure to secondhand smoke (SHS).
- Educate the client and family about the significance of changes in sputum characteristics, including color, character, amount, and odor. With this knowledge, the client and family can identify early the signs of infection and seek treatment before acute illness occurs.
- Teach the client/family the importance of taking antibiotics as prescribed, consuming all tablets until the prescription has run out. Taking the entire course of antibiotics helps eradicate bacterial infection, which decreases lingering, chronic infection.
- Teach the family of the dying client in hospice with a death rattle that rarely are clients aware of the fluid that has accumulated, and help them find evidence of comfort in the client's nonverbal behavior (Kolb et al, 2018).

# Risk for Allergy Reaction

**Domain 11** Safety/protection    **Class 5** Defensive processes
## NANDA-I Definition

Susceptible to an exaggerated immune response or reaction to substances, which may compromise health.

## Risk Factors

Exposure to allergen; exposure to environmental allergen; exposure to toxic chemicals; inadequate knowledge about avoidance of relevant allergens; inattentive to potential allergen exposure

## At-Risk Population

Individuals with history of food allergy; individuals with history of insect sting allergy; individuals with repeated exposure to allergen-producing environmental substance

## Client Outcomes

**Client Will (Specify Time Frame)**
- State risk factors for allergies
- Demonstrate knowledge of plan to treat allergic reaction

## Nursing Interventions

- A careful history is important in detecting allergens and avoidance of these allergens.
- Obtain a precise history of allergies, as well as medications taken and foods ingested before surgery.

• = Independent          ▲ = Collaborative

▲ Teach the client about the correct use of the injectable epinephrine and have the client do a return demonstration.

▲ Carefully assess the client for allergies.

**Causes**

Common allergens include animal dander; bee stings or stings from other insects; foods, especially nuts, fish, and shellfish; insect bites; medications; plants; pollens

**Symptoms**

Common symptoms of a mild allergic reaction include hives (especially over the neck and face); itching; nasal congestion; rashes; watery, red eyes

Symptoms of a moderate or severe reaction include cramps or pain in the abdomen; chest discomfort or tightness; diarrhea; difficulty breathing; difficulty swallowing; dizziness or lightheadedness; fear or feeling of apprehension or anxiety; flushing or redness of the face; nausea and vomiting; palpitations; swelling of the face, eyes, or tongue; weakness; wheezing; unconsciousness

**First Aid**

For a mild to moderate reaction: calm and reassure the person having the reaction because anxiety can worsen symptoms.

1. Try to identify the allergen and have the person avoid further contact with it. If the allergic reaction is from a bee sting, scrape the stinger off the skin with something firm (e.g., fingernail or plastic credit card). Do not use tweezers; squeezing the stinger will release more venom.

2. Apply cool compresses and over-the-counter hydrocortisone cream for itchy rash.

3. Watch for signs of increasing distress.

4. Get medical help. For a mild reaction, a health care provider may recommend over-the-counter medications (e.g., antihistamines).

**For a Severe Allergic Reaction (Anaphylaxis)**

1. Check the person's airway, breathing, and circulation (the ABCs of Basic Life Support). A warning sign of dangerous throat swelling is a very hoarse or whispered voice or coarse sounds when the person is breathing in air. If necessary, begin rescue breathing and cardiopulmonary resuscitation.

2. Call 911.

3. Calm and reassure the person.

4. If the allergic reaction is from a bee sting, scrape the stinger off the skin with something firm (e.g., fingernail or plastic credit card). Do not use tweezers; squeezing the stinger will release more venom.

• = Independent          ▲ = Collaborative

5. If the person has emergency allergy medication on hand, help the person take or inject the medication as soon as possible. Avoid oral medication if the person is having difficulty breathing.

6. Take steps to prevent shock. Have the person lie flat, raise the person's feet about 12 inches, and cover him or her with a coat or blanket. Do NOT place the person in this position if a head, neck, back, or leg injury is suspected or if it causes discomfort.

## Do NOT

- Do NOT assume that any allergy shots the person has already received will provide complete protection.
- Do NOT place a pillow under the person's head if he or she is having trouble breathing. This can block the airways.
- Do NOT give the person anything by mouth if the person is having trouble breathing.

## When to Contact a Medical Professional

Call for immediate medical emergency assistance if:

- The person is having a severe allergic reaction—always call 911. Do not wait to see if the reaction is getting worse.
- The person has a history of severe allergic reactions (check for a medical ID tag).

## Prevention

- Avoid triggers such as foods and medications that have caused an allergic reaction (even a mild one) in the past. Ask detailed questions about ingredients when you are eating away from home. Carefully examine ingredient labels.
- If you have a child who is allergic to certain foods, introduce one new food at a time in limited amounts so you can recognize an allergic reaction.
- People who know that they have had serious allergic reactions should wear a medical ID tag.
- Preoperative clients should be closely assessed for allergies.
- For clients with a history of serious allergic reactions, counsel to carry emergency medications (e.g., a chewable form of diphenhydramine and injectable epinephrine or a bee sting kit) according to their health care provider's instructions.
- Instruct clients to not give their injectable epinephrine (or any other personal medication) to anyone else as they may have a condition (e.g., a heart problem) that could be negatively affected by this drug.
▲ Refer the client for skin testing to confirm IgE-mediated allergic response.

• = Independent          ▲ = Collaborative

- Provide all clients with a history of anaphylaxis with education about anaphylaxis, risk of recurrence, trigger avoidance, self-injectable epinephrine, and thresholds for further care.
▲ Refer all clients with a history of anaphylaxis to an allergist for follow-up evaluation.
- See care plan for Risk for **Latex Allergy** Reaction.

**Pediatric**
- Teach parents and children with allergies to peanuts and tree nuts to avoid them and to identify them.
- Teach parents and children with asthma about modifiable risk factors, which include allergy triggers.
- Counsel parents to limit infant exposure to traffic and cigarette carbon monoxide pollution.
▲ Refer clients for food protein–induced enterocolitis syndrome (FPIES) in formula-fed infants with repetitive emesis, diarrhea, dehydration, and lethargy 1 to 5 hours after ingesting the offending food (the most common are cow's milk, soy, and rice). Remove the offending food.
▲ Children should be screened for seafood allergies and if an allergy is detected, avoid seafood and any foods containing seafood.

# Anxiety

**Domain 9** Coping/stress tolerance    **Class 2** Coping responses

## NANDA-I Definition

An emotional response to a diffuse threat in which the individual anticipates nonspecific impending danger, catastrophe, or misfortune.

## Defining Characteristics

### Behavioral/Emotional

Crying; decrease in productivity; expresses anguish; expresses anxiety about life event changes; expresses distress; expresses insecurity; expresses intense dread; helplessness; hypervigilance; increased wariness; insomnia; irritable mood; nervousness; psychomotor agitation; reduced eye contact; scanning behavior; self-focused

### Physiological Factors

Altered respiratory pattern; anorexia; brisk reflexes; chest tightness; cold extremities; diarrhea; dry mouth; expresses abdominal pain; expresses feeling faint; expresses muscle weakness; expresses tension; facial flushing; increased blood pressure; increased heart rate; increased sweating; nausea; pupil dilation; quivering voice; reports altered sleep-wake cycle; reports heart palpitations; reports tingling in extremities; superficial vasoconstriction; tremors; urinary frequency; urinary hesitancy

• = Independent          ▲ = Collaborative

## Cognitive Factors

Altered attention; confusion; decreased perceptual field; expresses forget-fulness; expresses preoccupation; reports blocking of thoughts; rumination

## Related Factors

Conflict about life goals; interpersonal transmission; pain; stressors; substance misuse; unfamiliar situation; unmet needs; value conflict

## At-Risk Population

Individuals experiencing developmental crisis; individuals experiencing situational crisis; individuals exposed to toxins; individuals in the perioperative period; individuals with family history of anxiety; individuals with hereditary predisposition

## Associated Conditions

Mental disorders

## Client Outcomes

### Client Will (Specify Time Frame)

- Identify and verbalize symptoms of anxiety
- Identify, verbalize, and demonstrate techniques to manage anxiety
- Verbalize absence of or decrease in subjective distress
- Have vital signs that reflect baseline or decreased sympathetic stimulation
- Have posture, facial expressions, gestures, and activity levels that reflect decreased distress or a more tolerable level of anxiety
- Demonstrate improved concentration and accuracy of thoughts
- Demonstrate return of basic problem-solving skills
- Demonstrate increased external focus
- Demonstrate some ability to reassure self

## Nursing Interventions

- Assess the client's level of anxiety by noticing the physiologic, emotional, cognitive, and behavioral symptoms associated with the feeling state of anxiety.
- Introduce yourself and your role, explain what you will be doing and why, and explain usual hospital procedures.
- Intervene when possible to remove sources of anxiety.
- Explain all activities, procedures, and issues that involve the client; use nonmedical terms and calm, slow speech; and then validate the client's understanding.
- ▲ Use massage therapy to reduce anxiety.
- ▲ Consider massage therapy for preoperative clients.
- Use guided imagery to decrease anxiety.

- Suggest yoga to the client.
- Provide clients with a means to listen to music of their choice or audiotapes.
▲ Refer to cognitive behavioral therapy (CBT).

**Pediatric**
- The previously mentioned interventions may be adapted for the pediatric client.

**Geriatric**
▲ Monitor the client for depression. Use appropriate interventions and referrals.
- Limit the use of benzodiazepines and nonbenzodiazepine agents for anxiety in the older adult. If these drugs must be used, give the lowest dose possible for short-term use only.

**Multicultural**
- Identify how anxiety is manifested in the culturally diverse client.
▲ Refer to culturally adapted CBT.

**Home Care**
- The previously mentioned interventions may be adapted for home care use.
- Encourage effective communication between family members.
- Assist family in being supportive of the client in the face of anxiety symptoms.
▲ Consider referral for the prescription of antianxiety or antidepressant medications for clients who have panic disorder or other anxiety-related psychiatric disorders.
▲ Assist the client/family to institute the medication regimen appropriately. Instruct in side effects and the importance of taking medications as ordered.

**Client/Family Teaching and Discharge Planning**
- Provide basic teaching information about anxiety and anxiety disorders that includes signs and symptoms, risk factors, treatments, and therapies.
- Provide client education about medications that includes side effects, ways to manage side effects, special administration issues (e.g., take with food, take at night), including which medications to avoid using concurrently. Education should also include a list of adverse effects that should be reported to the health care practitioner.
▲ Teach use of appropriate community resources in emergency situations (e.g., suicidal thoughts), such as hotlines, emergency departments, law enforcement, and judicial systems.

• = Independent          ▲ = Collaborative

**A**

- Teach the client to visualize or fantasize about the absence of anxiety or pain, successful experience of the situation, resolution of conflict, or outcome of procedure.
- Teach the relationship between a healthy physical and emotional lifestyle and a realistic mental attitude.

## Death Anxiety

**Domain 9** Coping/stress tolerance    **Class 2** Coping responses

### NANDA-I Definition

Emotional distress and insecurity, generated by anticipation of death and the process of dying of oneself or significant others, which negatively effects one's quality of life.

### Defining Characteristics

Dysphoria; expresses concern about caregiver strain; expresses concern about the impact of one's death on significant other; expresses deep sadness; expresses fear of developing terminal illness; expresses fear of loneliness; expresses fear of loss of mental abilities when dying; expresses fear of pain related to dying; expresses fear of premature death; expresses fear of prolonged dying process; expresses fear of separation from loved ones; expresses fear of suffering related to dying; expresses fear of the dying process; expresses fear of the unknown; expresses powerlessness; reports negative thoughts related to death and dying

### Related Factors

Anticipation of adverse consequences of anesthesia; anticipation of impact of death on others; anticipation of pain; anticipation of suffering; awareness of imminent death; depressive symptoms; discussions on the topic of death; impaired religiosity; loneliness; low self-esteem; nonacceptance of own mortality; spiritual distress; uncertainty about encountering a higher power; uncertainty about life after death; uncertainty about the existence of a higher power; uncertainty of prognosis; unpleasant physical symptoms

### At-Risk Population

Individuals experiencing terminal care of significant others; individuals receiving terminal care; individuals with history of adverse experiences with death of significant others; individuals with history of near-death experience; older adults; women; young adults

### Associated Conditions

Depression; stigmatized illnesses with high fear of death; terminal illness

### Client Outcomes

**Client Will (Specify Time Frame)**

- Express feelings associated with death and the process of dying

• = Independent                    ▲ = Collaborative

- State concerns about impact of death on others
- Seek help in dealing with feelings
- Discuss realistic goals
- State concerns about the impact of death on significant others
- Use strategies to lessen anxiety surrounding death and dying including spiritual intelligence and finding meaning in one's life
- Use spiritual support for comfort

## Nursing Interventions

- Complete a comprehensive nursing assessment on individuals with life-limiting illnesses.
- Assess family and caregivers' responses to death and dying, looking for symptoms of death anxiety.
- Assess for the development of new maladaptive coping in response to the powerful sense of fear or meaninglessness that is associated with awareness of death.
- Develop a trusting therapeutic relationship with the client and family.
- Continue to remain available and to use empathetic communication skills so that the client and family will continue to feel comfortable discussing ongoing concerns.
- Assess clients for pain and provide pain relief measures.
- Assess client for fears related to death.
- Use psychosocial techniques to decrease distress.
- Assist clients with life planning: consider and redefine main life goals, focus on areas of strength and/or goals that will provide satisfaction, adopt realistic goals, and recognize those that are impossible to achieve.
- Assist clients with life review and reminiscence.
- Provide music of the client's choosing.
- Provide social support for families: understanding what is most important to families who are caring for clients at the end of life.
- Encourage clients to use spiritual supports.
- Explore ways to provide spiritual support by asking clients what is important to them and what you can do to help and refer as needed.
- As a nurse, be aware of your own increased risk of experiencing symptoms of death anxiety and the negative impact this may have on your well-being. Seek support as needed.

## Geriatric

- Carefully assess older adults for issues regarding death anxiety.
- Assess the individual's resolution of Erikson's developmental stage of integrity versus despair. In this stage those age 65 and older reflect on

**A**

their life and either move into feeling satisfied and happy with one's life or feel a deep sense of regret.

- Teach components of spiritual intelligence (the adaptive use of spiritual information to facilitate everyday problem solving and goal attainment).
- Use strategies to strengthen the individual's spiritual health and support use of religion as a coping strategy when applicable.
- Refer to care plan for Maladaptive **Grieving.**

**Multicultural**
- Assist clients to identify with their culture and its values.
- Refer to care plans for **Anxiety** and Maladaptive **Grieving.**

**Home Care**
- The previously mentioned interventions may be adapted for home care.
▲ Support and facilitate a discussion of advance care plans/advanced directives as another strategy to lessen verbalized fears and concerns about death and the dying process. Document decisions.
▲ Make referrals to mental health professionals for CBT or logotherapy.
▲ Refer to appropriate medical services, social services, and/or mental health services, as needed.
▲ Identify the client's preferences for end-of-life care; aid in honoring preferences as much as practicable.
- Refer to care plan for **Powerlessness.**

**Client/Family Teaching and Discharge Planning**
- Give information and reassurance to clients and families that distressing symptoms can often be anticipated and prevented and, when present, can be treated by health care professionals.
- Keep client and families informed about current health status and what to expect in the future.
- Promote more effective communication to family members engaged in the caregiving role.

## Risk for Aspiration

**Domain 11** Safety/protection    **Class 2** Physical injury
**NANDA-I Definition**

Susceptible to entry of gastrointestinal secretions, oropharyngeal secretions, solids, or fluids to the tracheobronchial passages, which may compromise health.

• = Independent          ▲ = Collaborative

**A**

## Risk Factors

Barrier to elevating upper body; decreased gastrointestinal motility; difficulty swallowing; enteral nutrition tube displacement; inadequate knowledge of modifiable factors; increased gastric residue; ineffective airway clearance

## At-Risk Population

Older adults; premature infants

## Associated Conditions

Chronic obstructive pulmonary disease; critical illness; decreased level of consciousness; delayed gastric emptying; depressed gag reflex; enteral nutrition; facial surgery; facial trauma; head and neck neoplasms; incompetent lower esophageal sphincter; increased intragastric pressure; jaw fixation techniques; medical devices; neck surgery; neck trauma; neurological diseases; oral surgical procedures; oral trauma; pharmaceutical preparations; pneumonia; stroke; treatment regimen

## Client Outcomes

### Client Will (Specify Time Frame)

- Maintain patent airway and clear lung sounds
- Swallow and digest oral, nasogastric, or gastric feeding without aspiration

## Nursing Interventions

- Monitor respiratory rate, depth, and effort. Note any signs of aspiration such as dyspnea, cough, cyanosis, wheezing, hoarseness, foul-smelling sputum, or fever. If there is a new onset of symptoms, perform oral suction and notify provider immediately.
- Auscultate lung sounds frequently and before and after feedings, note any new onset of crackles or wheezing.
- Take vital signs frequently, noting onset of a fever, increased respiratory rate, and increased heart rate.
- Use of a bedside-aspiration risk screening process along with dysphagia therapists for acutely ill clients is a factor in decreasing client mortality from acquired aspiration.
- Before initiating oral feeding, check client's gag reflex and ability to swallow by feeling the laryngeal prominence as the client attempts to swallow (American Association of Critical Care Nurses, 2016; Wangen, et al, 2019). If client is having problems swallowing, see nursing interventions for Impaired **Swallowing.**
- If client needs to be fed, feed slowly and allow adequate time for chewing and swallowing.
- Have suction machine available when feeding high-risk clients. If aspiration does occur, suction immediately.

• = Independent        ▲ = Collaborative

**A**

- Keep the head of the bed (HOB) elevated at 30 to 45 degrees, preferably with the client sitting up in a chair at 90 degrees when feeding. Keep head elevated for an hour after eating.
- Note presence of nausea, vomiting, or diarrhea. Treat nausea promptly with antiemetics.
- If the client shows symptoms of nausea and vomiting, position on side.
- Assess the abdomen and listen to bowel sounds frequently, noting if they are decreased, absent, or hyperactive.
- Note new onset of abdominal distention or increased rigidity of abdomen.
- If client has a tracheostomy, ask for referral to speech pathologist for swallowing studies before attempting to feed.
- Provide meticulous oral care including brushing of teeth at least two times per day.
- Sedation agents can reduce cough and gag reflexes as well as interfere with the client's ability to manage oropharyngeal secretions.

**Enteral Feedings**

- Insert nasogastric feeding tube using the internal nares to distal-lower esophageal-sphincter distance, an updated version of the Hanson method. The ear-to-nose-to-xiphoid process is often inaccurate.
- Before instilling medication or enteral feeding, ensure proper gastric/ duodenal tube placement.
- After radiographic verification of correct placement of the tube or the intestines, mark the tube's exit site clearly with tape or a permanent marker.
- Secure the nasogastric tube securely to the nose using a skin protectant under the tape or commercially available securement device.
- Measure and record the length of the tube that is outside of the body at defined intervals to help ensure correct placement.
- Note the placement of the tube on any chest or abdominal radiographs that are obtained for the client.
- Check the pH of the aspirate.
- Do not rely on the air insufflation method to assess correct tube placement.
- Follow unit policy regarding checking for gastric residual volume during continuous feedings or before feedings and holding feedings if increased residual is present.
- The practice of holding tube feedings if there is increased residual reduces the amount of calories given to the client.

• = Independent          ▲ = Collaborative

- Follow unit protocol regarding returning or discarding gastric residual volume. At this time there is not a definitive research base to guide practice.
- Do not use blue dye to tint enteral feedings.
- During enteral feedings, position client with HOB elevated 30 to 45 degrees (Schallom et al, 2015; American Association of Critical Care Nurses, 2016).
- Nursing ventilated premature infants in right lateral position is associated with decreased aspiration of gastric secretions (Imam et al, 2019).
- Take actions to prevent inadvertent misconnections with enteral feeding tubes into intravenous (IV) lines or other harmful connections. Safety actions that should be taken to prevent misconnections include the following:
  - Trace tubing back to origin. Recheck connections at time of client transfer and at change of shift.
  - Label all tubing.
  - Use oral syringes for medications through the enteral feeding; do not use IV syringes.
  - Teach nonprofessional personnel "Do Not Reconnect" if a line becomes dislodged; rather, find the nurse instead of taking the chance of plugging the tube into the wrong place.

**Critical Care**
- Recognize that critically ill clients are at an increased risk for aspiration because of severe illness and interventions that compromise the gag reflex.
- Recognize that intolerance to feeding as defined by increased gastric residual is more common early in the feeding process.
- Avoid bolus feedings in tube-fed clients who are at high risk for aspiration (American Association of Critical Care Nurses, 2016).
- Maintain endotracheal cuff pressures at an appropriate level to prevent leakage of secretions around the cuff (American Association of Critical Care Nurses, 2016).

**Geriatric**
- Carefully check older client's gag reflex and ability to swallow before feeding.
- Watch for signs of aspiration pneumonia in older adults with cerebrovascular accidents, even if there are no apparent signs of difficulty swallowing or of aspiration.

• = Independent ▲ = Collaborative

- Recognize that older adults with aspiration pneumonia have fewer symptoms than younger people; repeat cases of pneumonia in older adults are generally associated with aspiration.
- Continually assess for the presence of gag reflex after critical illness that required mechanical ventilation.
- Use central nervous system depressants cautiously; older clients may have an increased incidence of aspiration with altered levels of consciousness.
- Keep an older, mostly bedridden client sitting upright for 45 minutes to 1 hour after meals.
- Recommend to families that enteral feedings may or may not be indicated for clients with advanced dementia. Instead, if possible, use hand-feeding assistance, modified food consistency as needed, and feeding favorite foods for comfort.

**Home Care**
- The above interventions may be adapted for home care use.
- For clients at high risk for aspiration, obtain complete information from the discharging institution regarding institutional management.
- Assess the client and family for willingness and cognitive ability to learn and cope with swallowing, feeding, and related disorders.
- Assess caregiver understanding and reinforce teaching regarding positioning and assessment of the client for possible aspiration.
- Provide the client with emotional support in dealing with fears of aspiration. Refer to care plan for Anxiety.
- Establish emergency and contingency plans for care of the client.
- Have a speech and occupational therapist assess the client's swallowing ability and other physiological factors and recommend strategies for working with the client in the home (e.g., pureeing foods served to the client; providing adequate adaptive equipment for independence in eating).
- Obtain suction equipment for the home as necessary.
- Teach caregivers safe, effective use of suctioning devices. Inform the client and family that only individuals instructed in suctioning should perform the procedure.
- Institute case management of frail elderly to support continued independent living.

**Client/Family Teaching and Discharge Planning**
- Teach the client and family signs of aspiration and precautions to prevent aspiration.
- Teach the client and family how to safely administer tube feeding.

• = Independent          ▲ = Collaborative

- Teach the family about proper client positioning to facilitate feeding and reduce risk of aspiration.
- Verify client family/caregiver knowledge about feeding, aspiration precautions, and signs of aspiration.

# Risk for Impaired Attachment

**Domain 7** Role relationship    **Class 2** Family relationships

## NANDA-I Definition

Susceptible to disruption of the interactive process between parent or significant other and child that fosters the development of a protective and nurturing reciprocal relationship.

## Risk Factors

Anxiety; child's illness prevents effective initiation of parental contact; disorganized infant behavior; inability of parent to meet personal needs; insufficient privacy; parent's illness prevents effective initiation of infant contact; parent-child separation; parental conflict resulting from disorganized infant behavior; physical barrier; substance misuse

## At-Risk Population

Premature infants

## Client Outcomes

### Parent(s)/Caregiver(s) Will (Specify Time Frame)

- Be willing to consider pumping breast milk (and storing appropriately) or breastfeeding, if feasible
- Demonstrate behaviors that indicate secure attachment to infant/child
- Provide a safe environment, free of physical hazards
- Provide nurturing environment sensitive to infant/child's need for nutrition/feeding, sleeping, comfort, and social play
- Read and respond contingently to infant/child's distress
- Support infant's self-regulation capabilities, intervening when needed
- Engage in mutually satisfying interactions that provide opportunities for attachment
- Give infant nurturing sensory experiences (e.g., holding, cuddling, stroking, rocking)
- Demonstrate an awareness of developmentally appropriate activities that are pleasurable, emotionally supportive, and growth fostering
- Avoid physical and emotional abuse and/or neglect as retribution for parent's perception of infant/child's misbehavior
- State appropriate community resources and support services

## Nursing Interventions

### Mother–Baby Dyad Interventions

- Establish a trusting relationship with parent/caregiver in the perinatal and postnatal period.
- Educate parents about the importance of the infant–caregiver relationship as a foundation for the development of the infant's self-regulation capacities.
- Educate parents in reading/responding sensitively to their infant's unique "body language" (behavior cues), which communicates approach ("I'm ready to play"), avoidance/stress ("I'm unhappy. I need a change."), and self-calming ("I'm helping myself").
- Encourage physical closeness using skin-to-skin experiences as appropriate.

### Maternal/Parental Interventions

- Identify factors related to postpartum depression (PPD)/major depression and offer appropriate interventions/referrals.
- Assess for additional comorbid factors related to depression and offer appropriate interventions/referrals.
- Nurture parents so that they in turn can nurture their infant/child.
- Offer parents opportunities to verbalize their childhood fears associated with attachment.
- Identify mothers who may need assistance in enhancing maternal role attainment (MRA).
- Encourage positive involvement and relationship development between children and fathers.

### Premature Infants/Infants Requiring Specialty or Intensive Care

- Support mothers of preterm infants in providing pumped breast milk for their babies until they are ready for oral feedings and transitioning from gavage to breast.
- Suggest journaling or scrapbooking as a way for parents of hospitalized infants to cope with stress and emotions.
- Offer parent-to-parent support to parents of infants in the NICU.
- Plan ways for parents and their support system to interact/assist with infant/child caregiving.
- Educate and support parents' ability to relieve the infant/child's stress, distress, or pain.
- Guide parents in adapting their behaviors/activities with infant/child cues and changing needs.
- Attend to both parents and infant/child to strengthen high-quality interactions.

• = Independent          ▲ = Collaborative

- Encourage opportunities for physical closeness.
- Recognize that fathers, compared with mothers, may have different starting points in the attachment process in the NICU because nurses encourage parents to have early skin-to-skin contact (SSC).

**Pediatric**

- Recognize and support infant/child's capacity for self-regulation and intervene when appropriate.
- Provide lyrical, soothing music in the nursery and at home that is age appropriate (i.e., corrected, in the case of premature infants) and contingent with state or behavioral cues.
- Recognize and support infant/child's attention capabilities.
- Encourage opportunities for mutually satisfying interactions between infant and parent.
- Encourage parents and caregivers to massage their infants and children.

**Multicultural**

- Provide culturally sensitive parent support to new immigrant families and other non–native-English-speaking mothers and families.
- Discuss cultural norms with families to provide care that is appropriate for enhancing attachment with the infant/child.

**Home Care**

- The previously mentioned interventions may be adapted for home care use.
- Observe the attachment style and pattern during all clinical encounters with infants and parents.
- Assess for social and environmental risk factors.
- Assess quality of interaction between parent and infant/child.
- Assess for PPD at the pediatric primary care visit at 1-, 2-, 4-, and 6-month visits.
- Empower family members to draw on personal strengths in which multiple worldviews/values are recognized, incorporated, and negotiated.

**Special Considerations**

- Promote attachment process/development of maternal sensitivity in incarcerated women.
- Promote the attachment process in women who have abused substances by providing a culturally based, family-centered, supportive treatment environment.
- Encourage custodial grandparents to use support groups available for caregivers of children.
- Provide options for communication for infants and children whose parents have been separated for military or work deployment.

# Autonomic Dysreflexia

**Domain 9** Coping/stress tolerance    **Class 3** Neurobehavioral stress

## NANDA-I Definition

Life-threatening, uninhibited sympathetic response of the nervous system to a noxious stimulus after a spinal cord injury at the 7th thoracic vertebra (T7) or above.

## Defining Characteristics

Blurred vision; bradycardia; chest pain; chilling; conjunctival congestion; diaphoresis above the injury; diffuse pain in different areas of the head; Horner's syndrome; metallic taste in mouth; nasal congestion; pallor below injury; paresthesia; paroxysmal hypertension; pilomotor reflex; red blotches on skin above the injury; tachycardia

## Related Factors

### Gastrointestinal Stimuli

Bowel distention; constipation; difficult passage of feces; digital stimulation; enemas; fecal impaction; suppositories

### Integumentary Stimuli

Cutaneous stimulation; skin irritation; sunburn; wound

### Musculoskeletal-Neurological Stimuli

Irritating stimuli below level of injury; muscle spasm; painful stimuli below level of injury; pressure over bony prominence; pressure over genitalia; range of motion exercises

### Regulatory-Situational Stimuli

Constrictive clothing; environmental temperature fluctuations; positioning

### Reproductive-Urological Stimuli

Bladder distention; bladder spasm; instrumentation; sexual intercourse

### Other Factors

Inadequate caregiver knowledge of disease process; inadequate knowledge of disease process

## At-Risk Population

Individuals exposed to environmental temperature extremes; men with spinal cord injury or lesion who are experiencing ejaculation; women with spinal cord injury or lesion who are experiencing labor; women with spinal cord injury or lesion who are menstruating; women with spinal cord injury or lesion who are pregnant

## Associated Conditions

Bowel fractures; detrusor sphincter dyssynergia; digestive system diseases; epididymitis; heterotopic bone; ovarian cyst; pharmaceutical preparations; renal calculi; substance withdrawal; surgical procedures; urinary catheterization; urinary tract infection; venous thromboembolism

• = Independent          ▲ = Collaborative

**A**

## Client Outcomes

### Client Will (Specify Time Frame)

- Maintain baseline blood pressure
- Remain free of dysreflexia symptoms
- Explain symptoms, treatment, and prevention of dysreflexia

### Nursing Interventions

- Teach clients with a spinal cord injury (SCI) about potential causes, symptoms, treatment, and prevention of autonomic dysreflexia (AD).
- Monitor the client for symptoms of dysreflexia, particularly those with high-level and more complete SCIs. See Defining Characteristics.
- ▲ Collaborate with providers and caregivers to identify the cause of dysreflexia. AD is triggered by a stimulus from below the level of injury, leading to systemic vasoconstriction. The most common triggers are bladder distention, kidney stones, kink in urinary catheter, urinary tract infection, fecal impaction, pressure ulcer, ingrown toenail, menstruation, hemorrhoids, tight clothing, invasive testing, and sexual intercourse (ACOG Committee on Obstetric Practice, 2020; Perkins, 2020).
- If dysreflexia symptoms are present, immediately place client in high Fowler's position, remove all support hoses or binders, loosen clothing, check the urinary catheter for kinks, and attempt to determine the noxious stimulus causing the response. Check the client's blood pressure every 3 to 5 minutes. If blood pressure cannot be decreased following these initial interventions, notify the provider emergently (i.e., STAT).
  - ○ First, assess bladder function. Check for distention, and if present, catheterize the client using an anesthetic jelly as a lubricant. Do not use the Valsalva maneuver or Crede's method to empty the bladder because this form of reflex voiding could worsen AD. Ensure existing catheter patency and irrigate if necessary. Also assess for signs of urinary tract infection.
  - ○ Second, assess bowel function. Numb the bowel area with a topical anesthetic as ordered and gently check for impaction.
  - ○ Third, assess the skin. Look for any pressure points, wounds, and ingrown toenails.
- ▲ Initiate antihypertensive therapy as soon as ordered and monitor for cardiac dysrhythmias.
- Monitor vital signs every 3 to 5 minutes during an acute event; continue to monitor vital signs after event is resolved (e.g., symptoms resolve and vital signs return to baseline, usually up to 2 hours after the event).

• = Independent        ▲ = Collaborative

- Watch for complications of dysreflexia, including signs of cerebral hemorrhage, seizures, cardiac dysfunction, or intraocular hemorrhage.
- Accurately and completely record any incidences of dysreflexia; especially note the precipitating stimuli.
- Use the following interventions to prevent dysreflexia:
  - ○ Ensure catheter patency and empty urinary catheter bags frequently. Assess the client for signs and symptoms of urinary tract infection during every shift.
  - ○ Ensure a regular pattern of defecation to prevent fecal impaction.
  - ○ Frequently change position of client to relieve pressure and prevent formation of pressure injuries.
- ▲ Notify all health care team members of recurrent AD episodes.
- ▲ For female clients with SCI, assess the client for AD during menstrual cycle. If the client becomes pregnant, collaborate with obstetrical health care practitioners to monitor for signs and symptoms of dysreflexia.

**Home Care**
- The previously mentioned interventions may be adapted for home care use.
- Provide the client and caregiver with written information on common causes of AD and initial treatment.
- Provide resources to clients with any known proclivity toward dysreflexia. Advise them to wear a medical alert bracelet and carry a medical alert wallet card when not accompanied by knowledgeable caregivers.
- ▲ Establish an emergency plan: maintain a current prescription of antihypertensive medication, and administer antihypertensives when dysreflexia is refractory to nonmedicinal interventions. If SBP remains over 150 mm Hg following the previously mentioned interventions, go to the nearest ED and present the AD wallet card on arrival.
- When an episode of dysreflexia has resolved, continue to monitor blood pressure every 30 to 60 minutes for the next 2 hours or admit to an institution for observation.

**Client/Family Teaching and Discharge Planning**
- Teach recognition of early dysreflexia symptoms, appropriate interventions, and the need to obtain help immediately. Give client a written card describing signs and symptoms of AD and initial actions.
- Teach steps to prevent dysreflexia episodes: routine bladder and bowel care, pressure injury prevention, and preventing other forms of noxious stimuli (e.g., not wearing clothing that is too tight, nail care). Discuss the potential impact of sexual intercourse and pregnancy on AD.

• = Independent          ▲ = Collaborative

# Risk for Autonomic Dysreflexia    A

**Domain 9** Coping/stress tolerance    **Class 3** Neurobehavioral stress

## NANDA-I Definition

Susceptible to life-threatening, uninhibited response of the sympathetic nervous system post–spinal shock, in an individual with spinal cord injury or lesion at the 6th thoracic vertebra (T6) or above (has been demonstrated in clients with injuries at the 7th thoracic vertebra [T7] and the 8th thoracic vertebra [T8]), which may compromise health.

## Risk Factors

### Gastrointestinal Stimuli

Bowel distention; constipation; difficult passage of feces; digital stimulation; enemas; fecal impaction; suppositories

### Integumentary Stimuli

Cutaneous stimulations; skin irritation; sunburn; wound

### Musculoskeletal-Neurological Stimuli

Irritating stimuli below level of injury; muscle spasm; painful stimuli below level of injury; pressure over bony prominence; pressure over genitalia; range of motion exercises

### Regulatory-Situational Stimuli

Constrictive clothing; environmental temperature fluctuations; positioning

### Reproductive-Urological Stimuli

Bladder distention; bladder spasm; instrumentation; sexual intercourse

### Other Factors

Inadequate caregiver knowledge of disease process; inadequate knowledge of disease process

## At-Risk Population

Individuals with spinal cord injury or lesion exposed to extremes of environmental temperature; men with spinal cord injury or lesion who are experiencing ejaculation; women with spinal cord injury or lesion who are experiencing labor; women with spinal cord injury or lesion who are menstruating; women with spinal cord injury or lesion who are pregnant

## Associated Conditions

Bone fractures; detrusor sphincter dyssynergia; digestive system diseases; epididymitis; heterotopic bone; ovarian cyst; pharmaceutical preparations; renal calculi; substance withdrawal; surgical procedures; urinary catheterization; urinary tract infection; venous thromboembolism

## Client Outcomes, Nursing Interventions, and Client/Family Teaching and Discharge Planning

Refer to care plan for **Autonomic Dysreflexia.**

• = Independent    ▲ = Collaborative

# Risk for Bleeding

**B**

**Domain 11** Safety/projection     **Class 2** Physical injury

## NANDA-I Definition

Susceptible to a decrease in blood volume, which may compromise health.

## Risk Factors

Inadequate knowledge of bleeding precautions

## At-Risk Population

Individuals with a history of falls

## Associated Conditions

Aneurysm; circumcision; disseminated intravascular coagulopathy; gastrointestinal condition; impaired liver function; inherent coagulopathy; postpartum complication; pregnancy complication; trauma; treatment regimen

## Client Outcomes

**Client Will (Specify Time Frame)**

- Identify clients at risk for bleeding and implement precautions to prevent bleeding and subsequent complications
- Identify and implement interventions to alleviate bleeding episodes
- Discuss precautions to prevent bleeding complications
- Explain actions that should be taken if bleeding happens
- Maintain adherence to mutually agreed upon anticoagulant medication and follow-up laboratory regimen
- Monitor for signs and symptoms of bleeding

## Nursing Interventions

- Identify clients at risk for bleeding episodes. Consider client-related and procedure-related risk factors.
- Perform admission fall risk assessment. Safety precautions should be implemented for all at-risk clients.
- Monitor the client at increased risk for bleeding for signs or symptoms of bleeding, including bleeding of the gums; nosebleed; blood in sputum, emesis, urine, or stool; bleeding from a wound or site of invasive procedure; petechiae; ecchymosis; and purpura.
- ▲ Clients with a history of cancer, current cancer, or leukemias are at a higher risk of bleeding associated with the disease and/or interplay of treatment-related factors. Risk of bleeding may be higher because of associated thrombocytopenia, platelet dysfunction, infection, and liver disease.
- If bleeding develops, apply pressure over the site or appropriate artery as needed. Apply pressure dressing; if unable to stop the bleeding, then consider a tourniquet if indicated.

• = Independent          ▲ = Collaborative

▲ Collaborate on an appropriate bleeding management plan, including nonpharmacological and pharmacological measures to stop bleeding based on the antithrombotic used.

▲ Monitor coagulation studies, including prothrombin time, INR, activated partial thromboplastin time (aPTT), fibrinogen, fibrin degradation/split products, and platelet counts as appropriate.

• Assess vital signs at frequent intervals to assess for physiological evidence of bleeding, such as tachycardia, tachypnea, and hypotension. Symptoms may include dizziness, shortness of breath, altered mental status, and fatigue.

▲ Monitor all medications for potential to increase bleeding, including antiplatelets, NSAIDs, selective serotonin reuptake inhibitors (SSRIs), and complementary and alternative therapies such as coenzyme Q10 and ginger.

**Safety Guidelines for Anticoagulant Administration: The Joint Commission National Patient Safety Goals**

• Follow approved protocol for anticoagulant administration:
• Use prepackaged medications and prefilled or premixed parenteral therapy as ordered.
• Check laboratory tests (i.e., INR) before administration.
• Use programmable pumps when using parenteral administration.
• Ensure appropriate education for client/family and all staff concerning anticoagulants used.
• Notify dietary services when warfarin is prescribed (to provide consistent vitamin K in diet).
• Monitor for any symptoms of bleeding before administration.
• Anticoagulation therapy is complex and requires consistent implementation of medication reconciliation in all settings.

▲ Before administering anticoagulants, assess the clotting profile of the client. If the client is on warfarin, assess the INR. If the INR is outside of the recommended parameters, notify the provider.

▲ Recognize that vitamin K for vitamin K antagonists (e.g., warfarin, phenprocoumon, Sinthrome, and phenindione) may be given orally or intravenously as ordered for INR levels greater than 4.5 without signs of bleeding. In the case of major bleeding, prohemostatic therapies may be warranted for the rapid reversal of vitamin K antagonists (tranexamic acid, fresh frozen plasma, cryoprecipitate, platelet transfusion, fibrinogen concentrate, factor IV prothrombin complex concentrate [Kcentra], and activated prothrombin complex concentrate) (Witt et al, 2016; Corbitt et al, 2019).

▲ Manage fluid resuscitation and volume expansion as ordered.

• = Independent          ▲ = Collaborative

**B**

▲ Consider use of permissive hypotension and restrictive transfusion strategies when treating bleeding episodes.

▲ Consider discussing the coadministration of a proton-pump inhibitor alongside traditional NSAIDs or with the use of a cyclooxygenase 2 inhibitor with the prescriber.

• Ensure adequate nurse staffing to provide a high level of surveillance capability.

**Pediatric**

▲ Recognize that prophylactic vitamin K administration should be used in neonates for vitamin K deficiency bleeding (VKDB).

▲ Recognize warning signs of VKDB, including minimal bleeds, evidence of cholestasis (icteric sclera, dark urine, and irritability), and failure to thrive.

▲ Use caution in administering NSAIDs in children.

▲ Monitor children and adolescents for potential bleeding after blunt trauma.

**Client/Family Teaching and Discharge Planning**

• Teach client and family or significant others about any anticoagulant medications prescribed, including when to take, how often to have laboratory tests done, signs of bleeding to report, dietary consistency, and need to wear medic alert bracelet and precautions to be followed. Instruct the client to report any adverse side effects to his or her health care provider.

• Instruct the client and family on the disease process and rationale for care. When clients and their family members have sufficient understanding of their disease process, they can participate more fully in care and healthy behaviors. Knowledge empowers clients and family members, allowing them to be active participants in their care.

• Provide client and family or significant others with both oral and written educational materials that meet the standards of client education and health literacy.

# Risk for Unstable Blood Pressure

**Domain 4** Activity/rest     **Class 4** Cardiovascular/pulmonary responses

**NANDA-I Definition**

Susceptible to fluctuating forces of blood flowing through arterial vessels, which may compromise health.

**Risk Factors**

Inconsistency with medication regimen; orthostasis

• = Independent          ▲ = Collaborative

## Associated Conditions

Adverse effects of pharmaceutical preparations; adverse effects of cocaine; cardiac dysrhythmia; Cushing's syndrome; fluid retention; fluid shifts; hormonal change; hyperparathyroidism; hyperthyroidism; hypothyroidism; increased intracranial pressure; pharmaceutical preparations; rapid absorption and distribution of pharmaceutical preparations; sympathetic responses

## Client Outcomes

### Client Will (Specify Time Frame)

- Maintain vital signs within normal range
- Remain asymptomatic with cardiac rhythm (have absence of arrhythmias, tachycardia, or bradycardia)
- Be free from dizziness with changes in positions (lying to standing)
- Deny fatigue, nausea, vomiting
- Deny chest pain

## Nursing Interventions

▲ Hypertension (HTN) is a major risk factor for cardiovascular disease, placing the client at increased risk of myocardial infarction and stroke (Whelton et al, 2017).

• Provide client-specific education about the importance of a healthy lifestyle to reduce complications associated with HTN.

• Provide drug- and client-specific education if medications are prescribed to manage the client's HTN.

▲ Screen clients for secondary causes of HTN with abrupt onset or age <30 years.

▲ Review the client's medical history.

• Explore the client's subjective statements concerning poor sleep, report of snoring, and daytime fatigue.

• Review the client's history of arrhythmias, especially a history of atrial fibrillation.

• Review the client's current medications, both prescribed and over the counter.

• Steroid agents, administered at higher doses (e.g., 80–200 mg/day), can trigger HTN.

• Ask the client if they are prescribed antidepressant agents.

• Nonsteroidal antiinflammatory drugs (NSAIDs) can induce HTN and/or interfere with antihypertensive therapy.

• Overconsumption of caffeine stimulates sympathetic activity, which causes a rise in blood pressure that can be followed by a decrease in blood pressure once the effects of the caffeine have worn off.

• = Independent          ▲ = Collaborative

**B**

- Licorice consumption may trigger HTN in some clients.
- Some herbal products may induce HTN and/or interfere with antihypertensive treatment.
- Alcohol is known to elevate blood pressure and increases the client's risk of HTN.
- Blood pressure may be unstable with substance abuse disorders (SUDs). Certain drugs have specific effects on the cardiovascular system.
- Cocaine use causes increased alertness and feelings of euphoria, along with dilated pupils, increased body temperature, tachycardia, and increased blood pressure.
- Cocaine overdose is a medical emergency because of the risk of cardiac toxicity.
- Opioid intoxication results in changes in heart rate, slowed breathing, and decrease in blood pressure leading to loss of alertness.
- Synthetic cannabinoids are man-made, mind-altering chemicals that may be added to foods or inhaled. There is a growing availability of these designer drugs in which adverse effects are not well known.
- Explore client use of wearable technology for self-monitoring heart rhythm irregularities.

**Critical Care**

- Monitor the client for symptoms associated with chest pain, myocardial infarction, acute HTN, and hypotension.
- Clients with hypertensive crisis will require close monitoring for signs and symptoms consistent with acute renal failure, stroke, myocardial infarction, and acute heart failure.
- Myxedema coma is an acute emergency associated with hypothyroidism that manifests with severe hypotension, bradycardia, hypothermia, seizures, and coma.
- Thyroid storm (thyrotoxicosis) is an acute, life-threatening, hypermetabolic state induced by excessive release of thyroid-stimulating hormone (TSH). Symptoms are severe and include fever, tachycardia, HTN, congestive heart failure leading to hypotension and shock, profuse sweating, respiratory distress, nausea and vomiting, diarrhea, abdominal pain, jaundice, anxiety, seizures, and coma.

**Pediatric**

- HTN is an underrecognized disease in children. Current recommendations include annual blood pressure monitoring with more focused monitoring in high-risk children.
- ▲ Secondary causes of HTN should be explored in the absence of childhood obesity, known cardiovascular disease, and family history.

• = Independent            ▲ = Collaborative

**B**

- Normal ranges for child and adolescent blood pressure measurements were recently updated to reflect age, gender, and weight considerations.

**Geriatric**

- Risk of cardiac arrhythmias increases with advanced age, placing the client at increased risk of HTN and hypotension.
- Comorbid cardiovascular disease risks increase with advanced age.
- Polypharmacy is a risk for both hypotension and HTN in older clients.

**Client/Family Teaching and Discharge Planning**

- Nutritional education has been found to be an important variable in an individual maintaining cardiovascular health.
- Teach the client to monitor blood pressure and to report changes in blood pressure to the provider and with each health care visit.

# Disturbed Body Image

**Domain 6** Self-perception     **Class 3** Body image

## NANDA-I Definition

Negative mental picture of one's physical self.

## Defining Characteristics

Altered proprioception; altered social involvement; avoids looking at one's body; avoids touching one's body; consistently compares oneself with others; depressive symptoms; expresses concerns about sexuality; expresses fear of reaction by others; expresses preoccupation with change; expresses preoccupation with missing body part; focused on past appearance; focused on past function; focused on past strength; frequently weighs self; hides body part; monitors changes in one's body; names body part; names missing body part; neglects nonfunctioning body part; nonverbal response to body changes; nonverbal response to perceived body changes; overexposes body part; perceptions that reflect an altered view of appearance; refuses to acknowledge change; reports feeling one has failed in life; social anxiety; uses impersonal pronouns to describe body part; uses impersonal pronouns to describe missing body part

## Related Factors

Body consciousness; conflict between spiritual beliefs and treatment regimen; conflict between values and cultural norms; distrust of body function; fear of disease recurrence; low self-efficacy; low self-esteem; obesity; residual limb pain; unrealistic perception of treatment outcome; unrealistic self-expectations

• = Independent      ▲ = Collaborative

**B**

## At-Risk Population

Cancer survivors; individuals experiencing altered body weight; individuals experiencing developmental transition; individuals experiencing puberty; individuals with altered body function; individuals with scars; individuals with stomas; women

## Associated Conditions

Binge-eating disorder; chronic pain; fibromyalgia; human immunodeficiency virus infections; impaired psychosocial functioning; mental disorders; surgical procedures; treatment regimen; wounds and injuries

## Client Outcomes

### Client Will (Specify Time Frame)

- Demonstrate adaptation to changes in physical appearance or body function as evidenced by adjustment to lifestyle change
- Identify and change irrational beliefs and expectations regarding body size or function
- Recognize health-destructive behaviors and demonstrate willingness to adhere to treatments or methods that will promote health
- Verbalize congruence between body reality and body perception
- Describe, touch, or observe affected body part
- Demonstrate social involvement rather than avoidance and use adaptive coping and/or social skills
- Use cognitive strategies or other coping skills to improve perception of body image and enhance functioning
- Use strategies to enhance appearance (e.g., wig, clothing)

## Nursing Interventions

- Incorporate psychosocial questions related to body image as part of nursing assessment to identify clients at risk for body image disturbance.
- Maintain awareness of conditions or changes that are likely to cause a disturbed body image: removal of a body part or change/loss of body function such as blindness or hearing loss, cancer survivors, clients with eating disorders, burns, skin disorders, or those with stomas or other disfiguring conditions, or a loss of perceived attractiveness such as hair loss.
- Incorporate an appropriate body image assessment tool or questions to identify clients at risk for body image disturbance.
- Assess the impact of body image on sexual function and sexuality.
- Be aware of the impact of treatments and surgeries that involve the face and neck and be prepared to address the client's psychosocial needs.
- Maintain understanding that age, gender, and other demographic identifiers may be associated with higher degrees of body image disturbance.

• = Independent          ▲ = Collaborative

B

- Consideration should be given to providing counseling for women with breast cancer to assist with acceptance of the reality of the disease and to increase their resilience against breast surgery.
- Offer breast cancer clients with appearance-related treatment side effects a beauty care intervention. Beauty care interventions can consist of make-up, hair care, or a photo shoot.
- Encourage individuals to express self-compassion related to their body image through writing.
- Nurses and other health professionals should support clients with stomas in problem-focused coping strategies.

**Pediatric**
- Many of the previously mentioned interventions are appropriate for the pediatric client.
- Educate parents on the role their own attitudes play in a child's body perception and acceptance.
- Avoid or redirect fat talk or negative comments about one's body.
- For adolescent clients, incorporate media literacy interventions to promote a healthy body image. Media literacy interventions are designed to influence media-related beliefs and attitudes to prevent risky behaviors.
- When caring for adolescents, be aware of the impact of acne vulgaris on body image and mental health. Assess for symptoms of social withdrawal, limited eye contact, and expressions of low self-esteem. Provide education on skin care and hygiene, and assist with referrals to a dermatologist as needed.

**Geriatric**
- Assess older adults with chronic illness for body image issues.

**Multicultural**
- Acknowledge that body image disturbances can affect all individuals regardless of culture, race, or ethnicity. Assess for the influence of cultural beliefs, regional norms, and values on the client's body image.

**Home Care**
- The previously mentioned interventions may be adapted for home care use.
- Assess client's level of social support. Social support is one of the determinants of the client's recovery and emotional health.
- Assess family/caregiver level of acceptance of the client's body changes.
- Encourage clients to discuss concerns related to sexuality and provide support or information as indicated. Many conditions that affect body image also affect sexuality.

• = Independent ▲ = Collaborative

**B**

- Teach all aspects of care. Involve clients and caregivers in self-care as soon as possible. Do this in stages if clients still have difficulty looking at or touching a changed body part.

**Client/Family Teaching and Discharge Planning**

- Advise clients with a stoma about the support available to them.

# Insufficient Breast Milk Production

**Domain 2** Nutrition    **Class 1** Ingestion

## NANDA-I Definition

Inadequate supply of maternal breast milk to support nutritional state of an infant or child.

## Defining Characteristics

Absence of milk production with nipple stimulation; breast milk expressed is less than prescribed volume for infant; delayed milk production; infant constipation; infant frequently crying; infant frequently seeks to suckle at breast; infant refuses to suckle at breast; infant voids small amounts of concentrated urine; infant weight gain <500 g in a month; prolonged breastfeeding time; unsustained suckling at breast

## Related Factors

Ineffective latching on to breast; ineffective sucking reflex; infant's refusal to breastfeed; insufficient maternal fluid volume; insufficient opportunity for suckling at the breast; insufficient suckling time at breast; maternal alcohol consumption; maternal malnutrition; maternal smoking; maternal treatment regimen

## At-Risk Population

Women who become pregnant while breastfeeding

## Client Outcomes

**Client Will (Specify Time Frame)**

- State knowledge of indicators of adequate milk supply
- State and demonstrate measures to ensure adequate milk supply

## Nursing Interventions

- Provide lactation support at all phases of lactation.
- Assess maternal intention regarding breastfeeding and communicate routine advice to mothers without making them feel pressured or guilty.
- Verify mothers' understanding and reinforce critical information.
- Initiate skin-to-skin holding at birth and undisturbed contact for the first hour following birth.

• = Independent     ▲ = Collaborative

B

- Encourage postpartum women to start breastfeeding based on infant need as early as possible and reduce formula use to increase breastfeeding frequency. Use nonnarcotic analgesics as early as possible.
- Provide suggestions for mothers on how to increase milk production and how to determine the infant is receiving sufficient milk.
- Instruct mothers that breastfeeding frequency, sucking times, and volume produced are variable and normal.
- ▲ Consider the use of medication for mothers of preterm infants with insufficient expressed breast milk.

**Pediatric**
- Provide individualized follow-up with extra home visits or outpatient visits for teen mothers within the first few days after hospital discharge and encourage schools to be more compatible with breastfeeding.

**Multicultural**
- Provide information and support to mothers on benefits of breastfeeding at antenatal visits.
- Refer to care plans Interrupted **Breastfeeding** and Readiness for Enhanced **Breastfeeding** for additional interventions.

# Ineffective Breastfeeding

**Domain 2** Nutrition    **Class 1** Ingestion
## NANDA-I Definition
Difficulty providing milk from the breast, which may compromise nutritional status of the infant/child.

## Defining Characteristics
### Infant or Child
Arching at breast; crying at breast; crying within 1 hour after breastfeeding; fussing within one hour after breastfeeding; infant inability to latch on to maternal breast correctly; inadequate stooling; inadequate weight gain; resisting latching on to breast; sustained weight loss; unresponsive to other comfort measures; unsustained suckling at breast

### Mother
Insufficient emptying of each breast during feeding; insufficient signs of oxytocin release; perceived inadequate milk supply; sore nipples persisting beyond first week

## Related Factors
Delayed stage II lactogenesis; inadequate family support; inadequate parental knowledge regarding breastfeeding techniques; inadequate parental knowledge regarding importance of breastfeeding; ineffective infant

• = Independent                    ▲ = Collaborative

**B**

suck-swallow response; insufficient breast milk production; insufficient opportunity for suckling at breast; interrupted breastfeeding; maternal ambivalence; maternal anxiety; maternal breast anomaly; maternal fatigue; maternal obesity; maternal pain; pacifier use; supplemental feedings with artificial nipple

## At-Risk Population

Individuals with history of breast surgery; individuals with history of breastfeeding failure; premature infants; women with short maternity leave

## Associated Conditions

Oropharyngeal defect

## Client Outcomes

**Client Will (Specify Time Frame)**

- Achieve effective milk transfer (dyad)
- Verbalize/demonstrate techniques to manage breastfeeding problems (mother)
- Manifest signs of adequate intake at the breast (infant)
- Manifest positive self-esteem in relation to the infant feeding process (mother)
- Explain alternative method of infant feeding if unable to continue exclusive breastfeeding (mother)

## Nursing Interventions

- Identify women with risk factors for lower breastfeeding initiation and continuation rates, as well as factors contributing to ineffective breastfeeding (see conditions listed in the section Related Factors) as early as possible in the perinatal experience.
- Provide time for clients to express expectations and concerns, and provide emotional support as needed.
- Encourage skin-to-skin holding, beginning immediately after delivery.
- Use valid and reliable tools to assess breastfeeding performance and identify dyads at risk for breastfeeding failure.
- Promote comfort and relaxation to reduce pain and anxiety.
- Avoid supplemental feedings.
- Teach mother to observe for infant behavioral cues and responses to breastfeeding.
- ▲ Provide necessary equipment/instruction/assistance for milk expression as needed.
- ▲ Provide referrals and resources: lactation consultants, nurse and peer support programs, community organizations, and written and electronic sources of information.
- See care plan for Readiness for Enhanced **Breastfeeding.**

• = Independent          ▲ = Collaborative

**B**

**Multicultural**

- Assess whether the client's cultural beliefs about breastfeeding are contributing to ineffective breastfeeding.
- Assess the influence of family support on the decision to continue or discontinue breastfeeding.
- See care plan for Readiness for Enhanced **Breastfeeding**.

**Home Care**

- The previously mentioned interventions may be adapted for home care use.
- Provide anticipatory guidance in relation to home management of breastfeeding.
- ▲ Investigate availability of support services and refer to public health department, hospital home follow-up breastfeeding program, or other postdischarge support.
- See care plan for Risk for Impaired **Attachment**.

**Client/Family Teaching and Discharge Planning**

- Instruct the client on maternal breastfeeding behaviors/techniques (preparation for, positioning, initiation of/promoting latch-on, burping, completion of session, and frequency of feeding) using a variety of strategies such as written materials, videos, and online resources.
- Teach the mother self-care measures (e.g., breast care, management of breast/nipple discomfort, nutrition/fluid, rest/activity).
- Provide information regarding infant feeding cues and behaviors and appropriate maternal responses, as well as measures of infant feeding adequacy.
- Provide education to partner/family/significant others as needed.

## Interrupted Breastfeeding

**Domain 2** Nutrition    **Class 1** Ingestion

### NANDA-I Definition

Break in the continuity of feeding milk from the breasts, which may compromise breastfeeding success and/or nutritional status of the infant/child.

### Defining Characteristics

Nonexclusive breastfeeding

### Related Factors

Abrupt weaning of infant; maternal-infant separation

### At-Risk Population

Employed mothers; hospitalized children; hospitalized infants; premature infants

• = Independent          ▲ = Collaborative

### Associated Conditions

**B** Contraindications to breastfeeding; infant illness; maternal illness

### Client Outcomes

**Client Will (Specify Time Frame)**

**Infant**

• Receive mother's breast milk if not contraindicated by maternal conditions (e.g., certain drugs, infections) or infant conditions (e.g., galactosemia)

**Maternal**

• Maintain lactation
• Achieve effective breastfeeding or satisfaction with the breastfeeding experience
• Demonstrate effective methods of breast milk collection and storage

### Nursing Interventions

• Provide information and support to mother and partner/family regarding mother's desire/intention to begin or resume breastfeeding.
• Clarify the indication for interrupting breastfeeding is warranted.
• Provide anticipatory guidance to the mother/family regarding potential duration of the interruption when possible/feasible, ensuring that measures to sustain or restart lactation and promote parent–infant attachment can make it possible to resume breastfeeding when the condition/situation requiring interruption is resolved.
• Reassure the mother/family that the infant will benefit from any amount of breast milk provided.
• Assess mother's concerns, and observe mother performing psychomotor skills (expression, storage, alternative feeding, skin-to-skin care, and/or breastfeeding) and assist as needed.
• Collaborate with mother/family/health care providers (as needed) to develop a plan for skin-to-skin contact.
• Collaborate with the mother/family/health care provider/employer (as needed) to develop a plan for expression/pumping of breast milk and/or infant feeding.
• Monitor for signs indicating infant's ability to breastfeed and interest in breastfeeding.
▲ Use formula supplementation only as medically indicated.
• Provide anticipatory guidance for common problems associated with interrupted breastfeeding (e.g., incomplete emptying of milk glands, diminishing milk supply, infant difficulty with resuming breastfeeding, or infant refusal of alternative feeding method).
▲ Initiate follow-up and make appropriate referrals.

• = Independent          ▲ = Collaborative

**B**

- Provide emotional support for the mother if effective breastfeeding is not achieved and assist with learning an alternative method of infant feeding.
- See care plans for Readiness for Enhanced **Breastfeeding** and Ineffective **Breastfeeding.**

**Multicultural**
- Assess the client's cultural beliefs about breastfeeding and the ability to exclusively breastfeed.
- See care plans for Readiness for Enhanced **Breastfeeding** and Ineffective **Breastfeeding.**

**Home Care**
- The previously mentioned interventions may be adapted for home care use.

**Client/Family Teaching and Discharge Planning**
- Teach mother effective methods to express breast milk.
- Teach mother/parents about skin-to-skin care.
- Instruct mother on safe breast milk handling and storage.
- See care plans for Readiness for Enhanced **Breastfeeding** and Ineffective **Breastfeeding.**

# Readiness for Enhanced Breastfeeding

**Domain 2** Nutrition    **Class 1** Ingestion

## NANDA-I Definition

A pattern of providing milk from the breasts to an infant or child, which can be strengthened.

## Defining Characteristics

Expresses desire to enhance ability to exclusively breastfeed; expresses desire to enhance ability to provide breast milk for child's nutritional needs

## Client Outcomes

Client Will (Specify Time Frame)
- Maintain effective breastfeeding
- Maintain normal growth patterns (infant)
- Verbalize satisfaction with breastfeeding process (mother)

## Nursing Interventions

- Encourage expectant mothers to learn about breastfeeding during pregnancy.
- Encourage and facilitate early skin-to-skin contact.
- Encourage breastfeeding on demand and rooming-in.

• = Independent          ▲ = Collaborative

**B**

- Monitor the breastfeeding process, identify opportunities to enhance knowledge and experience, and provide direction as needed.
- Provide encouragement and positive feedback to mothers as they learn to breastfeed.
- Discuss prevention and treatment of common breastfeeding problems, such as nipple pain and/or trauma.
- Teach mother to observe for infant behavioral cues and responses to breastfeeding.
- Identify current support-person network and opportunities for continued breastfeeding support.
- Use formula supplementation only as medically indicated, and do not provide samples of formula on discharge from hospital.

**Multicultural**
- Assess for the influence of cultural beliefs, norms, and values on current breastfeeding practices.

**Home Care**
- The previously mentioned interventions may be adapted for home care use.

**Client/Family Teaching and Discharge Planning**
- Include the partner and other family members in education about breastfeeding.
- Teach the client the importance of maternal nutrition and self-care.
- Teach mother to observe for the infant's hunger cues (e.g., rooting, sucking, mouthing, hand-to-mouth and hand-to-hand activity) and encourage her to breastfeed on demand.
- Review guidelines for frequency of feeds (at least every 2–3 hours, or 8–12 feedings per 24 hours) and feeding duration (until suckling and swallowing slow down and satiety is reached).
▲ Provide referrals and resources: lactation consultants, nurse and peer support programs, community organizations, and written and electronic sources of information.

# Ineffective Breathing Pattern

**Domain 4** Activity/rest    **Class 4** Cardiovascular/pulmonary responses
**NANDA-I Definition**

Inspiration and/or expiration that does not provide adequate ventilation.
**Defining Characteristics**

Abdominal paradoxical respiratory pattern; altered chest excursion; altered tidal volume; bradypnea; cyanosis; decreased expiratory pressure; decreased inspiratory pressure; decreased minute ventilation; decreased vital capacity; hypercapnia; hyperventilation; hypoventilation; hypoxemia; hypoxia; increased anterior-posterior chest diameter; nasal flaring; orthopnea; prolonged expiration phase; pursed-lip breathing; subcostal retraction; tachypnea; use of accessory muscles to breathe; use of three-point position

**Related Factors**

Anxiety; body position that inhibits lung expansion; fatigue; increased physical exertion; obesity; pain

**At-Risk Population**

Young women

**Associated Conditions**

Bony deformity; chest wall deformity; chronic obstructive pulmonary disease; critical illness; heart diseases; hyperventilation syndrome; hypoventilation syndrome; increased airway resistance; increased serum hydrogen concentration; musculoskeletal impairment; neurological immaturity; neurological impairment; neuromuscular diseases; reduced pulmonary complacency; sleep-apnea syndromes; spinal cord injuries

**Client Outcomes**

Client Will (Specify Time Frame)

- Demonstrate a breathing pattern that supports blood gas results within the client's normal parameters
- Report ability to breathe comfortably
- Demonstrate ability to perform pursed-lip breathing and controlled breathing
- Identify and avoid specific factors that exacerbate episodes of ineffective breathing patterns

**Nursing Interventions**

- Monitor respiratory rate, depth, and ease of respiration.
- Note pattern of respiration. If client is dyspneic, note what seems to cause the dyspnea, the way in which the client deals with the condition, and how the dyspnea resolves or gets worse.
- Note amount of anxiety associated with the dyspnea.
- Attempt to determine if client's dyspnea is physiological or psychological in cause.
- The rapidity of which the onset of dyspnea is noted is also an indicator of the severity of the pathological condition.

**Psychological Dyspnea—Hyperventilation**

- Monitor for symptoms of hyperventilation, including rapid respiratory rate, sighing breaths, lightheadedness, numbness and tingling of hands and feet, palpitations, and sometimes chest pain (Bickley et al, 2020a).
- Assess cause of hyperventilation by asking client about current emotions and psychological state.

• = Independent ▲ = Collaborative

**B**

- Pulmonary rehabilitation programs that contain components of behavioral, cognitive, or psychosocial components have been shown to improve dyspnea and reduce anxiety and depression, particularly in clients with COPD (GOLD, 2020).
- Pharmacological treatment to reduce anxiety and panic disorders that likely increase dyspnea may not be recommended for clients with asthma and COPD (GOLD, 2020).
- Ask the client to breathe with you to slow down respiratory rate.
- ▲ Consider having the client breathe in and out of a paper bag as tolerated.
- ▲ If client has chronic problems with hyperventilation, numbness and tingling in extremities, dizziness, and other signs of panic attacks, refer for counseling or pulmonary rehabilitation.

**Physiological Dyspnea**

- ▲ Ensure that clients in acute dyspneic state have received any ordered medications, oxygen, and any other treatment needed.
- Use valid and reliable tools to evaluate perceived dyspnea.
- Ask the client to describe the quality of breathing effort.
- Acute onset of dyspnea is often accompanied by signs of respiratory distress, which include tachypnea, cough, stridor, wheezing, cyanosis, impaired speech, tachycardia, hypotension, peripheral edema, frothy sputum, pursed-lip breathing, accessory respiratory muscle use, crackles, tripod positioning, and other signs.
- Observe color of tongue, oral mucosa, and skin for signs of cyanosis.
- Auscultate breath sounds, noting decreased or absent sounds, crackles, or wheezes.
- Assess for hemodynamic stability for the client with acute dyspnea.
- Monitor oxygen saturation continuously using pulse oximetry. Note blood gas results as available.
- Using touch on the shoulder, coach the client to slow respiratory rate, demonstrating slower respirations, making eye contact with the client, and communicating in a calm, supportive fashion. The nurse's presence, reassurance, and help in controlling the client's breathing can be beneficial in decreasing anxiety.
- Support the client in using pursed-lip and controlled breathing techniques.
- If the client is acutely dyspneic, consider having the client lean forward over a bedside table, resting elbows on the table if tolerated.
- Position the client in a semi-Fowler's position to address dyspnea symptoms.
- ▲ Administer oxygen as ordered.

• = Independent          ▲ = Collaborative

- Opioids may be used for both acute and terminal dyspnea, considering careful safe dosing for relief and side effect of constipation (Baldwin & Cox, 2016; Campbell, 2017).
- Use of music as a distraction may reduce the perception of dyspnea.
- Increase client's activity to walking three times per day as tolerated. Assist the client in using oxygen during activity as needed.
- Schedule rest periods before and after activity.
▲ Evaluate the client's nutritional status. Refer to a dietitian if needed. Use nutritional supplements to increase nutritional level if needed.
- Provide small, frequent feedings.
- Encourage the client to take deep breaths at prescribed intervals and do controlled coughing.
- Help the client with chronic respiratory disease to evaluate dyspnea experience to determine whether previous incidences of dyspnea were similar and to recognize that the client survived those incidences. Encourage the client to be self-reliant if possible, use problem-solving skills, and maximize use of social support.
- See care plan for Ineffective **Airway** Clearance if client has a problem with increased respiratory secretions.
▲ Refer the client with COPD for pulmonary rehabilitation.

**Geriatric**
- Assess respiratory systems in older adults with the understanding that inspiratory muscles weaken, resulting in a slight barrel chest.
- Encourage ambulation as tolerated.
- Encourage older clients to sit upright or stand and to avoid lying down for prolonged periods during the day.

**Home Care**
- Work with the client to determine what strategies are most helpful during times of dyspnea. Educate and empower the client to self-manage the disease associated with impaired gas exchange.
- Assist the client and family with identifying other factors that precipitate or exacerbate episodes of ineffective breathing patterns (e.g., stress, allergens, stairs, activities that have high energy requirements).
- Assess client knowledge of and compliance with medication regimen.
▲ Refer the client for telemonitoring with a pulmonologist as appropriate, with use of an electronic spirometer or an electronic peak flowmeter.
- Teach the client and family the importance of maintaining the therapeutic regimen and having as-needed drugs easily accessible at all times.

• = Independent          ▲ = Collaborative

**C**

- Provide the client with emotional support in dealing with symptoms of respiratory difficulty. Provide family with support for care of a client with chronic or terminal illness. Refer to care plan for **Anxiety.**
- When electrically based equipment for respiratory support is being implemented, evaluate home environment for electrical safety, such as proper grounding. Ensure that notification is sent to the local utility company, the emergency medical team, and police and fire departments.
- Support clients' efforts at self-care. Ensure they have all the information they need to participate in care.
▲ Referral for in-home occupational therapy evaluation and teaching of energy conservation techniques and appropriate home safety (GOLD, 2020).
▲ Institute case management of frail elderly to support continued independent living (Mahler, 2017).

**Client/Family Teaching and Discharge Planning**
- Teach pursed-lip and controlled breathing techniques.
- Teach about dosage, actions, and side effects of medications.
- Teach client progressive muscle relaxation techniques.
- Teach the client to identify and avoid specific factors that exacerbate ineffective breathing patterns, such as exposure to other sources of air pollution, especially smoking. If client smokes, refer to a smoking cessation program.

# Decreased Cardiac Output

**Domain 4** Activity/rest   **Class 4** Cardiovascular/pulmonary responses
## NANDA-I Definition
Inadequate volume of blood pumped by the heart to meet the metabolic demands of the body.
## Defining Characteristics
### Altered Heart Rate/Rhythm
Bradycardia, electrocardiogram change; heart palpitations; tachycardia
### Altered Preload
Decrease in central venous pressure; decrease in pulmonary artery wedge pressure; edema; fatigue; heart murmur; increased central venous pressure; increased pulmonary artery wedge pressure; jugular vein distention; weight gain
### Altered Afterload
Abnormal skin color; altered blood pressure; clammy skin; decreased peripheral pulses; decreased pulmonary vascular resistance; decreased systemic

• = Independent          ▲ = Collaborative

vascular resistance; dyspnea; increased pulmonary vascular resistance; increased systemic vascular resistance; oliguria; prolonged capillary refill

**Altered Contractility**

Adventitious breath sounds; coughing; decreased cardiac index; decreased ejection fraction; decreased left ventricular stroke work index; decreased stroke volume index; orthopnea; paroxysmal nocturnal dyspnea; presence of S3 heart sound; presence of S4 heart sound

**Behavioral/Emotional**

Anxiety; psychomotor agitation

**Related Factors**

To be developed

**Associated Conditions**

Altered afterload, altered contractility; altered heart rate; altered heart rhythm; altered preload; altered stroke volume

**Client Outcomes**

**Client Will (Specify Time Frame)**

- Demonstrate adequate cardiac output as evidenced by blood pressure, pulse rate, and rhythm within normal parameters for client; strong peripheral pulses; maintained level of mentation; lack of chest discomfort, dyspnea, or edema; maintain adequate urinary output; maintain an ability to tolerate activity without symptoms of dyspnea, syncope, or chest pain
- Remain free of side effects from the medications used to achieve adequate cardiac output
- Explain actions and precautions to prevent primary or secondary cardiac disease

**Nursing Interventions**

- Recognize characteristics of decreased cardiac output including, but not limited to, fatigue, dyspnea, edema, orthopnea, paroxysmal nocturnal dyspnea, chest pain, decreased exercise capacity, weight gain, hepatomegaly, jugular venous distention, palpitations, lung rhonchi, cough, clammy skin, skin color changes, dysuria, altered mental status, anemia, and hemodynamic changes.
- Monitor and report presence and degree of symptoms including dyspnea at rest, reduced exercise capacity, difficulty with activities of daily living, orthopnea, paroxysmal nocturnal dyspnea, cough, palpitations, chest pain, distended abdomen, early satiety, fatigue, presyncope/syncope, or weakness. Monitor and report signs including jugular vein distention, peripheral edema, firm or distended abdomen, prominent S2, S3 gallop, rales, positive hepatojugular reflux, ascites,

**C**

laterally displaced or pronounced point of maximal impact, holosystolic murmur, narrow pulse pressure, cool extremities, tachycardia with pulsus alternans, pulsus paradoxus, and irregular heartbeat.
- Monitor orthostatic blood pressures, oxygenation, hemodynamic values, urine output, and daily weights.
- Recognize that decreased cardiac output can occur in a number of noncardiac disorders such as septic shock, electrolyte imbalances, and hypovolemia. Expect variation in orders for differential diagnoses related to decreased cardiac output, because orders will be distinct to address the primary cause of the altered cardiac output.
- Obtain a thorough client-specific and familial history.
▲ Monitor pulse oximetry and administer oxygen as needed per health care provider's order. Supplemental oxygen increases oxygen availability to the myocardium and can relieve symptoms of hypoxemia. Resting hypoxia or oxygen desaturation may indicate fluid overload or concurrent pulmonary disease.
- Place client in semi-Fowler's or high Fowler's position with legs down or in a position of comfort. Elevating the head of the bed and legs in the down position may decrease the work of breathing and may decrease venous return and preload.
- During acute events, ensure client remains on short-term bed rest or maintains activity level that does not compromise cardiac output.
- Provide a restful environment by minimizing controllable stressors and unnecessary disturbances. Reducing stressors decreases cardiac workload and oxygen demand.
▲ Apply graduated compression stockings or intermittent pneumatic compression (IPC) leg sleeves as ordered. Ensure proper fit by measuring accurately. Remove stockings at least twice a day, and then reapply. Assess the condition of the extremities frequently. Graduated compression stockings may be contraindicated in clients with peripheral arterial disease.
▲ Check blood pressure, pulse, and condition before administering cardiac medications (e.g., angiotensin-converting enzyme inhibitors, angiotensin receptor blockers, angiotensin receptor-neprilysin inhibitors, calcium channel blockers, diuretics, digoxin, and beta-blockers). Notify health care provider if heart rate or blood pressure is low before holding medications. It is important that the nurse evaluate how well the client is tolerating current medications before administering cardiac medications; do not hold medications without health care provider input. The health care provider may decide to

• = Independent    ▲ = Collaborative

C

have medications administered even though the blood pressure or pulse rate has lowered.

- Observe for and report chest pain or discomfort; note location, radiation, severity, quality, duration, and associated manifestations such as nausea, indigestion, or diaphoresis; also note precipitating and relieving factors. Chest pain/discomfort may indicate an inadequate blood supply to the heart, which can further compromise cardiac output.

▲ If chest pain is present, refer to the interventions in Risk for Decreased **Cardiac** Tissue Perfusion care plan.

- Recognize the effect of sleep disordered breathing in HF and that sleep disorders are common in clients with HF (Yancy et al, 2013, 2017).

- Administer CPAP or supplemental oxygen at night as ordered for management of suspected or diagnosed sleep disordered breathing.

▲ Closely monitor fluid intake, including intravenous lines. Maintain fluid restriction if ordered. Clients with decreased cardiac output, poorly functioning ventricles, and ventricular dysfunction may not tolerate increased fluid volumes.

- Monitor intake and output (I&O). If client is acutely ill, measure hourly urine output and note decreases in output. Decreased cardiac output results in decreased perfusion of the kidneys, with a resulting decrease in urine output.

▲ Note results of initial diagnostic studies, including electrocardiography, echocardiography, and chest radiography.

▲ Note results of further diagnostic imaging studies such as radionuclide imaging, stress echocardiography, cardiac catheterization, computed tomography (CT), or magnetic resonance imaging (MRI).

▲ Review laboratory data as needed, including arterial blood gases, complete blood count, serum electrolytes (sodium, potassium, magnesium, and calcium), blood urea nitrogen, creatinine, iron studies, urinalysis, glucose, fasting lipid profile, liver function tests, thyroid-stimulating hormone, B-type natriuretic peptide assay (BNP), or N-terminal pro-B-type natriuretic peptide (NTpro-BNP). Routine blood work can provide insight into the etiology of HF and extent of decompensation.

- Gradually increase activity when the client's condition is stabilized by encouraging slower-paced activities, or shorter periods of activity, with frequent rest periods after exercise prescription; observe for symptoms of intolerance. Take blood pressure and pulse before and after activity

• = Independent          ▲ = Collaborative

**C**

and note changes. Activity of the cardiac client should be closely monitored. See care plan Decreased **Activity** Tolerance.

▲ Encourage a diet that promotes cardiovascular health and reduces risk of hypertension, atherosclerotic disease, renal impairment, insulin resistance, and hypervolemia, within the context of an individual's cultural preferences (Van Horn et al, 2016; Whelton et al, 2018; Arnett et al, 2019).

▲ Monitor bowel function. Provide stool softeners as ordered. Caution client not to strain when defecating, as this may cause vasovagal syncope. Decreased activity, pain medication, and diuretics can cause constipation.

• Weigh the client at the same time daily (after voiding). Daily weight is a good indicator of fluid balance. Use the same scale if possible when weighing clients for consistency. Increased weight and severity of symptoms can signal decreased cardiac function with retention of fluids.

▲ Provide influenza and pneumococcal vaccines as needed before client discharge for those who have yet to receive those inoculations (Centers for Disease Control and Prevention, 2020a).

• Evaluate a client's social determinants of health (SDOH), including race, gender identity, socioeconomic position, insurance coverage, living condition, food security, access to transportation, social support, and health literacy, among other factors.

• Assess for presence of depression and/or anxiety and refer for treatment if present. See Nursing Interventions for **Anxiety** to facilitate reduction of anxiety in clients and family.

▲ Refer to a cardiac rehabilitation program for education and monitored exercise.

▲ Refer to an HF program for education, evaluation, and guided support to increase activity and rebuild quality of life. Support for the HF client should be client centered, culturally sensitive, and include family and social support.

**Critically Ill**

▲ Observe for symptoms of cardiogenic shock, including impaired mentation, hypotension, decreased peripheral pulses, cold clammy skin, signs of pulmonary congestion, and decreased organ function. If present, notify the health care provider immediately. Cardiogenic shock is a state of circulatory failure from loss of cardiac function associated with inadequate organ perfusion and a high mortality rate.

▲ If shock is present, monitor hemodynamic parameters for an increase in pulmonary wedge pressure, an increase in systemic vascular

• = Independent            ▲ = Collaborative

resistance, or a decrease in stroke volume, cardiac output, and cardiac index.

▲ Titrate inotropic and vasoactive medications within defined parameters to maintain contractility, preload, and afterload per health care provider's order. By following parameters, the nurse ensures maintenance of a delicate balance of medications that stimulate the heart to increase contractility while maintaining adequate perfusion of the body.

▲ Identify significant fluid overload and initiate intravenous diuretics as ordered. Monitor I&O, daily weight, and vital signs, as well as signs and symptoms of congestion. Watch laboratory data, including cardiac biomarkers, serum electrolytes, creatinine, and urea nitrogen.

▲ When using pulmonary arterial catheter technology, be sure to appropriately level and zero the equipment, use minimal tubing, maintain system patency, perform square wave testing, position the client appropriately, and consider correlation to respiratory and cardiac cycles when assessing waveforms and integrating data into client assessment.

▲ Observe for worsening signs and symptoms of respiratory compromise. Recognize that invasive or noninvasive ventilation may be required for clients with acute cardiogenic pulmonary edema.

▲ Monitor client for signs and symptoms of fluid and electrolyte imbalance when clients are receiving ultrafiltration or continuous renal replacement therapy (CRRT). Clients with refractory HF may have ultrafiltration or CRRT ordered as a mechanical method to remove excess fluid volume.

• Recognize that hypoperfusion from low cardiac output can lead to altered mental status and decreased cognition.

• Recognize that clients with severe HF may undergo additional therapies, such as internal pacemaker or defibrillator placement, and/or placement of a ventricular assist device (VAD).

**Geriatric**

• Recognize that older clients may demonstrate fatigue and depression as signs of HF and decreased cardiac output.

• Recognize that older adults in the critical care setting often have geriatric syndromes such as polypharmacy, multimorbidity, cognitive decline, and frailty that can be exacerbated in the critical care setting and contribute to prolonged hospitalization, increased mortality, increased HF, increased disability, and decreased quality of life (Damluji et al, 2019).

**C**

▲ If the client has heart disease–causing activity intolerance, refer for cardiac rehabilitation.

▲ Recognize that edema can present differently in the older population.

▲ Recognize that blood pressure control is beneficial for older clients to reduce the risk of worsening HF.

▲ Recognize that renal function is not always accurately represented by serum creatinine in the older population because of less muscle mass (Yancy et al, 2013).

▲ Observe for side effects from cardiac medications. Older adults can have difficulty with metabolism and excretion of medications because of decreased function of the liver and kidneys; therefore, toxic side effects are more common.

▲ Older adults may require more frequent visits, closer monitoring of medication dose changes, and more gradual increases in medications.

▲ Recognize that older adults still benefit from smoking cessation.

▲ As older adults approach end of life, clinicians should help to facilitate a comprehensive plan of care that incorporates the client and family's values, goals, and preferences (Allen et al, 2012; National Consensus Project for Quality Palliative Care, 2018).

**Home Care**

• Some of the previously mentioned interventions may be adapted for home care use. Home care agencies may use specialized staff and methods to care for chronic HF clients.

• Assess for fatigue and weakness frequently. Assess home environment for safety, as well as resources/obstacles to energy conservation.

• Help family adapt daily living patterns to establish life changes that will maintain improved cardiac functioning in the client. Take the client's perspective into consideration and use a holistic approach in assessing and responding to client planning for the future.

• Assist client to recognize and exercise power in using self-care management to adjust to health change. Refer to care plan for **Powerlessness.**

▲ Refer to medical social services, cardiac rehabilitation, telemonitoring, and case management as necessary for assistance with home care, access to resources, and counseling about the impact of severe or chronic cardiac diseases.

▲ As the client chooses, refer to palliative care, which can begin earlier in the care of the HF client. Palliative care can be used to increase comfort and quality of life in the HF client before end-of-life care.

▲ If the client's condition warrants, refer to hospice.

• = Independent          ▲ = Collaborative

**C**

**Client/Family Teaching and Discharge Planning**

- Begin discharge planning as soon as possible on admission to the emergency department (ED) if appropriate with a case manager or social worker to assess home support systems and the need for community or home health services.
- Discharge education should be comprehensive, evidence based, culturally sensitive, and include both the client and family (Yancy et al, 2013).
- Teach the client about any medications prescribed. Medication teaching includes the drug name; its purpose; administration instructions, such as taking it with or without food; and any side effects. Instruct the client to report any adverse side effects to his or her health care provider.
- Teach the importance of performing and recording daily weights on arising for the day, and to report weight gain. Ask if client has a scale at home; if not, assist in getting one.
- Teach the types and progression patterns of worsening HF symptoms, when to call a health care provider for help, and when to go to the hospital for urgent care (Yancy et al, 2013).
- Stress the importance of ceasing tobacco use (Whelton et al, 2018).
- ▲ Individuals should be screened for electronic cigarette use (e-cigarette).
- On hospital discharge, educate clients about low-sodium, low–saturated fat diet, with consideration of client education, literacy, and health literacy level.
- Educate clients that comorbidities, including obesity, hypertension, metabolic syndrome, diabetes mellitus, and hyperlipidemia, are common in individuals with HF and can affect clinical outcomes related to HF if not controlled (Bozkurt et al, 2016).
- For clients with diabetes mellitus, educate about the importance of glycemic control.
- Instruct client and family on the importance of regular follow-up care with health care providers.
- ▲ Teach stress reduction (e.g., meditation, imagery, controlled breathing, muscle relaxation techniques).
- Discuss advance directives with the HF client, including resuscitation preferences.
- Clients should be provided with education regarding the influenza vaccine and pneumococcal vaccine before discharge.
- Teach the importance of physical activity as tolerated.

• = Independent          ▲ = Collaborative

# Risk for Decreased Cardiac Output

**Domain 4** Activity/rest **Class 4** Cardiovascular/pulmonary responses

**C**

## NANDA-I Definition

Susceptible to inadequate blood pumped by the heart to meet metabolic demands of the body, which may compromise health.

## Risk Factors

To be developed

## Associated Conditions

Altered afterload; altered contractility; altered heart rate; altered heart rhythm; altered preload; altered stroke volume

## Client Outcomes, Nursing Interventions, and Client/Family Teaching and Discharge Planning

Refer to care plan for Decreased **Cardiac** Output.

# Risk for Decreased Cardiac Tissue Perfusion

**Domain 4** Activity/rest **Class 4** Cardiovascular/pulmonary responses

## NANDA-I Definition

Susceptible to a decrease in cardiac (coronary) circulation, which may compromise health.

## Risk Factors

Inadequate knowledge of modifiable factors; substance misuse

## At-Risk Population

Individuals with a family history of cardiovascular disease

## Associated Conditions

Cardiac tamponade; cardiovascular surgery; coronary artery spasm; diabetes mellitus; elevated C-reactive protein; hyperlipidemia; hypertension; hypovolemia; hypoxemia; hypoxia; pharmaceutical preparations

## Client Outcomes

**Client Will (Specify Time Frame)**

- Maintain vital signs within normal range
- Retain an asymptomatic cardiac rhythm (have absence of arrhythmias, tachycardia, or bradycardia)
- Be free from chest and radiated discomfort as well as associated symptoms related to acute coronary syndromes (ACSs)
- Deny nausea and be free of vomiting or gastrointestinal distress
- Have skin that is dry and of normal temperature
- Maintain normal cognition

• = Independent ▲ = Collaborative

- Maintain healthy lifestyle behaviors that promote primary prevention of cardiovascular disease

**Nursing Interventions**

- Be aware that the primary cause of ACS which include unstable angina (UA), non–ST-elevation myocardial infarction (NSTEMI), and ST-elevation myocardial infarction (STEMI), is an imbalance between myocardial oxygen consumption and demand that is associated with partially or fully occlusive thrombus development in coronary arteries (Amsterdam et al, 2014).
- Assess for symptoms of coronary hypoperfusion and possible ACS, including chest discomfort (pressure, tightness, crushing, squeezing, dullness, or achiness), with or without radiation (or originating) in the retrosternal area, back, neck, jaw, shoulder, or arm discomfort or numbness; shortness of breath (SOB); associated diaphoresis; abdominal pain; dizziness, lightheadedness, loss of consciousness, or unexplained fatigue; nausea or vomiting with chest discomfort, heartburn, or indigestion; and associated anxiety.
- Evaluate client for noncardiac causes of chest pain, other than psychiatric disorders, including gastrointestinal disorders (reflux disease, esophagitis), pleuritic pain (secondary to pulmonary embolus, infection), costochondritis, and musculoskeletal disorders.
- Consider atypical presentations of ACS for women, older adults, and individuals with diabetes mellitus, impaired renal function, and dementia.
- Evaluate the client for socioeconomic or race/ethnicity factors that put them at higher risk for atherosclerotic cardiovascular disease (ASCVD).
- Review the client's medical, surgical, social, and familial history.
- Perform physical assessments for both coronary artery disease (CAD) and noncoronary findings related to decreased coronary perfusion, including vital signs, pulse oximetry, equal blood pressure in both arms, heart rate, respiratory rate, and pulse oximetry. Check bilateral pulses for quality and regularity. Report tachycardia, bradycardia, hypotension or hypertension, pulsus alternans or pulsus paradoxus, tachypnea, or abnormal pulse oximetry reading. Assess cardiac rhythm for arrhythmias; skin and mucous membrane color, temperature, and dryness; and capillary refill. Assess for peripheral vascular disease. Assess neck veins for elevated central venous pressure, cyanosis, and pericardial or pleural friction rub. Examine client for cardiac S4 gallop, new heart murmur, lung crackles, altered mentation, pain on

abdominal palpation, abdominal distention, decreased bowel sounds, or decreased urinary output.

▲ Administer supplemental oxygen as ordered and needed for clients presenting with ACS, respiratory distress, or other high-risk features of hypoxemia to maintain a $Po_2$ of at least 90%.

▲ Use continuous pulse oximetry as ordered.

▲ Insert one or more large-bore intravenous catheters to keep the vein open. Routinely assess saline locks for patency. Clients who come to the hospital with possible decrease in coronary perfusion or ACS may have intravenous fluids and medications ordered routinely or emergently to maintain or restore adequate cardiac function and rhythm.

▲ Observe the cardiac monitor for hemodynamically significant arrhythmias, ST depressions or elevations, T-wave inversions, and/or Q-waves as signs of ischemia or injury. Be aware that clients with prior cardiothoracic surgery may have abnormal electrocardiogram (ECG) changes at baseline. Report abnormal findings.

• Have emergency equipment and defibrillation capability nearby and be prepared to defibrillate immediately if ventricular tachycardia with clinical deterioration or ventricular fibrillation occurs.

▲ Perform a 12-lead ECG as ordered to be interpreted within 10 minutes of emergency department arrival and during episodes of chest discomfort or angina equivalent.

▲ Administer non–enteric-coated aspirin as ordered, as soon as possible after presentation and for maintenance.

▲ Administer nitroglycerin tablets sublingually as ordered, every 5 minutes until the chest pain is resolved while monitoring the blood pressure for hypotension, for a maximum of three doses as ordered. Administer nitroglycerin paste or intravenous preparations as ordered.

• Do not administer nitroglycerin preparations to individuals with hypotension, or individuals who have received phosphodiesterase type 5 inhibitors, such as sildenafil, tadalafil, or vardenafil, in the last 24 hours (48 hours for long-acting preparations).

▲ Administer morphine intravenously as ordered, every 5 to 30 minutes until pain is relieved while monitoring blood pressure when nitroglycerin alone does not relieve chest discomfort.

▲ Assess and report abnormal laboratory work results of cardiac enzymes, specifically troponin I or high-sensitivity troponin T, B-type natriuretic peptide, chemistries, hematology, coagulation studies, arterial blood gases, finger stick blood sugar, elevated C-reactive protein, or drug screen.

C

- Assess for individual risk factors for CAD, such as hypertension, dyslipidemia, cigarette smoking, diabetes mellitus, metabolic syndrome, obesity, or family history of heart disease. Other risk factors including socioeconomic factors, sedentary lifestyle, obesity, or cocaine or amphetamine use. Note age and gender as risk factors.
▲ Administer additional heart medications as ordered, including beta-blockers, calcium channel blockers, angiotensin-converting enzyme inhibitors, angiotensin II receptor blockers, aldosterone antagonists, antiarrhythmics, diuretics, antiplatelet agents, and anticoagulants. Always check blood pressure and pulse rate before administering these medications. If the blood pressure or pulse rate is low, contact the health care provider to establish whether the medication should be withheld. Also check platelet counts, renal function, and coagulation studies as ordered to assess proper effects of these agents.
▲ Administer lipid-lowering therapy as ordered.
▲ Prepare client with education, withholding of meals and/or medications, and intravenous access for early invasive therapy with cardiac catheterization, reperfusion therapy, and possible percutaneous coronary intervention in individuals with refractory angina or hemodynamic or electrical instability, and first medical contact to device time of less than 90 minutes if STEMI is suspected.
▲ Prepare clients with education, withholding of meals and/or medications, and intravenous access for noninvasive cardiac diagnostic procedures such as echocardiogram, exercise, or pharmacological stress test, and cardiac computed tomography scan as ordered.
▲ Request a referral to a cardiac rehabilitation program.

**Geriatric**
- Consider atypical presentations of possible ACS in older adults.
▲ Ask the prescriber about possible reduced dosage of medications for older clients, considering weight, creatinine clearance, and glomerular filtration rate.
- Consider issues such as quality of life, palliative care, end-of-life care, and differences in sociocultural aspects for clients and families when supporting them in decisions regarding aggressiveness of care. Ask about living wills, as well as medical and durable power of attorney.

**Client/Family Teaching and Discharge Planning**
▲ Client and family education regarding a multiprofessional plan of care should start early. Special attention to client and family education should occur during transitions of care.

• = Independent          ▲ = Collaborative

**C**

- Teach the client and family to call 911 for symptoms of new angina, existing angina unresponsive to rest and sublingual nitroglycerin tablets, or heart attack, or if an individual becomes unresponsive.
- On discharge, instruct clients about symptoms of ischemia, when to cease activity, when to use sublingual nitroglycerin, and when to call 911.
- Teach client about any medications prescribed. Medication teaching includes the drug name, its purpose, administration instructions such as taking it with or without food, and any side effects. Instruct the client to report any adverse side effects to the health care provider.
- On hospital discharge, educate clients and significant others about discharge medications, including nitroglycerin sublingual tablets or spray, with written, easy to understand, culturally sensitive information.
- Provide client education related to risk factors for decreased cardiac tissue perfusion, such as hypertension, hyperlipidemia, metabolic syndrome, diabetes mellitus, tobacco use, obesity, advanced age, and female gender.
- Instruct the client on antiplatelet and anticoagulation therapy, and about signs of bleeding, need for ongoing medication compliance, and international normalized ratio monitoring.
- After discharge, continue education and support for client blood pressure and diabetes control, weight management, and resumption of physical activity.
- ▲ Clients should be provided with education regarding the influenza vaccine and pneumococcal vaccine before hospital discharge.
- ▲ Stress the importance of ceasing tobacco use.
- ▲ Individuals should be screened for electronic cigarette (e-cigarette) use.
- ▲ On hospital discharge, educate clients about a low-sodium, low–saturated fat diet, with consideration to client education, literacy, and health literacy level.
- Teach the importance of exercise and physical activity as tolerated.

# Risk for Impaired Cardiovascular Function

**Domain 4** Activity/rest     **Class 4** Cardiovascular/pulmonary responses
**NANDA-I Definition**

Susceptible to disturbance in substance transport, body homeostasis, tissue metabolic residue removal, and organ function, which may compromise health.

• = Independent          ▲ = Collaborative

## Risk Factors

Anxiety; average daily physical activity is less than recommended for age and gender; body mass index above normal range for age and gender; excessive accumulation of fat for age and gender; excessive alcohol intake; excessive stress; inadequate dietary habits; inadequate knowledge of modifiable factors; inattentive to second-hand smoke; ineffective blood glucose level management; ineffective blood pressure management; ineffective lipid balance management; smoking; substance misuse

## At-Risk Population

Economically disadvantaged individuals; individuals with family history of diabetes mellitus; individuals with family history of dyslipidemia; individuals with family history of hypertension; individuals with family history of metabolic syndrome; individuals with family history of obesity; individuals with history of cardiovascular event; men; older adults; postmenopausal women

## Associated Conditions

Depression; diabetes mellitus; dyslipidemia; hypertension; insulin resistance; pharmaceutical preparations

## Client Outcomes, Nursing Interventions, and Client/Family Teaching and Discharge Planning

See the care plans for Decreased **Cardiac** Output; Risk for Decreased **Cardiac** Tissue Perfusion; Risk for **Metabolic Syndrome;** and Risk for **Thrombosis**

# Caregiver Role Strain

**Domain 7** Role relationship    **Class 1** Caregiving roles

## NANDA-I Definition

Difficulty in fulfilling care responsibilities, expectations and/or behaviors for family or significant others.

## Defining Characteristics

### Caregiving Activities

Apprehensive about future ability to provide care; apprehensive about future health of care receiver; apprehensive about potential institutionalization of care receiver; apprehensive about well-being of care receiver if unable to provide care; difficulty completing required tasks; difficulty performing required tasks; dysfunctional change in caregiving activities; preoccupation with care routine

### Caregiver Health Status

**Physiological:** Fatigue; gastrointestinal distress; headache; hypertension; rash; reports altered sleep-wake cycle; weight change

• = Independent        ▲ = Collaborative

**C**

**Emotional:** Depressive symptoms; emotional lability; expresses anger; expresses frustration; impatience; insufficient time to meet personal needs; nervousness; somatization

**Socioeconomic:** Altered leisure activities; isolation; low work productivity; refuses career advancement

### Caregiver-Care Receiver Relationship

Difficulty watching care receiver with illness; sadness about altered interpersonal relations with care receiver; uncertainty about alteration in interpersonal relations with care receiver

### Family Processes

Family conflict; reports concern about family member(s)

## Related Factors

### Caregiver

Competing role commitments; depressive symptoms; inadequate fulfillment of others' expectations; inadequate fulfillment of self-expectations; inadequate knowledge about community resources; inadequate psychological resilience; inadequate recreation; ineffective coping strategies; inexperience with caregiving; insufficient physical endurance; insufficient privacy; not developmentally ready for caregiver role; physical conditions; social isolation; stressors; substance misuse; unrealistic self-expectations

### Care Receiver Factors

Discharged home with significant needs; increased care needs; loss of independence; problematic behavior; substance misuse; unpredictability of illness trajectory; unstable health status

### Caregiver-Care Receiver Relationship

Abusive interpersonal relations; codependency; inadequate interpersonal relations; unaddressed abuse; unrealistic care receiver expectations; violent interpersonal relations

### Caregiving Activities

Altered nature of care activities; around-the-clock care responsibilities; complexity of care activities; excessive caregiving activities; extended duration of caregiving required; inadequate assistance; inadequate equipment for providing care; inadequate physical environment for providing care; inadequate respite for caregiver; insufficient time; unpredictability of care situation

### Family Processes

Family isolation; ineffective family adaptation; pattern of family dysfunction; pattern of family dysfunction prior to the caregiving situation; pattern of ineffective family coping

• = Independent          ▲ = Collaborative

**Socioeconomic**

Difficulty accessing assistance; difficulty accessing community resources; difficulty accessing support; inadequate community resources; inadequate social support; inadequate transportation; social alienation

C

### At-Risk Population

Care receiver with developmental disabilities; caregiver delivering care to partner; caregiver with developmental disabilities; female caregiver; individuals delivering care to infants born prematurely; individuals experiencing financial crisis

### Associated Conditions

**Care Receiver**

Impaired health status; psychological disorder

**Caregiver**

Chronic disease; congenital disorders; illness severity; mental disorders

### Client Outcomes

**Throughout the Care Situation, the Caregiver Will**

- Be able to express feelings of strain
- Feel supported by health care professionals, family, and friends; feel they have adequate information to provide care
- Report reduced or acceptable feelings of burden or distress
- Take part in self-care activities to maintain own physical and psychological/emotional health; identify resources (family and community) available to help in giving care
- Verbalize mastery of the care activities; feel confident and competent to provide care; have the skills to provide care
- Ask for help when needed
- Not refuse help when offered

**Throughout the Care Situation, the Care Recipient Will**

- Obtain quality and safe physical care and emotional care
- Be treated with respect and dignity

### Nursing Interventions

- Assess for caregiver role strain at the onset of the care situation, at regular intervals throughout the care situation, at care transitions, and with changes in care recipient status.
- Monitor overall health of the caregiver at regular intervals for signs and symptoms of depression, anxiety, role strain, hopelessness, posttraumatic stress, and deteriorating physical health, particularly their control over chronic diseases and comorbid conditions.
- Identify caregiver personal resources such as resilience, proficiency in caregiving skills, social support, optimism, positive aspects of care

• = Independent          ▲ = Collaborative

**C**

and resilience, and utilization or availability of social services (e.g., state-funded senior services, veterans' services, Area Agency on Aging resources).
- Encourage the caregiver to share feelings, concerns, uncertainties, and fears; support groups, including Internet-based ones, can be helpful to gain support.
- Regularly assess for any evidence of caregiver or care recipient violence or abuse, especially emotional and verbal abuse; risk factors include substance abuse, poor premorbid relationship, and psychiatric illness.
- Ensure appropriate referrals for physical, occupational, and speech-language therapy, as well as social work, including referrals for outpatient therapy or skilled home health care if needed (including therapy needed to maintain functional abilities and prevent decline).
- Talk with caregivers early and often about palliative care as a means of symptom management for the care recipient.
- Help the caregiver learn mindfulness stress management techniques, which can reduce psychological distress.
- Assist the client to identify spiritual beliefs and engage in spiritual practices.
- Encourage regular and open communication with the care recipient and with the health care team.

**Geriatric**
- The interventions described previously may be adapted for use with geriatric clients.
- Monitor the caregiver for psychological distress and signs of depression, especially if there was an unsatisfactory family relationship before caregiving.
- To improve the ability to provide safe care: assess caregiver's support and learning needs and provide skills training related to direct care, perform complex monitoring tasks, supervise, and interpret client symptoms, assist with decision-making, assist with medication adherence.

**Pediatric**
- Assess parents for perceived self-blame or worsened relationship with their child, especially if their child's condition is psychiatric in nature, and assist them to seek social support, instill hope, and identify how they might grow.
- Assess for partner support of the caregiver in dual-earning households, and provide resources related to couples' or family therapy if needed.

**Multicultural**
- Assess for cultural and spiritual needs of client and caregiver.

• = Independent    ▲ = Collaborative

**Home Care**

• Assess the client and caregiver at every visit for the quality of their relationship and for the quality and safety of the care provided.

• Encourage use of respite care, which may include regular care and assistance at home, or a brief period of total care (24/7) at home or in an inpatient facility to allow the caregiver to recover from an illness, attend a wedding, or go on a short vacation.

**Client/Family Teaching and Discharge Planning**

• Identify client and caregiver factors that necessitate the use of skilled home health care services or need to be addressed before the client can be safely discharged.

• Collaborate with the caregiver and discuss the care needs of the client, disease processes, medications, and what to expect as part of discharge planning and transition care.

• Involve the family caregiver in care transitions and discharge from institutions; use a multiprofessional team to provide medical and social services for detailed instruction and planning specific to the care need.

# Risk for Caregiver Role Strain

**Domain 7** Role relationship     **Class 1** Caregiving roles

**NANDA-I Definition**

Susceptible to difficulty in fulfilling care responsibilities, expectations, and/or behaviors for family or significant others, which may compromise health.

**Risk Factors**

**Caregiver Factors**

Competing role commitments; depressive symptoms; inadequate fulfillment of others' expectations; inadequate fulfillment of self-expectations; inadequate knowledge about community resources; inadequate psychological resilience; inadequate recreation; ineffective coping strategies; inexperience with caregiving; insufficient physical endurance; insufficient privacy; not developmentally ready for caregiver role; physical conditions; stressors; substance misuse; unrealistic self-expectations; unstable health status

**Care Receiver Factors**

Discharged home with significant needs; increased care needs; loss of independence; problematic behavior; substance misuse; unpredictability of illness trajectory; unstable health condition

**Caregiver-Care Receiver Relationship**

Abusive interpersonal relations; codependency; inadequate interpersonal relations; unaddressed abuse; unrealistic care receiver expectations; violent interpersonal relations

                    • = Independent                    ▲ = Collaborative

**Caregiving Activities**

Altered nature of care activities; around-the-clock care responsibilities; complexity of care activities; excessive caregiving activities; extended duration of caregiving required; inadequate assistance; inadequate equipment for providing care; inadequate physical environment for providing care; inadequate respite for caregiver; insufficient time; unpredictability of care situation

**Family Processes**

Family isolation; ineffective family adaptation; pattern of family dysfunction; pattern of family dysfunction prior to the caregiving situation; pattern of ineffective family coping

**Socioeconomic**

Difficulty accessing assistance; difficulty accessing community resources; difficulty accessing support; inadequate community resources; inadequate social support; inadequate transportation; social alienation; social isolation

## At-Risk Population

Care receiver with developmental disabilities; care receiver's condition inhibits conversation; caregiver delivering care to partner; caregiver with developmental disabilities; female caregiver; individuals delivering care to infants born prematurely; individuals experiencing financial crisis

## Associated Conditions

**Caregiver Factors**

Impaired health status; psychological disorder

**Care Receiver Factors**

Chronic disease; congenital disorders; illness severity; mental disorders

## Client Outcomes, Nursing Interventions, and Client/Family Teaching

Refer to care plan for **Caregiver** Role Strain.

# Risk for Ineffective Cerebral Tissue Perfusion

**Domain 4** Activity/rest     **Class 4** Cardiovascular/pulmonary responses

## NANDA-I Definition

Susceptible to a decrease in cerebral tissue circulation, which may compromise health.

## Risk Factors

Substance misuse

## At-Risk Population

Individuals with history of recent myocardial infarction

## Associated Conditions

Abnormal serum partial thromboplastin time; abnormal serum prothrombin time; akinetic left ventricular wall segment; atherosclerosis; atrial fibrillation; atrial myxoma; brain injuries; brain neoplasm; carotid stenosis; cerebral aneurysm; coagulopathy; dilated cardiomyopathy; disseminated intravascular coagulopathy; embolism; hypercholesterolemia; hypertension; infective endocarditis; mechanical prosthetic valve; mitral stenosis; pharmaceutical preparations; sick sinus syndrome; treatment regimen

**C**

## Client Outcomes

### Client Will (Specify Time Frame)

- State stable or improved headache
- Demonstrate appropriate orientation to person, place, time, and situation
- Demonstrate ability to follow simple commands
- Demonstrate equal bilateral motor strength
- Demonstrate adequate swallowing ability
- Maintain (or improve) neurological examination

## Nursing Interventions

- To decrease risk of reduced cerebral perfusion related to stroke or transient ischemic attack (TIA):
  - ○ Obtain a family history of hypertension, diabetes, and stroke to identify persons who may be at increased risk of stroke.
  - ○ Monitor BP regularly because hypertension is a major risk factor for both ischemic and hemorrhagic stroke.
  - ○ Teach hypertensive clients the importance of taking their health care provider–ordered antihypertensive agent to prevent stroke.
  - ○ Stress smoking cessation at every encounter with clients, using multimodal techniques to aid in quitting, such as counseling, nicotine replacement, and oral smoking cessation medications. Provide client and family education to reduce lifestyle-associated risk factors for stroke.
  - ○ Teach clients who experience a transient TIA that they are at increased risk for a stroke. Instruct clients that adherence to medication therapy decreases recurrent TIA/stroke risk.
  - ○ Screen clients 65 years of age and older for atrial fibrillation with pulse assessment.
  - ○ Instruct the client regarding the appropriate use and side effects of anticoagulation in the prevention of cardioembolic stroke.
  - ○ Call 911 or activate the rapid response team of a hospital immediately when clients display symptoms of stroke as determined by the Cincinnati Stroke Scale (F: facial drooping; A: arm drift on one side; S: speech slurred), being careful to note the time of symptom appearance. Additional symptoms of stroke include sudden numbness/weakness of face, arm, or leg, especially

• = Independent ▲ = Collaborative

**C**

on one side; sudden confusion; trouble speaking or understanding; sudden difficulty seeing with one or both eyes; sudden trouble walking, dizziness, loss of balance, or coordination; or sudden severe headache (Jauch et al, 2013).

○ Use clinical practice guidelines for glycemic control and BP targets to guide the care of clients with diabetes who have had a stroke or TIA.

○ Maintain head of bed less than 30 degrees in the acute phase (<72 hours of symptom onset) of ischemic stroke.

○ Head of bed may be elevated to sitting position without detrimental effect to cerebral blood flow in clients with ischemic stroke or hemorrhagic stroke at 72 hours after symptom onset.

○ Administer enteric/oral nimodipine as prescribed by the health care provider after aneurysmal subarachnoid hemorrhage for 21 days.

○ Monitor neurological function frequently in the first 2 weeks after subarachnoid hemorrhage because subtle declines may be related to cerebral vasospasm.

○ Maintain cerebral perfusion pressure (CPP) 60 to 70 mm Hg in clients with traumatic brain injury.

▲ To decrease risk of reduced CPP: CPP = Mean arterial pressure – intracranial pressure (CPP = MAP – ICP)

○ Maintain euvolemia.

▲ To treat decreased CPP:

○ Clients with subarachnoid hemorrhagic stroke experiencing delayed cerebral ischemia, as evidenced by declining neurological examination, should undergo a stepwise trial of induced hypertension up to 220 mm Hg.

○ Administer vasopressor infusions to raise MAP per collaborative protocol.

○ Mobilize clients with subarachnoid hemorrhage as early as 1 day after aneurysm is secured.

# Ineffective Childbearing Process

**Domain 8** Sexuality    **Class 3** Reproduction
## NANDA-I Definition

Inability to prepare for and/or maintain a healthy pregnancy, childbirth process, and care of the newborn for ensuring well-being.

• = Independent                     ▲ = Collaborative

## Defining Characteristics

### During Pregnancy

Failure to utilize social support; inadequate attachment behavior; inadequate prenatal care; inadequate prenatal lifestyle; inadequate preparation of newborn care items; inadequate preparation of the home environment; inadequate respect for unborn baby; ineffective management of unpleasant symptoms in pregnancy; unrealistic expectations about labor and delivery

### During Labor and Delivery

Decreased proactivity during labor and delivery; failure to utilize social support; inadequate attachment behavior; inadequate lifestyle for stage of labor; inappropriate response to onset of labor

### After Birth

Failure to utilize social support; inadequate attachment behavior; inadequate baby care techniques; inadequate infant clothing; inappropriate baby feeding techniques; inappropriate breast care; inappropriate lifestyle; unsafe environment for an infant

## Related Factors

Domestic violence; inadequate knowledge of childbearing process; inadequate mental preparation for parenting; inadequate parental role model; inadequate prenatal care; inadequate social support; inconsistent prenatal health visits; low maternal confidence; maternal malnutrition; maternal powerlessness; maternal psychological distress; substance misuse; unrealistic birth plan; unsafe environment

## At-Risk Population

Individuals experiencing unplanned pregnancy; individuals experiencing unwanted pregnancy

## Client Outcomes

### Client Will (Specify Time Frame)

#### Antepartum

- Obtain early prenatal care in the first trimester and maintain regular visits
- Demonstrate appropriate care of oneself during pregnancy including good nutrition and psychological health
- Attend prenatal education either virtual or in person with significant other or involved family member
- Understand the risks of substance abuse and resources available
- Feel empowered to seek social and spiritual support for emotional well-being during pregnancy
- Prepare home for baby (e.g., crib, diapers, infant car seat, outfits, blankets) before due date
- Use support systems for emotional support

• = Independent  ▲ = Collaborative

- Develop a realistic birth plan, taking into account any high-risk pregnancy issues before due date
- Understand the labor and delivery process and comfort measures to manage labor pain before due date

**Intrapartum**

- Use support system for emotional support during labor and delivery
- Demonstrate appropriate understanding of choices in labor and delivery
- Demonstrate effective coping strategies during labor and delivery

**Postpartum**

- Provide a safe environment for self and infant
- Demonstrate appropriate newborn care and postpartum care of self
- Demonstrate appropriate bonding and parenting skills

## Nursing Interventions

- Encourage early prenatal care and regular prenatal visits.
- Identify any high-risk factors that may require additional surveillance, such as preterm labor, hypertensive disorders of pregnancy, diabetes, depression, other chronic medical conditions, presence of fetal anomalies, virus exposure, homelessness (resources can be accessed through the HUD exchange [https://www.hudexchange.info/resources] and Homeless Prenatal Program [www.homelessprenatal.org]), or other high-risk factors.
- ▲ Assess and screen for signs and symptoms of depression during pregnancy and in the postpartum period and refer for behavioral-cognitive counseling and/or medication.
- ▲ Observe for signs of alcohol misuse and counsel women to stop drinking during pregnancy. Give appropriate referral for treatment if needed.
- ▲ Obtain a smoking history and counsel women to stop smoking for the safety of the baby. Give appropriate referral to a smoking cessation program if needed.
- ▲ Monitor for substance misuse with recreational drugs. Refer to a treatment program as needed. Refer opiate-dependent women to methadone clinics to improve maternal and fetal pregnancy outcomes.
- Monitor for psychosocial issues, including lack of social support system, loneliness, depression, lack of confidence, maternal powerlessness, and socioeconomic problems.
- ▲ Monitor for signs of domestic violence. Refer to a community program for abused women that provides safe shelter as needed.
- Provide antenatal education to increase the woman's knowledge needed to make informed choices during pregnancy, labor,

• = Independent        ▲ = Collaborative

and delivery and to promote a healthy lifestyle. Encourage pregnant women to use digital resources such as Text4Baby (see https://www.text4baby.org or https://www.whattoexpect.com) to track pregnancy progress and provide education and motivation to make healthy lifestyle choices in nutrition (abstinence from poor nutrition, smoking, and alcohol, and illicit drugs).

- Encourage expectant parents to prepare a realistic birth plan or "birth preferences" to prepare for the physical and emotional aspects of the birth process and to plan ahead for how they want various situations handled.
- Encourage good nutritional intake during pregnancy to facilitate proper growth and development of the fetus. Women should consume an additional 300 calories per day during pregnancy, take a multimicronutrient supplement containing at least 400 µg folic acid, and achieve a total weight gain of 25 to 30 pounds.

**Multicultural**

▲ Provide for a translator as needed.

▲ Provide depression screening.

- Perform a cultural assessment and provide care that is culturally appropriate.

**Postpartal**

- Assess client's beliefs and concerns about the postpartum period to provide culturally appropriate health and nutrition information and guidance on contemporary postpartum practices.

## Readiness for Enhanced Childbearing Process

**Domain 8** Sexuality    **Class 3** Reproduction

### NANDA-I Definition

A pattern of preparing for and maintaining a healthy pregnancy, childbirth process and care of the newborn for ensuring well-being which can be strengthened.

### Defining Characteristics

**During Pregnancy**

Expresses desire to enhance knowledge of childbearing process; expresses desire to enhance management of unpleasant pregnancy symptoms; expresses desire to enhance prenatal lifestyle; expresses desire to enhance preparation for newborn

• = Independent          ▲ = Collaborative

**C**

## During Labor and Delivery

Expresses desire to enhance lifestyle appropriate for stage of labor; expresses desire to enhance proactivity during labor and delivery

## After Birth

Expresses desire to enhance attachment behavior; expresses desire to enhance baby care techniques; expresses desire to enhance baby feeding techniques; expresses desire to enhance breast care; expresses desire to enhance environmental safety for the baby; expresses desire to enhance postpartum lifestyle; expresses desire to enhance use of support system

## Client Outcomes

**Client Will (Specify Time Frame)**

### Antepartum

- Attend all scheduled prenatal visits and attend prenatal education either with significant other or involved family member
- Use appropriate self-care for discomforts of pregnancy
- Prepare home for baby (e.g., crib, diapers, infant car seat, outfits, blankets) before due date
- Develop a realistic birth plan, taking into account any high-risk pregnancy issues before due date
- Feel empowered to seek social and spiritual support for emotional well-being during pregnancy
- Make healthy lifestyle choices prenatally: activity and exercise/healthy nutritional practices
- Use strategies to balance activity and rest

### Intrapartum

- Demonstrate appropriate lifestyle choices during labor
- State knowledge of birthing options, signs and symptoms of labor before due date
- Demonstrate effective labor techniques
- Use support systems for labor and emotional support

### Postpartum

- Demonstrate appropriate lifestyle choices postpartum
- Report normal physical sensations after delivery
- State understanding of recommended nutrient intake, strategies to balance activity and rest, appropriate exercise, time frame for resumption of sexual activity, strategies to manage stress
- Demonstrate bonding with infant
- Demonstrate proper handling and positioning of infant/infant safety
- Demonstrate feeding technique and bathing of infant

• = Independent        ▲ = Collaborative

## Nursing Interventions

▲ Refer to care plans Risk for Impaired **Attachment;** Readiness for Enhanced **Breastfeeding;** Readiness for Enhanced Family **Coping;** Readiness for Enhanced **Family** Processes; Readiness for Enhanced **Nutrition;** Readiness for Enhanced **Parenting;** and Ineffective **Role** Performance.

**Prenatal Care**

• Encourage early prenatal care (PNC) and regular prenatal visits.
▲ Ensure that pregnant clients have an adequate diet and take multimicronutrient supplements containing at least 400 µg of folic acid, especially during early pregnancy.
• Assess smoking status of pregnant clients and offer effective smoking-cessation interventions.
▲ Assess all pregnant clients for signs of depression and make appropriate referral for inadequate weight gain, underutilization of PNC, substance misuse, and premature birth.
• Provide the pregnant client with breastfeeding education.

**Intrapartal Care**

• Provide a calm, relaxing, and supportive birth environment.
• Offer the client in labor a clear liquid diet and water if allowed.

**Multicultural**
**Prenatal**

▲ Provide for an appropriate translator if needed.
• Assess the client's beliefs and concerns to inform culturally appropriate PNC.

**Intrapartal**

• Assess client's beliefs and concerns about labor.

**Postpartal**

• Assess client's beliefs and concerns about the postpartum period to provide culturally appropriate health and nutrition information and guidance on contemporary postpartum practices.

**Home Care**
**Prenatal**

▲ As needed refer pregnant clients to drug treatment programs that include coordinated interventions in several areas, such as drug misuse, infectious diseases, mental health, personal and social welfare, and gynecological/obstetric care.

**Postpartal**

• Provide information about parenting websites approved by the health care provider to support new parents with postpartum advice, newborn care, and breastfeeding.

• = Independent          ▲ = Collaborative

C

### Client/Family Teaching and Discharge Planning
**Prenatal**
- Provide dietary and lifestyle counseling as part of PNC to pregnant women.

**Postpartal**
- Encourage physical activity in postpartum women, after being cleared by the health care provider.
▲ Provide breastfeeding mothers contact information for a lactation consultant, phone numbers, and website information for the La Leche League (http://www.lalecheleague.org), and local breastfeeding support groups.
- Teach mothers of young children principles to substitute foods high in saturated fat with foods moderate in PUFAs such as avocados, tuna, walnuts, and olive oil. Include lean protein, fruits and vegetables, and complex carbohydrates.

# Risk for Ineffective Childbearing Process

**Domain 8** Sexuality  **Class 3** Reproduction
## NANDA-I Definition

Susceptible to an inability to prepare for and/or maintain a healthy pregnancy, childbirth process and care of the newborn for ensuring well-being.

## Risk Factors

Inadequate knowledge of childbearing process; inadequate mental preparation for parenting; inadequate parental role model; inadequate prenatal care; inadequate social support; inconsistent prenatal health visits; low maternal confidence; maternal malnutrition; maternal powerlessness; maternal psychological distress; substance misuse; unaddressed domestic violence; unrealistic birth plan; unsafe environment

## At-Risk Population

Individuals experiencing unplanned pregnancy; individuals experiencing unwanted pregnancy

## Client Outcomes, Nursing Interventions, and Client/Family Teaching

Refer to care plan for Ineffective **Childbearing** Process.

# Impaired Comfort

**Domain 12** Comfort  **Class 1** Physical comfort

• = Independent  ▲ = Collaborative

## NANDA-I Definition

Perceived lack of ease, relief, and transcendence in physical, psychospiritual, environmental, cultural, and/or social dimensions.

## Defining Characteristics

Anxiety; crying; difficulty relaxing; expresses discomfort; expresses discontentment with situation; expresses fear; expresses feeling cold; expresses feeling warm; expresses itching; expresses psychological distress; irritable mood; moaning; psychomotor agitation; reports altered sleep-wake cycle; reports hunger; sighing; uneasy in situation

## Related Factors

Inadequate control over environment; inadequate health resources; inadequate situational control; insufficient privacy; unpleasant environmental stimuli

## Associated Conditions

Illness-related symptoms; treatment regimen

## Client Outcomes

### Client Will (Specify Time Frame)

- Provide evidence for improved comfort compared to baseline
- Identify strategies, with or without significant others, to improve and/or maintain acceptable comfort level
- Perform appropriate interventions, with or without significant others, as needed to improve and/or maintain acceptable comfort level
- Evaluate the effectiveness of strategies to maintain/and or reach an acceptable comfort level
- Maintain an acceptable level of comfort when possible

## Nursing Interventions

- Assess client's understanding of ranking his or her comfort level.
- Ask about client's current level of comfort. This is the first step in helping clients achieve improved comfort.
- Comfort is a holistic state under which pain management is included.
- Manipulate the environment as necessary to improve comfort.
- Encourage early mobilization and provide routine position changes. Range of motion and weight-bearing decrease physical discomforts and disability associated with bed rest.
- Provide simple massage. Massage has many therapeutic effects, including improved relaxation, circulation, and well-being.
- Provide a healing touch, which is well suited for clients who cannot tolerate more stimulating interventions.
- Encourage clients to use relaxation techniques to reduce pain, anxiety, depression, and fatigue.

• = Independent          ▲ = Collaborative

**C**

## Geriatric

- Use hand massage for older adults. Most older adults respond well to touch and the health care provider's presence. Lines of communication open naturally during hand massage.
- Discomfort from cold can be treated with warmed blankets. There are physiological dangers associated with hypothermia.
- Use complementary therapies such as doll therapy in clients with dementia to increase comfort and reduce stress.
- Address any unmet physical, psychological, emotional, spiritual, and environmental needs when attempting to mediate the behavior of an older client with dementia.

## Multicultural

- Identify and clarify cultural language used to describe pain and other discomforts. Expressions of pain and discomfort vary across cultures.
- Encourage and allow clients to practice their own cultural beliefs and recognize the impact that diverse cultures have on a client's belief about health care, comforting measures, and decision-making.
- Assess for cultural and religious beliefs when providing care.

## Client/Family Teaching and Discharge Planning

- Teach techniques to use when the client is uncomfortable, including relaxation techniques, guided imagery, hand massage, and music therapy.
- At end of life, the dying client is comforted by having a companion.
- Teach the client to follow up with the health care provider if problems persist.
- Use nonpharmacological strategies to enhance comfort.
- Encourage clients to use the Internet as a means of providing education to complement medical care for those who may be homebound or unable to attend face-to-face education.
- Encourage clients to use guided imagery techniques. Guided imagery helps distract clients from stressful situations and facilitates relaxation.
- Provide psychospiritual support and a comforting environment to enhance comfort during emotional crises.
- When nurses attend to the comfort of perioperative clients, the clients' sense of hope for a full recovery increases.
- Providing music and verbal relaxation therapy enhances holistic comfort by reducing anxiety.
- Caregivers should not hesitate to use humor when caring for their clients.

• = Independent     ▲ = Collaborative

# Readiness for Enhanced Comfort

**Domain 12** Comfort    **Class 2** Environmental comfort

**NANDA-I Definition**

A pattern of ease, relief, and transcendence in physical, psychospiritual, environmental, and/or social dimensions, which can be strengthened.

**Defining Characteristics**

Expresses desire to enhance comfort; expresses desire to enhance feelings of contentment; expresses desire to enhance relaxation; expresses desire to enhance resolution of complaints

**Client Outcomes**

**Client Will (Specify Time Frame)**

- Assess current level of comfort as acceptable
- Express the need to achieve an enhanced level of comfort
- Identify strategies to enhance comfort
- Perform appropriate interventions as needed for increased comfort
- Evaluate the effectiveness of interventions at regular intervals
- Maintain an enhanced level of comfort when possible

**Nursing Interventions**

- Assess clients' comfort needs and current level of comfort in various contexts, as outlined in Kolcaba's comfort theory and practice: physical, psychospiritual, sociocultural, and environmental.
- Educate clients about the various contexts of comfort and help them understand that enhanced comfort is a desirable, positive, and achievable goal.
- Enhance feelings of trust between the client and the health care provider to maintain an effective and therapeutic relationship.
- Maintain an open and effective communication with clients and keep them informed about their health, their plan of care, and their environment.
- Implement comfort rounds that regularly assess for clients' comfort needs.
- Collaborate with other health care professionals, such as health care providers, pharmacists, social workers, chaplains, occupational and physical therapists, and dietitians, among others, in planning interventions that address comfort needs in various contexts: physical, psychospiritual, sociocultural, and environmental.
- Educate clients about and encourage the use of various integrative therapies and modalities to provide options that enhance comfort, beyond the traditional plan of care:
  ○ Massage.

• = Independent          ▲ = Collaborative

- ○ Guided imagery.
- ○ Mindfulness and mindfulness-based interventions.
- ○ Energy therapy or biofield therapy such as healing touch, therapeutic touch, and Reiki.
- ○ Acupuncture and auricular acupuncture.
- ○ Aromatherapy.
- ○ Music.
- ○ Other mind–body therapies such as meditation or yoga.
- Foster and instill hope in clients whenever possible. See the care plan for **Hopelessness.**
- Provide opportunities for and enhance spiritual care activities.
- ▲ Enhance social support and family involvement.
- ▲ Promote participation in creative arts and activity programs.
- ▲ Encourage clients to use health information technology (HIT) as needed.
- Evaluate the effectiveness of all comfort interventions at regular intervals and adjust therapies as necessary.

**Geriatric**
- Refer to previously mentioned interventions for geriatric interventions.

**Pediatric**
- Assess and evaluate the child's level of comfort at frequent intervals. With assessment of pain in children, it is best to use input from the parents or a primary caregiver.
- Skin-to-skin contact (SSC) in the comfort of newborns, especially those at risk.
- Encourage parental presence whenever possible.
- Promote use of alternative comforting strategies such as positioning, presence, massage, spiritual care, music therapy, art therapy, and storytelling to enhance comfort when needed.
- Support the child's spirituality.

**Multicultural**
- Identify cultural beliefs, values, lifestyles, practices, and problem-solving strategies when assessing a client's comfort.
- Enhance cultural knowledge by actively seeking out information regarding different cultural and ethnic groups.
- ▲ Recognize the impact of culture on communication styles and techniques.

**Home Care**
- The nursing interventions described for Readiness for Enhanced **Comfort** may be used with clients in the home care setting. When

• = Independent          ▲ = Collaborative

needed, adaptations can be made to meet the needs of specific clients, families, and communities.

▲ Make appropriate referrals to other organizations or health care providers as needed to enhance comfort.

▲ Promote a multiprofessional (e.g., home care nurses, physicians, pharmacy) approach to home care.

• Evaluate regularly if enhanced comfort is attainable in the home care setting.

**Client/Family Teaching and Discharge Planning**

• Teach client how to regularly assess levels of comfort.

• Instruct client that a variety of interventions may be needed at any given time to enhance comfort.

# Readiness for Enhanced Communication

**Domain 5** Perception/cognition    **Class 5** Communication

## NANDA-I Definition

A pattern of exchanging information and ideas with others, which can be strengthened.

## Defining Characteristics

Expresses desire to enhance communication

## Client Outcomes

Client Will (Specify Time Frame)

• Express willingness to enhance communication
• Demonstrate ability to speak or write a language
• Form words, phrases, and language
• Express thoughts and feelings
• Use and interpret nonverbal cues appropriately
• Express satisfaction with ability to share information and ideas with others

## Nursing Interventions

• Assess the client's health literacy level so information can be tailored accordingly.

▲ Provide resources for communication for those who are deaf or hard of hearing, ensuring applications are HIPAA compliant. For a comprehensive list of available resources, see http://connect-hear.com/.

▲ Refer clients with autism spectrum disorder (ASD) to augmentative and alternative communication (AAC) specialists for employment, as appropriate.

• = Independent          ▲ = Collaborative

**C**

▲ Refer couples in maladjusted relationships for psychosocial intervention and social support to strengthen communication; consider nurse specialists.
▲ Encourage communication partner training.
• Use social media as a means to facilitate communication.
• Teach clients mindfulness meditation.
• Use photographs as a communication aid.
• Encourage clients with aphasia to join communication groups.
▲ Use telephonic (with or without video) health care to promote communication, especially in areas with lower access or when infection control precautions are in place.
▲ Refer transgender clients for voice therapy if the client desires voice modification.
• See care plan for Impaired Verbal **Communication.**

**Pediatric**
• Use social media as appropriate.
• Implement a collaborative approach to communication.
• See care plan for Impaired Verbal **Communication.**

**Geriatric**
• Facilitate communication through reminiscence.
▲ Encourage group singing activities and music therapy interventions in clients with dementia.
• Encourage drawing by caregivers of clients with dementia.
• See care plan for Impaired Verbal **Communication.**

**Multicultural**
• See care plan for Impaired Verbal **Communication.**

**Home Care and Client/Family Teaching and Discharge Planning**
• The interventions described previously may be used in home care, discharge planning, and client and family teaching.
• See care plan for Impaired Verbal **Communication.**

## Impaired Verbal Communication

**Domain 5** Perception/cognition    **Class 5** Communication
**NANDA-I Definition**
Decreased, delayed, or absent ability to receive, process, transmit, and/or use a system of symbols.
**Defining Characteristics**
Absence of eye contact; agraphia; alternative communication; anarthria; aphasia; augmentative communication; decline of speech productivity; decline of speech rate; decreased willingness to participate in social

• = Independent          ▲ = Collaborative

interaction; difficulty comprehending communication; difficulty establishing social interaction; difficulty maintaining communication; difficulty using body expressions; difficulty using facial expressions; difficulty with selective attention; displays negative emotions; dysarthria; dysgraphia; dyslalia; dysphonia; fatigued by conversation; impaired ability to speak; impaired ability to use body expressions; impaired ability to use facial expressions; inability to speak language of caregiver; inappropriate verbalization; obstinate refusal to speak; slurred speech

## Related Factors

Altered self-concept; dyspnea; emotional lability; environmental constraints; inadequate stimulation; low self-esteem; perceived vulnerability; psychological barriers; values incongruent with cultural norms

## At-Risk Population

Individuals facing physical barriers; individuals in the early postoperative period; individuals unable to verbalize; individuals with communication barriers; individuals without a significant other

## Associated Conditions

Altered perception, developmental disabilities; flaccid facial paralysis; hemifacial spasm; motor neuron disease; neoplasms; neurocognitive disorders; oropharyngeal defect; peripheral nervous system diseases; psychotic disorders; respiratory muscle weakness; sialorrhea; speech disorders; tongue diseases; tracheostomy; treatment regimen; velopharyngeal insufficiency; vocal cord dysfunction

## Client Outcomes

### Client Will (Specify Time Frame)

- Use effective communication techniques
- Use alternative methods of communication effectively
- Demonstrate congruency of verbal and nonverbal behavior
- Demonstrate understanding even if not able to speak
- Express desire for social interactions

## Nursing Interventions

- Use a comprehensive nursing assessment to determine the language spoken, cultural considerations, satisfaction with communication, literacy level, cognitive level, and use of glasses and/or hearing aids; avoid making assumptions about clients' communication preferences.
- Determine client's own perception of communication difficulties and potential solutions, in accordance with the Healthy People 2030 goal to decrease the number of clients who report poor client–provider communication.
- Involve a familiar person when attempting to communicate with a client who has difficulty with communication, if accepted by the client.

• = Independent ▲ = Collaborative

- Listen carefully and validate verbal and nonverbal expressions particularly when dealing with pain and use appropriate scales for pain when appropriate.
- Use communication programs to improve communication in clients who are nonvocal and mechanically ventilated.
- Be mindful of word choice when communicating with clients.
- Avoid ignoring the client with verbal impairment and place call light within reach of client who cannot verbally call for help, in order to promote safety and concern.
- Validate clients' feelings, focus on their strengths, and assist them in gaining confidence in identifying needs.
- Explain all health care procedures, be persistent in deciphering what the client is saying, and do not pretend to understand when the message is unclear.
- ▲ Use an individualized and creative multiprofessional approach to augmentative and alternative communication (AAC) assistance and other communication interventions.
- Use consistent nursing staff for those with communication impairments.
- ▲ Consult communication specialists from various disciplines as appropriate. SLPs, audiologists, and translators provide comprehensive communication assistance for those with impaired communication.
- ▲ When the client is having difficulty communicating, assess and refer for audiology consultation for hearing loss (American Academy of Audiology, 2021). Suspect hearing loss when:
  - ○ Client frequently complains that people mumble and that others' speech is not clear.
  - ○ Client often asks people to repeat what they said and hears only parts of conversations.
  - ○ Client's friends or relatives state that the client does not seem to hear very well or plays the television or radio too loudly.
  - ○ Client does not laugh at jokes because of missing too much of the story.
  - ○ Client needs to ask others about the details of a meeting that the client attended.
  - ○ Client cannot hear the doorbell or the telephone.
  - ○ Client finds it easier to understand others when facing them, especially in a noisy environment.
- When communicating with a client with a hearing loss:
  - ○ Obtain client's attention before speaking and face toward his or her unaffected side or better ear while allowing client to see the speaker's face at a reasonably close distance, provide sufficient light,

do not stand in front of a window, use gestures as appropriate to aid in communication, do not raise voice or over enunciate, and minimize extraneous noise.

○ Encourage the client to wear hearing aids, if appropriate.

○ Remove masks if safe, or use see-through anti-fog masks to allow for visibility of the mouth and less muffling of sound which enhances communication.

## Pediatric

* Observe behavioral communication cues in infants.
* Identify and define at least two forms of augmentative and alternative communication modalities that may be used by children with significant disabilities.
* Teach children with severe disabilities functional communication skills.
▲ Refer children with primary speech and language delay/disorder for speech and language therapy interventions.

## Geriatric

* Be aware of nonverbal communication.
* Perform hearing screenings and refer for hearing evaluations in accordance with Healthy People 2030 goal to encourage increasing both the proportion of older adults having hearing examination and the number of referrals for hearing evaluation and treatment.
* Avoid use of "elderspeak," which is a speech style similar to baby talk.
* Initiate communication with the client with dementia and give client time to respond, use eye contact, speak in shorter sentences, and use music.
* Use touch, a therapeutic communication strategy, as appropriate.

## Multicultural

▲ Attend to the meaning of a culture's nonverbal communication modes, such as eye contact, facial expression, touch, and body language.
▲ Use instruments to determine culturally appropriate therapeutic communication.
▲ Assess for the influence of cultural beliefs, norms, and values on the client's communication process.
▲ Assess personal space needs, acceptable communication styles, acceptable body language, interpretation of eye contact, perception of touch, and use of paraverbal modes when communicating with the client.
▲ Assess how language barriers contribute to health disparities among ethnic and racial minorities.

• = Independent            ▲ = Collaborative

**C**

▲ The Office of Minority Health of the U.S. Department of Health and Human Services' national standards on culturally and linguistically appropriate services (CLAS) in health care should be used.

**Home Care**

• The interventions described previously may be adapted for home care use.

**Client/Family Teaching and Discharge Planning**

▲ Refer the client to a speech-language pathologist (SLP) or audiologist. Audiological assessment quantifies and qualifies hearing in terms of the degree of hearing loss, the type of hearing loss, and the configuration of the hearing loss. Once a particular hearing loss has been identified, a treatment and management plan can be put into place by an SLP.

# Acute Confusion

**Domain 5** Perception/cognition     **Class 4** Cognition
## NANDA-I Definition

Reversible disturbances of consciousness, attention, cognition, and perception that develop over a short period of time, and which last less than 3 months.

## Defining Characteristics

Altered psychomotor functioning; difficulty initiating goal-directed behavior; difficulty initiating purposeful behavior; hallucinations; inadequate follow-through with goal-directed behavior; inadequate follow-through with purposeful behavior; misperception; neurobehavioral manifestations; psychomotor agitation

## Related Factors

Altered in sleep-wake cycle; dehydration; impaired physical mobility, inappropriate use of physical restraint; malnutrition, pain, sensory deprivation; substance misuse; urinary retention

## At-Risk Population

Individuals aged ≥60 years; individuals with history of cerebral vascular accident; men

## Associated Conditions

Decreased level of consciousness; impaired metabolism; infections; neurocognitive disorders; pharmaceutical preparations

## Client Outcomes

**Client Will (Specify Time Frame)**

• Demonstrate restoration of cognitive status to baseline
• Be oriented to time, place, and person

• = Independent          ▲ = Collaborative

- Demonstrate appropriate motor behavior
- Maintain functional capacity
- Remain free from injury

**Nursing Interventions**

- Recognize that delirium is characterized by an acute onset, a fluctuating course, inattention, and disordered thinking.
- Use a validated screening tool to assess for delirium.
- Identify the three distinct types of delirium: hyperactive (easy to recognize), hypoactive (commonly missed), and mixed (the most commonly occurring) (Wilson et al, 2020).
  - Hyperactive: delirium characterized by restlessness, agitation, irritability, hypervigilance, hallucinations, and delusions; client may be combative or may attempt to remove tubes, lines.
  - Hypoactive: delirium characterized by decreased motor activity, decreased vocalization, detachment, apathy, lethargy, somnolence, reduced awareness of surroundings, and confusion.
  - Mixed: delirium characterized by the client fluctuating between periods of hyperactivity and agitation and hypoactivity and sedation.
- Perform a comprehensive nursing assessment and mental status examination that includes the following assessment (Solà-Miravete et al, 2018):
  - History from a reliable source that documents an acute and fluctuating change in cognitive function, attention, and behavior from baseline.
  - Cognition as evidenced by level of consciousness; orientation to time, person, and place; thought process (thinking may be disorganized, distorted, fragmented, slow, or accelerated with delirium; conversation may be irrelevant or rambling); and content (perceptual disturbances such as visual, auditory, or tactile delusions or hallucinations).
  - Level of attention (may be decreased or may fluctuate with delirium; may be unable to focus, shift, or sustain attention; may be easily distracted or may be hypervigilant).
  - Behavior characteristics and level of psychomotor behavior (activity may be increased or decreased and may include restlessness, finger tapping, picking at bedclothes, changing position frequently, spastic movements or tremors, or decreased psychomotor activity such as sluggishness, staring into space, remaining in the same position for prolonged periods).

• = Independent          ▲ = Collaborative

**C**

- ○ Level of consciousness (may be easily aroused, lethargic, drowsy, difficult to arouse, unarousable, hyperalert, easily startled, and overly sensitive to stimuli).
- ○ Mood and affect (may be paranoid or fearful with delirium; may have rapid mood swings).
- ○ Insight and judgment (may be impaired).
- ○ Memory (recent and immediate memory is impaired with delirium; unable to register new information).
- ○ Language (may have rapid, rambling, slurred, incoherent speech).
- ○ Altered sleep-wake cycle (insomnia, excessive daytime sleepiness).
- ○ Nutrition status.
- ○ Bowel and bladder elimination habits.
- ○ Mobility status.
- Identify predisposing factors that may precede the development of delirium: dementia, cognitive impairment, functional impairment, visual impairment, alcohol misuse, multiple comorbidities, severe illness, history of transient ischemic attack or stroke, depression, history of delirium, and advanced age (older than 65).
- Surgical procedures increase the risk of delirium postoperatively.
- Identify iatrogenic factors that may precede the development of delirium, especially for individuals with predisposing factors: use of restraints, indwelling bladder catheter, metabolic disturbances, polypharmacy, pain, infection, dehydration, blood loss, constipation, electrolyte imbalances, immobility, general anesthesia, mechanical ventilation, hospital admission for fractures or hip surgery, anticholinergic medications, anxiety, sleep deprivation, lack of use of vision and/or hearing aids, and environmental factors.
- Facilitate appropriate extended visitation for clients at risk of delirium.
- ▲ Assess for and report possible physiological alterations (e.g., sepsis, hypoglycemia, hypoxia, hypotension, infection, changes in temperature, fluid and electrolyte imbalance, use of medications with known cognitive and psychotropic side effects).
  - ○ Treat the underlying risk factors or the causes of delirium in collaboration with the health care team: establish/maintain normal fluid and electrolyte balance, normal body temperature, normal oxygenation (if the client experiences low oxygen saturation, deliver supplemental oxygen), normal blood glucose levels, and normal blood pressure, and address malnutrition and anemia.
  - ○ Monitor for any trends occurring in these manifestations, including laboratory tests.

• = Independent         ▲ = Collaborative

▲ Conduct a medication review and eliminate unnecessary medications; potentially inappropriate medications for older adults at risk for delirium include anticholinergics, benzodiazepines, corticosteroids, $H_2$ receptor antagonists, sedative hypnotics, and tricyclic antidepressants (American Geriatrics Society, 2015).

▲ Recognize that delirium is frequently treated with antipsychotic medications or sedatives; if there is no other way to keep the client safe, administer these medications cautiously, as ordered, while monitoring for medication side effects.

• Locate at risk-clients in private (single-bed) rooms when possible.

• Identify, evaluate, and treat pain quickly and adequately (see care plans for Acute **Pain** or Chronic **Pain**).

• Facilitate sleep hygiene. Establish day/night routines and plan care to allow for appropriate sleep-wake cycles (Lu et al, 2019).

• Promote regulation of bowel and bladder function; use bladder scanning to identify retention, avoid prolonged insertion of urinary catheters, and remove catheters as soon as possible (Bounds et al, 2016).

• Ensure adequate nutritional and fluid intake.

• Promote early mobilization and rehabilitation in a progressive manner.

• Promote continuity of care; avoid frequent changes in staff and surroundings.

• Facilitate appropriate sensory input by having clients use aids (e.g., glasses, hearing aids, dentures) as needed; check for impacted ear wax.

• Modulate sensory exposure; eliminate excessive noise, use appropriate lighting based on the time of day, and establish a calm environment.

• Provide cognitive stimulation through conversation about current events, viewpoints, and relationships and encourage reminiscence or word games.

• Provide reality orientation, including identifying self by name at each encounter with the client, calling the client by their preferred name, and the gentle use of orientation techniques; when reorientation is not effective, use distraction. Gently correct misperceptions.

• Provide clocks and calendars, update dry erase white boards each shift, encourage family to visit regularly and to bring familiar objects from home, such as family photos or an afghan.

• Use gentle, caring communication; provide reassurance of safety; and give simple explanations of procedures.

• Provide supportive nursing care, including meeting basic needs, such as feeding, regular toileting, and ensuring adequate hydration; closely observe behaviors that provide clues as to what might be distressing

• = Independent          ▲ = Collaborative

**C**

the client. Delirious clients are unable to care for themselves because of their confusion.

- If clients know that they are not thinking clearly, acknowledge the concern. Fear is frequently experienced by people with delirium.

**Critical Care**
- Recognize admission risk factors for delirium.
- Assess level of arousal using the Richmond Agitation Sedation Scale (RASS); clients receiving a score of –5 to –4 are comatose and unable to be assessed for delirium.
- Assess for pain every 2 to 3 hours or more frequently as needed with a standardized assessment tool, which includes either a numerical rating scale or one with behavioral indicators, such as the Behavioral Pain Scale (BPS) or Critical Care Pain Observation Tool (CPOT).
- ▲ Incorporate the Awakening and Breathing Coordination, Delirium Monitoring and Management, and Early Mobility (ABCDE) ICU delirium and weakness prevention bundle in conjunction with the multiprofessional team.
  - ○ Assess safety and implementation of a spontaneous awakening trial (SAT) using an established protocol.
  - ○ Assess sedation and agitation level using a valid and reliable tool; titrate sedation to target sedation level.

**Geriatric**
- The interventions described previously are relevant to the geriatric client.
- Recognize that delirium may be superimposed on dementia; the nurse must be aware of the client's baseline cognitive function.
- Understand that delirium is common in frail, older adults and leads to increased lengths of stay and mortality.
- Provide feeding assistance as needed. See care plan for Imbalanced **Nutrition**: Less than Body Requirements.
- Promote adequate hydration; keep a glass of water within easy reach of the client and offer fluids frequently.
- Avoid use of restraints; remove all nonessential equipment such as telemetry, blood pressure cuffs, catheters, and intravenous lines as soon as possible.
- Consider use of music to decrease the development of delirium, especially in surgical clients.
- ▲ Assess risk for falls and implement fall prevention strategies.
- ▲ Determine whether the client is nourished; watch for protein-calorie malnutrition. Consult with health care provider or dietitian as needed.

• = Independent          ▲ = Collaborative

- Explain hospital routines and procedures slowly and in simple terms; repeat information as necessary.
- Educate family members about delirium assessment and strategies to use to prevent and lessen delirium.

**Home Care**

- The interventions described previously are relevant to home care use.
- Assess and monitor for acute changes in cognition and behavior.
- Recognize that delirium is reversible but can contribute to early cognitive decline in many clients (Goldberg et al, 2020).
- Avoid preconceptions about the source of acute confusion; assess each occurrence on the basis of available evidence.
- ▲ Institute case management of frail elderly clients to support continued independent living if possible once delirium has resolved.

**Client/Family Teaching and Discharge Planning**

- Teach the family to recognize signs of early confusion and seek medical help.
- Counsel the client and family regarding the management of delirium and its sequelae. Increased care requirements at discharge may be needed for clients who have experienced delirium.

# Chronic Confusion

**Domain 5** Perception/cognition     **Class 4** Cognition

## NANDA-I Definition

Irreversible, progressive, insidious disturbances of consciousness, attention, cognition, and perception, which last more than 3 months.

## Defining Characteristics

Altered personality; difficulty retrieving information when speaking; difficulty with decision-making; impaired executive functioning skills; impaired psychosocial functioning; inability to perform at least one daily activity; incoherent speech; long-term memory loss; marked change in behavior; short-term memory loss

## Related Factors

Chronic sorrow; sedentary lifestyle; substance misuse

## At-Risk Population

Individuals aged ≥60 years

## Associated Conditions

Human immunodeficiency virus infections; mental disorders; neurocognitive disorders; stroke

• = Independent          ▲ = Collaborative

## Client Outcomes

### Client Will (Specify Time Frame)

- Remain content and free from harm
- Function at maximal cognitive level
- Participate in activities of daily living at the maximum of functional ability
- Have minimal episodes of agitation (agitation occurs in up to 70% of clients with dementia)

## Nursing Interventions

Note: Nursing science has a rich history of conceptualizing behavioral and psychological symptoms of dementia (BPSD), which include delusions, hallucinations, misidentification of depression, sleeplessness, anxiety, physical aggression, wandering, restlessness, agitation, pacing, screaming, culturally inappropriate behavior, sexual disinhibition, crying, cursing, apathy, repetitive questioning, and shadowing (stalking), as expressions of unmet pathophysiological and psychological needs related to environmental and caregiver factors (Kolanowski et al, 2017).

- Assess for BPSD using the BEHAVE-AD or Neuropsychiatry Inventory (NPI-Q), and determine cause(s) of symptoms, which may include changes in the environment, caregiver, or routine; demands to perform beyond capacity; multiple competing stimuli, including discomfort.
- Assess the client for delirium (physiological causes of delirium include acute hypoxia, pain, medication effects, malnutrition, and infections such as urinary tract infection, fatigue, electrolyte disturbances, constipation, and urinary retention).
- If the client is suspected of delirium (presenting as inattention, and impaired arousal or vigilance), initiate three-part delirium screener, which includes questions: "What are the days of the week backward?" and "What type of place is this?" If either question is incorrect or the client appears sleepy proceed to diagnostic delirium testing such as the Confusion Assessment Method (CAM).
- Assess the client for signs of depression and anxiety (including sadness, irritability, agitation, somatic complaints, tension, loss of concentration, insomnia, poor appetite, apathy, flat affect, and withdrawn behavior) with an instrument appropriate for the cognitive level.
- Assess for pain, including pain with movement, using a method appropriate to the client's level of cognition.
- Begin each interaction with the client calmly and empathetically, maintain eye contact, identify yourself, and call the client by their name;

• = Independent          ▲ = Collaborative

**C**

talk slowly, keep communication simple, give clear choices, and one-step instructions; if indicated, use gestures, prompts, cues, or visual aids.

- To promote completion of activity of daily living tasks, focus on what the client can still do (e.g., comb their hair, brush their teeth), as opposed to what they cannot do. Using a hand-under-hand technique, a caregiver can guide the client to complete tasks with less challenging behaviors exhibited, giving the client a sense of independence and completion of a task.
- Promote person-centered care, which includes getting to know the unique and complete person, recognizing/accepting the person's reality, supporting their ongoing opportunities for meaningful engagement, and evaluating care practices regularly.
- Obtain information about the client's life history, interests, routines, needs, and preferences from the family or significant others to plan care and facilitate reminiscence and validation therapy; collaborate with family members to engage in reminiscence using personal photographs and belongings to stimulate memories and improve sense of self.
- Utilize validation therapy techniques to meet clients where they are in their mind; instead of correcting their thoughts, guide them through the reminiscence of that thought.
- Facilitate the use of music therapy via activities staff, or electronic sources (e.g., Amazon Echo/Alexa and Google Home); identify the client's music preferences and interview family members if necessary.
- Use multisensory stimulation (e.g., exercise, nature, arts, group activities, music, aromas) to improve mood, behavior, and quality of life; engage assistance of volunteers and family caregivers in one-on-one activities.
- Promote regular, supervised physical activity and exercise.
- Provide opportunities for contact with nature gardens or nature-based stimuli, such as facilitating time spent outdoors with a safe walking path or indoor gardening.
- Facilitate the use of doll therapy for clients with advanced dementia and challenging dementia related behaviors.
- Provide pet therapy and other animal-assisted activities when possible.
- Use individual or group reminiscence therapy.
- Use an environmental audit tool to evaluate and optimize the living environment in group home and assisted living facilities (e.g., provide unobtrusive safety features, reduce unnecessary stimulation, enhance useful stimulation, provide wayfinding cues, and encourage safe wandering).

• = Independent        ▲ = Collaborative

**C**

- Use appropriate lighting to support regulation of sleep-wake patterns and associated behavioral issues.
- Provide the client and family information regarding advance directives, palliative and hospice care options, and discuss/document goals of care in the early stages of illness when further cognitive decline is anticipated.
- Refer to the care plans for Impaired **Memory, Wandering,** Feeding **Self-Care** Deficit; Dressing **Self-Care** Deficit; Toileting **Self-Care** Deficit; and Bathing **Self-Care** Deficit as needed.

**Geriatric**

Note: All interventions are appropriate for geriatric clients.

**Multicultural**

- Provide culturally and linguistically appropriate care.
- Facilitate cultural congruity, defined as the match of the client's cultural values, preferences (language, food, music, customs), and traditions within the care environment, which may include companion care, adult day care, board and care homes, or nursing homes, including state veterans' homes.
- Assess for the influence of cultural beliefs, norms, and values on the client and the family's understanding of chronic confusion or dementia; assist the family or caregiver in identifying and accessing available social services or other supportive services.

**Home Care**

- The interventions described previously may be adapted for home care use.
- Provide education and support to the family regarding effective communication, home safety, fall prevention, engagement in meaningful activities, ways to manage cognitive and behavioral changes, and comprehensive health care for both client and caregiver(s), including screening for depression and caregiver role strain.
- Provide information about respite care to family caregivers.
- Refer to the care plans for Feeding **Self**-Care Deficit; Dressing **Self-Care** Deficit; Toileting **Self-Care** Deficit; Bathing **Self-Care** Deficit; and **Caregiver** Role Strain, as needed.

**Client/Family Teaching and Discharge Planning**

- In the client's early stages of dementia, provide the caregiver with information on illness processes, needed care, available services, role changes, and importance of advance directives discussion; facilitate family cohesion.
- Provide education and support to the family regarding effective communication, home safety, fall prevention, engagement in

meaningful activities, ways to manage cognitive and behavioral changes, and comprehensive health care, including screening for depression. Be prepared to offer support and information to family members who also live at a distance.

• Refer for home care services before discharge as needed.

## Risk for Acute Confusion

**Domain 5** Perception/cognition     **Class 4** Cognition
### NANDA-I Definition

Susceptible to reversible disturbances of consciousness, attention, cognition, and perception that develop over a short period of time, which may compromise health.

### Risk Factors

Alteration in sleep-wake cycle; dehydration; impaired physical mobility; inappropriate use of physical restraint; malnutrition; pain; sensory deprivation; substance misuse; urinary retention

### At-Risk Population

Individuals aged ≥60 years; individuals with history of cerebral vascular accident; men

### Associated Conditions

Decreased level of consciousness; impaired metabolism; infections; neurocognitive disorders; pharmaceutical preparations

### Client Outcomes, Nursing Interventions, and Client/Family Teaching

Refer to care plan for Acute **Confusion**.

## Constipation

**Domain 3** Elimination and exchange     **Class 2** Gastrointestinal function
### NANDA-I Definition

Infrequent or difficult evacuation of feces.

### Defining Characteristics

Evidence of symptoms in standardized diagnostic criteria; hard stools; lumpy stools; need for manual maneuvers to facilitate defecation; passing fewer than three stools a week; sensation of anorectal obstruction; sensation of incomplete evacuation; straining with defecation

### Related Factors

Altered regular routine; average daily physical activity is less than recommended for age and gender; communication barriers; habitually suppresses urge to defecate; impaired physical mobility; impaired postural balance; inadequate knowledge of modifiable factors; inadequate toileting

• = Independent          ▲ = Collaborative

habits; insufficient fiber intake; insufficient fluid intake; insufficient privacy; stressors; substance misuse

## At-Risk Population

Individuals admitted to hospital; individuals experiencing prolonged hospitalization; individuals in aged care settings; individuals in the early postoperative period; older adults; pregnant women; women

## Associated Conditions

Blockage in the colon; blockage in the rectum; depression; developmental disabilities; digestive system diseases; endocrine diseases; heart diseases; mental disorders; muscular diseases; nervous system diseases; neurocognitive disorders; pelvic floor disorders; pharmaceutical preparations; radiotherapy; urogynecological disorders

## Client Outcomes

Client Will (Specify Time Frame)

- Maintain passage of soft, formed stool (i.e., Bristol Stool Scale Type 4) every 1 to 3 days without straining
- State relief from discomfort of constipation
- Identify measures that prevent or treat constipation

## Nursing Interventions

- Introduce yourself to the client and any companions and inform them of your role.
- Gain consent to perform care before proceeding further with the assessment.
- Wash hands using a recognized technique.
- Assess usual pattern of defecation and establish the extent of the constipation problem.
- Assess the client's bowel habits:
  ○ Time of day of bowel evacuation
  ○ Amount and frequency of stool
  ○ Consistency of stool (using the Bristol Stool Scale)
  ○ Bleeding/passing mucus on defecation
  ○ History of bowel habits and/or laxative use
- Assess the client's lifestyle factors that may influence constipation:
  ○ Fiber content in diet
  ○ Daily fluid intake
  ○ Exercise patterns
  ○ Personal remedies for constipation
  ○ Recently stopped smoking
  ○ Alcohol consumption/recreational drug use

• = Independent        ▲ = Collaborative

**C**

- Review the client's medical history:
  - ○ Obstetrical/gynecological/urological history and surgeries
  - ○ Diseases that affect bowel motility
  - ○ Bleeding/passing mucus on defecation
  - ○ Current medications
- Assess the client for emotional influences that may be contributing to constipation:
  - ○ Anxiety and depression
  - ○ Long-term defecation issues
  - ○ Stress
- Complete a physical examination (palpation for abdominal distention, percussion for dullness, and auscultation for bowel sounds).
- Complete a digital rectal examination (DRE) if competent and suitably trained to do so, to identify hemorrhoids, rectal prolapse, anal fissure, rectocele, the anal tone, and fecal impaction.
- Check for impaction; if present, use a combination of oral laxatives and enemas initially to remove fecal loading and impaction (National Institute for Health and Care Excellence, 2020). Clients with neurogenic bowel dysfunction (e.g., spinal cord injury) commonly require manual evacuation of stool (McClurg & Norton, 2016).
- Encourage the client or family to keep a 7-day diary of bowel habits, including time of day, length of time spent on the toilet, consistency, amount and frequency of stool, and any straining (using the Bristol Stool Scale).
- Encourage the client or family to keep a 7-day diary of lifestyle issues in relation to bowel habits, including fluid consumption, fiber content in diet, usual bowel stimulus, and exercise regimen.
- Use the Bristol Stool Scale to assess stool consistency.
▲ Review the client's current medications.
- Discuss with clients already taking opioids (temporarily or long term) that constipation is a common side effect. If the client is receiving temporary opioids (e.g., for acute postoperative pain), request an order for routine stool softeners from the primary care provider, monitor bowel movements, and request a laxative for the client if constipation develops. If the client is receiving around-the-clock opiates (e.g., for palliative care), laxatives, then softeners, stimulants, or osmotic laxatives should be requested.
▲ If the client is terminally ill and is receiving around-the-clock opioids for palliative care, speak with the prescribing health care provider about ordering low-dose naloxone, which is a drug that blocks opioid

• = Independent          ▲ = Collaborative

effects on the gastrointestinal tract without interfering with analgesia (Sanders et al, 2015).

- If new onset of constipation, determine whether the client has recently stopped smoking.
- ▲ Advise a fiber intake of 18 to 25 g daily and suggest foodstuffs high in fiber (e.g., prune juice, leafy green vegetables, whole meal bread and pasta).
- Add fiber gradually to the diet to decrease bloating and flatus.
- Recommend prunes or prune juice daily. Each 100 g of prunes contains about 6 g of fiber, 15 g of sorbitol, and 184 mg of polyphenol, which all have laxative effects.
- Advise a fluid intake of 1.5 to 2 L of fluid per day (ideally, 6–8 glasses of water), unless contraindicated by comorbidities, such as kidney or heart disease.
- ▲ If the client is uncomfortable or in pain because of constipation or has acute or chronic constipation that does not respond to increased fiber, fluid, activity, and appropriate toileting, refer the client to the primary care provider for an evaluation of bowel function and health status.
- Encourage physical activity within the client's current ability to mobilize. Encourage turning and changing position in bed if immobile. For clients with reduced mobility, encourage knee to chest raises, waist twists, and stretching the arms away from the body. For fully mobile clients, encourage walking and swimming.
- Demonstrate the use of gentle external abdominal massage, following the direction of colon activity.
- Recommend that clients establish a regular elimination routine that includes activity, diet and fluids, and scheduled toilet visits. If required, assist clients to the bathroom at the same time every day; always be mindful of the need for privacy (closing of bathroom doors).
- Educate the client about how to adopt the best posture for defecation. Keep knees slightly higher than hips, keep feet flat on the floor, and lean forward, putting elbows onto knees, thus adopting a squatting position.
- Teach clients about the importance of responding promptly to the urge to defecate.
- Consider the use of laxatives, suppositories, enemas, and bowel irrigation as required if other more natural interventions are not effective.
- Discourage the use of long-term laxatives and enemas and advise clients to gradually reduce their use if taken regularly.

• = Independent          ▲ = Collaborative

**Geriatric**

- Assess older adults for the presence of factors that contribute to constipation, including dietary fiber and fluid intake (<1.5 L/day), physical activity, use of constipating medications, and diseases that are associated with constipation.
- Explain the importance of adequate fiber intake, fluid intake, activity, and established toileting routines to ensure soft, formed stool.
- Determine the client's perception of normal bowel elimination and laxative use; promote adherence to a regular schedule.
- Explain why straining (Valsalva maneuver) should be avoided.
- Respond quickly to the client's call for assistance with toileting.
- Offer food, fluids, activity, and toileting opportunities to older clients who are cognitively impaired.
- Avoid regular use of enemas in older adults.
- Advise the client against attempting to remove impacted feces on his or her own.
▲ Use opioids cautiously.
- Position the client on the toilet or commode and place a small footstool under the feet.

**Home Care**

- The interventions described previously may be adapted for home care use.
- Take complaints seriously and evaluate claims of constipation in a matter-of-fact manner.
- Assess the self-care management activities the client is already using.
- Offer the following treatment recommendations:
  ○ Acknowledge the client's lifelong experience of bowel function; respect beliefs, attitudes, and preferences, and avoid patronizing responses.
  ○ Make available comprehensive, useful written information about constipation and possible solutions.
  ○ Make available empathetic and accessible professional care to provide treatment and advice; a multiprofessional approach (including health care provider, nurse, and pharmacist) should be used.
  ○ Institute a bowel management program.
  ○ Consider affordability when suggesting solutions to constipation; discuss cost-effective strategies.
  ○ Discuss a range of solutions to constipation and allow the client to choose the preferred options.

• = Independent          ▲ = Collaborative

**C**

○ Have orders in place for a suppository and enema as needed. As part of a bowel management program, suppositories or enemas may become necessary.
- Although the use of a bedside commode may be necessitated by the client's condition, allow the client to use the toilet in the bathroom when possible and provide assistance.
- In older clients, routinely advise consumption of fluids, fruits, and vegetables as part of the diet, and ambulation if the client is able.
▲ Refer for consideration of the use of polyethylene glycol 3350 (PEG-3350) for constipation.
- Use a bowel program to establish a pattern that is regular, thereby allowing the client to be part of the family unit.

**Client/Family Teaching and Discharge Planning**
- Instruct the client on normal bowel function and the need for adequate fluid and fiber intake, activity, and a defined toileting pattern in a bowel program.
- Encourage the client to heed defecation warning signs and develop a regular schedule of defecation by using a stimulus such as a warm drink or prune juice.
- Encourage the client to avoid long-term use of laxatives and enemas and to gradually withdraw from their use if they are used regularly.
- If not contraindicated, teach the client how to do bent-leg sit-ups to increase abdominal tone; also encourage the client to contract the abdominal muscles frequently throughout the day. Help the client develop a daily exercise program to increase peristalsis.
- Provide client with comprehensive written information about constipation and its management.
▲ Collaborate with members of the multiprofessional team to provide treatment and advice to clients and caregivers.
▲ Consider referral to other specialist practitioners if constipation persists.
- Document all care and advice given in a factual and comprehensive manner.

## Risk for Constipation

**Domain 3** Elimination and exchange    **Class 2** Gastrointestinal function
**NANDA-I Definition**

Susceptible to infrequent or difficult evacuation of feces, which may compromise health.

• = Independent          ▲ = Collaborative

## Risk Factors

Altered regular routine; average daily physical activity is less than recommended for age and gender; communication barriers; habitually suppresses urge to defecate; impaired physical mobility; impaired postural balance; inadequate knowledge of modifiable factors; inadequate toileting habits; insufficient fiber intake; insufficient fluid intake; insufficient privacy; stressors; substance misuse

## At-Risk Population

Individuals admitted to hospital; individuals experiencing prolonged hospitalization; individuals in aged care settings; individuals in the early postoperative period; older adults; pregnant women; women

## Associated Conditions

Blockage in the colon; blockage in the rectum; depression; developmental disabilities; digestive system diseases; endocrine system diseases; heart diseases; mental disorders; muscular diseases; nervous system diseases; neurocognitive disorders; pelvic floor disorders; pharmaceutical preparations; radiotherapy; urogynecological disorders

## Client Outcomes, Nursing Interventions, and Client/Family Teaching

Refer to care plan for **Constipation.**

# Perceived Constipation

**Domain 3** Elimination and exchange    **Class 2** Gastrointestinal function

## NANDA-I Definition

Self-diagnosis of infrequent or difficult evacuation of feces combined with abuse of methods to ensure a daily bowel movement.

## Defining Characteristics

Enema misuse; expects bowel movement at same time daily; laxative misuse; suppository misuse

## Related Factors

Cultural health beliefs; deficient knowledge about normal evacuation patterns; disturbed thought processes; family health beliefs

## Client Outcomes

Client Will (Specify Time Frame)
- Regularly defecate soft, formed stool without use of aids (i.e., Bristol Stool Scale Type 4) every 1 to 3 days without straining
- Understand the need to decrease or eliminate the use of stimulant laxatives, suppositories, and enemas
- Identify alternatives to stimulant laxatives, enemas, and suppositories for ensuring defecation
- Understand that defecation does not have to occur every day

• = Independent            ▲ = Collaborative

## Nursing Interventions

- Introduce yourself to the client and any companions and inform them of your role.

**C**

- Gain consent to perform care before proceeding further with the assessment.
- Wash hands using a recognized technique.
- Assess usual pattern of defecation and establish the extent of the perceived constipation problem. Assess the client's bowel habits:
  - Time of day
  - Amount and frequency of stool
  - Consistency of stool (using the Bristol Stool Scale)
  - Bleeding/passing mucus on defecation
  - Client history of bowel habits and/or laxative use
  - Family history of bowel habits and/or laxative use
- ▲ Assess the client's lifestyle factors that may affect bowel function:
  - Fiber content in diet
  - Daily fluid intake
  - Exercise patterns
  - Personal remedies for constipation
  - Cultural remedies for constipation
  - Recently stopped smoking
  - Alcohol consumption/recreational drug use
- ▲ Review the client's medical history:
  - Obstetrical/gynecological/urological history and surgeries
  - Diseases that affect bowel motility
  - Bleeding/passing mucus on defecation
  - Current medications
- ▲ Emotional influences:
  - Anxiety and depression/psychological disorders
  - History of eating disorders
  - History of physical/or sexual abuse
  - Long-term defecation issues
  - Stress
- Encourage the client or family to keep a 7-day diary of bowel habits, including time of day, length of time spent on the toilet, consistency, amount and frequency of stool, and any straining (using the Bristol Stool Scale).
- Encourage the client or family to keep a 7-day diary of lifestyle issues in relation to bowel habits, including fluid consumption, fiber content in diet, usual bowel stimulus, and exercise regimen.

• = Independent          ▲ = Collaborative

- Educate the client that it is not necessary to have a daily bowel movement.
- Encourage the client to record use of laxatives, suppositories, or enemas, and suggest replacing them with an increase in fluid and fiber intake.
- Advise a fiber intake of 18 to 30 g daily in adults and suggest foodstuffs high in fiber (e.g., prune juice, leafy green vegetables, whole meal bread and pasta).
- Advise a fluid intake of 1.5 to 2 L of fluid per day (ideally, 6–8 glasses of water), unless contraindicated by comorbidities, such as kidney or heart disease.
- Obtain a referral to a dietitian for analysis of the client's diet and fluid intake.
- Encourage physical activity within the client's current ability to mobilize. Encourage turning and changing position in bed if immobile. For clients with reduced mobility, encourage knee to chest raises, waist twists, and stretching the arms away from the body. For fully mobile clients, encourage walking and swimming.
- Demonstrate the use of gentle external abdominal massage, using aroma therapy oils, following the direction of colon activity.
- Recommend that clients establish a regular elimination routine that includes activity, diet and fluids, and scheduled toilet visits. If required, assist clients to the bathroom at the same time every day; always be mindful of the need for privacy (closing of bathroom doors).
- Observe for the presence of an eating disorder by using laxatives to control or decrease weight; refer for counseling if needed.
- Observe family cultural patterns related to eating and bowel habits. Cultural patterns may control bowel habits.

**Client/Family Teaching and Discharge Planning**
- Educate the client about how to adopt the best posture for defecation. Keep knees slightly higher than hips, keep feet flat on the floor, and lean forward putting elbows onto knees, thus adopting a squatting position.
- Teach clients about the importance of responding promptly to the urge to defecate.
- Discourage the use of long-term laxatives and enemas and explain the potential harmful effects of the continual use of defecation aids such as laxatives and enemas.
- Discourage the long-term use of laxatives and enemas and advise clients to gradually reduce their use if taken regularly.

• = Independent ▲ = Collaborative

**C**

- Provide client with comprehensive written information about constipation and its management.
- Collaborate with members of the multiprofessional team to provide treatment and advice to clients and caregivers.
- Document all care and advice given in a factual and comprehensive manner.

## Chronic Functional Constipation

**Domain 3** Elimination and exchange    **Class 2** Gastrointestinal function

### NANDA-I Definition

Infrequent or difficult evacuation of feces, which has been present for at least 3 of the prior 12 months.

### Defining Characteristics

#### General

Distended abdomen; fecal impaction; leakage of stool with digital stimulation; pain with defecation; palpable abdominal mass; positive fecal occult blood test; prolonged straining; Type 1 or 2 on Bristol Stool Chart

*Adult: Presence of ≥2 of the following symptoms on Rome III classification system:* Lumpy or hard stools in ≥25% defecations; manual maneuvers to facilitate ≥25% of defecations (digital manipulation, pelvic floor support); sensation of anorectal obstruction/blockage for ≥25% of defecations; sensation of incomplete evacuation for ≥25% of defecations; ≤3 evacuations per week

*Child >4 years; Presence of ≥2 criteria on the Rome III Pediatric classification system for ≥2 months:* Large diameter stools that may obstruct the toilet; painful or hard bowel movements; presence of large fecal mass in the rectum; stool retentive posturing; ≤2 defecations per week; ≥1 episode of fecal incontinence per week

*Child ≤4 years; Presence of ≥2 criteria on the Rome III Pediatric classification system for ≥1 month:* Large diameter stools that may obstruct the toilet; painful or hard bowel movements; presence of large fecal mass in the rectum; stool retentive posturing; ≤2 defecations per week; ≥1 episode of fecal incontinence per week

### Related Factors

Decreased food intake; dehydration; diet disproportionally high in fat; diet disproportionally high in protein; frail elderly syndrome; habitually suppresses urge to defecate; impaired physical mobility; inadequate dietary intake; inadequate knowledge of modifiable factors; insufficient fiber intake; insufficient fluid intake; low caloric intake; sedentary lifestyle

• = Independent        ▲ = Collaborative

## At-Risk Population
Older adults; pregnant women

## Associated Conditions

Amyloidosis; anal fissure; anal stricture; autonomic neuropathy; chronic intestinal pseudo-obstruction; chronic renal insufficiency; colorectal cancer; depression; dermatomyositis; diabetes mellitus; extra intestinal mass; hemorrhoids; Hirschsprung's disease; hypercalcemia; hypothyroidism; inflammatory bowel disease; ischemic stenosis; multiple sclerosis; myotonic dystrophy; neurocognitive disorders; panhypopituitarism; paraplegia; Parkinson's disease; pelvic floor disorders; perineal damage; pharmaceutical preparations; polypharmacy; porphyria; postinflammatory stenosis; proctitis; scleroderma; slow colon transit time; spinal cord injuries; stroke; surgical stenosis

## Client Outcomes

### Client Will (Specify Time Frame)

- Maintain passage of soft, formed stool (i.e., Bristol Stool Scale Type 4) every 1 to 3 days without straining.
- Identify measures that prevent or treat constipation

## Nursing Interventions

### All Client Ages

- Introduce yourself to the client and any companions and inform them of your role.
- Gain consent to perform care before proceeding further with the assessment.
- Wash hands using a recognized technique.
- Assess usual pattern of defecation and establish the extent of the constipation problem.
- Assess bowel habits:
  - Time of day
  - Amount and frequency of stool
  - Consistency of stool (using the Bristol Stool Scale)
  - Bleeding/passing mucus on defecation
  - History of bowel habits and/or laxative use
  - Assess children younger than 4 years using the Rome III pediatric classification (for at least 1 month)
  - Assess children older than age 4 years using the Rome III pediatric classification (for at least 2 months)
- ▲ Assess the client's lifestyle factors that may affect bowel function:
  - Fiber content in diet
  - Daily fluid intake
  - Exercise patterns

• = Independent          ▲ = Collaborative

**C**

- ○ Personal remedies for constipation
- ○ Recently stopped smoking
- ○ Alcohol consumption/recreational drug use
- ○ Personal habits related to defecation
▲ Review the client's medical history:
  - ○ Obstetrical/gynecological/urological history and surgeries
  - ○ Existing anatomical anomalies (e.g., anal fissures, anal strictures and hemorrhoids)
  - ○ Diseases that affect bowel motility (e.g., colorectal cancer, chronic intestinal pseudo-obstruction, and Hirschsprung's disease)
  - ○ Bleeding/passing mucus on defecation
  - ○ Current medications
▲ Review emotional influences with the client:
  - ○ Anxiety and depression
  - ○ Long-term defecation issues
  - ○ Stress
- • Complete a physical examination (palpation for abdominal distention, percussion for dullness, and auscultation for bowel sounds).
- • Encourage the client or family to keep a 7-day diary of bowel habits, including time of day, length of time spent on the toilet, consistency, amount and frequency of stool, and any straining (using the Bristol Stool Scale).
- • Encourage the client or family to keep a 7-day diary of lifestyle issues in relation to bowel habits, including fluid consumption, fiber content in diet, usual bowel stimulus, and exercise regimen.
- • Actively encourage children and families to attend bowel management programs to aid the establishment of regular bowel routines.
- • Discuss with clients already taking opioids (temporarily or long term) that constipation is a common side effect. If the client is receiving temporary opioids (e.g., for acute postoperative pain), request an order for routine stool softeners from the primary care provider, monitor bowel movements, and request a laxative for the client if constipation develops. If the client is receiving around-the-clock opiates (e.g., for palliative care), laxatives, then softeners, stimulants, or osmotics, should be requested.
- • Advise a fiber intake of 18 to 30 g of fiber daily in adults and suggest foodstuffs to facilitate this diet (e.g., prune juice, leafy green vegetables, whole meal bread and pasta).
- • Advise clients to drink at least 6–8 glasses of water a day, unless contraindicated by comorbidities, such as kidney or heart disease.

• = Independent          ▲ = Collaborative

- Encourage physical activity within the client's current ability to mobilize. Encourage turning and changing position in bed if immobile. For clients with reduced mobility, encourage knee to chest raises, waist twists, and stretching the arms away from the body. For fully mobile clients, encourage walking and swimming.
- Demonstrate the use of gentle external abdominal massage, following the direction of colon activity.
- Recommend that clients establish a regular elimination routine that includes activity, diet and fluids, and scheduled toilet visits. If required, assist clients to the bathroom at the same time every day; always be mindful of the need for privacy (closing of bathroom doors).
- Educate the client about how to adopt the best posture for defecation. Keep knees slightly higher than hips, keep feet flat on the floor, and lean forward putting elbows onto knees, thus adopting a squatting position.
- Consider the teaching of biofeedback therapy to encourage a "new normal" bowel routine for clients to adopt.
- Teach clients about the importance of responding promptly to the urge to defecate.
- Consider the use of laxatives, suppositories, enemas, and bowel irrigation as required if other more natural interventions are not effective.
- Discourage the long-term use of laxatives and enemas and advise clients to gradually reduce their use if taken regularly.
- Provide client with comprehensive written information about constipation and its management.
- Provide written instructions for children about taking their medication and about how the bowel works.
- Collaborate with members of the multiprofessional team to provide treatment and advice to clients and caregivers.
- Consider referral to other specialist practitioners if constipation persists.
- Document all care and advice given in a factual and comprehensive manner.

# Risk for Chronic Functional Constipation

**Domain 3** Elimination and exchange    **Class 2** Gastrointestinal function

• = Independent                ▲ = Collaborative

## NANDA-I Definition

Susceptible to infrequent or difficult evacuation of feces, which has been present nearly 3 of the prior 12 months, which may compromise health.

**C**

### Risk Factors

Decreased food intake; dehydration; diet disproportionally high in fat; diet disproportionally high in protein; frail elderly syndrome; habitually suppresses urge to defecate; impaired physical mobility; inadequate dietary intake; inadequate knowledge of modifiable factors; insufficient fiber intake; insufficient fluid intake; low caloric intake; sedentary lifestyle

### At-Risk Population

Older adults; pregnant women

### Associated Conditions

Amyloidosis; anal fissure; anal stricture; autonomic neuropathy; chronic intestinal pseudo-obstruction; chronic renal insufficiency; colorectal cancer; depression; dermatomyositis; diabetes mellitus; extra intestinal mass; hemorrhoids; Hirschsprung's disease; hypercalcemia; hypothyroidism; inflammatory bowel disease; ischemic stenosis; multiple sclerosis; myotonic dystrophy; neurocognitive disorders; panhypopituitarism; paraplegia; Parkinson's disease; pelvic floor disorders; perineal damage; pharmaceutical preparations; polypharmacy; porphyria; postinflammatory stenosis; proctitis; scleroderma; slow colon transit time; spinal cord injuries; stroke; surgical stenosis

### Client Outcomes, Nursing Interventions, and Client/Family Teaching and Discharge Planning

Refer to care plan for Chronic Functional **Constipation.**

## Contamination

**Domain 11** Safety/protection    **Class 4** Environmental hazards

## NANDA-I Definition

Exposure to environmental contaminants in doses sufficient to cause adverse health effects.

### Defining Characteristics

#### Pesticides

Dermatological effects of pesticide exposure; gastrointestinal effects of pesticide exposure; neurological effects of pesticide exposure; pulmonary effects of pesticide exposure; renal effects of pesticide exposure

#### Chemicals

Dermatological effects of chemical exposure; gastrointestinal effects of chemical exposure; immunological effects of chemical exposure;

neurological effects of chemical exposure; pulmonary effects of chemical exposure; renal effects of chemical exposure

**Biologics**

Dermatological effects of biologic exposure; gastrointestinal effects of biologic exposure; neurological effects of biologic exposure; pulmonary effects of biologic exposure; renal effects of biologic exposure

**Pollution**

Neurological effects of pollution exposure; pulmonary effects of pollution exposure

**Waste**

Dermatological effects of waste exposure; gastrointestinal effects of waste exposure; hepatic effects of waste exposure; pulmonary effects of waste exposure

**Radiation**

Genetic effects of radiotherapy exposure; immunological effects of radiotherapy exposure; neurological effects of radiotherapy exposure; oncological effects of radiotherapy exposure

## Related Factors

**External Factors**

Carpeted flooring; chemical contamination of food; chemical contamination of water; flaking, peeling surface in presence of young children; inadequate breakdown of contaminant; inadequate household hygiene practices; inadequate municipal services; inadequate personal hygiene practices; inadequate protective clothing; inappropriate use of protective clothing; individuals who ingested contaminated material; playing where environmental contaminants are used; unprotected exposure to chemical; unprotected exposure to heavy metal; unprotected exposure to radioactive material; use of environmental contaminant in the home; use of noxious material in inadequately ventilated area; use of noxious material without effective protection

**Internal Factors**

Concomitant exposure; malnutrition; smoking

## At-Risk Population

Children aged <5 years; economically disadvantaged individuals; individuals exposed perinatally; individuals exposed to areas with high concomitant level; individuals exposed to atmospheric pollutants; individuals exposed to bioterrorism; individuals exposed to disaster; individuals with history of exposure to contaminant; older adults; pregnant women; women

## Associated Conditions

Pre-existing disease; radiotherapy

• = Independent          ▲ = Collaborative

## Client Outcomes

### Client Will (Specify Time Frame)

C

- Have minimal health effects associated with contamination
- Cooperate with appropriate decontamination protocol
- Participate in appropriate isolation precautions
- Use health surveillance data system to monitor for contamination incidents
- Use disaster plan to evacuate and triage affected members
- Have minimal health effects associated with contamination
- Use measures to reduce household environmental risks

## Nursing Interventions

▲ Help individuals cope with contamination incident by doing the following:
  ○ Use organizations and groups that have survived terrorist attacks as a useful resource for victims
  ○ Provide accurate information on risks involved, preventive measures, and use of antibiotics and vaccines
  ○ Assist to deal with feelings of fear, vulnerability, and grief
  ○ Encourage individuals to talk to others about their fears
  ○ Assist victims to think positively and to move toward the future
▲ In a crisis situation, interventions aimed at supporting an individual's coping help the person deal with feelings of fear, helplessness, and loss of control that are normal reactions in a crisis situation.
- Triage, stabilize, transport, and treat affected community members.
- Prioritize mental health care for highly vulnerable risk groups or those with special needs (women, older persons, children and adolescents, displaced persons, especially those living in shelters; persons with preexisting mental health disorders, including those living in institutions, those significantly exposed to contaminants).
- Collaborate with members of the health care delivery system and outside agencies (local health department, emergency medical services [EMS], state and federal agencies).
- Use approved procedures for decontamination of persons, clothing, and equipment.
- Use appropriate isolation precautions: universal, airborne, droplet, and contact isolation to prevent cross-contamination by contaminating agents (U.S. Army Medical Research Institute of Infectious Diseases, 2014).
- Monitor individuals for therapeutic effects, side effects, and compliance with postexposure drug therapy that may extend over

• = Independent          ▲ = Collaborative

a long period of time and require monitoring for compliance and for therapeutic and side effects (Adalja, Toner, & Inglesby, 2015; Goodwin Veenema, 2019).

- Perform effective handwashing using 60% to 90% alcohol-based hand rub before and after touching a client, after touching client's immediate environment, aseptic tasks, contact with body fluids or contaminated surfaces, and immediately after glove removal (CDC, 2020b).
- Prevent cross-contamination by systematically disinfecting stethoscopes (diaphragm and tubing) after each use.
- Minimize occupational exposure to antineoplastic agents by following National Institute for Occupational Safety and Health (NIOSH) guidelines regarding personal protective equipment and correct handling of hazardous drugs.
- Adhere to standards and transmission-based precautions when caring for clients with SARS-CoV-2 and use correct donning and doffing procedure with PPE (CDC, 2020c).
- Follow institutional policy and procedure for optimizing supply of PPE during surges or instances of low or inadequate PPE (CDC, 2020c).

**Geriatric**
- Help the client identify age-related factors that may affect response to contamination incidents.
- Advise older adults to follow public notices related to drinking water.
- Encourage older adults to receive influenza vaccination when it is available, beginning as early as late August and continuing through the end of February.
- Instruct older adults with special needs or chronic conditions to create and share a plan with family and friends for emergencies and keep medications, prescriptions, and special devices on hand.

**Pediatric**
- Provide environmental health hazard information.
- Reduce risks from exposure to environmental contaminants by identifying the ages and life stages of children.
- Screen newly arrived immigrant and refugee children, adolescents, pregnant and lactating women, and children for elevated blood lead levels secondary to lead hazards in country of origin and residence in older housing.
- Be aware that the risk for lead exposure is much higher in many countries from which children are adopted than in the United States; screening should then be conducted for those identified from 6 months and up to 16 years of age (CDC, 2019a).

• = Independent          ▲ = Collaborative

- The current reference level of 5 μg/dL is used to identify children and environments associated with lead-exposure hazards.

**C**
- Encourage flu vaccination among children.

**Multicultural**
- Ask about use of imported or culture-specific products that contain lead, such as greta and azarcon (Hispanic folk medicine for upset stomach and diarrhea), ghasard (Indian folk medicine tonic), ba-baw-san (Chinese herbal remedy), and daw-tway (Thai and Myanmar [Burmese] remedy).
- Nurses need to consider the cultural and social factors that affect access to and understanding of the health care system, particularly for groups such as migrant workers who do not have consistent health care providers.

**Home Care**
- Assess current environmental stressors and identify community resources.
- Recognize that relocated and unemployed individuals/families are at risk for psychological distress.
- Support policy and program initiatives that integrate case identification, triage, and mental health interventions into emergency care response following large scale disaster events.
- Instruct community members concerned about lead in drinking water from plumbing pipes and fixtures to have the water tested by calling the US Environmental Protection Agency (EPA) drinking water hotline at 1-800-424-8802.
- Educate community members to reduce exposure to lead by inquiring about lead-based paint before buying a home or renting an apartment built before 1978.
- Instruct individuals and families that food contamination occurs through a variety of mechanisms and that food safety is associated with proper washing of hands, surfaces, and utensils; prompt refrigeration of food; and cooking foods at the correct temperature.

**Client/Family Teaching and Discharge Planning**
- Provide truthful information to the person or family affected.
- Discuss signs and symptoms of contamination.
- Explain decontamination protocols.
- Explain need for isolation procedures.
- Emphasize the importance of prehospital exposure and postexposure treatment of contamination.
- Provide parents with actionable information to reduce environmental contamination in the home.

• = Independent          ▲ = Collaborative

# Risk for Contamination

**Domain 11** Safety/protection    **Class 4** Environmental hazards

**C**

## NANDA-I Definition

Susceptible to exposure to environmental contaminants, which may compromise health.

## Risk Factors

### External Factors

Carpeted flooring; chemical contamination of food; chemical contamination of water; flaking, peeling surface in presence of young children; inadequate breakdown of contaminant; inadequate household hygiene practices; inadequate municipal services; inadequate personal hygiene practices; inadequate protective clothing; inappropriate use of protective clothing; individuals who ingested contaminated material; playing where environmental contaminants are used; unprotected exposure to chemical; unprotected exposure to heavy metal; unprotected exposure to radioactive material; use of environmental contaminant in the home; use of noxious material in inadequately ventilated area; use of noxious material without effective protection

### Internal Factors

Concomitant exposure; malnutrition; smoking

## At-Risk Population

Children aged <5 years; economically disadvantaged individuals; individuals exposed perinatally; individuals exposed to areas with high contaminant level; individuals exposed to atmospheric pollutants; individuals exposed to bioterrorism; individuals exposed to disaster; individuals with history of exposure to contaminant; older adults; pregnant women; women

## Associated Conditions

Preexisting disease; radiotherapy

## Client Outcomes, Nursing Interventions, and Client/Family Teaching

Refer to care plan for **Contamination.**

# Impaired Bowel Continence

**Domain 3** Elimination and exchange    **Class 2** Gastrointestinal function

## NANDA-I Definition

Inability to hold stool, to sense the presence of stool in the rectum, to relax and store stool when having a bowel movement is not convenient.

## Defining Characteristics

Abdominal discomfort; bowel urgency; fecal staining; impaired ability to expel formed stool despite recognition of rectal fullness; inability to delay

• = Independent          ▲ = Collaborative

defecation; inability to hold flatus; inability to reach toilet in time; inattentive to urge to defecate; silent leakage of stool during activities

**Related Factors**

Avoidance of non-hygienic toilet use; constipation; dependency for toileting; diarrhea; difficulty finding the bathroom; difficulty obtaining timely assistance to bathroom; embarrassment regarding toilet use in social situations; environmental constraints that interfere with continence; generalized decline in muscle tone; impaired physical mobility; impaired postural balance; inadequate dietary habits; inadequate motivation to maintain continence; incomplete emptying of bowel; laxative misuse; stressors

**At-Risk Population**

Older adults; women giving birth vaginally; women giving birth with obstetrical extraction

**Associated Conditions**

Anal trauma; congenital abnormalities of the digestive system; diabetes mellitus; neurocognitive disorders; neurological diseases; physical inactivity; prostatic diseases; rectum trauma; spinal cord injuries; stroke

**Client Outcomes**

**Client Will (Specify Time Frame)**

- Have regular, complete evacuation of fecal contents from the rectal vault (pattern may vary from every day to every 3 days)
- Have regulation of stool consistency (soft, formed stools)
- Reduce or eliminate frequency of incontinent episodes
- Exhibit intact skin in the perianal/perineal area
- Demonstrate the ability to isolate, contract, and relax pelvic muscles (when incontinence related to sphincter incompetence or high-tone pelvic floor dysfunction)
- Increase pelvic muscle strength (when incontinence related to sphincter incompetence)
- Identify triggers that precipitate change in bowel continence

**Nursing Interventions**

- In a private setting, directly question client about the presence of fecal incontinence. If the client reports altered bowel elimination patterns, problems with bowel control, or "uncontrollable diarrhea," complete a focused nursing history including previous and present bowel elimination routines, dietary history, frequency and volume of uncontrolled stool loss, and aggravating and alleviating factors.
- Recognize that risk factors for fecal incontinence include older individuals, female sex, impaired mobility, cognitive impairment, obesity, individuals who have undergone pelvic surgery, diabetes,

• = Independent ▲ = Collaborative

C

and structural or functional impairment of bowel function and medications (Young et al, 2017; Menees et al, 2018).

- Physiological changes of the female pelvis that occur with aging, along with those that occur with childbirth and anoreceptive intercourse increase the risk of elimination problems, both constipation and incontinence (Young et al, 2017; Brown et al, 2020).
- Recognize that additional risk factors for bowel incontinence in hospitalized clients include antibiotic therapy, medications, enteral feeding, indwelling urinary catheter placement, immobility, inability to communicate elimination needs, acute disease processes and procedures (e.g., cancer, abdominal surgery), sedation, and mechanical ventilation (Eman & Lohrmann, 2015; Pitta et al, 2019).
▲ Conduct a health history assessment that includes a review of current bowel patterns/habits, including constipation and use of laxatives; diarrhea; pelvic floor injury with childbirth; acute trauma to organs, muscles, or nerves involved in defecation; gastrointestinal inflammatory disorders; functional disability; and medications (Whitehead et al, 2016; Musa et al, 2019).
- Closely inspect the perineal skin and skinfolds for evidence of skin breakdown in clients with incontinence.
- Use a validated tool that focuses on bowel elimination patterns.
- Complete a focused physical assessment, including inspection of perineal skin, pelvic muscle strength assessment, digital examination of the rectum for the presence of impaction and anal sphincter strength, and evaluation of functional status (mobility, dexterity, and visual acuity).
- Complete an assessment of cognitive function; explore for a history of dementia, delirium, or acute confusion (Bliss et al, 2015; Blekken et al, 2018).
- Document patterns of stool elimination and incontinent episodes through a bowel record, including frequency of bowel movements, stool consistency, frequency and severity of incontinent episodes, precipitating factors, and dietary and fluid intake.
- Assess stool consistency and its influence on risk for stool loss. Several classification systems for stool exist and may assist the nurse and client to differentiate among normal soft, formed stool, hardened stools associated with constipation, and liquid stools associated with diarrhea.
- Identify conditions contributing to or causing fecal incontinence.
- Improve access to toileting:
  ○ Identify usual toileting patterns and plan opportunities for toileting accordingly.

• = Independent    ▲ = Collaborative

C

- ○ Provide assistance with toileting for clients with limited access or impaired functional status (mobility, dexterity, and access).
- ○ Institute a prompted toileting program for persons with impaired cognitive status.
- ○ Provide adequate privacy for toileting.
- ○ Respond promptly to requests for assistance with toileting.
- Review the client's nutritional history and evaluate methods to normalize stool consistency with dietary adjustments (e.g., avoiding high-fat foods) and use of fiber along with assessing for use of caffeine, lactose, and sugar replacements (Paquette et al, 2017; Da Silva & Sirany, 2019; International Foundation for Functional Gastrointestinal Disorders [IFFGD], 2019; O'Donnell, 2020).
- Encourage the client to keep a nutrition log to track foods that irritate the bowel (Paquette et al, 2017).
- For hospitalized clients with tube feeding–associated fecal incontinence, involve the nutrition specialist to evaluate the formula composition, osmolality, and fiber content.
- For the client with intermittent episodes of fecal incontinence related to acute changes in stool consistency, begin a bowel reeducation program consisting of the following:
  - ○ Cleansing the bowel of impacted stool if indicated
  - ○ Normalizing stool consistency by adequate intake of fluids (30 mL/kg of body weight per day) and dietary or supplemental fiber
  - ○ Establishing a regular routine of fecal elimination based on established patterns of bowel elimination (patterns established before onset of incontinence)
- Implement a scheduled stimulation defecation program for persons with neurological conditions causing fecal incontinence:
  - ○ Cleanse the bowel of impacted fecal material before beginning the program.
  - ○ Implement strategies to normalize stool consistency, including adequate intake of fluid and fiber and avoidance of foods associated with diarrhea.
  - ○ Determine a regular schedule for bowel elimination (typically every day or every other day) based on prior patterns of bowel elimination.
  - ○ Provide a stimulus before assisting the client to a position on the toilet; digital stimulation, a stimulating suppository, "mini-enema," or pulsed evacuation enema may be used for stimulation.
- Begin a reeducation or pelvic floor muscle exercise program for the person with sphincter incompetence or high-tone pelvic floor

muscle dysfunction of the pelvic muscles, or refer persons with fecal incontinence related to sphincter dysfunction to a nurse specialist or other therapist with clinical expertise in these techniques of care.

▲ Consider a sacral nerve stimulation program in clients with urgency to defecate and fecal incontinence related to weakened sphincter muscles or sphincter defect.

• Institute a structured skin care regimen that incorporates three essential steps: cleanse, moisturize, and protect:
  ○ Select a cleanser with a pH range comparable to that of normal skin (usually labeled "pH balanced").
  ○ Moisturize with an emollient to replace lipids removed with cleansing and protect with a skin. Products containing petrolatum, dimethicone, or zinc oxide base or a no-sting skin barrier should be used.
  ○ Routine incontinence care should include daily perineal skin cleansing and after each episode of incontinence.
  ○ When feasible, select a product that combines two or all three of these processes into a single step. Ensure that products are available at the bedside when caring for a client with total incontinence in an inpatient facility.

• Use of absorptive pads or adult containment briefs that are applied next to the client's skin increases the risk of IAD. Absorbent underpads that wick moisture away from skin may be used with immobile clients.

▲ Consult the provider if a fungal infection is suspected. An antifungal cream or powder beneath a protective ointment may be indicated (Gray et al, 2016; Coyer et al, 2017).

• Assist the client to select and apply a containment device for occasional episodes of fecal incontinence. A fecal containment device will prevent soiling of clothing and reduce odors in the client with uncontrolled stool loss.

• In the client with frequent episodes of fecal incontinence and limited mobility, monitor the sacrum and perineal area for pressure ulcerations.

• With acutely ill clients, anticipate and evaluate the cause of acute diarrhea. Anticipate diarrhea associated with treatment or specific interventions (e.g., medications, initiation of tube feedings).

▲ Consult a provider or the standing orders before inserting a bowel management system (BMS) in the critically ill client when conservative measures have failed and fecal incontinence is excessive and/or produces perianal skin injury or IAD.

• = Independent          ▲ = Collaborative

C

**Geriatric**
- Evaluate all older clients for established or acute fecal incontinence when the older client enters the acute or long-term care facility and intervene as indicated.
- Determine the client's cognitive level using a screening tool such as the Mini-Mental State Exam (MMSE), Montreal Cognitive Assessment (MoCA), the Confusion Assessment Method (CAM), or Mini-Cog.
- Teach nursing colleagues, nonprofessional care providers, family, and clients the importance of providing toileting opportunities and adequate privacy for the client in an acute or long-term care facility.

**Home Care**
- The preceding interventions may be adapted for home care use.
- Assess and teach a bowel management program to support continence. Address timing, diet, fluids, and actions taken independently to deal with bowel incontinence.
- Instruct the caregiver to provide clothing that is nonrestrictive, can be manipulated easily for toileting, and can be changed with ease.
- Evaluate self-care strategies of community-dwelling older adults, strengthen adaptive behaviors, and counsel older adults about altering strategies that compromise general health.
- Assist the family in arranging care in a way that allows the client to participate in family or favorite activities without embarrassment.
- ▲ If the client is limited to bed (or bed and chair), provide a commode or bedpan that can be easily accessed. Involve occupational and physical therapy services as indicated to promote safe transfers.
- ▲ If the client is frequently incontinent, refer for home health aide services to assist with hygiene and skin care.
- ▲ Refer the family to support services to assist with in-home management of fecal incontinence as indicated.
- Refer to care plans for **Diarrhea** and **Constipation** for detailed management of these related conditions.

# Risk for Adverse Reaction to Iodinated Contrast Media

**Domain 11** Safety/protection    **Class 5** Defensive processes
**NANDA-I Definition**

Susceptible to noxious or unintended reaction that can occur within seven days after contrast agent injection, which may compromise health.

• = Independent          ▲ = Collaborative

**C**

## Risk Factors
Dehydration; generalized weakness

## At-Risk Population
Individuals at extremes of age; individuals with history of adverse effect from iodinated contrast media; individuals with a history of allergy

## Associated Conditions
Chronic disease; concurrent use of pharmaceutical preparations; decreased level of consciousness; individuals with fragile veins

## Client Outcomes
### Client Will (Specify Time Frame)
- Maintain normal blood urea nitrogen and serum creatinine levels
- Maintain urine output of 0.5 mL/kg/hr
- Maintain serum electrolytes ($K^+$, $PO_4$, $Na^+$) within normal limits

## Nursing Interventions
Recognize that iodinated contrast media can be harmful to clients in a number of ways, including onset of contrast-induced nephropathy (CIN), allergic reactions to the dye, and damage to veins and vascular access devices.

### Contrast-Induced Nephropathy
Protect clients from contrast media-induced nephropathy by taking the following actions:
- Advocate for high-risk clients who are prone to develop contrast-induced acute kidney injury.
- Assess client's baseline kidney function, including serum creatinine, creatinine clearance, estimated glomerular filtration rate, and blood urea nitrogen (Nahar, 2017).
▲ Assess clients for risk factors for adverse reactions to contrast media: preexisting renal insufficiency, diabetes mellitus, dehydration, cardiovascular disease, diuretic use, advanced age, multiple myeloma, hypertension, hyperuricemia, multiple doses of iodinated contrast media in less than 24 hours (American College of Radiology, 2021).
- Communicate information about at-risk clients to provider and procedure team in the hand-off report and electronic medical record.
▲ Ensure that clients having diagnostic testing with contrast are well hydrated with isotonic intravenous (IV) fluids for volume expansion as ordered before and after the examination.
▲ Assess clients with symptoms of heart failure on an individual basis to determine tolerance for IV fluids used for hydration in the periprocedure period (Lambert et al, 2017).
▲ Monitor for and report signs of acute kidney injury for 48 hours after iodinated contrast administration in clients at risk: absolute

• = Independent　　　　▲ = Collaborative

**C**

serum creatinine increase ≥0.3 mg/dL, percentage increase in serum creatinine ≥50%, or urine output reduced to ≤0.5 mL/kg/hr for at least 6 hours. (Refer to your institution policy for specific clinical parameters.)

▲ Clients known to have acute kidney injury who are taking metformin should temporarily discontinue its use at the time of or before the procedure using contrast media, withhold metformin for 48 hours following, and reinstitute use only when renal function is found to be normal (Rose & Choi, 2015; American College of Radiology, 2021).

**Allergic Reaction to Contrast Media**

▲ Previous allergic reactions to contrast material, history of asthma, and other allergies are factors that may increase the client's risk of developing an adverse reaction. Discuss premedication with prednisone, methylprednisolone, or hydrocortisone with the provider for clients who have had previous reactions to contrast media or known asthma or allergies.

▲ Monitor carefully for symptoms of a hypersensitivity reaction, which can be mild, moderate, or severe. Report all symptoms to the provider because symptoms can advance rapidly from mild to severe.

○ *Mild reactions:* Nausea, vomiting, headache, itchy throat or eyes, flushing, mild skin rash, or hives.

○ *Moderate reactions:* Diffuse skin rash or hives, itchiness, erythema, wheezing but no hypoxia, facial edema but no dyspnea, throat tightness but no dyspnea.

○ *Severe reactions:* Diffuse hives with hypotension, diffuse itchiness or erythema with hypotension, diffuse edema including facial edema, wheezing with hypoxia, laryngeal edema with stridor and or hypoxia, anaphylactic shock (hypotension and tachycardia).

○ Both allergic and allergic-like (anaphylactoid) reactions can occur. Life-threatening events usually occur within 20 minutes after injection. Delayed reactions may occur with rash that appears hours or days afterward (American College of Radiology, 2021).

**Vein Damage and Damage to Vascular Access Devices**

• Recognize that *only* vascular access devices labeled "power injectable" can be used to administer power-injected contrast media. These include a power port, a power peripherally inserted central catheter (PICC) line, and a power central venous catheter (UCSF Department of Radiology and Biomedical Imaging, 2020a).

• Reduce the risk of vein and vascular access device damage with the following:

• = Independent          ▲ = Collaborative

- ○ Maintain constant communication with the client during the injection and monitor client for report of pain or swelling at the injection site, paresthesia, or tenderness.
- ○ Monitor access site for extravasation during and after the procedure; be vigilant for clients at increased risk of extravasation.
- ○ Assess for venous backflow before injecting contrast.
- ○ Directly monitor and palpate the venipuncture site during the first 15 seconds of injection.

**Geriatric**
- Screen the older client thoroughly before diagnostic testing using contrast media.

**Pediatric**
- Contrast medium can be safely administered intravenously by power injector at high flow rates of up to 2 mL/second (depending on size of client). A short peripheral IV catheter in the antecubital or forearm is the preferred route for intravenous contrast administration (UCSF Department of Radiology and Biomedical Imaging, 2020b).

**Client/Family Teaching and Discharge Teaching**
- Discharge instructions should include the importance of self-hydration after the procedure; reporting of symptoms of fluid retention or decrease in urine output; identifying which medications to take, withhold, or discontinue; scheduling laboratory evaluation 48 to 72 hours after the procedure; and scheduling follow-up with the provider (Lambert et al, 2017).

# Readiness for Enhanced Community Coping

**Domain 9** Coping/stress tolerance    **Class 2** Coping responses

## NANDA-I Definition

A pattern of community activities for adaptation and problem-solving for meeting the demands or needs of the community, which can be strengthened.

## Defining Characteristics

Expresses desire to enhance availability of community recreation programs; expresses desire to enhance availability of community relaxation programs; expresses desire to enhance communication among community members; expresses desire to enhance communication between groups and larger community; expresses desire to enhance community planning for predictable stressors; expresses desire to enhance community resources for managing stressors; expresses desire to enhance community responsibility

• = Independent    ▲ = Collaborative

for stress management; expresses desire to enhance problem-solving for identified issue

**C**

## Community Outcomes

**Community Will (Specify Time Frame)**
- Develop enhanced coping strategies
- Maintain effective coping strategies for management of stress

## Nursing Interventions

Note: Interventions depend on the specific aspects of community coping that can be enhanced (e.g., planning for stress management, communication, development of community power, community perceptions of stress, community coping strategies).

▲ Establish a collaborative partnership with the community.
- Assess community needs with the use of concept mapping methodology.
- Assess for the impact of social determinants of health on community health.
- Encourage participation in faith-based organizations that want to improve community stress management.
- Identify the health services and information resources that are currently available in the community through network analysis.
- Work with community members to increase problem-solving abilities.
- Provide support to the community and help community members identify and mobilize additional supports.
- Advocate for the community in multiple arenas (e.g., multimedia, social media, and governmental agencies).
- Work with communities to ensure that vulnerable individuals with access and functional needs are included in preparations for, response to, and recovery from disasters.
- Partner with community pharmacies to provide community education and health prevention services.

### Pediatric
- Protect children and adolescents from exposure to community violence.
- Assess children and adolescents for the effects of direct and indirect crime exposure rather than only focusing solely on violent victimization.

### Multicultural
- Acknowledge the stressors unique to racial/ethnic communities.
- Identify community strengths with community members.
- Use an empowerment approach to address health behaviors in diverse communities. An empowerment approach includes increasing clients' self-efficacy and capacity to make informed decisions about their health care.

• = Independent          ▲ = Collaborative

- Work with members of the community to prioritize and target health goals specific to the community.
- Establish and sustain partnerships with key individuals within communities when developing and implementing programs.
- Use mentoring strategies for community members.
- Use community church settings as a forum for advocacy, teaching, and program implementation.

## Defensive Coping

**Domain 9** Coping/stress tolerance     **Class 2** Coping responses

### NANDA-I Definition

Repeated projection of falsely positive self-evaluation based on a self-protective pattern that defends against underlying perceived threats to positive self-regard.

### Defining Characteristics

Altered reality testing; denies problems; denies weaknesses; difficulty establishing interpersonal relations; difficulty maintaining interpersonal relations; grandiosity; hostile laughter; hypersensitivity to a discourtesy; hypersensitivity to criticism; inadequate follow through with treatment regimen; inadequate participation in treatment regimen; projection of blame; projection of responsibility; rationalization of failures; reality distortion; ridicules others; superior attitude toward others

### Related Factors

Conflict between self-perception and value system; fear of failure; fear of humiliation; fear of repercussions; inadequate confidence in others; inadequate psychological resilience; inadequate self-confidence; inadequate social support; uncertainty; unrealistic self-expectations

### Client Outcomes

**Client Will (Specify Time Frame)**

- Acknowledge need for change in coping style
- Accept responsibility for own behavior
- Establish realistic goals with validation from caregivers
- Solicit caregiver validation in decision-making

### Nursing Interventions

- Assess for possible symptoms associated with defensive coping: depressive symptoms, excessive self-focused attention, negativism and anxiety, hypertension, posttraumatic stress disorder (e.g., exposure to terrorism), substance use symptoms, unjust world beliefs.

• = Independent          ▲ = Collaborative

**C**

▲ Use cognitive behavioral interventions.
• Ask appropriate questions to assess whether denial (defensive coping) is being used in association with health problems including alcoholism, myocardial infarction (MI), or other diagnoses.
• Promote interventions with multisensory stimulation approaches (MSA).
• Empower the client/caregiver's self-knowledge.

**Geriatric**
▲ Identify problems with alcohol in older adults with the appropriate tools and make suitable referrals.
• Encourage exercise for positive coping.
• Use individual and/or group reminiscence therapy (RT).

**Multicultural**
• Acknowledge racial/ethnic differences at the onset of care.
• Assess an individual's sociocultural backgrounds in teaching self-management and self-regulation.
• Encourage the client to use spiritual coping mechanisms such as faith and prayer.
• Encourage spirituality as a source of support for coping.

**Home Care**
▲ Refer the client for programs that teach coping skills.

**Client/Family Teaching and Discharge Planning**
• Teach coping skills to clients and caregivers.
• Teach reflexive and expressive writing to address emotions.

# Ineffective Coping

**Domain 9** Coping/stress tolerance    **Class 2** Coping responses
## NANDA-I Definition

A pattern of invalid appraisal of stressors, with cognitive and/or behavioral efforts, that fails to manage demands related to well-being.
## Defining Characteristics

Altered affective responsiveness; altered attention; altered communication pattern; destructive behavior toward others; destructive behavior toward self; difficulty organizing information; fatigue; frequent illness; impaired ability to ask for help; impaired ability to attend to information; impaired ability to deal with a situation; impaired ability to meet basic needs; impaired ability to meet role expectation; inadequate follow-through with goal-directed behavior; inadequate problem resolution; inadequate problem-solving skills; reports altered sleep-wake cycle; reports inadequate sense of control; risk-taking behavior; substance misuse

• = Independent    ▲ = Collaborative

## Related Factors

High degree of threat; inability to conserve adaptive energies; inaccurate threat appraisal; inadequate confidence in ability to deal with a situation; inadequate health resources; inadequate preparation for stressor; inadequate sense of control; inadequate social support; ineffective tension release strategies

## At-Risk Population

Individuals experiencing maturational crisis; individuals experiencing situational crisis

## Client Outcomes

### Client Will (Specify Time Frame)

- Use effective coping strategies
- Use behaviors to decrease stress
- Remain free of destructive behavior toward self or others
- Report decrease in physical symptoms of stress
- Report increase in psychological comfort
- Seek help from a health care professional as appropriate

## Nursing Interventions

- Appraise the presence of contributing factors for ineffective coping such as poor self-concept, grief, lack of problem-solving skills, lack of support, recent change in life situation, and maturational or situational crises.
- Use presence and other verbal and nonverbal therapeutic communication approaches including empathy, active listening, calm approach, and acceptance.
- Collaborate with the client to identify strengths such as the ability to relate the facts and to recognize the source of stressors.
- Explore the client's previous stressors and coping methods.
- Provide opportunities to discuss the meaning the situation might have for the client.
- Assist the client to set realistic goals and identify personal skills and knowledge.
- Provide information regarding care, including diagnoses, treatments, and anticipated expectations.
- Discuss changes with the client before making them.
- Provide mental and physical activities within the client's ability (e.g., reading, television, radio, crafts, outings, movies, dinners out, social gatherings, exercise, sports, games).
- Discuss the power of the client and family to change a situation or the need to accept a situation.
- Offer instruction regarding alternative coping strategies.

• = Independent        ▲ = Collaborative

- Encourage use of spiritual resources as desired.
- Encourage use of social support resources.
- ▲ Refer for additional or more intensive therapies as needed.

**Pediatric**

- Monitor the client's risk of harming self or others and intervene appropriately. **QSEN:** See care plan for Risk for **Suicidal Behavior.**
- Monitor pediatric clients for exposure to community violence.

**Geriatric**

- ▲ Assess and report possible physiological alterations (e.g., sepsis, hypoglycemia, hypotension, infection, changes in temperature, fluid and electrolyte imbalances, use of medications with known cognitive and psychotropic side effects).
- Screen for elder neglect or other forms of elder mistreatment.
- Encourage the client to make choices (as appropriate) and participate in planning care and scheduled activities.
- Target selected coping mechanisms for older persons based on client features, use, and preferences.
- Increase and mobilize support available to older persons by encouraging a variety of mechanisms involving family, friends, peers, and health care providers.
- Actively listen to complaints and concerns.
- Engage the client in reminiscence.

**Multicultural**

- Assess for the influence of cultural beliefs, norms, and values on the client's perceptions of effective coping.
- Assess for intergenerational family problems that can overwhelm coping abilities.
- Negotiate with the client regarding aspects of coping behavior that will need to be modified.
- Refer families experiencing race-based stress and trauma to evidence-based programs.
- Identify which family members the client can count on for support.
- Support the inner resources that clients use for coping.
- Use an empowerment framework to redefine coping strategies.

**Home Care**

- The interventions described previously may be adapted for home care use.
- Assess for suicidal tendencies. Refer for mental health care immediately if indicated.
- Identify an emergency plan should the client become suicidal. Ineffective coping can occur in a crisis situation and can lead to

suicidal ideation if the client sees no hope for a solution. A suicidal client is not safe in the home environment unless supported by professional help. Refer to the care plan for Risk for **Suicidal Behavior.**
- Discuss preferred coping strategies of family caregivers.
- Encourage clients to participate knowingly in their care. Refer to the care plan for **Powerlessness.**
▲ Refer the client and family to support groups.
▲ If monitoring medication use, discuss the barriers and facilitators to adapting and coping with the regimen.
▲ Institute case management for frail elderly clients to support continued independent living.

**Client/Family Teaching and Discharge Planning**
- Teach the client to problem solve. Have the client define the problem and cause, and list the advantages and disadvantages of the options.
- Teach relaxation techniques.
- Work closely with the client to develop appropriate educational tools that address individualized needs.
▲ Teach the client about available community resources (e.g., therapists, ministers, counselors, self-help groups).

# Readiness for Enhanced Coping

**Domain 9** Coping/stress tolerance  **Class 2** Coping responses
## NANDA-I Definition
A pattern of valid appraisal of stressors with cognitive and/or behavioral efforts to manage demands related to well-being, which can be strengthened.
## Defining Characteristics
Expresses desire to enhance knowledge of stress management strategies; expresses desire to enhance management of stressors; expresses desire to enhance social support; expresses desire to enhance use of emotion-oriented strategies; expresses desire to enhance use of problem-oriented strategies; expresses desire to enhance use of spiritual resource
## Client Outcomes
Client Will (Specify Time Frame)
- Acknowledge personal power
- State awareness of possible environmental changes that may contribute to decreased coping
- State that stressors are manageable
- Seek new effective coping strategies

          • = Independent          ▲ = Collaborative

- Seek social support for problems associated with coping
- Demonstrate ability to cope, using a broad range of coping strategies
- Use spiritual support of personal choice

**C**

## Nursing Interventions

- Assess and support positive psychological strengths, that is, hope, optimism, self-efficacy, resiliency, and social support.
- Be physically and emotionally present for the client while using a variety of therapeutic communication techniques.
- Empower the client to set realistic goals and to engage in problem-solving.
- Encourage expression of positive thoughts and emotions.
- Encourage the client to use spiritual coping mechanisms such as faith and prayer.
- Help the client with serious and chronic conditions such as depression, cancer diagnosis, and chemotherapy treatment to maintain social support networks or assist in building new ones.
- ▲ Refer for cognitive-behavioral therapy (CBT) to enhance coping skills.

### Pediatric

- Encourage children and adolescents to engage in diversional activities and exercise to promote self-esteem, enhance coping, and prevent behavioral and other physical and psychosocial problems.
- Provide families of children with chronic illness with education, transitional assistance, and psychosocial support to enhance coping.

### Geriatric

- Encourage active, meaning-based coping strategies for older adults with chronic illness.
- Consider the use of Web-based and technological resources for older adults in the community.
- Refer the older client to self-help support groups that address health, psychosocial, and/or social support.

### Multicultural

- Assess an individual's sociocultural backgrounds to identify factors that support coping.
- Encourage spirituality as a source of support for coping.
- Facilitate positive ethnocultural identity to enhance coping.
- Foster family support.

### Home Care

- The interventions described previously may be adapted for home care use.
- Engage both clients and their caregivers as a dyad.

• = Independent ▲ = Collaborative

C

▲ Institute case management for frail elderly clients to support continued independent living.
• Refer the client and family to support groups.
• Refer prostate cancer clients and their spouses to family programs that include family-based interventions of communication, hope, coping, uncertainty, and symptom management.
▲ Refer military members, veterans, and family members for appropriate health services.

**Client/Family Teaching and Discharge Planning**
• Teach the client about available community resources (e.g., therapists, ministers, counselors, self-help groups, family education groups).
• Teach caregivers using a variety of interventions that contribute to coping.
• Teach expressive writing, journaling, and education about emotions.

# Ineffective Community Coping

**Domain 9** Coping/stress tolerance    **Class 2** Coping responses

## NANDA-I Definition

A pattern of community activities for adaptation and problem-solving that is unsatisfactory for meeting the demands or needs of the community.

## Defining Characteristics

Community does not meet expectations of its members; deficient community participation; elevated community illness rate; excessive community conflict; excessive community stress; high incidence of community problems; perceived community powerlessness; perceived community vulnerability

## Related Factors

Inadequate community problem-solving resources; inadequate community resources; nonexistent community systems

## At-Risk Population

Community that has experienced a disaster

## Community Outcomes

**A Broad Range of Community Members Will (Specify Time Frame)**
• Participate in community actions to improve power resources
• Develop improved communication among community members
• Participate in problem-solving
• Demonstrate cohesiveness in problem-solving
• Develop new strategies for problem-solving
• Express power to deal with change and manage problems

• = Independent        ▲ = Collaborative

## Nursing Interventions

Note: The diagnosis of Ineffective **Coping** does not apply and should not
be used when stress is being imposed by external sources or circumstance.
If the community is a victim of circumstances, using the nursing diagnosis
Ineffective **Coping** is equivalent to blaming the victim. See the care plan
for Readiness for Enhanced Community **Coping**.

▲ Establish a collaborative partnership with the community (see the
care plan for Readiness for Enhanced Community **Coping** for
additional references).
• Assess community needs with the use of concept mapping methodology.
• Assess for the impact of social determinants of health on community
health.
• Encourage participation in faith-based organizations that want to
improve community stress management.
▲ Identify the health services and information resources that are
currently available in the community through network analysis.
• Work with community members to increase problem-solving abilities.
• Provide support to the community and help community members
identify and mobilize additional supports.
• Advocate for the community in multiple arenas (e.g., multimedia,
social media, governmental agencies).
• Work with communities to ensure that vulnerable individuals with
access and functional needs are included in preparations for, response
to, and recovery from disasters.
• Partner with community pharmacies to provide community education
and health prevention services.

### Pediatric
• Protect children and adolescents from exposure to community violence.
• Assess children and adolescents for the effects of direct and
indirect crime exposure rather than only focusing solely on violent
victimization.

### Multicultural
• Acknowledge the stressors unique to racial/ethnic communities.
• Identify community strengths with community members.
• Use an empowerment approach to address health behaviors in diverse
communities. An empowerment approach includes increasing clients'
self-efficacy and capacity to make informed decisions about their
health care.
• Work with members of the community to prioritize and target health
goals specific to the community.

• = Independent          ▲ = Collaborative

- Establish and sustain partnerships with key individuals within communities when developing and implementing programs.
- Use mentoring strategies for community members.
- Use community church settings as a forum for advocacy, teaching, and program implementation.

## Compromised Family Coping

**Domain 9** Coping/stress tolerance    **Class 2** Coping responses
### NANDA-I Definition
An usually supportive primary person (family member, significant other, or close friend) provides insufficient, ineffective, or compromised support, comfort, assistance, or encouragement that may be needed by the client to manage or master adaptive tasks related to his or her health challenge.
### Defining Characteristics
Client complaint about support person's response to health problem; client reports concern about support person's response to health problem; limitation in communication between support person and client; protective behavior by support person incongruent with client's abilities; protective behavior by support person incongruent with client's need for autonomy; support person reports inadequate knowledge; support person reports inadequate understanding; support person reports preoccupation with own reaction to client's need; support person withdraws from client; unsatisfactory assistive behaviors of support person
### Related Factors
Coexisting situations affecting support person; depleted capacity of support person; family disorganization; inaccurate information presented by others; inadequate information available to support person; inadequate reciprocal support; inadequate support given by client to support person; inadequate understanding of information by support person; misunderstanding of information by support person; preoccupation by support person with concern outside of family
### At-Risk Population
Families with member with altered family role; families with support person experiencing depleted capacity due to prolonged disease; families with support persons experiencing developmental crisis; families with support persons experiencing situational crisis

• = Independent    ▲ = Collaborative

**C**

## Client Outcomes

### Family/Significant Person Will (Specify Time Frame)

- Verbalize internal resources to help deal with the situation
- Verbalize knowledge and understanding of illness, disability, or disease
- Provide support and assistance as needed
- Identify need for and seek outside support

## Nursing Interventions

- Assess the strengths and deficiencies of the family system. Consider using Family Systems Nursing, which emphasizes collaboration and a strength-focused relationship between health care professionals and the entire family as a unit of care.
- Establish rapport with families by providing accurate communication.
- Assist family members to recognize the need for help and teach them how to ask for it.
- Encourage family members to verbalize feelings. Spend time with them, sit down and make eye contact, and offer coffee and other nourishment.
- Provide family support interventions in situations in which caregiving is involved in the family.
- Provide privacy during family visits. If possible, maintain flexible visiting hours to accommodate more frequent family visits. If possible, arrange staff assignments so the same staff members have contact with the family. Familiarize other staff members with the situation in the absence of the usual staff member.
- Provide education to clients regarding active coping strategies to use in situations involving chronic illnesses.
- Provide psychoeducation interventions and support for families providing palliative care to help reduce caregiver stress and burden.
- Refer the family with ill family members to appropriate resources for assistance as indicated (e.g., counseling, psychotherapy, financial assistance, spiritual support).

### Pediatric

- Provide screening for postpartum depression (PPD) during the prenatal period and during the 6-week postpartum checkup to identify symptoms of depression in mothers.
- Consider medication management and psychosocial interventions, including individual therapy, group therapy, support groups, and brief psychotherapy.
- ▲ Use preventive strategies, such as screening, psychoeducation, postpartum debriefing, and companionship in the delivery room (e.g.,

community volunteer). Continuing education is also recommended for health care professionals to improve knowledge regarding PPD.

- Use technology-based education to help increase knowledge and support for parents performing care procedures for their children.
- Use best practices and participate in training to help make communication and environmental adaptations when interacting with children with autism spectrum disorder (ASD) to enhance communication, improve quality of care, and reduce behavioral problems and frustration.
- Effectively engaging and collaborating with parents is essential for supporting parents of children with long-term health conditions, and it may enhance the parent–professional relationship and communication.
- Provide evidence-based psychological therapies for parents with children with chronic conditions.
- When performing pediatric diabetes care, be attentive to the mother's experience, including burnout experienced as a result of caregiving for the child.
- Provide options for home-based interventions when severe childhood illnesses make it difficult for children and families to participate in interventions. In-home visits, assessments, and interventions may help improve self-management among the client and family and reduce emergency department visits and inpatient hospitalizations.

### Geriatric

▲ Perform a holistic assessment of all needs of informal family caregivers.

▲ Assist informal caregivers with reducing unmet needs by helping them obtain the information, education, and support necessary for caring for an older adult with a chronic health condition.

- In situations in which familial caregiving is being provided, assess current coping strategies utilized within the family. Provide interventions for family caregivers that are designed specifically to enhance coping skills, including problem-solving strategies and emotional support.

### Multicultural

- Acknowledge sociocultural differences and health care disparities at the onset of care.
- Use valid and culturally competent assessment tools and procedures when working with families with different racial/ethnic backgrounds.

• = Independent       ▲ = Collaborative

- Assess for the influence of cultural beliefs, norms, and values on the individual/family/community's perceptions of coping.
- Provide opportunities for clients and families to discuss spirituality.
- Ensure culturally responsive approaches to end-of-life care.

**Home Care**

- The interventions described previously may be adapted for home care use.
- Assess the reason behind the breakdown of family coping.
- ▲ During the time of compromised coping, increase visits to ensure the safety of the client, support of the family, and reassurance regarding expectations for prognosis as appropriate.
- ▲ Assess the needs of the caregiver in the home, and intervene to meet needs as appropriate; explore all available resources that may be used to provide adequate home care (e.g., parish nursing as an effective adjunct, home health aide services to relieve the caregiver's fatigue).
- ▲ Encourage caregivers to attend to their own physical, mental, and spiritual health, and give more specific information about the client's needs and ways to meet them.
- ▲ Refer the family to medical social services for evaluation and supportive counseling. Serve as an advocate, mentor, and role model for caregiving; provide written information for the care needed by the client.
- ▲ A positive approach and caring by the nurse and concrete task definition and assignment reinforce positive coping strategies and allow caregivers to feel less guilty when tasks are delegated to multiple caregivers.
- ▲ When a terminal illness is the precipitating factor for ineffective coping, offer hospice services and support groups as possible resources.
- Encourage the client and family to discuss changes in daily functioning and routines created by the client's illness, and validate discomfort resulting from changes.
- Support positive individual and family coping efforts.
- Screen for mental health disorders (MHDs) in the elderly home care population.
- During home care visits and assessments, provide individuals and families with information for Internet-based interventions, including information on using social media as a health communications tool.

• = Independent                    ▲ = Collaborative

**C**

## Client/Family Teaching and Discharge Planning

- Assess grief in parents who have lost a child to help determine parental needs, especially in the first year after the death of a child.
▲ Refer women with breast cancer and their family caregivers to support groups (including social network sites and online communities), and to other services that provide assistance with daily coping.
▲ For families dealing with childhood illnesses, developmental disorders, or other psychosocial stressors, refer parents to training, support, and education groups to provide opportunities for parents to access support, learn new parenting skills, and obtain additional coping resources.
- Provide comprehensive discharge planning for individuals and families to help improve quality of life at home.
- Individuals diagnosed with a developmental disability and a mental illness and their families frequently experience multiple challenges and insufficient resources and support.
- Nurses can help clients with type 2 diabetes with self-management education and support (DSME/S), which includes the facilitation of knowledge, skills, and abilities necessary to manage diabetes, as well as obtaining the support necessary for executing and maintaining the coping and behavioral skills needed for self-management.

# Disabled Family Coping

**Domain 9** Coping/stress tolerance    **Class 2** Coping responses
## NANDA-I Definition

Behavior of primary person (family member, significant other, or close friend) that disables his or her capacities and the client's capacities to effectively address tasks essential to either person's adaptation to the health challenge.

## Defining Characteristics

Abandons client; adopts illness symptoms of client; aggressive behaviors; depressive symptoms; difficulty structuring a meaningful life; disregards basic needs of client; disregards family relations; distorted reality about client's health problem; expresses feeling abandoned; family behaviors detrimental to well-being; hostility; impaired individualism; inadequate ability to tolerate client; loss of client independence; neglects treatment regimen;

• = Independent          ▲ = Collaborative

performing routines without regard for client's needs; prolonged hyperfocus on client; psychomotor agitation; psychosomatic symptoms

## Related Factors

Ambivalent family relationships; chronically unexpressed feelings by support person; differing coping styles between support person and client; differing coping styles between support persons

## Client Outcomes

### Family/Significant Person Will (Specify Time Frame)

- Identify normal family routines that will need to be adapted
- Participate positively in the client's care within the limits of his or her abilities
- Identify responses that may be harmful
- Acknowledge and accept the need for assistance with circumstances
- Identify appropriate activities for affected family member

## Nursing Interventions

- Families dealing with acute trauma are susceptible to mild to very severe levels of anxiety. Support should be offered through necessary channels, which are appropriate to the situation, such as providing frequent information, offering social services, or counseling.
- Assess coping strategies of family members.
- Cancer caregiving interventions should include communication skill building, including strategies for self-care.
- Provide ideas for positive child coping and consider collaboration with mental health providers for children with chronic illnesses who are facing emotional problems.
- Assess social support of family members caring for survivors of traumatic brain injuries (TBIs). Facilitate realistic expectations about caregiving.
- Respect and promote the spiritual needs of the client and family.

### Pediatric

- Assist parents and children suffering from chronic illness to develop accommodative coping skills (adapting to stressors rather than attempting to change the stressors).
- Assess discharge readiness of parents of ill children and construct high-quality parent teaching to address educational attainment.

### Geriatric

- Assess the emotional well-being of family members who are caring for clients with long-term illnesses, such as stroke.
- Be aware of age-related deterioration in coping skills.

**Multicultural**
- Acknowledge racial/ethnic differences at the onset of care.
- Be sensitive to the stigma attached to particular illness in various cultures.

**Home Care**

The interventions described previously may be adapted for home care use:
- Assess for strain in family caregivers.
- Assess for "caregiver fatigue" and provide information related to available respite care.
- Consult social services for available home resources related to the client's age and illness.

**Client/Family Teaching and Discharge Planning**
- Provide psychoeducational family teaching for families impacted by mental illness.
- Involve the client and family in the planning of care as often as possible.
- Recognize that family decision makers may need additional psychosocial support services.

## Readiness for Enhanced Family Coping

**Domain 9** Coping/stress tolerance    **Class 2** Coping responses

### NANDA-I Definition

A pattern of management of adaptive tasks by primary person (family member, significant other, or close friend) involved with the client's health challenge, which can be strengthened.

### Defining Characteristics

Expresses desire to acknowledge growth impact of crisis; expresses desire to choose experiences that optimize wellness; expresses desire to enhance connection with others who have experienced a similar situation; expresses desire to enhance enrichment of lifestyle; expresses desire to enhance health promotion

### Client Outcomes

**Client Will (Specify Time Frame)**
- State a plan indicating coping strengths, abilities, and resources, as well as areas for growth and change

• = Independent          ▲ = Collaborative

- Perform tasks and engage resources needed for growth and change
- Evaluate changes and continually reevaluate plan for continued growth

**C**

## Nursing Interventions

▲ Assess the structure, resources, and coping abilities of families and use these assessments in selecting interventions and formulating care plans.

▲ Acknowledge, assess, and support the spiritual needs and resources of families and clients.

▲ Establish rapport with families and empower their decision-making through effective communication and person/family-centered care.

▲ Provide family members with educational and skill-building interventions to alleviate caregiving stress and to facilitate adherence to prescribed plans of care.

▲ Develop, provide, and encourage family members to use counseling services and interventions.

▲ Identify and refer to support programs that discuss experiences and challenges similar to those faced by the family (e.g., cancer support groups).

▲ Incorporate the use of emerging technologies to increase the reach of interventions to support family coping.

▲ Refer to Compromised Family **Coping** for additional interventions.

### Pediatric

▲ Identify and assess the management styles of families and facilitate the use of more effective ways of coping with childhood illness.

▲ Provide educational and supportive interventions for families caring for children with illness and disability.

### Geriatric

▲ Encourage family caregivers to participate in counseling and support groups.

▲ Provide educational and therapeutic interventions to family caregivers that focus on knowledge and skill building.

### Multicultural

- Acknowledge and understand the importance of cultural influences in families and ensure that assessments and assessment tools account for such cultural differences.
- Understand and incorporate cultural differences into interventions to enhance the impact of family interventions.

• = Independent          ▲ = Collaborative

# Readiness for Enhanced Decision-Making

**Domain 10** Life principles    **Class 3** Value/belief/action congruence

**D**

## NANDA-I Definition

A pattern of choosing a course of action for meeting short- and long-term health-related goals, which can be strengthened.

## Defining Characteristics

Expresses desire to enhance congruency of decisions with sociocultural goal; expresses desire to enhance congruency of decisions with sociocultural value; expresses desire to enhance congruency of decisions with goal; expresses desire to enhance congruency of decisions with values; expresses desire to enhance decision-making; expresses desire to enhance risk-benefit analysis of decisions; expresses desire to enhance understanding of choices; expresses desire to enhance understanding of meaning of choices; expresses desire to enhance use of reliable evidence for decisions

## Client Outcomes

### Client Will (Specify Time Frame)

- Review treatment options with providers
- Ask questions about the benefits and risks of treatment options
- Communicate decisions about treatment options to providers in relation to personal preferences, values, and goals

## Nursing Interventions

- Support and encourage clients and their representatives to engage in health care decisions.
- Provide information that is appropriate, relevant, and timely.
- Determine the health literacy of clients and their representatives before helping with decision-making.
- Tailor information to the specific needs of individual clients, according to principles of health literacy.
- Motivate clients to be as independent as possible in decision-making.
- Facilitate communication between the client and family members regarding the final decision; offer support to the person actually making the decision.
- Design educational interventions for decision support.

### Geriatric

- The previously mentioned interventions may be adapted for geriatric use.
- Facilitate collaborative decision-making.

### Multicultural

- Use existing decision aids for particular types of decisions or develop decision aids as indicated.

• = Independent          ▲ = Collaborative

**D**

### Home Care

- The previously mentioned interventions may be adapted for home care use.
- Develop clinical practice guidelines that include shared decision-making.

### Client/Family Teaching and Discharge Planning

- Instruct the client and family members to provide advance directives in the following areas:
  - ○ Person to contact in an emergency
  - ○ Preference (if any) to die at home or in the hospital
  - ○ Desire to initiate advance directives, such as a living will or medical power of attorney
  - ○ Desire to donate an organ
  - ○ Funeral arrangements (i.e., burial, cremation)

## Decisional Conflict

**Domain 10** Life principles     **Class 3** Value/belief/action congruence

### NANDA-I Definition

Uncertainty about course of action to be taken when choice among competing actions involves risk, loss, or challenge to values and beliefs.

### Defining Characteristics

Delayed decision-making; expresses distress during decision making; physical sign of distress; physical sign of tension; questions moral principle while attempting a decision; questions moral rule while attempting a decision; questions moral values while attempting a decision; questions personal beliefs while attempting a decision; questions personal values while attempting a decision; recognizes undesired consequences of potential actions; reports uncertainty about choices; self-focused; vacillating among choices

### Related Factors

Conflict with moral obligation; conflicting information sources; inadequate information; inadequate social support; inexperience with decision-making; interference in decision-making; moral principle supports mutually inconsistent actions; moral rule supports mutually inconsistent actions; moral value supports mutually inconsistent actions; unclear personal beliefs; unclear personal values

### Client Outcomes

**Client Will (Specify Time Frame)**

- State the advantages and disadvantages of choices
- Share fears and concerns regarding choices and responses of others

• = Independent          ▲ = Collaborative

- Seek resources and information necessary for making an informed choice
- Make an informed choice

**Nursing Interventions**

**D**

- Observe for factors causing or contributing to conflict (e.g., value conflicts, fear of outcome, poor problem-solving skills).
- Provide emotional support.
- Use decision aids or computer-based decision aids to assist clients in making decisions.
- Facilitate communication between the client and family members regarding the final decision; offer support to the person actually making the decision.

**Geriatric**

- Carefully assess clients with dementia regarding ability to make decisions.
- Discuss the purpose of advance directives such as a living will or medical power of attorney.

**Multicultural**

- Assess for the influence of cultural beliefs, norms, and values on the client's decision-making conflict.

**Home Care**

- The interventions described previously may be adapted for home care use.
- Encourage discussion of life-sustaining treatments and advance directives.

**Client/Family Teaching and Discharge Planning**

- Instruct the client and family members to provide advance directives in the following areas:
  ○ Person to contact in an emergency
  ○ Preference (if any) to die at home or in the hospital
  ○ Desire to initiate advance directives, such as a living will or medical power of attorney
  ○ Desire to donate an organ
  ○ Funeral arrangements (i.e., burial, cremation)
- Inform the family of treatment options; encourage and defend self-determination.
- Recognize and allow the client to discuss the selection of complementary therapies available, such as spiritual support, relaxation, imagery, exercise, lifestyle changes, diet (e.g., macrobiotic, vegetarian), and nutritional supplementation.
- ▲ Provide the POLST form for clients and families faced with end-of-life choices across the health care continuum.

• = Independent        ▲ = Collaborative

# Impaired Emancipated Decision-Making

**Domain 10** Life principles    **Class 3** Value/belief/action congruence

**D**

## NANDA-I Definition

A process of choosing a health care decision that does not include personal knowledge and/or consideration of social norms, or does not occur in a flexible environment, resulting in decisional dissatisfaction.

## Defining Characteristics

Delayed enactment of health care option; difficulty choosing a health care option that best fits current lifestyle; expresses constraint in describing own opinion; expresses distress about others' opinion; expresses excessive concern about others' opinions; expresses excessive fear of what others think about a decision; impaired ability to describe how option will fit into current lifestyle; limited verbalization about health care option in others' presence

## Related Factors

Decreased understanding of available health care options; difficulty adequately verbalizing perceptions about health care options; inadequate confidence to openly discuss health care options; inadequate information regarding health care options; inadequate privacy to openly discuss health care options; inadequate self-confidence in decision-making; insufficient time to discuss health care options

## At-Risk Population

Individuals with limited decision making experience; women accessing health care from systems with patriarchal hierarchy; women living in families with patriarchal hierarch

## Client Outcomes

**Client Will (Specify Time Frame)**

- Verbalize option outcomes freely before making a health care decision
- Freely verbalize own opinion with health care providers before making a health care decision
- Choose the health care option that fits his or her lifestyle within an appropriate amount of time that allows enactment of the choice
- Describe how the chosen option fits into his or her current lifestyle before or after the decision has been made
- Verbalizes appropriate concern about others' opinions before making the health care choice
- Remains stress-free when listening to others' opinions before making the health care choice
- Arrives at a decision in a timely manner

• = Independent        ▲ = Collaborative

## Nursing Interventions

- Assess client's readiness to openly discussing the decision-making process.
- Use active listening in a nonjudgmental manner to provide the client with a flexible decision-making environment.
- Use anticipatory guidance by proactively providing the client with information.
- Establish a purposeful provider–client relationship.
- ▲ Refer to counseling as needed.
- Provide decision-making support.
- Provide a flexible environment by encouraging others to accept the client's choice.
- Encourage the client to use personal knowledge as part of the decision-making process to increase decisional satisfaction.

### Pediatric

- When able, involve the client in health care decision-making when possible.
- Provide parental information in the decision-making process.
- Enhance client decision-making in the critical care setting.

### Geriatric

- Include geriatric clients in the decisional process.

### Multicultural

- Consider cultural influences on decision-making.

### Home Care

- Use open communication to assist clients to develop health care plans to which they can adhere.

# Readiness for Enhanced Emancipated Decision-Making

**Domain 10** Life principles    **Class 3** Value/belief/action congruence

## NANDA-I Definition

A process of choosing a health care decision that includes personal knowledge and/or consideration of social norms, which can be strengthened.

## Defining Characteristics

Expresses desire to enhance ability to choose health care options that enhance current lifestyle; expresses desire to enhance ability to enact chosen health care option; expresses desire to enhance ability to understand all available health care options; expresses desire to enhance ability to verbalize own opinion without constraint; expresses desire to enhance comfort to verbalize health care options in the presence of others; expresses desire to enhance

• = Independent                ▲ = Collaborative

confidence in decision-making; expresses desire to enhance confidence to discuss health care options openly; expresses desire to enhance decision-making; expresses desire to enhance privacy to discuss health care options

**Client Outcomes**

**D**

**Client Will (Specify Time Frame)**

- Verbalize option of outcomes freely before making a health care decision
- Freely verbalize own opinion with health care providers before making a health care decision
- Choose the health care option that best fits his or her lifestyle within an appropriate amount of time that allows enactment of the choice
- Describe how the chosen option fits into his or her current lifestyle before or after the decision has been made
- Verbalizes appropriate concern about others' opinions before making the health care choice
- Remains stress-free when listening to others' opinions before making the health care choice
- Arrives at a decision in a timely manner

**Nursing Interventions**

- Assess client's readiness to choose through active listening.
- Use anticipatory guidance by proactively providing the client with information. (Refer to Impaired Emancipated **Decision-Making.**)
- Establish a purposeful provider–client relationship.
- ▲ Include multiprofessional health care team members as needed to increase knowledge of chosen option.
- Provide decision-making support. (Refer to Impaired Emancipated **Decision-Making.**)
- Continue to provide a flexible environment for client to enact choice.
- Encourage the client to use personal knowledge as part of the decision-making process to increase decisional satisfaction.

**Pediatric**

- Understand interventions that parents prefer when in the decision-making process.

**Multicultural**

- Use open communication to assist clients to develop health care plans to which they can adhere.

**Home Care/Nursing Home Care**

- Optimize self-care personal knowledge for home care.
- Refer to care plan Impaired Emancipated **Decision-Making** for additional interventions for pediatric, critical care, geriatric, and multicultural care.

• = Independent ▲ = Collaborative

# Risk for Impaired Emancipated Decision-Making

**Domain 10** Life principles    **Class 3** Value/belief/action congruence

**D**

## NANDA-I Definition

Susceptible to a process of choosing a health care decision that does not include personal knowledge and/or consideration of social norms, or does not occur in a flexible environment, resulting in decisional dissatisfaction.

## Risk Factors

Decreased understanding of available health care options; difficulty adequately verbalizing perceptions about health care options; inadequate confidence to openly discuss health care options; inadequate information regarding health care options; inadequate privacy to openly discuss health care options; inadequate self-confidence in decision-making; insufficient time to discuss health care options

## At-Risk Population

Individuals with limited decision making experience; women accessing health care from systems with patriarchal hierarchy; women living in families with patriarchal hierarchy

## Client Outcomes

**Client Will (Specify Time Frame)**

- Verbalize option outcomes freely before making a health care decision in a private setting with in which they feel comfortable
- Freely verbalize own opinion with health care providers before making a health care decision
- Discuss how options fit or hinder his or her lifestyle within an appropriate amount of time that allows enactment of the choice
- Discuss concerns about others' opinions before making the health care choice
- Decrease stress about others' opinions by placing options in perspective through informational resources
- Discuss the time frame in which the decision needs to be made

## Nursing Interventions

- Assess client's vulnerability for an impaired decision-making process.
- Assess the client's experience with decision-making.
- Recognize the traditional hierarchical family and health care system.
- Provide privacy to discuss health care options.
- Allow the client time to choose.
- ▲ Understand the primary health care providers' role in the decision-making process.
- Provide informational resources.

• = Independent      ▲ = Collaborative

D

• Provide encouragement so clients increase their confidence in the decision-making process.

**Pediatric**

• Understand the parent/guardian's vulnerability when making health care decisions for their children.
• Understand the adolescent decision-making processes.
• Refer to care plan Impaired **Emancipated Decision-Making** for additional interventions for critical care, geriatric, multicultural care, and home care.

# Ineffective Denial

**Domain 9** Coping/stress tolerance     **Class 2** Coping responses

## NANDA-I Definition

Conscious or unconscious attempt to disavow the knowledge or meaning of an event to reduce anxiety and/or fear, leading to the detriment of health.

## Defining Characteristics

Delayed search for health care; denies fear of death; denies fear of disability; displaced source of symptoms; does not admit impact of disease on life; does not perceive relevance of danger; does not perceive relevance of symptoms; fear displacement regarding impact of condition; inappropriate affect; minimizes symptoms; refuses health care; uses dismissive comments when speaking of distressing event; uses dismissive gestures when speaking of distressing event; uses treatment not advised

## Related Factors

Anxiety; excessive stress; fear of death; fear of losing personal autonomy; fear of separation; inadequate emotional support; inadequate sense of control; ineffective coping strategies; perceived inadequacy in dealing with strong emotions; threat of unpleasant reality

## Outcomes

Client Will (Specify Time Frame)

• Demonstrate understanding of a crisis event or change in health status
• Seek out appropriate health care attention when needed
• Demonstrate adherence to treatment regimen
• Display appropriate affect and verbalize fears
• Actively engage in treatment program related to substance misuse as needed
• Remain substance free
• Demonstrate alternate adaptive coping mechanism

• = Independent          ▲ = Collaborative

## Nursing Interventions

- Establish a trusting nurse–client relationship.
- Assess the client's and family's understanding of the illness the person is experiencing and the feeling states evoked.
- Express empathetic concern for the anxiety that can be evoked as a person considers the forced adjustments and potential limitations imposed due to the development of a chronic illness or stressful event that leads to a change in lifestyle.
- Function as a knowledgeable resource for clients who rely on home remedies or complementary and alternative medicine.
- ▲ Support referral to a medical or mental health professional when the use of denial or extreme levels of anxiety significantly interfere with health care needs; the use of motivational interviewing is one counseling method to facilitate change.
- Aid the client in making choices regarding treatment and actively involve him or her in the decision-making process.
- Allow the client to express and use denial as a coping mechanism if appropriate to treatment.
- Assist the client in using existing and additional sources of support.
- Refer to care plans for Defensive **Coping** and Dysfunctional **Family** Processes.

### Geriatric

- Engage the person in any decision making about health care issues.
- Enlist the family and significant others to help support the individual.
- Allow the client to explain his or her concepts of health care needs, and then use reality-focused techniques whenever possible to provide feedback.
- Encourage communication among family members.

### Multicultural

- Discuss with the client those aspects of his or her health behavior/lifestyle that will remain unchanged by health status and those aspects of health behavior that need to be modified to improve health status.
- Establish a trusting relationship. Recognize the role that *medical mistrust* plays in the client's and family's ability to acknowledge health status. Groups who have faced exploitation and discrimination at the hands of the medical/health care community are at greater risk of struggling with this potential barrier.
- Support the client's spiritual coping.

### Home Care

- Previously mentioned interventions may be adapted for home care utilization.

• = Independent          ▲ = Collaborative

**D**

- Provide family with education about the individual's disease process, the grief process, and how to support a loved one through a difficult situation to encourage meaningful family support.
- Observe family interaction and roles. Encourage effective communication between family members.
- Support the use of peer support networks, including formal support groups, community group-based programs, and online social media platforms.
▲ Observe family interaction and roles. Refer the client/family for follow-up if prolonged denial is a risk.

**Client/Family Teaching and Discharge Planning**
- Instruct client and family to recognize the signs and symptoms of recurring illness and the appropriate responses to alterations in client's health status.
▲ Inform family of available community support resources.

## Impaired Dentition

**Domain 11** Safety/protection   **Class 2** Physical injury
### NANDA-I Definition

Disruption in tooth development/eruption pattern or structural integrity of individual teeth.

### Defining Characteristics

Abraded teeth; absence of teeth; dental caries; enamel discoloration; eroded enamel; excessive oral calculus; excessive oral plaque; facial asymmetry; halitosis; incomplete tooth eruption for age; loose tooth; malocclusion; premature loss of primary teeth; root caries; tooth fracture; tooth misalignment; toothache

### Related Factors

Difficulty accessing dental care; difficulty performing oral self-care; excessive intake of fluoride; excessive use of abrasive oral cleaning agents; habitual use of staining substance; inadequate dietary habits; inadequate knowledge of dental health; inadequate oral hygiene habits; malnutrition

### At-Risk Population

Economically disadvantaged individuals; individuals with genetic predisposition to dental disorders

### Associated Conditions

Bruxism; chronic vomiting; oral temperature sensitivity; pharmaceutical preparations

• = Independent          ▲ = Collaborative

## Client Outcomes
### Client Will (Specify Time Frame)
- Have clean teeth, healthy pink gums
- Be free of halitosis
- Explain and demonstrate how to perform oral care
- Demonstrate ability to masticate foods without difficulty
- State absence of pain in mouth

## Nursing Interventions
▲ Inspect oral cavity/teeth/gingiva at least once daily and note any discoloration, presence of debris, amount of plaque buildup, presence of lesions such as white lesions or patches, edema, or bleeding, and intactness of teeth. Refer to a dentist or periodontist as appropriate.

- If the client is free of bleeding disorders and able to swallow, encourage toothbrushing with a soft toothbrush using fluoride-containing toothpaste at least two times per day. Do not use foam swabs or lemon glycerin swabs to clean the teeth.

- The toothbrush is the most important tool for oral care. Twice daily mechanical toothbrushing is the most effective method of reducing plaque and controlling periodontal disease (Pitchika et al, 2019).

- Normal gums should be pink and firm.

- Encourage the client to perform interdental hygiene by flossing or cleaning between teeth with interdental brushes, woodsticks, or oral irrigation at least once per day if free of a bleeding disorder. If the client is unable to floss, assist with flossing or encourage the use of an oral irrigator (i.e., "water flossing").

- Use a rotation-oscillation power toothbrush for removal of dental plaque. If the client has a fixed orthodontic appliance, particularly any appliance that limits access or toothbrushing motion, a manual toothbrush may be used.

- Determine the client's mental status and manual dexterity; if the client is unable to care for self, nursing personnel must provide dental hygiene. The nursing diagnosis Bathing **Self-Care** Deficit is then applicable.

- If the client is unable to brush his or her own teeth, follow this procedure:
  ○ Position the client sitting upright or on side.
  ○ Use a soft bristle toothbrush.
  ○ Use fluoride toothpaste and tap water or saline as a solution.
  ○ Brush teeth with a manual toothbrush by positioning the brush at a 45-degree angle and directing the bristle tips just below the gingival margin.

**D**

- ○ Brush teeth with an oscillating toothbrush by positioning the brush over the teeth and directing the edge of the oscillating bristle head just below the gingival margin.
  ○ Suction as needed.
- Monitor the client's nutritional and fluid status to determine if adequate. Recommend the client eat a balanced diet and limit between-meal snacks.
- Recommend that the client maintain a healthy diet with limited sugar intake; in particular, the client should limit sugary beverages and snacks.
- Instruct the client with halitosis to clean the tongue when performing oral hygiene. Brush tongue with a tongue scraper or toothbrush and follow with a mouth rinse.
- Determine the client's usual method of oral care. Whenever possible, build on the client's existing knowledge base and current practices to develop an individualized plan of care, including strategies to support oral hygiene as a routine habit.
- Instruct the client on effective toothbrushing technique. A manual toothbrush should be held at a 45-degree angle to the gums; clients should brush using short lateral strokes, gently directing the bristle tips just below the gingival margin, brushing all surfaces of each tooth. An oscillating toothbrush should be placed directly over each tooth with the bristled head just below the gingival margin; the client should brush all surfaces of each tooth.
- Instruct the client to use a soft-bristled toothbrush, which should be replaced every 3 to 4 months or sooner if bristles begin to appear splayed or worn.
- Recommend appropriate therapeutic mouthwashes to prevent or reduce symptoms of periodontal disease, including plaque, gingivitis, caries, and halitosis. Over-the-counter mouthwashes containing mint or essential oils may be used in combination with toothbrushing and interdental cleaning to maintain oral health. Avoid routine use of hydrogen peroxide, chlorhexidine, or alcohol-based mouthwashes.
- Recommend client see a dentist at prescribed intervals, generally two times per year (recommended frequency depends on overall oral health and potential comorbidities).
- If there are any signs of bleeding when the teeth are brushed, refer the client to a dentist. If bleeding accompanies apparently inflamed gums, refer client to a periodontist.
- If platelets are low, use a soft-bristled toothbrush with a fluoride-containing toothpaste to maintain oral hygiene. Flossing should

• = Independent          ▲ = Collaborative

be avoided if it stimulates gingival bleeding. Moistened toothettes and mild cleaning fluids (e.g., saline rinse) may be used if thrombocytopenia is severe.

- Provide meticulous dental care/oral care to prevent hospital-acquired (or extended care–acquired) pneumonia.
- Provide scrupulous dental care to critically ill clients, including ventilated clients to prevent ventilator-associated pneumonia.
- If teeth are nonfunctional for chewing, modification of oral intake (e.g., edentulous diet, soft diet) may be necessary. The nursing diagnosis Imbalanced **Nutrition:** Less Than Body Requirements may apply.
- If the client is unable to swallow, keep suction nearby when providing oral care.
- See care plan for Impaired **Oral Mucous Membrane** Integrity.

**Pregnant Client**

- Encourage the expectant mother to eat a healthy, balanced diet that is rich in calcium and abstain from alcohol during pregnancy. The teeth usually start to form in the gums during the second trimester of pregnancy..
- Instruct the pregnant mother to perform twice-daily meticulous oral care.
- Advise the pregnant mother not to smoke.

**Infant Oral Hygiene**

- Gently wipe the infant's gums with a clean washcloth or sterile gauze at least once a day.
- Never allow the infant to fall asleep with a bottle containing milk, formula, fruit juice, or sweetened liquids. Instead, parents may give the infant a bottle filled with cool water or provide a clean pacifier recommended by the dentist or health care provider. Do not dip pacifiers in sweet liquids. Avoid filling the infant's bottle with liquids such as sugar water and soft drinks.
- Maintain meticulous parental and infant oral hygiene and avoid use of shared utensils or prechewing food when feeding the infant.
- Instruct parents to begin toothbrushing at first tooth eruption, twice daily using a small, soft toothbrush with a rice grain–sized amount of fluoride-containing toothpaste (a pea-sized amount should be used in children older than 3 years of age).
- Advise parents to begin regular dental visits at 12 months; parents should establish a "dental home" for routine care, including early application of dental fluoride.

• = Independent ▲ = Collaborative

**Older Children**
▲ Encourage the family to talk with the dentist about dental sealants or fluoride varnishes, which can help reduce biofilm and prevent cavities in permanent teeth.
• Teach children to brush teeth twice a day and begin flossing when directed by their dentist; instruct parents to provide support and guidance as needed until children are independent in the task.
• Recommend that parents should not allow the child to smoke or chew tobacco, and stress the importance of setting a good example by not using tobacco products themselves.
• Recommend the child drink fluoridated water when possible and use fluoride-containing toothpaste.

**Geriatric**
• Provide dentists with accurate medication history to avoid drug interactions and client harm. If the client is taking anticoagulants, laboratory values should be reviewed before providing dental care.
• Help clients brush their own teeth twice daily; if clients lack dexterity, provide assistance or modified equipment to support self-care.
• If the client has dementia or delirium and exhibits care-resistant behavior such as fighting, biting, or refusing care, use the following method:
  ○ Ensure client is in a quiet environment, such as his or her own bathroom, and sitting or standing at the sink to prime memory for appropriate actions.
  ○ Approach the client at eye level within his or her range of vision.
  ○ Approach with a smile, and begin conversation with a touch of the hand and gradually move up.
  ○ Use mirror–mirror technique, standing behind the client, and brush and floss teeth.
  ○ Use respectful adult speech. Avoid "elderspeak," a style of speech characterized by short phrases and questions uttered in a sing-song voice and use of collective pronouns and intimate terms (e.g., first name, nicknames, "deary" or "honey").
  ○ Promote self-care when client brushes own teeth if possible.
  ○ Use distractors when needed: talking, reminiscing, singing.
▲ Ensure that dentures are removed and cleaned regularly, after each meal and before bedtime. Brush and rinse dentures to remove debris and soak overnight in a peroxide-based cleaning solution. Dentures left in the mouth at night impede circulation to the palate and predispose the client to oral lesions.

• = Independent          ▲ = Collaborative

▲ Support other caregivers by providing oral hygiene. Physical and cognitive impairment in older adults can interfere with the client's ability to perform oral hygiene, and oral hygiene should be provided by a caregiver. If no caregiver is available, the client is prone to dental problems such as dental caries, tooth abscess, tooth fracture, and gingival and periodontal disease.

**Multicultural**

- Assess for the influence of cultural beliefs, norms, and values on the client's understanding of dental care.
- Assess for barriers to access to dental care, such as lack of insurance.

**Home Care**

- Assess client patterns for daily and professional dental care and related patterns (e.g., smoking, nail biting). Assess for environmental influences on dental status (e.g., fluoride).
- Assess client facilities and financial resources for providing dental care.
- Request dietary log from the client, adding column for type of food (i.e., soft, pureed, regular).
- Observe a typical meal to assess first-hand the effect of impaired dentition on nutrition.
- Assist the client with accessing financial or other resources.

**Client/Family Teaching and Discharge Planning**

- Teach how to inspect the oral cavity and monitor for problems with the teeth and gums.
- Teach clients to implement a personal plan of dental hygiene, including appropriate toothbrushing and interdental cleaning. Consider motivational interviewing sessions to promote self-care.
- Educate clients to change their toothbrush every 3 to 4 months to ensure effective plaque removal.
- Teach the client the value of having an optimal fluoride concentration in drinking water and to brush teeth twice daily with toothpaste containing fluoride.
- Teach clients of all ages about the need to decrease intake of sugary foods and to brush teeth regularly.
- Inform individuals who are considering oral piercing or body modification of the potential complications such as infection, development of oral "tic" behaviors, tooth chipping, or gingival recession. If client undergoes oral body modification, teach the client how to care for the wound and prevent complications.
- Advise clients to avoid smoking.

• = Independent          ▲ = Collaborative

# Delayed Child Development

**Domain 13** Growth/development    **Class 2** Development
## NANDA-I Definition
Child who continually fails to achieve developmental milestones within the expected timeframe.
## Defining Characteristics
Consistent difficulty performing cognitive skills typical of age group; consistent difficulty performing language skills typical of age group; consistent difficulty performing motor skills typical of age group; consistent difficulty performing psychosocial skills typical of age group
## Related Factors
### Infant or Child Factors
Inadequate access to health care provider; inadequate attachment behavior; inadequate stimulation; unaddressed abuse; unaddressed psychological neglect
### Caregiver Factors
Anxiety; decreased emotional support availability; depressive symptoms; excessive stress; unaddressed domestic violence
## At-Risk Population
Children aged 0-9 years; children born to economically disadvantaged families; children exposed to community violence; children exposed to environmental pollutants; children whose caregivers have developmental disabilities; children whose mothers had inadequate prenatal care; children with below normal growth standards for age and gender; institutionalized children; low birth weight infants; premature infants
## Associated Conditions
Antenatal pharmaceutical preparations; congenital disorders; depression; inborn genetic diseases; maternal mental disorders; maternal physical illnesses; prenatal substance misuse; sensation disorders
## Client Outcomes
### Client/Parents/Primary Caregiver Will (Specify Time Frame)
- Child will achieve expected milestones in all areas of development (physical, cognitive, academic, and psychosocial)
- Parent/caregiver will verbalize understanding of potential impediments to normal development and demonstrate actions or environmental/lifestyle changes necessary to provide appropriate care in a safe, nurturing environment
## Nursing Interventions
### Preconception/Pregnancy
- Assess for nutritional status during pregnancy. Review the importance of iron, folate, iodine, choline, and essential fatty acids.

• = Independent          ▲ = Collaborative

- Assess for alcohol/drug use during pregnancy. Expectant mothers should be instructed that no amount of alcohol consumption is safe during pregnancy.
- Assess and educate about consumption of marijuana use in pregnancy.
- Educate expectant mothers to stop smoking and assist with methods of smoking cessation. Smoking is an avoidable risk factor for low birth weight and other significant prenatal issues.
- Educate that it is recommended that women of childbearing age take 400 mcg of folic acid daily, along with a healthy, well-balanced diet, to reduce the risk of neural tube and other birth defects.

**Neonate/Infant**
- Educate new mothers about the importance of breastfeeding.
- Assess the neonate/infant for age-appropriate milestones.
- Assess for maternal depression when caring for a newborn infant.
- Provide information to parents about the importance of health supervision visits at the following intervals: first week of life, 1 month, 2 months, 4 months, 6 months, 9 months, and 12 months, with standardized developmental screen at 9 months old.
- Teach parents about the necessity of daily tummy time for infants less than 6 months old.
- Explain the use of developmentally appropriate toys for play.
- Monitor mother–baby interactions when caring for premature infants.

**Toddler/Preschooler/School-Age**
- Assess for the effects of social disruption on cognitive abilities.
- Educate about the importance of eating a well-balanced diet in early childhood.
- Assess for age-appropriate milestones and developmental history at every visit.
- Autism spectrum disorder (ASD) screening should be conducted at the 18-month and 24-month visits.
- Educate parents about the importance of health supervision visits yearly with standardized developmental screening at 30 months' old and then again at the 4- to 5-year-old visit.
- Monitor preterm infants more closely for developmental delays.
- Provide support and education to parents of toddlers with developmental disabilities (e.g., Down's syndrome [DS], cerebral palsy).
- Provide parents and caregivers with information about speech-language development, play development, and speech-language stimulation strategies for children with language delay. Refer to speech and language specialists as needed.

• = Independent          ▲ = Collaborative

---

- Monitor for maternal eating disorders because they have a direct effect on childhood development.
- Educate parents about the importance of avoiding lead-based paints in the home and other sources of lead in the environment.
▲ Refer parents and caregivers of children with language delays to Enhanced Milieu Teaching (EMT).

**D**

## Risk for Delayed Child Development

**Domain 13** Growth/development    **Class 2** Development

### NANDA-I Definition

Child who is susceptible to failure to achieve developmental milestones within the expected timeframe.

### Risk Factors

**Infant or Child Factors**

Inadequate access to health care provider; inadequate attachment behavior; inadequate stimulation; unaddressed abuse; unaddressed psychological neglect

**Caregiver Factors**

Anxiety; decreased emotional support availability; depressive symptoms; excessive stress; unaddressed domestic violence

### At-Risk Population

Children aged 0-9 years; children born to economically disadvantaged families; children exposed to community violence; children exposed to environmental pollutants; children whose caregivers have developmental disabilities; children whose mothers had inadequate prenatal care; children with below normal growth standards for age and gender; institutionalized children; low birth weight infants; premature infants

### Associated Conditions

Antenatal pharmaceutical preparations; congenital disorders; depression; inborn genetic diseases; maternal mental disorders; maternal physical illnesses; prenatal substance misuse; sensation disorders

### Client Outcomes, Nursing Interventions, and Client/Family Teaching

Refer to care plan for Delayed Child **Development**.

## Delayed Infant Motor Development

**Domain 13** Growth/development    **Class 2** Development

• = Independent           ▲ = Collaborative

## NANDA-I Definition

Individual who consistently fails to achieve developmental milestones related to the normal strengthening of bones, muscles and ability to move and touch one's surroundings.

## Defining Characteristics

Difficulty lifting head; difficulty maintaining head position; difficulty picking up blocks; difficulty pulling self to stand; difficulty rolling over; difficulty sitting with support; difficulty sitting without support; difficulty standing with assistance; difficulty transferring objects; difficulty with hand-and-knee crawling; does not engage in activities; does not initiate activities

## Related Factors

### Infant Factors

Difficulty with sensory processing; insufficient curiosity; insufficient initiative; insufficient persistence

### Caregiver Factors

Anxiety about infant care; carries infant in arms for excessive time; does not allow infant to choose physical activities; does not allow infant to choose toys; does not encourage infant to grasp; does not encourage infant to reach; does not encourage sufficient infant play with other children; does not engage infant in games about body parts; does not teach movement words; insufficient fine motor toys for infant; insufficient gross motor toys for infant; insufficient time between periods of infant stimulation; limits infant experiences in the prone position; maternal postpartum depressive symptoms; negative perception of infant temperament; overstimulation of infant; perceived infant care incompetence

## At-Risk Population

Boys; infants aged 0-12 months; infants born to economically disadvantaged families; infants born to large families; infants born to parents with low educational levels; infants in intensive care units; infants living in home with inadequate physical space; infants whose mothers had inadequate antenatal diet; infants with below normal growth standards for age and gender; low birth weight infants; premature infants; premature infants who do not receive physiotherapy during hospitalization

## Associated Conditions

5 Minute Appearance, Pulse, Grimace, Activity, & Respiration (APGAR) score < 7; antenatal pharmaceutical preparations; complex medical conditions; failure to thrive; maternal anemia in late pregnancy; maternal mental health disorders in early pregnancy; maternal prepregnancy obesity; neonatal abstinence syndrome; neurodevelopmental disorders; postnatal infection of preterm infant; sensation disorders

• = Independent          ▲ = Collaborative

## Client Outcomes

**Client/Parents/Primary Caregiver Will (Specify Time Frame)**

- Infant will achieve expected milestones in all areas of physical and motor development

**D**

- Parent/caregiver will verbalize understanding of potential impediments to normal development and demonstrate actions or environmental/lifestyle changes necessary to provide appropriate care in a safe, nurturing environment

## Nursing Interventions

**Preconception/Pregnancy**

- Assess for nutritional status during pregnancy. Review the importance of iron, folate, iodine, choline, and essential fatty acids.
- Assess for alcohol/drug use during pregnancy. Expectant mothers should be instructed that no amount of alcohol consumption is safe during pregnancy.
- Assess and educate about consumption of marijuana use in pregnancy.
- Educate expectant mothers to stop smoking and assist with methods of smoking cessation. Smoking is an avoidable risk factor for low birth weight and other significant prenatal issues.
- Educate that it is recommended that women of childbearing age take 400 mcg of folic acid daily, along with a healthy, well-balanced diet, to reduce the risk of neural tube and other birth defects.

**Neonate/Infant**

- Educate new mothers about the importance of breastfeeding.
- Assess the neonate/infant for age-appropriate milestones.
- Assess for maternal depression.
- Provide information to parents about the importance of health supervision visits at the following intervals: first week of life, 1 month, 2 months, 4 months, 6 months, 9 months, and 12 months, with standardized developmental screen at 9 months old.
- Teach parents about the necessity of daily tummy time for infants less than 6 months old.
- Explain the use of developmentally appropriate toys for play.
- Monitor mother–baby interactions when caring for premature infants.
- Educate about the importance of eating a well-balanced diet in early childhood.
- Monitor preterm infants more closely for developmental delays.
- Provide parents or caregiver with teaching to provide postural support and opportunities for movement with support during parent–infant interactions with the goal of increasing infant movement quality and quantity.

• = Independent          ▲ = Collaborative

- Provide support and education to parents of infants with developmental disabilities (c.g., Down's syndrome [DS], cerebral palsy).
- Provide education and support for parents of infants with tracheostomy to promote early motor development.
- Monitor for maternal eating disorders because they have a direct effect on childhood development.
- Educate parents about the importance of avoiding lead-based paints in the home and other sources of lead in the environment.

# Risk for Delayed Infant Motor Development

**Domain 13** Growth/development     **Class 2** Development

## NANDA-I Definition

Individual susceptible to fails to achieve developmental milestones related to the normal strengthening of bones, muscles and ability to move and touch one's surroundings.

## Risk Factors

### Infant Factors

Difficulty with sensory processing; insufficient curiosity; insufficient initiative; insufficient persistence

### Caregiver Factors

Anxiety about infant care; carries infant in arms for excessive time; does not allow infant to choose physical activities; does not allow infant to choose toys; does not encourage infant to grasp; does not encourage infant to reach; does not encourage sufficient infant play with other children; does not engage infant in games about body parts; does not teach movement words; insufficient fine motor toys for infant; insufficient gross motor toys for infant; insufficient time between periods of infant stimulation; limits infant experiences in the prone position; maternal postpartum depressive symptoms; negative perception of infant temperament; overstimulation of infant; perceived infant care incompetence

### At-Risk Population

Boys; infants aged 0-12 months; infants born to economically disadvantaged families; infants born to large families; infants born to parents with low educational levels; infants in intensive care units; infants living in home with inadequate physical space; infants whose mothers had inadequate antenatal diet; infants with below normal growth standards for age and gender; low birth weight infants; premature infants; premature infants who do not receive physiotherapy during hospitalization

• = Independent          ▲ = Collaborative

D

## Associated Conditions

5 Minute Appearance, Pulse, Grimace, Activity, & Respiration (APGAR) score <7; antenatal pharmaceutical preparations; complex medical conditions; failure to thrive; maternal anemia in late pregnancy; maternal mental health disorders in early pregnancy; maternal prepregnancy obesity; neonatal abstinence syndrome; neurodevelopmental disorders; postnatal infection of preterm infant; sensation disorders

## Client Outcomes, Nursing Interventions, and Client/Family Teaching

Refer to care plan for Delayed Infant Motor **Development.**

# Diarrhea

**Domain 3** Elimination and exchange   **Class 2** Gastrointestinal function

## NANDA-I Definition

Passage of three or more loose or liquid stools per day.

## Defining Characteristics

Abdominal cramping; abdominal pain; bowel urgency; dehydration; hyperactive bowel sounds

## Related Factors

Anxiety; early formula feeding; inadequate access to safe drinking water; inadequate access to safe food; inadequate knowledge about rotavirus vaccine; inadequate knowledge about sanitary food preparation; inadequate knowledge about sanitary food storage; inadequate personal hygiene practices; increased stress level; laxative misuse; malnutrition; substance misuse

## At-Risk Population

Frequent travelers; individuals at extremes of age; individuals exposed to toxins

## Associated Conditions

Critical illness; endocrine system diseases; enteral nutrition; gastrointestinal diseases; immunosuppression; infections; pharmaceutical preparations; treatment regimen

## Client Outcomes

**Client Will (Specify Time Frame)**

- Defecate formed, soft stool every 1 to 3 days
- Maintain the perirectal area free of irritation
- State relief from cramping and less or no diarrhea
- Explain cause of diarrhea and rationale for treatment
- Maintain good skin turgor and weight at usual level
- Have negative stool cultures

• = Independent        ▲ = Collaborative

## Nursing Interventions

- Recognize that diarrhea is defined as the passage of three or more loose or liquid stools in a 24-hour period (Shane et al, 2017).
- Assess pattern of defecation or have the client keep a diary that includes the following: time of day defecation occurs; usual stimulus for defecation; consistency, amount, and frequency of stool; type of, amount of, and time food consumed; fluid intake; history of bowel habits and laxative use; diet; exercise patterns; obstetrical/gynecological, medical, and surgical histories; medications; alterations in perianal sensations; and present bowel regimen.
- Recommend use of standardized tool to consistently assess, quantify, and then treat diarrhea.
- Although the abdominal examination has been historically performed in the order of inspection, auscultation, palpation, and percussion, recent scientific investigations have found that palpation and percussion do not affect the number of bowel sounds (Çalış et al, 2019; Vizioli et al, 2020).
- ▲ Use an evidence-based bowel management protocol that includes identifying and treating the cause of the diarrhea, obtaining a stool specimen if infectious etiology is suspected, evaluating current medications and osmolality of enteral feedings, assessing and treating hydration status of client, reviewing and stopping ordered and/or over-the-counter (OTC) laxatives, assessing food preparation practices, assessing home environment, providing good skin care and applying barrier creams to prevent skin irritation from diarrhea, and evaluating the need for antidiarrheal agents and possible fecal containment device with provider.
- Identify the cause of diarrhea if possible based on history (e.g., infection, gastrointestinal inflammation, medication effect, malnutrition or malabsorption, laxative abuse, osmotic enteral feedings, anxiety, stress).
- Identification of the underlying cause is important because the treatment is determined based on the cause of diarrhea.
- ▲ Testing for diarrhea may consist of laboratory work such as a complete blood count with differential and blood cultures if the client is febrile. Also obtain stool specimens as ordered to either rule out or diagnose an infectious process (e.g., ova and parasites, *Clostridioides [Clostridium] difficile* infection [CDI], bacterial cultures for food poisoning).
- Consider the possibility of CDI if the client over the age of 2 years has any of the following: watery diarrhea, low-grade fever, abdominal

**D**

cramps, history of antibiotic therapy, history of gastrointestinal tract surgery, and if the client is taking medications that reduce gastric acid, including proton-pump inhibitors (PPIs), or if diarrhea occurs in the hospital setting. Any antibiotic can cause CDI, but clindamycin, cephalosporins, β-lactam/β-lactamase inhibitors, and fluoroquinolones pose the greatest risk, as do multiple antibiotics and longer duration of antibiotics (Shane et al, 2017; McDonald et al, 2018).

- Use standard precautions when caring for clients with diarrhea to prevent spread of infectious diarrhea; for individuals with a CDI, employ contact precautions until 48 hours after diarrhea has resolved; use gloves, gowns, and, when able, disposable equipment; perform handwashing with soap and water; perform routine room and equipment decontamination with a *C. difficile* sporicidal agent; provide a private room or cohort with other clients with a CDI; and provide a dedicated toilet to reduce transmission. *C. difficile* and viruses causing diarrhea have been shown to be highly contagious. *C. difficile* is difficult to eradicate because of spore formation (Shane et al, 2017; McDonald et al, 2018).

▲ Antibiotic stewardship is an important aspect in the prevention of *C. difficile* infections. If the client has diarrhea associated with antibiotic therapy, consult with the health care provider regarding the use of probiotics, such as yogurt with active cultures, to treat diarrhea, or probiotic dietary supplements, or preferably use probiotics to prevent diarrhea when first beginning antibiotic therapy.

▲ Probiotics may also be ordered for immunocompetent clients to prevent a CDI when high-risk antibiotics are prescribed; if a probiotic is ordered, administer it with food. Recommend that it should be taken through the antibiotic course and 10 to 14 days afterward.

▲ Recognize that a CDI can commonly recur and that reculturing of stool is often required before initiating retreatment.

- Have the client complete a diet diary for 7 days and monitor the intake of high-fructose corn syrup and fructose sweeteners in relation to onset of diarrhea symptoms. If diarrhea is associated with fructose ingestion, intake should be limited or eliminated.

▲ If the client has infectious diarrhea, consider avoiding use of medications that slow peristalsis.

- Assess for dehydration by observing skin turgor over sternum or delayed capillary refill and inspecting for longitudinal furrows of the tongue. Watch for excessive thirst, fever, dizziness, lightheadedness, palpitations, excessive cramping, bloody stools, hypotension, and symptoms of shock.

• = Independent        ▲ = Collaborative

▲ Administer oral rehydration solution, consisting of a balanced sodium, potassium, and glucose solution, for individuals with mild to moderate dehydration or in individuals with mild dehydration associated with vomiting or severe diarrhea; provide isotonic intravenous solutions for severe dehydration, shock, or altered mental states (Shane et al, 2017; Ofei & Fuchs, 2019).

• Refer to care plans for Deficient **Fluid** Volume and Risk for Imbalanced **Fluid** Volume if appropriate.

▲ If the client has frequent or chronic diarrhea, consider suggesting use of dietary fiber after consultation with a nutritionist and/or provider.

▲ If diarrhea is chronic and there is evidence of malnutrition, consult with the provider for a dietary consultation and possible nutrition supplementation to maintain nutrition while the gastrointestinal system heals (Pitta et al, 2019).

• Encourage the client to eat small, frequent meals, eating foods that are easy to digest at first (e.g., bananas, crackers, pretzels, rice, potatoes, clear soups, applesauce), but switch to a regular diet as soon as tolerated. Also recommend avoiding milk products, foods high in fiber, and caffeine (dark sodas, tea, coffee, chocolate).

• Provide a readily available bathroom, commode, or bedpan; provide individuals with a CDI with a dedicated toilet to reduce transmission to other clients (McDonald et al, 2018).

• Thoroughly cleanse and dry the perianal and perineal skin daily as needed using a cleanser capable of stool removal. Apply skin moisture barrier cream as needed. Refer to perirectal skin care in the care plan for Impaired Bowel **Continence.**

▲ If the client has enteral tube feedings and diarrhea, consider infusion rate; position of feeding tube; tonicity of formula; fiber content in the formula; possible formula contamination; and excessive intake of hyperosmolar medications, such as sorbitol commonly found in the liquid version of medications; administer antidiarrheal medications such as loperamide as prescribed (Tatsumi, 2019; Pitta et al, 2019). Consider changing the formula to a lower osmolarity, lactose-free, or high-fiber feeding.

• Avoid administering bolus enteral feedings or hyperosmolar formulas directly into the small bowel.

▲ Dilute liquid medications before administration through the enteral tube and flush the enteral feeding tube with sufficient water before and after medication administration.

• Teach clients with cancer the types of diarrhea they may encounter, emphasizing not only chemotherapy- and radiation-induced diarrhea

• = Independent          ▲ = Collaborative

D

but also *C. difficile,* along with associated signs and symptoms and treatments.

▲ For chemotherapy-induced diarrhea (CID) and radiation-induced diarrhea (RID), review rationale for pharmacological interventions, along with soluble fiber and probiotic supplements. Consult a registered dietitian to assist with recommendations to alleviate diarrhea, decrease dehydration, and maintain nutritional status.

▲ Acute traveler's diarrhea is the most common illness affecting individuals traveling to, usually, low-income regions of the world.

**Pediatric**

▲ Assess for mild or moderate signs of dehydration with both acute and persistent diarrhea: mild (increased thirst and dry mouth or tongue) and moderate (decreased urination; no wet diapers for 3+ hours; feeling of weakness/lightheadedness, irritability, or listlessness; few or no tears when crying) (Gupta, 2016). Refer to primary care provider for treatment.

▲ Recommend that parents give the child oral rehydration fluids to drink in the amounts specified by the health care provider, especially during the first 4 to 6 hours to replace lost fluid; avoid sodas, fruit juices, and clear liquids such as water and chicken broth. Once the child is rehydrated, an orally administered maintenance solution should be used along with food. Continue even if child vomits.

• Recommend that the mother resume breastfeeding as soon as possible.

• Recommend that parents avoid giving the child flat soda, fruit juices, sports drinks, gelatin dessert, broth, or instant fruit drink.

• Recommend that parents give children foods with complex carbohydrates, such as potatoes, rice, bread, cereal, yogurt, fruits, and vegetables. Avoid fatty foods, foods high in simple sugars, and milk products.

• Advise parents to return for assistance if fever, bloody diarrhea, or signs of severe dehydration such as decreased urine output, lightheadedness, or lethargy occur.

• Recommend CDC principles of safe food preparation, which include clean, separate, cook, chill, and report, particularly for children under the age of 5 years (US Department of Health and Human Services, 2019).

▲ Recommend rotavirus vaccine within the child's vaccination schedule.

**Geriatric**

▲ Evaluate medications the client is taking. Recognize that many medications can result in diarrhea, including digitalis, propranolol, angiotensin-converting enzyme inhibitors, histamine-receptor antagonists, nonsteroidal antiinflammatory drugs, anticholinergic agents, oral hypoglycemia agents, antibiotics, and so forth.

▲ Monitor the client closely to detect whether an impaction is causing diarrhea; remove impaction as ordered. Clients with fecal impaction commonly experience leakage of mucus or liquid stool from the rectum, rectal irritation, distention, and impaired anal sensation (Schiller, Pardi, & Sellin, 2017; Pitta et al, 2019).

▲ Seek medical attention if diarrhea is severe or persists for more than 24 hours, or if the client has a history of dehydration or electrolyte disturbances, such as lassitude, weakness, or prostration.

• Provide emotional support for clients who are having trouble controlling unpredictable episodes of diarrhea.

**Home Care**

• Previously mentioned interventions may be adapted for home care use to keep the client well hydrated.

• Assess the home for general sanitation and methods of food preparation. Reinforce principles of sanitation for food handling.

• Assess for methods of handling soiled laundry if the client is bed bound or has been incontinent. Instruct or reinforce universal precautions with family and bloodborne pathogen precautions with agency caregivers.

• When assessing medication history, include OTC drugs, both general and those currently being used to treat the diarrhea. Instruct clients not to mix OTC medications when self-treating.

• Evaluate current medications for indications that specific interventions are warranted. Blood levels of medications may increase during prolonged episodes of diarrhea, indicating the need for close monitoring of the client or direct intervention.

• Teach client importance of food safety practices and hand hygiene after using the toilet, changing a diaper, handling garbage or soiled laundry, and touching animals or their feces or their environment (Shane et al, 2017).

• Teach the client experiencing diarrhea to avoid swimming, water-related activities, and sex with other people while symptomatic (Shane et al, 2017).

▲ Evaluate the need for a home health aide or homemaker service referral. Caregiver may need support for maintaining client cleanliness to prevent skin breakdown.

• Evaluate the need for durable medical equipment in the home. The client may need a bedside commode, call bell, or raised toilet seat to facilitate prompt toileting.

• = Independent          ▲ = Collaborative

**D**

**Client/Family Teaching and Discharge Planning**
- Encourage avoidance of coffee, spices, milk products, and foods that irritate or stimulate the gastrointestinal tract.
- Teach the appropriate method of taking ordered antidiarrheal medications; explain side effects.
- Explain how to prevent the spread of infectious diarrhea (e.g., careful handwashing, appropriate handling and storage of food, and thoroughly cleaning the bathroom and kitchen).
- Help the client to determine stressors and set up an appropriate stress reduction plan, if stress is the cause of diarrhea.
- Teach signs and symptoms of dehydration and electrolyte imbalance.
- Teach perirectal skin care.
▲ Consider teaching clients about complementary therapies, such as probiotics, after consultation with primary care provider.

# Risk for Disuse Syndrome

**Domain 4** Activity/rest    **Class 2** Activity/exercise
## NANDA-I Definition

Susceptible to deterioration of body systems as the result of prescribed or unavoidable musculoskeletal inactivity, which may compromise health.

## Risk Factors

Pain

## Associated Conditions

Decreased level of consciousness; immobilization; paralysis; prescribed movement restrictions

## Client Outcomes

**Client Will (Specify Time Frame)**
- Express pain level that is tolerable to allow for desired mobility
- Maintain full range of motion in joints
- Maintain intact skin, good peripheral blood flow, and normal pulmonary function
- Maintain normal bowel and bladder function
- Express feelings about imposed immobility
- Explain methods to prevent complications of immobility

## Nursing Interventions

- Screen for mobility skills in the following order: (1) bed mobility; (2) supported and unsupported sitting; (3) transitional movements such as sit to stand, stand to sit, and transfers to chair from bed, from chair to bed, and so forth; and (4) standing and walking activities. Use a mobility assessment tool such as the Banner Mobility Assessment

Tool (Boynton et al, 2014) or the ICU Mobility Scale (Hodgson et al, 2014).

- Assess the level of assistance needed by the client and express in terms of amount of effort expended by the person assisting the client. The range is as follows: total assist, meaning client performs 0% to 25% of task and, if client requires the help of more than one caregiver, it is referred to as a dependent transfer; maximum assist, meaning client gives 25% of effort while the caregiver performs the majority of the work; moderate assist, meaning client gives 50% of effort; minimal assist, meaning client gives 75% of effort; contact guard assist, meaning no physical assist is given but caregiver is physically touching client for steadying, guiding, or in case of loss of balance; standby assist, meaning caregiver's hands are up and ready in case needed; supervision, meaning supervision of task is needed even if at a distance; modified independent, meaning client needs assistive device or extra time to accomplish task; and independent, meaning client is able to complete task safely without instruction or assistance.
▲ Request a referral to a physical therapist (PT) as needed so that client's range of motion, muscle strength, balance, coordination, endurance, and early mobilization can be part of the initial evaluation. The PT may provide the client with bed exercises, including stretching, flexing/extending muscle groups, or using bands to maintain muscle strength and tone. Collaboration with nursing staff, therapy, and respiratory therapy as needed to mobilize clients as early and as safely possible.
- Passive range of motion can be done as the client tolerates.
- Use specialized boots to prevent pressure injury on the heels and foot drop; remove boots twice daily to assess the skin and to provide foot care as needed. Elevate heels off the bed as the client tolerates when boots are not in place.
- When positioning a client on the side, tilt client 30 degrees or less while lying on the side.
- Assess skin condition every shift and more frequently if needed. Use a risk assessment tool such as the Braden Scale or Waterlow scale to predict the risk of developing pressure ulcers (now referred to as pressure injury).
- Discuss with staff and management a "safe client handling" policy that may include a "no lift" policy to prevent staff injury.
- Turn clients at high risk for pressure/shear/friction frequently and apply pressure-relieving devices when able.

• = Independent        ▲ = Collaborative

**D**

- Provide the client with appropriate pressure-relieving devices. For further interventions on skin care, refer to the care plan for Impaired **Skin** Integrity.
- Help the client out of bed as soon as able.
- When getting the client up after bed rest, do so slowly and watch for signs and symptoms of postural (orthostatic) hypotension, including dizziness, tachycardia, nausea, diaphoresis, or syncope.
- Obtain assistive devices such as braces, crutches, or canes to help the client reach and maintain as much mobility as possible.
▲ Apply graduated compression stockings as ordered, if indicated for orthostatic hypotension. Ensure proper fit by measuring accurately. Remove the stockings at least twice a day, in the morning with the bath and in the evening to assess the condition of the extremity and skin, then reapply. Knee length is preferred rather than thigh length.
- Observe for signs of DVT, including pain, tenderness, redness, and swelling in the calf and thigh. Also observe for signs and symptoms of pulmonary embolism, including sudden onset of dyspnea, chest pain, syncope, dizziness, tachycardia, or tachypnea.
- Have the client cough and deep breathe or use incentive spirometry every 2 hours while awake.
- Monitor respiratory functions, noting breath sounds, work of breathing, and respiratory rate. Percuss for new onset of dullness in lungs.
- Note bowel function daily. Provide fluids, fiber, and natural laxatives such as prune juice as needed.
- Increase fluid intake to 2000 mL/day within the client's cardiac and renal reserve.
- Encourage intake of a balanced diet with adequate amounts of fiber and protein. Consider recommending Practical Interventions to Achieve Therapeutic Lifestyle Changes (TLC), which includes monounsaturated and polyunsaturated fats, oils, margarines, beans, peas, lentils, soy, skinless poultry, lean fish, trimmed cuts of meat, fat-free and low-fat dairy foods, omega-3 polyunsaturated fat sources, and whole grains, including soluble fiber sources such as oats, oat bran, and barley (Osborne et al, 2013).

**Critical Care**

▲ Recognize that the client who has been in an intensive care environment may develop a neuromuscular dysfunction acquired in the absence of causative factors other than the underlying critical illness and its treatment, resulting in ICU-acquired weakness, with an approximate incidence of 40% requiring more than 1 week of mechanical ventilation (Appleton, Kinsella, & Quasim, 2015). The client may need a workup to determine the cause before satisfactory ambulation can begin.

▲ Consider the use of a continuous lateral rotation therapy bed.

▲ For the stable client in the ICU, consider mobilizing the client in a four-phase method from dangling at the side of the bed to walking if there is sufficient knowledgeable staff available to protect the client from harm. Even ICU clients receiving mechanical ventilation can be mobilized safely if a multiprofessional team is present to support, protect, and monitor the client for intolerance to activity (Green et al, 2016; Agency for Healthcare Research and Quality, 2017).

**Geriatric**

• Get the client out of bed as early as possible and ambulate frequently after consultation with the health care provider.

• Consider physical and occupational therapy referrals to guide with environmental safety assessment and home exercise programs.

• Monitor nutrition status in the elderly to prevent malnutrition.

• Monitor for signs of depression: flat affect, poor appetite, insomnia, and many somatic complaints.

• Keep careful track of bowel function in older adults; do not allow the client to become constipated.

**Home Care**

• Some of the previous interventions may be adapted for home care use.

▲ Begin discharge planning at time of admission with case manager or social worker and input from physical and occupational therapy as appropriate to assess need for home support systems and community or home health services.

▲ Become oriented to all programs of care for the client before discharge from institutional care.

▲ Confirm the immediate availability of all necessary assistive devices for home.

• Perform complete physical assessment and recent history at initial home visit.

▲ Refer to physical and occupational therapies for immediate evaluations of the client's potential for independence and functioning in the home setting and for follow-up care.

• Allow the client to have as much input and control of the plan of care as possible.

• Assess knowledge of all care with caregivers. Review as necessary.

• = Independent          ▲ = Collaborative

▲ Support the family of the client in the assumption of caregiver activities. Refer for home health aide services for assistance and respite as appropriate. Refer to medical social services as appropriate.

▲ Institute case management of frail elderly to support continued independent living, if possible in the home environment.

**Client/Family Teaching and Discharge Planning**

• Teach client/family how to perform range-of-motion exercises in bed if not contraindicated; this is referred to as a home exercise program.

• Teach the family how to turn and position the client and provide all care necessary.

Note: Nursing diagnoses that are commonly relevant when the client is on bed rest include **Constipation,** Risk for Impaired **Skin** Integrity, Disturbed **Sleep** Pattern, **Frail Elderly** Syndrome, and **Powerlessness.**

# Decreased Diversional Activity Engagement

**Domain 1** Health promotion    **Class 1** Health awareness

## NANDA-I Definition

Reduced stimulation, interest, or participation in recreational or leisure activities.

## Defining Characteristics

Alteration in mood; boredom; expresses discontentment with situation; flat affect; frequent naps; physical deconditioning

## Related Factors

Current setting does not allow engagement in activities; environmental constraints; impaired physical mobility; inadequate available activities; inadequate motivation; insufficient physical endurance; physical discomfort; psychological distressdeco

## At-Risk Population

Individuals at extremes of age; individuals experiencing prolonged hospitalization; individuals experiencing prolonged institutionalization

## Associated Conditions

Prescribed movement restrictions; therapeutic isolation

## Client Outcomes

Client Will (Specify Time Frame)

• Engage in personally satisfying diversional activities

## Nursing Interventions

• Assess the client's needs through mapping to assess existing networks, current activities, and the impact on well-being.

• Encourage the client to share feelings of boredom.

• = Independent                    ▲ = Collaborative

D

- Encourage the client to participate in any available social or recreational opportunities in the health care environment.
- Promote relaxation through guided imagery, visual imagery, and music interventions.
- Use art making and music listening.
- Be creative, for example, use of the activity pillowcases with soft fabric pieces, plastic zipper, and a pouch to hold a picture as a diversional intervention that could be used in inpatient and hospice care settings.
- Engage clients in physical activity or exercise programs as an adjunct treatment modality for a variety of mental illnesses; for example, depression, schizophrenia, anxiety, disorders, posttraumatic stress disorders, and substance abuse.
- Engage clients in leisure activities such as art and coloring; puzzles, games, and reading; meditation, deep breathing, and relaxation techniques; and music as ways to reduce screen time during hospitalization.
- Engage antepartum women and families in diversional fun promoting activities including scrapbooking, game night, book clubs, movie night, and prayer services during hospitalization.
▲ Hospitalized clients, particularly quarantined clients, are at risk for isolation and boredom and must be engaged in meaningful activities including technology-based (iPad with games or reactional-based applications) and non–technology-based (e.g., books, magazines, crafts, puzzles, games, adult coloring books, mind-stimulating activity books) activities.
▲ Refer to recreational, occupational, or art therapist to assist with activities.

**Pediatric**
- Assess for the child's interests, preferences, and hobbies.
- Engage preschool children in play therapy.
- Engage school-age children in origami during hospitalization.
▲ Refer to a music therapist.
- Provide technology access for children to connect with family and friends, play computer games, and engage in virtual reality experiences for children.
- Provide animal-assisted therapy for hospitalized children.
▲ Refer to a child life specialist, play therapist, recreational therapist, or occupational therapist.

**Geriatric**
- Many of the previously listed interventions may be used with geriatric clients.

• = Independent ▲ = Collaborative

E

- If the client is able, arrange for participation in group community activities.
- Promote activity for older adults through the use of emerging information and communication technologies.
- Engage nursing home residents with dementia in music therapy.
- Engage hospitalized clients with dementia/delirium in a person-centered activity program including (1) the use of "Pleasant Events Schedule," (2) implementation of "Identity Cards," and (3) engaging in "Occupational Workstations and Programs."

**Home Care**
- Many of the previously listed interventions may be administered in the home setting.

**Client/Family Teaching and Discharge Planning**
- Offer group-based educational workshops such as the "Creative Ways to Care" for family and friends to learn strategies to engage their family or friends with dementia in diversional activities. "Creative Ways to Care" is a series of a total of seven workshops: (1) Introduction Session, (2) Dementia Behavior and Activities, (3) Reminiscence, (4) Stimulating and Soothing the Senses, (5) Music, (6) Creative Activities, and (7) Review Session.
- If the client is in isolation, give the client complete information on why isolation is needed and how it should be accomplished, especially guidelines for visitors; provide diversional activities and encourage visitation.

# Ineffective Adolescent Eating Dynamics

**Domain 2** Nutrition    **Class 1** Ingestion
## NANDA-I Definition

Altered eating attitudes and behaviors resulting in over or under eating patterns that compromise nutritional health.

## Defining Characteristics

Avoids participation in regular mealtimes; complains of hunger between meals; depressive symptoms; food refusal; frequent snacking; frequently consumes fast food; frequently eating processed food; frequently eats low quality food; inadequate appetite; overeating; undereating

## Related Factors

Altered family relations; anxiety; changes to self-esteem upon entering puberty; eating disorder; eating in isolation; excessive family mealtime control; excessive stress; inadequate dietary habits; irregular mealtime;

• = Independent                    ▲ = Collaborative

media influence on eating behaviors of high caloric unhealthy foods; media influence on knowledge of high caloric unhealthy foods; negative parental influences on eating behaviors; psychological neglect; stressful mealtimes; unaddressed abuse

## Associated Conditions

Depression; parental psychiatric disorder; physical challenge with eating; physical challenge with feeding; physical health issue of parent; psychological health issue of parent

## Client Outcomes

### Client Will (Specify Time Frame)

- Maintain weight within normal range for height and age
- Eat breakfast daily
- Participate in meal planning and preparation
- Consume healthy and nutritious foods

## Nursing Interventions

- Assess for goals and motives related to eating behaviors.
- Assess the adolescent client for comorbid psychological disorders and make appropriate referrals for treatment.
- Assess the adolescent for experiences of cyberbullying and the strength of friendship dynamics.
- Offer obese or overweight adolescents healthy methods for weight loss.
- Offer families of obese or overweight adolescents bias-free, individually accepting, and supportive interventions to address weight loss.
- Recommend that families eat together for at least one meal per day.
- Recommend involving the adolescents in planning family meals and food preparation.
- Assist parents at being good role models of healthy eating.
- Recommend that the family try new foods, such as either a new food or recipe every week.
- Frame healthy eating as consistent with the adolescent values of autonomy from adult control and the pursuit of social justice.
- Explore the adolescent's friendship dynamics.

### Multicultural

- Assess racial-ethnic minority overweight adolescents for disordered eating behaviors.
- Encourage racial-ethnic minority families to refrain from weight-based teasing.

### Home Care

- The interventions previously described may be adapted for home care use.

• = Independent          ▲ = Collaborative

E

**Client/Family Teaching and Discharge Planning**
- Refer the adolescent and family to family treatment-behavior (FT-B) for treatment of eating disorders.
- Teach the family that hospitalization of the adolescent may be indicated for medical stabilization of serious physical complications and refer as needed.

# Ineffective Child Eating Dynamics

**Domain 2** Nutrition    **Class 1** Ingestion

## NANDA-I Definition

Altered attitudes, behaviors, and influences on child eating patterns resulting in compromised nutritional health.

## Defining Characteristics

Avoids participation in regular mealtimes; complains of hunger between meals, food refusal, frequent snacking; frequently consumes fast food; frequently eating processed food; frequently eats low quality food; inadequate appetite; overeating; undereating

## Related Factors

### Eating Habit

Abnormal eating habit patterns; bribing child to eat; consumption of large volumes of food in a short period of time; eating in isolation; excessive parental control over child's eating experience; excessive parental control over family mealtime; forcing child to eat; inadequate dietary habits; lack of regular mealtimes; limiting child's eating; rewarding child to eat; stressful mealtimes; unpredictable eating patterns; unstructured eating of snacks between meals

### Family Process

Abusive interpersonal relations; anxious parent-child relations; disengaged parenting; hostile parent-child relations; insecure parent-child relations; intrusive parenting; tense parent-child relations; uninvolved parenting

### Parental

Anorexia; inability to divide eating responsibility between parent and child; inability to divide feeding responsibility between parent and child; inability to support healthy eating patterns; ineffective coping strategies; lack of confidence in child to develop healthy eating habits; lack of confidence in child to grow appropriately; substance misuse

### Unmodified Environmental Factors

Media influence on eating behaviors of high caloric unhealthy foods; media influence on knowledge of high caloric unhealthy foods

• = Independent                    ▲ = Collaborative

## At-Risk Population

Children born to economically disadvantaged families; children experiencing homelessness; children experiencing life transition; children living in foster care; children whose parents are obese

## Associated Conditions

Depression; parental psychiatric disorder; physical challenge with eating; physical challenge with feeding; physical health issue of parent; psychological health issue of parent

## Client Outcomes

### Client Will (Specify Time Frame)

- Identify hunger and satiety cues
- Consume healthy and nutritious foods
- Consume adequate calories to support growth and development
- Engage in positive interactions with caregiver during meals

## Nursing Interventions

- Use a nutritional screening tool designed for nurses, such as Subjective Global Nutrition Assessment (SGNA), and refer to a dietitian for scores of moderate or severe.
- Assess parents for food or eating concerns, aberrant feeding behavior, or inappropriate feeding practices.
- Assess child for type of eating difficulty. Children can present with limited appetite, food selectivity, and fear of feeding.
- Assess the caregiver's feeding style by asking three questions: How anxious are you about your child's eating? How would you describe what happens during mealtime? What do you do when your child will not eat?
- Assess the child for persistent picky eating with three questions/ answers: Is your child a picky eater? (yes). Does she or he have strong likes with regard to food? (yes). Does your child accept new foods readily? (no).
- Assess child for symptoms of malnutrition, including short stature, thin arms and legs, poor condition of skin and hair, visible vertebrae and rib cage, wasted buttocks, wasted facial appearance, lethargy, and, in extreme cases, edema.
- Assess weight and height of the child and use a growth chart to help determine growth pattern, which reflects nutrition. Age-related growth charts are available from www.cdc.gov/growthcharts/ (Centers for Disease Control and Prevention, 2016).
- Recommend that families turn off the television during meal times.
- Recommend that families eat together for at least one meal per day.
- Encourage parent–child interactions that promote attachment.

• = Independent ▲ = Collaborative

E

- Recommend that the child eats breakfast daily.
- Recommend involving the family in planning meals and food preparation. Children can learn about nutrition as they help plan and make meals.
- Assist parents at being good role models of healthy eating.
- Recommend that the family try new foods, either a new food or recipe every week.
- ▲ Refer children with highly selective food behaviors and sensory food aversion to a nutritional specialist.
- ▲ Refer children with feeding difficulties caused by a medical condition to the appropriate specialist.

**Multicultural**

- Assess for the meanings, attitudes, and behaviors related to feeding practices in culturally diverse families.
- Assess the feeding styles of Hispanic and African American mothers for congruence with current child feeding recommendations.

**Home Care**

- The interventions previously described may be adapted for home care use.

**Client/Family Teaching and Discharge Planning**

- Provide parents with the following guidelines: avoid distractions during mealtimes (e.g., television, cell phones), maintain a pleasant neutral attitude throughout meal, feed to encourage appetite, limit meal duration (20–30 minutes), limit to 4 to 6 meals/snacks a day with only water in between, serve age-appropriate foods, systematically introduce new foods (up to 8–15 times), encourage self-feeding, and tolerate age-appropriate mess.
- Teach families to provide a feeding environment that sets boundaries around food, through meal timing and the types of foods offered.
- Teach parents to recognize the difference between hunger and satiety in their children.
- Teach parents of children with limited appetites to establish a feeding schedule with a maximum of five meals per day and nothing but water in between. Parents must be taught to model healthy eating, adhere to the established feeding schedule, and set limits/consequences for mealtime behavior.
- Teach parents of children with food selectivity to refrain from coercive and indulgent feeding practices.
- Teach parents to use nondirective feeding strategies such as repeatedly offering foods, offering a familiar and accepted food (e.g., ketchup) alongside novel or refused foods, and having family and/or peers model eating the food with enjoyment.

• = Independent          ▲ = Collaborative

- Teach parents to avoid restrictive feeding practices such as limiting intakes of certain foods.
- Teach parents the concept of being a responsive feeder, in which the parent determines where, when, and what the child is fed and the child determines how much to eat. Responsive feeders guide the child's eating, set limits, model appropriate eating, talk positively about food, and respond appropriately to the child's feeding cues.

# Risk for Electrolyte Imbalance

**Domain 2** Nutrition   **Class 5** Hydration

## NANDA-I Definition

Susceptible to changes in serum electrolyte levels, which may compromise health.

## Risk Factors

Diarrhea; excessive fluid volume; inadequate knowledge of modifiable factors; insufficient fluid volume; vomiting

## Associated Conditions

Compromised regulatory mechanism; endocrine regulatory dysfunction; renal dysfunction; treatment regimen

## Client Outcomes

Client Will (Specify Time Frame)

- Maintain a normal sinus heart rhythm with a regular rate
- Have a decrease in edema
- Maintain an absence of muscle cramping
- Maintain normal serum potassium, sodium, calcium, magnesium and phosphorus
- Maintain normal serum pH

## Nursing Interventions

▲ Monitor vital signs at least three times a day, or more frequently as needed. Notify health care provider of significant deviation from baseline.

▲ Monitor cardiac rate and rhythm. Report changes to provider. Hypokalemia and hyperkalemia can result in electrocardiogram (ECG) changes that can lead to cardiac arrest and ventricular dysrhythmias.

- Monitor intake and output and daily weights using a consistent scale.
- Monitor for abdominal distention and discomfort. A focused assessment should be done on any client presenting with hepatic, gastrointestinal, or pancreatic dysfunction (Shrimanker & Bhattarai, 2020).

• = Independent          ▲ = Collaborative

**E**

- Monitor the client's respiratory status and muscle strength. Phosphorus is an essential element in cell structure, metabolism, and maintenance of acid-base processes.
- Assess cardiac status and neurological alterations.
- Imbalances of sodium, potassium, calcium, and magnesium all can cause neurological disturbances (Kear, 2017).
- ▲ Review laboratory data as ordered and report deviations to provider. Laboratory studies may include serum electrolytes potassium, chloride, sodium, bicarbonate, magnesium, phosphate, and calcium; serum pH; comprehensive metabolic panel; and arterial blood gases.
- Review the client's medical and surgical history for possible causes of altered electrolytes.
- ▲ Complete pain assessment. Assess and document the onset, intensity, character, location, duration, aggravating factors, and relieving factors. Notify the provider of any increase in pain or discomfort or if comfort measures are not effective.
- ▲ Monitor the effects of ordered medications such as diuretics and heart medications.
- ▲ Administer parenteral fluids as ordered and monitor their effects.

**Geriatric**
- Monitor electrolyte levels carefully, including sodium levels and potassium levels, with both increased and decreased levels possible.

**Client/Family Teaching and Discharge Planning**
- Teach client/family the signs of low potassium and the risk factors.
- Teach client/family the signs of high potassium and the risk factors.
- Teach client/family the signs of low sodium and the risk factors.
- Teach client/family the signs of high sodium and the risk factors.
- Teach client/family the importance of hydration during exercise. Dehydration occurs when the amount of water leaving the body is greater than the amount consumed.
- Teach client/family the warning signs of dehydration. Early signs of dehydration include thirst and decreased urine output. As dehydration increases, symptoms may include dry mouth, muscle cramps, nausea and vomiting, lightheadedness, and orthostatic hypotension.
- Teach client about any medications prescribed. Medication teaching includes the drug name, its purpose, administration instructions such as taking it with or without food, and any side effects.
- ▲ Instruct the client to report any adverse medication side effects to his or her health care provider. Assessing and instructing clients about medications and focusing on important details can help prevent client medication errors.

# Risk for Elopement Attempt

**Domain 1** Health promotion     **Class 2** Health management

### NANDA-I Definition

Susceptible to leaving a health care facility or a designated area against recommendation or without communicating to health care professionals or caregivers, which may compromise safety and/or health.

### Risk Factors

Anger behaviors; exit-seeking behavior; frustration about delay in treatment regimen; inadequate caregiver vigilance; inadequate interest in improving health; inadequate social support; perceived complexity of treatment regimen; perceived excessive family responsibilities; perceived excessive responsibilities in interpersonal relations; perceived lack of safety in surrounding environment; persistent wandering; psychomotor agitation; self-harm intent; substance misuse

### At-Risk Population

Economically disadvantaged individuals; homeless individuals; individuals brought to designated area against own wishes; individuals frequently requesting discharge; individuals hospitalized <3 weeks; individuals with history of elopement; individuals with history of non-adherence to treatment regimen; individuals with history of self-harm; individuals with impaired judgment; men; older adults with cognitive disorders; unemployed individuals; young adults

### Associated Conditions

Autism spectrum disorder; developmental disabilities; mental disorders

### Client Outcomes

**Client Will (Specify Time Frame)**
- Remain safely and securely in treatment area
- Remain at scheduled activities
- Identify the consequences of leaving treatment
- Make a commitment to continuing treatment
- Accept discharge date and process

### Nursing Interventions

- Identify client factors associated with elopement risk and implement appropriate precautions.
- Assess the client's stress level and coping.
- Assess for and ask about the client's responsibilities and commitments outside of the hospital setting.
- Offer the client time and information so they can be involved in decision-making related to their care.
- For clients admitted involuntarily to a psychiatric setting, implement elopement precautions to maintain client safety.

• = Independent          ▲ = Collaborative

**E**

**Pediatric**

- Assess for factors associated with risk for elopement.
- Counsel families of children diagnosed with autism spectrum disorder (ASD) about the danger related to elopement.
▲ If interested, refer families of children diagnosed with ASD for a consultation regarding electronic tracking device (ETD) technology.

**Geriatric**

- Many of the previous interventions can be adapted for use with geriatric clients.
- Assess for behaviors that may indicate the client with dementia may elope or wander away.
- Implement elopement precautions for clients who exhibit critical wandering behaviors.
- Use a unique room door design for individuals living with dementia in a residential care.
- Implement a structured physical activity program for with dementia.
- Refer to occupational therapy for assistive technology to address elopement safety for clients diagnosed with dementia.
- See the care plan for **Wandering.**

**Multicultural**

- The previous interventions can be adapted for use with multicultural clients.

**Home Care**

- The previous interventions can be adapted for use with home care clients.
▲ Refer families of clients with dementia to smart home technologies to manage nighttime wandering.

**Client/Family Teaching and Discharge Planning**

- Assess family reactions to the client's elopement attempts or wandering behavior.
- Provide family and caregivers information about elopement precautions.

## Labile Emotional Control

**Domain 5** Perception/cognition    **Class 4** Cognition
**NANDA-I Definition**

Uncontrollable outbursts of exaggerated and involuntary emotional expression.

• = Independent    ▲ = Collaborative

### Defining Characteristics

Absence of eye contact; crying; excessive crying without feeling sadness; excessive laughing without feeling happiness; expresses embarrassment regarding emotional expression; expression of emotion incongruent with triggering factor; impaired nonverbal communication; involuntary crying; involuntary laughing; social alienation; uncontrollable crying; uncontrollable laughing; withdrawal from occupational situation

### Related Factors

Altered self-esteem; excessive emotional disturbance; fatigue; inadequate knowledge about symptom control; inadequate knowledge of disease; insufficient muscle strength; social distress; stressors; substance misuse

### Associated Conditions

Brain injuries; functional impairment; mental disorders; mood disorders; musculoskeletal impairment; pharmaceutical preparations; physical disability

### Client Outcomes

**Client Will (Specify Time Frame)**

- Improve coping strategies
- Improve knowledge about disease process, signs and symptoms, triggers, symptom control
- Use mechanisms to control impulses and ask for help when feeling impulses
- Improve feelings of dignity
- Enhance and improve response to social and environmental stimuli

### Nursing Interventions

- Identify clients at risk of having labile emotional control.
- Assess clients with an appropriate screening tool such as the Pathological Laughter and Crying Scale (PLACS), Center for Neurologic Study-Lability Scale (CNS-LS), or the Emotional Lability Questionnaire (ELQ).
- Offer client the choice of email and/or videoconferencing for delivery of therapy.
- Assess clients for use of experiential avoidance, which is the process of negatively evaluating, escaping, or avoiding unwanted thoughts, emotions, or sensations.
- Offer the client choices when possible in emotional situations.
- Encourage clients to verbalize their emotional reactions and lability.
- Encourage clients to talk about their emotional reactions and acknowledge that the unpredictable and uncontrollable nature of emotional lability can be embarrassing and cause distress.

• = Independent        ▲ = Collaborative

- Encourage the client to use distraction, humor, optimism, and social support as a way to manage the episodes.
- Consider using motive-oriented therapeutic relationship (MOTR).
- Provide progressive muscle relaxation (PMR) exercise and guided imagery (GI) techniques.
- Consider using cognitive-behavioral therapy (CBT).

**Pediatric**
- Assess adolescents with high emotional dysregulation for substance use disorders.
- Teach parents that their reactions to their children's emotions play a critical role in teaching children effective emotion regulation.
- Provide parents with emotion coaching strategies to manage their children's emotional outbursts. Emotion coaching includes fostering parental awareness and acceptance of their children's emotions with behaviors that acknowledge their children's emotions and teaches understanding, coping with, and appropriately expressing emotion.
- ▲ Refer adolescent clients to a dialectical behavior therapy (DBT) group.

**Geriatric**
- Many of the previous interventions may be adapted for geriatric use.
- Evaluate geriatric clients suspected of PBA with the following three-step model: (1) crying inconsistent with environment/stimuli; (2) diagnosis of any of the following neurological disorders: TBI, PD, MS, ALS; or (3) at least two of the following disorders: stroke, schizophrenia (including schizoaffective and schizophreniform disorders), or documentation of spinal cord injury (SCI) as most closely associated with the PBA diagnosis.

**Multicultural and Home Care**
- The previous interventions may be adapted for multicultural and home care.

**Client/Family Teaching and Discharge Planning**
- Instruct client and family to monitor for cutaneous adverse effects of the neurological medications used to treat PBA and report occurrence to their health care provider.
- Inform client and family about the emotional lability and talk with them about how to cope with the situation.
- For clients with neurological disorders, provide teaching that emotionalism is a neurological condition and not a clinical mood disorder to promote better understanding for clients, their families, and significant others.

• = Independent          ▲ = Collaborative

- Use verbal and nonverbal therapeutic communication approaches including empathy, active listening, and confrontation to encourage the client and family to express emotions such as sadness, guilt, and anger (within appropriate limits); verbalize fears and concerns; and set goals.
- Offer instruction to the client and family to wait for emotional episodes to pass.

**E**

# Imbalanced Energy Field

**Domain 4** Activity/rest    **Class 3** Energy balance
## NANDA-I Definition
A disruption in the vital flow of human energy that is normally a continuous whole and is unique, dynamic, creative and nonlinear.
## Defining Characteristics
Arrhythmic energy field patterns; blockage of the energy flow; congested energy field patterns; congestion of the energy flow; dissonant rhythms of the energy field patterns; energy deficit of the energy flow; expression of the need to regain the experience of the whole; hyperactivity of the energy flow; irregular energy field patterns; magnetic pull to an area of the energy field; pulsating to pounding frequency of the energy field patterns; pulsations sensed in the energy flow; random energy field patterns; rapid energy field patterns; slow energy field patterns; strong energy field patterns; temperature differentials of cold in the energy flow; temperature differentials of heat in the energy flow; tingling sensed in the energy flow; tumultuous energy field patterns; unsynchronized rhythms sensed in the energy flow; weak energy field patterns
## Related Factors
Anxiety; discomfort; excessive stress; interventions that disrupt the energetic pattern or flow; pain
## At-Risk Population
Individuals experiencing life transition; individuals experiencing personal crisis
## Associated Conditions
Impaired health status; injury
## Nursing Interventions
- Consider using complementary health approaches (CHAs) such as energy medicine (TT/healing touch, hope inspiration, and reiki) for clients with anxiety, tension, pain, or other conditions that indicate a disruption in the flow of energy.
- Refer to care plans for **Anxiety,** Acute **Pain,** and Chronic **Pain.**

• = Independent          ▲ = Collaborative

**Guidelines for Complementary Health Approaches**
- CHAs may be practiced by anyone with the requisite preparation, desire, and commitment.
- Volunteers who are not licensed health care professionals may practice in the home, but not in the health care setting unless they undertake a rigorous training program.

**Pediatric**
- Consider using CHAs for pediatric clients with adjunct therapies to decrease stress, anxiety, and pain.

**Geriatric**
- Consider CHAs for elderly with pain.

**Multicultural**
- Assess for the influence of cultural beliefs, norms, and values on the client's use of CAM.

**Home Care**
- Help the client and family accept CAM therapies as natural healing interventions.
- ▲ In the presence of a psychiatric disorder, refer for psychiatric home health care services for client reassurance and implementation of therapeutic regimens.

**Client/Family Teaching and Discharge Planning**
- Teach the client how to use guided imagery.
- Consider the use of progressive muscle relaxation, autogenic training, relaxation response, biofeedback, emotional freedom technique, guided imagery, diaphragmatic breathing, transcendental meditation, cognitive behavioral therapy, mindfulness-based stress reduction, and emotional freedom technique.
- The practice of CAM therapies, both giving and receiving, can improve well-being.

# Readiness for Enhanced Exercise Engagement

**Domain 1** Health promotion   **Class 2** Health management

**NANDA-I Definition**

A pattern of attention to physical activity characterized by planned, structured, repetitive body movements, which can be strengthened.

**Defining Characteristics**

Expresses desire to enhance autonomy for activities of daily living; expresses desire to enhance competence to interact with physical and social environments; expresses desire to enhance knowledge about environmental conditions for participation in physical activity; expresses desire to enhance knowledge about group opportunities for participation in physical activity; expresses desire to enhance knowledge about physical settings for participation in physical activity; expresses desire to enhance knowledge about the need for physical activity; expresses desire to enhance physical abilities; expresses desire to enhance physical appearance; expresses desire to enhance physical conditioning; expresses desire to maintain motivation to participate in a physical activity plan; expresses desire to maintain physical abilities; expresses desire to maintain physical well-being through physical activity; expresses desire to meet others' expectations about physical activity plans

**Client Outcomes**

**Client Will (Specify Time Frame)**

- Engage in purposeful moderate-intensity cardiorespiratory (aerobic) exercise for 30 to 60 minutes/day on 5 or more days per week for a total of 2 hours and 30 minutes (150 minutes) per week
- Increase pedometer step counts by 1000 steps per day every 2 weeks to reach a daily step count of at least 7000 steps per day, with a daily goal for most healthy adults of 10,000 steps per day
- Perform resistance exercises that involve all major muscle groups (legs, hips, back, chest, abdomen, shoulders, and arms) performed 2 to 3 days/week
- Perform flexibility exercise (stretching) for each of the major muscle-tendon groups 2 days/week for 10 to 60 seconds to improve joint range of motion; greatest gains occur with daily exercise

**Nursing Interventions**

- * Determine whether the client needs a physical examination, with a focus on cardiac health, before engaging in additional exercise.
- ▲ Highlight benefits of exercise on health outcomes to increase motivation.
- ▲ Use theories to guide increasing motivation and engagement in physical activity.
- Support the client's autonomous (internal) motivation with regard to physical activity by discussing the value of positive health behaviors.
- Provide motivational support and encourage positive thinking to facilitate exercise engagement.
- Encourage activities the client finds enjoyable, to promote continued engagement.
- Develop exercise plans that allow for flexibility for the client.
- ▲ Provide resources for technology options, such as phone applications (which continue to be developed and tested), to increase exercise engagement.

• = Independent ▲ = Collaborative

- Administer the Physical Self-Description Questionnaire short form (PSDQ-s) to assess physical self-concept.
▲ Consider sports programs to increase motivation regarding exercise.
- Write a "prescription" for exercise for the client.
▲ Educate clients about modified or adaptive activities available.
▲ Incorporate genetically tailored physical activity interventions to individualize plan.

**Pediatric**
- Assess the child's current activity status using the Pediatric Inactivity Triad (Faigenbaum et al, 2018).
- Assess parent's perceptions of children's screen time and active play.
- Children and adolescents should participate in 60 minutes (1 hour) or more of physical activity daily.
  o Aerobic: Sixty or more minutes a day should be either moderate-intensity or vigorous-intensity aerobic physical activity, and should include vigorous-intensity physical activity at least 3 days a week.
  o Muscle-strengthening: As part of daily physical activity, children and adolescents should include muscle-strengthening physical activity at least 3 days of the week.
  o Bone-strengthening: As part of daily physical activity, children and adolescents should include bone-strengthening physical activity at least 3 days of the week.
  o Providing activities that are age appropriate, enjoyable, and varied will encourage young people to participate in physical activities (US Department of Health and Human Services, 2018).
- Assist families to develop family-based interventions to increase child physical activity.
- Encourage participation in youth sports.
- Encourage parents and caregivers to adhere to the following American Academy of Pediatrics guidelines for children's media use (Chassiakos et al, 2016):
  o For children younger than 18 months, avoid use of screen media other than video-chatting.
  o Parents of children 18 to 24 months of age who want to introduce digital media should choose high-quality programming and watch it with their children to help them understand what they are seeing.
  o For children ages 2 to 5 years, limit screen use to 1 hour/day of high-quality programs. Parents should co-view media with children to help them understand what they are seeing and apply it to the world around them.

• = Independent          ▲ = Collaborative

◌ For children ages 6 and older, place consistent limits on the time spent using media, and the types of media, and make sure media does not take the place of adequate sleep, physical activity, and other behaviors essential to health.

◌ Designate media-free times together, such as dinner or driving, and media-free locations at home, such as bedrooms.

◌ Have ongoing communication about online citizenship and safety, including treating others with respect online and off-line.

◌ Encourage parents and caregivers to create their personalized family media plan from the American Academy of Pediatrics (see https://www.healthychildren.org/English/media/Pages/default.aspx).

**Geriatric**

• Engage older adults in determining creative ways to exercise.

• Explain that shorter periods of activity can still be beneficial, to increase engagement in exercise.

▲ Encourage participation in physical activity programs to increase motivation and engagement, even when living in a facility.

▲ Educate older men about testosterone to increase physical activity.

**Multicultural**

▲ Incorporate spirituality into physical activity plans to individualize them to the client's culture, to facilitate continued engagement.

**Home Care**

• The interventions described previously may be used in home care.

**Client/Family Teaching and Discharge Planning**

▲ Refer clients returning to sports after an injury for on-field physical therapy rehabilitation after gym rehabilitation is completed.

▲ Encourage activity programs after the cardiac rehabilitation phase to increase physical activity.

# Ineffective Dry Eye Self-Management

**Domain 11** Safety/protection    **Class 2** Physical injury

**NANDA-I Definition**

Unsatisfactory management of symptoms, treatment regimen, physical, psychosocial, and spiritual consequences and lifestyle changes inherent in living with inadequate tear film.

## Defining Characteristics

### Dry Eye Signs

Chemosis; conjunctival hyperemia; epiphora; filamentary keratitis; keratoconjunctival staining with fluorescein; low aqueous tear production according to Schirmer I Test; mucous plaques

### Dry Eye Symptoms

Expresses dissatisfaction with quality of life; reports blurred vision; reports eye fatigue; reports feeling of burning eyes; reports feeling of ocular dryness; reports feeling of ocular foreign body; reports feeling of ocular itching; reports feeling of sand in eye

### Behaviors

Difficulty performing eyelid care; difficulty reducing caffeine consumption; inadequate maintenance of air humidity; inadequate use of eyelid closure device; inadequate use of prescribed medication; inappropriate use of contact lenses; inappropriate use of fans; inappropriate use of hairdryer; inappropriate use of moisture chamber goggles; inattentive to dry eye signs; inattentive to dry eye symptoms; inattentive to second-hand smoke; insufficient dietary intake of omega-3 fatty acids; insufficient dietary intake of vitamin A; insufficient fluid intake; nonadherence to recommended blinking exercises; nonadherence to recommended eye breaks; use of products with benzalkonium chloride preservatives

## Risk Factors

Competing demands; competing lifestyle preferences; conflict between health behaviors and social norms; decreased perceived quality of life; difficulty accessing community resources; difficulty managing complex treatment regimen; difficulty navigating complex health care systems; difficulty with decision-making; inadequate commitment to a plan of action; inadequate health literacy; inadequate knowledge of treatment regimen; inadequate number of cues to action; inadequate role models; inadequate social support; limited ability to perform aspects of treatment regimen; low self efficacy; negative feelings toward treatment regimen; nonacceptance of condition; perceived barrier to treatment regimen; perceived social stigma associated with condition; unrealistic perception of seriousness of condition; unrealistic perception of susceptibility to sequelae; unrealistic perception of treatment benefit

## At-Risk Population

Children; economically disadvantaged individuals; individuals experiencing prolonged hospitalization; individuals with history of ineffective health self-management; individuals with limited decision-making experience; individuals with low educational level; older adults; women experiencing menopause

• = Independent          ▲ = Collaborative

## Associated Conditions

Allergies; autoimmune diseases; chemotherapy; developmental disabilities; graft versus host disease; incomplete eyelid closure; leukocytosis; metabolic diseases; neurological injury with motor reflex loss; neurological injury with sensory reflex loss; oxygen therapy; pharmaceutical preparations; proptosis; radiotherapy; reduced tear volume; surgical procedures

## Client Outcomes

### Client Will (Specify Time Frame)

- State eyes are comfortable with no itching, burning, or dryness
- Have corneal surface that is intact and without injury
- Demonstrate self-administration of eye drops if ordered
- State vision is clear

## Nursing Interventions

▲ Assess for symptoms of dry eyes, such as "irritation, tearing, burning, stinging, dry or foreign body sensation, mild itching, photophobia, blurry vision, contact lens intolerance, redness, mucus discharge, increased frequency of blinking, eye fatigue, diurnal fluctuation, symptoms that worsen later in the day" (Boyd, 2018; Mukamal, 2020).

▲ If symptoms are present, refer client to an ophthalmologist for diagnosis and treatment.

▲ Administer ordered eye drops.

• Consider use of eyeglass side shields or moisture chambers.

▲ Watch for symptoms of blepharitis including crusting and irritation at the base of the lashes and adjacent redness of the eyelid, which may accompany dry eye; refer for treatment as needed.

▲ Discuss use of caffeine with client's health care provider.

• Provide education to the client about how limiting screen time, computers, smart devices, and television can assist with reducing eyestrain and dry eyes.

### Critical Care

▲ Provide regular cleaning of the eyes, lubricating eye drops and ointments, and consultation with an ophthalmologist if infection is suspected in clients in the intensive care unit (ICU). ICU staff may miss ocular complications while caring for life-threatening conditions. Ocular complications can seriously impair vision and quality of life.

• Avoid using adhesive tape to keep eyes closed in sedated clients.

### Geriatric

• Recognize that symptoms of dry eye are more common in menopausal women and geriatric clients.

• Many clients as they age develop comorbidities in which the treatments can cause dry eyes.

• = Independent          ▲ = Collaborative

**Client/Family Teaching and Discharge Planning**
- Teach client conditions that can exacerbate dry eye symptoms.
- Teach client good eye hygiene:
  - Apply warm compresses for 10-minute intervals using a clean cloth and water that has been boiled and cooled (or sterile water).
  - Gently massage around eyelids.
  - Gently clean eyelids to remove excess oil, crusts, and bacteria. Use a few drops of baby shampoo in water that has been boiled and cooled, or in sterile water.
  - Good hygiene can help improve dry eyes, especially dry eye associated with blepharitis (NHS, 2018).
- Teach client methods to decrease problems with dry eye, including the following:
  - Avoid drafty (e.g., ceiling fans) and low-humidity environments.
  - Avoid smoking and exposure to secondhand smoke.
- ▲ Discuss avoidance of offending medications with health care provider.
- Drink plenty of water to keep well hydrated.
- Teach client to lower the computer screen to below eye level and to blink more frequently.
- ▲ Teach client to consult with the health care provider regarding use of omega-3 supplements to decrease dry eye.
- Teach client how to self-administer eye drops.
- Warn client with dry eyes that driving at night can be dangerous. Clients with dry eyes have light sensitivity and decreased refraction.

## Risk for Dry Eye

**Domain 11** Safety/protection    **Class 2** Physical injury

### NANDA-I Definition

Susceptible to inadequate tear film, which may cause eye discomfort and/or damage ocular surface, which may compromise health.

### Risk Factors

Air conditioning; air pollution; caffeine consumption; decreased blinking frequency; excessive wind; inadequate knowledge of modifiable factors; inappropriate use of contact lenses; inappropriate use of fans; inappropriate use of hairdryer; inattentive to second-hand smoke; insufficient fluid intake; low air humidity; omega-3 fatty acids deficiency; smoking; sunlight exposure; use of products with benzalkonium chloride preservatives; vitamin A deficiency

• = Independent          ▲ = Collaborative

## At-Risk Population

Contact lens wearer; individuals experiencing prolonged intensive care unit stay; individuals with history of allergy; older adults; women

## Associated Conditions

Artificial respiration; autoimmune disease; chemotherapy; decreased blinking; decreased level of consciousness; hormonal change; incomplete eyelid closure; leukocytosis; metabolic diseases; neurological injury with sensory or motor reflex loss; neuromuscular blockade; oxygen therapy; pharmaceutical preparations; proptosis; radiotherapy; reduced tear volume; surgical procedures

## Client Outcomes, Nursing Interventions, and Client/Family Teaching and Discharge Planning

Refer to care plan for Ineffective Dry Eye Self-Management.

# Risk for Adult Falls

**Domain 11** Safety/protection    **Class 2** Physical injury

## NANDA-I Definition

Adult susceptible to experiencing an event resulting in coming to rest inadvertently on the ground, floor, or other lower level, which may compromise health.

## Risk Factors

### Physiological Factors

Chronic musculoskeletal pain; decreased lower extremity strength; dehydration; diarrhea; faintness when extending neck; faintness when turning neck; hypoglycemia; impaired physical mobility; impaired postural balance; incontinence; obesity; sleep disturbances; vitamin D deficiency

### Psychoneurological Factors

Agitated confusion; anxiety; depressive symptoms; fear of falling; persistent wandering; substance misuse

### Unmodified Environmental Factors

Cluttered environment; elevated bed surface; exposure to unsafe weather-related condition; inadequate anti-slip material in bathroom; inadequate anti-slip material on floors; inadequate lighting; inappropriate toilet seat height; inattentive to pets; lack of safety rails; objects out of reach; seats without arms; seats without backs; uneven floor; unfamiliar setting; use of throw rugs

### Other Factors

Factors identified by standardized, validated screening tool; getting up at night without help; inadequate knowledge of modifiable factors; inappropriate clothing for walking; inappropriate footwear

• = Independent        ▲ = Collaborative

## At-Risk Population

Economically disadvantaged individuals; individuals aged ≥60 years; individuals dependent for activities of daily living; individuals dependent for instrumental activities of daily living; individuals experiencing prolonged hospitalization; individuals in aged care settings; individuals in palliative care settings; individuals in rehabilitation settings; individuals in the early postoperative period; individuals living alone; individuals receiving home-based care; individuals with history of falls; individuals with low educational level; individuals with restraints

## Associated Conditions

Anemia; assistive devices for walking; depression; endocrine system diseases; lower limb prosthesis; major injury; mental disorders; musculoskeletal diseases; neurocognitive disorders; orthostatic hypotension; pharmaceutical preparations; sensation disorders; vascular disease

## Client Outcomes

### Client Will (Specify Time Frame)

- Remain free of falls
- Have a decreased risk of injury if sustains a fall
- Adapt environment to minimize the incidence of falls
- Explain methods to prevent injury

## Nursing Interventions

- Safety guidelines suggest a fall-risk assessment be completed for older adults in any health care setting with national guidelines and action plans such as the Falls Free Initiative (National Council on Aging, 2021).
- Use a valid and reliable fall risk assessment tool to assess the client's risk for falling; for example, in the acute care setting use the Hendrich II Model (Hendrich, 2013). Recognize that risk factors for falling include recent history of falls, fear of falling, confusion, depression, altered elimination patterns, cardiovascular/respiratory disease impairing perfusion or oxygenation, postural hypotension, dizziness or vertigo, primary cancer diagnosis, and altered mobility (National Council on Aging, 2021; Gray-Miceli & Quigley, 2021).
- Screen all clients for balance and mobility skills (i.e., supine to sit, sitting supported and unsupported, sit to stand, standing, walking and turning around, transferring, stooping to floor and recovering, and sitting down). Use tools such as the Balance Scale by Tinetti, the Performance-Oriented Mobility Assessment (POMA), or the Timed Up & Go Test.
- Identify client mobility function deficits and consider appropriate equipment needed to safely mobilize clients while promoting self-

• = Independent          ▲ = Collaborative

care. The Bedside Mobility Assessment Tool 2.0 (BMAT 2.0) helps nurses assess client mobility status and standardize safe client handling and mobility equipment use.

- Older adults and others who may have been immobile due to acute illnesses and changing medications may be at risk for orthostatic hypotension. This is a drop in systolic blood pressure of 20 mm Hg or more or a drop in diastolic blood pressure of 10 mm Hg or more when changing from lying to sitting or sitting to standing. A concurrent rise in heart rate may occur as well. The client may or may not experience lightheadedness or dizziness.
- Carefully assist a mostly immobile client up. Be sure to lock the bed and wheelchair and have sufficient personnel to protect the client from falls. When rising from a lying position, have the client change positions slowly, dangle legs, and stand next to the bed before walking to prevent orthostatic hypotension.
- Use a "high-risk fall" armband/bracelet and fall risk room sign to alert staff for increased vigilance and mobility assistance.
- ▲ Evaluate the client's medications to determine whether medications increase the risk of falling. Consult with health care provider regarding the client's need for medication if appropriate.
- Orient the client to the environment. Place the call light within reach and show how to call for assistance; answer call light promptly.
- Use one-fourth to one-half length side rails only, and maintain bed in a low position. Ensure that wheels are locked on the bed and commode. Keep dim light in the room at night.
- Routinely assist the client with toileting on his or her own schedule. Take the client to the bathroom on awakening and before bedtime (Goodwin et al, 2014).
- Keep the path to the bathroom clear, label the bathroom, and leave the door open.
- ▲ Avoid use of restraints if possible. Obtain health care provider's order if restraints are deemed necessary, and use the least restrictive device.
- In place of restraints, use the following:
  - ○ Well-staffed and educated nursing personnel with frequent client contact with careful consideration during shift changes
  - ○ Nursing units designed to care for clients with cognitive and/or functional impairments
  - ○ Nonskid footwear, sneakers preferable
  - ○ Glasses and/or hearing aids, as needed
  - ○ Adequate lighting, night-light in bathroom

• = Independent      ▲ = Collaborative

- ○ Frequent toileting
- ○ Frequently assess need for invasive devices, tubes, intravenous (IV) access
- ○ Hide tubes with bandages to prevent pulling of tubes
- ○ Consider alternative IV placement site to prevent pulling out IV line
- ○ Alarm systems with ankle, above-the-knee, or wrist sensors
- ○ Bed or wheelchair alarms
- ○ Wedge cushions on chairs to prevent slipping
- ○ Increased observation of the client
- ○ Locked doors to unit
- ○ Low- or very-low-height beds
- ○ Border-defining pillow/mattress to cue the client to stay in bed

- If the client has an acute change in mental status (delirium), recognize that the cause is usually physiological and is a medical emergency. Consider possible causes for delirium. Consult with the health care provider immediately. See interventions for Acute **Confusion.**
- If the client has chronic confusion caused by dementia, implement individualized strategies to enhance communication. Assessment of specific receptive and expressive language abilities is needed to understand the client's communication difficulties and facilitate communication. See interventions for Chronic **Confusion.**
- Ask family to stay with the client to assist with activities of daily living and prevent the client from accidentally falling or pulling out tubes.
- ▲ If the client is unsteady on his or her feet, have two nursing staff members alongside when walking the client. Use facility-approved mobility devices to assist with client ambulation (e.g., gait belts, walkers). Consider referral to physical therapy for gait training and strengthening.
- Place a fall-prone client in a room that is near the nurses' station.
- Help clients sit in a stable chair with armrests. Avoid use of wheelchairs except for transportation as needed. Clients are likely to fall when left in a wheelchair because they may stand up without locking the wheels or removing the footrests.
- ▲ Refer to physical therapy or other programs for exercise programs that target strength, balance, flexibility, or endurance.

**Geriatric**
- Assess mobility and gait speed using the Timed Up & Go Test. Ask the client to stand up from a standard arm chair, walk 10 feet (or 3

meters), turn around, walk back to the chair, and sit down (Podsiadlo & Richardson, 1991). This should be done with the client wearing usual footwear.

- Mobility assessment and acting on findings are crucial in care of older adults. This is embedded in the Age-Friendly Health System's Model of Care, an initiative of the John A. Hartford Foundation and the Institute of Healthcare Improvement (IHI) in partnership with the American Hospital Association and the Catholic Health Association of the United States that began in 2017. The Age-Friendly Health System model promotes the evidence-based 4Ms framework: (1) **What Matters** to the older adult, considering what is most important to the older adult, family, and caregivers, in terms of goals and preferences; (2) **Medication**, making sure all medications have a clear indication, prescribed at the lowest effective dosage and frequency; (3) **Mentation**, assessing and managing dementia, delirium, and/or depression; and (4) **Mobility**, maintaining or improving mobility and function (Institute for Healthcare Improvement, 2020).

- Complete a fall risk assessment for older adults in acute care using a valid and reliable tool such as the Hendrich II Fall Risk Model.

- ▲ If there is new onset of falling, assess for laboratory abnormalities, signs and symptoms of infection and dehydration, and blood glucose level for diabetics, and check blood pressure and pulse rate with client in supine, sitting, and standing positions for hypotension and orthostatic hypotension. If the client has borderline high blood pressure, the risk of falling because of the administration of antihypertensives may outweigh the benefits of the antihypertensive medication. Discuss with the health care provider on a client-to-client basis.

- Complete a fear of falling assessment for older adults. This includes measuring fear of falling, or the level of concern about falling, and falls self efficacy, which is the degree of confidence a person has in performing common activities of daily living without falling. Fear of falling may be measured by a single-item question asking about the presence of fear of falling or rating severity of fear of falling on a 1 to 4 Likert scale as is commonly done in studies. Falls self-efficacy may be measured using a valid and reliable tool such as the Falls Efficacy Scale—International (Yardley et al, 2005; Greenberg, 2012; Greenberg et al, 2016; Greenberg 2019).

- Encourage the client to wear glasses and use walking aids when ambulating.

• = Independent          ▲ = Collaborative

- If the client experiences dizziness because of orthostatic hypotension when getting up, teach methods to decrease dizziness, such as rising slowly, remaining seated several minutes before standing, flexing feet upward several times while sitting, sitting down immediately if feeling dizzy, and trying to have someone present when standing.
▲ If the client is experiencing syncope, determine symptoms that occur before syncope and note medications that the client is taking. Refer for medical care. The circumstances surrounding syncope often suggest the cause.
▲ Observe client for signs of anemia, and refer to health care provider for testing if appropriate.
- Evaluate client for chronic alcohol intake and mental health and neurological function.
▲ Refer to physical therapy for strength training, using free weights or machines, and suggest participation in exercise programs.
▲ Evidence-based guidelines for preventing falls in older adults were published by the American Geriatrics Society (AGS) and British Geriatrics Society (BGS) collaboratively and specify recommendations for all clinical settings. The Centers for Disease Control and Prevention's Stopping Elderly Accidents, Deaths, & Injuries (STEADI) initiative related to older adult fall prevention provides implementation strategies. These recommendations include screening and assessment and interventions. Examples of interventions include (1) exercise for balance and for gait and strength training, such as tai chi or physical therapy; (2) environmental adaptation to reduce fall risk factors in the home and in daily activities; (3) cataract surgery when indicated; (4) medication reduction with particular attention to medications that affect the brain such as sleeping medications and antidepressants; (5) assessment and treatment of postural hypotension; (6) identification and appropriate treatment of foot problems; and (7) vitamin D supplementation for those with vitamin D deficiency (American Geriatrics Society [AGS], 2011; Centers for Disease Control and Prevention, & National Center for Injury Prevention and Control, 2020d; Centers for Disease Control and Prevention, 2021a)
▲ Refer community-dwelling older adults to evidence-based community-based programs (National Council on Aging, 2021).

**Home Care**
- Some of the previously mentioned interventions may be adapted for home care use.

• = Independent          ▲ = Collaborative

- Implement evidence-based fall prevention practices in community settings and home health care programs for older adults (National Council on Aging, 2021).
- ▲ If delirium is present, assess for cause of delirium and/or falls with the use of a multiprofessional team. Consult with the health care provider immediately. Assess and monitor for acute changes in cognition and behavior.
- Assess home environment for threats to safety, including clutter, slippery floors, scatter rugs, and other potential hazards. Additionally, assess external environment (e.g., uneven pavement, unleveled stairs/steps).
- ▲ Institute a home-based, nurse-delivered exercise program to reduce falls or refer to physical therapy services for client and family education of safe transfers and ambulation and for strengthening exercises for the client (Grabiner, 2014; National Council on Aging, 2021).
- ▲ Instruct the client and family or caregivers on how to correct identified hazards for those with visual impairment. Refer to physical and occupational therapy services for assistance if needed.
- ▲ Use a multifactorial assessment along with interventions targeted to the identified risk factors. Key components of the interventions include evaluating need for all medications, balance, gait, and strength training, use of strategies to deal with postural hypotension if present, home safety evaluation with needed modifications, and any needed cardiovascular treatment.
- If the client lives alone or spends a great deal of time alone, teach the client what to do if he or she falls and cannot get up, and make sure he or she has a personal emergency response system or a mobile phone that is available from the floor (AGS, 2011; National Council on Aging, 2021).
- Ensure appropriate nonglare lighting in the home. Ask the client to install indoor strip or "runway" type of lighting to baseboards to help clients balance. Install motion-sensitive lighting that turns on automatically when the client gets out of bed to go to the bathroom.
- Have the client wear supportive, low-heeled shoes with good traction when ambulating. Avoid use of slip-on footwear. Wear appropriate footwear in inclement weather.
- Provide a signaling device for clients who wander or are at risk for falls. Orienting a vulnerable client to a safety net relieves the anxiety of the client and caregiver and allows for rapid response to a crisis situation.

• = Independent ▲ = Collaborative

- Provide medical identification bracelet for clients at risk for injury from dementia, diabetes, seizures, or other medical disorders.
- Suggest a tai chi class designed for older adults and selected clients who have sufficient balance to participate.

**Client/Family Teaching and Discharge Planning**
- Teach the client and the family about the fall reduction measures that are being used to prevent falls (The Joint Commission, 2020).
- Providing education on safety guidelines to prevent falls is an important nursing intervention that should be completed as part of discharge planning (National Council on Aging, 2021)
- Teach the client how to safely ambulate at home, including using safety measures such as handrails in bathroom, reaching for items on high shelves, and avoiding carrying things or performing other tasks while walking.
- Teach the client the importance of maintaining a regular exercise program. If the client is afraid of falling while walking outside, suggest that he or she walk the length of a local mall.

# Risk for Child Falls

**Domain 11** Safety/protection    **Class 2** Physical injury
## NANDA-I Definition

Child susceptible to experiencing an event resulting in coming to rest inadvertently on the ground, floor, or other lower level, which may compromise health.

## Risk Factors

### Caregiver Factors

Changes diapers on raised surfaces; exhaustion; fails to lock wheels of child equipment; inadequate knowledge of changes in developmental stages; inadequate supervision of child; inattentive to environmental safety; inattentive to safety devices during sports activities; places child in bouncer seat on raised surfaces; places child in infant walkers; places child in mobile seat on raised surfaces; places child in seats without a seat belt; places child in shopping cart basket; places child on play equipment unsuitable for age group; postpartum depressive symptoms; sleeps with child in arms without protective measures; sleeps with child on lap without protective measures

### Physiological Factors

Decreased lower extremity strength; dehydration; hypoglycemia; hypotension; impaired physical mobility; impaired postural balance; incontinence; malnutrition; neurobehavioral manifestations; obesity; sleep disturbances

• = Independent                    ▲ = Collaborative

## Unmodified Environmental Factors

Absence of stairway gate; absence of stairway handrail; absence of wheel locks on child equipment; absence of window guard; cluttered environment; furniture placement facilitates access to balconies; furniture placement facilitates access to windows; high chairs positioned near tables or counters; inadequate anti-slip material on floors; inadequate automobile restraints; inadequate lighting; inadequate maintenance of play equipment; inadequate restraints on elevated surfaces; inattentive to pets; objects out of reach; seats without arms; seats without backs; uneven floor; unfamiliar setting; use of furniture without anti-tipping devices; use of non–age appropriate furniture; use of throw rugs

## Other Factors

Factors identified by standardized, validated screening tool; inappropriate clothing for walking; inappropriate footwear

## At-Risk Population

Boys; children <12 years of age; children born to economically disadvantaged families; children experiencing prolonged prescribed fasting period; children exposed to overcrowded environment; children in the labor force; children whose caregivers have low educational level; children whose caregivers have mental health issues; children with history of falls; children with stressed caregivers; children with young caregivers; children within the first week of hospitalization

## Associated Conditions

Assistive devices for walking; feeding and eating disorders; musculoskeletal diseases; neurocognitive disorders; pharmaceutical preparations; sensation disorders

## Client Outcomes

### Client Will (Specify Time Frame)

- Remain free of falls
- Verbalize environmental conditions to prevent falls
- Have a decreased risk of injury if sustains a fall
- Adapt environment to minimize the incidence of falls
- Explain methods to prevent injury

## Nursing Interventions

- Provide and review home safety plans with parents.
- Follow national guidelines to teach parents and guardians about fall safety for children.
  - ○ Playground safety includes ensuring surfaces under equipment are soft and well maintained.
  - ○ Home safety addresses guards on windows that are above ground level and use of stair gates and guard rails.

• = Independent        ▲ = Collaborative

○ Use helmets and wrist, knee, and elbow pads/protective gear during recreation and sports activities.

○ Keep fire safety ladder available near window on floors above ground level.

○ Close supervision of young children is essential to reduce fall risks.

- Explore possible concerns of harm indirectly or directly resulting in a child fall.

- Children younger than 4 years of age and those with special needs that increase caregiver burden are at greater risk of harm from unintentional falls (Chaudhary et al, 2018; CDC, 2021b).

- Assess height from which the child fell and possible impact.

- Safety guidelines suggest that a pediatric fall risk assessment tool should be completed to assess fall risk.

- Use a valid and reliable fall risk assessment tool to assess the client risk for falling (DiGerolamo & Davis, 2017).

- Screen children for balance and mobility skills (i.e., supine to sit, sitting supported and unsupported, sit to stand, standing, walking and turning around, transferring, stooping to floor and recovering, and sitting down). Use tools such as the Pediatric Balance Scale (Franjoine et al, 2003) or the Performance-Oriented Mobility Assessment–Gait (POMA-G) (Phillips et al, 2018).

- Keep the path to the bathroom clear, label the bathroom, and leave the door open.

▲ Refer to physical therapy or other programs for exercise programs that target strength, balance, flexibility, or endurance.

**Home Care**

- Some of the previously mentioned interventions may be adapted for home care use.

- Encourage the child to engage in exercise and activities that are appropriate for development age to strengthen balance and muscles.

- Assess home environment for threats to safety, including clutter, slippery floors, scatter rugs, and other potential hazards. Additionally, assess external environment (e.g., uneven pavement, unleveled stairs/steps).

▲ Institute a home-based, balance performance program to improve youth core strength and balance.

▲ Use a multifactorial assessment along with interventions targeted to the identified risk factors. Key components of the interventions include evaluating all medications, balance, gait and strength training, home safety evaluation with needed modifications, and any needed safety equipment.

• = Independent          ▲ = Collaborative

- Ensure appropriate nonglare lighting in the home. Ask the client to install indoor strip or "runway" type of lighting to baseboards to help clients balance. Install motion-sensitive lighting that turns on automatically when the client gets out of bed to go to the bathroom.
- Provide medical identification bracelet for clients at risk for injury from diabetes, seizures, or other medical disorders.

**Client/Family Teaching and Discharge Planning**

- Teach the client and the family about the fall reduction measures that are being used to prevent falls (CDC, 2019b).
- Providing education on safety guidelines to prevent falls is an important nursing intervention that should be completed as part of discharge planning (CDC, 2019b)
- Teach the child and parent how to safely ambulate at home, including using safety measures such as handrails, avoid reaching for items or performing other tasks while walking.

## Dysfunctional Family Processes

**Domain 7** Role relationship    **Class 2** Family relationships

### NANDA-I Definition

Family functioning which fails to support the well-being of its members.

### Defining Characteristics

#### Behavioral

Altered academic performance; altered attention; conflict avoidance; contradictory communication pattern; controlling communication pattern; criticizing others; decreased physical contact; denies problems; difficulty accepting a wide range of feelings; difficulty accepting help; difficulty adapting to change; difficulty dealing constructively with traumatic experiences; difficulty expressing a wide range of feelings; difficulty having fun; difficulty meeting the emotional needs of members; difficulty meeting the security needs of members difficulty meeting the spiritual needs of its members; difficulty receiving help appropriately; difficulty with intimate interpersonal relations; difficulty with life-cycle transition; enabling substance misuse pattern; escalating conflict; harsh self-judgment; immaturity; inadequate communication skills; inadequate knowledge about substance misuse; inappropriate anger expression; loss of independence; lying; maladaptive grieving; manipulation; nicotine addiction; orientation favors tension relief rather than goal attainment; paradoxical communication pattern; pattern of broken promises; power struggles; psychomotor agitation; rationalization; refuses to accept personal responsibility; refuses to get help; seeks affirmation; seeks approval; self-blame; social isolation;

• = Independent      ▲ = Collaborative

special occasions centered on substance misuse; stress-related physical illness; substance misuse; unreliable behavior; verbal abuse of children; verbal abuse of parent; verbal abuse of partner

**Feelings**

Anxiety; confuses love and pity; confusion; depressive symptoms; dissatisfaction; emotionally controlled by others; expresses anger; expresses distress; expresses embarrassment; expresses fear; expresses feeling abandoned; expresses feeling of failure; expresses feeling unloved; expresses frustration; expresses insecurity; expresses lingering resentment; expresses loneliness; expresses shame; expresses tension; hopelessness; hostility; loss; loss of identity; low self-esteem; mistrust of others; moodiness; powerlessness; rejection; reports feeling different from others; reports feeling emotionally isolated; reports feeling guilty; reports feeling misunderstood; repressed emotions; taking responsibility for substance misuser's behavior; unhappiness; worthlessness

**Roles and Relationships**

Altered family relations; altered role function; chronic family problems; closed communication system; conflict between partners; deterioration in family relations; diminished ability of family members to relate to each other for mutual growth and maturation; disrupted family rituals; disrupted family roles; family denial; family disorganization; inadequate family cohesiveness; inadequate family respect for autonomy of its members; inadequate family respect for individuality of its members; inadequate interpersonal relations skills; inconsistent parenting; ineffective communication with partner; neglects obligation to family member; pattern of rejection; perceived inadequate parental support; triangulating family relations

**Related Factors**

Addictive personality; inadequate problem-solving skills; ineffective coping strategies; perceived vulnerability

**At-Risk Population**

Economically disadvantaged families; families with history of resistance to treatment regimen; families with member with history of substance misuse; families with members with genetic predisposition to substance misuse

**Associated Conditions**

Depression; developmental disabilities; intimacy dysfunction; surgical procedures

**Client Outcomes**

**Family/Client Will (Specify Time Frame)**

• State one way that alcoholism has affected the health of the family
• Identify three healthy coping behaviors that family members can use to facilitate a shift toward improved family functioning

• = Independent         ▲ = Collaborative

- Express feelings
- Meet physical, psychosocial, and spiritual needs of members
- Seek appropriate assistance
- Participate in the development of the plan of care

## Nursing Interventions

- Refer to care plans for Interrupted **Family** Process, Ineffective **Denial,** and Defensive **Coping** for additional interventions.
- Assess family members for adverse childhood experiences (ACEs).
- Acknowledge the range of emotions and feelings that may be experienced when the health status of a family member changes.
- Adopt a strength-oriented psychoeducational approach to assist family functioning.
- Allow and encourage family members to assist in the client's treatment.
- Support family members during emotional and conflict-type situations in the clinical setting.
- Screen clients for at-risk drinking during routine primary care visits and before surgery using the US Alcohol Use Disorders Identification Test (USAUDIT).
- ▲ Refer for family therapy and other family-oriented resources.
- ▲ Behavioral screening and intervention (BSI) should be integrated into all health care settings. Different terminology has evolved for screening, intervention, and referral for various behavioral issues. The five As—ask, advise, assess, assist, and arrange—apply to tobacco use. Screening, brief intervention, and referral to treatment (SBIRT) pertains to alcohol and drug use.

### Pediatric

- ▲ Encourage early intervention. When parental depression, childhood exposure to conflict and violence, and childhood experience with abuse and neglect coexist with parental substance abuse, their children are more likely to engage in increased teacher-rated unfavorable student behavioral problems.
- Assess for the illness beliefs of the pediatric client as well as illness beliefs of the family.
- Educate family members about available educational and support programs and encourage no/limited alcohol use in the home.
- Encourage adolescents to attend a 12-step program as needed.
- Provide interactive school-based drug-prevention program to middle school students.

### Geriatric

- Include the assessment of possible alcohol abuse when assessing older family members.

**Multicultural**
- Acknowledge racial/ethnic differences at the onset of care.
- Assess lesbian, gay, bisexual, or transgender (LGBTQ) youth for factors that contribute to family rejection.

**Home Care**

Note: In the community setting, alcoholism as a cause of dysfunctional family processes must be considered in two categories: (1) when the client suffers personally from the illness, and (2) when a significant other suffers from the illness, that is, the client is not the active alcoholic but may depend on the alcoholic for caregiving. The following considerations apply to both situations with appropriate adaptation for the circumstances.
- The previous interventions may be adapted for home care use.

**Client/Family Teaching and Discharge Planning**
- Provide education for the family.
- Facilitate participation in mutual help groups (MHGs).

## Interrupted Family Processes

**Domain 7** Role relationship  **Class 2** Family relationships

**NANDA-I Definition**

Break in the continuity of family functioning which fails to support the well-being of its members.

**Defining Characteristics**

Altered affective responsiveness; altered communication pattern; altered family conflict resolution; altered family satisfaction; altered interpersonal relations; altered intimacy; altered participation in decision-making; altered participation in problem-solving; altered somatization; altered stress-reduction behavior; assigned tasks change; decreased emotional support availability; decreased mutual support; ineffective task completion; power alliance change; reports conflict with community resources; reports isolation from community resources; ritual change

**Related Factors**

Altered community interaction; altered family role; difficulty dealing with power shift among family members

**At-Risk Population**

Families with altered finances; families with altered social status; families with member experiencing developmental crisis; families with member experiencing developmental transition; families with member experiencing situational transition

**Associated Conditions**

Altered health status

• = Independent  ▲ = Collaborative

## Client Outcomes

**Family/Client Will (Specify Time Frame)**
- Express feelings (family)
- Identify ways to cope effectively and use appropriate support systems (family)
- Treat impaired family member as normally as possible to avoid overdependence (family)
- Meet physical, psychosocial, and spiritual needs of members or seek appropriate assistance (family)
- Demonstrate knowledge of illness or injury, treatment modalities, and prognosis (family)
- Participate in the development of the plan of care to the best of ability (significant person)

## Nursing Interventions

- Recognize informal roles in medical decision-making by family members.
- Acknowledge the range of emotions and feelings that may be experienced when the health status of a family member changes.
- Adopt a strength-oriented psychoeducational approach to assist family functioning.
- Establish relationships among clients, their families, and health care professionals.
- Encourage family to visit the client; adjust visiting hours to accommodate the family's schedule.
- Allow and encourage family members to assist in the client's treatment.
- Support family members during emotional and conflict-type situations in the clinical setting
- Anticipate and implement family reunification efforts after a disaster.
- Refer to the care plan Readiness for Enhanced **Family** Processes for additional interventions.

### Pediatric
- Carefully assess potential for reunifying children placed in foster care with their birth parents.
- Assess for the influence of family socioeconomic status on family processes.
- Provide prebirth risk assessments to identify prebirth and postbirth supports for high-risk pregnant women.
- Provide parents with both general information and professional support by family-centered early childhood intervention services to their families.

• = Independent        ▲ = Collaborative

F

- Encourage and support parents/family to assist in client's care.
- Assess military families for the influence of deployment on family functioning.
▲ Refer parents and other primary caregivers to a mindfulness-based stress reduction (MBSR) program.

**Geriatric**

- Encourage family members to be involved in the care of relatives who are in residential care settings.
▲ Refer for Family Life Review (FLR) therapy.
▲ Refer family for counseling with a psychotherapist who is knowledgeable about gerontology.
- Refer to care plan for Readiness for Enhanced **Family** Processes for additional interventions.

**Multicultural**

- Assess lesbian, gay, bisexual, transgender, and queer (LGBTQ) youth for factors that contribute to family rejection.
- Refer to the care plan Readiness for Enhanced **Family** Processes for additional interventions.

**Home Care**

- The nursing interventions described in the care plan for Compromised Family **Coping** should be used in the home environment with adaptations as necessary.
- Encourage family members to find meaning in life with a serious illness.

**Client/Family Teaching and Discharge Planning**

- Refer to Client/Family Teaching and Discharge Planning in Compromised Family **Coping** and Readiness for Enhanced Family **Coping** for suggestions that may be used with minor adaptations.

# Readiness for Enhanced Family Processes

**Domain 7** Role relationship    **Class 2** Family relationships

## NANDA-I Definition

A pattern of family functioning to support the well-being of members, which can be strengthened.

## Defining Characteristics

Expresses desire to enhance balance between personal autonomy and family cohesiveness; expresses desire to enhance communication pattern; expresses desire to enhance energy level of family to support activities of daily living; expresses desire to enhance family adaptation to change;

• = Independent                    ▲ = Collaborative

expresses desire to enhance family dynamics; expresses desire to enhance family psychological resilience; expresses desire to enhance growth of family members; expresses desire to enhance interdependence with community; expresses desire to enhance maintenance of boundaries between family members; expresses desire to enhance respect for family members; expresses desire to enhance safety of family members

## Client Outcomes

### Family/Client Will (Specify Time Frame)

- Identify ways to cope effectively and use appropriate support systems (family)
- Meet physical, psychosocial, and spiritual needs of members or seek appropriate assistance (family)
- Demonstrate knowledge of potential environmental, lifestyle, and genetic risks to health and use appropriate measures to decrease possibility of risk (family)
- Focus on wellness, disease prevention, and maintenance (family and individual)
- Seek balance among exercise, work, leisure, rest, and nutrition (family and individual)

## Nursing Interventions

- Assess the structure, resources, and coping abilities of families and use these assessments in selecting interventions and formulating care plans.
- Acknowledge, assess, and support the spiritual needs and resources of families and clients.
- Develop, provide, and encourage family members to use counseling services and interventions.
- Consider the use of family-centered theory as the conceptual foundation to help guide interventions.
- Establish rapport with families and empower their decision-making through effective communication and person- and family-centered care.
- Provide family members with educational and skill-building interventions to alleviate caregiving stress and to facilitate adherence to prescribed plans of care.

### Pediatric

- Provide educational and supportive interventions for families caring for children with illness and disability.
- Encourage participation in virtual support groups.
- Encourage families with children and adolescents to have family meals.

• = Independent          ▲ = Collaborative

**Geriatric**
- Provide educational and therapeutic interventions to family caregivers that focus on knowledge and skill building.
- Encourage use of information and communications technologies (ICT) for social networking; social integration; and social engagement with friends, children, and relatives.

**Multicultural**
- Understand and incorporate cultural differences into interventions to enhance the impact of family interventions.
- With the client's consent, facilitate a group meeting for family members to discuss how the family is functioning.
- Facilitate modeling and role playing for the client and family regarding healthy ways to start a discussion about the client's prognosis.
- Encourage family mealtimes.

**Home Care**
- The previous nursing interventions should be used in the home environment with adaptations as necessary.
▲ Encourage participation in virtual support groups to family caregivers.

**Client/Family Teaching and Discharge Planning**
- Refer to Client/Family Teaching and Discharge Planning for Readiness for Enhanced Family **Coping** for suggestions that may be used with minor adaptations.

# Fatigue

**Domain 4** Activity/rest     **Class 3** Energy balance
**NANDA-I Definition**

An overwhelming sustained sense of exhaustion and decreased capacity for physical and mental work at the usual level.

**Defining Characteristics**

Altered attention; apathy; decreased aerobic capacity; decreased gait velocity; difficulty maintaining usual physical activity; difficulty maintaining usual routines; disinterested in surroundings; drowsiness; expresses altered libido; expresses demoralization; expresses frustration; expresses lack of energy; expresses nonrelief through usual energy-recovery strategies; expresses tiredness; expresses weakness; inadequate role performance; increased physical symptoms; increased rest requirement; insufficient physical endurance; introspection; lethargy; tiredness

• = Independent          ▲ = Collaborative

## Related Factors

Altered sleep-wake cycle; anxiety; depressive symptoms; environmental constraints; increased mental exertion; increased physical exertion; malnutrition; nonstimulating lifestyle; pain; physical deconditioning; stressors

## At-Risk Population

Individuals exposed to negative life event; individuals with demanding occupation; pregnant women; women experiencing labor

## Associated Conditions

Anemia; chemotherapy; chronic disease; chronic inflammation; dementia; fibromyalgia; hypothalamus-pituitary-adrenal axis dysregulation; myasthenia gravis; neoplasms; radiotherapy; stroke

## Client Outcomes

**Client Will (Specify Time Frame)**

- Identify potential etiology of fatigue
- Identify potential factors that precipitate, aggravate, and relieve fatigue
- Describe ways to assess and monitor patterns of fatigue over time (e.g., within a day, a few days, a week, a month)
- Describe ways in which fatigue affects the ability to accomplish activities of daily living (ADLs)
- Verbalize increased energy and improved vitality
- Explain energy conservation plan to offset fatigue
- Verbalize ability and capacity to concentrate and make decisions
- Verbalize strategies for energy restorative activities

## Nursing Interventions

- Assess severity of fatigue on a scale of 0 to 10 (average fatigue, worst and best levels); assess frequency of fatigue (number of days per week and time of day), activities and symptoms associated with increased fatigue (e.g., pain), activities that relieve, ability to perform ADLs and instrumental ADLs, interference with social and role function, times of the day for increased energy, ability to concentrate, mood, usual pattern of physical activity, and interference with sleep cycles. Consider use of an instrument such as the Profile of Mood State Short Form Fatigue Subscale (PROMIS), the Multidimensional Assessment of Fatigue, the Lee Fatigue Scale, the Fatigue Symptom Inventory, the Multidimensional Fatigue Inventory, the HIV Related Fatigue Scale, the Brief Fatigue Inventory, Short Form Vitality Subscale, Fatigue Impact Scale, Fatigue Assessment Instrument, or Nottingham of Chronic Illness Therapy Fatigue Scale, Fatigue Severity Scale.
- Evaluate adequacy of nutrition and sleep hygiene (weight loss, anorexia, napping throughout the day, inability to fall asleep

**F**

or stay asleep). Encourage the client to get adequate rest, limit naps (particularly in the late afternoon or evening), use a routine sleep/wake schedule, plan and prioritize for daily activities as tolerated, allow exposure to bright light during daytime hours, use relaxation techniques before bedtime such as meditation, music, or guided imagery (Dikmen & Terzioglu, 2019), avoid caffeine in the late afternoon or evening, and eat a well-balanced diet that includes fresh fruits, vegetables, and lean meats. Mindfulness interventions also result in improved sleep quality (Gok Metin et al, 2019).

- Refer to Imbalanced **Nutrition**: Less Than Body Requirements or **Insomnia** if appropriate.
- Evaluate fluid status and assess for dehydration. Encourage at least eight glasses of water a day. Avoid caffeine, which can cause further dehydration.
▲ Collaborate with the primary provider to identify physiological and/or psychological causes of fatigue that could be treated, such as nutritional deficit, pain, electrolyte imbalance (e.g., altered potassium levels, vitamin D deficiency), dehydration, thyroid disorders, anemia, arthritis, depression, anxiety, sleep disturbances (insomnia/sleep deprivation), acute or chronic infection, medication use or side effects, alcohol use/abuse, metabolic disorders (diabetes), or a preexisting comorbidity or disease (multiple sclerosis, cancer or cancer treatment, respiratory disease, fibromyalgia, cardiac disease, renal disease, Parkinson's disease).
▲ Work with the primary care or specialty provider to determine if the client has chronic fatigue syndrome. Chronic fatigue syndrome is unexplained fatigue lasting 6 months or longer that is not associated with a diagnosed physical or psychological condition but may include muscle pain, memory problems, headaches, sleep problems, joint pain, and diarrhea (Milrad et al, 2018).
- Encourage clients to express feelings, attribution of cause, and behaviors about fatigue, including potential causes of fatigue, and interventions that they use to alleviate or moderate the fatigue. Such interventions could include setting small, easily achieved short-term goals and developing energy management and energy conservation techniques; use active listening techniques to help identify sources of hope. In addition, help them determine the time of day when they have the most energy to do important things. Assess clients' level of motivation and willingness to adopt new behaviors or change behaviors that can improve symptoms of fatigue.

• = Independent          ▲ = Collaborative

- Encourage the client to keep a journal of activities (or record using one of the many apps available) that contribute to symptoms of fatigue, patterns of symptoms across days/weeks/months, and feelings, including how fatigue affects the client's normal daily activities and roles. Have client identify the activities that contribute the most to fatigue.
- Assist the client to identify sources of support and prioritize essential and nonessential tasks to determine which tasks need to be completed and which can be delegated and to whom. Give the client permission to limit or change or remove social and role demands if needed (e.g., switch to part-time employment, simplify meal preparation, give up activities for a short period, hire cleaning service).
▲ Collaborate with the primary provider regarding the appropriateness of referrals to physical therapy for carefully monitored and prescribed aerobic exercise program.
- Encourage the client to use complementary and alternative therapies such as relaxation, meditation, and mindfulness to support other strategies.
▲ Refer the client to diagnosis-appropriate support groups such as the American Parkinson Disease Association, National Chronic Fatigue Syndrome Association, National Parkinson Foundation, PatientsLikeMe, National Multiple Sclerosis Society, American Heart Association, American Cancer Society, National Comprehensive Cancer Network, Chronic Myalgic Encephalomyelitis, and Chronic Fatigue Society.
▲ For an individual with cardiac disease, recognize that fatigue is common with myocardial infarction, congestive heart failure, or chronic cardiac insufficiency (Matura et al, 2018). Refer to cardiac rehabilitation for a carefully prescribed and monitored exercise and rehabilitation program.
- If fatigue is associated with cancer or cancer-related treatment, assess for other symptoms that may increase fatigue (e.g., pain, insomnia, anemia, emotional distress, electrolyte imbalance [nausea, vomiting, diarrhea], or depression).
▲ Refer the client for cognitive behavioral therapy (CBT) to improve coping and self-management of fatigue.
▲ Collaborate with primary provider to identify attentional fatigue, which may manifest itself as the inability to direct attention necessary to perform usual activities. Attentional fatigue is associated with sleep disturbances, depressive symptoms, anxiety, and psychosocial stressors

• = Independent ▲ = Collaborative

and can lead to inability to concentrate, plan goals, control emotions, or engage in social interactions.

▲ Collaborate with primary providers to identify potential pharmacological treatment for fatigue.

**Geriatric**

• Evaluate fatigue in geriatric clients routinely, particularly in clients with limited physical function and lower levels of social support.

• Review medications to determine possible side effects or interaction effects that could cause fatigue.

• Review comorbid conditions that may contribute to fatigue, such as congestive heart failure, pulmonary disease, cardiac disease, multiple sclerosis, arthritis, obesity, anemia, depression, Parkinson's disease, insomnia, cancer, and viral infections (e.g., COVID-19).

• Identify recent losses, even loss of physical function; monitor for depression or loneliness as a possible contributing factor to fatigue.

• Review other symptoms the client may be experiencing. Fatigue is often associated with other symptom clusters such as depression and sleep disturbances (National Comprehensive Cancer Network, 2021a).

▲ Review medications for side effects.

**Home Care**

• The previously mentioned interventions may be adapted for home care use as well.

• Assess the client's history and current patterns of fatigue as they relate to the home environment and environmental and behavioral triggers of increased fatigue.

▲ Encourage planned exercise regimens or physical activities such as walking or light aerobic exercises. This activity can be organized in the home, mall, on a treadmill, or in a setting such as senior centers or wellness facilities.

▲ Refer to occupational and/or physical therapy if substantial intervention is needed to assist the client in adapting to home and daily patterns.

• For clients receiving chemotherapy, intervene to:
  ○ Relieve symptom distress (anxiety, nausea and vomiting, diarrhea, lack of appetite, emotional distress, difficulty sleeping)
  ○ Encourage as much physical activity as possible with a specific recommendation (Hoffman et al, 2017)

• Teach the client and family the importance of and methods for setting priorities for activities, especially those with high energy demand (e.g., home or family events). Instruct in realistic expectations and behavioral pacing.

• = Independent          ▲ = Collaborative

○ Identify with clients ways in which they continue to be a valued part of their social environment.

○ Identify with clients ways in which they continue to maintain daily activity or social activities.

○ Encourage the client to maintain regular family routines (e.g., meals, daily activities, sleep patterns), as well as physical activity, as much as possible.

**F**

### Client/Family Teaching and Discharge Planning

• Help the client to reframe cognitively; share information about fatigue, how to live with it, and how to moderate it, including need for positive self-talk.

• Teach strategies for energy conservation that can result in improved fatigue level (e.g., sitting instead of standing during showering, limiting trips up and down stairs).

• Teach the client to carry a pocket calendar, make lists of required activities, use electronic reminders, and post reminders around the house.

• Teach the importance of following a healthy lifestyle with adequate nutrition, fluids, and rest; pain relief; insomnia correction; and appropriate exercise to decrease fatigue (i.e., energy restoration).

• Engage in outdoor relaxation and use of nature as an option to relieve fatigue.

## Fear

**Domain 9** Coping/stress tolerance     **Class 2** Coping responses

### NANDA-I Definition

Basic, intense emotional response aroused by the detection of imminent threat, involving an immediate alarm reaction (American Psychological Association).

### Defining Characteristics

#### Physiological Factors

Anorexia; diaphoresis; diarrhea; dyspnea; increased blood pressure; increased heart rate; increased respiratory rate; increased sweating; increased urinary frequency; muscle tension; nausea; pallor; pupil dilation; vomiting; xerostomia

#### Behavioral/Emotional

Apprehensiveness; concentration on the source of fear; decreased self-assurance; expresses alarm; expresses fear; expresses intense dread; expresses tension; impulsive behaviors; nervousness; psychomotor agitation

• = Independent          ▲ = Collaborative

## Related Factors

Communication barriers; learned response to threat; response to phobic stimulus; unfamiliar situation

## At-Risk Population

Children; individuals exposed to traumatic situation; individuals living in areas with increased violence; individuals receiving terminal care; individuals separated from social support; individuals undergoing surgical procedure; individuals with family; individuals with history of falls; older adults; pregnant women; women; women experiencing childbirth

## Associated Conditions

Sensation disorders

## Client Outcomes

**Client Will (Specify Time Frame)**

- Verbalize known fears
- State accurate information about the situation
- Identify, verbalize, and demonstrate those coping behaviors that reduce own fear
- Report and demonstrate reduced fear

## Nursing Interventions

- Assess the source of fear in the client.
- Assess for presence of fear avoidance beliefs.
- Provide counseling to enhance client's self-efficacy.
- Engage clients in skills that promote and contribute to their psychological flexibility, such as acceptance and openness to one's experience; cognitive defusion, or holding one's thoughts lightly; flexible attention to the here and now; having a stable and transcendental sense of self; clarification of and living based on deeply meaningful chosen values; and committed purposeful action.
- Engage clients with a fear of cancer recurrence about cognitive-behavioral therapies that include teaching skills to identify patterns of thoughts, emotions, and behaviors; skills to identify triggers of fear of cancer recurrence; reframing skills to cope with cognitive appraisals of uncontrollability to make them as less threatening; skills for problem-solving; and behavioral exposure skills to confront avoidance of cancer-related stimuli.
- Engage clients in a mindfulness-based training program.
- Engage pregnant women with fear of childbirth in individual or group psychoeducation sessions or therapeutic conversations during pregnancy.
- Provide antenatal education to women with fear of childbirth.
- Provide brief psychoeducation to a client who has fear about surgery.

• = Independent            ▲ = Collaborative

- Offer psychological interventions for clients with a fear of public speaking. The psychological interventions can be delivered through traditional (face-to-face) or technology-assisted formats.
- Assist clients with fear of lower back pain through a combination of strategies focused on reconceptualizing clients' knowledge about their lower back pain (e.g., "explain pain" and exposure in vivo). Strategies are targeted to assist clients to gain control over pain and responses to pain as a way to make sense of their lower back pain experience.
- Integrate psychologically informed practices for athletes who experience fear of reinjury through self-report questionnaires to quantify fear of reinjury at various key points of rehabilitation journey, education to reduce fear-avoidance beliefs, quota-based exercise, and graded exposure.
▲ Refer client for cognitive behavioral therapy (CBT).
- See care plan for **Anxiety.**

**Pediatric**
- Use distraction techniques to reduce fear of painful procedures.
- Incorporate play therapy as an intervention to reduce fears during painful procedures.
- For adolescents with disordered eating behaviors, assess for a fear of food.
▲ For children with cancer, refer children and families to screening for cancer-related posttraumatic stress symptoms (PTSS) and other stressors.

**Geriatric**
- Engage clients with a fear of falling in CBT-based multicomponent interventions, including cognitive restructuring, motivational interviewing, or goal-setting.
- Engage clients with a fear of falling in an intervention program that includes both CBT and exercise (focused primarily on balance and strength training or tai chi).
- Provide mind-body interventions involving meditative movements (e.g., tai chi, qigong, yoga, and Pilates) for clients with fear of falling.
- Pair cognitive-behavioral strategies with exercises to improve physical skills and mobility to decrease fear of falling.
- Engage clients with the fear of death and dying in intervention strategies including psychotherapy, mindfulness exercises, and virtual reality.
- See care plan for **Anxiety** or Death **Anxiety.**

**Multicultural**
- Assess for fears of racism in culturally diverse clients.

• = Independent          ▲ = Collaborative

- Assess for fear of health care providers.
- Provide education, support, and guidance to engage clients in their care.

**Home Care**
- The previous interventions may be adapted for home care use.
- Refer to care plan for **Anxiety.**

**Client/Family Teaching and Discharge Planning**
- Assess for fears related to discharge from hospital.
- See care plan for **Anxiety.**

# Ineffective Infant Feeding Dynamics

**Domain 2** Nutrition    **Class 1** Ingestion

## NANDA-I Definition

Altered parental feeding behaviors resulting in over or under eating patterns.

## Defining Characteristics

Food refusal; inadequate appetite; inappropriate transition to solid foods; overeating; undereating

## Related Factors

Abusive interpersonal relations; attachment issues; disengaged parenting; intrusive parenting; lack of confidence in child to develop healthy eating habits; lack of confidence in child to grow appropriately; lack of knowledge of appropriate methods of feeding infant for each stage of development; lack of knowledge of infant's developmental stages; lack of knowledge of parent's responsibility in infant feeding; media influence on feeding infant high caloric unhealthy foods; media influence on knowledge of high caloric unhealthy foods; multiple caregivers; uninvolved parenting

## At-Risk Population

Abandoned infants; infants born to economically disadvantaged families; infants experiencing homelessness; infants experiencing life transition; infants experiencing prolonged hospitalization; infants living in foster care; infants who are small for gestational age; infants with history of hospitalization in neonatal intensive care; infants with history of unsafe eating and feeding experiences; premature infants

## Associated Conditions

Chromosomal disorders; cleft lip; cleft palate; congenital heart disease; inborn genetic diseases; neural tube defects; parental psychiatric disorder; physical challenge with eating; physical challenge with feeding; physical health issue of parent; prolonged enteral nutrition; psychological health issue of parent; sensory integration dysfunction

• = Independent          ▲ = Collaborative

## Client Outcomes

### Client Will (Specify Time Frame)

- Infant will consume adequate calories to support growth and development
- Caregiver will follow healthy infant feeding practices
- Caregiver will identify infant behavioral cues related to hunger and satiety
- Caregiver and infant will engage in positive interactions during feeding

## Nursing Interventions

- Assess weight and height of the infant and use a growth chart to help determine growth pattern, which reflects nutrition. Age-related growth charts are available from www.cdc.gov/growthcharts/ (Centers for Disease Control and Prevention, 2016).
- Assess mothers for symptoms of postpartum depression.
- Encourage parent–child interactions that promote attachment.
- Encourage overweight and obese mothers to follow current infant feeding guidelines.
- Encourage individualized breastfeeding support as appropriate.
- Teach infant caregivers to recognize the following infant communication: infants signal appetite through interest or disinterest in food; infants use rapid and transient facial expressions to signal liking; and they use subtle or potent gestures, body movements, and vocalizations to express wanting.
- Provide teaching and resources during pregnancy about recommended infant feeding practices.
- Provide caregivers of infants with teaching to encourage the early development of healthy eating patterns.
- Provide caregivers of infants with teaching on the importance of synchrony (offering the infant food and their willingness to eat) during the infant feeding time.
- Encourage caregiver co-eating during infant feeding times.
- Provide caregivers of infants with teaching about the strong association between sugar-sweetened beverages, obesity, and related chronic diseases.
- Assist mothers to identify infant engagement and disengagement cues during breastfeeding or formula feeding.
- Provide mothers with unconditional positive regard in their choice of breast, formula, or mixed feeding of their infant.

### Multicultural

- Assess for cultural beliefs, values, and practices related to the feeding of infants.

• = Independent ▲ = Collaborative

- Identify the support persons of the infant caregiver and extend healthy infant feeding education and information to those support persons.

**Home Care**
- The interventions previously described may be adapted for home care use.

**Client/Family Teaching and Discharge Planning**
- Many of the interventions previously described involve teaching.

## Risk for Female Genital Mutilation

**Domain 11** Safety/protection    **Class 3** Violence
### NANDA-I Definition

Susceptible to full or partial ablation of the female external genitalia and other lesions of the genitalia, whether for cultural, religious or any other non-therapeutic reasons, which may compromise health.

### Risk Factors

Lack of family knowledge about impact of practice on physical health; lack of family knowledge about impact of practice on psychosocial health; lack of family knowledge about impact of practice on reproductive health

### At-Risk Population

Women belonging to ethnic group in which practice is accepted; women belonging to family in which any female member has been subjected to practice; women from families with favorable attitude towards practice; women planning to visit family's country of origin in which practice is accepted; women residing in country where practice is accepted; women whose family leaders belong to ethnic group in which practice is accepted

### Client/Family Outcomes

Client Will (Specify Time Frame)
- Express effects of family/culture on beliefs about female genital mutilation (FGM)
- Demonstrate evidence that FGM has not occurred
- Express/implement a plan for avoiding FGM
- Maintain safety of female children
- Demonstrate the ability to make decisions independent of cultural group
- Demonstrate self-advocacy skills

### Nursing Interventions

- Use therapeutic and culturally competent communication when asking women about FGM.
- Identify the decision-making process related to the practice of FGM.
- Identify the type of FGM for which the female client is at risk.

• = Independent          ▲ = Collaborative

- Assess and identify geographic, environmental, familial, religious, and/or other cultural factors that increase risk for FGM.
- Encourage the mothers of at-risk daughters to express their beliefs and attitudes toward FGM.
- Assess the mothers of at-risk daughters for positive affect (expression of feelings) and attitudes toward FGM.
- In a respectful and nonjudgmental manner, provide men, fathers, and male partners with health education to address beliefs about FGM and provide information about the negative health outcomes associated with FGM.
- In a respectful and nonjudgmental manner, convey accurate and clear information about FGM, using language and methods that can be readily understood by clients.
- In a respectful and nonjudgmental manner, provide the client, the client's parents, and the client's family with information that FGM is not a universal practice and that it is an illegal practice in many parts of the world.
- In a respectful and nonjudgmental manner, provide the client, the client's parents, and the client's family with health education to address false beliefs about female and clitoral anatomy and the physiology of women.
- In a respectful and nonjudgmental manner, provide the client, the client's parents, and the client's family with health education to inform about the negative health outcomes associated with FMG.
- In a respectful and nonjudgmental manner, address false ideas or beliefs about FGM.
- In a respectful and nonjudgmental manner, provide the client, the client's parents, and the client's family with health education to inform about the negative birth outcomes associated with mothers who have had FMG.
- In a respectful and nonjudgmental manner, provide the client, the client's parents, and the client's family with health education to inform about the negative mental health outcomes associated with FGM.
- Use therapeutic and culturally competent communication to focus on the current and future safety of the female child at risk for FGM.
- Use a cultural mediator to interpret cross-cultural norms about FGM.
- In a respectful and nonjudgmental manner, provide fathers with health education to address beliefs about FGM and provide information about the negative health outcomes associated with FGM.

• = Independent          ▲ = Collaborative

▲ Refer families to counseling services.

• See care plans for **Post-Trauma** Syndrome, Impaired **Parenting,** and **Social** Isolation.

**Pediatric**

• Identify a system for assessment and referral of female infants at risk of FGM born to mothers who have undergone FGM.

• For female children who may be survivors of FGM, or are at risk of FGM, notify Child Protective Services and other law enforcement authorities.

• Implement a school-based intervention to provide FGM health education to adolescent females.

# Risk for Imbalanced Fluid Volume

**Domain 2** Nutrition    **Class 5** Hydration

## NANDA-I Definition

Susceptible to a decrease, increase, or rapid shift from one to the other of intravascular, interstitial, and/or intracellular fluid, which may compromise health.

## Risk Factors

Altered fluid intake; difficulty accessing water; excessive sodium intake; inadequate knowledge about fluid needs; ineffective medication self-management; insufficient muscle mass; malnutrition

## At-Risk Population

Individuals at extremes of weight; individuals with external conditions affecting fluid needs; individuals with internal conditions affecting fluid needs; women

## Associated Conditions

Active fluid volume loss; deviations affecting fluid absorption; deviations affecting fluid elimination; deviations affecting fluid intake; deviations affecting vascular permeability; excessive fluid loss through normal route; fluid loss through abnormal route; pharmaceutical preparations; treatment regimen

## Client Outcomes

**Client Will (Specify Time Frame)**

• Lung sounds clear, respiratory rate 12 to 20 and free of dyspnea

• Urine output greater than 0.5 mL/kg/hr

• Blood pressure, pulse rate, temperature, and oxygen saturation within expected range

• Laboratory values within expected range, that is, normal serum sodium, hematocrit, and osmolarity

• = Independent          ▲ = Collaborative

- Extremities and dependent areas free of edema
- Mental orientation appropriate based on previous condition

## Nursing Interventions
### Surgical Clients
- Monitor the fluid balance. If there are symptoms of hypovolemia, refer to the interventions in the care plan for Deficient **Fluid** Volume. If there are symptoms of hypervolemia, refer to the interventions in the care plan for Excess **Fluid** Volume.

### Preoperative
- Collect a thorough history and perform a preoperative assessment to identify clients with increased risk for hemorrhage or hypovolemia, that is, clients who take herbal supplements; those with recent traumatic injury, abnormal bleeding or altered clotting times, complicated kidney or liver disease, diabetes, cardiovascular disease, major organ transplant, history of aspirin and/or nonsteroidal antiinflammatory drug (NSAID) use, or anticoagulant therapy; or history of hemophilia, von Willebrand's disease, or disseminated intravascular coagulation. Assess the client's use of over-the-counter agents, including herbal products.
- Recognize that nothing per mouth (NPO) at midnight may or may not be appropriate for each surgical client. Guidelines from the American Society of Anesthesiologists Committee (2011) recommended that healthy clients having elective surgery should be allowed to have clear liquids up to 2 hours before surgery.
- Determine length of time the client has been without normal intake, been NPO, or experienced fluid loss (e.g., vomiting, diarrhea, bleeding).
- Assess and document the client's mental status. A baseline assessment is important so that changes in mental status during the postoperative period can be easily identified.
- Recognize that there is conflicting evidence regarding liberal intraoperative fluid management versus restrictive fluid management. Fluid administration during surgery is more restrictive to prevent pulmonary complications associated with excessive fluid administration (Myles et al, 2017).
- To reduce fluid administration volume, colloids rather than crystalloid fluids may be administered during surgery (Myles et al, 2017).
- Recognize that an individualized fluid management plan would be developed incorporating client-specific assessment parameters (e.g., existing comorbid diseases, age) and type of surgical procedure (Myles et al, 2017; Lindahl, 2020).

• = Independent ▲ = Collaborative

**F**

- Recognize the effects of general anesthetics, inhalational agents, and regional anesthesia on perfusion in the body and the potential for decreasing the blood pressure.
- Monitor for signs of intraoperative hypovolemia such as dry skin, dry mucous membranes, tachycardia, decreased urinary output, decreased CVP, hypotension, increased pulse, and/or deep rapid respirations.
- Monitor for signs of intraoperative hypervolemia such as dyspnea, coarse crackles, increased pulse and respirations, decreased oxygenation, and decreased urinary output, all of which could progress to pulmonary edema.
- In the critically ill surgical client a pulmonary artery catheter or other minimally invasive CO monitoring device may be used to determine fluid balance and guide fluid and vasoactive intravenous (IV) drip administration.
- Monitor the client for hyponatremia with symptoms such as headache, anorexia, nausea and vomiting, diarrhea, tachycardia, general malaise, muscle cramps, weakness, lethargy, change in mental status, disorientation, seizures, and death.
- Monitor clients undergoing laparoscopic or hysteroscopic procedures for the development of hyponatremia, hypervolemia, and pulmonary edema when an irrigation fluid is used.
- Monitor clients undergoing transurethral resection of the prostate (TURP) procedures for development of hyponatremia and hypervolemia with symptoms of TURP syndrome including headache, visual changes, agitation, lethargy, vomiting, muscle twitching, bradycardia, diminished pupillary reflexes, hypertension, and respiratory distress.
- Measure the irrigation fluid used during urological and gynecological procedures accurately for volume deficit such as amount of irrigation used minus amount of irrigation recovered via suction.
- Monitor intraoperative intake and output including blood loss, urine output, and third-space losses to provide an estimate of fluid volume.
- Observe the surgical client for hyperkalemia with symptoms including dysrhythmias, heart block, asystole, abdominal distention, and weakness.
- Maintain the client's core temperature at normal levels, using warming devices as needed.
- Fluids administration during surgery can increase risk of hypothermia.

**Postoperative**
- Continue to monitor fluids postoperatively.

• = Independent ▲ = Collaborative

- Assess the client for development of tissue edema, especially after cataract surgery in clients with comorbidities such as diabetes.
- Recognize that IV fluid replacement decisions incorporate multiple assessment parameters such as hourly urine output, blood pressure, heart rate, respiratory rate, lung sounds, output from drains, and changes in laboratory results (e.g., hemoglobin/hematocrit, serum electrolytes).

**F**

**Geriatric**
- Check skin turgor of older clients on the forehead, subclavian area, or inner thigh; also look for the presence of longitudinal furrows on the tongue and dry mucous membranes.
- Closely monitor urine output, concentration of urine, and serum BUN/creatinine results.
- Monitor older clients for excess fluid volume during the treatment of deficient fluid volume: auscultate lung sounds, assess for edema, and trend vital signs.
- Assess the older client's cognitive status.

**Pediatric**
- Assess the pediatric client's weight, length of NPO status, and underlying illness, and the surgical procedure to be performed.
- Recognize that newborns require very little fluid replacement when undergoing major surgical procedures during the first few days of life.
- Monitor pediatric surgical clients closely for signs of fluid loss.
- Administer fluids preoperatively until NPO status must be initiated so that fluid deficit is decreased.
- Perform an assessment for signs of fluid responsiveness in the pediatric client.

## Deficient Fluid Volume

**Domain 2** Nutrition    **Class 5** Hydration
### NANDA-I Definition

Decreased intravascular, interstitial, and/or intracellular fluid. This refers to dehydration, water loss alone without change in sodium
### Defining Characteristics

Altered mental status; altered skin turgor; decreased blood pressure; decreased pulse pressure; decreased pulse volume; decreased tongue turgor; decreased urine output; decreased venous filling; dry mucous membranes; dry skin; increased body temperature; increased heart rate; increased serum hematocrit levels; increased urine concentration; sudden weight loss; thirst; weakness

• = Independent        ▲ = Collaborative

### Related Factors

Difficulty meeting increased fluid volume requirement; inadequate access to fluid; inadequate knowledge about fluid needs; ineffective medication self-management; insufficient fluid intake; insufficient muscle mass; malnutrition

### At-Risk Population

Individuals at extremes of weight; individuals with external conditions affecting fluid needs; individuals with internal conditions affecting fluid needs; women

### Associated Conditions

Active fluid volume loss; deviations affecting fluid absorption; deviations affecting fluid elimination; deviations affecting fluid intake; excessive fluid loss through normal route; fluid loss through abnormal route; pharmaceutical preparations; treatment regimen

### Client Outcomes

**Client Will (Specify Time Frame)**

- Maintain urine output of 0.5 to 1.5 mL/kg/h or at least more than 1300 mL/day
- Maintain normal blood pressure, heart rate, and body temperature
- Maintain elastic skin turgor; moist tongue and mucous membranes; and orientation to person, place, and time
- Explain measures that can be taken to treat or prevent fluid volume loss
- Describe symptoms that indicate the need to consult with health care provider

### Nursing Interventions

- Watch for early signs of hypovolemia, including thirst, restlessness, headaches, and inability to concentrate.
- Recognize symptoms of cyanosis, cold clammy skin, weak thready pulse, confusion, and oliguria as late signs of hypovolemia.
- Monitor pulse, respiration, and blood pressure of clients with deficient fluid volume every 15 minutes to 1 hour for the unstable client and every 4 hours for the stable client.
- Check orthostatic blood pressures with the client lying, sitting, and standing.
- Note skin turgor over bony prominences such as the hand or shin.
- Monitor for the existence of factors causing deficient fluid volume (e.g., hypovolemia from vomiting, diarrhea, difficulty maintaining oral intake, fever, uncontrolled type 2 diabetes, diuretic therapy).
- Observe for dry tongue and mucous membranes and longitudinal tongue furrows.

• = Independent          ▲ = Collaborative

- Recognize that checking capillary refill is an assessment of peripheral perfusion and may not be helpful in identifying fluid volume deficit.
- Weigh client daily and watch for sudden decreases, especially in the presence of decreasing urine output or active fluid loss.
- Monitor total fluid intake and output every 4 hours (or every hour for the unstable client or the client who has urine output equal to or less than 0.5 mL/kg/h).
- A urine output of less than 0.5 mL/kg/h for more than 6 hours may be indicative of acute kidney injury (Dean, 2020; Molinari et al, 2020). Nevertheless, in any condition of hypovolemia, renal perfusion pressure falls. If it falls below the level of autoregulation (blood pressure [BP] <80 mm Hg), renal blood flow and glomerular filtration will fall (Andreucchi et al, 2017).
- Note the color of urine, urine osmolality, and specific gravity.
- Provide fresh water and oral fluids preferred by the client (distribute over 24 hours [e.g., 1200 mL during days, 800 mL during evenings, and 200 mL during nights]), provide prescribed diet, offer snacks (e.g., frequent drinks, fresh fruits, fruit juice), and instruct significant other to assist the client with feedings as appropriate.
- ▲ Provide oral replacement therapy as ordered and tolerated with a hypotonic glucose-electrolyte solution when the client has acute diarrhea or nausea/vomiting. Provide small, frequent quantities of slightly chilled solutions.
- ▲ Administer antidiarrheals and antiemetics as ordered and appropriate. Consider what the client is eating to prevent further diarrhea (Bolen, 2020). The goal is to stop the loss that results from vomiting or diarrhea. Refer to care plan for **Diarrhea** or **Nausea.**
- If the client is on enteral feedings, evidence has shown either continuous or intermittent feedings had similar results regarding diarrhea and nausea (Houston & Fuldauer, 2017).
- ▲ Hydrate the client with isotonic IV solutions as prescribed.
- Assist with ambulation if the client has postural hypotension.

**Critically Ill**
- ▲ Monitor stroke volume, passive leg lift, and ultrasound as trends for more accurate fluid volume status.
- ▲ Monitor serum and urine osmolality blood urea nitrogen (BUN)/creatinine ratio and hematocrit for elevations.
- ▲ Insert an indwelling urinary catheter if ordered and measure urine output hourly. Notify health care provider if urine output is less than 0.5 mL/kg/h.

• = Independent          ▲ = Collaborative

**F**

▲ When ordered, initiate a fluid challenge of crystalloids (e.g., lactated Ringer's or 0.9% normal saline) for replacement of intravascular volume.

▲ Monitor the client's response to prescribed fluid therapy and fluid challenge, especially noting vital signs (mean arterial pressure [MAP] >65 mm Hg in the first 6 hours of treatment, systolic blood pressure >100 mm Hg) (Singer, 2016; Rhodes et al, 2017), urine output, blood lactate concentrations, and lung sounds.

• Position the client flat with legs elevated when hypotensive, if not contraindicated.

▲ Monitor trends in serum lactic acid levels and base deficit obtained from blood gases as ordered.

▲ Consult provider if signs and symptoms of deficient fluid volume persist or worsen.

**Pediatric**

• Monitor the child for signs of deficient fluid volume, including sunken eyes, decreased tears, dry mucous membranes, poor skin turgor, and decreased urine output (Hockenberry et al, 2019).

▲ Reinforce the health care provider recommendation for the parents to give the child oral rehydration fluids to drink in the amounts specified, especially during the first 4 to 6 hours to replace fluid losses. Consider using diluted oral rehydration fluids. Once the child is rehydrated, an orally administered maintenance solution should be used along with food.

• Recommend that the mother resume breastfeeding as soon as possible.

• Recommend that parents not give the child carbonated soda, fruit juices, gelatin dessert, or instant fruit drink mix; instead, give the child oral rehydration fluids ordered and, when tolerated, food.

• Once the child has been rehydrated, begin feeding regular food, but avoid milk products (Guandalini et al, 2020).

**Geriatric**

• Monitor older clients for deficient fluid volume carefully, noting new onset of headache, weakness, dizziness, and postural hypotension.

• Implement fall precautions for clients experiencing weakness, dizziness, and/or postural hypotension.

• Dehydration in the older adult is associated with poor health outcomes, including fractures, heart disease, infections, and drug toxicity (Lešnik et al, 2017).

• Evaluate the risk for dehydration using the Dehydration Risk Appraisal Checklist.

• = Independent          ▲ = Collaborative

- Check skin turgor of older clients on the forehead and axilla; check for dry mucous membranes and dry tongue.
- Encourage fluid intake by offering fluids regularly to cognitively impaired clients.
- Because older clients have low water reserves, they should be encouraged to drink regularly even when not thirsty. Frequent and varied beverage offerings should be made available by hydration assistants to routinely offer increased beverages to clients in extended care.
- Flag the food tray of clients with chronic dehydration to indicate if the client is identified as having chronic dehydration and indicate that they should finish 75% to 100% of their food and fluids.
- Recognize that lower blood pressures and monitoring of an intake record over 24 hours are recommended to track oral intake and possible dehydration (Oates & Price, 2017).
- A higher BUN/creatinine ratio can be significant signs of dehydration in older adults.
- In the United States, more than 50% of seniors over the age of 75 are believed to have kidney disease (National Kidney Foundation, 2021).
- Monitor older clients for excess fluid volume during the treatment of deficient fluid volume: auscultate lung sounds, assess for edema, and note vital signs.

**Home Care**

- Teach family members how to monitor output in the home (e.g., use of commode "hat" in the toilet, urinal, or bedpan, or use of catheter and closed drainage system). Instruct them to monitor both intake and output. Use common terms such as "cups" or "glasses of water a day" when providing education.
- When weighing the client, use same scale each day. Be sure scale is on a flat, not cushioned, surface. Do not weigh the client with a scale placed on any type of rug because scales provide more accurate readings when used on a hard surface.
- Teach family about complications of deficient fluid volume and when to call the health care provider.
- Teach the family the signs of hypovolemia, especially in older adults, and how to monitor for dizziness or unsteady gait.
- If the client is receiving IV fluids, there must be a responsible caregiver in the home. Teach caregiver about administration of fluids, complications of IV administration (e.g., fluid volume overload, development of phlebitis, speed of medication reactions), and when to call for assistance. Assist caregiver with administration for as long

• = Independent          ▲ = Collaborative

F

as necessary to maintain client safety. Administration of IV fluids in the home is a high-technology procedure and requires sufficient professional support to ensure safety of the client.

- Identify an emergency plan, including when to call 911. Some complications of deficient fluid volume cannot be reversed in the home and are life-threatening. Clients progressing toward hypovolemic shock will need emergency care.

- Deficient fluid volume may be a symptom of impending death in terminally ill clients. In palliative care situations, treatment of deficient fluid volume should be determined based on client/family goals. Information and support should be provided to assist the client/family in this decision. Support the family/client in a palliative care situation to decide if it is appropriate to intervene for deficient fluid volume or to allow the client to die without fluids.

**Client/Family Teaching and Discharge Planning**

- Instruct the client to avoid rapid position changes, especially from supine to sitting or standing.

- Teach the client and family about appropriate diet, fluid intake, and how to weight self weekly.

- Teach the client and family how to measure and record intake and output accurately.

- Teach the client and family about measures instituted to treat hypovolemia and to prevent or treat fluid volume loss.

- Instruct the client and family about signs of deficient fluid volume that indicate they should contact health care provider.

# Excess Fluid Volume

**Domain 2** Nutrition    **Class 5** Hydration

## NANDA-I Definition

Surplus retention of fluid.

## Defining Characteristics

Adventitious breath sounds; altered blood pressure; altered mental status; altered pulmonary artery pressure; altered respiratory pattern; altered urine specific gravity; anxiety; azotemia; decreased serum hematocrit levels; decreased serum hemoglobin level; edema; hepatomegaly; increased central venous pressure; intake exceeds output; jugular vein distention; oliguria; pleural effusion; positive hepatojugular reflex; presence of S3 heart sound; psychomotor agitation; pulmonary congestion; weight gain over short period of time

• = Independent          ▲ = Collaborative

## Related Factors

Excessive fluid intake; excessive sodium intake; ineffective medication self-management

## Associated Conditions

Deviations affecting fluid elimination; pharmaceutical preparations

## Client Outcomes

### Client Will (Specify Time Frame)

**F**

- Remain free of edema, effusion, and anasarca
- Maintain body weight appropriate for the client
- Maintain clear lung sounds; no evidence of dyspnea or orthopnea
- Remain free of jugular vein distention, positive hepatojugular reflex, and S3 heart sound
- Maintain normal central venous pressure, pulmonary artery pressure, cardiac output, and vital signs
- Maintain urine output of 0.5 mL/kg/h or more with normal urine osmolality and specific gravity
- Explain actions that are needed to treat or prevent excess fluid volume including fluid and dietary restrictions, and medications
- Describe symptoms that indicate the need to consult with health care provider

## Nursing Interventions

- Monitor location and extent of edema using the 1+ to 4+ scale to quantify edema; also measure the legs using a millimeter tape in the same area at the same time each day. Note differences in measurement between extremities.
- Monitor daily weight for sudden increases; use same scale and type of clothing at same time each day, preferably before breakfast.
- Monitor intake and output; note trends reflecting decreasing urine output in relation to fluid intake.
- Chronic HF is characterized by neurohormonal activation and sodium retention that leads to excessive fluid accumulation in the systemic and pulmonary circulations.
- Auscultate lung sounds for crackles, monitor respiration effort, and determine the presence and severity of orthopnea.
- Monitor serum and urine osmolality, serum sodium, blood urea nitrogen (BUN)/creatinine ratio, and hematocrit for abnormalities.
- BUN and creatinine are monitored currently as biomarkers of kidney injury and failure.
- With head of bed elevated 30 to 45 degrees, monitor jugular veins for distention with the client in the upright position; assess for positive hepatojugular reflex.

 • = Independent           ▲ = Collaborative

- Monitor the client's behavior for restlessness, anxiety, or confusion; use safety precautions if symptoms are present.

▲ Monitor for the development of conditions that increase the client's risk for excess fluid volume, including HF, kidney failure, and liver failure, all of which result in decreased glomerular filtration rate and fluid retention.

**F**

▲ Provide a restricted-sodium diet as appropriate if ordered.

▲ Monitor serum albumin level and provide protein intake as appropriate.

▲ Administer prescribed diuretics as appropriate; ensure adequate blood pressure before administration. If diuretic is administered intravenously, note and record the blood pressure and urine output after the dose. Monitor serum sodium for hyponatremia.

- Monitor for side effects of diuretic therapy, including orthostatic hypotension (especially if the client is also receiving angiotensin-converting enzyme [ACE] inhibitors), hypovolemia, and electrolyte imbalances (hypokalemia and hyponatremia).

- Implement fluid restriction as ordered, especially when serum sodium is low; include all routes of intake. Schedule limited intake of fluids around the clock, and include the type of fluids preferred by the client. Fluid restriction may decrease intravascular volume and myocardial workload. Overzealous fluid restriction should not be used because hypovolemia can worsen HF. Client involvement in planning will enhance participation in the necessary fluid restriction.

- Maintain the rate of all IV infusions, using an IV pump.

- Turn clients with dependent edema at least every 2 hours and monitor for areas that may develop pressure ulcers.

▲ Provide ordered care for edematous extremities, including compression, elevation, and muscle exercises.

- Promote a positive body image and good self-esteem. Visible edema may alter the client's body image. Refer to the care plan for Disturbed **Body** Image.

▲ Consult with the health care provider if signs and symptoms of excess fluid volume persist or worsen.

**Critically Ill**

- Insert an indwelling urinary catheter if ordered and measure urine output hourly. Notify health care provider if output is less than 0.5 mL/kg/h.

▲ Monitor blood pressure, heart rate, passive leg lift, mean arterial pressure, central venous pressure, pulmonary artery pressure, and cardiac output/index; note and report trends of increasing or decreasing pressures over time.

▲ Monitor the effects of infusion of diuretic drips. Perform continuous renal replacement therapy (CRRT) as ordered if the client is critically ill and hemodynamically unstable and excessive fluid must be removed.

**F**

**Geriatric**

• Recognize that the presence of fluid volume excess is particularly serious in older adults.

• Monitor electrolyte levels carefully, including sodium levels and potassium levels, with both increased and decreased levels possible.

**Home Care**

• Assess client and family knowledge of disease processes causing excess fluid volume.

▲ Teach about disease process and complications of excess fluid volume, including when to contact the health care provider.

• Assess client and family knowledge and compliance with medical regimen, including medications, diet, rest, and exercise. Assist family with integrating restrictions into daily living. Assistance with integration of cultural values, especially those related to foods, with medical regimen promotes compliance and decreased risk of complications.

▲ Teach and reinforce knowledge of medications. Instruct the client not to use over-the-counter medications (e.g., diet medications) without first consulting the provider.

▲ Instruct the client to make the primary health care provider aware of medications ordered by other health care providers.

• Identify emergency plan for rapidly developing or critical levels of excess fluid volume when diuresing is not safe at home. Excess fluid volume can be life-threatening.

▲ Teach about signs and symptoms of both excess and deficient fluid volume, such as darker urine, dry mouth, and peripheral edema, and when to call the health care provider.

**Client/Family Teaching and Discharge Planning**

• Describe signs and symptoms of excess fluid volume and actions to take if they occur.

▲ Teach client on diuretics to weigh self daily in the morning and to notify the health care provider if there is a 2.2 pound (1 kg) or more weight gain (Walsh-Irwin, 2021).

▲ Teach the importance of fluid and sodium restrictions. Help the client and family devise a schedule for intake of fluids throughout the entire

• = Independent ▲ = Collaborative

day. Refer to a dietitian concerning implementation of a low-sodium diet.
- Teach clients how to measure and document intake and output with common household measurements, such as cups.
▲ Teach how to take diuretics correctly: take one dose in the morning and second dose (if taken) no later than 4 p.m.
- For the client undergoing hemodialysis, teach client the required restrictions in dietary electrolytes, protein, and fluid. Spend time with the client to detect any factors that may interfere with the client's compliance with the fluid restriction or restrictive diet.

# Risk for Deficient Fluid Volume

**Domain 2** Nutrition    **Class 5** Hydration

## NANDA-I Definition

Susceptible to experiencing decreased intravascular, interstitial, and/or intracellular fluid volumes, which may compromise health.

## Risk Factors

Difficulty meeting increased fluid volume requirement; inadequate access to fluid; inadequate knowledge about fluid needs; ineffective medication self-management; insufficient fluid intake; insufficient muscle mass; malnutrition

## At-Risk Population

Individuals at extremes of weight; individuals with external conditions affecting fluid needs; individuals with internal conditions affecting fluid needs; women

## Associated Conditions

Active fluid volume loss; deviations affecting fluid absorption; deviations affecting fluid elimination; deviations affecting fluid intake; excessive fluid loss through normal route; fluid loss through abnormal route; pharmaceutical preparations; treatment regimen

## Client Outcomes, Nursing Interventions, and Client/Family Teaching

Refer to care plan for Deficient **Fluid** Volume.

# Frail Elderly Syndrome

**Domain 1** Health promotion    **Class 2** Health management

## NANDA-I Definition

Dynamic state of unstable equilibrium that affects the older individual experiencing deterioration in one or more domains of health (physical,

• = Independent          ▲ = Collaborative

functional, psychological, or social) and leads to increased susceptibility to adverse health effects, in particular disability.

## Defining Characteristics

Bathing self-care deficit (00108); decreased activity tolerance (00298); decreased cardiac output (00029); dressing self-care deficit (00109); fatigue (00093); feeding self-care deficit (00102); hopelessness (00124); imbalanced nutrition: less than body requirements (00002); impaired memory (00131); impaired physical mobility (00085); impaired walking (00088); social isolation (00053); toileting self-care deficit (00110)

## Related Factors

Anxiety; decreased energy; decreased muscle strength; exhaustion; fear of falling; impaired postural balance; inadequate knowledge of modifiable factors; inadequate social support; malnutrition; neurobehavioral manifestations; obesity; sadness; sedentary lifestyle

## At-Risk Population

Economically disadvantaged individuals; individuals aged >70 years; individuals experiencing prolonged hospitalization; individuals for whom walking 15 feet requires > 6 seconds (4 meters >5 seconds); individuals living alone; individuals living in constricted spaces; individuals with history of falls; individuals with low educational level; individuals with unintentional loss of 25% of body weight over one year; individuals with unintentional weight loss >10 pounds (>4.5 kg) in one year; socially vulnerable individuals; women

## Associated Conditions

Anorexia; blood coagulation disorders; chronic disease; decreased serum 25-hydroxyvitamin D concentration; depression; endocrine regulatory dysfunction; mental disorders; sarcopenia; sarcopenic obesity; sensation disorders; suppressed inflammatory response

## Client Outcomes

### Client Will (Specify Time Frame)

- Remain living as independently as possible in the home or care setting of his or her choice
- Maintain safety when engaging in activities of daily living and ambulation
- Increase exercise and/or daily physical activity to build muscle strength
- Maintain a healthy weight

## Nursing Interventions

- Establish a trusting relationship with the client.
- Assess frailty with a tool such as the Frailty Index or the Edmonton Frail Scale.
- Perform a fall risk assessment on frail clients.

• = Independent     ▲ = Collaborative

**F**

- Assess nutritional status using a validated nutritional screening assessment tool such as the Malnutrition Universal Screening Tool (MUST).
- Assess for loneliness and implement measures to reduce feelings of loneliness.
- Encourage clients to engage in active lifestyles.
- Recognize that balance and gait impairment are features of frailty and are risk factors for falls.
- Address balance and gait impairments with a resistance based exercise program.
- Preserve physical functioning through individualized physical activity plans.
- Assess risk of fracture using tools such as the Cardiovascular Health Study (CHS) or Study of Osteoporotic Fracture (SOF) indicators.
- Evaluate the client's medications to determine whether medications increase the risk of frailty and/or are potentially inappropriate medications (PIMs), and if appropriate, consult with the client's health care provider regarding the client's medications.
- Use the Screening Tool of Older People's Prescriptions (STOPP) and the Screening Tool to Alert Right Treatment (START) to avoid omissions and inappropriateness in prescription.
- Assess and monitor vitamin D levels.
- ▲ Refer client to an exercise-training program.
- Monitor weight loss.
- Use an multiprofessional and person-centered approach for supporting frail older adults.
- Refer to care plan for Readiness for Enhanced **Nutrition** for additional interventions.

**Multicultural, Home Care, and Client/Family Teaching**
- The previously mentioned interventions may be adapted for multicultural, home care, and client family teaching.
- Provide a home-based exercise-training program.

# Risk for Frail Elderly Syndrome

**Domain 1** Health promotion　　**Class 2** Health management
## NANDA-I Definition

Susceptible to a dynamic state of unstable equilibrium that affects the older individual experiencing deterioration in one or more domain of health (physical, functional, psychological, or social) and leads to increased susceptibility to adverse health effects, in particular disability.

• = Independent　　　　　　　▲ = Collaborative

## Risk Factors

Anxiety; decreased energy; decreased muscle strength; exhaustion; fear of falling; impaired postural balance; inadequate knowledge of modifiable factors; inadequate social support; malnutrition; neurobehavioral manifestations; obesity; sadness; sedentary lifestyle

## At-Risk Population

Economically disadvantaged individuals; individuals aged >70 years; individuals experiencing prolonged hospitalization; individuals for whom walking 15 feet requires > 6 seconds (4 meters >5 seconds); individuals living alone; individuals living in constricted spaces; individuals with history of falls; individuals with low educational level; individuals with unintentional loss of 25% of body weight over one year; individuals with unintentional weight loss >10 pounds (>4.5 kg) in one year; socially vulnerable individuals; women

**G**

## Associated Conditions

Anorexia; blood coagulation disorders; chronic disease; decreased serum 25-hydroxyvitamin D concentration; depression; endocrine regulatory dysfunction; mental disorders; sarcopenia; sarcopenic obesity; sensation disorders; suppressed inflammatory response

## Client Outcomes and Nursing Interventions

Refer to care plan for **Frail Elderly** Syndrome.

# Impaired Gas Exchange

**Domain 3** Elimination and exchange    **Class 4** Respiratory function

## NANDA-I Definition

Excess or deficit in oxygenation and/or carbon dioxide elimination.

## Defining Characteristics

Abnormal arterial pH; abnormal skin color; altered respiratory depth; altered respiratory rhythm; bradypnea; confusion; decreased carbon dioxide levels; diaphoresis; headache upon awakening; hypercapnia; hypoxemia; hypoxia; irritable mood; nasal flaring; psychomotor agitation; somnolence; tachycardia; tachypnea; visual disturbances

## Related Factors

Ineffective airway clearance; ineffective breathing pattern; pain

## At-Risk Population

Premature infants

## Associated Conditions

Alveolar-capillary membrane changes; asthma; general anesthesia; heart diseases; ventilation-perfusion imbalance

• = Independent    ▲ = Collaborative

## Client Outcomes

**Client Will (Specify Time Frame)**

- Demonstrate improved ventilation and adequate oxygenation as evidenced by blood gas levels within normal parameters for that client
- Maintain clear lung fields and remain free of signs of respiratory distress
- Verbalize understanding of oxygen supplementation and other therapeutic interventions

**G**

## Nursing Interventions

- Monitor respiratory rate, depth, and ease of respiration. Watch for use of accessory muscles and nasal flaring.
- Auscultate breath sounds every 1 to 2 hours. The presence of crackles and wheezes may alert the nurse to airway obstruction, which may lead to or exacerbate existing hypoxia.
- The nurse should consider respiratory rate, work of breathing, and lung sounds along with $Pao_2$ values, $SaO_2$, $SpO_2$, client tidal volume, and minute ventilation.
- Monitor the client's behavior and mental status for the onset of restlessness, agitation, confusion, and (in the late stages) extreme lethargy.
- ▲ Monitor oxygen saturation continuously using pulse oximetry. Note blood gas results as available to determine correlation of pulse oximetry value with arterial blood gas oxygen saturation.
- Monitor venous oxygen saturation to determine an index of oxygen balance to reflect between oxygen delivery and oxygen consumption (Dirks, 2017).
- Measurements of oxygenation supply in the macrocirculation include those made upstream from the tissue level. The parameters measured are arterial partial pressure of oxygen ($Pao_2$), arterial oxygen saturation ($SaO_2$) determined on the basis of arterial blood gas (ABG) analysis and pulse oximetry ($SpO_2$), and ratio of $Pao_2$ to fraction of inspired oxygen ($FiO_2$), or the P:F ratio. Measurements of oxygenation or oxygen extraction or consumption in the macrocirculation made downstream from tissues include tissue oxygen consumption, mixed venous oxygen saturation ($SvO_2$) or central venous oxygen saturation ($ScvO_2$), and blood levels of lactate (Siela & Kidd, 2017; Şanci, Coşkun, & Bayram, 2020).
- Observe for cyanosis of the skin; especially note color of the tongue and oral mucous membranes.
- Position the client in a semirecumbent position with the head of the bed at a 30- to 45-degree angle to decrease the aspiration of gastric, oral, and nasal secretions.

• = Independent        ▲ = Collaborative

- If the client has unilateral lung disease, position with head of bed at 30 to 45 degrees with "good lung down" in a side-lying position and affected lung up (Barton, Vanderspank-Wright, & Shea, 2016).
▲ If the client is acutely dyspneic, consider having the client lean forward over a bedside table, resting elbows on the table if tolerated.
- Help the client deep breathe and perform controlled coughing. Have the client inhale deeply, hold the breath for several seconds, and cough two or three times with the mouth open while tightening the upper abdominal muscles as tolerated. Controlled coughing uses the diaphragmatic muscles, which makes the cough more forceful and effective.
▲ If the client has excessive fluid in the respiratory system based on auscultation, inform the prescribing provider to appropriate interventions.
▲ Monitor the effects of sedation and analgesics on the client's respiratory pattern; use judiciously.
- Schedule nursing care to provide rest and minimize fatigue.
▲ Administer humidified oxygen through an appropriate device (e.g., nasal cannula or venturi mask per the provider's order); aim for an oxygen ($O_2$) saturation level of 90% or above. Oxygen should be titrated to target an $SpO_2$ of >94%, except with carbon monoxide poisoning (100% oxygen), acute respiratory distress syndrome (ARDS) (88%–95%), those at risk for hypercapnia (88%–92%), and premature infants (88%–94%) (Bickley et al, 2020b). Watch for onset of hypoventilation as evidenced by increased somnolence.
- Once oxygen is started, arterial blood gases should be checked 30 to 60 minutes later to ensure satisfactory oxygenation without carbon dioxide retention or acidosis (GOLD, 2020).
- Supplemental oxygen can cause toxicity and should be administered at the lowest level that achieves an arterial saturation appropriate for a given client (Helmerhorst et al, 2015; Drake, 2018).
- Assess nutritional status including serum albumin level and body mass index (BMI).
▲ Assist the client to eat small meals frequently and use dietary supplements as necessary. Engage dietary in evaluating and creating an optimal nutrition plan. For some clients, drinking 30 mL of a supplement every hour while awake can be helpful.
▲ If the client is severely debilitated from chronic respiratory disease, consider the use of a wheeled walker to help in ambulation. Request a physical therapy consultation to assist with mobility and strength training.

• = Independent         ▲ = Collaborative

- Assess for signs of psychological distress, including anxiety, agitation, and insomnia.
▲ Refer the client with respiratory diseases, especially COPD, to a pulmonary rehabilitation program. Pulmonary rehabilitation is now considered a standard of care for the client with respiratory diseases (GOLD, 2020).

## Critical Care

▲ Assess and monitor oxygen indices such as the P:F ratio ($Pao_2$ to $FiO_2$), venous oxygen saturation/oxygen consumption ($SvO_2$ or $ScvO_2$) (Dirks, 2017; Siela & Kidd, 2017; Lough et al, 2022).
▲ Turn the client every 2 hours. Monitor oxygen saturation closely after turning. If it drops by 10% or fails to return to baseline promptly, turn the client back into the supine position and evaluate oxygen status. If the client does not tolerate turning, consider use of a kinetic bed that rotates the client from side to side in a turn of at least 40 degrees (St. Clair & MacDermott, 2017).
▲ If the client has ARDS with difficulty maintaining oxygenation, consider positioning the client prone with the upper thorax and pelvis supported. Monitor oxygen saturation and turn the client back to supine position if desaturation occurs.
▲ High levels of positive end-expiratory pressures may be prescribed to improve oxygenation and gas exchange (Barton, Vanderspank-Wright, & Shea, 2016).

## Geriatric

- Use central nervous system depressants and other sedating agents carefully to avoid decreasing respiration rate.
- Teach the client how to cough and perform deep breathing exercises to enhance gas exchange.
- Maintain appropriate levels of supplemental oxygen therapy for clients with impaired gas exchange and hypoxemia (GOLD, 2020).

## Home Care

- Work with the client to determine what strategies are most helpful during times of dyspnea. Educate and empower the client to self-manage the disease associated with impaired gas exchange.
- Collaborate with health care providers regarding long-term oxygen administration for chronic respiratory failure clients with severe resting hypoxemia. Administer long-term oxygen therapy for $Pao_2$ less than 55 or $SaO_2$ at or below 88% (GOLD, 2020).
- Assess the home environment for irritants that impair gas exchange. Help the client adjust the home environment as necessary (e.g., install an air filter to decrease the level of dust).

• = Independent          ▲ = Collaborative

▲ Refer the client to occupational therapy as necessary to assist the client in adapting to the home and environment and in energy conservation (GOLD, 2020).

• Assist the client with identifying and avoiding situations that exacerbate impairment of gas exchange (e.g., stress-related situations, exposure to pollution of any kind, proximity to noxious gas fumes such as chlorine bleach). Irritants in the environment decrease the client's effectiveness in accessing oxygen during breathing.

• Instruct the client to keep the home temperature above 68°F (20°C) and to avoid cold weather.

• Instruct the client to limit exposure to persons with respiratory infections.

• Instruct the family on the complications of the disease and the importance of maintaining the medical regimen, including when to call a health care provider.

▲ Refer the client for home health aide services as necessary for assistance with activities of daily living.

• When respiratory procedures are being implemented, explain equipment and procedures to family members, and provide needed emotional support. Family members assuming responsibility for respiratory monitoring often find this stressful.

• When electrically based equipment for respiratory support is being implemented, evaluate home environment for electrical safety, proper grounding, and so on. Ensure that notification is sent to the local utility company, the emergency medical team, and police and fire departments. Notification is important to provide for priority service. Work with the family to have an emergency plan and ensure all individuals in the home are aware of the plan.

▲ Assess family role changes and coping ability. Refer the client to medical social services as appropriate for assistance in adjusting to chronic illness.

• Support the family of the client with chronic illness.

**Client/Family Teaching and Discharge Planning**

• Teach the client how to perform pursed-lip breathing and inspiratory muscle training, and how to use the tripod position. Have the client watch the pulse oximeter to note improvement in oxygenation with these breathing techniques.

• Teach the client energy conservation techniques and the importance of alternating rest periods with activity. See nursing interventions for **Fatigue.**

        • = Independent                    ▲ = Collaborative

▲ Teach the importance of not smoking. Refer to smoking cessation programs, and encourage clients who relapse to keep trying to quit. Ensure that clients receive appropriate medications to support smoking cessation from the primary health care provider.

▲ Instruct the family regarding home oxygen therapy if ordered (e.g., delivery system, liter flow, safety precautions).

▲ Teach the client the need to receive a yearly influenza vaccine.

• Teach the client relaxation techniques to help reduce stress responses and panic attacks resulting from dyspnea.

• Teach the client to use music, along with a rest period, to decrease dyspnea and anxiety (Loscalzo, 2018; Ergin et al, 2018).

# Dysfunctional Gastrointestinal Motility

**Domain 3** Elimination and exchange     **Class 2** Gastrointestinal function

## NANDA-I Definition

Increased, decreased, ineffective, or lack of peristaltic activity within the gastrointestinal tract.

## Defining Characteristics

Abdominal cramping; abdominal pain; absence of flatus; acceleration of gastric emptying; altered bowel sounds; bile-colored gastric residual; diarrhea; difficulty with defecation; distended abdomen; hard, formed stool; increased gastric residual; nausea; regurgitation; vomiting

## Related Factors

Altered water source; anxiety; eating habit change; impaired physical mobility; malnutrition; sedentary lifestyle; stressors; unsanitary food preparation

## At-Risk Population

Individuals who ingested contaminated material; older adults; premature infants

## Associated Conditions

Decreased gastrointestinal circulation; diabetes mellitus; enteral nutrition; food intolerance; gastroesophageal reflux disease; infections; pharmaceutical preparations; treatment regimen

## Client Outcomes

**Client Will (Specify Time Frame)**

• Be free of abdominal distention and pain
• Have normal bowel sounds
• Pass flatus rectally at intervals
• Defecate formed, soft stool every day to every third day

• = Independent          ▲ = Collaborative

- State has an appetite
- Be able to eat food without nausea and vomiting

## Nursing Interventions

- Monitor for abdominal distention and presence of abdominal pain, weight loss, nausea, vomiting, obstipation, or diarrhea.
- Inspect, auscultate for bowel sounds noting characteristics and frequency; palpate and percuss the abdomen. Hypoactive bowel sounds are found with decreased motility as with peritonitis from paralytic ileus or from late bowel obstruction.
- Review history noting any anorexia or nausea and vomiting. Other symptoms may include relation of symptoms to meals, especially if aggravated by food, satiety, postprandial fullness/bloating, and weight loss or weight loss with severe gastroparesis.
- Monitor for fluid deficits by checking skin turgor and moisture of tongue, daily weights, input and output, and electrolyte values. Refer to care plan for Deficient **Fluid** Volume if relevant.
- ▲ Monitor for nutritional deficits by keeping close track of food intake. Review laboratory studies that affirm nutritional deficits, such as decreased albumin and serum protein levels, liver profile, glucose, fecal analysis, and an electrolyte panel. Refer to care plan for Imbalanced **Nutrition:** Less Than Body Requirements or Risk for **Electrolyte** Imbalance as appropriate.

### Slowed Gastric Motility

- Monitor the client for signs and symptoms of decreased gastric motility, which may include nausea after meals, vomiting, early satiety, postprandial fullness, abdominal bloating, and abdominal pain (Grover et al, 2019; Vavricka & Greuter, 2019).
- ▲ Monitor daily laboratory studies and point of care testing blood glucose levels, ensuring ordered glucose levels are performed and evaluated.
- Obtain a thorough gastrointestinal history if the client has diabetes because he or she is at high risk for gastroparesis and gastric reflux.
- ▲ If client has nausea and vomiting, provide an antiemetic and intravenous fluids as ordered. Offer or perform oral hygiene after vomiting. Refer to the care plan for **Nausea.**
- ▲ Administer prokinetic, antisecretory, fundic relaxant, and neuromodulator medications as prescribed (Grover et al, 2019; Sullivan et al, 2020).
- ▲ Evaluate medications the client is taking. Recognize that opioids, calcium channel blockers, GLP-1 analogs, diphenhydramine, and anticholinergic medications can cause gastric slowing (Onyimba & Clarke, 2019; Shen et al, 2019).

• = Independent ▲ = Collaborative

▲ Review laboratory and other diagnostic tools, including complete blood count, amylase, and thyroid-stimulating hormone level, glucose with other metabolic studies, upper endoscopy, and gastric-emptying scintigraphy.

▲ Recognize that endoscopic and surgical therapies for severe gastroparesis include pyloric disruption, electrical stimulation, venting or bypass, and gastric resection (Onyimba & Clarke, 2019; Sullivan et al, 2020).

▲ Alternative and complementary therapies such as acupuncture, electroacupuncture, ginger, and massage may offer symptom relief for gastroparesis (Onyimba & Clarke, 2019).

▲ Obtain a nutritional consultation, considering a small particle size diet or diets lower or higher in liquids or solids, depending on gastric motility.

▲ If the client is unable to eat or retain food, consult with the registered dietitian and health care provider, considering further nutritional support in the form of enteral or parenteral feedings for the client with gastroparesis.

▲ If the client is receiving gastric enteral nutrition, see the care plan Risk for **Aspiration.**

▲ Administer bulk-forming or osmotic laxative medications that increase gastrointestinal motility as ordered (Nagarwala, Dev, & Markin, 2016; Coutts, 2019).

• Advise client to eat small meals low in fat and fiber four to five times each day to allow for adequate nutritional intake while limiting the sensation of fullness; avoid spicy food, carbonated beverages, alcohol, and acidic foods; avoid smoking (Grover et al, 2019; Sullivan et al, 2020).

**Postoperative Ileus**

• Observe for complications of delayed intestinal motility. Symptoms include vague abdominal pain and distention, nausea, vomiting, anorexia, sometimes bloating, and tympany to percussion. Clients may or may not pass flatus and some stool (Eamudomkarn et al, 2018; Hedrick et al, 2018).

▲ Encourage the client to drink coffee three times per day postoperatively to decrease the time to first flatus and defecation after abdominal surgery (Eamudomkarn et al, 2018; Hedrick et al, 2018).

▲ Recommend chewing gum for the abdominal surgery client who is not at risk for aspiration and has normal dentition, particularly if oral intake is limited.

• = Independent          ▲ = Collaborative

G

▲ Limit preoperative fasting to 6 hours for solid food and 2 hours for liquids; discontinue fasting and reintroduce oral nutrition postoperatively; if the client has difficulty with oral intake or experiences nonbilious emesis postoperatively, provide a clear liquid diet and advance as tolerated (Hedrick et al, 2018; Taurchini et al, 2018).

• A preoperative walking program helps reduce time to first postoperative flatus and defecation for clients undergoing surgery for gynecological cancer (Özdemir et al, 2019). Assist the client with early mobilization after surgery; encourage client to eat all meals in a chair. Exercise may increase gastrointestinal motility.

▲ Minimize the use of opioids and use a multimodal analgesic approach for pain as feasible (Hedrick et al, 2018; Özdemir et al, 2019).

▲ Administer alvimopan, a mu opioid receptor antagonist medication, as prescribed (Venara et al, 2016; Hedrick et al, 2018).

▲ Avoid routine use of prophylactic nasogastric tubes (Hedrick et al, 2018; Taurchini et al, 2018).

▲ Administer an antiemetic for nausea and nonbilious emesis; for clients experiencing bilious emesis with abdominal distention, tympany, and intolerance of oral intake, insert a nasogastric tube as prescribed and consider other etiologies for the symptoms (Hedrick et al, 2018).

▲ Maintain euvolemia and replace electrolytes as needed (Hedrick et al, 2018; Taurchini et al, 2018).

**Increased Gastrointestinal Motility**

▲ Observe for complications of gastric surgeries such as dumping syndrome. This syndrome is the effect of changes in size and function of the stomach, with rapid dumping of hyperosmolar food into the intestines (Vavricka & Greuter, 2019).

• Watch for signs and symptoms of early dumping syndrome that occur within 15 minutes to 1 hour after a meal, which might include nausea, vomiting, bloating, cramping, abdominal pain, epigastric fullness, borborygmi, diarrhea, dizziness, desire to lie down, palpitations, tachycardia, syncope, perspiration, headache, hypotension, flushing, pallor, and fatigue (Vavricka & Greuter, 2019).

• Monitor for low blood sugar, fatigue, weakness, confusion, hunger, syncope, perspiration, palpitations, tremor, irritability, and dizziness 1 to 3 hours after eating because this is when late rapid gastric emptying may occur; late rapid gastric emptying is associated with low blood sugar (Vavricka & Greuter, 2019).

• = Independent          ▲ = Collaborative

▲ Order a nutritional consultation to discuss diet changes; the diet may vary depending on the kind of surgery causing dumping syndrome.

• Encourage client to lie down for 30 minutes after a meal to delay gastric emptying (Vavricka & Greuter, 2019).

▲ Administer acarbose to decrease intraluminal digestion of carbohydrates and somatostatin to delay gastric emptying and decrease the release of insulin as prescribed (Vavricka & Greuter, 2019).

▲ Administer antiemetics and antidiarrhea medications as prescribed (Vavricka & Greuter, 2019).

▲ Give intravenous fluids as ordered for the client complaining of diarrhea with weakness and dizziness. Monitor electrolyte panel and acid-base balance. Severe diarrhea can cause deficient fluid volume with extreme weakness and metabolic acidosis.

• Offer bathroom, commode, or bedpan assistance, depending on frequency, amount of diarrhea, and condition of client.

• Monitor rectal area for altered skin integrity and apply barrier creams as needed to protect and treat skin.

• Consider a fecal management system for bedbound clients with frequent loose stools to protect the perineal skin and minimize spread of infection.

• Refer to the care plans for the nursing diagnoses of Deficient **Fluid** Volume, **Nausea,** Impaired **Skin** Integrity, and **Diarrhea** as relevant.

**Pediatric**

• Assess infants and children with suspected delayed gastric emptying for fullness and vomiting.

▲ Observe for nutritional and fluid deficits with assessment of skin turgor, mucous membranes, fontanels, furrows of the tongue, electrolyte panel, fluid status, input and output, and daily weights (Islam, 2015).

▲ For pediatric clients age 6 months to 21 years with uncomplicated gastroenteritis, initiate oral rehydration therapy for mild (<5%) and moderate (5%–10%) dehydration with small, frequent volumes replacing ongoing losses with 2 ounces or 8 milliliters per kilogram for each episode of diarrhea or emesis; administer intravenous fluids as prescribed for severe (>10%) dehydration as prescribed; administer ondansetron for vomiting as prescribed (Carson et al, 2017).

▲ Recommend gentle massage for preterm infants as appropriate and to treat acute diarrhea in children.

• = Independent          ▲ = Collaborative

**Geriatric**

- Closely monitor diet and medication use/side effects because they affect the gastrointestinal system; watch for constipation.
- ▲ Watch for symptoms of dysphagia, gastroesophageal reflux disease, dyspepsia, chronic atrophic gastritis, peptic ulcer disease, mesenteric ischemia, irritable bowel syndrome, inflammatory bowel disease, maldigestion, diverticular disease, and reduced absorption of nutrients.

**Client/Family Teaching and Discharge Planning**

- Teach the client and caregivers about medications, reinforcing side effects as they relate to gastrointestinal function.
- Teach client and caregivers to report signs and symptoms that may indicate further complications, including increased abdominal girth, projectile vomiting, and unrelieved acute cramping pain (bowel obstruction).
- Review signs and symptoms of dehydration with client and caregivers.

G

## Risk for Dysfunctional Gastrointestinal Motility

**Domain 3** Elimination and exchange    **Class 2** Gastrointestinal function

### NANDA-I Definition

Susceptible to increased, decreased, ineffective, or lack of peristaltic activity within the gastrointestinal tract, which may compromise health.

### Risk Factors

Altered water sources; anxiety; eating habit change; impaired physical mobility; malnutrition; sedentary lifestyle; stressors; unsanitary food preparation

### At-Risk Population

Individuals who ingested contaminated material; older adults; premature infants

### Associated Conditions

Decreased gastrointestinal circulation; diabetes mellitus; enteral nutrition; food intolerance; gastroesophageal reflux disease; infections; pharmaceutical preparations; treatment regimen

### Client Outcomes, Nursing Interventions, and Client/Family Teaching and Discharge Planning

Refer to care plan for Dysfunctional **Gastrointestinal** Motility.

• = Independent        ▲ = Collaborative

# Risk for Unstable Blood Glucose Level

**Domain 2** Nutrition    **Class 4** Metabolism

## NANDA-I Definition

Susceptible to variation in serum levels of glucose from the normal range, which may compromise health.

## Risk Factors

Excessive stress; excessive weight gain; excessive weight loss; inadequate adherence to treatment regimen; inadequate blood glucose self-monitoring; inadequate diabetes self-management; inadequate dietary intake; inadequate knowledge of disease management; inadequate knowledge of modifiable factors; ineffective medication self-management; sedentary lifestyle

## At-Risk Population

Individuals experiencing rapid growth period; individuals in intensive care units; individuals of African descent; individuals with altered mental status; individuals with compromised physical health status; individuals with delayed cognitive development; individuals with family history of diabetes mellitus; individuals with history of autoimmune disorders; individuals with history of gestational diabetes; individuals with history of hypoglycemia; individuals with history of pre-pregnancy overweight; low birth weight infants; Native American individuals; pregnant women >22 years of age; premature infants; women with hormonal shifts indicative of normal life stage changes

## Associated Conditions

Cardiogenic shock; Diabetes mellitus; infections; pancreatic diseases; pharmaceutical preparations; polycystic ovary syndrome; pre-eclampsia; pregnancy-induced hypertension; surgical procedures

## Client Outcomes

### Client Will (Specify Time Frame)

- NOTE: All goals are general recommendations for most clients. Consult health care provider for client-specific goals.
- For most nonpregnant adults, maintain the following blood glucose targets (American Diabetes Association [ADA], 2021):
  - A1C less than 7% (normal level <5.7%) or lower if it can be safely achieved
  - A1C less than 8% in adults with limited life expectancy, or in those whom harms of treatment outweigh the benefits
  - Preprandial glucose between 80 and 130 mg/dL
  - Peak postprandial (1–2 hours after beginning of meal) glucose below 180 mg/dL

- For children and adolescents with diabetes, maintain the following blood glucose targets (ADA, 2021):
  - A1C less than 6.5% if it can be achieved without excessive hypoglycemia (types 1 and 2)
  - A1C less than 7% in most children (types 1 and 2)
  - A1C less than 7.5% in children who are at higher risk of hypoglycemia (types 1 and 2)
  - A1C less than 8% in children with history of severe life expectancy, short life expectancy, or in those whom harms of treatment outweigh the benefits (type 1)
- In pregnant mothers with gestational or preexisting type 1 or 2 diabetes, maintain blood glucose as follows (ADA, 2021):
  - A1C less than 6% for most women, less than 7% if necessary to prevent hypoglycemia
  - Fasting <95 mg/dL
  - One-hour postprandial ≤140 mg/dL
  - Two-hour postprandial ≤120 mg/dL
- In older adults, maintain blood glucose control as follows (ADA, 2021):
  - Healthy older adults: A1C < 7 .0 to 7.5; preprandial blood glucose 80 to 130 mg/dL; bedtime 80 to 180 mg/dL
  - Older adults with complex coexisting chronic illness, cognitive impairment, or functional dependence: A1C <8.0%, fasting or preprandial 90 to 150 mg/dL; bedtime 100 to 180 mg/dL
  - Older adult end-stage chronic illness or moderate to severe cognitive impairment: A1C not pertinent; preprandial 100 to 180 mg/dL; bedtime 110 to 200 mg/dL
- Maintain blood glucose in the majority of hospitalized clients between 140 and 180 mg/dL; more stringent goals may be appropriate if hypoglycemia can be avoided (ADA, 2021)

## Nursing Interventions

▲ Monitor blood glucose in hospitalized clients with diabetes who are eating, before meals; who are not eating, every 4 to 6 hours; and who are receiving intravenous (IV) insulin, every 30 minutes to 2 hours.

▲ In clients receiving multiple-dose insulin or insulin pump therapy, obtain blood glucose before meals and snacks, at bedtime, occasionally postprandially, before exercise or critical tasks such as driving, if low blood glucose is suspected, and after treatment for low blood glucose until normoglycemic. This may require checking up to 6 to 10 times daily.

• = Independent          ▲ = Collaborative

- ▲ Consider SMBG in clients with type 2 diabetes not using insulin.
- ▲ Consider continuous glucose monitoring in clients with type 1 diabetes on intensive insulin regimens.
- ▲ Evaluate A1C level for glucose control over previous 3 months.
- ▲ Consider monitoring 2 hours after the start of meals in individuals who have premeal glucose values within target but have A1C values above target.
- ▲ Consult provider for insulin therapy orders for any client whose glucose is consistently above 180 mg/dL.
- • Monitor for signs and symptoms of hypoglycemia, such as shakiness, irritability, confusion, tachycardia, hunger, headache, loss of consciousness, or seizures.
- • Identify level of hypoglycemia. Level 1 hypoglycemia is defined as a measurable glucose concentration <70 mg/dL (3.9 mmol/L) but ≥54 mg/dL (3.0 mmol/L) that can alert a person to take action" (Agiostratidou et al, 2017). Level 2 hypoglycemia is a blood glucose concentration <54 mg/dL (3.0 mmol/L), which is typically the threshold for neuroglycopenic symptoms. Level 3 hypoglycemia is a clinical event characterized by altered mental and/or physical functioning that requires assistance from another person for recovery. Levels 2 and 3 require immediate correction of low blood glucose (ADA, 2021).
- ▲ Raise glycemic targets in insulin-treated clients with hypoglycemia unawareness, one level 3 hypoglycemic event, or a pattern of unexplained level 2 hypoglycemia to strictly avoid hypoglycemia for at least several weeks.
- • If the client is experiencing signs and symptoms of hypoglycemia, test glucose; if the result is below 70 mg/dL (level 1), administer 15 to 20 g glucose if the client is conscious. Pure glucose (e.g., three to four glucose tablets) is the preferred treatment, but any form of carbohydrate that contains glucose will suffice (a cup of fruit juice or regular [not diet] soda, one cup of milk, a small piece of fruit). Avoid treating with foods that contain fat, or in type 2 diabetes, avoid foods high in protein. Repeat test in 15 minutes and repeat treatment if indicated. Once blood glucose returns to normal, the individual should consume a meal or snack to prevent recurrence of hypoglycemia.
- ▲ Treat severe (level 3) hypoglycemia as follows, if client is unable to swallow glucose:
  - ○ If the client has IV access, administer 25 g of 50% glucose IV (check agency protocol).

• = Independent                    ▲ = Collaborative

○ In the absence of IV access, administer 3 mg intranasal or 1 mg intramuscular or subcutaneous glucagon.

○ For the client at home with no IV glucose or glucagon access, contact emergency personnel and administer oral glucose or cake frosting into the buccal space. Tilt client's head to side to avoid aspiration.

▲ Monitor for and report signs and symptoms of hyperglycemia, such as increased thirst or urination, high blood glucose levels, or elevated A1C.

▲ Monitor fluid balance and replace fluids in clients with diabetic ketoacidosis.

▲ Avoid use of sliding scale insulin alone in hospitalized clients.

• Before administering IV insulin solution using polyethylene-lined tubing, precondition tubing with insulin solution and allow the solution to dwell for 30 minutes before completing a flush. Use an amount of solution equal to the volume of the tubing for the dwell and again for the flush.

▲ Evaluate the client's medication regimen for medications that can alter blood glucose.

▲ Refer client to a registered dietitian nutritionist (RDN) who is skilled in diabetes medical nutrition therapy (MNT) for individualized instruction.

▲ Refer people with type 1 diabetes and those with type 2 diabetes who are prescribed a flexible insulin therapy program for education on how to use carbohydrate counting (and in some cases fat and protein gram estimation) to determine mealtime insulin dosing.

▲ Refer overweight and obese clients with diabetes for diet and activity instruction.

• Assist clients with periodontal disease to access dental care.

▲ Assist clients with depression or mental illness to gain access to mental health services, and ensure collaboration with the diabetes treatment team.

▲ Advise all clients to avoid use of cigarettes and other tobacco products or e-cigarettes.

• For interventions regarding foot care, refer to the care plan Ineffective Peripheral **Tissue Perfusion.**

**Geriatric**

• Screen for geriatric syndromes (i.e., polypharmacy, cognitive impairment, depression, urinary incontinence, falls, and persistent pain) in older adults.

▲ In clients with diabetes who require tube feedings, use a diabetes-specific formulation.

▲ Refer older adults for diabetes self-management education and support.

▲ Collaborate with provider to ensure that diabetes treatment costs are affordable and cost-related nonadherence is avoided.

**Pediatric**

▲ Treat hypoglycemia in newborn infants with 0.5 mL/kg oral (buccal) dextrose gel.

▲ Teach parents of children with diabetes how to recognize and treat symptoms of hypoglycemia.

▲ Begin screening youth with type 1 diabetes for eating disorders between 10 and 12 years of age. The Diabetes Eating Problems Survey—Revised (DEPS-R) is a reliable, valid, and brief screening tool for identifying disturbed eating behavior.

• Teach children and adolescents (and their parents) with type 1 diabetes to self-monitor glucose (with meter or continuous glucose monitoring) multiple times daily: before meals and snacks, at bedtime, before exercise, when they suspect low blood glucose, after treating low blood glucose until they are normoglycemic, and before critical tasks such as driving.

• Teach parents and children that children and adolescents with type 1 and 2 diabetes should spend 60 minutes or more per day in moderate to vigorous aerobic activity, and at least 3 days/week in muscle/bone-strengthening activity.

**Home Care**

• Teach family and others having close contact with the person with diabetes how to use an emergency glucagon kit (intranasal, injection kit, or autoinjector, as prescribed).

**Multicultural**

▲ Assess social context, including potential food insecurity, housing stability, and financial barriers, and collaborate with provider to apply the information to treatment decisions.

• Provide ethnically and culturally appropriate content that is person centered, considering such things as literacy levels, ethnic foods, and traditional remedies.

**Client/Family Teaching and Discharge Planning**

• Provide "survival skills" education or review for hospitalized clients before discharge, including information about: (1) identification

---

• = Independent          ▲ = Collaborative

of the health care provider who will provide diabetes care after discharge; (2) level of understanding related to the diabetes diagnosis, self-monitoring of blood glucose, home blood glucose goals, and when to call the provider; (3) definition, recognition, treatment, and prevention of hyperglycemia and hypoglycemia; (4) information on making healthy food choices at home and referral to an outpatient RDN to guide individualization of meal plan, if needed. If relevant, when and how to take glucose-lowering medications, including insulin administration; (5) sick-day management; and (6) proper use and disposal of needles and syringes. Providing a structured discharge plan tailored to the individual client may reduce length of hospital stay and readmission rates and increase client satisfaction (ADA, 2021).

- Evaluate clients' monitoring technique and ability to use results to adjust therapy at regular intervals.
- Teach clients with type 2 diabetes the importance of reducing sedentary behavior, and to interrupt prolonged sitting at least every 30 minutes.
- Teach adults with type 1 and type 2 diabetes to engage in 150 min or more of moderate to vigorous-intensity aerobic activity per week, spread over at least 3 days/week, with no more than 2 consecutive days without activity. Shorter durations (minimum 75 min/week) of vigorous intensity or interval training may be sufficient for younger and more physically fit individuals. Adults with type 1 and type 2 diabetes should engage in 2–3 sessions/week of resistance exercise on nonconsecutive days.
▲ Discuss recommending resistance training with the client's provider.
- Teach clients with type 1 diabetes to test for urine or blood ketones if they are ill, if their blood glucose is >240 mg/dL, and before exercise if blood glucose is >250 mg/dL. Advise to increase fluid intake and contact provider at first detection of ketones.
▲ Teach clients taking insulin or secretagogue medication to check blood glucose before and after exercise. Blood glucose levels before exercise should ideally be >90 mg/dL. Discuss carbohydrate use in relation to exercise with provider.
- Teach clients to use alcohol with caution.
- Inform clients that use of smartphone applications may help them manage their diabetes care and glucose control.

• = Independent          ▲ = Collaborative

# Maladaptive Grieving

**Domain 9** Coping/stress response  **Class 2** Coping responses

## NANDA-I Definition

A disorder that occurs after the death of a significant other, in which the experience of distress accompanying bereavement fails to follow sociocultural expectations.

## Defining Characteristics

Anxiety; decreased life role performance; depressive symptoms; diminished intimacy levels; disbelief; excessive stress; experiencing symptoms the deceased experienced; expresses anger; expresses being overwhelmed; expresses distress about the deceased person; expresses feeling detached from others; expresses feeling of emptiness; expresses feeling stunned; expresses shock; fatigue; gastrointestinal symptoms; grief avoidance; increased morbidity; longing for the deceased person; mistrust of others; nonacceptance of a death; persistent painful memories; preoccupation with thoughts about a deceased person; rumination about deceased person; searching for a deceased person; self-blame

## Related Factors

Difficulty dealing with concurrent crises; excessive emotional disturbance; high attachment anxiety; inadequate social support; low attachment avoidance

## At-Risk Population

Economically disadvantaged individuals; individuals experiencing socially unacceptable loss; individuals experiencing unexpected sudden death of significant other; individuals experiencing violent death of significant other; individuals unsatisfied with death notification; individuals who witnessed uncontrolled symptoms of the deceased

## Client Outcomes

**Client Will (Specify Time Frame)**

- Express appropriate feelings of guilt, fear, anger, or sadness
- Identify somatic distress associated with grief (e.g., anxiety, changes in appetite, insomnia, nightmares, loss of libido, decreased energy, altered activity levels)
- Seek support in dealing with grief-associated issues
- Identify personal strengths and effective coping strategies
- Function at a normal developmental level and begin to successfully and increasingly perform activities of daily living

## Nursing Interventions

- Assess for signs of maladaptive grieving that include symptoms that persist at least 6 months after the death and are experienced at least

• = Independent  ▲ = Collaborative

daily or to a disabling degree. Symptoms include feeling emotionally numb, stunned, shocked, and that life is meaningless; dysfunctional thoughts and maladaptive behaviors; experiencing mistrust and estrangement from others; anger and bitterness over the loss; identity confusion; avoidance of the reality of the loss, or excessive proximity seeking to try to feel closer to the deceased, sometimes focused on wishes to die or suicidal statements and behavior; or difficulty moving on with life. Symptoms must be associated with psychosocial and physical impairments.

▲ Determine the client's state of grieving. Use a tool such as the Prolonged Grief Disorder (PGD) scale (Jordan & Litz, 2014), the Grief Support in Health Care Scale (Anderson et al, 2010), the Hogan Grief Reaction Checklist (Hogan, Worden, & Schmidt, 2004), and the Beck Depression Inventory.

▲ Determine whether the client is experiencing depression, suicidal tendencies, or other emotional disorders. Refer the client for counseling or therapy as appropriate.

• Educate the client and his or her support systems that grief resolution is not a sequential process and that the positive outcome of grief resolution is the integration of the deceased into the ongoing life of the griever.

▲ Assess caregivers, particularly younger caregivers, for pessimistic thinking and additional stressful life events. Refer for appropriate support.

• See the interventions in the care plans for Readiness for Enhanced **Grieving** and Chronic **Sorrow**.

**Pediatric/Parent**

▲ Refer grieving children and parents to a program to help facilitate grieving if desired, especially if the death was traumatic.

• Encourage grieving parents to take part in activities that are supportive, such as faith-based activities.

• Encourage grieving parents to seek mental health services as needed.

• Help the adolescent determine sources of support and how to use them effectively. If the client is an adolescent exposed to a peer's suicide, watch for symptoms of traumatic grief and posttraumatic stress disorder, which include numbness, preoccupation with the deceased, functional impairment, and poor adjustment to the loss.

**Geriatric**

• Assess for deterioration in bereaved older adults' self-care.

• Those who have lived with older adults with dementia and experienced significant feelings of loss before the loved one's death may be at risk for more intense feelings of grief after the death of the client with dementia.

- Monitor the older client for complicated grieving manifesting in physical and mental health problems.

**Multicultural**

- Assess for the influence of cultural beliefs, norms, and values on the client's grief and mourning practices.
- Encourage discussion of the grief process.
- Identify whether the client had been notified of the health status of the deceased and was able to be present during illness and death.

**Home Care**

- Previous interventions can be adapted for home care use.
- Consider providing support via the Internet.

# Risk for Maladaptive Grieving

**Domain 9** Coping/stress tolerance     **Class 2** Coping responses

**NANDA-I Definition**

Susceptible to a disorder that occurs after death of a significant other, in which the experience of distress accompanying bereavement fails to follow sociocultural expectations, which may compromise health.

**Risk Factors**

Difficulty dealing with concurrent crises; excessive emotional disturbance; high attachment anxiety; inadequate social support; low attachment avoidance

**At-Risk Population**

Economically disadvantaged individuals; individuals experiencing socially unacceptable loss; individuals experiencing unexpected sudden death of significant other; individuals experiencing violent death of significant other; individuals unsatisfied with death notification; individuals who witnessed uncontrolled symptoms of the deceased; individuals with history of childhood abuse; individuals with history of unresolved grieving; individuals with significant predeath dependency on the deceased; individuals with strong emotional proximity to the deceased; individuals with unresolved conflict with the deceased; individuals without paid employment; women

**Associated Conditions**

Anxiety disorders; depression

**Client Outcomes, Nursing Interventions, and Client/Family Teaching and Discharge Planning**

Refer to care plan for Maladaptive **Grieving**.

• = Independent          ▲ = Collaborative

# Readiness for Enhanced Grieving

**Domain 9** Coping/stress tolerance    **Class 2** Coping responses

## NANDA-I Definition

A pattern of integration of a new functional reality that arises after an actual, anticipated or perceived significant loss, which can be strengthened.

## Defining Characteristics

Expresses desire to carry on legacy of the deceased; expresses desire to engage in previous activities; expresses desire to enhance coping with pain; expresses desire to enhance forgiveness; expresses desire to enhance hope; expresses desire to enhance personal growth; expresses desire to enhance sleep-wake cycle; expresses desire to integrate feelings of anger; expresses desire to integrate feelings of despair; expresses desire to integrate feelings of guilt; expresses desire to integrate feelings of remorse; expresses desire to integrate positive feelings; expresses desire to integrate positive memories of deceased; expresses desire to integrate possibilities for a joyful life; expresses desire to integrate possibilities for a meaningful life; expresses desire to integrate possibilities for a purposeful life; expresses desire to integrate possibilities for a satisfactory life; expresses desire to integrate the loss; expresses desire to invest energy in new interpersonal relations

## Client/Family Outcomes

### Client/Family Will (Specify Time Frame)

- Express meaning of the loss to his or her life and the functioning of the family
- Identify ways to support family members and articulate methods of support he or she requires from family and friends
- Accept assistance in meeting the needs of the family from friends and/or extended family

## Nursing Interventions

### Anticipatory Grieving Interventions

- Acknowledge grieving of a critically ill or dying client and clients' family/relatives for the losses experienced during the deteriorating illness, and the future that will be filled with loss.
- Develop a trusting relationship both with the client and with the family by using presence and therapeutic communication techniques.
- Keep the family apprised of the client's ongoing condition as much as possible. Consult with the family for decision-making as appropriate.
- Keep the family informed of client's needs for physical care and support in symptom control, and inform them about health care options at the end of life, including palliative care, hospice care, and home care.

• = Independent          ▲ = Collaborative

- Ask family members about having adequate resources to care for themselves and the critically ill family member.
- Encourage family members to show their caring feelings and talk to the client.
- Recognize and respect different feelings and wishes from both the family members and the client.
- If necessary, refer a family member for counseling or to a minister/priest to help him or her cope with the existential questions and current overwhelming reality.
- Promote mutual goal setting in which decisions are made together that affect the family.

**Grieving Interventions When Death of a Loved One Occurs**

Use the following activities when interacting with the bereaved person:

- Be present and attentive; use active empathetic listening.
- Validate the client's feelings of grief and feeling hurt, stressful, anxious, out of control, and further symptoms of grieving with an appropriate tool.
- Provide time and space for the person to tell their story of loss.
- Offer condolences: "I am sorry that you lost your husband."
- Intentionally schedule meetings with family members to provide support during grieving.
- Help the client use a method to give voice to his or her unique story of loss. Methods include keeping a personal journal to record feelings and insights; retelling of the loss narrative to a caring person; music therapy techniques with a trained therapist or listening to music that has significance to the relationship; and use of the "virtual dream," which is a dreamlike short story written by the grieving person to tell the narrative of the loss.
- Discuss coping methods with the grieving person. Common coping techniques include exercise, telling the story of grief to a caring person, journaling, pets, and developing a legacy for the deceased.
- Encourage the family to create a quiet and comfortable healing environment, and follow comforting grief rituals such as prayer, interacting with nature, or lighting votive candles.
- Help the family determine the best way and place to find social support. Encourage family members to continue to use support for as long as needed.
- Identify available community resources, including bereavement groups at local hospitals and hospice centers. Volunteers who provide bereavement support can also be effective.

• = Independent ▲ = Collaborative

▲ Refer the family members for spiritual counseling as desired.
• Refer to Maladaptive **Grieving** if the experience of distress accompanying bereavement fails to follow sociocultural expectations.

**Pediatric/Parent**
• Treat the child/parents with respect, and give them the opportunity to talk about concerns and answer questions honestly.
• Listen to the child's expression of grief.
• Help parents recognize that the grieving child does not have to be "fixed"; instead they need support going through an experience of grieving just like adults.
• Consider the use of art for children in hospice care who are dying or dealing with the death of a parent, sibling, or other family member.
▲ Refer grieving children and parents to a program to help facilitate grieving if desired, especially if the death was traumatic.
• Help the adolescent determine sources of support and how to use them effectively.
• Encourage grieving parents to take good care of their own health.
▲ Refer grieving parents to seek mental health services as needed. The death of a child is regarded as among the most traumatic, incomprehensible, and devastating of losses, with the potential to precipitate a crisis of meaning for the bereaved parent.
• Recognize that men and women often grieve differently, and explain this to parents as needed.
• Recognize that mothers who have a miscarriage/stillbirth grieve and experience sorrow because of the loss of the child.

**Geriatric**
• Monitor an older adult who has been treated for bereavement-related depression for relapse or recurrence.
• Provide support for the family when the loss is associated with dementia of the family member.
• Determine the social supports of older adults.

**Multicultural**
• See interventions in care plans for Maladaptive **Grieving** and Chronic **Sorrow**.

**Home Care**
• The interventions previously described may be adapted for home care use. Assessment of activities of daily living (ADLs) and instrumental ADLs is essential as part of comprehensive care after a home care client has suffered the loss of a loved one.

• = Independent          ▲ = Collaborative

- Actively listen as the client grieves for his or her own death or for real or perceived loss. Normalize the client's expressions of grief for self. Demonstrate a caring and hopeful approach.
▲ Refer the client to social services as necessary for losses not related to death. Support is helpful to grief work for all types of losses. Social workers can help the client plan for financial changes as a result of job losses and help with community referrals as appropriate.
▲ Refer the bereaved to hospice bereavement programs or an Internet self-help group. Relief of the suffering of clients and families (physical, emotional, and spiritual) is the goal of hospice care.

**H**

# Deficient Community Health

**Domain 1** Health promotion    **Class 2** Health management

## NANDA-I Definition

Presence of one or more health problems or factors that deter wellness or increase the risk of health problems experienced by a group or population.

## Defining Characteristics

Health problem experienced by groups or populations; program unavailable to enhance wellness of a group or population; programs unavailable to eliminate health problems of a group or population; programs unavailable to prevent health problems of a group or population; programs unavailable to reduce health problems of a group or population; risk of hospitalization to a group or population; risk of physiological manifestations to a group or population; risk of psychological manifestations to a group or population

## Related Factors

Inadequate access to health care provider; inadequate consumer satisfaction with programs; inadequate expertise within the community; inadequate health resources; inadequate program budget; inadequate program evaluation plan; inadequate program outcome data; inadequate social support for programs; programs incompletely address health problems

## Client Outcomes

### Community/Adolescents/Minority Clients Will (Specify Time Frame)

- Provide programs for healthy behaviors
- Demonstrate goal setting
- Describe and comply with healthy behaviors

## Nursing Interventions

- Refer to care plans for Readiness for Enhanced Community **Coping**, Ineffective Community **Coping**, Ineffective **Health** Maintenance

• = Independent       ▲ = Collaborative

Behaviors, Ineffective **Home** Maintenance Behaviors, and Risk for Other-Directed **Violence.**

- Assess for the presence of social determinants associated with community mortality.
- Assess for needs related to the community's priority health concerns.
- Assess clients accessing health services for a history of military service and provide the necessary referrals and information.
- Implement community engagement techniques for collaboration with stakeholders to design, develop, and adapt relevant health interventions.
- Encourage attendance at community-based exercise programs.
- Implement community engagement techniques in conjunction with tailored interventions to address health deficiencies.
- Collaborate with other community-based programs to use text messaging to broadcast targeted health messages to reach large numbers of community members.

**Pediatric**

- Consider use of a clinical-community collaborative to address health deficiencies in underserved populations with children.
- Screen at-risk pediatric populations for lead exposure.

**Geriatric**

- Assess community-dwelling older individuals for cognitive impairment using the Brief Cognitive Assessment Tool-Short Form (BCAT-SF).
- Refer older clients with a diagnosis of dementia to a home-based missing incident prevention program (HMIPP).
- Assess community-dwelling older individuals with the Identification of Seniors at Risk (ISAR) screening tool when they present for treatment in the emergency department.
- Screen community-dwelling older individuals for fall risk with the Timed Up and Go Test (TUG) or the Functional Gait Assessment (FGA) and refer to a fall prevention program.

**Multicultural**

- Assess for the impact of race/ethnic-based segregation on health outcomes.
- Provide culturally and linguistically appropriate community health programs.
- Use decision aids (DAs) (personal counseling, multimedia, and print materials) to facilitate communication between patients and health care providers to determine a plan for health care.

• = Independent                    ▲ = Collaborative

**Home Care and Client/Family Teaching and Discharge Planning**
- The previously mentioned interventions may be adapted for home care and client/family teaching.

## Risk-Prone Health Behavior

**Domain 1** Health promotion    **Class 2** Health management
### NANDA-I Definition

Impaired ability to modify lifestyle and/or actions in a manner that improves the level of wellness.

### Defining Characteristics

Failure to achieve optimal sense of control; failure to take action that prevents health problem; minimizes health status change; nonacceptance of health status change; smoking; substance misuse

### Related Factors

Inadequate social support; inadequate understanding of health information; low self efficacy; negative perception of health care provider; negative perception of recommended health care strategy; social anxiety; stressors

### At-Risk Population

Economically disadvantaged individuals; individuals with family history of alcoholism

### Client Outcomes

**Client Will (Specify Time Frame)**
- State acceptance of change in health status
- Request assistance in altering behaviors to adapt to change
- State personal goals for dealing with change in health status and means to prevent further health problems
- State experience of a period of grief that is proportional to the actual or perceived effect of the loss
- Report and/or demonstrate behavior changes mutually agreed upon with nurse as evidence of positive adaptation

### Nursing Interventions

- Assess the client's perceptions of health, wellness, disability, and major barriers to health and wellness.
- Assess the client for adverse childhood experiences (ACEs) and refer for counseling and follow-up as appropriate.
- Assess the client for depression and refer for counseling and follow-up as appropriate.
- Use motivational interviewing to help the client identify and change unhealthy behaviors.

• = Independent        ▲ = Collaborative

- Encourage mindfulness and meditation to help the client cope with changes in health status.
- Allow the client adequate time to express feelings about the change in health status.
- Encourage participation in work-based wellness programs.
- Provide the client with positive feedback for accomplishments.
- Promote use of positive spiritual and religious experiences as appropriate.
- Discuss the client's current goals and assist in modification as needed. Use a goal attainment scaling (GAS) approach, which is a therapeutic method that refers to the development of a written follow-up guide between the client and the nurse and is used for monitoring client progress.
▲ Refer to community resources. Provide general and contact information for ease of use.

**Pediatric**

- Include social history in client assessment to help identify past abuse and traumatic experiences.
- Encourage participation in school-based wellness programs.
- Promote use of positive spiritual experiences and religious attendance, as appropriate.
- Encourage parents to process and express grief, uncertainty, and discouragement after learning about their child's diagnosis, prognosis, and treatments. Provide parents with resources and tools to help further their understanding of the illness.
- Provide parents of critically ill children with individualized coping resources.
- Use distraction with children undergoing procedures or treatment with unpleasant side effects.

**Geriatric**

▲ Assess for signs of depression resulting from illness-associated changes and make appropriate referrals.
- Support activities that promote a sense of purpose for older adults.
- Encourage social support.

**Multicultural**

- Assess for the influence of cultural beliefs, norms, and values on the client's ability to modify health behavior.
- Assess the client's readiness for change.
- Assess the role of fatalism on the client's ability to modify health behavior. Fatalistic perspectives, which involve the belief that you

cannot control your own fate, may influence health behaviors in some cultures.
- Encourage spirituality as a source of support for coping.
- Acknowledge client's identified gender and sexual orientation and refer client and family members to support networks that have experience with lesbian, gay, bisexual, or transgender (LGBT) issues, as appropriate.

**Home Care**
- The previously mentioned interventions may be adapted for home care use.
- Take the client's perspective into consideration and use a holistic approach in assessing and responding to client planning for the future.
- Assist the client/family to adapt to his or her diagnosis and to live with their disease.
- Ensure that evaluations of the client's ability to perform activities of daily living are age appropriate and consider existing, as well as new, diagnoses.
- Refer to care plan for **Powerlessness.**

**Client/Family Teaching and Discharge Planning**
- Assess family/caregivers for coping and teaching/learning styles.
- Foster communication between the client/family and medical staff.
- Educate and prepare families regarding the appearance and function of the client and the environment before initial exposure.
- Teach clients and their family relaxation techniques (controlled breathing, guided imagery) and help them practice.

# Ineffective Health Self-Management

**Domain 1** Health promotion    **Class 2** Health management
## NANDA-I Definition

Unsatisfactory management of symptoms, treatment regimen, physical, psychosocial, and spiritual consequences and lifestyle changes inherent in living with a chronic condition.
## Defining Characteristics

Difficulty with prescribed regimen; failure to include treatment regimen in daily living; failure to take action to reduce risk factor; ineffective choices in daily living for meeting health goal
## Related Factors

Competing demands; competing lifestyle preferences; conflict between cultural beliefs and health practices; conflict between health behaviors and social norms; conflict between spiritual beliefs and treatment regimen; decreased perceived quality of life; depressive symptoms; difficulty accessing community resources; difficulty managing complex treatment regimen; difficulty navigating complex health care systems; difficulty with decision-making; inadequate commitment to a plan of action; inadequate health literacy; inadequate knowledge of treatment regimen; inadequate number of cues to action; inadequate role models; inadequate social support; individuals with limited decision making experience; limited ability to perform aspects of treatment regimen; low self efficacy; negative feelings toward treatment regimen; neurobehavioral manifestations; nonacceptance of condition; perceived barrier to treatment regimen; perceived social stigma associated with condition; substance misuse; unrealistic perception of seriousness of condition; unrealistic perception of susceptibility to sequelae; unrealistic perception of treatment benefit

**H**

## At-Risk Population

Children; economically disadvantaged individuals; individuals experiencing adverse reactions to medications; individuals with caregiving responsibilities; individuals with history of ineffective health self-management; individuals with low educational level; older adults

## Associated Conditions

Asymptomatic disease; developmental disabilities; high acuity illness; neurocognitive disorders; polypharmacy; significant comorbidity

## Client Outcomes

### Client Will (Specify Time Frame)

- Describe daily food and fluid intake that meets therapeutic goals
- Describe activity/exercise patterns that meet therapeutic goals
- Describe scheduling of medications that meets therapeutic goals
- Verbalize ability to manage therapeutic regimens
- Collaborate with health professionals to decide on a therapeutic regimen that is congruent with health goals and lifestyle

## Nursing Interventions

- Establish a collaborative partnership with the client for purposes of meeting health-related goals.
- Explore the client's perception of their illness experience and identify uncertainties and needs through open-ended questions.
- Assist the client to enhance self-efficacy or confidence in his or her own ability to manage the illness.
- Review factors of the health belief model (HBM) (individual perceptions of seriousness and susceptibility, demographic and other modifying factors, and perceived benefits and barriers) with the client.

• = Independent ▲ = Collaborative

**H**

- Help the client identify and modify barriers to effective self-management.
- Help the client self-manage his or her own health through education about strategies for changing habits such as overeating, sedentary lifestyle, and smoking.
- Develop a contract with the client to maintain motivation for changes in behavior.
- Use focus groups to evaluate the implementation of self-management programs.
- Refer to the care plan Ineffective Family **Health** Self-Management.

**Geriatric**
- Identify the reasons for behaviors that are not therapeutic and discuss alternatives.

**Multicultural**
- Assess the influence of cultural beliefs, norms, and values on the individual's perceptions of the therapeutic regimen.
- Provide health information that is consistent with the health literacy of clients.
- Assess for barriers that may interfere with client follow-up of treatment recommendations.
- Validate the client's feelings regarding the ability to manage his or her own care and the impact on lifestyle.

**Home Care**
- Prepare and instruct clients and family members in the use of a medication box. Set up an appropriate schedule for filling the medication box, and post medication times and doses in an accessible area (e.g., attached by a magnet to the refrigerator).
- Refer to health care professionals for questions and self-care management.

**Client/Family Teaching and Discharge Planning**
- Identify the client's and/or family's current knowledge and adjust teaching accordingly. Teach the client and family about all aspects of the therapeutic regimen, providing as much knowledge as the client and family will accept, in a culturally congruent manner.
- Teach ways to adjust activities of daily living (ADLs) for inclusion in therapeutic regimens.
- Teach safety in taking medications.

• = Independent ▲ = Collaborative

# Readiness for Enhanced Health Self-Management

**Domain 1** Health promotion      **Class 2** Health management

## NANDA-I Definition

A pattern of satisfactory management of symptoms, treatment regimen, physical, psychosocial, and spiritual consequences and lifestyle changes inherent in living with a chronic condition, which can be strengthened.

## Defining Characteristics

Expresses desire to enhance choices of daily living for meeting goals; expresses desire to enhance immunization/vaccination status; expresses desire to enhance management of illness; expresses desire to enhance management of prescribed regimens; expresses desire to enhance management of risk factors; expresses desire to enhance management of symptoms

## Client Outcomes

### Client Will (Specify Time Frame)

- Describe integration of therapeutic regimen into daily living
- Demonstrate continued commitment to integration of therapeutic regimen into daily living routines

## Nursing Interventions

- Acknowledge the expertise that the client and family bring to health management.
- Review factors that contribute to the likelihood of health promotion and health protection. Use Pender's Health Promotion Model and Becker's Health Belief Model to identify contributing factors (Pender et al, 2015).
- Further develop and reinforce contributing factors that might change with ongoing self-management of the therapeutic regimen (e.g., knowledge, self-efficacy, self-esteem, and perceived benefits).
- Review the client's strengths in the management of the therapeutic regimen.
- Collaborate with the client to identify strategies to maintain strengths and develop additional strengths as indicated.
- Identify contributing factors that may need to be improved now or in the future.
- Help the client maintain existing support and seek additional supports as needed.

### Geriatric

- Facilitate the client and family to obtain health insurance and drug payment plans whenever needed and possible.

• = Independent          ▲ = Collaborative

**Multicultural**
- Assess client's cultural perspectives on health management.
- Assess health literacy in clients of diverse backgrounds.
- Validate the client's feelings regarding the ability to manage his or her own care and the impact on current lifestyle.

**Client/Family Teaching and Discharge Planning**
- Facilitate the client and family to obtain financial assistance in the form of health insurance and drug payment plans whenever needed and possible.
- Use electronic monitoring to improve medication adherence.
- Review therapeutic regimens and their optimal integration with daily living routines.
- Teach disease processes and therapeutic regimens to clients and peer supporters for management of disease processes.

# Ineffective Family Health Self-Management

**Domain 1** Health promotion    **Class 2** Health management

## NANDA-I Definition

Unsatisfactory management of symptoms, treatment regimen, physical, psychosocial and spiritual consequences and lifestyle changes inherent in living with one or more family members' chronic condition.

## Defining Characteristics

Caregiver strain; decrease in attention to illness in one or more family members; depressive symptoms of caregiver; exacerbation of disease signs of one or more family members; exacerbation of disease symptoms of one or more family members; failure to take action to reduce risk factor in one or more family members; ineffective choices in daily living for meeting health goal of family unit; one or more family members report dissatisfaction with quality of life

## Related Factors

Cognitive dysfunction of one or more caregivers; competing demands on family unit; competing lifestyle preferences within family unit; conflict between health behaviors and social norms; conflict between spiritual beliefs and treatment regimen; difficulty accessing community resources; difficulty dealing with role changes associated with condition; difficulty managing complex treatment regimen; difficulty navigating complex health care systems; difficulty with decision-making; family conflict; inadequate commitment to a plan of action; inadequate health literacy of caregiver; inadequate knowledge of treatment

• = Independent         ▲ = Collaborative

regimen; inadequate number of cues to action; inadequate social support; ineffective communication skills; ineffective coping skills; limited ability to perform aspects of treatment regimen; low self efficacy; negative feelings toward treatment regimen; nonacceptance of condition; perceived barrier to treatment regimen; perceived social stigma associated with condition; substance misuse; unrealistic perception of seriousness of condition; unrealistic perception of susceptibility to sequelae; unrealistic perception of treatment benefit; unsupportive family relations

### At-Risk Population

Economically disadvantaged families; families with member experiencing delayed diagnosis; families with members experiencing low educational level; families with members who have limited decision-making experience; families with premature infant

### Associated Conditions

Chronic disease; mental disorders; neurocognitive disorders; terminal illness

### Client Outcomes

**Client Will (Specify Time Frame)**

- Make adjustments in usual activities (e.g., diet, activity, stress management) to incorporate therapeutic regimens of its members
- Reduce illness symptoms of family members
- Express desire to manage therapeutic regimens of its members
- Describe a decrease in the difficulties of managing therapeutic regimens
- Describe actions to reduce risk factors

### Nursing Interventions

- Base family interventions on knowledge of the family, family context, family dynamics, family structure, and family function.
- Use a family approach when helping an individual with a health problem that requires therapeutic management.
- Review with family members the congruence and incongruence of family behaviors and health-related goals.
- Acknowledge the challenge of integrating therapeutic regimens with family behaviors.
- Review the symptoms of specific illnesses and work with the family toward development of greater self-efficacy in relation to these symptoms.
- Support family decisions to adjust therapeutic regimens as indicated.
- Help the family mobilize social supports.
- Help family members modify perceptions as indicated.

• = Independent ▲ = Collaborative

- Use one or more theories of family dynamics to describe, explain, or predict family behaviors (e.g., theories of Bowen, Satir, and Minuchin).
▲ Collaborate with expert nurses or other consultants regarding strategies for working with families.
- Coaching methods can be used to help families improve their health.

**Pediatric**

**H**

- Support skin-to-skin care for infants at risk at birth. Keep infants in an upright position in skin-to-skin contact until they no longer tolerate it.

**Geriatric**

- Recommend that clients use the "Ask Me 3" program when communicating with their health providers (What is my main problem? What do I need to do? Why is it important for me to do this?).

**Multicultural**

- Acknowledge racial and ethnic differences at the onset of care.
- Ensure that all strategies for working with the family are congruent with the culture of the family.
- Use the nursing intervention of cultural brokerage to help families deal with the health care system.

**Client/Family Teaching and Discharge Planning**

- Teach about all aspects of therapeutic regimens. Provide as much knowledge as family members will accept, adjust instruction to account for what the family already knows, and provide information in a culturally congruent manner.
- Teach ways to adjust family behaviors to include therapeutic regimens, such as safety in taking medications and teaching family members to act as self-advocates with health providers who prescribe therapeutic regimens.

# Ineffective Health Maintenance Behaviors

**Domain 1** Health promotion    **Class 2** Health management
**NANDA-I Definition**

Management of health knowledge, attitudes, and practices underlying health actions that is unsatisfactory for maintaining or improving well-being, or preventing illness and injury.

• = Independent                    ▲ = Collaborative

## Defining Characteristics

Failure to take action that prevents health problem; failure to take action that reduces risk factor; inadequate commitment to a plan of action; inadequate health literacy; inadequate interest in improving health; inadequate knowledge about basic health practices; ineffective choices in daily living for meeting health goal; pattern of lack of health-seeking behavior

## Related Factors

Competing demands; competing lifestyle preferences; conflict between cultural beliefs and health practices; conflict between health behaviors and social norms; conflicts between spiritual beliefs and health practices; depressive symptoms; difficulty accessing community resources; difficulty navigating complex health care systems; difficulty with decision-making; inadequate health resources; inadequate social support; inadequate trust in health care professional; individuals with limited decision making experience; ineffective communication skills; ineffective coping strategies; ineffective family coping; low self efficacy; maladaptive grieving; neurobehavioral manifestations; perceived prejudice; perceived victimization; spiritual distress

## At-Risk Population

Economically disadvantaged individuals; individuals from families with ineffective family coping; individuals with history of violence; men; older adults; young adult

## Associated Conditions

Chronic disease; developmental disabilities; mental disorders

## Client Outcomes

### Client Will (Specify Time Frame)

- Discuss fear of or blocks to implementing health regimen
- Follow mutually agreed on health care maintenance plan
- Meet goals for health care maintenance

## Nursing Interventions

- Provide support to clients in making their health care decisions and provide information about options and associated benefits/harms.
- Assess for family patterns, economic issues, and spiritual and cultural patterns that influence compliance with a given medical regimen.
- Involve the client in shared decision-making regarding health maintenance.
- Show genuine interest in the client's individual needs.
- Assist the client in finding methods to reduce stress.
- Identify complementary healing modalities, such as herbal remedies, acupuncture, healing touch, yoga, or cultural shamans that the client uses in addition to or instead of the prescribed allopathic regimen

• = Independent      ▲ = Collaborative

along with the client's perception of the complementary healing modalities.
▲ Refer the client to appropriate and accessible medical and social services as needed, providing adequate information on details about the service.
• Identify in-person and teleconferenced support groups related to the disease process.
• Use social media such as text messaging to remind clients of scheduled appointments.
• Use telehealth interventions to facilitate self-care.

**Geriatric**
• Assess the client's perception of health and health maintenance.
• Assist client to identify realistic health-related goals.
• Encourage and facilitate informed decision-making.
• Educate the client about the symptoms of life-threatening illness, such as myocardial infarction (MI), and the need for timeliness in seeking care.

**Multicultural**
• Assess influence of cultural beliefs, norms, and values on the client's ability to modify health behavior.
• Assess the effect of fatalism on the client's ability to modify health behavior.
• Clarify culturally related health beliefs and practices.
• Provide culturally appropriate education and health care services.

**Home Care**
• The interventions described previously may be adapted for home care use.
▲ Provide nurse-led case management.
• Provide a health promotion focus for the client with disabilities, with the goals of reducing secondary conditions (e.g., obesity, hypertension, pressure sores), maintaining functional independence, providing opportunities for leisure and enjoyment, and enhancing overall quality of life.
• Provide support and individual training for caregivers before the client is discharged from the hospital.

**Client/Family Teaching and Discharge Planning**
• Provide the patient and family with credible social media sources from which health information can be obtained.
▲ Develop collaborative multiprofessional partnerships.
• Tailor both the information provided and the method of delivery of information to the specific client and/or family.

• = Independent          ▲ = Collaborative

# Ineffective Home Maintenance Behaviors

**Domain 1** Health promotion    **Class 2** Health management

## NANDA-I Definition

An unsatisfactory pattern of knowledge and activities for the safe upkeep of one's residence.

## Defining Characteristics

Cluttered environment; difficulty maintaining a comfortable environment; failure to request assistance with home maintenance; home task-related anxiety; home task-related stress; impaired ability to regulate finances; negative affect toward home maintenance; neglected laundry; pattern of hygiene-related diseases; trash accumulation; unsafe cooking equipment; unsanitary environment

## Related Factors

Competing demands; depressive symptoms; difficulty with decision-making; environmental constraints; impaired physical mobility; impaired postural balance; inadequate knowledge of home maintenance; inadequate knowledge of social resources; inadequate organizing skills; inadequate role models; inadequate social support; insufficient physical endurance; neurobehavioral manifestations; powerlessness; psychological distress

## At-Risk Population

Economically disadvantaged individuals; individuals living alone; older adult

## Associated Conditions

Depression; mental disorders; neoplasms; neurocognitive disorders; sensation disorders; vascular diseases

## Client Outcomes

### Client Will (Specify Time Frame)

- Maintain a healthy home environment
- Use community resources to assist with home care needs
- Maintain a safe home environment

## Nursing Interventions

- Assess the knowledge and concerns of family members, especially the primary caregiver, about home care maintenance and management.
- Provide home safety education and safety equipment when possible.
- Assess injury prevention knowledge and practices of the client and caregivers and provide information as appropriate.
- ▲ Consider a predischarge home assessment referral to determine the need for accessibility and safety-related environmental changes.
- Use an assessment tool to identify environmental safety hazards in the home.

• = Independent          ▲ = Collaborative

- Establish an individualized plan of care for improved home maintenance with the client and family based on the client's needs and the caregiver's capabilities.
- Set up a system of relief for the main caregiver in the home and a plan for sharing household duties and/or outside assistance.
▲ Provide a multiprofessional approach to target the home environment and the client's ability to function in the home.

**Geriatric**

- All of the previously mentioned interventions are applicable for the geriatric population.
- Assess functional ability to manage safely after hospital discharge.
- Explore community resources to assist with home maintenance (e.g., senior centers, Department of Aging, hospital case managers, friends and relatives, the Internet, or church parish nurse).
- Provide education related to home modification.
- Focus on the interaction between the older client and the technology, assisting the client to be an active participant in choices of and uses for technology.
- See the care plans for Risk for **Injury** and Risk for **Falls**.

**Multicultural**

- Acknowledge the stresses unique to racial/ethnic communities.

**Home Care**

- The previously mentioned interventions incorporate these resources.
- See care plans **Contamination** and Risk for **Contamination**.

**Client/Family Teaching and Discharge Planning**

- Identify support groups within the community to assist families in the caregiver role.
- Incorporate the perspectives of patients and their caregivers in the definition and description of safety.
- Focus teaching on environmental hazards identified in the nursing assessment. Areas may include, but are not limited to, the following:
  ○ **Home Safety.** Identify the need for and use of common safety measures in the home.
  ○ **Food Safety.** Instruct client to avoid microbial foodborne illness by storing and cooking food at the proper temperature; regularly washing hands, food contact surfaces, and fruits and vegetables; and monitoring expiration dates.
- Teach clients to assess their homes for potential environmental health hazards in the home, including risks related to structure, moisture/mold, fire, pets, electrical, ventilation, pests, and lifestyle.

• = Independent        ▲ = Collaborative

- See care plans **Contamination,** Risk for **Contamination,** Risk for Adult **Falls,** Risk for Child **Falls,** Risk for **Infection,** and Risk for **Injury.**

# Readiness for Enhanced Home Maintenance Behaviors

**Domain 1** Health promotion    **Class 2** Health management

## NANDA-I Definition

A pattern of knowledge and activities for the safe upkeep of one's residence, which can be strengthened.

## Defining Characteristics

Expresses desire to enhance affect toward home tasks; expresses desire to enhance attitude toward home maintenance; expresses desire to enhance comfort of the environment; expresses desire to enhance home safety; expresses desire to enhance household hygiene; expresses desire to enhance laundry management skills; expresses desire to enhance organizational skills; expresses desire to enhance regulation of finances; expresses desire to enhance trash management

## Client Outcomes

Client Will (Specify Time Frame)

- Maintain a healthy home environment
- Use community resources to assist with home care needs
- Maintain a safe home environment

## Nursing Interventions

- Assess the client's level of readiness for change in home maintenance.
- Take the client's age and level of disability into account when determining need for housing adaptations.
- Engage the client in decisions related to home modifications.
- Consider the expectations of individuals living with/caring for the client in determining home adaptations.
- Reduce injury hazards for children in the home and implement use of safety devices.
- Encourage home rules regarding a smoke free environment.

**Geriatric**

- All of the previously mentioned interventions are applicable for the geriatric population.
- Provide information to older adults and their families to promote independent living.
- Focus on fall prevention in the home.

• = Independent                    ▲ = Collaborative

- Monitor the ways in which home adaptations and equipment are used in the home to ensure continuing safety.

**Multicultural**
- Encourage maintenance of personal and cultural possessions in the home even as adaptations are made to the structure and function of the home.

**Home Care**
- Use principles of client-centeredness in home care.

**Client/Family Teaching and Discharge Planning**
- Provide the patient and family with sufficient, quality information and resources before discharge to ensure a feeling of confidence in home care.
- Promote good communication between older persons, hospital providers, and home care providers to improve coordination of care and a seamless transition to home.

# Risk for Ineffective Home Maintenance Behaviors

**Domain 1** Health promotion    **Class 2** Health management

## NANDA-I Definition

Susceptible to an unsatisfactory pattern of knowledge and activities for the safe upkeep of one's residence, which may compromise health.

## Defining Characteristics

Competing demands; depressive symptoms; difficulty with decision-making; environmental constraints; impaired physical mobility; impaired postural balance; inadequate knowledge of home maintenance; inadequate knowledge of social resources; inadequate organizing skills; inadequate role models; inadequate social support; insufficient physical endurance; neurobehavioral manifestations; powerlessness; psychological distress

## At-Risk Population

Economically disadvantaged individuals; individuals living alone; older adults

## Associated Conditions

Depression; mental disorders; neoplasms; neurocognitive disorders; sensation disorders; vascular disease

## Client Outcomes, Nursing Interventions, and Client/Family Teaching and Discharge Planning

Refer to care plans for Ineffective **Home** Maintenance Behaviors and Readiness for Enhanced **Home** Maintenance Behaviors.

• = Independent            ▲ = Collaborative

# Readiness for Enhanced Hope

**Domain 6** Self-perception    **Class 1** Self-concept

## NANDA-I Definition

A pattern of expectations and desires for mobilizing energy to achieve positive outcomes, or avoid a potentially threatening or negative situation, which can be strengthened.

## Defining Characteristics

Expresses desire to enhance ability to set achievable goals; expresses desire to enhance belief in possibilities; expresses desire to enhance congruency of expectation with goal; expresses desire to enhance deep inner strength; expresses desire to enhance giving and receiving of care/love; expresses desire to enhance initiative; expresses desire to enhance involvement with self-care; expresses desire to enhance positive outlook on life; expresses desire to enhance problem-solving to meet goal; expresses desire to enhance sense of meaning in life; expresses desire to enhance spirituality

## Client Outcomes

**Client Will (Specify Time Frame)**

- Describe values, expectations, and meanings
- Set achievable goals that are consistent with values
- Design strategies to achieve goals
- Express belief in possibilities

## Nursing Interventions

- Spend one-on-one time with the client. Use empathy; try to understand what the client is saying and communicate this understanding to the client to create a nonjudgmental trusting environment to develop therapeutic relationships with the client.
- Assist clients to identify sources of gratitude in their lives.
- Screen the client for hope using a valid and reliable instrument as indicated.
- Focus on the positive aspects of hope.
- Assist the client to develop positive expectations outcomes and recognize the pathways to achieve the positive outcomes.
- Explore the meanings, functions, objects, sources, and nature of hope with patients as they relate to their current situation.
- Teach individuals how to become aware of attention that is focused on unwanted aspects of life and how to redirect attention toward things that feel more wanted or desired by using a future-directed approach.
- Review the client's strengths and resources in conjunction with the client.

• = Independent                  ▲ = Collaborative

- Assist the client to consider alternatives and set long- and short-term goals that are important to him or her.
- Encourage engagement in positive and pleasant events.
- Facilitate sources of the client's resilience.
- Implement social supports and reintegration programs for postdeployment soldiers and veterans in a timely fashion.
- Encourage the client to adopt active coping strategies.
- Identify spiritual beliefs and practices.

**H**

### Home Care
- The previously mentioned interventions may be adapted for home care use.

### Client/Family Teaching and Discharge Planning
- Assist families to identify sources of gratitude in their lives.
- Use a family-centered approach to provide information regarding the client's condition, treatment plan, and progress.
- Teach alternative coping strategies such as physical activity.
▲ Refer the client to self-help groups.

## Hopelessness

**Domain 6** Self-perception    **Class 1** Self-concept
### NANDA-I Definition

The feeling that one will not experience positive emotions, or an improvement in one's condition.

### Defining Characteristics

Anorexia; avoidance behaviors; decreased affective display; decreased initiative; decreased response to stimuli; decreased verbalization; depressive symptoms; expresses despondency; expresses diminished hope; expresses feeling of uncertain future; expresses inadequate motivation for the future; expresses negative expectations about self; expresses negative expectations about the future; expresses sense of incompetency in meeting goals; inadequate involvement with self care; overestimates the likelihood of unfortunate events; passivity; reports altered sleep-wake cycle; suicidal behaviors; unable to imagine life in the future; underestimates the occurrence of positive events

### Related Factors

Chronic stress; fear; inadequate social support; loss of belief in spiritual power; loss of belief in transcendent values; low self efficacy; prolonged immobility; social isolation; unaddressed violence; uncontrolled severe disease symptoms

• = Independent                    ▲ = Collaborative

## At-Risk Population

Adolescents; displaced individuals; economically disadvantaged individuals; individuals experiencing infertility; individuals experiencing significant loss; individuals with history of attempted suicide; individuals with history of being abandoned; older adults; unemployed individuals

## Associated Conditions

Critical illness; depression; deterioration in physiological condition; feeding and eating disorders; mental disorders; neoplasms; terminal illness

## Client Outcomes

### Client Will (Specify Time Frame)

**H**

- Verbalize feelings
- Participate in care
- Make positive statements (e.g., "I can" or "I will try")
- Set goals
- Make eye contact, focus on speaker
- Maintain appropriate appetite for age and physical health
- Sleep appropriate length of time for age and physical health
- Express concern for another
- Initiate activity

## Nursing Interventions

- Assess for, monitor, and document the potential for suicide. (Refer the client for appropriate treatment if a potential for suicide is identified.) Refer to the care plan Risk for **Suicidal** Behavior for specific interventions.
- Assess and monitor potential for depression. (Refer the client for appropriate treatment if depression is identified.)
- Assess for hopelessness with the modified Beck Hopelessness Scale.
- Assess and monitor family caregivers for symptoms of hopelessness.
- Assess for pain and respond with appropriate measures for pain relief.
- Facilitate sources of the client's resilience.
- Assist the adolescent client to develop positive expectations.
- Assist the client to explore the meaning of his or her life, satisfaction with his or her life, and life goals.
- Encourage adolescent clients to get 9 to 10 hours of sleep nightly.
- Assist the client in looking at alternatives and setting long- and short-term goals that are important to him or her.
- Explore the meanings, functions, objects, sources, and nature of hope with clients as they relate to their current situation.

- Spend one-on-one time with the client. Use empathy; try to understand what the client is saying and communicate this understanding to the client to create a nonjudgmental trusting environment to develop therapeutic relationships with the client.
- Teach alternative coping strategies such as physical activity.
- Use a future-directed approach that teaches individuals how to become aware of attention that is focused on unwanted aspects of life and how to redirect attention toward things that feel more wanted or desired.
- Review the client's strengths and resources in conjunction with the client.
- Encourage the client to adopt active coping strategies.
- Implement social supports and reintegration programs for postdeployment soldiers and veterans in a timely fashion.
- For additional interventions, see the care plans for Readiness for Enhanced **Hope, Spiritual** Distress, Readiness for Enhanced **Spiritual** Well-Being, and Disturbed **Sleep** Pattern.

**Geriatric**
- Previous interventions may be adapted for geriatric clients.
▲ If depression is suspected, confer with the primary health care provider regarding referral for mental health services.
- Take threats of self-harm or suicide seriously and intervene as needed.
- Encourage engagement in positive and pleasant events.

**Multicultural**
- Assess for the influence of cultural beliefs, norms, and values on the client's feelings of hopelessness.
- Assess for the effect of fatalism on the client's expression of hopelessness.
- Use caution when highlighting health disparities of multicultural populations through public health campaigns and media broadcasts.
- Encourage spirituality as a source of support for hopelessness.

**Home Care**
- Previously mentioned interventions may be adapted for home care use.
- Use in-person problem-solving therapy (PST) to address depressive symptoms and hopelessness.

**Client/Family Teaching and Discharge Planning**
- Provide information regarding the client's condition, treatment plan, and progress.
▲ Refer the client to self-help groups.

• = Independent      ▲ = Collaborative

# Risk for Compromised Human Dignity

**Domain 6** Self-perception    **Class 1** Self-concept

## NANDA-I Definition

Susceptible for perceived loss of respect and honor, which may compromise health.

## Risk Factors

Dehumanization; disclosure of confidential information; exposure of the body; humiliation; inadequate understanding of health information; insufficient privacy; intrusion by clinician; loss of control over body function; perceived social stigma; values incongruent with cultural norms

## At-Risk Population

Individuals with limited decision making experience

## Client Outcomes

**Client/Caregiver Will (Specify Time Frame)**

- Perceive that dignity is maintained throughout hospitalization/encounter
- Consistently call client by name and pronoun of choice
- Maintain client's privacy

## Nursing Interventions

- Use the person-centered approach for each client, while listening actively and addressing their individual needs.
- Encourage client to enter into and stay in communication with others. Encourage connections with the inner life world of meaning and spirit of the other. Join in a mutual search for meaning and wholeness of being and becoming to potentiate comfort measures, pain control, a sense of well-being, wholeness, or even spiritual transcendence of suffering.
- Determine the client's perspective about his or her health. Example questions include "Tell me about your health." "What is it like to be in your situation?" "Tell me how you perceive yourself in this situation." "What meaning are you giving to this situation?" "Tell me about your health priorities." "Tell me about the harmony you wish to reach."
- Determine the client's preferences for when and how nursing care is needed and follow the client's guidelines if possible.
- Maintain the client's privacy at all times.
- Encourage the client to share thoughts about spirituality and mortality as desired.
- Use interventions to instill increased hope; see the care plan for Readiness for Enhanced **Hope.**

• = Independent    ▲ = Collaborative

- Refer client for dignity therapy.
- See the care plan for Readiness for Enhanced **Spiritual** Well-Being.

**Geriatric**

- Always ask the client how he or she would like to be addressed. Avoid calling older clients "sweetie," "honey," "Gramps," "mama," or other terms that could be considered as demeaning unless this is acceptable in the client's culture or requested by the client. Appropriate forms of address and person-centered approaches must be used with older adults to maintain dignity.
- Treat the older client with the utmost respect, even if delirium or dementia is present with confusion.

**Multicultural**

- Assess for the influence of cultural beliefs, norms, and values on the client's way of communicating, and follow the client's lead in communicating in matters of eye contact, amount of personal space, voice tones, and amount of touching. If in doubt, ask the client.
- Provide diverse clients with person-centered care that is responsive, respectful, and individualized.

**Home Care**

- Many of the previous intervention may be adapted for home care use.
- Encourage client participation in self-care and the management of one's own care process.

**Client/Family Teaching and Discharge Planning**

- Teach and support family and caregiver actions that maintain the dignity of the client. How an individual cognitively perceives and emotionally deals with the illness can depend on the person's family and social relationships, and ultimately can affect the ability to heal.

# Neonatal Hyperbilirubinemia

**Domain 2** Nutrition    **Class 4** Metabolism

## NANDA-I Definition

The accumulation of unconjugated bilirubin in the circulation (less than 15 mL/dL) that occurs after 24 hours of life.

## Defining Characteristics

Abnormal liver function test results; bruised skin; yellow mucous membranes; yellow sclera; yellow-orange skin color

## Related Factors

Delay in meconium passage; inadequate paternal feeding behavior; malnourished infants

## At-Risk Population

East Asian neonates; low birth weight neonates; Native American neonates; Neonates aged ≤ 7 days; neonates who are breastfed; neonates whose blood groups are incompatible with mothers'; neonates whose mothers had gestational diabetes; neonates whose sibling had history of jaundice; neonates with significant bruising during birth; populations living at high altitudes; premature neonates

## Associated Conditions

Bacterial infections; enzyme deficiency; impaired metabolism; internal bleeding; liver malfunction; prenatal infection; sepsis; viral infection

## Client Outcomes

### Client (Infant) Will (Specify Time Frame)

- Establish effective feeding pattern (breast or bottle)
- Receive nursing assessments to determine risk for severity of jaundice
- Receive bilirubin assessment and screening within the first few days of life to identify potentially harmful levels of serum bilirubin
- Receive appropriate therapy to enhance indirect bilirubin excretion
- Maintain hydration: moist buccal membranes, four to six wet diapers in a 24-hour period, weight loss no greater than 10% of birth weight within the first week of life
- Evacuate stool within 48 hours of birth, and pass three or four stools per 24 hours by day 4 of life

### Client (Parent[s]) Will (Specify Time Frame)

- Receive information on neonatal jaundice before discharge from birth hospital
- Verbalize understanding of physical signs of jaundice prior to discharge
- Verbalize signs requiring immediate health practitioner notification: sleepy infant who does not awaken easily for feedings, fewer than four to six wet diapers in 24-hour period by day 4, fewer than three to four stools in 24 hours by day 4, breastfeeds fewer than eight times per day
- Demonstrate ability to operate home phototherapy unit if prescribed

## Nursing Interventions

- Evaluate maternal and delivery history for risk factors for neonatal jaundice (RhD, ABO, G6PD deficiency, direct Coombs).
- Perform neonatal gestational age assessment once the newborn has had an initial period of interaction with mother and father. Gestational age is calculated using completed weeks of age. There are two major categories, preterm and term newborns, with further subdivisions in each category. Infants born before 34 weeks' completed gestation will be admitted to the neonatal intensive care unit (NICU).

• = Independent ▲ = Collaborative

| Preterm Category | Term Category |
|---|---|
| Extremely preterm <28 weeks' completion | Early term 37 to 38 weeks' completion |
| Very preterm 28 to <32 weeks' completion | Term >38 to 42 weeks' completion |
| Late preterm 32 to <37 weeks' completion | Postterm >42 weeks' completion |

**H**

- Encourage breastfeeding within the first hour (otherwise known as the Golden Hour) of the neonate's life.
- Encourage skin-to-skin mother–newborn contact shortly after delivery to support the Golden Hour after birth.
- Encourage and assist mother with frequent breastfeeding.
- Assist parents who choose to bottle feed their neonate.
- Avoid feeding supplements such as water, dextrose water, or any other milk substitutes in breastfeeding neonate.
- Assess neonate's stooling pattern in first 48 hours of life.
- Monitor infant's neurological status for any signs of emerging bilirubin encephalopathy.
- ▲ Monitor transcutaneous bilirubin level in jaundiced neonate per unit protocol.
- ▲ Collect and evaluate laboratory blood specimens as prescribed or per unit protocol.
- Perform hour-specific total serum bilirubin (TSB) risk assessment before discharge from hospital or birth center and document the results.
- Monitor newborn for signs of inadequate breast milk or formula intake: dry oral mucous membranes, fewer than 4 to 6 wet diapers per 24 hours, no stool in 24 hours, and body weight loss greater than 10%.
- Assess late preterm infant (born between 34 and 37 weeks' gestation) for ability to breastfeed successfully and adequate intake of breast milk.
- Assist mother with breastfeeding and assess latch-on. See Readiness for Enhanced **Breastfeeding.**
- Encourage alternate methods for providing expressed breast milk if maternal health status is compromised, such as assisting the mother with collection of breast milk via use of breast pump or hand expression.
- Encourage partner's participation in newborn care by changing diapers, helping position newborn for breastfeeding, and holding newborn while mother rests.

• = Independent          ▲ = Collaborative

- Weigh newborn daily.
▲ When phototherapy is ordered, place seminude infant (diaper only) under prescribed amount of phototherapy lights.
- Protect infant's eyes from phototherapy light source with eye shields; remove eye shields periodically when infant is removed from light source for feeding and parent–infant interaction.
- Monitor infant's hydration status, fluid intake, skin status, and body temperature while undergoing phototherapy.
▲ Collect and evaluate laboratory blood specimens (TSB) while infant is undergoing phototherapy.
- Encourage continuation of breastfeeding and brief infant care activities such as changing diapers while the infant is being treated with phototherapy; phototherapy may be interrupted for breastfeeding.
- Provide emotional support for parents of infants undergoing phototherapy.
- Provide for novel therapies that can be used in tandem with phototherapy to support parent–infant interaction during treatment.

**Multicultural**
- Assess infants of Southeast Asian or Far East Asian and American Indian ethnicity for early rising bilirubin levels, especially when breastfeeding.

**Client/Family Teaching and Discharge Planning**
- Teach parents the signs of inadequate milk intake: fewer than three to four stools per day by day 4, fewer than four to six wet diapers in 24 hours, and dry oral mucous membranes; additional danger signs include a sleepy baby that does not awaken for breastfeeding or appears lethargic (decreased activity level from usual newborn pattern).
- Teach parents about the transition in stool color and consistency starting with meconium, followed by green, seedy stool, to mustard-colored, seedy stool by the fourth day of life.
▲ Teach parents and support persons about the appearance of jaundice (yellow or orange color of skin) after hospital or birth center discharge. Teach parents about the importance of medical follow-up in the first several days of life for the evaluation of jaundice.
- Teach parents about the use of phototherapy (hospital or home, as prescribed); the proper use of the phototherapy equipment; feedings; and assessment of hydration, body temperature, skin status, and urine and stool output.

• = Independent          ▲ = Collaborative

# Risk for Neonatal Hyperbilirubinemia

**Domain 2** Nutrition   **Class 4** Metabolism

## NANDA-I Definition

Susceptible to the accumulation of unconjugated bilirubin in the circulation (less than 15 ml/dl) that occurs after 24 hours of life, which may compromise health.

## Risk Factors

Delay in meconium passage; inadequate paternal feeding behavior; malnourished infants

## At-Risk Population

East Asian neonates; low birth weight neonates; Native American neonates; neonates aged ≤7 days; neonates who are breastfed; neonates whose blood groups are incompatible with mothers'; neonates whose mothers had gestational diabetes; neonates whose sibling had history of jaundice; neonates with significant bruising during birth; populations living at high altitudes; premature neonates

## Associated Conditions

Bacterial infections; enzyme deficiency; impaired metabolism; internal bleeding; liver malfunction; prenatal infection; sepsis; viral infection

## Client Outcomes

**Client Will (Specify Time Frame)**

- Neonatal total serum bilirubin (TSB) will be monitored and there will be no undetected TSB values in the high-risk (95th percentile or greater) or high-intermediate risk (75th to 94th percentile) zones (as determined by the hour-specific nomogram)
- Newborn will receive appropriate therapies to enhance bilirubin excretion
- Receive bilirubin assessment and screening within the first 24 hours of life with higher risk infants being reevaluated every 24 hours to detect increasing levels of serum bilirubin
- Receive nursing assessments to determine risk for severity of jaundice prior to discharge from birth hospital and schedule return clinic visit within 2 days of discharge for higher risk neonates
- Establish effective on-demand feeding pattern at least every 2 to 3 hours (breast or bottle)
- Maintain hydration: moist buccal membranes, four to six wet diapers in a 24-hour period, weight loss no greater than 10% of birth weight
- Evacuate stool within 48 hours of birth, and pass three to four stools per 24 hours by day 4 of life

• = Independent        ▲ = Collaborative

### Nursing Interventions

- Identify clinical risk factors that place the infant at greater risk for development of neonatal jaundice: exclusive breastfeeding, isoimmune or hemolytic disease, preterm birth (37{6/7} weeks' gestation or less), weight loss of 10% or more from birth weight within the first week, neonatal sepsis, maternal diabetes, maternal obesity, previous sibling with jaundice, East Asian ethnicity, and significant bruising or cephalohematoma.
- Measure transcutaneous bilirubin (TcB) of all newborns in the first 24 to 48 hours of life, using a noninvasive transcutaneous bilirubinometer. Plot TcB on a nomogram standardized for the appropriate client population; determine newborn's risk of subsequent significant hyperbilirubinemia.
- Refer to care plan for Neonatal **Hyperbilirubinemia** for additional interventions for multicultural and discharge planning.

### Client/Family Teaching and Discharge Planning

- Teach parents about the importance of medical follow-up in the first several days of life for the evaluation of jaundice, especially in the late preterm infant.
- Refer to care plan for Neonatal **Hyperbilirubinemia** for additional interventions.

## Hyperthermia

**Domain 11** Safety/protection    **Class 6** Thermoregulation

### NANDA-I Definition

Core body temperature above the normal diurnal range due to failure of thermoregulation.

### Defining Characteristics

Abnormal posturing; apnea; coma; flushed skin; hypotension; infant does not maintain suck; irritable mood; lethargy; seizure; skin warm to touch; stupor; tachycardia; tachypnea; vasodilation

### Related Factors

Dehydration; inappropriate clothing; vigorous activity

### At-Risk Population

Individuals exposed to high environmental temperature

### Associated Conditions

Decreased sweat response; impaired health status; increased metabolic rate; ischemia; pharmaceutical preparations; sepsis; trauma

• = Independent    ▲ = Collaborative

## Client Outcomes

### Client Will (Specify Time Frame)

- Maintain core body temperature within adaptive levels (<40°C [104°F])
- Remain free of complications of malignant hyperthermia
- Remain free of complication of neuroleptic malignant syndrome
- Remain free of dehydration
- Remain free from infection
- Verbalize signs and symptoms of heat stroke and actions to prevent heat stroke
- Verbalize personal risks for malignant hyperthermia and neuroleptic malignant syndrome to be reported during health history reviews to all health care professionals, including pharmacists

### Nursing Interventions

**Temperature Measurement**

- Recognize that hyperthermia is a rise in body temperature above 40°C (104°F) that is not regulated by the hypothalamus, resulting in an uncontrolled increase in body temperature exceeding the body's ability to lose heat.
- Continually measure a client's core temperature with a distal esophageal probe or obtain near core body temperature measurements with a rectal or bladder temperature probe and verify with a second method.
- Use the same site and method (device) for temperature measurement for a given client so that temperature trends are assessed accurately; record site of temperature measurement.
- ▲ Work with the health care provider to help determine the cause of the temperature increase (hyperthermia), which will often help direct appropriate treatment.
- Refer to care plan for Ineffective **Thermoregulation** for interventions managing fever (pyrexia).

**Heat Stroke**

- Recognize that heat stroke may be separated into two categories: classic and exertional.
- Watch for risk factors for classic heat stroke, which include the following (Gaudio & Grissom, 2016; Knapik & Epstein, 2019):
  - ○ Medications, especially diuretics, anticholinergic agents, beta-blockers, calcium channel blockers, anti-Parkinson's medications, antidepressants, thyroid agonists, and antihistamines
  - ○ City dwellers who reside on top floors of buildings
  - ○ Alcoholism

• = Independent        ▲ = Collaborative

- Diabetes mellitus
- Mental illness
- Obesity
- Heart disease
- Renal disease

- Risk factors of exertional heat stroke include the following (Gaudio & Grissom, 2016; Lipman et al, 2019):
  - Preexisting illness
  - Drug use (e.g., alcohol, amphetamines, ecstasy)
  - Wearing protective clothing (uniforms and athletic gear) that limits heat dissipation
  - Obesity
  - Low physical fitness
  - Lack of sleep

- Recognize that antipyretic agents are of little use in treatment of hyperthermia.

▲ Assess fluid loss and facilitate oral intake or administer intravenous fluids as prescribed to accomplish fluid replacement and support the cardiovascular system. Refer to the care plan for Deficient **Fluid** Volume.

▲ Recognize use of alpha-adrenergic agents should be avoided if possible.

- Remove clothing and immerse young and healthy clients who have suffered exertional heat stroke in a cold water bath ensuring the head does not go underwater, or continuously douse the client with cold water.

- For clients with classic heat stroke, remove clothes and spray or douse the skin with water and provide continual airflow over the body with a fan.

▲ Recognize adjunctive cooling measures include administering cold (4°C [39.2°F] ) intravenous fluids, ice sheeting (covering patient with bed linens that have been soaked in ice water), water circulating hydrogel coated pads placed over the chest and legs, ice packs over the entire body, intravascular cooling catheter, and cooling blankets.

▲ Continuously monitor the effects of cooling measures, stop cooling interventions once the body temperature is less than 39°C [102.2°F], and benzodiazepines may be administered to control shivering.

▲ Continually assess the client's neurologic and other organ function, especially kidney function (i.e., signs of rhabdomyolysis), for signs of injury from hyperthermia.

• = Independent    ▲ = Collaborative

**Malignant Hyperthermia**
▲ If the client has just received general anesthesia, especially halothane, sevoflurane, desflurane, enflurane, isoflurane, or succinylcholine, recognize that the hyperthermia may be caused by malignant hyperthermia and requires immediate treatment to prevent death.
• Monitor core temperature for all clients receiving general anesthetic agents for longer than 30 minutes.
• Recognize that signs and symptoms of malignant hyperthermia typically occur suddenly after exposure to the anesthetic agent and include rapid rise in core body temperature (as much as 1°C–2°C every 5 minutes [approximately 1.8°F–3.6°F]), hypercarbia (increase in end tidal carbon dioxide), muscle rigidity, masseter muscle spasm, dysrhythmias, tachycardia, tachypnea, rhabdomyolysis, acute kidney injury, and elevated serum calcium and potassium, progressing to disseminated intravascular coagulation and cardiac arrest (Riazi et al, 2018; Cieniewicz et al, 2019).
▲ If the client has malignant hyperthermia, begin treatment as prescribed, including cessation of the anesthetic agent and intravenous administration of dantrolene sodium, STAT, along with cooling measures, core body temperature monitoring, hyperventilation with 100% oxygen, antidysrhythmics, and continued support of the cardiovascular system.
▲ Recognize that dysrhythmias must not be treated with calcium channel blockers (e.g., verapamil) when the client has malignant hyperthermia.
▲ Recognize that antipyretics are not recommended.
• Monitor for reoccurrence of malignant hyperthermia symptoms that correlates with the half-life of dantrolene, typically within 16 hours (Cieniewicz et al, 2019; Malignant Hyperthermia Association of the United States [MHAUS], 2020).
• Provide client and family education when malignant hyperthermia occurs because it is an inherited muscle disorder.

**Neuroleptic Malignant Syndrome**
▲ Recognize that neuroleptic malignant syndrome is a rare condition associated with clients who are taking typical and atypical antipsychotic agents or after abrupt discontinuation of dopaminergic agonist agents used for Parkinson's disorder (Pileggi & Cook, 2016; Ware et al, 2018).
• Watch for signs and symptoms that can range from mild to severe and include a sudden change in mental status, rapid rise in body temperature, muscle rigidity (lead pipe), tachycardia, tachypnea,

• = Independent          ▲ = Collaborative

elevated or labile blood pressure, diaphoresis, urinary incontinence rhabdomyolysis, and acute kidney injury (Kollmann-Camaiora et al, 2017; van Rensburg & Decloedt, 2019).

▲ Begin treatment when diagnosed, including cessation of the neuroleptic or dopamine antagonist agent or resumption of dopamine agonist agent that may have been abruptly discontinued; order administration of dantrolene, bromocriptine, amantadine, or benzodiazepine; initiate cooling measures; continue support of the cardiovascular, pulmonary, and renal systems; and electroconvulsive therapy if drug therapy fails or for severe symptoms (Kollmann-Camaiora et al, 2017; van Rensburg & Decloedt; 2019).

• A client health history that reports extrapyramidal reaction to any medication should be further explored for risk of neuroleptic malignant syndrome because this syndrome can occur at any time during a client's treatment with typical and atypical antipsychotic agents (Kollmann-Camaiora et al, 2017; Ware et al, 2018).

• Recognize that clients receiving rapid dose escalation of antipsychotic agents (e.g., haloperidol) intramuscularly for acute treatment of delirium may be at increased risk for neuroleptic malignant syndrome (Kollmann-Camaiora et al, 2017; Ware et al, 2018).

**Drug Fever**

• Recognize an elevated body temperature in response to a medication ranges from 37.2°C to 42.2°C [98.7°F–108°F] with a typical onset from 7 to 10 days after initiating the medication (Maddock & Connor, 2020).

• Recognize individuals suffering from a drug fever will appear clinically well with a lower heart rate relative to the body temperature (relative bradycardia) but may have a maculopapular rash, headache, myalgias, and an elevated eosinophil count (Maddock & Connor, 2020).

▲ Medications most commonly responsible for a drug fever include antimicrobials, antineoplastic agents, anticonvulsants, antiarrhythmics, and dexmedetomidine.

**Pediatric**

• Assess risk factors of malignant hyperthermia, including a personal or family history of anesthesia-related complications or death or a history of muscle disorders.

▲ Administer dantrolene, provide oxygen and assist with ventilation, monitor heart rate and rhythm, and treat electrolyte and acid-base disorders (i.e., metabolic acidosis) as ordered if malignant hyperthermia is present.

• = Independent        ▲ = Collaborative

**Geriatric**

- Help the client seek medical attention immediately if elevated core temperature is present. To diagnose the hyperthermia, assess for possible precipitating factors, including changes in medication, environmental changes, and recent medical interventions or infectious exposures.
- In hot weather, encourage the client to wear lightweight cotton clothing (Jain et al, 2018; Leyk et al, 2019).
- Provide education on the importance of drinking eight glasses of fluid per day (within their cardiac and renal reserves) regardless of whether they are thirsty, wearing appropriate clothing for the environmental temperature, keeping the head covered, staying home in the afternoon, and avoiding direct sunlight and sitting in a parked vehicle in the sun; assess for the need for and presence of fans or air conditioning.
- In hot weather, monitor the older client for signs of heat stroke such as rising temperature, orthostatic blood pressure drop, weakness, restlessness, mental status changes, faintness, thirst, nausea, and vomiting. If signs are present, move the client to a cool place, have the client lie down, give sips of water, check orthostatic blood pressure, spray with lukewarm water, cool with a fan, and seek medical assistance immediately.
- During warm weather, help the client obtain a fan or an air conditioner to increase evaporation, as needed. Help the older client locate a cool environment to which they can go for safety in hot weather.
- Take the temperature of the older client in hot weather.

**Home Care**

- Some of the interventions described previously may be adapted for home care use.
- Determine whether the client or family has a functioning thermometer, and know how to use it. Refer to the previous interventions on taking a temperature.
- Help the client and caregivers prevent and monitor for heat stroke/hyperthermia during times of high outdoor temperatures.
- To prevent heat-related injury in athletes, laborers, and military personnel, instruct them to acclimate gradually to the higher temperatures, increase fluid intake, wear vapor-permeable clothing, and take frequent rests (Knapick & Epstein, 2019; CDC, 2020e).
- In the event of temperature elevation above the adaptive range, institute measures to decrease temperature (e.g., get the client out of the sun and into a cool place, remove excess clothing, have the client

• = Independent          ▲ = Collaborative

drink fluids, spray the client with lukewarm water, fan with cool air, initiate emergency transport).

**Client/Family Teaching and Discharge Planning**

▲ Instruct to increase fluids to prevent heat-induced hyperthermia and dehydration in the presence of fever.

• Teach the client to stay in a cooler environment during periods of excessive outdoor heat or humidity. If the client does go out, instruct them to avoid vigorous physical activity; wear lightweight, loose-fitting clothing; and wear a hat to minimize sun exposure.

H

# Hypothermia

**Domain 11** Safety/protection     **Class 6** Thermoregulation

## NANDA-I Definition

Core body temperature below normal diurnal range in individuals > 28 days of life.

## Defining Characteristics

Acrocyanosis; bradycardia; cyanotic nail beds; decreased blood glucose level; decreased ventilation; hypertension; hypoglycemia; hypoxia; increased metabolic rate; increased oxygen consumption; peripheral vasoconstriction; piloerection; shivering; skin cool to touch; slow capillary refill; tachycardia

## Related Factors

Alcohol consumption; excessive conductive heat transfer; excessive convective heat transfer; excessive evaporative heat transfer; excessive radiative heat transfer; inactivity; inadequate caregiver knowledge of hypothermia prevention; inadequate clothing; low environmental temperature; malnutrition

## At-Risk Population

Economically disadvantaged individuals; individuals at extremes of age; individuals at extremes of weight

## Associated Conditions

Damage to hypothalamus; decreased metabolic rate; pharmaceutical preparations; radiotherapy; trauma

## Client Outcomes

**Client Will (Specify Time Frame)**

• Maintain body temperature within normal range
• Identify risk factors of hypothermia
• State measures to prevent hypothermia
• Identify symptoms of hypothermia and actions to take when hypothermia is present

• = Independent          ▲ = Collaborative

- If hypothermia is medically induced client/family will state goals for hypothermia treatment

## Nursing Interventions

### Temperature Measurement

- Recognize hypothermia as a drop in core body temperature to 35°C (95°F) or lower (Zafren, 2017; Dow et al, 2019).
- Measure and record the client's temperature hourly or, if the client's temperature is less than 35°C (95°F), continuously.
- Select a core or a near core measurement site based on the clinical situation and ability to obtain an accurate measurement; verify the temperature reading with a second monitoring device as needed.
- Use the same site and method (device) for a given client so that temperature trends are accurately assessed.
- See the care plan for Ineffective **Thermoregulation** as appropriate.

### Accidental Hypothermia

- Recognize that there are three categories of hypothermia based on the core temperature (Dow et al, 2019): mild—35°C to 32°C (95°F–89.6°F), where the individual is conscious and shivering; moderate—32°C to 28°C (89.6°F–82.4°F), where the individual exhibits altered mental status, paradoxical undressing, and loss of shivering and where thermoregulatory mechanisms are less effective, necessitating the application of exogenous heat; and severe—less than 28°C (82.4°F), resulting in unconsciousness, loss of shivering, and increased risk of cardiac arrest.
- Remove the client from the cause of the hypothermic episode (e.g., cold environment, cold or wet clothing), bring into a warm environment, cover the client with warm blankets, and apply a covering to the head and neck to conserve body heat.
- Keep the moderately and severely hypothermic client horizontal, limit limb movement, and handle gently during movements.
- Monitor the client for signs of hypothermia: shivering, slurred speech, confusion, clumsy movements, fatigue progressing to a further decrease in level of consciousness, bradycardia, hypoventilation, hypotension, ventricular fibrillation, and asystole (Rischall & Rowland-Fisher, 2016; Zafren, 2017).
- Monitor the client's vital signs every hour and as appropriate, noting changes associated with hypothermia such as increased pulse rate, respiratory rate, and blood pressure, as well as diuresis with mild hypothermia, progressing to a decreased pulse rate, respiratory rate, and blood pressure, and oliguria with moderate to severe hypothermia.

▲ Attach electrodes and a cardiac monitor, increase the gain (QRS amplitude), and monitor for dysrhythmias.

▲ Recognize that clients with a core temperature less than 30°C (86°F) are at a higher risk for cardiac arrest; if the client arrests:

○ Check the pulse for up to 1 minute because the pulse may be slow and weak.

○ Provide chest compressions unless the client has a frozen noncompressible chest.

○ Deliver ventilations at the same rate as recommended for a normothermic client if an advanced airway is not in place. If an advanced airway is in place, use an end-tidal $CO_2$ monitor to guide ventilations or provide ventilations at half the rate recommended for a normothermic client to avoid hyperventilation.

○ Limit defibrillations to one attempt at maximal power for clients with ventricular fibrillation or pulseless ventricular tachycardia until the client's core temperature is at least 30°C (86°F).

○ Medications may be withheld until the client has a core temperature greater than 30°C (86°F); double the interval between doses once the temperature is above 30°C (86°F); resume normal doses of medications once the temperature reaches 35°C (95°F).

○ Recognize that prolonged cardiopulmonary resuscitation may be necessary as the client is rewarmed.

▲ Monitor for signs of coagulopathy (e.g., oozing of blood from any open areas or from intravascular catheter sites or mucous membranes) and note the results of clotting studies as available.

• Assess for localized cold injuries such as frostbite.

• For mild hypothermia (core temperature of 32.2°C–35°C [90°F–95°F]), rewarm client passively:

○ Set room temperature to 21°C to 24°C (70°F–75°F).

○ Keep the client dry; remove any damp or wet clothing.

○ Layer clothing and blankets and cover the client's head.

○ Offer warm fluids, particularly beverages high in carbohydrates for clients who are shivering and able to safely swallow; avoid alcohol or caffeine; avoid fluids that are so warm they might burn the esophagus (Zafren, 2017; Dow et al, 2019).

• For mild hypothermia, allow the client to rewarm at his or her own pace as heat is generated through the normal metabolism.

▲ For moderate hypothermia (core temperature 28°C–32.1°C [82.4°F–90°F]) or any client with a decreased level of consciousness, use active external rewarming methods, not exceeding an increase of more than 1°C to 2°C (approximately 1.8°F–3°F) per hour.

• = Independent          ▲ = Collaborative

- Methods to rewarm the client include the following (Dow et al, 2019; Rathjen et al, 2019):
  - Forced-air warming blankets
  - Circulation of warm water through external pads
  - Heated and humidified oxygen (42°C–46°C [107.6°F–114.8°F]) through the ventilator circuit as ordered
  - Warmed (40°C–42°C [104°F–107.6°F]) intravenous (IV) normal saline and blood products using a commercial IV fluid warmer (hypothermic clients cannot metabolize lactate so IV lactated Ringer's should not be administered)
  - Radiant heat sources; concentrate heat to axillae and upper torso
▲ For severe hypothermia (core temperature below 28°C [82.4°F]), use active core rewarming techniques as ordered (Dow et al, 2019; Rathjen et al, 2019):
  - Hemodialysis
  - Intravascular temperature management catheter
  - Body cavity (thorax, peritoneal, stomach, and bladder) lavage with warmed fluid
  - Recognize that warming by extracorporeal life support (ECLS) using venoarterial extracorporeal membrane oxygenation (ECMO) or cardiopulmonary bypass is essential for clients experiencing hemodynamic instability or hypothermic cardiac arrest
- Rewarm clients slowly, generally at a rate of 1°C to 2°C every hour (approximately 1.8°F–3.6°F).
- Measure the blood pressure frequently when rewarming and monitor for hypotension.
- After rewarming, monitor the client for afterdrop, or a decrease in body temperature due to return of colder blood from the periphery to the core.
▲ Administer isotonic IV normal saline warmed to 40°C to 42°C [104°F–107.6°F] as prescribed.
- Place a barrier between the client and the heating blanket and monitor the client's skin every 30 minutes.
- Determine the factors leading to the hypothermic episode, particularly if the client fails to rewarm, and treat the underlying condition; see Related Factors.
▲ Request a social service referral to help the client obtain the heat, shelter, and food needed to maintain body temperature.
▲ Encourage proper nutrition and hydration.

• = Independent          ▲ = Collaborative

**Targeted Temperature Hypothermia**

- Recognize that targeted temperature management, previously called therapeutic hypothermia, is the active lowering of the client's body temperature, in a controlled manner, to preserve neurological function after a cardiac arrest; targeted temperature management may also be considered for clients who have refractory intracranial hypertension.
- Recognize that controlled cooling of clients should be considered for all unconscious survivors of in-hospital or out-of-hospital cardiac arrest with an initial shockable (ventricular fibrillation or pulseless ventricular tachycardia) or nonshockable (asystole or pulseless electrical activity) rhythm; achieve and maintain a constant target temperature between 32°C and 36°C (89.6°F–96.8°F) for at least 24 hours.
- Monitor core or near core temperatures continuously using two methods of temperature monitoring.
- Recognize that cooling may be achieved noninvasively, using fluid-filled cooling pads or with an esophageal cooling catheter, or invasively, with an intravascular cooling catheter.
- Monitor for signs of infection and implement measures to prevent hospital-acquired infections.
- Obtain vital signs hourly (or via continuous monitoring) and include continuous electrocardiogram monitoring, and observe for signs of hypotension, bradycardia, and dysrhythmias. Mechanical ventilation is required to protect the client's airway and breathing during treatment.
- ▲ Observe for shivering using a tool such as the Bedside Shivering Assessment Scale (BSAS) and implement skin counter-warming with blankets or a forced warm-air device; administer sedatives, opioids, neuromuscular blocking agents, α-agonists, buspirone, acetaminophen, nonsteroidal antiinflammatory agents, or magnesium sulfate as prescribed.
- ▲ Closely inspect the skin before and throughout the cooling intervention and implement frequent turning and other pressure reduction interventions as indicated.
- ▲ Monitor and treat serum electrolytes (e.g., potassium, magnesium, calcium, phosphorus) and serum glucose closely during targeted hypothermia and during rewarming of the client; electrolytes will fluctuate as the client is rewarmed.
- ▲ Monitor blood cell counts and observe for signs and symptoms of coagulopathy during targeted hypothermia treatment.
- Rewarming should occur in a controlled manner, with a rise in body temperature no faster than 0.5°C (approximately 0.9°F) per hour and a targeted goal of normothermia, 37°C [98.6°F] for 48 hours.

• = Independent          ▲ = Collaborative

▲ Neurological and cognitive function should be assessed during targeted temperature treatment and after rewarming.

**Pediatric**

- Recognize that pediatric clients have a decreased ability to adapt to temperature extremes; take the following actions to maintain body temperature in the infant/child:
  ○ Keep the head covered.
  ○ Use blankets to keep the client warm.
  ○ Keep the client covered during procedures, transport, and diagnostic testing.
  ○ Keep the room temperature at 22.2°C (72°F) for children and between 23°C and 25°C[73.4°F–77°F] for infants less than 32 weeks' gestation.

- The combination of a relatively smaller body surface area, smaller body fluid volume, less well-developed temperature control mechanisms, and smaller amount of protective body fat limits the infant's and child's ability to maintain normal temperatures (Sgro et al, 2016; Shah & Madhok, 2019).

- For the preterm or low-birth-weight newborn, set the room temperature to 25°C (77°F) before the delivery; dry the infant; wrap in prewarmed, dry blankets; cover the infant's head with a wool or polyethylene cap; and use specially designed bags, skin-to-skin care, TransWarmer mattresses, radiant warmers, and thermal blankets to keep the infant warm.

- Avoid bathing neonates for at least 12 to 24 hours after birth when temperature stability is achieved; perform immersion bathing rather than sponge bathing for newborns and swaddled bathing for premature neonates; avoid removing the vernix caseosa and allow it to wear off with normal activity and handling; grossly contaminated vernix caseosa may be gently removed.

- Targeted hypothermia to 34°C (93.2°F) for 72 hours may be implemented in the treatment of neonates with hypoxic-ischemic encephalopathy (HIE).

- Measure the temperature of the neonate undergoing therapeutic hypothermia for HIE with a rectal or esophageal probe.

**Geriatric**

- Normal aging often includes changes in touch-related sensations, making it harder to differentiate cool and cold.

- Recognize that older adults can develop hypothermia even from exposure to mildly cold temperatures of 15.5°C to 18.3°C (60°F–65°F).

• = Independent        ▲ = Collaborative

○ Set the room temperature to 20°C to 21.1°C (68°F–70°F).

○ Instruct client to wear warm clothes as appropriate (long underwear, socks, slippers, and a cap or hat) and to use a blanket to keep shoulders and legs warm while indoors.

○ Instruct client to dress in loose layers and wear a hat, scarf, and gloves or mittens when going outside during cold weather.

○ Instruct client to maintain adequate calorie intake.

• Assess neurological signs frequently, watching for confusion and decreased level of consciousness.

**H**

### Home Care

• Hypothermia is not a symptom that appears in the normal course of home care, but when it occurs it is a clinical emergency, and the client/family should access emergency medical services immediately.

• Some of the interventions described earlier may be adapted for home care use.

• Before a medical crisis occurs, confirm that the client or family has a thermometer that registers accurately, and the client or family can read it.

• Instruct the client or family to take the temperature when the client displays cyanosis, pallor, or shivering.

▲ Monitor temperature every hour, as noted previously; if the temperature of the client begins dropping below the normal range, apply layers of clothing or blankets, or adjust environmental heat to the comfort level, being careful to not overheat the client. Passive rewarming is the only method of rewarming that is appropriate for home care under normal circumstances.

▲ If temperature continues to drop, activate the emergency system and notify a health care provider. Hypothermia is a clinically acute condition that cannot be managed safely in the home.

▲ If the client is in hospice care or is terminally ill, follow advance directives, client wishes, and the health care provider's orders; keep the client free of pain. The goal of terminal care is to provide dignity and comfort during the dying process.

### Client/Family Teaching and Discharge Planning

• Teach the client and family signs of hypothermia and the method of taking the temperature (age appropriate).

• Teach the client methods to prevent hypothermia: wearing adequate clothing, including a hat and mittens; heating the environment to a minimum of 20°C (68°F); and ingesting adequate food and fluid.

• = Independent          ▲ = Collaborative

- Teach clients who engage in cold weather outdoor activities the importance of appropriate clothing, survival skills, and emergency planning.
▲ Teach the client and family about medications such as sedatives, opioids, and anxiolytics that predispose the client to hypothermia (as appropriate).

## H | Risk for Hypothermia

**Domain 11** Safety/protection    **Class 6** Thermoregulation
### NANDA-I Definition
Susceptible to a failure of thermoregulation that may result in a core body temperature below the normal diurnal range, in individuals >28 days of life, which may compromise health.

### Risk Factors
Alcohol consumption; excessive conductive heat transfer; excessive convective heat transfer; excessive evaporative heat transfer; excessive radiative heat transfer; inactivity; inadequate caregiver knowledge of hypothermia prevention; inadequate clothing; low environmental temperature; malnutrition

### At-Risk Population
Economically disadvantaged individuals; individuals at extremes of age; individuals at extremes of weight

### Associated Conditions
Damage to hypothalamus; decreased metabolic rate; pharmaceutical preparations; radiotherapy; trauma

### Client Outcomes, Nursing Interventions, and Client/Family Teaching and Discharge Planning
Refer to care plan for **Hypothermia**.

## Neonatal Hypothermia

**Domain 11** Safety/protection    **Class 6** Thermoregulation
### NANDA-I Definition
Core body temperature of an infant below the normal diurnal range.

### Defining Characteristics
Acrocyanosis; bradycardia; decreased blood glucose level; decreased metabolic rate; decreased peripheral perfusion; decreased ventilation; hypertension; hypoglycemia; hypoxia; increased oxygen demand; insufficient energy to maintain sucking; irritability; metabolic acidosis; pallor; peripheral

vasoconstriction; respiratory distress; skin cool to touch; slow capillary refill; tachycardia; weight gain <30 g/day

## Related Factors

Delayed breastfeeding; early bathing of newborn; excessive conductive heat transfer; excessive convective heat transfer; excessive evaporative heat transfer; excessive radiative heat transfer; inadequate caregiver knowledge of hypothermia prevention; inadequate clothing; malnutrition

## At-Risk Population

Low birth weight neonates; neonates aged 0-28 days; neonates born by cesarean delivery; neonates born to an adolescent mother; neonates born to economically disadvantaged families; Neonates exposed to low environmental temperatures; Neonates with high-risk out-of-hospital birth; neonates with inadequate subcutaneous fat; neonates with increased body surface area to weight ratio; neonates with unplanned out-of-hospital birth; premature neonates

**H**

## Associated Conditions

Damage to hypothalamus; immature stratum corneum; increased pulmonary vascular resistance; ineffective vascular control; inefficient non-shivering thermogenesis; low Appearance, Pulse, Grimace, Activity, & Respiration (APGAR) scores; pharmaceutical preparations

## Client Outcomes

### Client Will (Specify Time Frame)

- Maintain a body temperature of 36.5°C to 37.5°C (97.7°F–99.5°F)
- Identify risk factors of hypothermia
- State measures to prevent hypothermia
- Identify symptoms of hypothermia and actions to take when hypothermia is present

## Nursing Interventions

- At delivery, neonates should be maintained at a temperature of 36.5°C to 37.5°C (97.7°F–99.5°F). Room temperature should be increased to 23°C to 25°C (74°F–77°F).
- Monitor infants at risk for hypothermia and cold stress.
- Monitor temperature by skin or axillary measurements using digital/electronic thermometers.
- Reduce risk of hypothermia by avoiding exposure to sources of heat loss, such as exposing wet skin to the air; direct contact with a cold surface; or placing close to a window or cold wall or near open doors or air conditioner vents.
- Infants with mild hypothermia (36°C–36.4°C [96.8°F–97.5°F]) can be warmed by being placed skin-to-skin with mother in a warm room.

• = Independent          ▲ = Collaborative

- Infants with moderate (32°C–35.9°C [89.6°F–96.6°F]) or severe (<32°C [<89.6°F]) hypothermia should be placed on a radiant warmer or a preheated, double-walled incubator set at 35°C to 36°C (95°F–96.8°F).
- Bathing or weighing the infant should be delayed if evidence of cold stress or hypothermia exists.
- Monitor the cold-stressed or hypothermic infant for respiratory distress (grunting, tachypnea, retractions) and hypoglycemia.

**H** **Multicultural**

- An occlusive plastic wrap or bag at birth can be used in resource-limited settings.

# Risk for Neonatal Hypothermia

**Domain 11** Safety/protection  **Class 6** Thermoregulation

## NANDA-I Definition

Susceptibility of an infant to a core body temperature below the normal diurnal range, which may compromise health.

## Risk Factors

Delayed breastfeeding; early bathing of newborn; excessive conductive heat transfer; excessive convective heat transfer; excessive evaporative heat transfer; excessive radiative heat transfer; inadequate caregiver knowledge of hypothermia prevention; inadequate clothing; malnutrition

## At-Risk Population

Low birth weight neonates; neonates aged 0-28 days; neonates born by cesarean delivery; neonates born to an adolescent mother; neonates born to economically disadvantaged families; neonates exposed to low environmental temperatures; neonates with high-risk out-of-hospital birth; neonates with inadequate subcutaneous fat; neonates with increased body surface area to weight ratio; neonates with unplanned out-of- hospital birth; premature neonates

## Associated Conditions

Damage to hypothalamus; immature stratum corneum; increased pulmonary vascular resistance; ineffective vascular control; inefficient non-shivering thermogenesis; low Appearance, Pulse, Grimace, Activity, & Respiration (APGAR) scores; pharmaceutical preparations

## Client Outcomes and Nursing Interventions

Refer to care plan for Neonatal **Hypothermia**.

• = Independent          ▲ = Collaborative

# Risk for Perioperative Hypothermia

**Domain 11** Safety/protection    **Class 6** Thermoregulation

## NANDA-I Definition

Susceptible to an inadvertent drop in core body temperature below 36°C/96.8°F occurring one hour before to 24 hours after surgery, which may compromise health.

## Risk Factors

Anxiety; body mass index below normal range for age and gender; environmental temperature <21°C/69.8°F; inadequate availability of appropriate warming equipment; wound area uncovered

## At-Risk Population

Individuals aged ≥60 years; individuals in environment with laminar air flow; individuals receiving anesthesia for a period >2 hours; individuals undergoing long induction time; individuals undergoing open surgery; individuals undergoing surgical procedure >2 hours; individuals with American Society of Anesthesiologists (ASA) Physical Status classification score >1; individuals with high Model for End-Stage Liver Disease (MELD) score; individuals with increased intraoperative blood loss; individuals with intraoperative diastolic arterial blood pressure <60 mm Hg; individuals with intraoperative systolic blood pressure <140 mm Hg; individuals with low body surface area; neonates <37 weeks gestational age; women

## Associated Conditions

Acute hepatic failure; anemia; burns; cardiovascular complications; chronic renal impairment; combined regional and general anesthesia; neurological disorder; pharmaceutical preparations; trauma

## Client Outcomes

**Client Will (Specify Time Frame)**

- Maintain body temperature within normal range
- Identify risk factors of hypothermia
- State measures to prevent hypothermia
- Identify symptoms of hypothermia and actions to take when hypothermia is present
- Be free of surgical site infection

## Nursing Interventions

**Temperature Measurement**

- Recognize perioperative hypothermia as a drop in core body temperature below 36°C (96.8°F). Hypothermia can be divided into mild (36°C–34°C [96.8°F–93.2°F]), moderate (33°C–28°C

[91.4°F–82.4°F]), and severe (≤28°C [<82.4°F]) (Granum et al, 2019; Centers for Disease Control and Prevention [CDC], 2020f; Nordgren et al, 2020).

- Measure the client's temperature frequently, at least every 15 minutes, while the client is undergoing general anesthesia and with changes in client condition (e.g., chills, change in mental status); if more than mild hypothermia is present (temperature lower than 36°C [96.8°F]), use a continuous temperature-monitoring device. Two modes of temperature monitoring may be indicated. Continuous temperature monitoring using an indwelling method of temperature measurement is usually indicated to monitor effectiveness of treating body alterations in core body temperature.
- Use the same site and method (device) for temperature measurement for a given client so that temperature trends are assessed accurately, and record site of temperature measurement.
- Bladder temperature may be used because an indwelling urinary catheter is often inserted in the management of hypothermia to monitor diuresis.

**Unintentional Perioperative Hypothermia**
- Keep the client warm throughout the perioperative period (preoperatively, intraoperatively, and postoperatively) to prevent unintentional perioperative hypothermia.
- Factors that increase the risk of perioperative hypothermia include anesthetic agents, ambient room air temperature, intravenous (IV) fluid infusion, cavity solution irrigation, blood product administration, duration and type of surgical procedure, anemia, extremes of age, neurological disorders, cachexia, minimal covering during surgery, and preexisting conditions (e.g., peripheral vascular disease, endocrine disease, pregnancy, burns, open wounds) (Brodshaug, Tettum, & Raeder, 2019; Bu et al, 2019; Link, 2020; American Society of PeriAnesthesia Nurses [ASPAN], 2021).
- Closely monitoring and preventing unintentional perioperative hypothermia is necessary to prevent adverse client outcomes.
- Several interventions should be implemented to prevent unintentional perioperative hypothermia:
  ○ Use warming booties perioperatively
  ○ Use warming blankets over and under the client perioperatively
  ○ Use warming blankets under the client on the operating table
  ○ Use of reflective blankets
  ○ Adjust environmental room controls to maintain ambient room temperature between 20°C (68°F) and 25°C (77°F)

- ○ Use humidified heated breathing circuit
- ○ Use warmed forced-air blankets preoperatively, during surgery, and in the postanesthesia care unit
- ○ Use circulating-water mattress
- ○ Use warmed IV fluids and irrigation solutions
- ○ Designate responsibility and accountability for thermoregulation
- Using warmed IV fluids and irrigation solutions during the operative period may assist with reducing the client's risk of unintentional perioperative hypothermia.
- Active warming interventions include the use of warm blankets and forced-air warming devices.
- A heated humidified breathing circuit can be used intraoperatively to decrease hypothermia.
- Watch the client for signs of hypothermia: shivering, slurred speech, confusion, clumsy movements, fatigue, and dehydration. Shivering increases oxygen consumption by about 40%. As hypothermia progresses, the skin becomes pale, muscles are tense, fatigue and weakness progress, breathing is decreased, and pulmonary congestion is present, compromising oxygenation. Pulses are decreased and blood pressure and heart rate decrease, progressing to lethal arrhythmias (e.g., ventricular fibrillation) (Torossian et al, 2016; Danzl, 2018).
- ▲ Administer oxygen as ordered.
- ▲ Attach electrodes and a cardiac monitor. Watch for dysrhythmias.
- ▲ Monitor for signs of coagulopathy (e.g., oozing of blood from any open areas or from intravascular catheter sites or mucous membranes). Also note results of clotting studies as available.
- ▲ Monitor for signs of surgical site infection (e.g., increased incisional pain, drainage, poor healing, poor incision approximation).
- See care plans for Ineffective **Thermoregulation** and **Hypothermia** as appropriate.

**Pediatric**
- Interventions implemented in the care of adult clients are similar when providing care to pediatric clients to prevent hypothermia.

**Home Care**
- ▲ Hypothermia is not a symptom that appears in the normal course of postoperative home care. If the client continues to complain of chills or feeling cold after discharge home from a surgical procedure, provide the client with warm blankets and, if the client is allowed to drink, provide warm fluids by mouth.
- ▲ Monitor temperature every hour, as noted previously. If the temperature of the client begins dropping below the normal range,

• = Independent          ▲ = Collaborative

apply layers of clothing or blankets, or adjust environmental heat to the comfort level. Do not overheat. Contact a health care provider.

▲ If temperature continues to drop, activate the emergency system and notify a health care provider.

**Client/Family Teaching and Discharge Planning**

• Teach the client/family signs of hypothermia and the method of taking the temperature (age appropriate).

▲ Teach the client and family about medications such as sedatives, opioids, and anxiolytics that predispose the client to hypothermia (as appropriate). If the client has had hypothermia in the past, using alternative medications is an option if there is no contraindication (Danzl, 2018).

# Disturbed Family Identity Syndrome

**Domain 7** Role relationship    **Class 2** Family relationships

## NANDA-I Definition

Inability to maintain an ongoing interactive, communicative process of creating and maintaining a shared collective sense of the meaning of the family.

## Defining Characteristics

Decisional conflict (00083); disabled family coping (00073); disturbed personal identity (00121); dysfunctional family processes (00063); impaired resilience (00210); ineffective childbearing process (00221); ineffective relationship (00223); ineffective sexuality pattern (00065); interrupted family processes (00060)

## Related Factors

Ambivalent family relations; different coping styles among family members; disrupted family rituals; disrupted family roles; excessive stress; inadequate social support; ineffective coping strategies; ineffective family communication; perceived social discrimination; sexual dysfunction; unaddressed domestic violence; unrealistic expectations; values incongruent with cultural norms

## At-Risk Population

Blended families; economically disadvantaged families; families experiencing infertility; families with history of domestic violence; families with incarcerated member; families with member experiencing alteration in health status; families with member experiencing developmental crisis; families with member living far from relatives; families with member with history of adoption; families with member with intimacy dysfunction; families with unemployed member; infertility treatment regimen

## Client Outcomes

### Client Will (Specify Time Frame)

- Identify communication strategies that family members can use to facilitate an improved sense of family identity
- Express feelings and share collective experiences
- Meet physical, psychosocial, and spiritual needs of members
- Support one another and family goals
- Work cooperatively to solve problems

## Nursing Interventions

- Provide family-centered care in all nursing settings to alleviate disturbed family identity.
- Include family assessment as part of comprehensive nursing assessment to guide appropriate interventions.
- Assess for clients' self-reports of family dysfunction, particularly noting any reports of abuse or self-injury.
- Apply theoretical models to understand family dynamics and communication patterns.
- Ascertain client's own meaning of family.
- Use established instruments to assess for family communication and functioning.
- ▲ Involve families, with client consent, in decision-making processes to facilitate family harmony.
- ▲ Consider novel family therapy interventions aimed at coping and reducing relational conflict during periods of extended isolation.
- ▲ Include early identification of family dysfunction in a comprehensive chronic pain treatment program.

### Pediatric

- Encourage families to maintain and develop family rituals and traditions.
- Encourage and support the family to have frequent and regular family meals.

### Geriatric

- Encourage intergenerational communication among family members.
- Incorporate family interventions for early-onset Alzheimer's disease.
- Conduct family life review with older adults as they transition to new environments to enhance family relations.
- ▲ Explore alternative means for family interaction if in-person visits are restricted or not feasible, to maintain connections.

• = Independent          ▲ = Collaborative

**Multicultural**

▲ Incorporate multicultural considerations into family therapy.

• Consider cultural factors in assessing family identity.

▲ Be aware of cultural considerations when using instruments to assess family functioning.

• Incorporate faith tenets, as relevant, to strengthen family dynamics.

• Encourage cultural rituals to enhance expression of family identity.

**Home Care**

▲ Refer clients with chronic pain and their families for occupational therapy (OT) interventions.

• Be sensitive about timing of a family coping intervention.

**Client/Family Teaching and Discharge Planning**

▲ Refer families experiencing substance use disorder for family counseling.

▲ Refer couples to relationship education that includes family social supports in its curriculum.

▲ Refer couples with infertility for specialist consultation.

# Risk for Disturbed Family Identity Syndrome

**Domain 7** Role relationship    **Class 2** Family relationships

## NANDA-I Definition

Susceptible to an inability to maintain an ongoing interactive, communicative process of creating and maintaining a shared collective sense of the meaning of the family, which may compromise family members' health

## Risk Factors

Ambivalent family relations; different coping styles among family members; disrupted family rituals; disrupted family roles; excessive stress; inadequate social support; ineffective coping strategies; ineffective family communication; perceived social discrimination; sexual dysfunction; unaddressed domestic violence; unrealistic expectations; values incongruent with cultural norm

## At-Risk Population

Blended families; economically disadvantaged families; families experiencing infertility; families with history of domestic violence; families with incarcerated member; families with member experiencing alteration in health status; families with member experiencing developmental crisis; families with member living far from relatives; families with member with history of adoption; families with member with intimacy dysfunction; families with unemployed member

• = Independent         ▲ = Collaborative

## Associated Conditions

Infertility treatment regimen

## Client Outcomes, Nursing Interventions, and Client/Family Teaching

Refer to care plan for Disturbed **Family** Identity Syndrome.

# Disturbed Personal Identity

**Domain 6** Self-perception   **Class 1** Self-concept

## NANDA-I Definition

Inability to maintain an integrated and complete perception of self.

## Defining Characteristics

Altered body image; confusion about cultural values; confusion about goals; confusion about ideological values; delusional description of self; expresses feeling of emptiness; expresses feeling of strangeness; fluctuating feelings about self; impaired ability to distinguish between internal and external stimuli; inadequate interpersonal relations; inadequate role performance; inconsistent behavior; ineffective coping strategies; reports social discrimination

## Related Factors

Altered social role; cult indoctrination; dysfunctional family processes; gender conflict; low self-esteem; perceived social discrimination; values incongruent with cultural norms

## At-Risk Population

Individuals experiencing developmental transition; individuals experiencing situational crisis; individuals exposed to toxic chemical

## Associated Conditions

Dissociative identity disorder; mental disorders; neurocognitive disorders; pharmaceutical preparations

## Client Outcomes

Client Will (Specify Time Frame)

- Demonstrate new purposes for life
- Show interests in surroundings
- Perform self-care and self-control activities appropriate for age
- Acknowledge personal strengths
- Engage in interpersonal relationships

## Nursing Interventions

- Assess and support family strengths of commitment, appreciation, and affection toward each other; positive communication; time together; a sense of spiritual well-being; and the ability to cope with stress and crisis.

• = Independent       ▲ = Collaborative

▲ Assess for suicidal ideation and make appropriate referral for clients dealing with mental illness or other risk factors.

▲ Assess clients with mood disorders and make appropriate referrals for treatment.

▲ Assess and make appropriate referrals for clients with physical or mental disabilities.

▲ Assess clients for substance misuse or addictive behaviors and make appropriate referrals.

• Use empathetic communication and encourage the client and family to verbalize fears, express emotions, and set goals.

• Be present for clients physically or by telephone.

• Encourage expression of positive thoughts and emotions.

• Encourage the client to use coping mechanisms.

• Help clients with serious and chronic conditions to maintain social support networks or assist in building new ones.

▲ Refer women facing diagnostic and curative breast cancer surgery for psychosocial support.

• Refer for cognitive behavioral therapy (CBT).

▲ Refer clients with borderline personality disorder (BPD) and dual-diagnosed BPD and substance misuse for dialectical behavior therapy (DBT) and psychoanalytical-orientated day-hospital therapy.

▲ Refer to the care plans for Readiness for Enhanced **Communication** and Readiness for Enhanced **Spiritual** Well-Being.

### Pediatric

• Encourage adolescents to promote positive self-esteem, to enhance coping, and to prevent behavioral and psychological problems.

▲ Evaluate and refer children and adolescents for eating disorder prevention programs that include medical care, nutritional intervention, and mental health treatment and care coordination.

• Use computer-mediated support groups to enhance identity formation.

### Geriatric

• Evaluate the effectiveness of nursing interventions used to promote positive self-identify in older adults.

• Encourage clients to discuss their "life histories." Life history–based interventions and self-esteem and life-satisfaction questionnaires may be used to reinforce personal identity and foster hope.

▲ Refer the older client to support groups.

▲ Refer the client with Alzheimer's disease who is terminally ill to hospice.

• = Independent      ▲ = Collaborative

**Multicultural**
- Assess an individual's sociocultural background in teaching self-management and self-regulation as a means of supporting hope and coping.
- Decrease discrimination to promote positive ethnic identity.
- Refer to care plan for Ineffective **Coping.**

**Home Care**
- The interventions described previously may be adapted for home care use.
- Provide an Internet-based health coach to encourage self-management for clients with chronic conditions such as depression, impaired mobility, and chronic pain. Use computer-mediated support groups to enhance identity formation.
- ▲ Refer the client to mutual health support groups. Participating in mutual health support groups led to enhanced coping by improving psychological and social functioning.
- ▲ Refer cancer clients and their spouses to family programs that include family-based interventions for communication, hope, coping, uncertainty, and symptom management.
- Refer combat veterans and service members directly involved in combat, as well as those providing support to combatants, including nurses, for mental health services.

**Client/Family Teaching and Discharge Planning**
- Teach the client about available community resources (e.g., therapists, ministers, counselors, self-help groups, family education groups).
- Teach coping skills to family caregivers of cancer clients.

# Risk for Disturbed Personal Identity

**Domain 6** Self-perception   **Class 1** Self-concept

## NANDA-I Definition

Susceptible to the inability to maintain an integrated and complete perception of self, which may compromise health.

## Risk Factors

Altered social role; cult indoctrination; dysfunctional family processes; gender conflict; low self-esteem; perceived social discrimination; values incongruent with cultural norms

## At-Risk Population

Individuals experiencing developmental transition; individuals experiencing situational crisis; individuals exposed to toxic chemicals

• = Independent          ▲ = Collaborative

## Associated Conditions

Dissociative identity disorder; mental disorders; neurocognitive disorders; pharmaceutical preparations

## Client Outcomes, Nursing Interventions, and Client/Family Teaching and Discharge Planning

Refer to care plan for Disturbed Personal **Identity**.

# Risk for Complicated Immigration Transition

**Domain 9** Coping/stress tolerance    **Class 1** Post-trauma responses

## NANDA-I Definition

Susceptible to experiencing negative feelings (loneliness, fear, anxiety) in response to unsatisfactory consequences and cultural barriers to one's immigration transition, which may compromise health.

## Related Factors

Abusive landlord; available work below educational preparation; communication barriers; cultural barriers; inadequate knowledge about accessing resources; inadequate social support; non-related persons within household; overcrowded housing; overt social discrimination; parent-child conflicts related to enculturation; unsanitary housing

## At-Risk Population

Individuals experiencing forced migration; individuals experiencing labor exploitation; individuals experiencing precarious economic situation; individuals exposed to hazardous work conditions with inadequate training; individuals living far from significant others; individuals with undocumented immigration status; individuals with unfulfilled expectations of immigration

## Client Outcomes

**Client Will (Specify Time Frame)**

- Participate in community activities
- State satisfaction with social relationships, living arrangements, and social integration
- State satisfaction with health status and access to health care
- Demonstrate actions that are congruent with expressed feelings and thoughts
- State sense of belonging
- Accept strengths and limitations of new environment

## Nursing Interventions

- Understand immigrants' perspectives/stories about their health maintenance and illness management.

• = Independent        ▲ = Collaborative

- Assess for use of acculturation strategies.
- Focus on providing holistic (physical, emotional, psychological, social, and spiritual) care while caring for immigrants. When appropriate, integrate the use of complementary and alternative approaches.
- Assess for intergenerational conflict and parental stress.
- Assist clients to identify coping strategies and sources of social support.
- Obtain a professional translator to enhance cross-cultural communication.
- Demonstrate cultural humility to achieve cultural competence to offer individualized discharge services to immigrant mothers with their preterm babies from the neonatal intensive care unit.
- Health care professionals need to identify risks and obstacles that migrant women transitioning to motherhood may be faced with, including poverty, language barriers, loneliness, and limited access to health care, which can contribute to mental health concerns such as stress, anxiety, depression, and social isolation.
- Nurses working with immigrant clients in psychiatric units need to (1) assess for posttraumatic stress syndrome and associated symptoms, (2) employ compassionate and trauma-informed care, (3) educate about early recognition of mental illness, (4) share information about psychiatric services, (5) use family-oriented and interpreter services often and as needed, and (6) create trusting relationship in the psychiatric community care.
- Actively engage in policy-driven solutions to mitigate structural racism. Such macrolevel factors shape the health of racial and ethnic minorities.
- Explore immigrant women's experience of menopause and self-management strategies for menopausal symptoms to be able to provide culturally relevant care and enhance their satisfaction with the specific care they received.

**Pediatric**

- Promote self-efficacy of the newly migrated adolescents by supporting their effort to learn and use the language of the migrated country.
- Assess for mental health consequences among youth from the ethnic and racial minorities of trauma experienced across the migration process (including before, during, and after migration) through the use of culturally sensitive diagnostic tools, and offer treatment services to facilitate a positive transition to healthy adulthood.
- Recognize and address the specific needs of both immigrant youths with disabilities transitioning to adulthood (e.g., autonomy) and their

• = Independent        ▲ = Collaborative

caregivers' needs (e.g., information about their youths' condition and of available health services).

**Home Care**
- Educate and encourage immigrants' family members to use available home care–specific support services as needed.

# Ineffective Impulse Control

**Domain 5** Perception/cognition   **Class 4** Cognition
## NANDA-I Definition
A pattern of performing rapid, unplanned reactions to internal or external stimuli without regard for the negative consequences of these reactions to the impulsive individual or to others.

## Defining Characteristics
Acting without thinking; asking personal questions despite discomfort of others; dangerous behavior; gambling addiction; impaired ability to regulate finances; inappropriate sharing of personal details; irritable mood; overly familiar with strangers; sensation seeking; sexual promiscuity; temper outbursts

## Related Factors
Hopelessness; mood disorder; neurobehavioral manifestations; smoking; substance misuse

## Associated Conditions
Altered development; developmental disabilities; neurocognitive disorders; personality disorders

## Client Outcomes
**Client Will (Specify Time Frame)**
- Be free from harm
- Cooperate with behavioral modification plan
- Verbalize adaptive ways to cope with stress by means other than impulsive behaviors
- Delay gratification and use adaptive coping strategies in response to stress
- Verbalize understanding that behavior is unacceptable
- Accept responsibility for own behavior

## Nursing Interventions
- Refer to mental health treatment for cognitive behavioral therapy (CBT).
- Assess individuals with impulsive behaviors for exposure to trauma and referral for mental health evaluation.

• = Independent        ▲ = Collaborative

- Implement motivational interviewing for clients with impulse control disorders.
- Teach client mindfulness meditation techniques. Mindfulness meditation includes observing experiences in the present moment, describing those experiences without judgments or evaluations, and participating fully in one's current context.
- Refer to self-help groups such as Gambler's Anonymous.
- Use a brief intervention model to screen and provide information and referral to services for clients that may experience at-risk gambling.
- Teach clients to use urge surfing techniques when impulses or urges are triggered.
- Teach client to use cue avoidance techniques to reduce impulsive behaviors.

**Pediatric**
- Assess children for environmental lead exposure.
- Refer to mental health treatment for CBT.
- Refer adolescent clients with impulsive symptoms at risk of self-harm to Dialectical Behavioral Therapy for Adolescents (DBT-A).

**Geriatric**
- Assess for impulsive symptoms and maintain increased surveillance of the client whenever the use of dopamine agonists has been initiated.
- Implement fall risk screening and precautions for geriatric clients with inattention and impulse control symptoms.
- Monitor caregivers for evidence of caregiver burden.

**Client/Family Teaching and Discharge Planning**
- Families should be encouraged to use practical measures to manage behavior such as limiting access to credit cards and restricting and monitoring Internet access gambling and casino websites, checking medication compliance, reporting behavior typical of impulse control disorders, and transferring control of financial affairs to a partner or other family members.

# Disability-Associated Urinary Incontinence

**Domain 3** Elimination and exchange    **Class 1** Urinary function

## NANDA-I Definition

Involuntary loss of urine not associated with any pathology or problem related to the urinary system.

• = Independent          ▲ = Collaborative

## Defining Characteristics

Adaptive behaviors to avoid others' recognition of urinary incontinence; mapping routes to public bathrooms prior to leaving home; time required to reach toilet is too long after sensation of urge; use of techniques to prevent urination; voiding prior to reaching toilet

## Related Factors

Avoidance of non-hygienic toilet use; caregiver inappropriately implements bladder training techniques; difficulty finding the bathroom; difficulty obtaining timely assistance to bathroom; embarrassment regarding toilet use in social situations; environmental constraints that interfere with continence; habitually suppresses urge to urinate; impaired physical mobility; impaired postural balance; inadequate motivation to maintain continence; increased fluid intake; neurobehavioral manifestations; pelvic floor disorders

## At-Risk Population

Children; older adults

## Associated Conditions

Heart diseases; impaired coordination; impaired hand dexterity; intellectual disability; neuromuscular diseases; osteoarticular diseases; pharmaceutical preparations; psychological disorder; vision disorders

## Client Outcomes

**Client Will (Specify Time Frame)**

- Eliminate or reduce incontinent episodes on a daily basis
- Eliminate or overcome environmental barriers to toileting on a daily basis
- Use adaptive equipment to reduce or eliminate incontinence related to impaired mobility or dexterity on a daily basis
- Use portable urinary collection devices or urine containment devices when access to the toilet is not feasible on a daily basis

## Nursing Interventions

- Introduce yourself to the client and anyone accompanying him or her and inform them of your role.
- Gain consent to provide care before proceeding further with the assessment. For clients unable to give consent, discuss permission with relevant health care professionals and/or family members.
- Wash hands using a recognized technique.
- Assess usual pattern of bladder management and establish the extent of the problem to include a detailed and accurate assessment of the client.
- Evaluate the client's bladder habits:
  - Episodes of incontinence during the day and night

• = Independent ▲ = Collaborative

○ Alleviating and aggravating factors
- Current management strategies include containing/collection devices, restriction of fluid intake, and avoidance of fluid/food groups that cause bladder irritation.
- Complete a Lifestyle and Risk Assessment that includes assessment of toilet access and ability to use, including the following:
  ○ Distance of the toilet from the bed, chair, and living quarters
  ○ Characteristics of the bed, including presence of side rails and distance of the bed from the floor
  ○ Characteristics of the pathway to the toilet, including barriers such as stairs, loose rugs on the floor, and inadequate lighting
  ○ Characteristics of the bathroom, including patterns of use, lighting, height of the toilet from the floor, the presence of handrails to assist transfers to the toilet, and breadth of the door and its accessibility for a wheelchair, walker, or other assistive devices
- Assess the client's physical and mental abilities:
  ○ Ability to rise from chair and bed, transfer to the toilet, and ambulate and the need for physical assistive devices such as a cane, walker, or wheelchair.
  ○ Ability to manipulate buttons, hooks, and zippers as needed to remove clothing.
  ○ Functional and cognitive status assessment should be done using a tool such as the Mini-Mental Status Examination for the older client with functional incontinence.
  ○ Daily fluid intake, including amount and types of fluids consumed.
  ○ Risk of falls caused by dizziness, impaired vision, and hearing.
  ○ Functional ability declines secondary to comorbidities (e.g., cerebrovascular incidents, amputation).
- Discuss quality-of-life issues relating to socialization and family events.
- Review the client's medical history:
  ○ Obstetrical/gynecological/urological history and surgeries
  ○ Relevant comorbidities such as cardiac, respiratory, renal, or neurological
  ○ Recurrent urinary tract infections
- Teach the client, the client's care providers, or the family to complete a bladder diary. Each 24-hour period should be subdivided into 1- to 2-hour periods and include number of urinations occurring in the toilet, actual episodes of incontinence and amount of urine leaked, reasons for episode of incontinence, type and amount of liquid intake, number of bowel movements, and incontinence pads or other products used.

• = Independent    ▲ = Collaborative

- Consult with the health care provider and complete a medication review relating to side effects and contraindications.
- Ensure that an appropriate, safe urinary receptacle such as a three-in-one commode, female or male handheld urinal, no-spill urinal, or containment device when toileting access is limited by immobility or environmental barriers is available to assist the client with elimination needs while other interventions are being implemented.
▲ Refer to occupational therapy for help in obtaining assistive devices and adapting the home for optimal toilet accessibility.
- Provide advice to clients relating to loose-fitting clothing with stretch waistbands rather than buttoned or zippered waist; minimize buttons, snaps, and multilayered clothing; and substitute a loop-and-pile closure or other easily loosened systems such as Velcro for buttons, hooks, and zippers in existing clothing.
- Work with the client on retraining the bladder by regularly timed toileting regimens (every 2 hours). For the older client in the home or a long-term care facility who has functional incontinence and dementia:
  - ○ Determine the frequency of current urination using an alarm system or check-and-change device.
  - ○ Record urinary elimination and incontinent patterns in a bladder log to use as a baseline for assessment and evaluation of treatment efficacy.
  - ○ Begin a prompted toileting program based on the results of this program; toileting frequency may vary from every 1.5 to 2 hours to every 4 hours.
  - ○ Provide positive reinforcement.
- Monitor older clients in a long-term care facility, acute care facility, or home for dehydration.
- Inspect the perineal and perianal skin for evidence of incontinence-associated dermatitis, including inflammation, vesicles in skin exposed to urinary leakage, and especially skinfolds or denudation of the skin, particularly when incontinence is managed by absorptive pads or containment briefs.
- Begin a preventive skin care regimen for all clients with urinary incontinence and treat clients with incontinence-associated dermatitis or related skin damage.
- Advise the client about the advantages of using disposable or reusable insert pads, pad-pant systems, or replacement briefs specifically designed for urinary incontinence as indicated for short-term/long-term use, including social events.

• = Independent        ▲ = Collaborative

- Consider the use of an indwelling catheter for continuous drainage in the client who is both homebound and bedbound and is receiving palliative or end-of-life care (requires a health care provider's order). At end of life, they may be the best choice.
- When an indwelling urinary catheter is in place, follow prescribed maintenance protocols for managing the catheter, taping and replacing the catheter, the drainage bag, and care of perineal skin and urethral meatus. Teach infection control measures adapted to the home care setting.
- Assist the client in adapting to the catheter. Encourage discussion of the client's response to the catheter. Research has consistently shown that indwelling catheter users need to be given more information, but some clients still feel poorly informed.
- Provide clients with comprehensive written information about the management of continence-related problems.
- Document all care and advice given in a factual and comprehensive manner.

## Mixed Urinary Incontinence

**Domain 3** Elimination and exchange    **Class 1** Urinary function

### NANDA-I Definition

Involuntary loss of urine in combination with or following a strong sensation or urgency to void, and also with activities that increase intra-abdominal pressure.

### Defining Characteristics

Expresses incomplete bladder emptying; involuntary loss of urine upon coughing; involuntary loss of urine upon effort; involuntary loss of urine upon laughing; involuntary loss of urine upon physical exertion; involuntary loss of urine upon sneezing; nocturia; urinary urgency

### Related Factors

Incompetence of the bladder neck; incompetence of the urethral sphincter; overweight; pelvic organ prolapse; skeletal muscular atrophy; smoking; weak anterior wall of the vagina

### At-Risk Population

Individuals with chronic cough; individuals with one type of urinary incontinence; multiparous women; older adults; women experiencing menopause; women giving birth vaginally

### Associated Conditions

Diabetes mellitus; estrogen deficiency; motor disorders; pelvic floor disorders; prolonged urinary incontinence; surgery for stress urinary incontinence; urethral sphincter injury

• = Independent          ▲ = Collaborative

## Client Outcomes

### Client Will (Specify Time Frame)

- Follow prescribed schedule for bladder emptying on a daily basis
- Have intact perineal skin on a daily basis
- Remain clear of symptomatic urinary tract infection on a daily basis
- Demonstrate how to apply containment device or insert intermittent catheter or be able to provide caregiver with instructions for performing these procedures as per individual needs on a daily basis

## Nursing Interventions

- Introduce yourself to the client and anyone accompanying him or her and inform them of your role.
- Gain consent to provide care before proceeding further with the assessment.
- Wash hands using a recognized technique.
- Assess the usual pattern of bladder management and establish the extent of the problem.
- Ask the client to complete a bladder diary/log to determine the pattern of urine elimination, any incontinence episodes, and current bladder management program. An electronic voiding diary may be kept whenever feasible.
- ▲ Consult with the health care provider concerning current bladder function and the potential of the bladder to produce hydronephrosis, vesicoureteral reflux, febrile urinary tract infection, or compromised renal function.
- ▲ Consult with the health care provider and physical therapist concerning the neuromuscular ability to perform bladder management. The type of neurological disorder, as well as the level of neurological impairment and the ability to use the hands effectively, determines the method of urine management in reflex incontinence.
- Inspect the perineal and perigenital skin for signs of incontinence-associated dermatitis and pressure ulcers (Beeckman, 2017).
- ▲ In consultation with the rehabilitation team, counsel the client and family concerning the merits and potential risks associated with each possible bladder management program, including spontaneous voiding, intermittent self-catheterization (ISC), and reflex voiding with condom catheter containment and in some cases, indwelling suprapubic catheterization.
- Ensure the client is aware of when and how to report any problems and/or complications of reflex incontinence care when at home.
- Provide clients with comprehensive written information about the management of continence-related problems.

• = Independent          ▲ = Collaborative

- Assist the family with arranging care in a way that allows the client to participate in family or favorite activities without embarrassment. Elicit discussion of the client's concerns about the social or emotional burden of incontinence.
- Teach the client to ensure good hydration.
- Teach the client with a spinal injury the signs of autonomic dysreflexia, its relationship to bladder fullness, and management of the condition. Refer to the care plan for **Autonomic Dysreflexia.**

**Intermittent Self-Catheterization**

- Begin intermittent catheterization as ordered using sterile technique; the client may be taught to use clean technique in the home situation.
- Adopt a person-centered ISC approach to motivate and schedule the frequency of intermittent catheterization based on the frequency/volume records of previous catheterizations, functional bladder capacity, and the impact of catheterization on the quality of the client's life.
- Teach the client to recognize signs of symptomatic urinary tract infection and to seek care promptly when these signs occur. The signs of symptomatic infection include the following:
  ○ Discomfort over the bladder or during urination
  ○ Acute onset of urinary incontinence
  ○ Fever
  ○ Markedly increased spasticity of muscles below the level of the spinal lesion
  ○ Malaise, lethargy
  ○ Hematuria
  ○ Autonomic dysreflexia (hyperreflexia) symptoms
- Recognize that intermittent catheterization is typically associated with asymptomatic bacteriuria, and the indwelling catheter is routinely associated with asymptomatic colonization.
- Teach intermittent catheterization as the client approaches discharge as per operational guidelines and best practices. Instruct the client and at least one family member in the performance of catheterization. Teach the client with quadriplegia how to instruct others to perform this procedure.
- Clients using ISC may experience bladder spasms that hinder the insertion process.

**Condom Catheter/Sheath System**

- For a male client with reflex incontinence who does not have urinary retention and cannot manage the condition effectively with spontaneous voiding, who does not choose to perform intermittent catheterization, or who cannot perform catheterization, teach the client and his family to obtain, select, and apply an external collective device and urinary drainage system. Assist the client and family to choose a product that adheres to the glans penis or penile shaft without allowing seepage of urine onto surrounding skin or clothing, which avoids provoking hypersensitivity reactions on the skin, and that includes a urinary drainage reservoir that is easily concealed under the clothing and does not cause irritation to the skin of the thigh.

• Teach the client whose incontinence is managed by a condom catheter to routinely inspect the skin with each catheter change for evidence of lesions caused by pressure from the containment device or by exposure to urine, to cleanse the penis thoroughly, and to reapply a new device daily or every other day.

• Document all care and advice given in a factual and comprehensive manner.

# Stress Urinary Incontinence

**Domain 3** Elimination and exchange    **Class 1** Urinary function

## NANDA-I Definition

Involuntary loss of urine with activities that increase intra-abdominal pressure, which is not associated with urgency to void.

## Defining Characteristics

Involuntary loss of urine in the absence of detrusor contraction; involuntary loss of urine the absence of overdistended bladder; involuntary loss of urine upon coughing; involuntary loss of urine upon effort; involuntary loss of urine upon laughing; involuntary loss of urine upon physical exertion; involuntary loss of urine upon sneezing

## Related Factors

Overweight; pelvic floor disorders; pelvic organ prolapse

## At-Risk Population

Individuals who perform high-intensity physical exercise; multiparous women; pregnant women; women experiencing menopause; women giving birth vaginally

## Associated Conditions

Damaged pelvic floor muscles; degenerative changes in pelvic floor muscles; intrinsic urethral sphincter deficiency; nervous system diseases; prostatectomy; urethral sphincter injury

• = Independent        ▲ = Collaborative

## Client Outcomes
Client Will (Specify Time Frame)
- Report no stress incontinence episodes and/or a decrease in the severity of urine loss over a 24-hour period
- Experience no episodes of urinary incontinence as recorded on voiding diary (bladder log) over a 24-hour period
- Identify containment devices that assist in management of stress incontinence over a 24-hour period

## Nursing Interventions
- Introduce yourself to the client and anyone accompanying him or her and inform them of your role.
- Gain consent to provide care before proceeding further with the assessment. In clients unable to give consent, discuss permission with relevant health care professionals and/or family members.
- Wash hands using a recognized technique.
- Assess usual pattern of bladder management to understand the extent of the problem and establish pattern of bladder management. Explore factors provoking urine loss (diuretics, bladder irritants, alcohol), focusing on the differential diagnosis of stress, urge or mixed stress, and urge urinary symptoms. Consider using a symptom questionnaire that elicits relevant lower urinary tract symptoms and provides differentiation between stress and urge incontinence symptoms.
- Review the client's medical history to identify possible risk factors for stress incontinence (i.e., pregnancy, parity, large babies, forceps or breech deliveries, obesity, chronic cough, physical activity, previous urinary tract or gynecological surgery, smoking history).
- Review the client's medication list (e.g., diuretics, lithium, adrenergic blockers, diabetes medications) to see what may exacerbate the client's urinary urgency.
- Review the client's bladder habits:
  - Onset and duration of urinary leakage
  - Related lower urinary tract symptoms, including voiding frequency (day/night) and urgency, severity (small, moderate, large amounts) of urinary leakage
- Assess for mixed urinary incontinence (a combination of stress and urge incontinence) by asking the client:
  - Can you delay urination for a 2-hour movie or car ride?
  - How often do you wake/arise at night to urinate?
  - When you have the urge to urinate, can you reach the toilet without leaking?

• = Independent      ▲ = Collaborative

- Complete a lifestyle assessment to understand the effect of stress urinary incontinence on an individual's lifestyle. Inquire about incontinence pad use and change in daily, social, or recreational activities, as well as emotional impact.
- Inspect the perineal skin for evidence of incontinence-associated dermatitis, including inflammation, vesicles in skin exposed to urinary leakage, and especially skinfolds or denudation of the skin, particularly when incontinence is managed by absorptive pads or containment briefs.
▲ Refer client for specific testing to confirm incontinence etiology and diagnosis. If trained to do so, perform the cough stress test and request a 24-hour pad test (if appropriate) and urodynamic studies (including urine speed and flow, postvoid residual measurement, leak point pressure, and pressure flow study).
- Establish with the client the current use of containment devices, for example, a well-fitted sheath; evaluate the devices for their ability to adequately contain urine loss, protect clothing, and control odor. Assist the client in identifying containment devices specifically designed to contain urinary leakage and not to use sanitary pads.
- Teach the client to complete a bladder diary by recording voiding frequency, the frequency and degree of urinary incontinence episodes, association with urgency (a sudden and strong desire to urinate that is difficult to defer), fluid intake, and pad usage over a 3- to 7-day period. An electronic voiding diary may be kept whenever feasible.
▲ With the client and in close consultation with the health care provider, review treatment options, including behavioral management; drug therapy; use of a pessary, vaginal device, or urethral insert; and surgery. Outline the potential benefits, efficacy, and side effects of each treatment option.
- Teach the client how to carry out pelvic floor muscle training. Teach the client to identify, contract, and relax the pelvic floor muscles without contracting distal muscle groups (e.g., abdominal muscles or gluteus muscles) using verbal feedback based on vaginal or anal palpation, biofeedback, or electrical stimulation and the assistance of an incontinence specialist or health care provider as necessary.
- Incorporate principles of exercise physiology into a pelvic muscle training program using the following strategies:
  ○ Begin a graded exercise program, usually starting with 5 to 10 repetitions and advancing gradually to no more than 35 to 50 repetitions every day or every other day based on baseline and ongoing evaluation of maximal strength and endurance.

• = Independent ▲ = Collaborative

- ○ Continue exercise sessions over a period of 3 to 6 months.
- ○ Integrate muscle training into activities of daily living.
- ○ Assess progress every 2 weeks during the first month and every 4 to 6 weeks thereafter.
- Work with the client on retraining the bladder by regularly timed toileting regimens (every 2 hours). For the older client in the home or a long-term care facility who has functional incontinence and dementia:
  - ○ Determine the frequency of current urination using an alarm system or check-and-change device.
  - ○ Record urinary elimination and incontinent patterns in a bladder log to use as a baseline for assessment and evaluation of treatment efficacy.
  - ○ Begin a prompted toileting program based on the results of this program; toileting frequency may vary from every 1.5 to 2 hours to every 4 hours.
  - ○ Provide positive reinforcement.
- ▲ Teach the client to self-administer duloxetine as ordered by the consulting health care provider and to monitor for adverse side effects.
- ▲ Teach the client to self-administer topical (vaginal) estrogens as directed and to monitor for adverse side effects.
- Refer the female client with stress urinary incontinence and pelvic organ prolapse who wishes to use a pessary to manage stress incontinence to a nurse specialist or gynecologist with expertise in the placement and maintenance of these devices.
- Discuss potentially reversible or controllable risk factors, such as weight loss, with the client with stress incontinence, and assist the client to formulate a strategy to eliminate these conditions.
- Refer the client with persistent stress incontinence to a continence service, health care provider, or nurse who specializes in the management of this condition.
- Teach the client to ensure good hydration.
- Provide client with comprehensive written information about bladder care and how to access relevant support resources (e.g., national associations).
- Encourage a program of self-care management.
- Assist the family with arranging care in a way that allows the client to participate in family or favorite activities without embarrassment. Elicit discussion of the client's concerns about the social or emotional burden of incontinence.

• = Independent          ▲ = Collaborative

- Document all care and advice given in a factual and comprehensive manner.
- Refer to the Disability-Associated Urinary **Incontinence** care plan.

# Urge Urinary Incontinence

**Domain 3** Elimination and exchange   **Class 1** Urinary function

## NANDA-I Definition

Involuntary loss of urine in combination with or following a strong sensation or urgency to void.

## Defining Characteristics

Decreased bladder capacity; feeling of urgency with triggered stimulus; increased urinary frequency; involuntary loss of urine before reaching toilet; involuntary loss of urine with bladder contractions; involuntary loss of urine with bladder spasms; involuntary loss of varying volumes of urine between voids, with urgency; nocturia

## Related Factors

Alcohol consumption; anxiety; caffeine consumption; carbonated beverage consumption; fecal impaction; ineffective toileting habits; involuntary sphincter relaxation; overweight; pelvic floor disorders; pelvic organ prolapse

## At-Risk Population

Individuals exposed to abuse; individuals with history of urinary urgency during childhood; older adults; women; women experiencing menopause

## Associated Conditions

Atrophic vaginitis; bladder outlet obstruction; depression; diabetes mellitus; nervous system diseases; nervous system trauma; overactive pelvic floor; pharmaceutical preparations; treatment regimen; urologic diseases

## Client Outcomes

**Client Will (Specify Time Frame)**

- Report relief from urge urinary incontinence or a decrease in the frequency of incontinent episodes on a daily basis
- Identify containment devices that assist in the management of urge urinary incontinence on a daily basis

## Nursing Interventions

- Introduce yourself to the client and anyone accompanying him or her and inform them of your role.
- Gain consent to perform care before proceeding further with the assessment.
- Wash hands using a recognized technique.

• = Independent          ▲ = Collaborative

- Assess the usual pattern of bladder management and establish the pattern of bladder management and extent of the problem.
- Assess bladder habits and quality-of-life issues:
  - Diurnal frequency (voiding more than once every 2 hours while awake)
  - Urgency, daytime frequency, and nocturia
  - Involuntary leakage and leakage accompanied by or preceded by urgency
  - Amount of urine loss, moderate or large volume
  - Severity of symptoms
  - Alleviating and aggravating factors
  - Effect on quality of life
- Ask specific questions relating to urge presentation:
  - Can you delay urination for a 2-hour movie or car ride?
  - How often do you wake at night to urinate?
  - When you have the urge to urinate, can you reach the toilet without leaking?
- Assess the severity of incontinence and the effect on the individual's lifestyle; inquire about incontinence pad use and change in daily, social, or recreational activities, and emotional impact.
- ▲ Perform a focused physical assessment, in close consultation with a health care practitioner or advanced practice nurse, including the following:
  - Bladder palpation after voiding to check for retention
  - Bladder scanning for postvoid residual
  - Inspection of the perineal skin
  - Vaginal examination to determine hypoestrogenic changes in the mucosa (may contribute to urge incontinence)
  - Pelvic examination to determine the presence, location, and severity of vaginal wall prolapse, and reproduction of stress urinary incontinence with the cough test
- Anal tone and constipation should be assessed.
- Inspect the perineal and perianal skin for evidence of incontinence-associated dermatitis, including inflammation, vesicles in skin exposed to urinary leakage, and especially skinfolds or denudation of the skin, particularly when incontinence is managed by absorptive pads or containment briefs.
- Teach the client to complete a bladder diary by recording voiding frequency, the frequency and degree of urinary incontinence episodes, their association with urgency (a sudden and strong desire to urinate that is difficult to defer), fluid intake, and pad usage over a 3- to 7-day period. An electronic voiding diary may be kept whenever

feasible. In addition to these parameters, the client may be asked to record voided volume and fluid intake.

- Review all medications the client is receiving, paying particular attention to sedatives, opioid analgesics, diuretics, antidepressants, psychotropic drugs, and cholinergics. Consult the health care practitioner or nurse practitioner about altering or eliminating these medications if they are suspected of affecting incontinence.
- Assess the client for urinary retention (see the care plan for **Urinary Retention**).
- Assess the client for functional limitations (environmental barriers, limited mobility or dexterity, and impaired cognitive function).
- Consult the health care practitioner concerning diabetic management or pharmacotherapy for urinary tract infection when indicated. In specific cases, urgency and an increased risk of urge incontinence may be related to bacteriuria or urinary tract infection.
- ▲ Assess for signs and symptoms of atrophic vaginal changes in the perimenopausal or postmenopausal woman, including vaginal dryness, tenderness to touch, mucosal dryness, friability, and discomfort with gentle palpation. Specifically query the woman with atrophic vaginitis concerning associated lower urinary tract symptoms (usually voiding frequency, urgency, and dysuria). Refer the woman with atrophic vaginal changes and bothersome lower urinary tract symptoms to a gynecologist, urologist, or women's health nurse practitioner for further evaluation and management.

**Pelvic Floor Training Program**

- Teach the client how to carry out pelvic floor muscle training. Teach the client to identify, contract, and relax the pelvic floor muscles without contracting distal muscle groups (e.g., abdominal muscles or gluteus muscles) using verbal feedback based on vaginal or anal palpation, biofeedback, or electrical stimulation and the assistance of an incontinence specialist or health care provider as necessary.
- Incorporate principles of exercise physiology into a pelvic muscle training program using the following strategies:
  - Begin a graded exercise program, usually starting with 5 to 10 repetitions and advancing gradually to no more than 35 to 50 repetitions every day or every other day based on baseline and ongoing evaluation of maximal strength and endurance.
  - Continue exercise sessions over a period of 3 to 6 months.
  - Integrate muscle training into activities of daily living.
  - Assess progress every 2 weeks during the first month and every 4 to 6 weeks thereafter.

• = Independent          ▲ = Collaborative

**Bladder Training Program**

- Assist the client in completing a voiding diary over a period of a minimum of 3 days or up to 7 days.
- Review the results with the client, determining typical voiding frequency and establishing goals for voiding frequency based on the longest time interval between voids that is comfortable for the client.
- Using baseline voiding frequency, as determined by the diary, teach the client to void first thing in the morning, every time the predetermined voiding interval passes, and before going to bed at night.
- Encourage adherence to the program with timing devices and verbal encouragement and support, and address individual reasons for schedule interruption.
- Teach distraction and urge suppression techniques (see later discussion) to control urgency while the client postpones urination.
- Gradually increase the time between urinations to the negotiated goal. Time intervals between voiding are typically increased in increments of 15 to 30 minutes for clients with a baseline frequency of less than every 60 minutes and increments of 25 to 30 minutes for clients with a baseline frequency of more than every 60 minutes. The voiding interval should be increased by 15 to 30 minutes each week (based on the client's tolerance) until a voiding interval of 3 to 4 hours is achieved. Use a bladder diary to monitor progress.
- Review with the client the types of beverages consumed, focusing on the intake of caffeine, which is associated with a transient effect on lower urinary tract symptoms. Advise all clients to reduce or eliminate intake of caffeinated beverages or over-the-counter medications of dietary aids containing caffeine. Identify and counsel the client to eliminate other bladder irritants that may exacerbate incontinence, such as smoking, carbonated beverages, citrus, sugar substitutes, and tomato products.
- Teach the client to ensure good hydration.
- Teach the client methods to avoid constipation such as increasing dietary fiber, moderately increasing fluid intake, exercising, and establishing a routine defecation schedule.

**Urge Suppression**

- Urge suppression skills are essential in helping clients learn a new way of responding to the sense of urgency.
- Teach the client the following techniques:
  - ○ When a strong or precipitous urge to urinate is perceived, teach the client to avoid running to the toilet.

• = Independent      ▲ = Collaborative

- ○ Pause, sit down, and relax the entire body.
- ○ Perform repeated, rapid pelvic muscle contractions until the urge is relieved.
- ○ Use distraction: count backward from 100 by sevens; recite a poem; write a letter; balance a checkbook; do handwork such as knitting; and take five deep breaths, focusing on breathing.
- ○ Relief is followed by micturition within 5 to 15 minutes, using nonhurried movements when locating a toilet and voiding.
- ○ Use urge suppression strategies on waking during the night. If the urge subsides, the client should be encouraged to go back to sleep. If after a minute or two the urge does not subside, clients should be instructed to get up to void to avoid sleep interruption.
- Teach the client to self-administer antimuscarinic (anticholinergic) drugs as directed. Teach dosage side effects and administration of the medication and the importance of combining pharmacotherapy with scheduled voiding, adequate fluid intake, restriction of bladder irritants, and urge suppression techniques.
- Assist the client in selecting, obtaining, and applying a containment device for urine loss as indicated.
- Provide client with comprehensive written information about bladder care and how to access relevant support resources (e.g., national associations).
- Assess the functional and cognitive status of all clients with urge incontinence; use interventions to improve mobility.
- Refer client for occupational therapy for help in obtaining assistive devices and adapting the home for optimal toilet accessibility.
- Encourage the client to develop an action plan for self-care management of incontinence. Making an action plan facilitates behavior change.
- Document all care and advice given in a factual and comprehensive manner.
- Refer to Disability-Associated Urinary **Incontinence** care plan.

# Risk for Urge Urinary Incontinence

**Domain 3** Elimination and exchange     **Class 1** Urinary function
**NANDA-I Definition**

Susceptible to involuntary passage of urine occurring soon after a strong sensation or urgency to void, which may compromise health.

• = Independent          ▲ = Collaborative

**Risk Factors**

Alcohol consumption; anxiety; caffeine consumption; carbonated beverage consumption; fecal impaction; ineffective toileting habits; involuntary sphincter relaxation; overweight; pelvic floor disorders; pelvic organ prolapse

**At-Risk Population**

Individuals exposed to abuse; individuals with history of urinary urgency during childhood; older adults; women; women experiencing menopause

**Associated Conditions**

Atrophic vaginitis; bladder outlet obstruction; depression; diabetes mellitus; nervous system diseases; nervous system trauma; overactive pelvic floor; pharmaceutical preparations; treatment regimen; urologic disease

**Client Outcomes, Nursing Interventions, and Client/Family Teaching and Discharge Planning**

Refer to care plan for Urge Urinary **Incontinence**.

# Disorganized Infant Behavior

**Domain 9** Coping/stress tolerance    **Class 3** Neurobehavioral stress

**NANDA-I Definition**

Disintegration of the physiological and neurobehavioral systems of functioning.

**Defining Characteristics**

**Attention-Interaction System**

Impaired response to sensory stimuli

**Motor System**

Altered primitive reflexes; exaggerated startle response; fidgeting; finger splaying; fisting; hands to face behavior; hyperextension of extremities; impaired motor tone; maintains hands to face position; tremor; twitching; uncoordinated movement

**Physiological**

Abnormal skin color; arrhythmia; bradycardia; inability to tolerate rate of feedings; inability to tolerate volume of feedings; oxygen desaturation; tachycardia; time-out signals

**Regulatory Problems**

Impaired ability to inhibit startle reflex; irritable mood

**State-Organization System**

Active-awake state; diffuse alpha electroencephalogram (EEG) activity with eyes closed; irritable crying; quiet-awake state; state oscillation

• = Independent    ▲ = Collaborative

## Related Factors

Caregiver misreading infant cues; environmental overstimulation; feeding intolerance; inadequate caregiver knowledge of behavioral cues; inadequate containment within environment; inadequate physical environment; insufficient environmental sensory stimulation; malnutrition; pain; sensory deprivation; sensory overstimulation

## At-Risk Population

Infants exposed to teratogen in utero; infants with low postmenstrual age; premature infants

## Associated Conditions

Congenital disorders; immature neurological functioning; impaired infant motor functioning; inborn genetic diseases; invasive procedure; oral impairment

## Client Outcomes

### Client Will (Specify Time Frame)

**Infant/Child**

- Display physiological/autonomic stability: cardiopulmonary, digestive functioning
- Display signs of organized motor system
- Display signs of organized state system: ability to achieve and maintain a state and transition smoothly between states
- Demonstrate progress toward effective self-regulation
- Demonstrate progress toward or ability to maintain calm attention
- Demonstrate progress or ability to engage in positive interactions
- Demonstrate ability to respond to sensory information (visual, auditory, tactile) in an adaptive way

**Parent/Significant Other**

- Recognize infant/child behaviors as a complex communication system that expresses specific needs and wants (e.g., hunger, pain, stress, desire to engage or disengage)
- Educate parents/caregivers to recognize infant's avenues of neurobehavioral communication: autonomic/physiological, motor, state, attention/interaction
- Recognize how infants respond to environmental sensory input through stress/avoidance and approach/engagement behaviors
- Recognize and support infant's self-regulatory, coping behaviors used to regain or maintain homeostasis
- Teach parents to "tune in" to their own interactive style and how that affects their infant's behavior
- Teach parents ways to adapt their interactive style in response to infant's style of communication appropriate for developmental stage and gestational age

• = Independent          ▲ = Collaborative

- Identify appropriate positioning and handling techniques that will enhance normal motor development
- Promote infant/child's attention capabilities that support visual and auditory development
- Engage parents in pleasurable parent–infant interactions that encourage bonding and attachment
- Structure and modify the environment in response to infant/child's behavior and personal needs; personalize their bed space
- Identify available community resources that provide early intervention services, emotional support, community health nursing, and parenting classes
- Communicate the infant's medical, nursing, and developmental needs to the family in a culturally sensitive and appropriate way that is understandable

## Nursing Interventions

- Sensitive nursing care must be implemented at the infant's admission to the neonatal intensive care unit (NICU), continued during the stay, and continued past discharge as the family adjusts to transitioning home and into the community.
- Assess the neurobehavior systems through which infants communicate organized and/or disorganized stress behaviors within the subsystems of functioning (i.e., physiological/autonomic, motor, states, attention/interactional, self-regulatory).
- Recognize and educate parents to recognize the behavior cues infants use to communicate stress/avoidance and approach/engagement.
- Provide high-quality individualized developmental care for low-birth-weight preterm infants in a family-centered care environment that promotes normal neurological, physical, and emotional developmental and prevents disabilities.
- Identify and manage pain using appropriate pain management techniques during invasive procedures (e.g., tube insertion, heel sticks, intravenous lines).
- Provide care that supports development state organization, such as the ability to achieve and maintain quiet sleep and awake states and transition smoothly between states.
- Encourage parents to speak slowly and/or sing to their babies during visits.
- Provide infants several opportunities for nonnutritive sucking (NNS).
- Provide parents opportunities to experience physical closeness through loving touch, massage, cuddling, and skin-to-skin contact (kangaroo care), which enhances parent–infant attachment.

• = Independent          ▲ = Collaborative

- Teach parents to use calming interventions that mimic the sensory environment in the womb such as swaddling, side position, sound (white noise), swinging, and sucking (5 S's).
- Encourage parental engagement and early interactions in the NICU to set the foundation for parent–infant attachment and social relationships.
- Support effective and pleasurable feeding practices, such as breast, bottle, or combination, as essential for healthy nutrition/calories, for mother–baby bonding and attachment, and for setting the foundation for successful feeding/eating patterns.
- Provide infants with positive sensory experiences (e.g., visual, auditory, tactile, olfactory, vestibular, proprioceptive) to enhance development of sensory pathways and avoid overstimulation of sensory systems.
- Incorporate parents as coparticipants of infant care by communicating daily progress of their infant's condition.
- Provide social support to parents including all members of the family.

**Multicultural**
- Identify cultural beliefs, norms, and values of family's perceptions of infant/child behavior.
- Recognize and support positive mother–infant interactive behaviors and be sensitive to cultural and ethnic backgrounds.

**Client/Family Teaching and Discharge Planning**
- Perform a family assessment to understand the family's specific needs and circumstances.
- Assess for any sociodemographic risks within the family.
- Educate parents on safe "back-to-sleep" practice before NICU discharge.
- ▲ Provide information or refer to community-based follow-up programs for preterm/at-risk infants and their families.
- ▲ Refer and support transition to early intervention services on discharge.

**Home Care**
- Assess for domestic violence risks in the home environment.
- Listening to fears, answering questions, and giving time to practice new skills before discharge may increase parents' confidence for NICU discharge.
- Encourage parents to use home visitation whenever possible because it enhances neonatal progress and parental support.
- Encourage families to teach extended family and support persons to recognize and respond appropriately to the infant's behavioral cues; supportive help may be most appreciated doing physical tasks.

• = Independent          ▲ = Collaborative

- Provide education on positioning and handling that supports optimal infant growth and development.
- Suggest babywearing. Babywearing holds babies in a kangaroo position to support caregivers and promote positive health outcomes after NICU discharge.
- Encourage home visitors to recognize maternal depression resulting from the NICU or new parent experiences.
- Provide families with information about community resources, developmental follow-up services, and parent-to-parent support programs, and request primary health care providers to follow developmental progress with parent-friendly developmental questionnaires.

# Readiness for Enhanced Organized Infant Behavior

**Domain 9** Coping/stress tolerance    **Class 3** Neurobehavioral stress
## NANDA-I Definition
An integrated pattern of modulation of the physiological and neurobehavioral systems of functioning, which can be strengthened.
## Defining Characteristics
Primary caregiver expresses desire to enhance cue recognition; primary caregiver expresses desire to enhance environmental conditions; primary caregiver expresses desire to enhance recognition of infant's self-regulatory behaviors
## Client Outcomes, Nursing Interventions, and Client/Family Teaching and Discharge Planning
Refer to care plans for Disorganized **Infant** Behavior and Risk for Disorganized **Infant** Behavior.

# Risk for Disorganized Infant Behavior

**Domain 9** Coping/stress tolerance    **Class 3** Neurobehavioral stress
## NANDA-I Definition
Susceptible to disintegration in the pattern of modulation of the physiological and neurobehavioral systems of functioning, which may compromise health.
## Risk Factors
Caregiver misreading infant cues; environmental overstimulation; feeding intolerance; inadequate caregiver knowledge of behavioral cues; inadequate containment within environment; inadequate physical environment;

• = Independent        ▲ = Collaborative

insufficient environmental sensory stimulation; malnutrition; pain; sensory deprivation; sensory overstimulation

## At-Risk Population

Infants exposed to teratogen in utero; infants with low postmenstrual age; premature infants

## Associated Conditions

Congenital disorders; immature neurological functioning; impaired infant motor functioning; inborn genetic diseases; invasive procedure; oral impairment

## Client Outcomes, Nursing Interventions, and Client/Family Teaching and Discharge Planning

Refer to Disorganized **Infant** Behavior.

# Risk for Infection

**Domain 11** Safety/protection    **Class 1** Infection

## NANDA-I Definition

Susceptible to invasion and multiplication of pathogenic organisms, which may compromise health.

## Risk Factors

Difficulty managing long-term invasive devices; difficulty managing wound care; dysfunctional gastrointestinal motility; exclusive formula feeding; impaired skin integrity; inadequate access to individual protective equipment; inadequate adherence to public health recommendations; inadequate environmental hygiene; inadequate health literacy; inadequate hygiene; inadequate knowledge to avoid exposure to pathogens; inadequate oral hygiene habits; inadequate vaccination; malnutrition; mixed breastfeeding; obesity; smoking; stasis of body fluid

## At-Risk Population

Economically disadvantaged individuals; individuals exposed to disease outbreak; individuals exposed to increased environmental pathogens; individuals with low level of education; infants who are not breastfed

## Associated Conditions

Altered pH of secretion; anemia; chronic illness; decrease in ciliary action; immunosuppression; invasive procedure; leukopenia; premature rupture of amniotic membrane; prolonged rupture of amniotic membrane; suppressed inflammatory response

## Client Outcomes

### Client Will (Specify Time Frame)

• Remain free from symptoms of infection during contact with health care providers

• = Independent    ▲ = Collaborative

- State symptoms of infection before initiating a health care–related procedure
- Demonstrate appropriate care of infection-prone sites within 48 hours of instruction
- Maintain white blood cell count and differential within normal limits within 48 hours of treatment initiation
- Demonstrate appropriate hygienic measures such as handwashing, oral care, and perineal care within 24 hours of instruction

## Nursing Interventions

- Maintain open communication with the infection prevention (IP) department. Inquire about facility-specific targeted multidrug-resistant organism (MDRO) surveillance. Learn which MDROs are of significant importance at your facility. Acquire a basic understanding of antibiotic stewardship through collaboration with IP and pharmacy.
- Obtain a travel history and history of any overnight stay in a hospital in a foreign country from clients presenting to the health care site (e.g., emergency department, clinic).
- Antimicrobial resistance and health care–associated infections (HAIs) are global health problems that increase social and economic burden and are associated with higher mortality and increased hospital stays. Inappropriate antimicrobial use is estimated to be at 20% to 50% and is believed to be a key contributor to antimicrobial resistance. The Centers for Disease Control and Prevention (CDC) and the American Nurses Association (ANA) identify staff nurses as critical players in antibiotic stewardship (AS) work. Nurses play a key role in ensuring client safety and quality (Olans et al, 2017; Jeffs et al, 2018; CDC, 2019c; Monsees et al, 2020).
- Sepsis is the body's overwhelming and life-threatening response to infection that can lead to tissue damage, organ failure, and death. Sepsis and septic shock are leading causes of death worldwide. Early identification and aggressive treatment are integral to sepsis survival. Nurses play a significant role in early identification of sepsis. Monitor vital signs and mental status.
- Assess temperature of neutropenic clients; report a single temperature of greater than 38°C (100.5°F).
- Oral, rectal, tympanic, temporal artery, or axillary thermometers may be used to assess temperature in adults and infants.
- ▲ Note and report laboratory values (e.g., white blood cell count and differential, serum protein, serum albumin, cultures).

• = Independent          ▲ = Collaborative

- Assess skin for color, moisture, texture, and turgor (elasticity). Keep accurate, ongoing documentation of changes.
- Carefully wash and pat dry skin, including skinfold areas. Use hydration and moisturization on all at-risk surfaces.
▲ Monitor client's vitamin D level.
- Use strategies to prevent health care–acquired pneumonia: implement an evidence-based pneumonia prevention bundle, aggressive mobilization, assess client risk for aspiration and request swallow evaluation as necessary, position client in an upright position for all meals, and provide aggressive oral care at least twice per day (Tablan et al, 2004; Gupta et al, 2019; Naik et al, 2019). Implementation of an evidence-based ventilator-associated pneumonia (VAP) bundle should be followed. Management of ventilated clients should include avoidance of benzodiazepines to manage agitation, daily interruption of sedation (sedation vacation), daily assessment of readiness to extubate (spontaneous breathing trials), use of endotracheal (ET) tubes that accommodate subglottic suctioning, and maintaining head of bed (HOB) at 30 to 45 degrees (Tablan et al, 2004; Klompas et al, 2014).
- Encourage fluid intake.
- Use appropriate hand hygiene (i.e., handwashing or use of alcohol-based hand rubs).
- When using an alcohol-based hand rub, apply an ample amount of product to the palm of one hand and rub hands together, covering all surfaces of hands and fingers, until hands are dry. Note that the volume needed to reduce the number of bacteria on hands varies by product.
- Follow standard precautions and wear gloves during any contact with blood, mucous membranes, nonintact skin, or any body substance except sweat. Use goggles and gowns when appropriate. Standard precautions apply to all clients. You must assume all clients are carrying blood-borne pathogens (Siegel et al, 2007).
- Implement respiratory hygiene/cough etiquette.
- Follow transmission-based precautions for airborne-, droplet-, and contact-transmitted microorganisms:
  ○ **Airborne:** Isolate the client in a room with monitored negative air pressure, with the room door closed and the client remaining in the room. Always wear appropriate respiratory protection when you enter the room. Limit the movement and transport of the client from the room to essential purposes only. Have the client wear a surgical mask during transport.

• = Independent          ▲ = Collaborative

○ **Droplet:** Keep the client in a private room, if possible. If not possible, maintain a spatial separation of 3 feet from other beds or visitors. The door may remain open. Wear a surgical mask when you must come within 3 feet of the client. Some hospitals may choose to implement a mask requirement for droplet precautions for anyone entering the room. Limit transport to essential purposes and have the client wear a mask, if possible.

○ **Contact:** Place the client in a private room, if possible, or with someone (cohorting) who has an active infection from the same microorganism. Wear clean, nonsterile gloves when entering the room. When providing care, change gloves after contact with any infective material such as wound drainage. Remove the gloves and clean your hands before leaving the room and take care not to touch any potentially infectious items or surfaces on the way out. Wear a gown before entering the contact precaution room. Remove the gown before leaving the room. Limit transport of the client to essential purposes and take care that the client does not contact other environmental surfaces along the way. Dedicate the use of noncritical client care equipment to a single client.

▲ Use alternatives to indwelling catheters whenever possible (external catheters, incontinence pads, and bladder control techniques).

• If a urinary catheter is necessary, follow catheter management practices. All indwelling catheters should be connected to a sterile, closed drainage system (i.e., not broken), except for good clinical reasons. Cleanse the perineum and meatus twice daily using soap and water.

• Use evidence-based practices and educate personnel in care of peripheral catheters: use aseptic technique for insertion and care, label insertion sites and all tubing with date and time of insertion, inspect every 8 hours for signs of infection, record, and report.

• Use sterile technique wherever there is a loss of skin integrity.

• Good personal hygiene is essential for skin health but it also has an important role in maintaining self-esteem and quality of life. Supporting clients to maintain personal hygiene is a fundamental aspect of nursing care. Personal hygiene includes hair, skin, nails, mouth, perineal areas, and facial shaving (Lawton & Shepherd, 2019). Ensure the client's daily personal needs are met by either the client, family, or nurse.

• Recommend responsible use of antibiotics; use antibiotics sparingly.

**Pediatric**

• Many of the preceding interventions are appropriate for the pediatric client.

• = Independent          ▲ = Collaborative

- Follow meticulous hand hygiene when working with children.
- Encourage early enteral feeding with human milk.
- ▲ Monitor recurrent antibiotic use in children.
- Instruct parents on appropriate indicators for medical visits and the risks associated with overuse of antibiotics.

**Geriatric**

- ▲ Suspect pneumonia when the client has symptoms of disorientation, confusion, respiratory rate of 30 or higher, and fever above 37.8°C (100°F). Offer clients influenza and pneumococcal vaccinations per national guidelines (CDC, 2021c). Assess response to treatment, especially antibiotic therapy.
- Most clients develop health care–associated pneumonia (HCAP) by either aspirating contaminated substances or inhaling airborne particles. Refer to care plan for Risk for **Aspiration.**
- ▲ Carefully screen older women with incontinence for urinary tract infections.
- Observe and report if the client has a low-grade fever or new onset of confusion.
- Recognize that chronically ill geriatric clients have an increased susceptibility to *C. difficile* infection; practice meticulous hand hygiene and monitor antibiotic response to antibiotics.

**Home Care**

- Adapt the previously mentioned interventions for home care as needed.
- Assess and treat wounds in the home.
- Review standards for surveillance of infections in home care.
- Maintain infection-prevention standards of practice.
- Refer for nutritional evaluation; implement dietary changes to support recovery and maintain health.

**Client/Family Teaching and Discharge Planning**

- Teach the client risk factors contributing to surgical wound infection.
- Teach the client and family the importance of hand hygiene in preventing postoperative infections.
- ▲ Encourage high-risk persons, including health care workers, to get vaccinated (CDC, 2019d; CDC, 2021d).
- ▲ Influenza: Teach symptoms of influenza and the importance of vaccination for influenza. Provide client education using the CDC Vaccine Information Sheets (VISs).

• = Independent      ▲ = Collaborative

# Risk for Surgical Site Infection

**Domain 11** Safety/protection    **Class 1** Infection
## NANDA-I Definition
Susceptible to invasion of pathogenic organisms at surgical site, which may compromise health.
## Risk Factors
Alcoholism, obesity, smoking
## At-Risk Population
Individuals exposed to excessive number of personnel during surgical procedure; individuals exposed to increased environmental pathogens; individuals with American Society of Anesthesiologists (ASA) Physical health status score ≥2
## Associated Conditions
Diabetes mellitus; extensive surgical procedures; general anesthesia; hypertension; immunosuppression; inadequate antibiotic prophylaxis; ineffective antibiotic prophylaxis; infections at other surgical sites; invasive procedure; post-traumatic osteoarthritis; prolonged duration of surgical procedure; prothesis; rheumatoid arthritis; significant comorbidity; surgical implant; surgical wound contamination
## Client Outcomes
**Client Will (Specify Time Frame)**
- Remain free from symptoms of surgical site infections (SSIs)
- Identify personal risk factors associated with increased SSI risk
- Modify personal behaviors that increase SSI risk
- Demonstrate appropriate hygienic practices to reduce infection risk such as handwashing
## Nursing Interventions
▲ The number of surgical procedures performed in the United States continues to rise, and surgical clients often have comorbidities that increase the complexity. It is estimated that approximately half of SSIs are deemed preventable using evidence based strategies (World Health Organization [WHO], 2018). SSIs are a complication of surgical care and are associated with significant morbidity, mortality, and cost (Preas, O'Hara, & Thom, 2017).

▲ Optimizing the client's medical condition before surgery and eliminating or even diminishing modifiable risk factors for infection can lower the risk of SSIs (Hutzler & Williams, 2017).

▲ SSI prevention, known as surgical care bundles, consists of evidence-based interventions that, when implemented together, can reduce the risk of infection. There are different surgical care bundles for specific

• = Independent        ▲ = Collaborative

high-risk surgical procedures, for example, colorectal surgery bundle, pediatric spinal surgery bundle, total joint arthroplasty surgery bundle, and cardiothoracic surgery bundle.

▲ SSIs can occur because of either client-related (endogenous) or procedure-related (exogenous) risk factors. Risk factors are further stratified into preoperative, intraoperative, and postoperative risk.

• Review endogenous client-related risk factors.

**Compromised Host Defenses**

• Age: Extremes of ages and advanced age increase client risk.

• Wound: A wound classification scoring system is used to identify the degree of surgical site skin integrity at the time of surgery. Assess and document skin integrity during the preoperative period to identify classification of surgical site.

• Smoking: The nicotine in tobacco products results in microvascular vasoconstriction, in addition to tissue hypoxia, which can contribute to the development of SSI. Surgical complications, such as SSI, can be decreased by 50% in clients who successfully stop smoking before surgery (Anderson et al, 2017).

▲ Assess client's smoking status and offer smoking cessation information to the receptive client. Seek nicotine patch order for client use during hospital admission.

▲ Educate the client on smoking risks using the CDC Fact Sheet on Health Effects of Cigarette Smoking (CDC, 2020g).

• Nutrition status: Assess the client's nutrition status. Preoperative risk factors include albumin less than 3.5 mg/dL or total bilirubin greater than 1.0 mg/dL (Ban et al, 2017; Tsantes et al, 2020). Malnutrition leads to less competent immune response and increased risk of acquiring infections (Tsantes et al, 2020).

• Immunocompromised/immunosuppression: Clients who are immunocompromised or who have immunosuppression are at increased risk of developing infection because of their weakened immune system and inability to mount a defense against pathogenic organisms. Clients who may be immunocompromised or immunosuppressed include clients receiving cancer treatment, organ transplant recipients, clients taking steroids, and clients with HIV.

• Review the client's medical history and current medications. Medications that compromise the client's immune response may increase the risk of SSI.

• Diabetes mellitus: Monitor blood glucose levels with the goal to maintain normoglycemia in the perioperative period. Educate the client of the increased risk for SSI with episodes of hyperglycemia.

• = Independent          ▲ = Collaborative

When available, coordinate referral to a diabetic educator as part of the discharge education.

- Preexisting infection: Be aware of all preoperative laboratory work, positive cultures, and actions taken to treat the infection (e.g., was the client started on oral antibiotics).
- Obesity: Obesity is defined as a body mass index (BMI) greater than 30 kg/m$^2$. Obese clients are at significant risk for SSI, more surgical blood loss, and a longer operation time.

**Procedure-Related Risk Factors—Exogenous**

- SSI pathogenic microbes may originate from exogenous sources such as the operating room environment, members of the surgical team, and instruments and material brought within the surgical field during the procedure (Khan et al, 2020). Observe clients identified as being at increased risk for SSI because of modifiable risk factors for signs and/or symptoms of postoperative SSI.
- Extended procedure time may increase SSI risk.
- Estimated blood loss greater than 1 L requiring blood transfusion increases the risk of SSI.
- Suboptimal timing of prophylactic antibiotic places the client at increased risk of SSI.
- Preoperative infections place the client at increased risk of SSI before elective surgery.
- Preoperative interventions: Establish a protocol for procedure-specific preoperative testing to detect medical conditions that increase the risk of SSI. The protocol should focus on nutritional counseling, glycemic control, smoking cessation, preadmission infections, and reconciling medications with adjustments before surgery as indicated (Anderson et al, 2017; Khan et al, 2020).
  - Identify high risks: diabetes, history of transplant, chemotherapy, immunosuppressed or immunocompromised, elderly, poor dentition, obese, and malnourished. Clients having a high-risk procedure with an extended surgical procedure time (e.g., cardiac surgery, joint replacement, major abdominal surgery) are at increased risk of SSI.
  - Maintain glycemic control for clients with and without diabetes.
  - *Staphylococcus aureus* (SA) is the most frequent pathogen causing about 50% of SSIs. MRSA accounts for up to 35% of SA infections in primary cases and up to 48% in revision surgery. Studies show that 18% to 25% of clients undergoing elective spine and orthopedic surgery are colonized with methicillin-sensitive SA (MSSA) and 3% to 5% are MRSA carriers. Carriers of MSSA

are 2 to 3 times and MRSA 8 to 10 times more likely to have an SSI. Perform SA intranasal decolonization by using cotton-tipped applicators to apply a 2% mupirocin ointment in each nostril and with 2% chlorhexidine gluconate (CHG) showers for up to 5 days before surgery (Anderson et al, 2017).

○ Provide education on preoperative bathing with soap (antimicrobial or nonantimicrobial) or an antiseptic agent on at least the night before and morning of the day of surgical intervention.

○ Address preexisting dental and nutritional status.

○ Nutrition consultation as needed.

○ Prepare the surgical site using an alcohol-based antiseptic agent unless contraindicated to reduce SSI risk.

○ Proper hair removal.

• If possible, educate the client preoperatively on the risk of shaving the surgical site, or the area near in which the surgical incision will be, because of the risk for microscopic cuts and abrasions. These cuts and abrasions increase the risk of developing an SSI. For example, for breast surgery, instruct the client not to shave underarms because the underarm is potentially in close proximity to the surgical site. Another example is instructing the client having a total knee replacement not to shave the leg involved in the surgery.

• Intraoperative interventions:

○ Maintain glycemic control.

○ Maintain normothermia (temperature of 35.5°C [95.9°F] or above) during the perioperative period in surgical clients who have an anesthesia duration of at least 60 minutes (Anderson et al, 2017). WHO defines hypothermia as a core temperature less than 36°C (WHO, 2018).

○ Provide supplemental oxygenation, during surgery for intubated clients and in the immediate postoperative period for 2 to 6 hours via a nonrebreathing mask for procedures performed under general anesthesia to ensure Hgb saturation of greater than 95% is maintained.

• Postoperative interventions:

○ Discharge instructions: Teach the client postoperative self-care after discharge. Provide written instructions that include information on how and when to contact the provider, date and time for the scheduled follow-up visit, and signs and symptoms of infection.

○ Wound care: Wound care instructions will be based on the type of surgical wound closure.

• = Independent ▲ = Collaborative

○ Nutrition follow-up: For the malnourished and obese clients, provide written dietary instructions by the registered dietitian, if appropriate. Encourage a diet that supports wound healing (high protein) and glycemic control. If appropriate, provide written information on community nutrition support group options and contact information.

○ Bathing/showering instructions: Review instructions with client and family on timing to shower and if/when the client can take a bath. Explain to the client that taking a bath is generally discouraged, at a minimum, for the first week after surgery.

○ Physical therapy (PT): For clients prescribed PT after discharge, review options to access services, provide contact phone numbers to call and schedule therapy, and review options for transportation to PT appointments (e.g., spouse, family, friend, senior center transport, cab, Uber, Lyft). Work with the discharge coordinator for client assistance with transport options as needed.

○ Medications: Review discharge medication prescription(s). Provide written instructions on medication(s) ordered, how often to take them, and side effects of the prescribed medication(s). Reinforce with client and family that client should not be driving if taking prescription narcotic medications. Review with client and family pain relief expectations, explaining that 100% postoperative pain relief is not realistic, but adequate pain relief should allow the client to function, to ambulate, and to perform activities of daily living (ADLs) with minimal pain.

**Pediatric**
- SSI prevention measures deemed effective in adults are also indicated in the pediatric surgical population (Berríos-Torres et al, 2017).

**Geriatric**
- The most common cause of postoperative complication in the frail elderly is delirium (Ersan & Schwer, 2021).
- For the frail, elder client who lived independently in a private home before surgical procedure, work with the discharge coordinator to assess appropriate client placement in the immediate postoperative period. Explore independent living, acute rehabilitation facility, or skilled nursing facility.
- For the cognitively impaired client being discharged back to independent living (private home or home with a family member), identify a key contact person who will participate in discharge education. Assess for any need of community services (e.g., food

• = Independent          ▲ = Collaborative

assistance, meal prep, transport, home health care) at time of discharge.
- Nutritional deficiencies can be common in elderly clients. Monitor laboratory tests; an albumin level less than 3.2 mg/dL and a cholesterol level of less than 160 mg/dL in the frail elderly are indicators for increased mortality.
- As part of the discharge process, ask the client how they will be obtaining groceries: Will they be cooking? Will they need assistance with meal prep? Do they have someone (friend or family member) who can come into the home to assist with cooking? Does the client need to have a food service (i.e., Meals on Wheels) set up for the immediate postdischarge period? Refer client to community services as necessary.

**Multicultural**
- Consider race and ethnicity as a key factor when developing the client's plan of care.
- In the case of a language barrier, use a qualified interpreter rather than family members, unless as a last resort, to communicate with the non–English-speaking client. The use of family members to translate health care–specific information may risk client privacy issues and interpretation bias. Nurses must be attentive to nonverbal cues, such as effective listening, attentive body language, and use of eye contact.
- Cultural nonverbal communication may also include values of modesty, touch, silence, and provider gender (Douglas et al, 2014). Identify the need for an interpreter at time of admission and schedule an interpreter to be available, either by phone or in person, for discussions with providers and for education sessions.
- Identify and accommodate the client who prefers same-gender providers. Effective communication may be affected in the client assigned opposite-gender caregivers, which may negatively affect recovery.

**Home Care**
- Previously listed interventions appropriately pertain to home care.
- Coordinate with discharge planner, as necessary, for assessment of the client's home care situation that suggests potential safety and mobility concerns.
- Clients discharged back to independent living with new use of walker, crutches, wheelchair, oxygen, and so forth should have egress access evaluated, and bathing/showering options and potential need for grab bars.

• = Independent     ▲ = Collaborative

# Risk for Injury

**Domain 11** Safety/protection   **Class 2** Physical injury

## NANDA-I Definition

Susceptible to physical damage due to environmental conditions interacting with the individual's adaptive and defensive resources, which may compromise health.

## Risk Factors

Exposure to toxic chemicals; immunization level within community; inadequate knowledge of modifiable factors; malnutrition; neurobehavioral manifestations; nosocomial agent; pathogen exposure; physical barrier; tainted nutritional source; unsafe mode of transport

## Associated Conditions

Altered psychomotor performance; autoimmune diseases; biochemical dysfunction; effector dysfunction; hypoxia; immune system diseases; impaired primary defense mechanisms; sensation disorders; sensory integration dysfunction

## Client Outcomes

**Client Will (Specify Time Frame)**

- Remain free of injuries
- Explain methods to prevent injuries
- Demonstrate behaviors that decrease the risk for injury

## Nursing Interventions

- Prevent iatrogenic harm to the hospitalized client by following the National Patient Safety Goals.
- Accuracy of client identification:
  - ○ Use at least two methods (e.g., client's name and medical record number or birth date) to identify the client on initial entrance to a client's room and before administering medications, blood products, treatments, or procedures.
- Effectiveness of communication among care staff:
  - ○ Get important test results to the right staff person on time.
- Medication safety:
  - ○ Before a procedure, label medications that are not labeled. For example, medicines in syringes, cups, and basins.
  - ○ Take extra care with clients who take medications to thin their blood.
  - ○ Record and pass along correct information about a client's medications. Find out what medications the client is taking. Compare those medications to new medications given to the client.

• = Independent            ▲ = Collaborative

- ○ Give the client written information about the medicines they need to take.
  - ○ Tell the client it is important to bring their up-to-date list of medicines every time they visit a health care provider.
- Alarm safety:
  - ○ Make improvements to ensure that alarms on medical equipment are heard and responded to on time.
- Infection control:
  - ○ Use the hand cleaning guidelines from the Centers for Disease Control and Prevention (2020b) or the World Health Organization. Set goals for improving hand cleaning. Use the goals to improve hand cleaning.
- Identify clients with safety risks:
  - ○ Identify which clients are at risk for suicidal behavior.
- Prevent errors in surgery:
  - ○ Make sure that the correct surgery is done on the correct client and at the correct place on the client's body.
  - ○ Mark the correct place on the client's body where the surgery is to be done.
  - ○ Pause before the surgery to make sure that a mistake is not being made.
- See care plans for Risk for **Falls,** Risk for **Suicidal** Behavior, and Risk for **Poisoning.**
- Avoid use of physical and chemical restraints, if possible. Restraint free is now the standard of care for hospitals and long-term care facilities. Obtain a health care provider's order if restraints are necessary.
- Consider providing individualized music of the client's choice if a client is agitated.
- Review drug profile for potential side effects and interactions that may increase risk of injury.
- Provide a safe environment:
  - ○ Use one-fourth– to one-half–length side rails only and maintain bed in a low position. Ensure that wheels are locked on bed and commode. Keep dim light in room at night.
  - ○ Remove all possible hazards in environment such as razors, medications, room clutter, wet floors, and matches.
- If the client has a new onset of confusion (delirium), refer to the care plan for Acute **Confusion.** If the client has chronic confusion, see the care plan for Chronic **Confusion.**
- ▲ Refer the client for physical therapy for strengthening as needed.

• = Independent ▲ = Collaborative

- Use nonphysical forms of behavior management for the agitated client with psychosis disorder.

**Pediatric**

- Teach parents the need for close supervision of young children playing near water.
- Assess the client's socioeconomic status because financial hardship may correlate with increased rates of injury.
- Never leave young children unsupervised around cooking or open flames.
- Teach parents and children the need to maintain safety for the physically active child, including wearing helmets when biking and skateboarding.
- Encourage parents to insist on safety precautions in all phases of participation in sports involving children.
- Provide parents of children with traumatic brain injury with written instruction and emergency phone numbers. Ensure that instructions are understood before the child is discharged from a health care setting. Instruct parents to observe for the following symptoms: nausea, mild headache, dizziness, irritability, lethargy, poor concentration, loss of appetite, and insomnia.
- Teach both parents and children the need for gun safety.
- Educate parents regarding proper car safety seat use.

**Geriatric**

- Encourage the client to wear glasses and hearing aids and to use walking aids, including nonslip footwear when ambulating.
- Assess for orthostatic hypotension when getting up, and teach methods to decrease dizziness, such as rising slowly, remaining seated several minutes before standing, flexing feet upward several times while sitting, sitting down immediately if feeling dizzy, and trying to have someone present when standing.
- Discourage driving at night.

**Multicultural**

- Evaluate the influence of culture on the client's perceptions of risk for injury.
- Evaluate whether exposure to community violence is a contributor to a client's risk for injury.
- Use culturally relevant injury prevention programs when possible. Validate the client's feelings and concerns related to environmental risks.

**Home Care and Client/Family Teaching and Discharge Planning**

- Previous interventions can be adapted for home care use.
- See Risk for Physical **Trauma** for Nursing Interventions.

• = Independent ▲ = Collaborative

# Risk for Corneal Injury

**Domain 11** Safety/protection    **Class 2** Physical injury

## NANDA-I Definition

Susceptible to infection or inflammatory lesion in the corneal tissue that can affect superficial or deep layers, which may compromise health.

## Risk Factors

Exposure of the eyeball; inadequate knowledge of modifiable factors

## At-Risk Population

Individuals experiencing prolonged hospitalization

## Associated Conditions

Artificial respiration; Blinking <5 times per minute; Glasgow Coma Scale score <6; oxygen therapy; periorbital edema; pharmaceutical preparations; tracheostomy

## Client Outcomes

**Client Will (Specify Time Frame)**

• Demonstrate relaxed facial expressions and grimacing reduction
• Remain as independent as possible
• Remain free of physical harm resulting from vision injury risk
• Demonstrate improvement in visual acuity

## Nursing Interventions

**Emergency Department Visit or Primary Care Office Visit**

▲ Perform a standard ophthalmic examination or examine eye with a slit lamp using fluorescein stain to optimize visualization of the abrasion injury if available.

• Attempt visual acuity measuring using the Snellen eye chart (corrected with glasses).

• Ensure immunization status is current, namely tetanus-diphtheria-pertussis status (every 10 years).

• Teach the client that foreign body corneal abrasions are one of the most common eye injuries and are at risk for complications (Zimmerman et al, 2019).

• Topical anesthetics such as tetracaine may be used to provide pain relief for corneal abrasions (Fusco et al, 2019).

▲ Clients will require topical antibiotics to reduce the risk of infection (Thiel, Sarau, & Ng, 2017; Fusco et al, 2019). Nonsteroidal antiinflammatory drugs (NSAIDs) may be prescribed to facilitate healing and reduce pain.

• Injuries that penetrate the cornea are more serious. The outcome depends on the specific injury. Corneal abrasions usually heal quickly and without vision concerns. Even after the original injury is healed,

• = Independent    ▲ = Collaborative

however, the surface of the cornea is sometimes not as smooth as before.

**Hospitalization**

- Traumatic corneal abrasions are common ophthalmic injuries, accounting for 8% of emergency department visits, with fingernail-induced corneal abrasions being common (Gotekar, 2017; Wakai et al, 2017).
- Perioperative corneal abrasions typically heal within 72 hours. Risk factors include advanced age, prominent eyes (proptosis, exophthalmos), ocular surface abnormalities (dry eye, recurrent erosion syndrome), surgery greater than 60 to 90 minutes, prone/lateral and Trendelenburg positions, operations on the head and neck body regions, intraoperative hypotension, and preoperative anemia. Potential sources of corneal injury in the surgical client are after induction (laryngoscope, name badge, watch band), before incision (surgical preparation, gauze/sponges/drapes), during the procedure (instruments, chemical solutions, heat sources, pressure on globe, eye shields), and awakening/recovery (oxygen face mask, fingernails) (Malafa et al, 2016; Kaye et al, 2019).
- ▲ All surgical clients should have eyelids secured in the closed position immediately after induction. A strip of tape is generally sufficient; however, in high-risk cases with Trendelenburg position clients may benefit from use of transparent bio-occlusive dressing, which can span the entire lid and provide strong uniform closure, minimizing tear evaporation and acting as a barrier to trauma (Malafa et al, 2016).
- Ocular lubricants support surface moisture, but studies comparing different types of lubricants fail to demonstrate differences in efficacy. However, preservative-free methylcellulose-based ointments are preferred because they are retained in the eye longer than aqueous solutions. Paraffin-based (petroleum) ointments disrupt tear film stability, carry a higher risk of eye irritation, and are flammable (Malafa et al, 2016).
- Assess for corneal abrasion and eye dryness, which are common problems in clients in the intensive care unit. Eye dryness is the main risk factor for the development of corneal abrasions.

**Client/Family Teaching and Discharge Planning**

- ▲ First-aid principles should be reinforced in the event of an eye injury. Clients should not attempt to remove any object in the eye; reserve this for the provider. A referral to an ophthalmologist may be required (Jacobs, 2021).

• = Independent          ▲ = Collaborative

- Teach clients to use caution when using household cleaners. Many household products contain strong acids, alkalis, or other chemicals. Drain and oven cleaners are particularly dangerous and can lead to blindness if not used correctly.
- If chemical exposure has occurred, flush the eye immediately with clean water for 10 minutes. Seek prompt health care attention.
- Wear safety goggles at all times when using hand or power tools or chemicals, during high-impact sports, or in other situations when eye injury is more likely.
- Most fingernail injuries to the cornea are preventable, and health teaching should be provided about the importance of supervision in children (Gotekar, 2017).
- Wear sunglasses that screen ultraviolet light when outdoors, even in winter.
- Pain is usually improved within 3 days. If pain becomes intolerable, an analgesic may be prescribed short term. Seek medical attention if pain is not resolving.
- Driving should be restricted for safety until client's visual acuity is evaluated.

# Risk for Occupational Injury

**Domain 11** Safety/projection    **Class 4** Environmental hazards
**NANDA-I Definition**

Susceptible to a work-related accident or illness, which may compromise health.

**Risk Factors**

**Individual**

Distraction from interpersonal relations; excessive stress; improper use of personal protective equipment; inadequate knowledge; inadequate time management skills; ineffective coping strategies; misinterpretation of information; psychological distress; unhealthy habits; unsafe work behaviors

**Unmodified Environmental Factors**

Environmental constraints; exposure to biological agents; exposure to chemical agents; exposure to noise; exposure to radiotherapy; exposure to teratogenic agents; exposure to vibration; inadequate access to individual protective equipment; inadequate physical environment; labor relationships; night shift work rotating to day shift work; occupational burnout; physical workload; shift work

• = Independent      ▲ = Collaborative

## At-Risk Population

Individuals exposed to environmental temperature extremes

## Client Outcomes

### Client Will (Specify Time Frame)

- Attend and participate in all required health and safety training activities
- Demonstrate safe and healthy work behaviors to reduce the risk of occupational injuries and illnesses
- Comply with the organization's health and safety policies and procedures
- Report to management any work hazards, such as facility, tools, and equipment that needs to be repaired
- Demonstrate healthy personal habits, such as healthy nutritional choices, regular exercise, smoking cessation, and effective sleep patterns

## Nursing Interventions

- Interventions to reduce the risks of occupational injury focus on providing resources for safe work and education to the individual to know safety rules and procedures. Occupational safety requires the individual to engage in safe acts, proper use of equipment (including personal protective equipment [PPE]), cognitive focus during work, and self-identification of stressors that may adversely affect the individual's personal safety during work.
- Encourage employee compliance with safety policies and procedures to reduce the opportunity for slips, trips, and falls; breaks in skin integrity through chemical exposure, mechanical means (trauma, friction, pressure), physical exposure (heat, cold, radiation), and exposure to biological elements (viruses, bacteria, fungi); musculoskeletal injuries; and misuse of equipment and tools.
- Enforce compliance with organizational and regulatory health and safety policies and procedures, demonstrating at least adequate training and the proper use of appropriate tools, equipment, and PPE to reduce risk of injury and illness and ensure that the client receives appropriate training and education on occupational tasks and equipment.
- Assist the client in reduction of personal and work stress to increase coping skills, improve interpersonal relationships, and avoid burnout.
- Educate clients to engage in active coping strategies to reduce work-related stress.
- Promote good sleep hygiene, which will result in increased alertness and decreased occupational injuries and illnesses.

• = Independent ▲ = Collaborative

- Educate client on the detrimental effects of shift work, atypical working time, and nonstandard work schedules.
- Provide medical screening, surveillance, and postexposure testing for symptomatic employees to identify exposure and control effects that can lead to illness and injury.
- Assist in the integration of personal health behaviors that promote total worker health and safety for the employee, which translates to a more productive worker generating better quality products, resulting in fewer occupational injuries and illnesses for the workers.
- Identify client risk factors that can lead to occupational injury and address them with health coaching techniques.
- Provide resources to assist with smoking/vaping cessation.
- Implement environmental and behavioral strategies to aid workers in maintaining a healthy weight.
- Promote a drug-free workplace through education, training, policy development, and evaluation.
- Identify high-risk work areas and environmental hazards by conducting periodic walkthroughs of the workplace for unsafe acts and conditions. Possible risks include excessive noise, poorly maintained equipment, lack of PPE, uneven or poorly designed workspaces, inadequate lighting, environmental toxins, and lack of safety training.
- Ensure that appropriate respiratory protection is available and used when workers can be potentially exposed to transmissible respiratory infections.
- Ensure that infection prevention and control policies and procedures are enforced. Blood-borne pathogen risks are inherent when providing nursing care in health care facilities for injured or ill employees, and appropriate measures must be taken to avoid contact with and spread of infectious organisms.
- Implement measures to prevent occupational back pain, which can be prevented or limited in its severity.
- Ensure workers have access to and use PPE to reduce noise exposure. Engineering and administrative controls should be considered before the use of PPE.
- Health professionals should understand potential interruptions and cognitive distractions to adopt a task-design–oriented approach that focuses on aspects of the work environment that can be observed, measured, and controlled.
- Provide multiprofessional collaboration to reduce occupational risks to health and safety.

• = Independent            ▲ = Collaborative

- Implement an early reporting system that allows workers to safely report injuries or illness.
- Ensure appropriate medical referrals and communication with health care providers to achieve safe work environment goals and include follow-up assessment to ensure that the worker is not further injured by the accommodated work situation.
- Provide accurate and legal documentation for medical and exposure records with adverse health effects from health and safety exposures, maintaining confidentiality of personal medical issues. Legal requirements for documentation ensure correct communication of all aspects of the injury or illness and protects the nurse in case of litigation.

## Geriatric

- Consider the physiological changes in the aging population.
- Although older clients may experience fewer occupational injuries and illnesses, the aging workforce may take longer to heal and return to work.

## Multicultural

- Address differences in cultures that affect attitudes toward health care professionals and treatment modalities.
- According to the Centers for Disease Control and Prevention (CDC, 2021e), young workers have high rates of job-related injury. These injuries are often the result of the many hazards present in the places they typically work, such as sharp knives and slippery floors in restaurants. Limited or no prior work experience and a lack of safety training also contribute to high injury rates. Middle and high school workers may be at increased risk for injury because they may not have the strength or cognitive ability needed to perform certain job duties.
- The US workforce is becoming more diverse (National Center for Public Policy and Higher Education, 2005). Baby boomers are remaining in the workforce past traditional retirement age because their health is better, and they need or want additional income (Bureau of Labor Statistics, 2008).
- The size of the minority workforce is growing, and more women are entering the workforce (Thompson & Wachs, 2012) There is greater diversity in the workplace, and people from different backgrounds and cultures are working alongside each other, often speaking different languages with different educational and literacy backgrounds.
- Depending on the setting, comprehensive health care, including, for example, smoking cessation and early diagnosis and treatment

of depression, could be provided to high-risk populations using culturally sensitive outreach and motivational interviewing strategies.

• The Americans with Disabilities Act (ADA) requires that public buildings be designed to accommodate wheelchairs and other accommodations and that jobs be modified if accommodation is reasonable so that people with disabilities can gain access to buildings and jobs (see https://www.ada.gov/ada_req_ta.htm).

# Nipple-Areolar Complex Injury

**Domain 11** Safety/protection    **Class 2** Physical injury

## NANDA-I Definition

Localized damage to nipple-areolar complex as a result of the breastfeeding process.

## Defining Characteristics

Abraded skin; altered skin color; altered thickness of nipple-areolar complex; blistered skin; discolored skin patches; disrupted skin surface; ecchymosis; eroded skin; erythema; expresses pain; hematoma; macerated skin; scabbed skin; skin fissure; skin ulceration; skin vesicles; swelling; tissue exposure below the epidermis

## Related Factors

Breast engorgement; hardened areola; improper use of milk pump; inadequate latching on; inappropriate maternal hand support of breast; inappropriate positioning of the infant during breastfeeding; inappropriate positioning of the mother during breastfeeding; ineffective infant sucking reflex; ineffective non-nutritive sucking; mastitis; maternal anxiety about breastfeeding; maternal impatience with the breastfeeding process; mother does not wait for the infant to spontaneously release the nipple; mother withdraws infant from breast without breaking the suction; nipple confusion due to use of artificial nipple; postprocedural pain; prolonged exposure to moisture; supplementary feeding; use of products that remove the natural protection of the nipple

## At-Risk Population

Primiparous women; sole mother; women aged < 19 years; women breastfeeding for the first time; women with depigmented nipple areolar complex; women with history of inadequate nipple-areolar preparation during prenatal care; women with history of nipple trauma in breastfeeding; women with non-protruding nipples; women with pink nipple-areolar complex

## Associated Conditions

Ankyloglossia; maxillofacial abnormalities

• = Independent    ▲ = Collaborative

## Client Outcomes

### Client Will (Specify Time Frame)
- Avoid artificial nipple use with infant
- Use techniques to prevent nipple tenderness
- Establish a position of comfort during nursing
- Recognize infant swallowing

## Nursing Interventions

- Nipple trauma and sore nipples are common complaints among breastfeeding women and are a leading cause of breastfeeding discontinuation.
- Identify clients at risk for nipple trauma.
- Evaluate the nipple for five signs of nipple trauma in order to help reduce pain and further trauma and to promote continuation of breastfeeding.
- Use a valid and reliable tool for assessing nipple trauma associated with breastfeeding.
- Help to correct any factors that may be contributing to nipple trauma.
- Offer options to promote healing.
- Offer instruction on latch in order to promote effective milk transfer and decrease potential nipple trauma.
- Usage of a breast pump to express milk can be beneficial to promote feeding an infant breast milk when feeding at the breast is causing nipple trauma.
- Assist the client in alternative feeding methods if nipple trauma is severe in order to promote healing and prevent further damage.

### Home Care

- Assess availability of and refer client to lactation support if nursing interventions and self-management are not alleviating the nipple trauma.
- Refer client to pediatrician to assess if the infant has an upper, anterior, or submucosal tongue and/or lip-tie.
- Assess clients' emotional state as nipple trauma can lead to inefficient breastfeeding, which can account for unstable mood and postpartum depression.
- Encourage family participation and provide information to the father as appropriate in order to support the breastfeeding mother.

# Risk for Nipple-Areolar Complex Injury

**Domain 11** Safety/protection    **Class 2** Physical injury

• = Independent                    ▲ = Collaborative

## NANDA-I Definition

Susceptible to localized damage to nipple-areolar complex as a result of the breastfeeding process.

## Related Factors

Breast engorgement; hardened areola; improper use of milk pump; inadequate latching on; inadequate nipple-areolar preparation during prenatal care; inappropriate maternal hand support of breast; inappropriate positioning of the infant during breastfeeding; inappropriate positioning of the mother during breastfeeding; ineffective infant sucking reflex; ineffective non-nutritive sucking; mastitis; maternal anxiety about breastfeeding; maternal impatience with the breastfeeding process; mother does not wait for the infant to spontaneously release the nipple; mother withdraws infant from breast without breaking the suction; nipple confusion due to use of artificial nipple; postprocedural pain; prolonged exposure to moisture; supplementary feeding; use of products that remove the natural protection of the nipple

## At-Risk Population

Primiparous women; sole mother; women aged < 19 years; women breastfeeding for the first time; women with depigmented nipple areolar complex; women with history of nipple trauma in breastfeeding; women with non-protruding nipples; women with pink nipple-areolar complex

## Associated Conditions

Ankyloglossia; maxillofacial abnormalities

## Client Outcomes and Nursing Interventions

Refer to care plan for Nipple-Areolar Complex **Injury**.

# Risk for Urinary Tract Injury

**Domain 11** Safety/protection   **Class 2** Physical injury

## NANDA-I Definition

Susceptible to damage of the urinary tract structures from use of catheters, which may compromise health.

## Risk Factors

Confusion; inadequate caregiver knowledge regarding urinary catheter care; inadequate knowledge regarding urinary catheter care; neurobehavioral manifestations; obesity

## At-Risk Population

Individuals at extremes of age

## Associated Conditions

Anatomical variation in the pelvic organs; condition preventing ability to secure catheter; detrusor sphincter dyssynergia; latex allergy; long-term

• = Independent        ▲ = Collaborative

use of urinary catheter; medullary injury; prostatic hyperplasia; repetitive catheterizations; retention balloon inflated to ≥30 mL; use of large caliber urinary catheter

## Client Outcomes

### Client Will (Specify Time Frame)

- Remain free of urinary tract injury
- State absence of pain with catheter care and during urination
- Experience unobstructed urination after removal of catheter
- Identify signs and symptoms of urinary obstruction and urinary tract injury after removal of catheter
- Identify interventions to prevent catheter-associated urinary tract infection (CAUTI)
- Maintain adequate urine volume (0.5–1.0 mL/kg/h for adult); urine without odor; urine clear
- Maintain adequate fluid intake considering client age and comorbidities

## Nursing Interventions

- Monitor urinary elimination, including frequency, consistency, odor, volume, and color, as appropriate.
- Teach the client and caregiver signs and symptoms of urinary tract infection and CAUTI.
- Assess for appropriate use of an indwelling urinary catheter. Insert urinary catheters only when indicated and leave in only as long as clinically necessary.
- To prevent injury, educate the client and family and/or caregiver regarding the use of an indwelling urinary catheter (AHRQ, 2015; Mody et al, 2017).
- Assess clinical indications for urinary catheter use daily.
- To avoid catheterizations, evaluate alternative strategies for managing urine output for the client.
- If an indwelling urinary catheter is determined to be clinically indicated in the care of a client, proper selection of the right catheter, technique during insertion, and evidence-based care management are needed to reduce infection and injury to the urinary tract structures.
  - ○ Perform hand hygiene and use Standard Precautions before and after insertion of the urinary catheter and any time the catheter, catheter site, or collection system is accessed (AHRQ, 2015; Gould et al, 2019).
  - ○ Ensure that only properly trained personnel familiar with appropriate catheter care techniques are used for inserting and maintaining the catheter (AHRQ, 2015; Gould et al, 2019).

• = Independent          ▲ = Collaborative

- Selecting the smallest catheter size (e.g., smaller than 18 French) reduces irritation and inflammation of the urethra and reduces infection risk (Gould et al, 2019).
- Insert the catheter using aseptic technique in the acute care setting. Wash hands and use sterile technique when opening the catheterization kit and cleansing the urethral meatus and perineal area with an antiseptic solution. Insert the catheter using a no-touch technique (AHRQ, 2015; Gould et al, 2019).
- If a urine sample is needed from the urinary collection system sampling port, disinfect the sampling port and allow disinfectant to dry before accessing the port.
- Provide routine hygiene care; once a urinary catheter is placed, optimal management includes care of the urethral meatus according to "routine hygiene" (e.g., daily cleansing of the meatal surface during bathing with soap and water and as needed, such as following a bowel movement) (AHRQ, 2015; Gould et al, 2019).
- Secure the catheter after placement to reduce friction and pain from movement (Gould et al, 2019; Kranz et al, 2020).
  - ❍ Disruptions in aseptic technique, disconnection, or leakage require the catheter and collection system to be replaced using aseptic technique and sterile equipment (AHRQ, 2015; Gould et al, 2019).
  - ❍ Maintain unobstructed urine flow; maintain the catheter and collecting tube below the level of the bladder and free of kinks. Do not rest the collection bag on the floor.
- Establish workflow protocols to routinely empty the drainage bag frequently and before transport to reduce urine reflux and opportunities for infection.
- Change urinary catheters and drainage systems based on clinical indications such as infection, obstruction, or when the drainage system is not adequately maintained.
- Monitor the client with an indwelling urinary catheter for increased temperature (>38°C; 100.4°F), suprapubic pain, frequency, urgency, and flank pain; monitor the skin around the catheter for redness, drainage, or swelling.
- Consider an ultrasound scanner for clients who require intermittent catheterization to assess urine volume and reduce unnecessary catheter insertion (Gould et al, 2019; Meddings et al, 2015).
- ▲ Implement systemwide quality improvement programs, including the following interventions to decrease CAUTI:

• = Independent          ▲ = Collaborative

- o Establish health care provider alerts or reminders for all clients with catheters regarding the need for continued catheterization.
- o Provide performance feedback and education to personnel responsible for catheter care (Gould et al, 2019; Mody et al, 2017).
- o Establish evidence-based "bladder bundles" as part of a multimodal approach to preventing CAUTI. "Bladder bundles" may include educational interventions aimed at health care providers for appropriate use of urinary catheters, use of appropriately trained personnel to insert and care for the catheter, catheter restriction and removal protocols, and the use of bladder ultrasound to assess urine volume (Saint et al, 2016; Mody et al, 2017).

**Home Care and Client/Family Teaching and Discharge Planning**

- Teach the client and family discharged with an indwelling urinary catheter or performing intermittent catheterization at home techniques for care of urinary catheter and collection bag using the interventions listed above (AHRQ, 2015).
- Ensure client has adequate supplies at home for catheter insertion and care.
- Teach the client and family to contact the health care provider regarding symptoms of CAUTI, including increased temperature (>38°C; 100.4°F), suprapubic pain, frequency, urgency, and flank pain; no drainage of urine in the collection bag; inability to perform activities of daily living; delirium; and foul-smelling, cloudy, or bloody urine (Blodgett et al, 2015; Gbinigie et al, 2018; Shah, 2019).
- Teach client and family to monitor for signs of obstruction such as decreased urine output after catheter is removed.

## Insomnia

**Domain 4** Activity/rest   **Class 1** Sleep/rest
**NANDA-I Definition**

Inability to initiate or maintain sleep, which impairs functioning.

**Defining Characteristics**

Altered affect; altered attention; altered mood; early awakening; expresses dissatisfaction with quality of life; expresses dissatisfaction with sleep; expresses forgetfulness; expresses need for frequent naps during the day; impaired health status; increased absenteeism; increased accidents; insufficient physical endurance; nonrestorative sleep-wake cycle

**Related Factors**

Anxiety; average daily physical activity is less than recommended for age and gender; caffeine consumption; caregiver role strain; consumption of

• = Independent          ▲ = Collaborative

sugar-sweetened beverages; depressive symptoms; discomfort; dysfunctional sleep beliefs; environmental disturbances; fear; frequent naps during the day; inadequate sleep hygiene; lifestyle incongruent with normal circadian rhythms; low psychological resilience; obesity; stressors; substance misuse; use of interactive electronic devices

## At-Risk Population

Adolescents; economically disadvantaged individuals; grieving individuals; individuals undergoing changes in marital status; night shift workers; older adults; pregnant women in third trimester; rotating shift workers; women

## Associated Conditions

Chronic disease; hormonal change; pharmaceutical preparations

## Client Outcomes

### Client Will (Specify Time Frame)

- Verbalize plan to implement sleep-promoting routines
- Fall asleep with less difficulty a minimum of four nights out of seven
- Wake up less frequently during night a minimum of four nights out of seven
- Sleep a minimum of 6 hours most nights and more if needed to meet next stated outcome
- Awaken refreshed and not be fatigued during day most of the time

## Nursing Interventions

- Obtain a sleep history including amount of time needed to initiate sleep, duration of any awakenings after sleep onset, total nighttime sleep amounts, and dissatisfaction with daytime energy levels and alertness.
- From the history, assess client's current ability to initiate and maintain sleep and the short-term versus chronic nature of inability to initiate and maintain sleep.

### For Short-Term Insomnia

- For clients historically able to initiate and maintain sleep but unable to do so in the current situation: (1) minimize sleep disruptions (see Nursing Interventions for Disturbed **Sleep** Pattern) and (2) promote sleep hygiene practices (see Nursing Interventions for Readiness for Enhanced **Sleep**).
- Also attend to the following factors often associated with short-term insomnia:
  - Assess pain medication use and, when feasible, advocate for pain medications that promote rather than interfere with sleep. (See Nursing Interventions for Acute **Pain** and Chronic **Pain**.)
  - Assess level of tension and encourage use of relaxation techniques as needed.

○ Assess level of distress and use therapeutic communication to increase comfort. (See further Nursing Interventions for Readiness for Enhanced **Comfort.**)

▲ Assess for signs of overactive bladder.

**For Chronic Insomnia**

▲ Rule out and/or address any disorders and syndromes associated with chronic insomnia (e.g., addiction to alcohol or other psychoactive substances, anxiety and depressive disorders, chronic pain syndrome, or other sleep disorders).

• Monitor for uncomfortable sensations in legs and involuntary leg movements during sleep.

• Be aware that clients diagnosed with chronic insomnia may have a low pain threshold.

• Encourage use of the following stimulus control strategies in addition to any relaxation and sleep hygiene interventions recommended for short-term insomnia that the client finds helpful; (1) if feasible, have client arise from bed to participate in calming activities whenever anxious about failure to fall asleep; (2) if not feasible for client to get out of bed when unable to sleep, encourage sitting up in bed to engage in calming activities or simply resting in bed without attempting to fall asleep; (3) avoid a focus on what time it is and subsequent worry about amount of sleep time lost to sleeplessness; and (4) distract from sleeplessness with a focus on positive aspects of life.

• Consider use of warm foot baths.

• For clients whose chronic inability to initiate and maintain sleep has led to sleep deprivation, see Nursing Interventions for **Sleep** Deprivation.

• For clients with unremitting chronic insomnia, refer to a nurse practitioner trained in cognitive behavioral therapies for insomnia (CBT-I).

• Assist clients diagnosed with chronic insomnia who have been treated with CBT-I to limit use of sleeping medications and to select intermittent nights for sleeping pill use if complete discontinuance of sleeping pills is not feasible.

• Supplement other interventions with teaching about sleep and sleep promotion. (See further Nursing Interventions for Readiness for Enhanced **Sleep.**)

**Geriatric**

• Most interventions discussed above may be used with geriatric clients. In addition, see the Geriatric section of Nursing Interventions for (1) Readiness for Enhanced **Sleep** and (2) Disturbed **Sleep**, and **Sleep** Deprivation.

• = Independent          ▲ = Collaborative

- Note that it is especially helpful for the elderly client with short-term or chronic insomnia to engage in routine exercise unless contraindicated by health status.

**Home Care**
- Assessments and interventions discussed previously can all be adapted for use in home care.
- In addition, see the Home Care section of Nursing Interventions for Readiness for Enhanced **Sleep.**

**Client/Family Teaching**
- Teach family about normal sleep and promote adoption of behaviors that enhance it. See Nursing Interventions for Readiness for Enhanced **Sleep.**
- Teach family about sleep deprivation and how to avoid it. See Nursing Interventions for **Sleep** Deprivation.
- Advise family of importance of not disrupting sleep of others unnecessarily. See Nursing Interventions for Disturbed **Sleep** Pattern.
- Advise family about the importance of minimizing noise and light, including light from electronic devices, in the sleep environment. See Nursing Interventions for Disturbed **Sleep** Pattern.
- Help family members understand the difference between the two major precursors of sleep deprivation, that is, insomnia versus externally caused sleep disruptions.

# Deficient Knowledge

**Domain 5** Perception/cognition    **Class 4** Cognition
## NANDA-I Definition
Absence of cognitive information related to a specific topic, or its acquisition.
## Defining Characteristics
Inaccurate follow-through of instruction; inaccurate performance on a test; inaccurate statements about a topic; inappropriate behavior
## Related Factors
Anxiety; depressive symptoms; inadequate access to resources; inadequate awareness of resources; inadequate commitment to learning; inadequate information; inadequate interest in learning; inadequate knowledge of resources; inadequate participation in care planning; inadequate trust in health care professional; low self efficacy; misinformation; neurobehavioral manifestations

• = Independent        ▲ = Collaborative

## At-Risk Population

Economically disadvantaged individuals; illiterate individuals; individuals with low educational level

## Associated Conditions

Depression; developmental disabilities; neurocognitive disorders

## Client Outcomes

### Client Will (Specify Time Frame)

- Explain disease state, recognize need for medications, and understand treatments
- Describe the rationale for therapy/treatment options
- Incorporate knowledge of health regimen into lifestyle
- State confidence in one's ability to manage health situation and remain in control of life
- Demonstrate how to perform health-related procedure(s) satisfactorily
- Identify resources that can be used for more information or support after discharge

## Nursing Interventions

- Health care providers who are nonjudgmental and supportive can assist clients to be involved in planning individual intervention strategies that can increase compliance.
- Consider the health literacy and the readiness to learn for all clients and caregivers (e.g., mental acuity, ability to see or hear, existing pain, emotional readiness, motivation, previous knowledge).
- Focus on the nature of spoken and written communication when teaching clients and caregivers, especially those who may have health literacy needs.
- Consider the context, timing, and order of how information is presented.
- Use person-centered approaches that engage clients and caregivers as active versus passive learners.
- Reinforce learning through frequent repetition and follow-up sessions.
- Use electronic methods for delivery of information when appropriate.
- Help the client and caregivers locate appropriate postdischarge groups and resources.
- Encourage clients and caregivers to maintain and/or expand supportive social networks as self-care learning resources when appropriate.

### Pediatric

- Use family-centered approaches when teaching children and adolescents.

• = Independent          ▲ = Collaborative

- Guide children and adolescents to credible information about their condition.

**Geriatric**

- Educate all older clients on safety issues, including fall prevention and medication management.
- Use multiprofessional teams to enhance client education.
- Consider using teaching methods and materials appropriate for older adults, especially those with cognitive challenges.
- Assess readiness of older adults for use of technological resources.

**Multicultural**

- Use educational interventions that are culturally tailored to the health literacy needs of the client.
- Assess for cultural/ethnic self-care practices.
- Consider the potential influence of medical interpreters in information sharing and decision-making and of the possible difficulties for clients when using medical interpreters.
- Consider involving bilingual members of a community who are considered outside the traditional health care system who may assist in the teaching of community health issues.

**Home Care**

- All of the previously mentioned interventions are applicable to the home setting.
- Use telehealth and technology-enhanced practices as appropriate.

## Readiness for Enhanced Knowledge

**Domain 5** Perception/cognition    **Class 4** Cognition

### NANDA-I Definition

A pattern of cognitive information related to a specific topic, or its acquisition, which can be strengthened.

### Defining Characteristics

Expresses desire to enhance learning

### Client Outcomes

Client Will (Specify Time Frame)

- Meet personal health-related goals
- Explain how to incorporate new health regimen into lifestyle
- List sources to obtain information

### Nursing Interventions

- Assume a facilitator role versus an authority role when engaging clients seeking health-related knowledge.

• = Independent      ▲ = Collaborative

- Consider "health coaching" and motivational interviewing techniques when focusing on health-related goals, priorities, and preferences.
- Seek teachable moments for those with chronic conditions to enhance their knowledge of health promotion.
- Refer clients to interactive and Web-based technological resources as appropriate.
- Refer to Deficient **Knowledge** care plan.

**Pediatric**
- Consider the use of mobile text messaging as a resource for delivery of health promotion information.
- Involve children and especially adolescents in designing health promotion programs and teaching methods.
- Refer to Deficient **Knowledge** care plan.

**Geriatric**
- Discuss healthy lifestyle changes that promote safety, health promotion, and health maintenance for older clients.
- Consider involving bilingual members of a community who are considered outside the traditional health care system who may assist in the teaching of community health issues.

**Multicultural**
- Refer to Geriatric interventions.
- Refer to Deficient **Knowledge** care plan.

# Risk for Latex Allergy Reaction

**Domain 11** Safety/protection   **Class 5** Defensive processes

## NANDA-I Definition

Susceptible to a hypersensitive reaction to natural latex rubber products or latex reactive foods, which may compromise health.

## Risk Factors

Inadequate knowledge about avoidance of relevant allergens; inattentive to potential environmental latex exposure; inattentive to potential exposure to latex reactive foods

## At-Risk Population

Individuals frequently exposed to latex product; individuals receiving repetitive injections from rubber topped bottles; individuals with family history of atopic dermatitis; individuals with history of latex reaction; infants undergoing numerous operations beginning soon after birth

• = Independent     ▲ = Collaborative

## Associated Conditions

Asthma; atopy; food allergy; hypersensitivity to natural latex rubber protein; multiple surgical procedures; poinsettia plant allergy; urinary bladder diseases

## Client Outcomes

### Client Will (Specify Time Frame)

- State risk factors for natural rubber latex (NRL) allergy
- Request latex-free environment
- Demonstrate knowledge of plan to treat NRL allergic reaction

## Nursing Interventions

- Clients at high risk for NRL allergy need to be identified.
- Clients with spina bifida are a high-risk group for NRL allergy and should remain latex free from the first day of life.
- Assess for NRL allergy in clients who are exposed to "hidden" latex.
- Assess for NRL allergy in clients with a history of multiple surgeries or other latex-exposing procedures.
- Assess for NRL allergy in atopic individuals (persons with a tendency to have multiple allergic conditions, including allergies to certain food products).
- Assess persons who have an ongoing occupational exposure to NRL.
- Assess for latex sensitization in older adults.
- Obtain a thorough history of the client at risk before performing procedures that may involve latex products, such as urinary catheter insertion or venipuncture.
- Have management protocols in place for treating anaphylaxis.
- Question the client about associated symptoms of itching, swelling, and redness after contact with rubber products such as rubber gloves, balloons, and barrier contraceptives, or swelling of the tongue and lips after dental examinations.
- Treat all latex-sensitive clients as if they have NRL allergy.
- Clients with spina bifida and others with a positive history of NRL sensitivity or NRL allergy should have all medical/surgical/dental procedures performed in a latex-controlled environment.
- In select high-risk atopic individuals, a specific immunotherapy regimen should be discussed with their health care provider.
- ▲ If latex gloves are chosen for protection from blood or body fluids, a reduced-protein, powder-free glove should be selected.
- Ensure that the client has a medical plan if a latex response develops.
- Note client history and environmental assessment.

• = Independent        ▲ = Collaborative

### Client/Family Teaching and Discharge Planning

▲ Instruct the client to inform health care professionals if he or she has an NRL allergy, particularly if the client is scheduled for surgery.

• Provide the client with written information about latex allergy and sensitivity.

• Teach clients that the most effective approach to preventing NRL anaphylaxis is complete latex avoidance.

▲ Teach clients that materials and items that contain NRL must be identified and latex-free alternatives must be substituted.

• Health care workers should avoid the use of latex gloves and seek alternatives such as unpowdered gloves made from nitrile.

• Institute measures that reduce or completely avoid any latex exposure to clients.

• Health care institutions should develop prevention programs and establish latex-safe areas in their facilities.

### Home Care

• Assess the home environment for presence of NRL products (e.g., balloons, condoms, gloves, and products of related allergies, such as bananas, avocados, and poinsettia plants).

• Ensure that the client has a medical plan if a response develops.

• Note client history and environmental assessment.

## Readiness for Enhanced Health Literacy

**Domain 1** Health promotion    **Class 1** Health awareness

### NANDA-I Definition

A pattern of using and developing a set of skills and competencies (literacy, knowledge, motivation, culture and language) to find, comprehend, evaluate and use health information and concepts to make daily health decisions to promote and maintain health, decrease health risks and improve overall quality of life, which can be strengthened.

### Defining Characteristics

Expresses desire to enhance ability to read, write, speak and interpret numbers for everyday health needs; expresses desire to enhance awareness of civic and/or government processes that impact public health; expresses desire to enhance health communication with health care providers; expresses desire to enhance knowledge of current determinants of health on social and physical environments; expresses desire to enhance personal health care decision-making; expresses desire to enhance social support for health; expresses desire to enhance understanding of customs and beliefs to

• = Independent                    ▲ = Collaborative

make health care decisions; expresses desire to enhance understanding of health information to make health care choices; expresses desire to obtain sufficient information to navigate the health care system

## Client Outcomes

**Client Will (Specify Time Frame)**

- Use reputable information sources
- Seek information from health care providers
- Communicate with health care provider about understanding of information provided

## Nursing Interventions

▲ Work collaboratively with multiprofessional groups to create and maintain health-literate health care organizations.
- Use a standard tool to identify the level of health literacy.
- Identify and take into consideration factors affecting health literacy such as age, ethnicity, education, and cognitive function.
- Implement health literacy universal precautions: assume that all clients may have difficulty understanding health information.
- Tailor health teaching and educational materials to accommodate the needs of those with low health literacy.
- Modify health teaching and educational materials to client preferences.
- Use empowerment to enhance health literacy and improve client outcomes.

### Geriatric

- The previous interventions may be adapted for geriatric use.
- Assess health literacy as it relates to health perceptions in older adults.
- Use simple educational materials targeted at health-promoting behaviors.

### Multicultural

- Take the client's culture into account when designing teaching and educational materials.
- Use educational strategies targeted at both the individual and the community.

### Client/Family Teaching and Discharge Planning

- Promote shared decision-making.

# Risk for Impaired Liver Function

**Domain 2** Nutrition   **Class 4** Metabolism

## NANDA-I Definition

Susceptible to a decrease in liver function, which may compromise health.

• = Independent          ▲ = Collaborative

## Risk Factors

Substance misuse

## Associated Conditions

Human immunodeficiency virus (HIV) coinfection; pharmaceutical preparations; viral infection

## Client Outcomes

### Client Will (Specify Time Frame)

- State the upper limit of the amount of acetaminophen safely taken per day
- Verbalize understanding that over-the-counter (OTC) medications may contain acetaminophen (e.g., OTC cold medicines)
- Have normal liver enzymes, serum and urinary bilirubin levels, white blood cell count, and red blood cell count
- Be free of unexplained weight loss, jaundice, pruritus, bruising, petechiae, gastrointestinal bleeding, and hemorrhage
- Be free of abdominal tenderness/pain, increased abdominal girth, and have normal colored stool and urine
- Be able to eat frequent small meals per day without nausea and/or vomiting
- If alcohol abuse is factor, state relationship between abuse and worsening gastrointestinal and liver disease

## Nursing Interventions

▲ Assess for signs of liver dysfunction including fatigue, nausea, jaundice of the eyes or skin, pruritus, gastrointestinal bleeding, coagulopathy, infections, increasing abdominal girth, fluid overload, shortness of breath, mental status changes, light-colored stools, dark urine, and increased serum and urinary bilirubin levels.

▲ Evaluate liver function tests. Standard liver panels include the serum enzymes aspartate transaminase (AST), alanine transaminase (ALT), alkaline phosphatase, and γ-glutamyl transferase; total, direct, and indirect serum bilirubin; and serum albumin.

▲ Discuss with the client/family preparations for other diagnostic studies, such as ultrasound, computed tomography, and magnetic resonance imaging (MRI) examinations.

▲ Evaluate coagulation studies such as international normalized ratio, prothrombin time, and partial thromboplastin time, especially when there is bleeding of the mouth or gums. Prolonged prothrombin time and decreased production of clotting factors can result in bleeding.

- Monitor for signs of hemorrhage, especially in the upper gastrointestinal tract, because it is the most frequent site.

• = Independent          ▲ = Collaborative

- Obtain a list of all medications, including OTC nonsteroidal antiinflammatory drugs, acetaminophen, herbal remedies, and dietary supplements. Review risk of drug-induced liver disease. The list includes some antibiotics, anticonvulsants, antidepressants, antiinflammatory drugs, antiplatelets, antihypertensives, calcium channel blockers, cyclosporine, lipid-lowering drugs, chemotherapy drugs, immunotherapy drugs, oral hypoglycemics, proton pump inhibitors, inhaled anesthetics, and tranquilizers, among others (Hamilton, Collins-Yoder, & Collins, 2016; Suzman et al, 2018). If client is taking either OTC medications or herbals, discuss signs and symptoms of toxic hepatitis.
- ▲ For clients receiving drugs associated with liver injury, review risk factors to prevent potentially severe drug reactions.
- ▲ Determine the total amount of acetaminophen the client is taking per day. The amount of acetaminophen ingested should not exceed 3.25 g/day, or even lower in the client with chronic alcohol intake (Hamilton, Collins-Yoder, & Collins, 2016).
- ▲ Evaluation of acetaminophen-associated drug-induced liver injury is done by client history of ingestion, time, and doses of the medication per weight calculation and serum level of acetaminophen.
- ▲ If the client is on statin medications, ensure that liver enzyme testing is done at intervals. Liver enzymes can become elevated from taking statin medications; it is rare but possible for statins to cause actual liver damage (Hamilton, Collins-Yoder, & Collins, 2016).
- ▲ If the client is an alcoholic, refer to a cessation program. It is essential the client stop drinking as soon as possible to allow the liver to heal. Alcoholism is associated with malnutrition, which is harmful to the liver (Fabrellas, 2017). Alcoholism is also associated with increased plasma endotoxins and disruption of the gut barrier, which cause inflammation and resultant damage to the liver (Cassard, Gérard, & Perlemuter, 2017). See care plans for Ineffective **Denial** and Dysfunctional **Family** Processes.
- ▲ Provide frequent smaller meals for easier digestion. Provide diet with optimal carbohydrates, proteins, and fats. Consult with a registered dietitian to discuss best nutritional support.
- ▲ Recognize that severe malnutrition may result in acute liver failure, which is reversible with improved nutrition.
- ▲ Review medical history with the client, recognizing that obesity and type 2 diabetes, along with hypertriglyceridemia and polycystic ovarian syndrome, are major risk factors in the development of liver disease, specifically nonalcoholic fatty liver disease.

• = Independent          ▲ = Collaborative

- Encourage vaccinations for hepatitis A and B for all ages.
- Measure abdominal girth if individual presents with abdominal distention and pain.
- Assess for tenderness and/or pain level in the right upper quadrant. Tenderness in this area is a symptom of biliary, liver, and/or pancreatic problems.
- Use standard precautions for handling of blood and body fluids. Review sterile techniques when giving intravenous solution and/or medications.
▲ Observe for signs and symptoms of mental status changes such as confusion from encephalopathy.

**Pediatric/Parents**

▲ Prescreen pregnant women for hepatitis B surface antigens. If found, recommend nursing case management during pregnancy.
▲ Recommend implementation of postexposure prophylaxis, including the hepatitis B virus vaccine for an infant born to a hepatitis B surface antigen–positive woman (CDC, 2020h).
- Encourage vaccinations for hepatitis A and B for all ages.
▲ Recognize that children can develop fatty liver disease, which can result in liver failure. Most children are asymptomatic, but others complain of malaise, fatigue, or vague recurrent abdominal pain. The development of NAFLD may be affected by perinatal and in utero stressors, with increased sensitivity to environmental and genetic factors (Goldner & Lavine, 2020).
▲ During a well-baby visit, assess for signs of potential liver problems. Observe for prolonged jaundice, pale stools, and urine that is anything other than colorless. Consult with health care provider to order a split bilirubin as needed (CDC, 2020h).

**Home Care**

- Encourage rest, optimal nutrition (high carbohydrates, sufficient protein, and essential vitamins and minerals) during initial inflammatory processes of the liver.
- The COVID-19 pandemic has increased the need for home care, telemedicine, and telephone visits for clients with chronic liver disease. Prioritization of client care is indicated, including transplantation, diagnostic evaluations, and hospitalization, with consideration for clients with NAFLD or NASH at higher risk for severity related to COVID-19 infections due to comorbidities (Boettler et al, 2020).
- Consider referral to palliative care for clients with end-stage liver disease.

• = Independent          ▲ = Collaborative

### Client/Family Teaching and Discharge Planning

- Teach the client and family to examine all medications the client is taking, looking for acetaminophen as an ingredient, and reinforce the 3.25-g upper limit of intake of acetaminophen to protect liver function (Hamilton, Collins-Yoder, & Collins, 2016).
- For the caregiver or client with hepatitis A, B, or C, teach the need for careful handwashing, use of gloves, and other precautions to prevent spread of any of these diseases.
- Teach avoidance of high-risk behaviors that cause hepatitis and ways to avoid those behaviors.
- For clients with chronic liver disease, provide education and support on lifestyle changes to prevent or delay disease progression. Structured follow-up may minimize readmission to the hospital (Hjorth et al, 2018).
- Educate clients and their caregivers about treatment options and interventions for hepatitis. Recommend other informational support: risk factors, side effects of the different treatment options, and dietary advice.
- Recommend psychological support if possible during education sessions.
- Assess for adherence to antiviral therapies for the treatment of hepatitis and institute nursing interventions such as client education, communication, and reminder tools to assist clients in medication adherence.
- For those clients with mental health problems, collaborate with outreach programs to teach signs/symptoms of hepatitis, risk factors, and factors that increase transmission.

## Risk for Loneliness

**Domain 12** Comfort    **Class 3** Social comfort

### NANDA-I Definition

Susceptible to experiencing discomfort associated with a desire or need for more contact with others, which may compromise health.

### Risk Factors

Affectional deprivation; emotional deprivation; physical isolation; social isolation

### Client Outcomes

**Client Will (Specify Time Frame)**

- Maintain one or more meaningful relationships (growth-enhancing versus codependent or abusive in nature)

• = Independent          ▲ = Collaborative

- Sustain relationships that allow self-disclosure and demonstrate a balance between emotional dependence and independence
- Participate in personally meaningful activities and interactions that are ongoing, positive, and relevant socially
- Demonstrate positive use of time alone when socialization is not possible

## Nursing Interventions

- Assess the client's perception of loneliness. (Is the person alone by choice, or are there other factors that contribute to the feelings of loneliness? Is the client in one of the at-risk populations for loneliness?)
- Assess the client's needs through mapping to assess existing networks, current activities, and the impact on well-being.
- Assess the client for signs of emotional distress.
- ▲ Assess the bereaved client for risk of suicide and make appropriate referrals as necessary.
- Evaluate the client's desire for social interaction.
- Teach the client problem-focused coping strategies.

### Pediatric

- Evaluate peer relationships.
- Encourage relationships with peers and involvement with groups and organizations.
- Encourage organized activity (OA) participation for adolescent clients with a diagnosis of autism spectrum disorder.
- ▲ Refer parents of disabled or seriously ill children to support groups.

### Geriatric

- Identify risk factors for loneliness in older persons.
- Practice laughter therapy with the client through laughter exercises or other humorous activities.
- Consider use of technology, such as computers, video conferencing, the Internet, and apps to alleviate or reduce loneliness or social isolation among older adults.
- Engage the client in positive reminiscence.
- Consider telephone outreach for isolated older individuals.
- ▲ Refer client to horticulture therapy.
- ▲ Refer client to pet therapy or consider pet ownership if feasible.
- Encourage support for the client when the decision to stop driving must be made.

### Multicultural

- The preceding interventions may be adapted for diverse clients. Refer to the care plan for **Social** Isolation.

• = Independent          ▲ = Collaborative

- Use a person-centered, biopsychosocial, health-focused approach to incorporate and address social determinants of health.

**Home Care**

▲ The preceding interventions may be adapted for home care use.

▲ Assess for depression with the lonely older client and make appropriate referrals.

- If the client has unexplained somatic complaints, evaluate these complaints to ensure that the client's physical needs are being met and assess for a possible relationship between somatic complaints and loneliness.

- Assist clients to interact with neighbors in the community when they move to supported housing.

- Refer to the care plan for **Social** Isolation.

**Client/Family Teaching and Discharge Planning**

- Provide appropriate education for clients and their support persons about disease transmission and treatment if applicable.

- Refer to the care plan for **Social** Isolation for additional interventions.

# Ineffective Lymphedema Self-Management

**Domain 4** Activity/rest     **Class 4** Cardiovascular/pulmonary responses

## NANDA-I Definition

Unsatisfactory management of symptoms, treatment regimen, physical, psychosocial, and spiritual consequences and lifestyle changes inherent in living with edema related to obstruction or disorders of lymph vessels or nodes.

## Defining Characteristics

### Lymphedema Signs

Fibrosis in affected limb; recurring infections; swelling in affected limb

### Lymphedema Symptoms

Expresses dissatisfaction with quality of life; reports feeling of discomfort in affected limb; reports feeling of heaviness in affected limb; reports feeling of tightness in affected limb

### Behaviors

Average daily physical activity is less than recommended for age and gender; inadequate manual lymph drainage; inadequate protection of affected area; inappropriate application of nighttime bandaging; inappropriate diet; inappropriate skin care; inappropriate use of compression garments; inattentive to carrying heavy objects; inattentive to extreme temperatures;

• = Independent          ▲ = Collaborative

inattentive to lymphedema signs; inattentive to lymphedema symptoms; inattentive to sunlight exposure; reduced range of motion of affected limb; refuses to apply night-time bandages; refuses to use compression garments

## Related Factors

Competing demands; competing lifestyle preferences; conflict between health behaviors and social norms; decreased perceived quality of life; difficulty accessing community resources; difficulty managing complex treatment regimen; difficulty navigating complex health care systems; difficulty with decision-making; inadequate commitment to a plan of action; inadequate health literacy; inadequate knowledge of treatment regimen; inadequate number of cues to action; inadequate role models; inadequate social support; limited ability to perform aspects of treatment regimen; low self efficacy; negative feelings toward treatment regimen; neurobehavioral manifestations; nonacceptance of condition; perceived barrier to treatment regimen; perceived social stigma associated with condition; unrealistic perception of seriousness of condition; unrealistic perception of susceptibility to sequelae; unrealistic perception of treatment benefit

## At-Risk Population

Adolescents; children; economically disadvantaged individuals; individuals with history of ineffective health self-management; individuals with limited decision making experience; individuals with low educational level; older adults

## Associated Conditions

Chemotherapy; chronic venous insufficiency; developmental disabilities; infections; invasive procedure; major surgery; neoplasms; obesity; radiotherapy; removal of lymph nodes; trauma

## Client Outcomes

### Client Will (Specify Time Frame)

- Monitor skin firmness of affected area
- Report numbness of affected area
- Report redness of affected area
- Report pain
- Report feelings of anxiety and/or depression

## Nursing Interventions

- Recognize individual client risk factors for development of immediate or delayed lymphedema and assess at-risk clients at each visit to promote early identification.
- At each visit, ask clients if they are experiencing any early symptoms of lymphedema, including swelling or a sense of heaviness, fullness, tightness, or pain in the at-risk limb. Assess signs of lymphedema, including observation of swelling, pitting, or fibrosis.

• = Independent          ▲ = Collaborative

- Perform detailed medication reconciliation, consider medications that may exacerbate lymphedema symptoms, and review concerning medications with client and ordering provider.
- Assess the client's skin and understanding of skin self-care regimen. Demonstrate and instruct the client in meticulous skin care in the at-risk limb.
- Review the client's dietary habits and encourage a healthy diet.
- If the client has experienced symptoms of lymphedema, assess the frequency, severity, and impact on activities of daily living, pain, range of motion, and strength. Inspect the at-risk limb for signs or symptoms of infection.
- Refer the client with lymphedema to a trained lymphedema specialist, if available.
- When possible, assist the client in establishing baseline limb measurements for comparison with subsequent posttreatment and interval measures. Advocate for client access to a trained lymphedema specialist, if available.
- Assess the client for psychosocial distress, including anxiety, depression, fear of cancer recurrence, body image disturbance, difficulty coping, financial challenges, and changes in sexuality. In cancer clients and survivors, use of a validated psychosocial screening tool may facilitate screening and assessment.
- Connect the client with appropriate, individualized resources and referrals for any psychosocial distress identified. For example, a client struggling to cope with adherence to self-management may benefit from motivational interviewing, whereas a client suffering from lymphedema-related body image disturbance may wish to connect with a lymphedema support group.
- Explore any client beliefs, priorities, support, and financial resources that may affect client's adherence to lymphedema self-management plan.
- Provide individualized lymphedema teaching, including basic explanation of the lymphatic system, personal risk factors, signs and symptoms of lymphedema, self-management, treatments, and potential psychosocial concerns.
- Confirm fit and demonstrate donning/doffing of compression garments and devices, when applicable. Assist the client with obtaining ordered compression garments and devices and connect client with referrals and resources to address client financial responsibility.
- Demonstrate self-massage and exercises (typically a combination of resistance and strength training) to promote lymphatic drainage, as

• = Independent          ▲ = Collaborative

instructed by a provider or lymphedema specialist. In postoperative clients at risk for lymphedema, delay start of exercises for 7 days or until cleared by the surgeon and lymphedema specialist.
• Provide dietary teaching.
• Assess impact of lymphedema on client's physiological, functional, and occupational status. Consider limitations in activities of daily living and work limitations, when appropriate.
• If lymphedema symptoms worsen or fail to improve with intervention, assess client's understanding of and adherence to treatment plan. Consider approaches to improve client adherence to self-management and health-promoting behaviors (e.g., motivational interviewing).
• Support client-provider interactions to identify some form of appropriate, active lymphedema treatment plan (e.g., complete decongestive therapy, resistance training, surgery) in addition to self-management if lymphedema cannot be managed by self-care alone.

**Pediatrics and Adolescents**
• Support caregivers of children and adolescents with lymphedema by teaching self-management techniques to both the child and caregiver, using flexible and individualized approaches, and addressing caregiver fears and anxiety over the child's health condition.

**Multicultural**
• In Latina cancer survivors, family involvement, peer-mentoring, culturally competent education, and self-care skills are important additions to the client's lymphedema self-management plan.

**Client/Family Teaching and Discharge Planning**
• Encourage the client to inform health care providers of any history of lymphedema, procedures that increase lymphedema risk, and contraindications against venipuncture or blood pressure in the at-risk/affected limb.
• Instruct the client to take medication only as ordered and review all medications with health care providers.
• Teach the client to self-monitor and report early signs or symptoms of lymphedema (e.g., swelling, fullness, tightness, heaviness, or pain in the at-risk limb).
• Instruct the client to observe the at-risk limb for signs of infection, including fever, warmth, redness, or swelling, and immediately report these to a health care provider if they occur.
• Teach meticulous skin care in the at-risk limb, including keeping skin clean and dry; applying lotion; using an electric razor versus a razor blade to shave; avoiding exposure of the limb to excessive heat, cold, or direct sunlight; and protecting skin from injury.

• = Independent    ▲ = Collaborative

- Emphasize the importance of regular exercise in reducing lymphedema risk and severity.
- Encourage the client to discuss any psychosocial concerns related to lymphedema, including anxiety, depression, body image disturbance, difficulty coping, financial challenges, and changes in sexuality.

# Risk for Ineffective Lymphedema Self-Management

**Domain 4** Activity/rest   **Class 4** Cardiovascular/pulmonary responses

## NANDA-I Definition

Susceptible to unsatisfactory management of symptoms, treatment regimen, physical, psychosocial, and spiritual consequences and lifestyle changes inherent in living with edema related to obstruction or disorders of lymph vessels or nodes which may compromise health.

## Related Factors

Competing demands; competing lifestyle preferences; conflict between health behaviors and social norms; decreased perceived quality of life; difficulty accessing community resources; difficulty managing complex treatment regimen; difficulty navigating complex health care systems; difficulty with decision-making; inadequate commitment to a plan of action; inadequate health literacy; inadequate knowledge of treatment regimen; inadequate number of cues to action; inadequate role models; inadequate social support; limited ability to perform aspects of treatment regimen; low self efficacy; negative feelings toward treatment regimen; neurobehavioral manifestations; nonacceptance of condition; perceived barrier to treatment regimen; perceived social stigma associated with condition; unrealistic perception of seriousness of condition; unrealistic perception of susceptibility to sequelae; unrealistic perception of treatment benefit

## At-Risk Population

Adolescents; children; economically disadvantaged individuals; individuals with history of ineffective health self-management; individuals with limited decision making experience; individuals with low educational level; older adults

## Associated Conditions

Chemotherapy; chronic venous insufficiency; developmental disabilities; infections; invasive procedure; major surgery; neoplasms; obesity; radiotherapy; removal of lymph nodes; trauma

## Client Outcomes and Nursing Interventions

Refer to care plan for Ineffective **Lymphedema** Self-Management.

• = Independent          ▲ = Collaborative

# Risk for Disturbed Maternal–Fetal Dyad

**Domain 8** Sexuality    **Class 3** Reproduction

## NANDA-I Definition

Susceptible to a disruption of the symbiotic mother-fetal relationship as a result of comorbid or pregnancy-related conditions, which may compromise health.

## Risk Factors

Inadequate prenatal care; substance misuse; unaddressed abuse

## Associated Conditions

Compromised fetal oxygen transport; glucose metabolism disorders; pregnancy complication; treatment regimen

## Client Outcomes

### Client Will (Specify Time Frame)

**During Pregnancy**

- Attend all scheduled prenatal visits and attend prenatal education either virtual or in person with significant other or involved family member
- Cope with fears and discomforts of high-risk pregnancy until delivery of baby
- Demonstrate emotional attachment to fetus during pregnancy
- Adhere to prescribed regimens to maintain homeostasis during pregnancy

## Nursing Interventions

**Prenatal**

- Encourage early prenatal care and regular prenatal visits.
- Determine the presence of medical factors that are related to poor pregnancy outcome (e.g., diabetes, hypertension, lupus erythematosus, herpes, hepatitis, HIV, multiple gestation, substance abuse, epilepsy, infection); provide educational materials that address the risk factors and usual surveillance tests and procedures.
- Assess the antenatal client for fear related to high-risk pregnancy and fetal outcomes.
- Assess antepartum clients for depression using a culturally competent tool that evaluates the bio-psycho-social-spiritual dimensions.
- Focus on the abilities of a pregnant woman with disabilities by encouraging identification of support systems, resources, and need for environmental modification.
- Assess for lack of social support system, loneliness, depression, lack of confidence, maternal powerlessness, domestic violence, and socioeconomic problems.

• = Independent          ▲ = Collaborative

- Identify patterns of intimate partner violence in all pregnant and postpartum women.
- Perform accurate blood pressure readings at each client's clinic encounter.
- Provide educational materials and support for personal autonomy about genetic counseling and testing options before pregnancy with preimplantation genetic testing or during pregnancy with fetal nuchal translucency ultrasound, quadruple screen, and cystic fibrosis screening.
- Ensure that pregnant clients have an adequate diet and take multimicronutrient supplements containing at least 400 µg of folic acid, especially during early pregnancy.
- Provide pregnant women diagnosed with gestational diabetes with education about management and treatment.
- Assess use of tobacco and, if positive for use, offer a tobacco cessation program and explain the health risks to the unborn fetus and mother.
- Assess for alcohol misuse and counsel women to stop drinking during pregnancy. Provide appropriate referral for treatment as needed.
- Screen for current illicit drug use. Emphasize the risks of drug exposure to the fetus/newborn and the potential for withdrawal.
- Refer clients who self-report drug misuse or have positive toxicology screens to a comprehensive treatment program designed for the pregnant woman.
- Encourage pregnant women to use digital resources, such as Text4Baby (see https://www.text4baby.org) or https://www.whattoexpect.com, to track pregnancy progress and provide education and motivation to make healthy lifestyle choices.

**Multicultural**
**Prenatal**
- Assess the client's beliefs and concerns about pregnancy.

## Impaired Memory

**Domain 5** Perception/cognition   **Class 4** Cognition
### NANDA-I Definition
Persistent inability to remember or recall bits of information or skills, while maintaining the capacity to independently perform activities of daily living.
### Defining Characteristics
Consistently forgets to perform a behavior at the scheduled time; difficulty acquiring a new skill; difficulty acquiring new information; difficulty

recalling events; difficulty recalling factual information; difficulty recalling familiar names; difficulty recalling familiar objects; difficulty recalling familiar words; difficulty recalling if a behavior was performed; difficulty retaining a new skill; difficulty retaining new information

## Related Factors

Depressive symptoms; inadequate intellectual stimulation; inadequate motivation; inadequate social support; social isolation; water-electrolyte imbalance

## At-Risk Population

Economically disadvantaged individuals; individuals aged 60 years; individuals with low educational level

## Associated Conditions

Anemia; brain hypoxia; cognition disorders

## Client Outcomes

### Client Will (Specify Time Frame)

- Demonstrate use of techniques to help with memory loss
- State he or she has improved memory for everyday concerns

## Nursing Interventions

- Determine whether onset of memory loss is gradual or sudden; if sudden, screen for delirium using the Confusion Assessment Method (CAM) (see digital resources).
- Assess overall cognitive function and memory. A brief screening instrument such as the short Montreal Cognitive Assessment (s-MoCA) or Revised Metamemory in Adulthood (MIA) Questionnaire (MIA-Revised) is useful as a first level of evaluation.
- Assess risk of B-vitamin deficiencies, including thiamine (vitamin $B_1$), associated with aging, chronic alcohol abuse, cancer, or bariatric surgery, and encourage a diet plan with adequate B vitamins.
- Assess risk of vitamin D deficiency associated with history of inadequate exposure to sunlight and associated with depression and impaired cognitive function in older adults.
- Determine the client's sleep quality and patterns; if sleep quantity and quality are insufficient and client shows symptoms of daytime sleepiness, or symptoms of sleep apnea are present, report to physician/primary care provider and refer to the care plan for Disturbed **Sleep** Pattern.
- Teach clients, including those with cognitive disorders, to use memory techniques such as concentrating and attending, repeating information, making mental associations, and placing items in strategic places so that they will not be forgotten.

• = Independent ▲ = Collaborative

- Encourage the client to incorporate daily meditation such as multimodal Kirtan Kriya or other mind-body interventions to improve memory functioning and health.
▲ Where available, refer for access to computer-based cognitive training or socially assistive robots.
▲ Where available and of interest to client, refer for regular yoga training and practice.
▲ Where available and of interest to client, refer for participation in calligraphy classes.
▲ Refer the client for participation in a multicomponent cognitive rehabilitation program that includes stress and relaxation training, physical activity, structured learning, and social interaction.
- For clients with memory impairments associated with dementia, also see care plan for Chronic **Confusion.**

**M**

### Geriatric
- All interventions are appropriate for geriatric clients.
- Assess for signs and symptoms of depression using an age-appropriate screening tool such as the Geriatric Depression Scale, and notify provider of results.

### Multicultural
- When using cognitive assessments translated into other languages, refer to translation-specific scoring instructions and any recommended adjustment for low levels of education.
- Visitation facilitation: stigma may result in social isolation, and older adults with memory impairment may need assistance to rebuild and strengthen their social network.

### Home Care
- The previously mentioned interventions may be adapted for home care use.
- Assist clients to select and use cuing strategies or assistive technology, such as a smart watch, smart phone, pill box, calendar, alarm clock, microwave oven, whistling tea kettle, sign, or written list, to cue behaviors at designated times.

### Client/Family Teaching and Discharge Planning
- Evaluate the need for skilled home health care (skilled nursing, occupational therapy).
- Discuss and assist with use of assistive technology to support client and caregiver with discharge plan: memory aids (e.g., medication reminders, pill box, timers, lists); orientation aids (e.g., electronic clocks and calendars, voice assistant, built-in "Remember This" feature); safety devices (e.g., nightlights, personal alarms);

communication aids (e.g., easy-to-use landline and mobile phones, speed dialing, voice-activated dialing, or photo dialing); other devices (e.g., easy-to-use TV remote controls, microwave oven, whistling tea kettle).

- Clarify instructions for medications, treatments, and exercises in writing.
- Assist with developing schedule/chart and reminder system for scheduled and as-needed medications and use of nonpharmacological strategies.

# Risk for Metabolic Syndrome

**Domain 2** Nutrition    **Class 4** Metabolism

## NANDA-I Definition

Susceptible to developing a cluster of symptoms that increase risk of cardiovascular disease and type 2 diabetes mellitus, which may compromise health.

## Risk Factors

Absence of interest in improving health behaviors; average daily physical activity is less than recommended for age and gender; body mass index above normal range for age and gender; excessive accumulation of fat for age and gender; excessive alcohol intake; excessive stress; inadequate dietary habits; inadequate knowledge of modifiable factors; inattentive to second-hand smoke; smoking

## At-Risk Population

Individuals aged >30 years; individuals with family history of diabetes mellitus; individuals with family history of dyslipidemia; individuals with family history of hypertension; individuals with family history of metabolic syndrome; individuals with family history of obesity; individuals with family history of unstable blood pressure

## Associated Conditions

Hyperuricemia; insulin resistance; polycystic ovary syndrome

## Client Outcomes

Client Will (Specify Time Frame)

- Maintain blood glucose within normal limits
- Explain actions and precautions to decrease cardiovascular risk
- Maintain waist circumference of less than 102 cm (40 inches) in men, or less than 88 cm (35 inches) in women
- Explain the risk factors associated with lipid disorders

• = Independent        ▲ = Collaborative

- Maintain normal laboratory results, specifically high-sensitivity C-reactive protein, triglycerides, fasting blood glucose, and high-density lipoprotein (HDL) cholesterol
- Design lifestyle modifications to meet individual long-term goal of health, using effective risk control strategies
- Maintain weight within normal range for height and age
- Develop a system of self-management for improved dietary intake and physical activity

### Nursing Interventions

- Assess for risk factors associated with metabolic syndrome. Risk factors for metabolic syndrome include central obesity, dyslipidemia, insulin resistance, and increased blood pressure.
- Assess clients for elevated waist circumference measures; greater than 102 cm/40 inches or more in men, or greater than 88 cm/35 inches or more in women.
- Assess clients for problematic eating behaviors and relationship with food.
- Assess for metabolic syndrome in adults with intellectual disabilities.
- Examine the client's skin for acanthosis nigricans, acrochordons, keratosis pilaris, hyperandrogenism, and hirsutism, which are skin diseases associated with insulin resistance and obesity.
- Assess and report abnormal laboratory results, specifically high-sensitivity C-reactive protein, triglycerides, fasting blood glucose, and HDL cholesterol.
- Screen clients who are prescribed antipsychotic medications for metabolic syndrome during routine health treatment.
- Screen clients with a family history of polycystic ovary syndrome for metabolic syndrome.
- Assist obese clients to develop a system of self-management, which may include self-monitoring of weight, body mass index (BMI), realistic goal setting, planning, and action planning for improved dietary intake and physical activity; problem-solving; and tracking dietary intake and exercise.
- Encourage strength training for the client to address modifiable risk factors of metabolic syndrome.
- Provide nutritional teaching targeted at reducing daily energy, fat intakes, and sugar intakes, and increasing the frequency of eating two portions of vegetables during each meal.
- Encourage the client to engage in vigorous-intensity physical activity for at least 150 minutes weekly or moderate-intensity physical activity for at least 300 minutes weekly to improve cardiorespiratory fitness and influence body shape and weight.

- Counsel clients to slow the pace of their eating during meals.
- Provide teaching about reducing intake of ultra-processed foods and increasing intake of minimally processed foods.
- Encourage once or more weekly consumption of lean fish.
- Use social media for communication with clients to implement social support and share information about lifestyle modifications.
- Refer clients with Class II and III obesity and diabetes for bariatric surgery consideration.

**Pediatric**
- Assess adolescent clients for vitamin D deficiency with additional screening for prediabetes if deficiencies are found.
- Assess and report uric acid levels in at-risk children.
- Provide preventive interventions for obesity during early childhood.

**Geriatric**
- Many of the preceding interventions also apply.
- Encourage strength training for older women.
- Encourage Tai chi training for older adults.

**Multicultural**
- Use criteria in addition to overweight and obesity when screening for cardiometabolic abnormalities in racial/ethnic minority populations.
- Provide African American women with community-based prevention education targeted toward improving knowledge, reducing clinical risk profiles, adoption of heart-healthy lifestyles, reducing inflammatory burden, and decreasing cardiometabolic risk.
- Provide Hispanic clients at risk of metabolic syndrome with cultural and language appropriate teaching and cooking demonstrations.

**Home Care**
- Previously discussed interventions may be adapted for home care use.
- Screen clients who are cancer caregivers for signs and symptoms of metabolic syndrome.

**Client/Family Teaching and Discharge Planning**
- Many of the preceding interventions involve teaching.
- Work with the family members regarding information on how to identify and reduce risk factors related to metabolic syndrome.

## Impaired Bed Mobility

**Domain 4** Activity/rest    **Class 2** Activity/exercise
**NANDA-I Definition**

Limitation in independent movement from one bed position to another.

• = Independent          ▲ = Collaborative

## Defining Characteristics

Difficulty moving between long sitting and supine positions; difficulty moving between prone and supine positions; difficulty moving between sitting and supine positions; difficulty reaching objects on the bed; difficulty repositing self in bed; difficulty returning to the bed; difficulty rolling on the bed; difficulty sitting on edge of bed; difficulty turning from side to side

## Related Factors

Decreased flexibility; environmental constraints; impaired postural balance; inadequate angle of headboard; inadequate knowledge of mobility strategies; insufficient muscle strength; obesity; pain; physical deconditioning

## At-Risk Population

Children; individuals experiencing prolonged bed rest; individuals in the early postoperative period; older adults

## Associated Conditions

Artificial respiration; critical illness; dementia; drain tubes; musculoskeletal impairment; neurodegenerative disorders; neuromuscular diseases; Parkinson's disease; pharmaceutical preparations; sedation

## Client Outcomes

**Client Will (Specify Time Frame)**

• Demonstrate optimal independence in positioning, exercising, and performing functional activities in bed
• Demonstrate ability to direct others on how to do bed positioning, exercising, and functional activities

## Nursing Interventions

▲ Normal bed mobility includes rolling, bridging, scooting, long sitting, and sitting upright. Begin with the client supine, flat in bed. Promote normal movements that are bilateral, segmental, and well-timed, with set positions using weight-bearing and trunk centering. Consult a physical therapist (PT) for individualized instructions and mobility strategies.
• Choose therapeutic beds and positions based on client's history and risk profile.
   ○ Advocate for specialty beds for bedbound clients incorporating low-air-loss pressure relief, shear reduction with position changes, turn assist, and moisture management.
   ○ Use devices such as trapeze, friction-reducing slide sheets, mechanical lateral transfer aids, or ceiling-mounted or floor lifts to move (rather than drag) clients in bed to prevent injury to caregivers.
   ○ Use a special bed and equipment, such as mattress overlay, sliding/

• = Independent        ▲ = Collaborative

roller board, trapeze, and stirrup with pulley attached to overhead traction system (holds one leg up during peri care).

- Place clients in free-standing or ceiling-mounted lifts with padded slings while changing bed linen.
- Many clients can benefit from a high sitting position to potentially minimize orthostatic intolerance (Khan et al, 2002).
- Assess to determine whether positioning for one condition may negatively affect another; use critical thinking skills for risk–benefit analysis. Use critical thinking to determine when specialty bed surfaces will help protect clients from tissue injury if frequent turning is contraindicated by client instability.
- Elevate head of bed (HOB) to 30 to 45 degrees unless contraindicated, and elevate HOB to 90 degrees during oral intake of fluids, solids, and oral medications.
- Raise HOB to 30 degrees for clients with acute increased intracranial pressure and brain injury. Refer to care plan for Decreased **Intracranial** Adaptive Capacity.
▲ Consult health care provider for HOB elevation for acute stroke and monitor response. Refer to care plan for Decreased **Intracranial** Adaptive Capacity.
- Raise HOB as close to 45 degrees as possible for critically ill ventilated clients to prevent pneumonia (this height may place clients at higher risk for pressure ulcers).
- Assist client with dysphagia to sit as upright as possible for oral intake, including solids, fluids, and oral medications. Refer to care plan for Impaired **Swallowing.**
- Periodically sit client upright as tolerated in bed; dangle client, if vital signs and oxygen saturation levels remain stable.
- To decrease risk of pressure injury, maintain HOB at lowest elevation that is medically possible and raise the foot of the bed to prevent shear-related injury. Assess the client's sacrum, ischial tuberosities, and heels at least every 2 hours.
- Try periods of prone positioning for clients and monitor their tolerance/response.
- Assess client's risk for falls using a valid fall risk assessment tool, such as the Morse Fall Scale (Morse, Tylko, & Dixon, 1987; Dykes, 2020) and implement specific measures to mitigate identified risk factors.
- Beds should be kept locked and in the lowest position when occupied.
▲ Although placing all four bed rails up is considered a form of restraint and requires a provider's prescription, two and even three rails up can be a support for bed mobility (Zhao et al, 2019).

• = Independent        ▲ = Collaborative

- Place frequently used items within client's reach; demonstrate use of call bell (Zhao et al, 2019).
- Use a formalized screening tool to identify clients who are at high risk for deep venous thrombosis (e.g., obesity, cancer diagnosis, pelvic surgery, immobility, prior history of deep vein thrombosis).
▲ Assess for injury associated with thromboembolism prophylaxis and other prescribed treatment (e.g., anticoagulants, compression stockings, elastic leg wraps, sequential compression devices, feet/ankle exercises, and hydration). Refer to care plan for Ineffective Peripheral **Tissue Perfusion.**
- Use a valid and reliable tool to assess a client's risk for pressure injury.
- Implement interventions to prevent pressure ulcers and complications of immobility.
- Refer to care plan for Risk for Impaired **Skin** Integrity.
- Explain importance of avoiding breath-holding (Valsalva maneuver) and straining during bed mobility.
- Reassess pain level, especially before movement and/or exercising, and accept clients' pain ratings and levels they think are appropriate for comfort. Administer analgesics based on clients' pain rating. Refer to Acute **Pain** or Chronic **Pain.**

**Exercise**
- Test strength in bilateral grips, arms at elbow flexion and extension, bilateral arm abduction and adduction, bilateral leg or thigh raise (one at a time in bed or chair), and quadriceps and hamstring strength to extend and flex at knee to assess baseline and interval strength gains.
- Perform passive range of motion (ROM) of three repetitions, at least twice a day, to immobile joints. Perform ROM slowly and rhythmically. Do not range beyond point of pain. Range only to point of resistance in those with loss of sensation and mentation. Fast, jerky ROM increases pain and tone. Slow, rhythmical movements relax/lengthen spastic muscles so they can be ranged further. For clients with neuromuscular conditions, consult with physical therapy for ROM exercises.
- Range or move a hemiplegic arm with the shoulder slightly externally rotated (hand up).
▲ Encourage client's practice of exercises taught by therapists (muscle setting, strengthening, contraction against resistance, and weight lifting).

**Bed Positioning**
- Incorporate the following measures to promote normal tone and prevent complications in clients with neurological impairment:

• = Independent          ▲ = Collaborative

○ Use a flat head pillow when clients are supine. Use a small pillow behind the head and/or between shoulder blades if neck extension occurs to prevent contractures of the cervical spine and abnormal tone of the neck.

○ Abduct the shoulders of clients with high paraplegia or quadriplegia horizontally to 90 degrees briefly two to three times a day while client is supine.

○ Position a hemiplegic shoulder fairly close to the client's body.

• Tilt hemiplegics onto both unaffected and affected sides with the affected shoulder slightly forward (e.g., move/lift the affected shoulder, not the forearm/hand).

▲ Elevate a client's paralyzed forearms on a pillow when client is supine. Elevate edematous legs on a pillow supporting the knees to prevent hyperextension. Apply resting wrist, hand, and foot/ankle splints and pressure garments or other devices as prescribed. Range joints before applying splints. Adhere to on/off schedule as prescribed by the PT. Remove splints and compression garments or devices to check underlying tissues for signs of pressure/poor circulation every 2 hours or more often if client resists or manipulates them.

### Geriatric

• Assess caregiver's strength, health history, and cognitive status to predict ability/risk for assisting bedbound clients at home. Refer to care plan for **Caregiver** Role Strain.

• Assess the client's stamina and energy level during bed activities/exercises; if limited, spread out activities and allow rest breaks.

### Home Care

▲ Collaborate with nurse case managers, care coordinators, social workers, visiting nurses, and physical/occupational therapists to assess home support systems and needs and to provide for home safety and access modifications, durable medical equipment as needed for condition (e.g., bariatric), handling equipment (e.g., friction pads, slide boards, lifts) needed for safe bed mobility, exercise, toileting, and bathing, ramps, rails, assistive technology, and home health follow-up.

• Encourage use of the client's own bed unless contraindicated. Raise HOB with commercial blocks or grooved-out pieces of wood under legs; set bed against walls in a corner. Emotionally, clients may benefit from sleeping in their own beds with familiar partners.

• Stress psychological/physical benefits of clients being as self-sufficient as possible with bed mobility/care even though it may be time-consuming. Allowing independence and autonomy may help prevent disuse syndromes and feelings of helplessness and low self-esteem.

• = Independent          ▲ = Collaborative

- Offer emotional support and help client identify usual coping responses to help with adjustment and loss issues. The home environment may trigger the reality of lost function and disability.
- Discuss support systems available for caregivers to help them cope. Refer to care plan for **Caregiver** Role Strain.
▲ Institute case management for frail older adults to support continued independent living as much as possible or as desired by the client.
- Refer to the home care interventions in the care plan for Impaired Physical **Mobility.**

**Client/Family Teaching and Discharge Planning**

- Teach client/caregivers correct ROM, exercises, positioning, self-care activities, and use of devices. Assess readiness and learning styles, which vary but may be enhanced with visual/auditory/tactile/cognitive stimuli such as the following:
   ○ Demonstrations, sketches, online resources (e.g., YouTube), written directions/schedules, notes
   ○ Verbal instructions, recorded audiotapes, timers, reading written directions aloud, and self-talk during activities
   ○ Motor task practice/repetition, return demonstrations, note taking, manual guidance, or staff's-hand-on-client's-hand technique
   ○ Referral to community group activities, support groups, parish nursing, adaptive recreation, or other out-of-the-home resources
▲ Schedule time with family/caregivers for education and practice for nursing, physical therapy, and occupational therapy. Suggest family come prepared with questions and wear comfortable, safe clothing/shoes. Practice provides opportunity for learning; repetition helps memory retention.
▲ Teach safe approaches for caregivers/home care staff and reinforce an adequate number of people to decrease risk of injury (Olinsky & Norton, 2017).

## Impaired Physical Mobility

**Domain 4** Activity/rest    **Class 2** Activity/exercise
### NANDA-I Definition

Limitation in independent, purposeful movement of the body or of one or more extremities.

### Defining Characteristics

Altered gait; decreased fine motor skills; decreased gross motor skills; decreased range of motion; difficulty turning; engages in substitutions for movement; expresses discomfort; movement-induced tremor; postural

• = Independent            ▲ = Collaborative

instability; prolonged reaction time; slowed movement; spastic movement; uncoordinated movement

**Related Factors**

Anxiety; body mass index >75th percentile appropriate for age and gender; cultural belief regarding acceptable activity; decreased activity tolerance; decreased muscle control; decreased muscle strength; disuse; inadequate environmental support; inadequate knowledge of value of physical activity; insufficient muscle mass; insufficient physical endurance; joint stiffness; malnutrition; neurobehavioral manifestations; pain; physical deconditioning; reluctance to initiate movement; sedentary lifestyle

**Associated Conditions**

Altered bone structure integrity; contractures; depression; developmental disabilities; impaired metabolism; musculoskeletal impairment; neuromuscular diseases; pharmaceutical preparations; prescribed movement restrictions; sensory-perceptual impairment

**Client Outcomes**

**Client Will (Specify Time Frame)**

- Meet mutually defined goals of increased ambulation and exercise that include individual choice, preference, and enjoyment in the exercise prescription
- Describe feeling stronger and more mobile
- Describe less fear of falling and pain with physical activity
- Demonstrate use of adaptive equipment (e.g., wheelchairs, walkers, gait belts, weighted walking vests) to increase mobility
- Increase exercise to 20 minutes/day for those who were previously sedentary (less than 150 minutes/week). Note: Light to moderate intensity exercise may be beneficial in deconditioned persons. In very deconditioned individuals exercise bouts of less than 10 minutes are beneficial
- Increase pedometer step counts with a daily goal for most healthy adults of at least 4400 steps per day (Harvard Women's Health Watch, 2019)
- Perform resistance exercises that involve all major muscle groups (legs, hips, back, chest, abdomen, shoulders, and arms) performed 2 or 3 days/week
- Perform flexibility exercise (stretching) for each of the major muscle-tendon groups 2 days/week for 10 to 60 seconds to improve joint range of motion (ROM); greatest gains occur with daily exercise
- Engage in neuromotor exercise 20 to 30 minutes/day including motor skills (e.g., balance, agility, coordination, gait), proprioceptive exercise training, and multifaceted activities (e.g., Tai chi, yoga) to improve and

• = Independent ▲ = Collaborative

maintain physical function and reduce falls in those at risk for falling (older persons)

- Engage in purposeful moderate-intensity cardiorespiratory (aerobic) exercise for 30 to 60 minutes/day at least 5 days/week for a total of 2 hours and 30 minutes (150 minutes) per week

### Nursing Interventions

- Adults should be as physically active as their abilities allow and avoid inactivity. Use "start low and go slow" approach for intensity and duration of physical activity if client is deconditioned, functionally limited, or has chronic conditions affecting performance of physical tasks. When progressing client's activities, use an individualized and tailored approach based on client's tolerance and preferences (US Department of Health and Human Services, 2018).
- Screen for mobility skills in the following order: (1) bed mobility; (2) dangling and supported and unsupported sitting; (3) weight-bearing for sit to stand, transfer to chair; (4) standing and walking with assistance; and (5) walking independently.
- Assess muscle strength and other factors affecting balance, mobility, and endurance. Immobility can affect tissue perfusion and increase risk of postural hypotension; shortness of breath decreases endurance and increases fear; bowel or bladder incontinence can decrease motivation to be mobile; cognitive and neuromuscular deficits, including side effects of medications that affect balance, coordination, and movement; and pain, fear, or sick role because expectations can decrease willingness to be mobile.
- Assess for fear of falling.
- ▲ Consult physical therapist (PT) for recommendations for assistive devices, such as gait belt, weighted vest, walker, cane, crutches, wheelchair, shower chairs; lifts; lateral transfer devices.
- Refer to care plans for Risk for **Falls,** Acute **Pain,** Chronic **Pain,** Ineffective **Coping,** or **Hopelessness.**
- Increase activity tolerance with graded increases in self-care (function-focused care [FFC]), such as bathing, walking to the bathroom instead of using a bedpan/urinal, and ROM.
- ▲ Before activity, observe for and, if possible, treat pain with massage, heat pack to affected area, or medication.
- Monitor and record the client's response to activity, such as pulse rate, blood pressure, dyspnea, skin color, subjective report. Refer to the care plan for **Activity** Intolerance.

### Special Considerations: Immobility

- Refer to the care plan for Impaired Bed **Mobility.**

• = Independent          ▲ = Collaborative

- Help the client achieve mobility and start walking as soon as possible if not contraindicated.
- Initiate a "no lift" policy where appropriate assistive devices are used for manual lifting. Refer to the care plan for Impaired Bed **Mobility**.

**Other Clinical Conditions**

▲ Osteoarthritis or rheumatoid arthritis: Consult with a physical therapist on ways to integrate aerobic exercise, resistance exercise, and flexibility exercise (stretching) into care.

▲ Cerebrovascular accident (CVA) with hemiparesis: Consult with physical therapist on constraint-induced movement therapy, in which the functional extremity is purposely constrained and the client is forced to use the involved extremity (Wattchow, McDonnell, & Hillier, 2018) or graded motor mirror therapy (Mekonen, 2019).

- If the client does not feed or groom self, sit side by side with the client, put your hand over the client's hand, support the client's elbow with your other hand, and help the client complete these simple movements.

**Geriatric**

- Assess ability to move using valid and reliable criterion-referenced standards for fitness testing that can predict the level of capacity associated with maintaining physical independence into later years of life (e.g., Get Up and Go test).
- Help the mostly immobile client achieve mobility as soon as possible, depending on physical condition.
- Use the FFC rehabilitative philosophy of care in older adults to prevent avoidable functional decline.
- If the client will have elective surgery that will result in immobility, initiate a rehabilitation program with warm-up, aerobic activity, strength, flexibility, neuromotor, and functional task work.
- Use gestures and nonverbal cues when helping clients move if they are anxious or have difficulty understanding and following verbal instructions. Nonverbal gestures are part of a universal language that can be understood when the client is having difficulty with communication.
- Recognize that wheelchairs are not a good mobility device and often serve as a mobility restraint.
- Ensure that chairs fit clients. Chair seat should be 3 inches above the height of the knee. Provide a raised toilet seat if needed. Raising the height of a chair can dramatically improve the ability of many older clients to stand up. Low, deep, soft seats with armrests that are far apart reduce a person's ability to get up and down without help.

• = Independent ▲ = Collaborative

- If the client is mainly immobile, provide opportunities for socialization and sensory stimulation. Refer to the care plan for Deficient **Diversional** Activity.
- Recognize that immobility and a lack of social support and sensory input may result in confusion or depression in older adults. Refer to nursing interventions for Acute **Confusion** or **Hopelessness** as appropriate.

**Home Care**

- All preceding interventions should be applied and used for home care.
- ▲ Begin discharge planning as soon as possible with a personal health navigator (e.g., nurse care coordinator or case manager) to assess need for and arrange home support systems, assistive devices, community or home health services, and provider follow-up.
- ▲ Assess home environment for factors that create barriers to physical mobility. Refer to occupational therapy for home safety evaluation and adaptive technology.
- ▲ Refer to home health services to support the client and family through changing levels of mobility. Reinforce need to promote independence in mobility as tolerated.
- ▲ Refer to home physical therapy for evaluation, gait training, strengthening, and balance training.
- Assess skin condition at every visit. Establish a skin care program that enhances circulation and maximizes position changes. Impaired mobility decreases circulation to dependent areas. Decreased circulation and shearing place the client at risk for skin breakdown.
- Once the client is able to walk independently, suggest that the client enter an exercise program or walk with a friend.
- Provide support to the client and family/caregivers during long-term impaired mobility. Long-term impaired mobility may necessitate role changes within the family and precipitate caregiver stress. Refer to the care plan for **Caregiver** Role Strain.

**Client/Family Teaching and Discharge Planning**

- Consider using motivational interviewing techniques to increase a client's activity. Refer to the care plan for **Sedentary** Lifestyle or Motivational Interviewing.
- Teach the client and caregivers processes and tools used during care to use at home to assess fall risk and promote progressive mobility. Involve them in planning for these activities at home.

• = Independent    ▲ = Collaborative

# Impaired Wheelchair Mobility

**Domain 4** Activity/rest    **Class 2** Activity/exercise

## NANDA-I Definition

Limitation of independent operation of wheelchair within environment.

## Defining Characteristics

Difficulty bending forward to pick up object from the floor; difficulty folding or unfolding wheelchair; difficulty leaning forward to reach for something above head; difficulty locking brakes on manual wheelchair; difficulty maneuvering wheelchair sideways; difficulty moving wheelchair out of an elevator; difficulty navigating through hinged door; difficulty operating battery charger of power wheelchair; difficulty operating power wheelchair on a decline; difficulty operating power wheelchair on an incline; difficulty operating power wheelchair on curbs; difficulty operating power wheelchair on even surface; difficulty operating power wheelchair on uneven surface; difficulty operating wheelchair backwards; difficulty operating wheelchair forward; difficulty operating wheelchair in corners; difficulty operating wheelchair motors; difficulty operating wheelchair on a decline; difficulty operating wheelchair on an incline; difficulty operating wheelchair on curbs; difficulty operating wheelchair on even surface; difficulty operating wheelchair on stairs; difficulty operating wheelchair on uneven surface; difficulty operating wheelchair while carrying an object; difficulty performing pressure relief; difficulty performing stationary wheelie position; difficulty putting feet on the footplates of the wheelchair; difficulty rolling across side-slope while in wheelchair; difficulty selecting drive mode on power wheelchair; difficulty selecting speed on power wheelchair; difficulty shifting weight; difficulty sitting on wheelchair without losing balance; difficulty stopping wheelchair before bumping something; difficulty transferring from wheelchair; difficulty transferring to wheelchair; difficulty turning in place while on wheelie position

## Related Factors

Altered mood; environmental constraints; inadequate adjustment to wheelchair size; inadequate knowledge of wheelchair use; insufficient muscle strength; insufficient physical endurance; neurobehavioral manifestations; obesity; pain; physical deconditioning; substance misuse; unaddressed inadequate vision

## At-Risk Population

Individuals using wheelchair for short time; individuals with history of fall from wheelchair; older adults

## Associated Conditions

Musculoskeletal impairment; neuromuscular diseases; vision disorders

• = Independent          ▲ = Collaborative

**M**

## Client Outcomes

**Client Will (Specify Time Frame)**

- Demonstrate independence in operating and moving a wheelchair or other wheeled device
- Demonstrate ability to direct others in operating and moving a wheelchair or other device
- Demonstrate therapeutic positioning, pressure relief, and safety principles while operating and moving a wheelchair or other wheeled device

## Nursing Interventions

- Assess the client's coccyx and encourage frequent repositioning.
- ▲ Refer to physical and occupational therapy or wheelchair seating clinic. Refer to care plan for Risk for Adult **Pressure Injury**; Risk for Child **Pressure Injury.**
- ▲ Support surfaces on chairs and beds should redistribute pressure and be used for at-risk clients as an adjunct to reduce risk of pressure injury.
- Tilt-in-space chairs are effective at off-loading pressure areas.
- Intervene to maintain continence or use air-permeable absorbent underpads or diapers to help prevent skin breakdown caused by excessive moisture and macerated skin. Some wheelchair cushions have moisture-wicking characteristics.
- Assess client's sitting posture frequently and reposition for alignment. Document specific measures to allow for reproducibility.
- Implement use of friction-coated projection hand rims and leather gloves for clients to propel manual wheelchairs. Friction-coated projection rims are less invasive and slippery than aluminum rims; gloves absorb forces of propulsion and help prevent nerve damage/ carpal tunnel injury.
- Manually guide or explain to the client to push forward on both wheel rims to move ahead, push the right rim to turn left and vice versa, and pull backward on both wheel rims to back up.
- Recommend that clients back wheelchair into an elevator. If entering face first, instruct them to turn chairs around to face the elevator doors and controls.
- ▲ In conjunction with physical therapy for teaching and assessment, reinforce principle of descending a curb backward ("popping a wheelie") if balance, trunk control, strength, and timing are adequate. Backward descent carries less risk of clients losing control and falling forward out of the wheelchair.

• = Independent        ▲ = Collaborative

- Ascend curbs in a forward position by popping a wheelie or having someone aid in tilting the chair back, place front wheels over curb, and roll chair up. If surface is muddy or sandy, ascend backward. Front casters will not roll on soft surfaces; a backward approach requires less energy and prevents getting stuck or falling forward.
- During assisted wheelies, helper must hold wheelchair until all four wheels are back on the ground and client has control of wheelchair. Releasing one's grip too soon may alter client's balance and cause injury.
▲ Follow therapist's recommendations for how clients should propel manual wheelchairs to prevent upper extremity pain and joint degeneration.
- Recognize that ultra-lightweight, push rim–activated, power-assisted, or powered wheelchairs may be indicated. Striking the balance between optimum independence and preventing injury (e.g., rotator cuff injury from years of manual propulsion) is a consideration. Consider push rim–activated power-assisted wheelchairs (manual wheelchairs with a motor linked to the push rim in each rear hub) because they reduce energy needed for propulsion and reserve energy for uneven terrain or obstacle negotiation. Recommend antirollback devices for inclined planes to decrease stress on shoulders.
▲ Reduce floor clutter and establish safety rules for drivers of electric/power mobility devices; make referrals to physical or occupational therapy for driver reevaluations if accidents occur or client's health deteriorates.
- Request and receive client's permission before moving an unoccupied wheelchair. Wheelchair dependent clients may view the chair as part of their identity and independence.
- Reinforce compensatory strategies for unilateral neglect and agnosia (e.g., visual scanning, self-talk, self-questioning as to what could be wrong) as clients propel wheelchair through doorways and around obstacles. Too often nurses physically move the wheelchair or obstacle instead of cueing the client to detect and solve problems. Refer to care plan for **Unilateral Neglect.**
- Offer support to help clients cope with issues related to physical disability. Depression and anxiety may occur with physical loss. Refer to care plan for Ineffective **Role** Performance.
- Provide information on support group and reliable Internet resource options.
- Provide information about advocacy, accessibility, assistive technology, and issues under the Americans with Disabilities Act as Amended (2008) (U.S. Department of Justice, Civil Rights Division, 2020).

**M**

• = Independent          ▲ = Collaborative

▲ Make social service or wheelchair clinic referral to educate clients on financial coverage/regulations of third-party payers and Health Care Financing Association for wheelchairs. It is wise to recognize cost, advantages, and durability of different wheelchair models before purchasing one.

• Recommend that clients test-drive wheelchairs and try out cushions/postural supports with the advice of a qualified seating professional, not a vendor, before purchasing. If a specialty chair is indicated, for example, for sports or outdoor use, having clients test-drive the wheelchair is especially important. Equipment is expensive, and different models have different advantages and disadvantages.

• Optimize nutrition and hydration for skin and tissue health.

**Pediatric**

• Consult physical or occupational therapist for special considerations for wheelchair fitting and positioning for pediatric client.

• Help client/family transition from a manual to a powered wheelchair/scooter if disability is severe.

**Geriatric**

• Avoid using restraints on fidgeting clients who slide down in a wheelchair. Instead, assess for deformities; spinal curvatures; abnormal tone; limited joint range; discomfort from clothing, pressure, or constriction areas; social isolation; and toileting needs.

• Ensure proper seat depth/leg positioning and use custom footrests (not elevated leg rests) to prevent older adults from sliding down in wheelchairs.

▲ Assess for side effects of medications and potential need for dosage readjustments to increase wheelchair tolerance. Give prescribed hydration and medications to treat orthostatic hypotension. Consider leg wraps. Assist client to perform warm-up bed exercises if possible. Cerebral hypoperfusion and prolonged bed rest are common causes of orthostatic intolerance and hypotension. Refer to the care plan for Impaired Bed **Mobility**.

• Allow client to control speed to propel wheelchair independently if possible. Older adults may move slowly because of diminished range of motion/strength, stiff/sore joints, and cardiopulmonary compromise. Observe carefully for fatigue, shoulder pain, or other signs of activity intolerance.

• Assess the client's ability to safely maneuver independently using a wheelchair.

## Home Care

▲ Establish a support system for emergency and contingency care (e.g., remote monitoring, emergency call system, alert local emergency medical system, smart speaker). Wheelchair dependence may be life-threatening during a crisis (e.g., fall, fire, or other environmental emergency).

- Recommend the following changes to the home to accommodate the use of a wheelchair:
  ○ Arrange traffic patterns so they are wide enough to maneuver a wheelchair.
  ○ Recognize that a 5-foot turning space is necessary to maneuver wheelchairs, doorways need to have 32 to 36 inches clear width, and entrance ramps/path slope should be assessed before permanent ramps are installed because standardized slopes may not be appropriate. Temporary ramps are cost-effective and easier to adjust.
  ○ Replace door hardware with fold-back hinges, remove doorway encasements (if too narrow), remove/replace thresholds (if too high), hang wall-mounted sinks/handrails, grade floors in showers for roll-in chairs, and use nonskid/nonslip floor coverings (e.g., nonwaxed wood, linoleum, or Berber carpet).
  ○ Rearrange room functions, furniture, and storage so that toileting, sleeping, bathing, and preparing/eating meals can safely take place on one level of the home.

▲ Request physical and occupational therapy referrals to evaluate wheelchair fitting, skills, safety, and maintenance. Suggest community resources for servicing and tuning up wheelchairs and/or locating parts so clients can service their own chairs; an annual tune-up is recommended.

## Client/Family Teaching and Discharge Planning

▲ Assess pain levels of long-term wheelchair users and make referrals to therapists or wheelchair clinics for modifications as needed. Have client check warranty information for servicing options.

- Instruct and have client return demonstrate reinflation of pneumatic tires; encourage client to monitor tire pressure every 2 to 3 weeks.
- Instruct family/clients to remove large wheelchair parts (leg rests, armrests) when lifting wheelchair into car for transport; when reassembling, check that all parts are fastened securely and temperature is tepid. This reduces weight that needs to be lifted; locked parts and a safe temperature prevent injury/thermal injury.

**M**

• = Independent          ▲ = Collaborative

- Teach the critical importance of using seatbelts and secure chair tie-downs when riding in motor vehicles in a wheelchair. Never transport a client in an unsecured wheelchair in any kind of vehicle or allow this to occur with any method of transport. Teach users and family to check safe tie-downs in any transport vehicle.
- For further information, refer to care plan for Impaired **Transfer** Ability.

# Impaired Mood Regulation

**Domain 9** Coping/stress tolerance    **Class 2** Coping response

### NANDA-I Definition

A mental state characterized by shifts in mood or affect and which is comprised of a constellation of affective, cognitive, somatic, and/or physiologic manifestations varying from mild to severe.

### Defining Characteristics

Altered verbal behavior; appetite change; disinhibition; dysphoria; excessive guilt; excessive self-awareness; flight of thoughts; hopelessness; impaired attention; irritable mood; psychomotor agitation; psychomotor retardation; sad affect; self-blame; social alienation

### Related Factors

Altered sleep-wake cycle; anxiety; difficulty functioning socially; external factors influencing self-concept; hypervigilance; loneliness; pain; recurrent thoughts of death; recurrent thoughts of suicide; social isolation; substance misuse; weight change

### Associated Conditions

Chronic disease; functional impairment; psychosis

### Client Outcomes

**Client Will (Specify Time Frame)**

- State feelings related to changes in mood
- Follow exercise plan
- Have no attempts at self-harm
- Attention during activities
- Have a regular sleep-wake cycle
- Have sense of self-efficacy
- Achieve a mindfulness-based awareness

### Nursing Interventions

- Monitor the client's mood with a rating scale.
- Enable the client to express his or her feelings and try to support the client emotionally if necessary.
- Promote the self-efficacy of the client.

• = Independent          ▲ = Collaborative

- Instill hopefulness in client about regaining his or her health.
- Encourage physical activities.
- Encourage regular physical exercise to increase physical mobility and independence in daily activities.
- Inform clients about the negative effects associated with excessive mobile phone and social media use.
- Avoid circadian rhythm disturbances.
- Encourage the client to practice dance therapy.
- Encourage the client to listen to music when in a negative mood.
▲ Refer to aromatherapy massage.
▲ Refer to cognitive behavior therapy.

# Moral Distress

**Domain 10** Life principles   **Class 3** Value/belief/action congruence

**M**

## NANDA-I Definition

Response to the inability to carry out one's chosen ethical or moral decision and/or action.

## Defining Characteristics

Reports anguish about acting on one's moral choice

## Related Factors

Conflict among decision-makers; difficulty making end-of-life decisions; difficulty making treatment decision; information available for decision making conflicts; time constraint for decision-making; values incongruent with cultural norms

## At-Risk Population

Individuals experiencing loss of personal autonomy; individuals physically distant of decision-maker

## Client Outcomes

**Client Will (Specify Time Frame)**
- Be able to act in accordance with values, goals, and beliefs
- Regain confidence in the ability to make decisions and/or act in accord with values, goals, and beliefs
- Express satisfaction with the ability to make decisions consistent with values, goals, and beliefs
- Have choices respected

## Nursing Interventions

- Assess if moral distress is present and its relationship to intrinsic or extrinsic factors.
- Affirm the distress, commitment "to take care of yourself," and your obligations. Validate feelings and perceptions with others.

• = Independent          ▲ = Collaborative

- Implement strategies to change situations causing moral distress.
- Assess sources and severity of distress.
- Give voice/recognition to moral distress and express concerns about constraints to supportive individuals.
- Engage in healthy problem-solving.
- Engage in multiprofessional problem-solving forums, including family meeting and/or multiprofessional rounds.
- Identify/use a support system.
- Initiate an ethics consultation or ethics committee review.

**Pediatric**
- Consider the developmental age of children when evaluating decisions and conflict.

**Multicultural**
- Acknowledge and understand cultural differences that may influence a client's moral choices.

**Geriatric and Home Care**
- Previous interventions may be adapted for geriatric or home care use.
- Assess for the effect of functional independence.
- Refer to a palliative care team as needed.

# Risk for Dry Mouth

**Domain 11** Safety/projection    **Class 2** Physical injury

## NANDA-I Definition

Susceptible to discomfort or damage to the oral mucosa due to reduced quantity or quality of saliva to moisten the mucosa, which may compromise health.

## Risk Factors

Dehydration; depressive symptoms; excessive stress; excitement; smoking

## At-Risk Population

Pregnant women

## Associated Conditions

Chemotherapy; depression; fluid restriction; inability to feed orally; oxygen therapy; pharmaceutical preparations; radiotherapy to the head and neck; systemic diseases

## Client Outcomes

**Client Will (Specify Time Frame)**
- Maintain intact, moist oral mucous membranes that are free of ulceration, inflammation, infection, and debris
- Demonstrate measures to maintain or regain oral health

• = Independent      ▲ = Collaborative

- Demonstrate oral hygiene knowledge and skills to maintain moisture within the mouth
- Be free of halitosis and oral discomfort
- State tolerable to no changes in taste sensation (dysgeusia)

## Nursing Interventions

- Perform a comprehensive extraoral and intraoral examination for associated conditions and risk factors that reduce quantity or quality of saliva and client complaints of oral dryness and difficulty speaking, eating, or swallowing.
- Assess for symptoms of dry mouth.
- Inspecting and palpating major salivary glands and lymph nodes for masses, enlargement, tenderness, purulent discharge, or absence of salivary pooling/secretions are components of a comprehensive head and neck examination to differentiate between salivary and nonsalivary causes of dry mouth (Plemons, Al-Hashimi, & Marek, 2014).
- Inspect nasal turbinates for enlargement, swelling, polyps, and nasal flow because nasal blockages increase mouth breathing, which may exacerbate oral dryness symptoms.
- Assess client for oral candidiasis, dental caries, and gingival recession (Plemons, Al-Hashimi, & Marek, 2014). Oral candidiasis may suggest the client is immunocompromised or on a treatment that increases the risk of fungal infection, which can lead to additional health care concerns.
- Assess client for dental caries and gingival recession.
- Assess client for difficulty chewing, swallowing (dysphagia), or speaking.
- Assess client for mouth breathing caused by functional impairment of the upper airway and/or presence of nasal, endotracheal, or orogastric tubes that may prevent mouth closure or irritate oral mucosa, which may contribute to an increase in dry mouth symptoms experienced by clients.
- Assess client hydration status. A dry tongue and mucous membranes are symptoms of decreased hydration status. Decreased hydration status can worsen symptoms of dry mouth.
- Assess fluid status because dehydration will also affect salivary flow (Plemons, Al-Hashimi, & Marek, 2014). Consider fluid loss associated with fever, cachexia, vomiting, or diarrhea. Recognize that dehydration is prevalent in older adults and may affect salivary flow (Plemons, Al-Hashimi, & Marek, 2014).

**M**

• = Independent          ▲ = Collaborative

▲ Dry mouth, mouth dryness, or oral dryness (xerostomia) is a dryness of the oral cavity resulting from insufficient or complete lack of saliva secretion. Although dry mouth is a common symptom of salivary gland hyposecretion, there is a distinction between dryness caused by malfunction of the salivary glands and the client's subjective report of oral dryness despite normal salivary gland function (Tanasiewicz, Hildebrandt, & Obersztyn, 2016).

▲ The client may require a dental referral to evaluate salivary flow rate as a tool to monitor dry mouth symptoms (Plemons, Al-Hashimi, & Marek, 2014).

▲ Consider use of oral screening, client self-report tool, and/or subjective questioning regarding dry mouth symptoms to assess client oral health and to predict need for dental intervention and degree of salivary hypofunction.

▲ Use client self-report to measure symptoms of dry mouth.

• Ask the client about symptoms of hyposalivation.

▲ Review client medication usage for dry mouth as a side effect of medication. If symptoms are present consult with provider, or refer client to see a dentist or specialist.

▲ Administer pilocarpine and cevimeline as prescribed because these medications are considered first-line therapy in Sjögren's syndrome and head and neck cancer clients with radiotherapy-induced dry mouth and hyposalivation.

▲ The American Dental Association (ADA) Council on Scientific Affairs report identifies that pilocarpine and cevimeline have US Food and Drug Administration approval for treating dry mouth caused by Sjögren's syndrome or radiation therapy (Plemons, Al-Hashimi, & Marek, 2014).

• Teach clients about conditions that can exacerbate dry mouth symptoms:
   ○ Avoidance of low-humidity environments
   ○ Avoidance of oral irritants: acidic fluids such as carbonated beverages and juices, caffeine, alcohol, tobacco
   ○ Avoidance of salty, spicy, acidic, or high-sucrose content foods
   ○ Avoidance of dry, hard, and sticky foods
   ○ Referral of client to smoking and/or alcohol cessation program

• Teach the client good oral hygiene:
   ○ Twice daily toothbrushing with regular topical fluoride toothpaste.
   ○ Use of soft bristle toothbrush.
   ○ Daily use of dental floss or another interdental cleaner.
   ○ Daily use of alcohol-free mouth rinse.

• = Independent        ▲ = Collaborative

- ○ Recommend use of prescription-strength fluoride toothpastes for severe salivary hypofunction.
- Provide instruction regarding cleaning, and assist with care of dental prosthesis as needed. Daily cleansing of a dental prosthetic is an accepted standard of care to maintain and promote oral health and dentition (ADA, 2020).
- ▲ Provide instruction on candidiasis prevention and control. Administer antifungal topical treatments as prescribed using available suspensions, pastilles, and lozenges for uncomplicated oral candidiasis. Systemic antifungal agents may be prescribed for complicated candidiasis mucosal infection (Baer & Sankar, 2020).
- ▲ Soak partial or complete dental prosthesis overnight in 0.2% chlorhexidine HCl.
- ▲ Recommend professional dental oral examination every 3 to 6 months. Recommend professional teeth cleaning at least every 6 months.
- Discuss selection and use of salivary substitutes with client and health care provider to assist in maintaining mouth moisture.
- Teach the client that any topical product that is acidic or contains sugar, or noted as sugarless with high fructose, should be avoided.
- Encourage the client to try several products, based on client preference, to find a suitable saliva substitute. Clients reported that use of saliva substitutes may be more helpful before sleep because of diurnal variation on reduction in salivary flow at night. It is also suggested that clients mix and match salivary agents based on their daily schedules or activities such as eating or public speaking (Baer & Sankar, 2020).
- Lubricate lips every 2 hours, while awake, and as needed. Apply moisturizer (e.g., lanolin) to dry lips every 2 hours, as needed to assist with dryness.
- Teach clients preventive measures to reduce oral dryness:
  - ○ Maintain adequate oral hydration by sipping water regularly and/or sucking on ice chips (AAOM, 2016).
  - ○ While eating, drink fluids carefully.
  - ○ Maintain an oral intake log.
  - ○ Rinse with normal saline or clean water as a part of daily oral care to prevent dry mouth, or sodium bicarbonate solution (1 teaspoon salt and 1 teaspoon baking soda to 1 L of water).
- Encourage the client to use sugar-free gum or sugar-free candy to promote salivary flow.

• = Independent          ▲ = Collaborative

- Encourage the client to use saline nasal sprays to maintain open nasal passages.
- The client may find the use of a humidifier during sleep at night helpful in reducing symptoms.
- ▲ Discuss with the client the use of acupuncture, electrical nerve stimulation, and powered versus manual toothbrushes to assist in maintaining mouth moisture.
- ▲ Encourage the client to discuss the use of emerging preventive treatments with the health care provider such as gene therapy, tissue engineering, stem cell therapy, and growth factors for etiologies associated with dry mouth.
- ▲ Discuss use of bethanechol HCl saliva stimulant in head and neck cancer clients with radiotherapy-induced dry mouth and hyposalivation with the client and health care provider.

**Geriatric**
- Recognize that symptoms of dry mouth are more common in menopausal women and geriatric clients.
- ▲ Age-associated increase of systemic disease and subsequent disease treatment are the primary causes of dry mouth.
- ▲ Older adults are at risk of xerostomia from a variety of etiologies.
- ▲ Review client medication list routinely.

**Multicultural and Home Care Considerations**
- The previously mentioned nursing interventions and client teaching may be adapted for multicultural and home care considerations. See care plan on Impaired **Oral Mucous Membrane** Integrity.

# Nausea

**Domain 12** Comfort    **Class 1** Physical comfort

## NANDA-I Definition

A subjective phenomenon of an unpleasant feeling in the back of the throat and stomach, which may or may not result in vomiting.

## Defining Characteristics

Food aversion; gagging sensation; increased salivation; increased swallowing; sour taste

## Related Factors

Anxiety; exposure to toxin; fear; noxious taste; unpleasant sensory stimuli

## At-Risk Population

Pregnant women

• = Independent          ▲ = Collaborative

## Associated Conditions

Abdominal neoplasms; altered biochemical phenomenon; esophageal disease; gastric distention; gastrointestinal irritation; intracranial hypertension; labyrinthitis; liver capsule stretch; localized tumor; Ménière's disease; meningitis; motion sickness; pancreatic diseases; pharmaceutical preparations; psychological disorder; splenetic capsule stretch; treatment regimen

## Client Outcomes

### Client Will (Specify Time Frame)

- State relief of nausea
- Explain methods clients can use to decrease nausea and vomiting (N&V)

## Nursing Interventions

▲ Determine cause or risk for N&V (e.g., medication effects, infectious causes [viral and bacterial gastroenteritis], disorders of the gut and peritoneum [mechanical obstruction, motility disorders, or other intraabdominal causes], central nervous system causes [including anxiety], endocrine and metabolic causes [including pregnancy], postoperative-related status).

▲ Evaluate and document the client's history of N&V, with attention to onset, duration, timing, volume of emesis, frequency of pattern, setting, associated factors, aggravating factors, and medical and social histories.

• Document each episode of nausea and/or vomiting separately and the effectiveness of interventions. Consider an assessment tool for consistency of evaluation.

• Identify and eliminate contributing causative factors. This may include eliminating unpleasant odors or medications that may be contributing to nausea. These interventions are theory based; however, there is no research evidence to support these interventions outside of expert opinion.

▲ Implement appropriate dietary measures such as nothing by mouth (NPO) status as appropriate; small, frequent meals; and low-fat, high-protein meals. It may be helpful to avoid foods that are spicy, fatty, or highly salty. Reverting to previous practices when ill in the past and consuming "comfort foods" may also be helpful at this time.

▲ Recognize and implement interventions and monitor complications associated with N&V. This may include administration of intravenous fluids and electrolytes.

▲ Administer appropriate antiemetics, according to guidelines, with consideration to emetic cause, most effective route, and side effects

• = Independent ▲ = Collaborative

of the medication, and with attention to and coverage for the time frames in which the nausea is anticipated.

- Consider nonpharmacological interventions such as acupressure, acupuncture, music therapy, distraction, and slow, deliberate movements.
- Provide oral care after the client vomits. Oral care helps remove the taste and smell of vomitus, reducing the stimulus for further vomiting.

**Nausea in Pregnancy**

- Early recognition and conservative measures are recommended to successfully manage nausea in pregnancy and to prevent progression to hyperemesis gravidarum. Dietary and lifestyle modifications should be implemented before pharmacological interventions. Avoidance of any aversive odors or foods is recommended. Eating multiple small meals per day is also recommended to have some food in the stomach at all times, avoiding hypoglycemia and gastric overdistention. Foods with higher protein (before bedtime) and carbohydrate and lower fat content are helpful (between meals and before getting out of bed early in the morning). Drinking smaller volumes of liquids at multiple times throughout the day is recommended.
- Recognize that certain maternal characteristics may be at higher risk for nausea and vomiting in pregnancy and hyperemesis gravidarum.
▲ It is well established that *Helicobacter pylori* infection is associated with hyperemesis gravidarum.
▲ Coexisting psychosocial factors may also influence the severity of N&V with pregnancy. Symptoms of anxiety and depression can occur in early pregnancy, especially when N&V is severe and can make the treatment of the N&V more challenging and even ineffective.
▲ The American College of Obstetricians and Gynecologists (ACOG) currently recommends converting the prenatal vitamin to folic acid only if nausea persists. Pharmacological options include a combination of oral pyridoxine hydrochloride (vitamin $B_6$, 10–25 mg) and doxylamine succinate (antihistamine 12.5 mg) to be used three to four times a day as first-line treatment for N&V of pregnancy after failure of pyridoxine alone. This combination agent of pyridoxine and doxylamine (Diclegis) is the only US Food and Drug Administration pregnancy Category A approved therapy for N&V of pregnancy. There are, however, several pharmacological treatments outlined by the ACOG.
▲ Nonpharmacological interventions that are recommended include P6 acupressure with wrist bands and ginger capsules, 250 mg four times a day.

• = Independent          ▲ = Collaborative

**Nausea After Surgery**

▲ Evaluate for risk factors for postoperative N&V (PONV).

▲ Reduction of risk factors associated with PONV is beneficial for both adults and children.

▲ Medicate the client prophylactically for nausea as ordered, throughout the period of risk.

▲ Alleviate postoperative pain using ordered analgesic agents (refer to the care plan for Acute **Pain**).

• Consider the use of nonpharmacological techniques, such as P6 acupoint stimulation, as an adjunct for controlling PONV, which has been shown to be effective in reducing PONV by 30%. Acupoint pressure is noninvasive, is inexpensive, and has no side effects; thus it is part of a combined approach with antiemetic medication.

• Include client education on the management of PONV for all outpatients and discuss key assessment criteria.

**Nausea After Chemotherapy**

• Perform risk assessment before chemotherapy administration. Risk factors include female gender, younger age, history of low alcohol consumption, history of morning sickness during pregnancy, anxiety, previous history of chemotherapy, client expectancy of nausea, and emetic potential of the regimen.

▲ Initiate antiemetic strategy prophylactically or when N&V occurs in accordance with evidence-based guidelines.

▲ Drug classes that are recommended for practice include serotonin receptor antagonists, NK-1 receptor antagonists, and cannabinoids.

▲ Consider the use of the following integrative therapies that are likely to be effective in reducing N&V: hypnosis with anticipatory N&V, and progressive muscle relaxation and guided imagery with antiemetics. Ginger may be effective for acute N&V and showed significant efficacy in a recent meta-analysis.

• Consider managing client expectations about CINV.

**Geriatric**

• There are no specific guidelines that address the prophylaxis of CINV in older adults. Risk still needs to be assessed, although many older clients are often treated with less emetic chemotherapy. Chemotherapy, however, can cause increased toxicity caused by age-related decreases in organ function, comorbidities, and drug–drug interactions secondary to polypharmacy. Additionally, adherence may be an issue because of cognitive decline, impaired senses, and economic issues.

N

• = Independent          ▲ = Collaborative

**Pediatric**
- Interventions for CINV should be implemented before and after chemotherapy.
- Use of a validated nausea tool in pediatrics for estimating incidence and severity of CINV is useful in clinical trials and standard practice. Examples include the PeNAT and pictorial scales (Sherani, Boston, & Mba, 2019).
- Relatively few systematic reviews exist examining the antiemetic medications used for CINV in children. It appears that a triple-drug regimen, including 5-HT3 antagonists, combined with dexamethasone and aprepitant, is recommended in children receiving highly emetogenic chemotherapy (Sherani, Boston, & Mba, 2019).
- Integrative therapies for control of nausea in children with cancer have not yet been studied as adequately as they have with adults. Some integrative therapies with potential include cognitive distraction, hypnosis, and acupressure (Momani & Berry, 2017).

**Home Care**
- Previously mentioned interventions may be adapted for home care use.
- ▲ In palliative care and hospice care clients, N&V is common and can considerably affect quality of life. Assessment is relevant in the management of N&V and should include history, physical examination, and evaluation of reversible causes.
- Assist the client and family with identifying and avoiding irritants in the home that exacerbate nausea (e.g., strong odors from food, plants, perfume, and room deodorizers). All medications except antiemetics should be given after meals to minimize the risk of nausea.

**Client/Family Teaching and Discharge Planning**
- Teach the client techniques to use before and after chemotherapy, including antiemetics/medication management schedules and dietary approaches, such as eating smaller meals, avoiding spicy and fatty foods, and avoiding an empty stomach before chemotherapy (Marx et al, 2016).

# Neonatal Abstinence Syndrome

**Domain 9** Coping/stress tolerance    **Class 3** Neurobehavioral stress
## NANDA-I Definition

A constellation of withdrawal symptoms observed in newborns as a result of in-utero exposure to addicting substances, or as a consequence of post-natal pharmacological pain management.

• = Independent        ▲ = Collaborative

## Defining Characteristics

Diarrhea (00013); disorganized infant behavior (00116); disturbed sleep pattern (00198); impaired comfort (00214); ineffective feeding pattern (00107); neurobehavioral stress; risk for aspiration (00039); risk for impaired attachment (00058); risk for impaired skin integrity (00047); risk for ineffective thermoregulation (00274); risk for injury (00035)

## Related Factors

To be developed

## At-Risk Population

Neonates exposed to maternal substance misuse in utero; neonates iatrogenically exposed to substance for pain control; premature neonates

## Client Outcomes

### Client Will (Specify Time Frame)

- Tolerate small frequent formula feedings or frequent breastfeedings
- Maintain weight and readjust feedings frequency as necessary for appropriate growth
- Provide calorie-dense formula, which is appropriate for weight gain
- Maintain proper hydration with elastic skin turgor and moist mucous membranes
- Maintain adequate nutrition, which will promote adequate growth
- Preserve skin integrity in perianal area

## Nursing Interventions

- Provide supportive nonpharmacological care with formula feeding as prescribed.
- Encourage breastfeeding for nutrition and nonpharmacological supportive care.
- Use nursing skills to provide supportive nonpharmacological care.
- Use vibrotactile stimulation (VS) as a nonpharmacological supportive care option.
- Practice supportive nursing interventions with an understanding of the levels of evidence.
- Provide pharmacological treatment as indicated for symptoms.
- Use of nonpharmacological and complementary therapy to comfort infants and provide relief of symptoms.
- Use of rooming-in and promotion of maternal–infant bonding for mother–infant dyad.
- Provide compassionate care, free of judgment, to substance-abusing mothers.

### Pediatric

- When available, consider professional, supportive programs for infants with a history of NAS.

• = Independent       ▲ = Collaborative

- Refer children and adolescents with a diagnostic history of NAS to educational supports and resources.

**Multicultural**

- Identify specific rural areas that are high risk for NAS.

**Client/Family Teaching and Discharge Planning**

- Develop plans of safe care for opioid-exposed mother–infant dyads before discharge.
- Provide parenting education before discharge that includes infant signs of hunger, infant feeding, ways to calm a fussy baby, the importance of never shaking a baby, safe sleep practices (including safe swaddling), and the importance of not co-sleeping.

**Home Care**

- Consider alternative models of care for treatment for infants with NAS.

# N Readiness for Enhanced Nutrition

**Domain 2** Nutrition    **Class 1** Ingestion

## NANDA-I Definition

A pattern of nutrient intake, which can be strengthened.

## Defining Characteristics

Expresses desire to enhance nutrition

## Client Outcomes

**Client Will (Specify Time Frame)**

- Explain how to eat according to the US Dietary Guidelines
- Design dietary modifications to meet individual long-term goal of health, using principles of variety, balance, and moderation
- Maintain weight within normal range for height and age

## Nursing Interventions

- Assess the meaning and importance of food in the client's life.
- Assess client readiness to determine whether he or she is ready to discuss enhanced nutrition and/or would like nutrition information.
- Use a motivational interviewing technique when working with clients to promote healthy eating and improved nutrition.
- Counsel the client to measure regularly consumed foods periodically. Help the client learn usual portion sizes. Measuring food alerts the client to normal portion sizes. Estimating amounts can be extremely inaccurate.
- Assist the client to develop a system of self-management, which may include self-monitoring of weight and BMI; realistic goal setting, planning, and action planning for improved dietary intake and

physical activity; problem-solving; and tracking dietary intake and exercise.

- Document the client's height and weight and teach the significance of his or her BMI in relation to current nutritional health. Use a chart or a website such as http://www.cdc.gov/healthyweight/assessing/bmi/index.html (Centers for Disease Control and Prevention [CDC], 2020i).
- Recommend that the client avoid eating in fast-food restaurants.
- Assist the client to reframe slips in nutrition or physical activity behavior as lapses that are a single event and not a full return to previous unhealthy behaviors. Relapse prevention strategies include managing lapses in healthy behavior, identifying high-risk situations for relapses, self-monitoring, providing social support, enhancing skills for coping, and increasing self-efficacy for avoiding relapse.
- Assist clients to engage their social support systems either digitally or face to face in ways that facilitate healthy eating and physical activity behavior change.
- Assist the client to implement informal and formal mindfulness-based interventions (MBIs). Informal MBIs include mindful eating, increasing awareness of hunger and satiety cues, taste satisfaction, and decreasing impulsive tendencies to overeat when experiencing negative emotions. Meditation practice is a formal MBI.
- Assist the client to develop stimulus control techniques designed to reduce environmental cues associated with eating behaviors. Specifically, clients should be taught to limit the presence of high-calorie/high-fat foods in the home; to reduce the visibility of unhealthy food choices in the home; to limit where and when they eat; to avoid distractions like reading, using the computer, or watching television when eating; and to eat more slowly.
- Encourage 7.5 to 8.5 hours of sleep nightly.
- Recommend the CDC behavior modification approach "reflect, replace, and reinforce" to improve eating habits.

**Pediatric**
- Offer obese or overweight adolescents healthy methods for weight loss.
- Offer families of obese or overweight children prejudice-free, individually accepting, and supportive interventions to address weight loss.
- Recommend that families eat together for at least one meal per day.

• = Independent          ▲ = Collaborative

- Recommend involving the family in planning meals and food preparation. Children can learn about nutrition as they help plan and make meals.
- Assist parents at being good role models of healthy eating.
- Recommend that the family try new foods, either a new food or recipe every week.

**Geriatric**
- Observe for social, psychological, and economic factors that influence diet quality.

**Multicultural**
- Tailor nutritional interventions to be consistent with cultural beliefs, norms, and values.
- Offer tailored lifestyle counseling via the telephone.
- Integrate weight loss and weight maintenance interventions with church faith-based supports for cultural congruence with African American clients.

**Client/Family Teaching and Discharge Planning**
- The majority of the preceding interventions involve teaching.
- Work with the family members regarding information on how to support and promote enhanced nutritional choices and healthy intakes.

# Imbalanced Nutrition: Less Than Body Requirements

**Domain 2** Nutrition     **Class 1** Ingestion

## NANDA-I Definition

Intake of nutrients insufficient to meet metabolic needs.

## Defining Characteristics

Abdominal cramping, abdominal pain; body weight below ideal weight range for age and gender; capillary fragility; constipation; delayed wound healing; diarrhea; excessive hair loss; food intake less than recommended daily allowance (RDA); hyperactive bowel sounds; hypoglycemia; inadequate head circumference growth for age and gender; inadequate height increase for age and gender; lethargy; muscle hypotonia; neonatal weight gain < 30 g per day; pale mucous membranes; weight loss with adequate food intake

## Related Factors

Altered taste perception; depressive symptoms; difficulty swallowing; food aversion; inaccurate information; inadequate food supply; inadequate interest in food; inadequate knowledge of nutrient requirements; injured buccal cavity; insufficient breast milk production; interrupted breastfeeding; misperception about ability to ingest food; satiety immediately upon ingesting food; sore buccal cavity; weakened muscles required for swallowing; weakened of muscles required for mastication

### At-Risk Population

Competitive athletes; displaced individuals; economically disadvantaged individuals; individuals with low educational level; premature infants

### Associated Conditions

Body dysmorphic disorders; digestive system diseases; immunosuppression; kwashiorkor; malabsorption syndromes; mental disorders; neoplasms; neurocognitive disorders; parasitic disorders

### Client Outcomes

### Client Will (Specify Time Frame)

- Promote weight gain of 5% to 10% of body weight
- Receive feeding assistance and texture modification as needed
- Identify factors contributing to being underweight
- Identify nutritional requirements based on specific client needs
- Increase overall intake
- Minimize further decline of weight status
- Be free of signs and symptoms of malnutrition

### Nursing Interventions

- Conduct a nutrition screen on all clients within 24 hours of admission and refer to a dietitian as deemed necessary.
- The screening tool should be based on the unique characteristics of the client population and the validity and reliability of the screening tool.
- Recognize the importance of rescreening and monitoring oral intake in hospitalized individuals to help facilitate the early identification and prevention of nutritional decline.
- Recognize the characteristics that classify individuals as malnourished and refer to a dietitian for a complex nutritional assessment and intervention.
- Recognize clients who are likely to experience malnutrition in the context of social or environmental circumstances, characterized by cachexia without the presence of an inflammatory process (chronic disease-related malnutrition: those with organ failure, pancreatic cancer, rheumatoid arthritis, sarcopenic obesity, acute disease, or injury-related malnutrition; those with major infection, burns, trauma, or closed-head injuries accompanied by a marked inflammatory response).

• = Independent ▲ = Collaborative

▲ Note laboratory values cautiously; decrease in albumin and prealbumin may be indicators of the inflammatory response that often accompanies acute malnutrition, but it should not be used to diagnose malnutrition. Other potential indicators of inflammatory response include C-reactive protein, white blood cell count, and blood glucose values.

• Weigh the client daily in acute care and weekly to monthly in extended care at the same time (usually before breakfast) with same amount of clothing.

• Observe for potential barriers to eating such as willingness, ability, and appetite.

• If the client is unable to feed self, refer to Feeding **Self-Care** Deficit. If the client has difficulty swallowing, refer to Nursing Interventions for Impaired **Swallowing.** If the client is receiving tube feedings, refer to the Nursing Interventions for Risk for **Aspiration.**

• Advocate for the implementation of a feeding protocol, if not already in place, to avoid unnecessary and/or prolonged nothing by mouth/clear liquid diet (NPO/CLD) status in hospitalized clients.

• For the client with anorexia nervosa, consider offering high-calorie foods and snacks often.

• For the client who is able to eat but has a decreased appetite, try the following activities:
   ○ Offer oral nutritional supplements (ONSs) based on client preference and indication of need.
   ○ Avoid interruptions during mealtimes and offer companionship; meals should be eaten in a calm and peaceful environment.
   ○ Allow for access to meals or snacks during "off times" if the client is not available at time of meal delivery, monitor food and ONS intake, and communicate with dietitian/health provider.
   ○ If the client lacks endurance, schedule rest periods before meals, and open packages and cut up food for the client.

• For the client who has had a stroke, repeat nutritional screenings weekly and provide timely interventions for those at risk or who may already be malnourished.

• Monitor state of oral cavity (gums, tongue, mucosa, and teeth). Provide good oral hygiene before each meal.

▲ Administer antiemetics and pain medications as ordered and needed before meals.

• If client is nauseated, remove cover of food tray before bringing it into the client's room.

• Work with the client to develop a plan for increased activity.

• = Independent        ▲ = Collaborative

**Critical Care**

- Recognize the need to begin enteral feeding within 24 to 48 hours of admission to the critical care environment, once the client is free of hemodynamic compromise, if the client is unable to eat.
- Recognize that it is important to administer feedings to the client and that frequently checking for gastric residual and fasting clients for procedures can be a limiting factor to adequate nutrition in the tube-fed client.
- Refer to care plan for Risk for **Aspiration.**

**Pediatric**

- ▲ Use a nutritional screening tool designed for nurses such as the Subjective Global Nutrition Assessment (SGNA), and if the child's malnutrition is identified as moderate or severe, refer to a dietitian.
- Watch for symptoms of malnutrition in the child, including short stature; thin arms and legs; poor condition of skin and hair; visible vertebrae and rib cage; wasted buttocks; wasted facial appearance; lethargy; and, in extreme cases, edema.
- Weigh and measure the length (height) of the child and use a growth chart to help determine growth pattern, which reflects nutrition. Age-related growth charts are available from https://www.cdc.gov/growthcharts/.
- ▲ Refer to a health provider and a dietitian a child who is underweight for any reason.
- Work with the child and parent to develop an appropriate weight gain plan.
- Recognize that a large percentage of girls and teenagers are dieting, which can result in nutritional problems.

**Geriatric**

- Screen for malnutrition in older clients.
- Screen for dysphagia in all older clients. See the care plan for Impaired **Swallowing.**
- Recognize that geriatric clients with moderate or severe cognition impairment have a significant risk for developing malnutrition.
- ▲ Interpret laboratory findings cautiously. Watch the color of urine for an indication of fluid balance; darker urine demonstrates dehydration. Low axillary moisture could indicate mild to moderate dehydration.
- Consider using dining assistants and trained nonnursing staff, to provide feeding assistance care in extended care facilities to ensure adequate time for feeding clients as needed.
- Encourage high-protein foods for the older client unless medically contraindicated by organ failure.

• = Independent            ▲ = Collaborative

- Recognize the implications of malnutrition on client strength and mobility.
- Monitor for onset of depression.
- If the client is unable to feed self, refer to Nursing Interventions for Feeding **Self-Care** Deficit. If client has impaired physical function, malnutrition, depression, or cognitive impairment, refer to care plan for **Frail Elderly** Syndrome.
- Emphasize the importance of good oral care in the older client.
- Initiate multiprofessional approach if the client is at high risk for pressure ulcers or has a pressure ulcer.

**Home Care**
- The preceding interventions may be adapted for home care use.
- Monitor food intake. Instruct the client in the intake of small frequent meals of foods with increased calories and protein.
- Assess the client's willingness and ability to eat.
- Consider social factors that may interfere with nutrition (e.g., lack of transportation, inadequate income, lack of social support).
- Continue to encourage intake of oral nutritional support to help optimize oral intake.
- ▲ Recognize that the client on home parenteral nutrition requires regularly scheduled laboratory work for electrolyte monitoring, increased risk of catheter-related complication, parenteral nutrition–associated liver disease (PNALD), and metabolic bone disease.

**Client/Family Teaching and Discharge Planning**
- Develop a client-centered nutrition plan with measurable goals.
- Amplify the identified strengths in the client/family's food habits. Select appropriate teaching aids for the client/family's background and educational level.
- Review food safety guidelines and hand hygiene when working with food.
- Implement instructional follow-up to answer the client/family's questions.
- Recommend that clients discuss with their primary health provider before taking any supplements such as vitamins, minerals, and botanicals.
- Suggest community resources for home-delivered or congregate meals.
- Encourage socialization at meal time.
- Teach the client and family how to manage tube feedings or parenteral therapy at home as needed.

• = Independent          ▲ = Collaborative

# Impaired Oral Mucous Membrane Integrity

**Domain 11** Safety/protection    **Class 2** Physical injury

## NANDA-I Definition

Injury to the lips, soft tissue, buccal cavity, and/or oropharynx.

## Defining Characteristics

Bad taste in mouth; bleeding; cheilitis; coated tongue; decreased taste perception; desquamation; difficulty eating; difficulty swallowing; dysphonia; enlarged tonsils; geographic tongue; gingival hyperplasia; gingival pallor; gingival pocketing deeper than 4 mm; gingival recession; halitosis; hyperemia; macroplasia; mucosal denudation; oral discomfort; oral edema; oral fissure; oral lesion; oral mucosal pallor; oral nodule; oral pain; oral papule; oral ulcer; oral vesicles; pathogen exposure; presence of mass; purulent oral-nasal drainage; purulent oral-nasal exudates; smooth atrophic tongue; spongy patches in mouth; stomatitis; white patches in mouth; white plaque in mouth; white, curd-like oral exudate; xerostomia

## Related Factors

Alcohol consumption; decreased salivation; dehydration; depressive symptoms; difficulty performing oral self-care; inadequate access to dental care; inadequate knowledge of oral hygiene; inadequate oral hygiene habits; inappropriate use of chemical agent; malnutrition; mouth breathing; smoking; stressors

## At-Risk Population

Economically disadvantaged individuals

## Associated Conditions

Allergies; autosomal disorder; behavioral disorder; chemotherapy; decreased female hormone levels; decreased platelets; depression; immune system diseases; immunosuppression; infections; loss of oral support structure; mechanical factor; nil per os (NPO) >24 hours; oral trauma; radiotherapy; Sjögren's syndrome; surgical procedures; trauma; treatment regimen

## Client Outcomes

**Client Will (Specify Time Frame)**

- Maintain intact, moist oral mucous membranes that are free of ulceration, inflammation, infection, and debris
- Demonstrate measures to maintain or regain intact oral mucous membranes
- Demonstrate oral hygiene knowledge and skills

• = Independent          ▲ = Collaborative

## Nursing Interventions

▲ Inspect the oral cavity/teeth/gingiva at least once daily and note any discoloration; presence of debris; amount of plaque buildup; presence of lesions such as white lesions or patches, edema, or bleeding; and intactness of teeth. Refer to a dentist or periodontist as appropriate.

• If the client is free of bleeding disorders and able to swallow, encourage toothbrushing with a soft toothbrush using fluoride-containing toothpaste at least two times per day.

• Recommend the use of a power, rotation-oscillation toothbrush for removal of dental plaque and prevention of gingivitis.

• Use foam sticks to moisten the oral mucous membranes, clean out debris, and swab out the mouth of the edentulous client. Do not use foam sticks to clean the teeth unless the platelet count is very low and the client is prone to bleeding gums.

• Avoid lemon-glycerin swabs for oral care.

• If the client does not have a bleeding disorder, encourage the client to perform interdental hygiene by flossing or cleaning between teeth with interdental brushes, woodsticks, or oral irrigation. If the client is unable to floss, assist with flossing or encourage the use of an oral irrigator (i.e., "water flossing").

• Over-the-counter mouthwashes containing mint or essential oils may be used in combination with toothbrushing and interdental cleaning to maintain oral health. Avoid routine use of hydrogen peroxide, chlorhexidine, or alcohol-based mouthwashes.

• Provide oral hygiene if the client is unable to care for himself or herself. The nursing diagnosis Bathing **Self-Care** Deficit is then applicable.

• If the client is unable to brush own teeth, follow this procedure:
  ○ Position the client sitting upright or on side.
  ○ Use a soft bristle toothbrush.
  ○ Use fluoride toothpaste and tap water or saline as a solution.
  ○ Brush teeth in an up-and-down manner.
  ○ Suction as needed.

• Monitor the client's nutritional and fluid status to determine whether it is adequate. Dehydration and malnutrition predispose clients to impaired oral mucous membranes. Refer to the care plan for Deficient **Fluid** Volume or Imbalanced **Nutrition:** Less Than Body Requirements if applicable.

• Encourage fluid intake of up to 3000 mL/day if not contraindicated by the client's medical condition. Fluids help increase moisture in the mouth, which protects the mucous membranes from damage.

• = Independent          ▲ = Collaborative

▲ Determine the client's usual method of oral care and address any concerns regarding oral hygiene. If the client has a dry mouth (xerostomia):

- ○ Recognize that more than 50 classes of medications may cause xerostomia, which is often exacerbated by polypharmacy. When feasible, medications can be discontinued or replaced to increase the client's comfort (Marcott et al, 2020).
- ○ Provide saliva substitutes as ordered.
- ○ Suggest the client chew sugarless gum or sugarless sour candy to promote salivary flow.
- ○ Examine the oral cavity for signs of caries, dental plaque, infection, mucositis ulceration, and oral candidiasis.

- Recommend that the client decrease or preferably stop intake of soft drinks. Sugar-containing soft drinks can cause cavities, and the low pH of the drink can cause erosion in teeth.
- If client has halitosis, review good oral care with the client including brushing teeth, using floss, and brushing the tongue.
- Instruct the client with halitosis to clean the tongue when performing oral hygiene; brush tongue with tongue scraper or toothbrush and follow with a mouth rinse.
- Assess the client for underlying medical conditions that may be causing halitosis. Causes of halitosis can be subdivided into three categories: oral origin, in which good mouth care can help prevent halitosis; halitosis from the upper respiratory tract, including the sinuses and nose; and halitosis from systemic diseases that are blood-borne, volatilized in the lungs, and expelled from the lower respiratory tract. Potential sources of blood-borne halitosis are some systemic diseases, metabolic disorders, medication, and certain foods such as onions and garlic (Raghu Ram, 2019).
- Keep the lips well lubricated using a water-based or aloe-based lip balm.

**Client Receiving Chemotherapy and/or Radiation**

- Ensure that the client receives a comprehensive oral examination before initiation of chemotherapy or radiation, with aggressive preventive dental care given as needed.
- Provide both verbal and written instruction about the need for and method of providing frequent oral care to the client before radiation therapy or chemotherapy. Assess the condition of the oral cavity daily in the client receiving radiation or chemotherapy.
- For measurement of presence or severity of mucositis, use the Oral Mucositis Assessment Scale (OMAS).

• = Independent          ▲ = Collaborative

- Use a protocol to prevent/treat mucositis that includes the following:
  - ○ Use a soft toothbrush that is replaced on a regular basis; brush teeth at least two times a day and for at least 90 seconds.
  - ○ Continue to floss teeth daily.
  - ○ Use a bland, alcohol-free rinse to remove debris and moisten the oral cavity. Rinse the mouth often (every 2 hours while awake) if the client has mouth sores.
  - ○ Avoid tobacco, alcohol, and irritating foods (hot, rough, acidic, or spicy).
  - ○ Use a valid and reliable pain assessment tool and treatment of pain as needed.
- Help the client use a mouth rinse of normal saline or salt and soda every 1 to 2 hours for prevention and treatment of stomatitis. A typical mixture is 1 teaspoon of salt or sodium bicarbonate per pint of water. Clients are directed to take a tablespoon of the rinse and swish it in the mouth for 30 seconds, then expectorate.
- ▲ If the mouth is severely inflamed and it is painful to swallow, contact the health care provider for a topical anesthetic or analgesic order. Modification of oral intake (e.g., soft or liquid diet) may also be necessary to prevent friction trauma.
- If the client's platelet count is lower than 50,000/mm³ or the client has a bleeding disorder, use a soft toothbrush or a toothette that is not soaked in glycerin or flavorings; if the client cannot tolerate a toothbrush or a toothette, a piece of gauze wrapped around a finger can be used to remove plaque and debris.

**Critical Care—Client on a Ventilator**

- Use a soft toothbrush to brush teeth to clean the client's teeth at least every 12 hours; use suction to remove secretions. Provide oral moisturizer to oral mucosa and lips every 4 hours. Recognize that good oral care is paramount in the prevention of ventilator-associated events (VAEs) and ventilator-associated pneumonia (VAP).
- ▲ Apply chlorhexidine gluconate mouthwash or gel in the oral cavity after performing tooth brushing, which may reduce the risk of the client developing VAEs and VAP.

**Geriatric**

- Determine the functional ability of the client to provide his or her own oral care. Interventions must be directed toward both treatment of the functional loss and care of oral health.
- Provide appropriate oral care to older adults with a self-care deficit, brushing the teeth after breakfast and in the evening.

• = Independent ▲ = Collaborative

- If the client has dementia or delirium and exhibits care-resistant behavior, such as fighting, biting, or refusing care, use the following method:
  - Ensure client is in a quiet environment such as own bathroom, sitting or standing at the sink to prime memory for appropriate actions.
  - Approach the client at eye level within his or her range of vision.
  - Approach with a smile and begin conversation with a touch of the hand and gradually move up.
  - Use mirror–mirror technique, standing behind the client, and brush and floss teeth.
  - Use respectful adult speech. Avoid "elderspeak," a style of speech characterized by short phrases and questions uttered in a sing-song voice and use of collective pronouns and intimate terms (e.g., first name, nicknames, "deary" or "honey").
  - Promote self-care in which client brushes own teeth if possible.
  - Use distractors when needed: talking, reminiscing, singing.
- Carefully observe the oral cavity and lips for abnormal lesions such as white or red patches, masses, ulcerations with an indurated margin, or a raised granular lesion.
- Ensure that dentures are removed and cleaned regularly, preferably after every meal and before bedtime. Dentures left in the mouth at night may impede circulation to the palate and predispose the client to oral lesions.

**Home Care**

- The interventions described previously may be adapted for home care use.
- Instruct the client in ways to soothe the oral cavity (e.g., cool beverages, popsicles, viscous lidocaine).
- ▲ If necessary, refer for home health aide services to support the family in oral care and observation of the oral cavity.

**Client/Family Teaching and Discharge Planning**

- Teach the client how to inspect the oral cavity and monitor for signs and symptoms of infection or complications and when to call the health care provider.
- Recommend the client not smoke, use chewing tobacco, or drink excessive amounts of alcohol.
- Teach the client and family, if necessary, how to perform appropriate mouth care. Use the motivational interviewing technique.

# Risk for Impaired Oral Mucous Membrane Integrity

**Domain 11** Safety/protection    **Class 2** Physical injury

## NANDA-I Definition

Susceptible to injury to the lips, soft tissues, buccal cavity, and/or oropharynx, which may compromise health.

## Risk Factors

Alcohol consumption; decreased salivation; dehydration; depressive symptoms; difficulty performing oral self-care; inadequate access to dental care; inadequate knowledge of oral hygiene; inadequate oral hygiene habits; inappropriate use of chemical agent; malnutrition; mouth breathing; smoking; stressors

## At-Risk Population

Economically disadvantaged individuals

## Associated Conditions

Allergies; autosomal disorder; behavioral disorder; chemotherapy; decreased female hormone levels; decreased platelets; depression; immune system diseases; immunosuppression; infections; loss of oral support structure; mechanical factor; nil per os (NPO) >24 hours; oral trauma; radiotherapy; Sjögren's syndrome; surgical procedures; trauma; treatment regimen

## Client Outcomes, Nursing Interventions, and Client/Family Teaching

Refer to care plan for Impaired **Oral Mucous Membrane** Integrity.

# Obesity

**Domain 2** Nutrition    **Class 1** Ingestion

## NANDA-I Definition

A condition in which an individual accumulates excessive fat for age and gender that exceeds overweight.

## Defining Characteristics

Adult: Body mass index >30 kg/m$^2$; Child 2 to 18 years: body mass index >30 kg/m$^2$ or >95th percentile or 30 kg/m$^2$ for age and gender; Child <2 years: term not used with children at this age

## Related Factors

Abnormal eating behavior patterns; abnormal eating perception patterns; average daily physical activity is less than recommended for age and gender; consumption of sugar-sweetened beverages; dyssomnias; energy expenditure below energy intake based on standard assessment; excessive alcohol consumption; fear regarding lack of food supply; frequent snacking; high

• = Independent          ▲ = Collaborative

frequency of restaurant or fried food; insufficient dietary calcium intake by children; portion sizes larger than recommended; sedentary behavior occurring for ≥2 hours/day; shortened sleep time; solid foods as major food source at <5 months of age

## At-Risk Population

Economically disadvantaged individuals; individuals who experienced premature pubarche; individuals who experienced rapid weight gain during childhood; individuals who experienced rapid weight gain during infancy; individuals who inherit interrelated factors; individuals who were not exclusively breastfed; individuals who were overweight during infancy; individuals whose mothers had gestational diabetes; individuals whose mothers have diabetes; individuals whose mothers smoke during childhood; individuals whose mothers smoke during pregnancy; individuals with high disinhibition and restraint eating behavior score; individuals with parents who are obese neonates whose mothers had gestational diabetes

## Associated Conditions

Inborn genetic diseases

## Client Outcomes

### Client Will (Specify Time Frame)

- Explain how to eat according to the US Dietary Guidelines
- Design dietary modifications to meet individual long-term goal of health, using principles of variety, balance, and moderation
- Maintain weight within normal range for height and age

## Nursing Interventions

- Assess the meaning and importance of food in the client's life.
- Assess client readiness to determine whether the client is ready to discuss weight loss and/or would like weight loss information.
- Use a motivational interviewing technique when working with clients to promote healthy eating and weight loss.
- Counsel the client to measure regularly consumed foods periodically. Help the client learn usual portion sizes. Measuring food alerts the client to normal portion sizes. Estimating amounts can be extremely inaccurate.
- Assist the client to develop a system of self-management, which may include self-monitoring of weight and BMI; realistic goal setting, planning, and action planning for improved dietary intake and physical activity; problem-solving; and tracking dietary intake and exercise.
- Encourage the client to adopt dietary as well as physical activity changes.

• = Independent          ▲ = Collaborative

- Document the client's height and weight and teach the significance of his or her BMI in relationship to current health. Use a chart or a website such as http://www.cdc.gov/healthyweight/assessing/bmi/index.html (Centers for Disease Control and Prevention [CDC], 2020i).
- Encourage the client to engage in moderate- to vigorous-intensity physical activity for at least 200 to 300 minutes weekly for weight loss.
- Recommend that the client limit fast food and take-out meals.
- Assist the client to reframe slips in weight loss or physical activity behavior as lapses that are a single event and not a full return to previous unhealthy behaviors. Relapse prevention strategies include managing lapses in healthy behavior, identifying high-risk situations for relapses, self-monitoring, providing social support, enhancing skills for coping, and increasing self-efficacy for avoiding relapse.
- Assist clients to engage their social support systems either digitally or face to face in ways that facilitate weight loss, healthy eating, and physical activity behavior change.
- Assist the client to reframe the goal from a focus on outcome (weight loss) to a focus on process (weight-loss behaviors) for weight loss.
- Assist the client to implement informal and formal mindfulness-based interventions (MBIs). Informal MBIs include mindful eating, increasing awareness of hunger and satiety cues, taste satisfaction, and decreasing impulsive tendencies to overeat when experiencing negative emotions. Meditation practice is a formal MBI.
- Assist the client to develop stimulus control techniques designed to reduce environmental cues associated with eating behaviors. Specifically, clients should be taught to limit the presence of high-calorie/high-fat foods in the home; to reduce the visibility of unhealthy food choices in the home; to limit where and when they eat; to avoid distractions such as reading, using the computer, or watching television when eating; and to eat more slowly.
- Encourage 7.5 to 8.5 hours of sleep nightly.
- Refer the client to a weight loss–related therapy group.
- Recommend that clients use dietary supplements such as vitamins and minerals after consulting with their primary health care provider.
- Recommend the CDC behavior modification approach "reflect, replace, and reinforce" to improve eating habits.
- Incorporate the following recommendations from the Academy of Nutrition and Dietetics "Interventions for the Treatment of Overweight and Obesity in Adults" (Raynor & Champagne, 2016):

• = Independent        ▲ = Collaborative

○ Assess food- and nutrition-related history; anthropometric measures; biochemical data, medical tests, and procedures; nutrition-focused physical findings; and client history.
○ Assess the energy intake and nutrient content of the diet.
○ Use height and weight to calculate BMI; use waist circumference to determine risk of cardiovascular disease, type 2 diabetes, and all-cause mortality.
○ Use a measured resting metabolic rate to determine energy needs.
○ Set a realistic weight-loss goal such as one of the following: up to 2 pounds/week, up to 10% of baseline body weight, or a total of 3% to 5% of baseline weight if cardiovascular risk factors (hypertension, hyperlipidemia, and hyperglycemia) are present.
○ To achieve weight loss, use an individualized diet, including client preferences and health status, to achieve and maintain nutrient adequacy and reduce caloric intake, based on one of the following caloric reduction strategies: 1200 to 1500 kcal/day for women and 1500 to 1800 kcal/day for men, with an energy deficit of approximately 500 or 750 kcal/day.
▲ Refer for medical management of obesity.

**Pediatric**
• Offer obese or overweight adolescents healthy methods for weight loss.
• Offer families of obese or overweight children prejudice-free, individually accepting, and supportive interventions to address weight loss.
• Recommend that families eat together for at least one meal per day.
• Recommend involving the family in planning meals and food preparation. Children can learn about nutrition as they help plan and make meals.
• Assist parents at being good role models of healthy eating.
• Recommend that the family try new foods, either a new food or recipe every week.

**Geriatric**
• Determine the risks and benefits of weight loss in the older client. A BMI greater than 30 in the older client suggests a moderate weight-loss approach.
• Observe for social, psychological, and economic factors that influence diet quality.

**Multicultural**
• Tailor nutritional interventions to be consistent with cultural beliefs, norms, and values.

• = Independent          ▲ = Collaborative

- Offer tailored lifestyle counseling via the telephone.
- Integrate weight loss and weight maintenance interventions with church faith–based supports for African American clients.

**Client/Family Teaching and Discharge Planning**
- The majority of the preceding interventions involve teaching.
- Work with the family members regarding information on how to support and promote weight loss and healthy intakes.

# Overweight

**Domain 2** Nutrition   **Class 1** Ingestion

## NANDA-I Definition

A condition in which an individual accumulates abnormal or excessive fat for age and gender.

## Defining Characteristics

Adult: Body mass index >25 kg/m$^2$; Child 2 to 18 years: Body mass index >85th percentile or 25 kg/m$^2$ but <95th percentile or 30 kg/m$^2$ for age and gender; Child <2 years: Weight-for-length >95th percentile

## Related Factors

Abnormal eating behavior patterns; abnormal eating perception patterns; average daily physical activity is less than recommended for age and gender; consumption of sugar-sweetened beverages; dyssomnias; energy expenditure below energy intake based on standard assessment; excessive alcohol consumption; fear regarding lack of food supply; frequent snacking; high frequency of restaurant or fried food; inadequate knowledge of modifiable factors; insufficient dietary calcium intake by children; portion sizes larger than recommended; sedentary behavior occurring for ≥2 hours/day; shortened sleep time; solid foods as major food source at <5 months of age

## At-Risk Population

ADULT: Body mass index approaching 25 kg/m$^2$; CHILD 2-18 years: Body mass index approaching 85th percentile or 25 kg/m$^2$; CHILD <2 years: Weight-for-length approaching 95th percentile; children with body mass index crossing percentiles upward; children with high body mass index percentiles for age and gender; economically disadvantaged individuals; individuals who experienced premature pubarche; individuals who experienced rapid weight gain during childhood; individuals who experienced rapid weight gain during infancy; individuals who inherit interrelated factors; individuals who were not exclusively breastfed; individuals who were obese during childhood; individuals whose mothers have diabetes; individuals whose mothers smoke during childhood; individuals whose mothers smoke during pregnancy; individuals with high disinhibition and restraint eating behavior score; individuals with parents who are obese

## Associated Conditions

Inborn genetic disorders

## Client Outcomes

### Client Will (Specify Time Frame)

- Explain how to eat according to the US Dietary Guidelines
- Design dietary modifications to meet individual long-term goal of health, using principles of variety, balance, and moderation
- Maintain weight within normal range for height and age

## Nursing Interventions

- Assess the meaning and importance of food in the client's life.
- Assess client readiness to determine whether the client is ready to discuss weight loss and/or would like weight-loss information.
- Use a motivational interviewing technique when working with clients to promote healthy eating and weight loss.
- Counsel the client to measure regularly consumed foods periodically. Help the client learn usual portion sizes. Measuring food alerts the client to normal portion sizes. Estimating amounts can be extremely inaccurate.
- Assist the client to develop a system of self-management, which may include self-monitoring of weight and BMI; realistic goal setting, planning, and action planning for improved dietary intake and physical activity; problem-solving; and tracking dietary intake and exercise.
- Document the client's height and weight and teach the significance of his or her BMI in relationship to current health. Use a chart or a website such as http://www.cdc.gov/healthyweight/assessing/bmi/index.html (Centers for Disease Control and Prevention [CDC], 2020i).
- Encourage the client to engage in vigorous-intensity physical activity for at least 150 minutes weekly or moderate-intensity physical activity for at least 300 minutes weekly.
- Recommend the client avoid eating in fast-food restaurants.
- Assist the client to reframe slips in weight loss or physical activity behavior as lapses that are a single event and not a full return to previous unhealthy behaviors. Relapse prevention strategies include managing lapses in healthy behavior, identifying high-risk situations for relapses, self-monitoring, providing social support, enhancing skills for coping, and increasing self-efficacy for avoiding relapse.

• = Independent          ▲ = Collaborative

- Assist clients to engage their social support systems either digitally or face to face in ways that facilitate weight loss, healthy eating, and physical activity behavior change.
- Assist the client to reframe the goal from a focus on outcome (weight loss) to a focus on process (eating behaviors) for weight loss.
- Assist the client to implement informal and formal mindfulness-based interventions (MBIs). Informal MBIs include mindful eating, increasing awareness of hunger and satiety cues, taste satisfaction, and decreasing impulsive tendencies to overeat when experiencing negative emotions. Meditation practice is a formal MBI.
- Assist the client to develop stimulus control techniques designed to reduce environmental cues associated with eating behaviors. Specifically, clients should be taught to limit the presence of high-calorie/high-fat foods in the home; to reduce the visibility of unhealthy food choices in the home; to limit where and when they eat; to avoid distractions such as reading, using the computer, or watching television when eating; and to eat more slowly.
- Encourage 7.5 to 8.5 hours of sleep nightly.
- Refer the client to a weight loss–related therapy group.
- Recommend that clients use dietary supplements such as vitamins and minerals after consulting with their primary health care provider.
- Recommend the CDC behavior modification approach "reflect, replace, and reinforce" to improve eating habits.
- Incorporate the following recommendations from the Academy of Nutrition and Dietetics "Interventions for the Treatment of Overweight and Obesity in Adults" (Raynor & Champagne, 2016):
  ○ Assess food- and nutrition-related history; anthropometric measures; biochemical data, medical tests, and procedures; nutrition-focused physical findings; and client history.
  ○ Assess the energy intake and nutrient content of the diet.
  ○ Use height and weight to calculate BMI and waist circumference to determine risk of cardiovascular disease, type 2 diabetes, and all-cause mortality.
  ○ Use a measured resting metabolic rate to determine energy needs.
  ○ Set a realistic weight-loss goal such as one of the following: up to 2 pounds/week, up to 10% of baseline body weight, or a total of 3% to 5% of baseline weight if cardiovascular risk factors (hypertension, hyperlipidemia, and hyperglycemia) are present.
  ○ To achieve weight loss, use an individualized diet, including client preferences and health status, to achieve and maintain nutrient adequacy and reduce caloric intake, based on one of the following

**O**

caloric reduction strategies: 1200 to 1500 kcal/day for women and 1500 to 1800 kcal/day for men, and energy deficit of approximately 500 or 750 kcal/day.

**Pediatric**
- Offer obese or overweight adolescents healthy methods for weight loss.
- Offer families of obese or overweight children prejudice-free, individually accepting, and supportive interventions to address weight loss.
- Recommend that families eat together for at least one meal per day.
- Recommend involving the family in planning meals and food preparation. Children can learn about nutrition as they help plan and make meals.
- Assist parents at being good role models of healthy eating.
- Recommend that the family try new foods, either a new food or recipe every week.

**Geriatric**
- Determine the risks and benefits of weight loss in the older client. A BMI greater than 30 in the older client suggests a moderate weight-loss approach.
- Observe for social, psychological, and economic factors that influence diet quality.

**Multicultural**
- Tailor nutritional interventions to be consistent with cultural beliefs, norms, and values.
- Offer tailored lifestyle counseling via the telephone.
- Integrate weight loss and weight maintenance interventions with church faith-based supports for African American clients.

**Client/Family Teaching and Discharge Planning**
- The majority of the preceding interventions involve teaching.
- Work with the family members regarding information on how to support and promote weight loss and healthy intakes.

# Risk for Overweight

**Domain 2** Nutrition    **Class 1** Ingestion
## NANDA-I Definition

Susceptible to excessive fat accumulation for age and gender, which may compromise health.

• = Independent          ▲ = Collaborative

## Risk Factors

Abnormal eating behavior patterns; abnormal eating perception patterns; average daily physical activity is less than recommended for age and gender; consumption of sugar-sweetened beverages; dyssomnias; energy expenditure below energy intake based on standard assessment; excessive alcohol consumption; fear regarding lack of food supply; frequent snacking; high frequency of restaurant or fried food; inadequate knowledge of modifiable factors; insufficient dietary calcium intake by children; portion sizes larger than recommended; sedentary behavior occurring for ≥ 2 hours/day; shortened sleep time; solid foods as major food source at < 5 months of age

## At-Risk Population

ADULT: Body mass index approaching 25 kg/m²; CHILD 2-18 years: Body mass index approaching 85th percentile or 25 kg/m²; CHILD <2 years: Weight-for-length approaching 95th percentile; children with body mass index crossing percentiles upward; children with high body mass index percentiles for age and gender; economically disadvantaged individuals; individuals who experienced premature pubarche; individuals who experienced rapid weight gain during childhood; individuals who experienced rapid weight gain during infancy; individuals who inherit interrelated factors; individuals who were not exclusively breastfed; individuals who were obese during childhood; individuals whose mothers have diabetes; individuals whose mothers smoke during childhood; individuals whose mothers smoke during pregnancy; individuals with high disinhibition and restraint eating behavior score; individuals with parents who are obese

## Associated Conditions

Inborn genetic diseases

## Client Outcomes

### Client Will (Specify Time Frame)

- Explain how to eat according to the US Dietary Guidelines
- Design dietary modifications to meet individual long-term goal of health, using principles of variety, balance, and moderation
- Maintain weight within normal range for height and age

## Nursing Interventions

- Assess the meaning and importance of food in the client's life.
- Assess client readiness to determine whether the client is ready to discuss weight loss and/or would like weight-loss information.
- Use a motivational interviewing technique when working with clients to promote healthy eating and weight loss.
- Counsel the client to measure regularly consumed foods periodically. Help the client learn usual portion sizes. Measuring food alerts the

client to normal portion sizes. Estimating amounts can be extremely inaccurate.

- Assist the client to develop a system of self-management, which may include self-monitoring of weight and BMI; realistic goal setting, planning, and action planning for improved dietary intake and physical activity; problem-solving; and tracking dietary intake and exercise.
- Document the client's height and weight and teach significance of his or her BMI in relationship to current health. Use a chart or a website such as http://www.cdc.gov/healthyweight/assessing/bmi/index.html (Centers for Disease Control and Prevention [CDC], 2020i).
- Encourage the client to engage in moderate-intensity physical activity (at least 150 minutes/week of moderate physical activity) to prevent weight gain.
- Recommend that the client avoid eating in fast-food restaurants.
- Assist the client to reframe slips in weight loss or physical activity behavior as lapses that are a single event and not a full return to previous unhealthy behaviors. Relapse prevention strategies include managing lapses in healthy behavior, identifying high-risk situations for relapses, self-monitoring, providing social support, enhancing skills for coping, and increasing self-efficacy for avoiding relapse.
- Assist clients to engage their social support systems either digitally or face to face in ways that facilitate weight loss, healthy eating, and physical activity behavior change.
- Assist the client to reframe the goal from a focus on outcome (weight loss) to a focus on process (eating behaviors) for weight loss.
- Assist the client to implement informal and formal mindfulness-based interventions (MBIs). Informal MBIs include mindful eating, increasing awareness of hunger and satiety cues, taste satisfaction, and decreasing impulsive tendencies to overeat when experiencing negative emotions. Meditation practice is a formal MBI.
- Assist the client to develop stimulus control techniques designed to reduce environmental cues associated with eating behaviors. Specifically, clients should be taught to limit the presence of high-calorie/high-fat foods in the home; to reduce the visibility of unhealthy food choices in the home; to limit where and when they eat; to avoid distractions such as reading, using the computer, or watching television when eating; and to eat more slowly.
- Encourage 7.5 to 8.5 hours of sleep nightly.
- Refer the client to a weight loss–related therapy group.

• = Independent          ▲ = Collaborative

- Recommend that clients use dietary supplements such as vitamins and minerals after consulting with their primary health care provider.
- Recommend the CDC behavior modification approach "reflect, replace, and reinforce" to improve eating habits.
- Incorporate the following recommendations from the Academy of Nutrition and Dietetics "Interventions for the Treatment of Overweight and Obesity in Adults" (Raynor & Champagne, 2016):
  - Assess food- and nutrition-related history; anthropometric measures; biochemical data, medical tests, and procedures; nutrition-focused physical findings; and client history.
  - Assess the energy intake and nutrient content of the diet.
  - Use height and weight to calculate BMI and waist circumference to determine risk of cardiovascular disease, type 2 diabetes, and all-cause mortality.
  - Use a measured resting metabolic rate to determine energy needs.
  - Set a realistic weight-loss goal such as one of the following: up to 2 pounds/week, up to 10% of baseline body weight, or a total of 3% to 5% of baseline weight if cardiovascular risk factors (hypertension, hyperlipidemia, and hyperglycemia) are present.
  - To achieve weight loss, use an individualized diet, including client preferences and health status, to achieve and maintain nutrient adequacy and reduce caloric intake, based on one of the following caloric reduction strategies: 1200 to 1500 kcal/day for women and 1500 to 1800 kcal/day for men and energy deficit of approximately 500 or 750 kcal/day.

**Pediatric**
- Offer obese or overweight adolescents healthy methods for weight loss.
- Offer families of obese or overweight children prejudice-free, individually accepting, and supportive interventions to address weight loss.
- Recommend that families eat together for at least one meal per day.
- Recommend involving the family in planning meals and food preparation. Children can learn about nutrition as they help plan and make meals.
- Assist parents at being good role models of healthy eating.
- Recommend that the family try new foods, either a new food or recipe every week.

**Geriatric**
- Determine the risks and benefits of weight loss in the older client. A BMI greater than 30 in the older client suggests a moderate weight-loss approach.
- Observe for social, psychological, and economic factors that influence diet quality.

• = Independent ▲ = Collaborative

**Multicultural**
- Tailor nutritional interventions to be consistent with cultural beliefs, norms, and values.
- Offer tailored lifestyle counseling via the telephone.
- Integrate weight loss and weight maintenance interventions with church faith–based supports for African American clients.

**Client/Family Teaching and Discharge Planning**
- The majority of the preceding interventions involve teaching.
- Work with the family members regarding information on how to support and promote weight loss and healthy intakes.

# Acute Pain

**Domain 12** Comfort    **Class 1** Physical comfort

## NANDA-I Definition

Unpleasant sensory and emotional experience associated with actual or potential tissue damage, or described in terms of such damage (International Association for the Study of Pain); sudden or slow onset of any intensity from mild to severe with an anticipated or predictable end, and with a duration of less than 3 months.

## Defining Characteristics

Altered physiological parameter; appetite change; diaphoresis; distraction behavior; evidence of pain using standardized pain behavior checklist for those unable to communicate verbally; expressive behavior; facial expression of pain; guarding behavior; hopelessness; narrow focus; positioning to ease pain; protective behavior; proxy report of activity changes; proxy report of pain behavior; pupil dilation; reports intensity using standardized pain scale; reports pain characteristics using standardized pain instrument; self-focused

## Related Factors

Biological injury agent; inappropriate use of chemical agent; physical injury agent

## Client Outcomes

**Client Will (Specify Time Frame)**

**For the Client Who Is Able to Provide a Self-Report**
- Use a self-report pain tool to identify current pain intensity level and establish a comfort-function goal
- Report that the pain management regimen achieves comfort-function goal without side effects

• = Independent    ▲ = Collaborative

- Notify member of the health care team promptly for pain intensity level that is consistently greater than the comfort-function goal, or occurrence of side effects
- Describe nonpharmacological methods that can be used to help achieve comfort-function goal
- Perform activities of recovery or activities of daily living (ADLs) easily
- Describe how unrelieved pain will be managed
- State ability to obtain sufficient amounts of rest and sleep

**For the Client Who Is Unable to Provide a Self-Report**

- Decrease in pain-related behaviors
- Perform activities of recovery or ADLs easily as determined by client condition
- Demonstrate the absence of side effects of analgesics
- No pain-related behaviors will be evident in the client who is completely unresponsive; demonstrate a reasonable absence of side effects related to the prescribed pain treatment plan

**Nursing Interventions**

- During the initial assessment and interview, if the client is experiencing pain, or when pain first occurs, conduct and document a comprehensive pain assessment, using appropriate pain assessment tools.
- Assess if the client is able to provide a self-report of pain intensity, and if so, assess pain intensity level using a valid and reliable self-report pain tool.
- Ask the client to describe prior experiences with pain, effectiveness of pain management interventions, responses to analgesic medications (including occurrence of side effects), and concerns about pain and its treatment (e.g., fear about addiction, worries, anxiety).
- Using a self-report pain tool, ask the client to identify a comfort-function goal that will allow the client to perform necessary or desired activities easily.
- Use the Hierarchy of Pain Measures as a framework for pain assessment: (1) consider the client's condition and search for possible causes of pain (e.g., presence of tissue injury, pathological conditions, exposure to procedures/interventions that are thought to result in pain); (2) attempt to obtain the client's self-report of pain; (3) observe for behaviors that may indicate pain presence (e.g., facial expressions, crying, restlessness, changes in activity); (4) speak with the client's significant others (i.e., parent, spouse, health care provider) about the client's customary behavioral responses to pain; and (5) conduct an analgesic trial.

• = Independent          ▲ = Collaborative

- Vital signs should not be used to determine or validate the presence or absence of pain.
- Assume that pain is present if the client is unable to provide a self-report and has tissue injury, has a pathological condition, or has undergone a procedure that is thought to produce pain, and conduct an analgesic trial.
- Obtain and review an accurate and complete list of medications the client is taking or has taken.
▲ Recognize the adverse effects of unrelieved pain.
▲ Explain to the client the pain management approach, including pharmacological and nonpharmacological interventions, the assessment and reassessment process, potential side effects, and the importance of prompt reporting of unrelieved pain.
▲ Reassure the client that pain will be regularly assessed and treated and that they will be observed for medication side effects and signs of opioid use disorder (OUD).
- Teach the client about pain and pharmacological and nonpharmacological interventions when pain is relatively well controlled.
▲ Regularly reassess the client for the presence of pain and response to pain management interventions, including effectiveness and the presence of adverse effects related to pain management interventions. Review the client's pain flow sheet and medication administration record to evaluate effectiveness of pain relief, previous 24-hour opioid requirements, and occurrence of side effects.
▲ Advocate for and manage acute pain using a multimodal, opioid-sparing approach.
▲ Select the route for administration of analgesics based on client condition and pain characteristics.
▲ Support the use of perineural infusions and intraspinal analgesia when appropriate and available.
▲ Use diverse analgesic delivery methods such as PCA to improve postoperative pain control and increase clients' satisfaction with pain management.
▲ Administer a nonopioid analgesic for mild to moderate pain and add an opioid analgesic if indicated for moderate to severe acute pain.
- Avoid administering analgesics based solely on a client's pain intensity rating.
- Administer nonopioid analgesics around the clock for acute postoperative pain and if necessary opioid analgesics for intermittent or breakthrough pain.

• = Independent      ▲ = Collaborative

- Prevent pain by administering analgesia before painful procedures whenever possible (e.g., endotracheal suctioning, wound care, heel puncture, venipunctures, and peripherally inserted IV catheters).
- Perform nursing care during the peak effect of analgesics to optimize client comfort and participation in care.
- Advocate for the use of "as needed" opioid range orders to provide effective and appropriate pain relief.
- Choose analgesic and dose based on orders that reflect the client's report of pain severity and response to the previous dose in terms of pain relief, occurrence of side effects, and ability to perform the activities of recovery or ADLs.
- ▲ When converting opioids from parenteral doses to oral doses (the preferred route when the client can tolerate and absorb oral medications), use equianalgesic dosing charts and carefully monitor the client's response to the new medication route and dose.
- ▲ Although all clients who are receiving opioids for acute pain are at risk for serious opioid-related adverse effects such as advancing sedation and respiratory depression, some are at even higher risk. Clients should have frequent respiratory assessment (rate, rhythm, noisiness, and depth) and systematic assessment of sedation level using a sedation scale.
- ▲ When opioids are included in the multimodal analgesic plan, clients need regular assessment for common side effects such as constipation, nausea, pruritus, lack of appetite, and changes in rest and sleep, and preventive measures are implemented when possible.
- Monitor frequency of bowel movements and alert the opioid prescriber when frequency is reduced.
- ▲ Support the client's use of nonpharmacological methods to supplement pharmacological analgesic approaches to help control pain, such as distraction, imagery, music therapy, simple massage, relaxation, and application of heat and cold.
- ▲ Assist client to identify resources for coping with psychological impact of pain.

**Pediatric**

- Assess for the presence of pain using a valid and reliable pain scale based on age, cognitive development, and the child's ability to provide a self-report. Pain intensity scales should be used in conjunction with valid and reliable tools that assess the impact of pain on the child's quality of life (Manworren & Stinson, 2016).
- ▲ Administer prescribed analgesics using a multimodal approach to treat pain in children, infants, and neonates.

• = Independent            ▲ = Collaborative

- Prevent procedural pain in neonates, infants, and children by using analgesics and sedatives as indicated.
- Use a topical local anesthetic treatment or other nonpharmacological treatment before performing venipuncture in neonates, infants, and children.
- For the neonate, use oral sucrose and nonnutritional sucking (NNS) or human milk for pain of short duration such as heel stick or venipuncture. Neonates, especially preterm neonates, are more sensitive to pain than older children.
- As with adults, use nonpharmacological analgesic interventions to supplement, not replace, pharmacological interventions in pediatric clients.

**Geriatric**
- Refer to the Nursing Interventions in the care plan for Chronic **Pain.**

**Multicultural**
- Refer to the Nursing Interventions in the care plan for Chronic **Pain.**

**Home Care**
▲ Develop the treatment plan with the client and caregivers.
- Assess the client's full medication profile, including medications prescribed by all health care providers and all over-the-counter (OTC) medications for drug interactions, and educate the client about the need to discuss use of all medications, including OTC medications, with the health care provider.
▲ Assess the client/family's knowledge of side effects and safety precautions associated with pain medications.
- If medication is administered using highly technological methods, assess the home for the necessary resources (e.g., electricity) and ensure that there will be responsible caregivers available to assist the client with administration.
- Assess the knowledge base of the client and family regarding highly technological medication administration and provide necessary education, including the procedure to follow if analgesia is unsatisfactory.

**Client/Family Teaching and Discharge Planning**
Note: To avoid the negative connotations associated with the words "drugs" and "narcotics," use the term "pain medicine" when teaching clients.
- Discuss the various discomforts encompassed by the word "pain" and ask the client to give examples of previously experienced pain. Explain the pain assessment process and the purpose of the pain rating scale.
- Teach the client to use the self-report pain tool to rate the intensity of past or current pain. Ask the client to set a comfort-function

goal by selecting a pain level on the self-report tool that will allow performance of desired or necessary activities of recovery with relative ease (e.g., turn, cough, deep breathe, ambulate, participate in physical therapy). If the pain level is consistently above the comfort-function goal, the client should take action that decreases pain or notify a member of the health care team so that effective pain management interventions may be implemented promptly.

• Provide written educational materials on various aspects of pain control to improve client understanding of pain and pain-related interventions.

• Discuss and evaluate the client's understanding of the total plan for pharmacological and nonpharmacological treatment, including the medications prescribed and their indication, proper dosing schedule, and adverse events and what to do should they occur.

• Teach basic principles of pain management using a variety of educational strategies, and evaluate learning.

▲ Reinforce the importance of taking pain medications to maintain the comfort-function goal.

▲ Reinforce that short-term use of opioids for acute pain relief is an appropriate part of their multimodal pain treatment plan.

▲ Reinforce the importance of safe storage of opioid medications out of the reach of others, and teach clients how to responsibly dispose of any unused opioids.

• Client education by nurses in the emergency department setting related to the use, storage, and disposal of pain medications may increase client knowledge and promote safety (Waszak et al, 2018).

▲ Demonstrate the use of appropriate nonpharmacological approaches in addition to pharmacological approaches to help control pain, such as application of heat and/or cold, distraction techniques, relaxation breathing, visualization, rocking, stroking, listening to music, and watching television.

## Chronic Pain

**Domain 12** Comfort    **Class 1** Physical comfort
### NANDA-I Definition

Unpleasant sensory and emotional experience associated with actual or potential tissue damage, or described in terms of such damage (International Association for the Study of Pain); sudden or slow onset of any intensity from mild to severe, constant or recurring without an anticipated or predictable end, and a duration of greater than 3 months.

• = Independent                    ▲ = Collaborative

## Defining Characteristics

Altered ability to continue activities; anorexia; evidence of pain using standardized pain behavior checklist for those unable to communicate verbally; expresses fatigue; facial expression of pain; proxy report of activity changes; proxy report of pain behavior; reports altered sleep-wake cycle; reports intensity using standardized pain scale; reports pain characteristics using standardized pain instrument; self-focused

## Related Factors

Body mass index above normal range for age and gender; fatigue; ineffective sexuality pattern; injury agent; malnutrition; prolonged computer use; psychological distress; repeated handling of heavy loads; social isolation; whole-body vibration

## At-Risk Population

Individuals aged >50 years; individuals with history of being abused; individuals with a history of genital mutilation; individuals with history of over indebtedness; individuals with history of static work postures; individuals with history of substance misuse; individuals with history of vigorous exercise; women

## Associated Conditions

Bone fractures; central nervous system sensitization; chronic musculoskeletal diseases; contusion; crush syndrome; imbalance of neurotransmitters, neuromodulators, and receptors; immune system diseases; impaired metabolism; inborn genetic diseases; ischemia; neoplasms; nerve compression syndromes; nervous system diseases; post-trauma related condition; prolonged increase in cortisol level; soft tissue injuries; spinal cord injuries

## Client Outcomes

**Client Will (Specify Time Frame)**

**For the Client Who Is Able to Provide a Self-Report**

- Provide a description of the pain experience including physical, social, emotional, and spiritual aspects
- Use a self-report pain tool to identify current pain level and establish a comfort-function goal
- Report that the pain management regimen achieves comfort-function goal without the occurrence of side effects
- Describe nonpharmacological methods that can be used to supplement, or enhance, pharmacological interventions and help achieve the comfort-function goal
- Perform necessary or desired activities at a pain level less than or equal to the comfort-function goal
- Demonstrate the ability to pace activity, taking rest breaks before they are needed

• = Independent        ▲ = Collaborative

- Describe how unrelieved pain will be managed
- State the ability to obtain sufficient amounts of rest and sleep
- Notify a member of the health care team for pain level consistently greater than the comfort-function goal or occurrence of side effect

**For the Client Who Is Unable to Provide a Self-Report**

- Demonstrate decrease or resolved pain-related behaviors
- Perform desired activities as determined by client condition
- Demonstrate the absence of side effects
- No pain-related behaviors will be evident in the client who is completely unresponsive; a reasonable outcome is to demonstrate the absence of side effects related to the prescribed pain treatment plan

## Nursing Interventions

▲ During the initial assessment and interview, if the client is experiencing pain, conduct and document a comprehensive pain assessment, using appropriate pain assessment tools.

▲ Determine the quality of the pain and whether the pain has persisted beyond the usual duration for tissue healing. Refer to the care plan for Acute **Pain** and discussion of the Hierarchy of Pain Measures for assessment approach in clients who are unable to provide self-report of pain.

▲ Perform a pain assessment using a reliable self-report pain tool.

▲ Ask the client to describe prior experiences with pain, effectiveness of pain management interventions, responses to analgesic medications (including occurrence of side effects), and concerns about pain and its treatment (e.g., fear about addiction, worries, anxiety) and informational needs.

• Using a self-report tool, ask the client to identify a comfort-function goal that will allow the client to perform necessary or desired activities easily.

▲ Assess chronic pain regularly, including the impact of chronic pain on activity; sleep; eating habits; and social conditions, including relationships, finances, and employment.

▲ Assess the client for the presence of psychiatric conditions, including anxiety and depression.

▲ If opioid therapy is considered, assist the provider with aspects of an opioid risk assessment, which includes a comprehensive client interview and examination with a pain focus, mental health screening, use of an opioid risk assessment tool, examination of prescription drug monitoring program results, and urine drug screening.

▲ For the client who is receiving outpatient opioid therapy, at each visit, assess effect of opioids on pain status, function, goal achievement,

• = Independent      ▲ = Collaborative

and presence of side effects, including sleep disturbance and sexual dysfunction; assessment for signs of misuse and OUD should be included, which may involve the use of random urine drug toxicology screening, pill counts, and review of prescription monitoring database.

• Ask the client to maintain a diary (if able) of pain ratings, timing, precipitating events, medications, and effectiveness of pain management interventions.

▲ Obtain and review an accurate and complete list of medications the client is taking or has taken.

• Medication review has been found to improve the quality of medication interventions, including client adherence, and outcomes (Rose et al, 2015).

▲ Explain to the client the pain management approach that has been ordered or revised, including therapies, medication administration, side effects, and complications.

• Discuss the client's fears of undertreated pain, side effects, OUD, and overdose and reassure the client that there will be regular assessment and treatment of pain and assessment for side effects and signs of OUD.

▲ Manage chronic pain using an individualized, multimodal nonopioid or opioid-sparing approach.

▲ When chronic pain has a neuropathic component, treat with adjuvant analgesics, such as anticonvulsants, antidepressants, and topical local anesthetics.

▲ Administer a nonopioid analgesic for mild to moderate chronic pain and as a component of the treatment for all levels of pain for clients with cancer pain.

▲ Recognize that opioid therapy may be indicated for some clients experiencing chronic pain.

▲ Administer analgesics around the clock for continuous pain and as needed (PRN) for intermittent or breakthrough pain as may be experienced by clients with cancer pain.

▲ Long-acting or extended-release opioids may be indicated for clients with cancer pain if clients require the regular use of short-acting opioids and receive adequate relief with them.

▲ At regular intervals, assess inpatient clients with chronic pain for opioid-related adverse events and include frequent assessment of pain level, assessment of respiratory status (including rate, rhythm, noisiness, and depth), and systematic assessment of sedation level using a sedation scale.

• = Independent          ▲ = Collaborative

▲ During outpatient follow-up, assess clients receiving opioids for risk factors that may increase opioid-related harm.

▲ Provide the client with a bowel regimen, including adequate hydration, fiber, and laxatives to prevent/treat opioid-related constipation. Ask about other opioid-related side effects including nausea, pruritus, lack of appetite, and changes in rest and sleep.

▲ In addition to administering analgesics, support the client's use of nonpharmacological methods to help control pain, such as distraction, imagery, relaxation, and application of heat and cold.

▲ Cognitive behavioral techniques have been shown to be useful in the management of chronic pain.

▲ Encourage the client to plan activities around periods of greatest comfort whenever possible.

▲ Explore appropriate resources for long-term management of chronic pain (e.g., hospice, pain care center).

▲ If the client has progressive cancer pain, assist the client and family with handling issues related to death and dying and provide access to palliative care programs and hospice services.

**P** **Pediatric**

• Assess for the presence of pain using a valid and reliable pain scale based on age, cognitive development, and the child's ability to provide a self-report.

▲ Manage chronic pain children, infants, and neonates with a multiprofessional and multimodal approach.

• Use a variety of nonpharmacological analgesic interventions to address chronic pain in pediatric clients.

**Geriatric**

▲ An older client's report of pain should be taken seriously and assessed and treated.

• When assessing pain, speak clearly, slowly, and loudly enough for the client to hear; ensure hearing aids and glasses are in place as appropriate; enlarge pain scales and written materials; and repeat information as needed.

• Handle the client's body gently and allow the client to move at his or her own speed.

▲ Use nonpharmacological approaches including physical therapy, exercise, or other movement-based programs as the core components to persistent pain management in the older adult.

▲ When pharmacological measures are needed to address chronic pain in the elderly, use a multimodal approach, including nonopioid analgesics for mild to moderate pain.

• = Independent                    ▲ = Collaborative

▲ Use opioids cautiously in the older client with chronic pain.

▲ Monitor for signs of depression in older clients and refer to specialists with relevant expertise.

**Multicultural**

▲ Assess for and identify the presence of pain disparities among clients and work to develop opportunities for equal care.

▲ Assess for the influence of cultural beliefs, norms, and values on the client's perception and experience of pain.

▲ Social support should be facilitated as it has a positive impact on the client's ability to cope with chronic pain.

▲ Use culturally relevant pain scales to assess pain in the client.

**Home Care**

• The interventions previously described may be adapted for home care use. Refer to the Nursing Interventions in the care plan for Acute **Pain.**

**Client/Family Teaching and Discharge Planning**

Note: To avoid the negative connotations associated with the words "drugs" and "narcotics," use the term "pain medicine" when teaching clients.

• Discuss the various discomforts encompassed by the word "pain" and ask the client to give examples of previously experienced pain. Explain the pain assessment process and the purpose of the pain rating scale.

• Teach the client that if the pain level is consistently above the comfort-function goal, the client should take action that decreases pain or should notify a member of the health care team so that effective pain management interventions may be implemented promptly. (See information on teaching clients to use the pain rating scale.)

• Provide educational materials on various aspects of pain control to improve client understanding of pain and pain-related interventions.

• Discuss and evaluate the client's understanding of the total plan for pharmacological and nonpharmacological treatment, including the medication plan, the maintenance of a pain diary, and the use of supplies and equipment.

▲ Reinforce that opioids, when prescribed for chronic pain, may be an appropriate component of multimodal pain treatment plan, but clients require knowledge of safe opioid use and potential adverse effects.

▲ Reinforce the importance of safe storage of opioid medications out of the reach of others and to responsibly dispose of any unused opioids.

• Demonstrate the use of appropriate nonpharmacological approaches in addition to pharmacological approaches for helping control pain, such as application of heat and/or cold, distraction techniques, relaxation breathing, visualization, rocking, stroking, listening to music, and watching television. Teach these methods when pain is relatively well controlled, because pain interferes with cognition.

▲ Emphasize to the client the importance of participating in a structured, individualized pacing activity and taking rest breaks before they are needed to reduce fatigue, reduce joint stiffness, and maintain physical activity.

• Teach nonpharmacological methods when pain is relatively well controlled.

## Chronic Pain Syndrome

**Domain 12** Comfort    **Class 1** Physical comfort
### NANDA-I Definition

Recurrent or persistent pain that has lasted at least 3 months and that significantly affects daily functioning or well-being.

### Defining Characteristics

Anxiety (00146); constipation (00011); disturbed sleep pattern (00198); fatigue (00093); fear (00148); impaired mood regulation (00241); impaired physical mobility (00085); insomnia (00095); social isolation (00053); stress overload (00177)

### Related Factors

Body mass index above normal range for age and gender; fear of pain; fear-avoidance beliefs; inadequate knowledge of pain management behaviors; negative affect; sleep disturbances

### Client Outcomes, Nursing Interventions, Client/Family Teaching and Discharge Planning

Refer to care plan for Acute **Pain** and Chronic **Pain.**

## Labor Pain

**Domain 12** Comfort    **Class 1** Physical comfort
### NANDA-I Definition

Sensory and emotional experience that varies from pleasant to unpleasant, associated with labor and childbirth.

### Defining Characteristics

Altered blood pressure; altered heart rate; altered muscle tension; altered neuroendocrine functioning; altered respiratory rate; altered urinary functioning; anxiety; appetite change; diaphoresis; distraction behavior; expressive behavior; facial expression of pain; narrow focus; nausea;

perineal pressure; positioning to ease pain; protective behavior; pupil dilation; reports altered sleep-wake cycle; self-focused; uterine contraction; vomiting

## Related Factors
### Behavioral Factors
Insufficient fluid intake; supine position
### Cognitive Factors
Fear of childbirth; inadequate knowledge about childbirth; inadequate preparation to deal with labor pain; low self efficacy; perception of labor pain as nonproductive; perception of labor pain as negative; perception of labor pain as threatening; perception of labor pain as unnatural; perception of pain as meaningful
### Social Factors
Interference in decision-making; unsupportive companionship
### Unmodified Environmental Factors
Noisy delivery room; overcrowded delivery room; turbulent environment

## At-Risk Population
Women experiencing emergency situation during labor; women from cultures with negative perspective of labor pain; women giving birth in a disease based health care system; women whose mothers have a high level of education; women with history of pre-pregnancy dysmenorrhea; women with history of sexual abuse during childhood; women without supportive companion

## Associated Conditions
Cervical dilation; depression; fetal expulsion; high maternal trait anxiety; prescribed mobility restriction; prolonged duration of labor

## Client Outcomes
### Client Will (Specify Time Frame)
- Recognize pharmacological and nonpharmacological interventions to address labor pain
- Demonstrate coping strategies to address labor pain
- Verbalize pain relief effectiveness throughout the labor process

## Nursing Interventions
- Initial assessment and interview, if the client is experiencing pain, conduct and document a comprehensive pain assessment, using appropriate pain assessment tools.
- Observe for nonverbal pain assessment such as grimacing, lackluster eyes, and fixed or scattered movements.
- Assess pain on pain level tool such as the 0 to 10 numerical pain rating scale (NRS) if appropriate or the CWLA (Fairchild et al, 2017). Discuss with client the desire for pain management for

• = Independent       ▲ = Collaborative

this labor, past experiences with labor and effectiveness of pain management techniques employed at that time, concerns about pain and its treatment, and information needs (e.g., pain coping techniques that are both analgesic and nonpharmaceutical).

- Goal is for the client to manage labor pain from admission until delivery of infant with either natural childbirth and associated pain management techniques or pharmaceutical measures to reduce pain experience.

- Based on the client's ability to cope with labor pain, discuss with client pain management options, including pharmacological and nonpharmacological interventions. Coping strategies women may implement include being still or rocking, focusing on breathing, relaxing muscles, changing position, listening to soothing music, making noises, and being in water (ACNM, 2020).

- Based on the client's ability to cope and their perception of labor pain, assess the physiological-natural process of labor, physical environment, and emotional/psychosocial dynamics and behaviors (Asl et al, 2018).

- Based on the client's ability to cope, offer intervention (either nonpharmacological or pharmacological).

- Nonpharmacological pain relief measures are low-risk and low-resource interventions (Caughey & Tilden, 2021). These approaches can encompass the physical sensation of pain and the psychoemotional and spiritual components of care. By addressing all aspects of client needs (physical, emotional, and spiritual), suffering can be reduced during labor (Caughey & Tilden, 2021).

  ○ Ambulation/rocking/swaying is a safe and effective coping measure for labor pain. This is usually a client-initiated response to labor pain; however, caregivers can encourage women to ambulate or change position to ease pain or allow clients to cope better with labor pain.

  ○ Hydrotherapy either as immersion in water or bathing can be used to promote relaxation, decrease acute anxiety, help cope with pain, promote greater maternal movement, reduce the need for pharmacological pain relief measures, and promote normal physiological labor (Shaw-Battista, 2017; Sidebottom et al, 2020).

  ○ TENS is a small, handheld device that transmits low-voltage electrical impulses to the skin (Caughey & Tilden, 2021). The device suppresses the conduction of pain through pain fibers by using small electrical impulses (Shahoei et al, 2017).

• = Independent          ▲ = Collaborative

- Pharmacological measures for pain relief are high resource and high risk; they require professional training for administration, incur cost, and have a greater risk to mother and baby (Caughey & Tilden, 2021).
- Nitrous oxide is a blend of 50% nitrous oxide with 50% oxygen. The use of nitrous oxide may not alleviate pain, but it may help with satisfaction of the birth experience (Richardson et al, 2019).
- IV medications for pain management are an alternative for some women who do not desire an epidural; IV medications are generally opioids.
- Epidural, combined spinal-epidural (CSE), and dural puncture epidural (DPE) are appropriate for laboring women when requested by the client (unless there is a contraindication).
- Account for clients' abilities to cope with labor pain regarding their psychosocial, cultural, and spiritual backgrounds. A woman's positive perceptions of how she will be able to cope with labor are associated with reduced anxiety, pain, and intervention during labor (Van der Gucht & Lewis, 2015; Caughey & Tilden, 2021).
- Document pain assessment through direct observation. Also document interventions to facilitate labor pain management through the continuum of the women's labor experience (Van der Gucht & Lewis, 2015).

**P**

# Impaired Parenting

**Domain 7** Role relationship    **Class 1** Caregiving roles

## NANDA-I Definition

Limitation of primary caregiver to nurture, protect, and promote optimal growth and development of the child, through a consistent, empathic exercise of authority and appropriate behavior in response to the child's needs.

## Defining Characteristics

### Parental Externalizing Symptoms

Hostile parenting behaviors; impulsive behaviors; intrusive behaviors; negative communication

### Parental Internalizing Symptoms

Decreased engagement in parent-child relations; decreased positive temperament; decreased subjective attention quality; extreme mood swings; failure to provide safe home environment; inadequate response to infant behavioral cues; inappropriate child-care arrangements; rejects child; social alienation

• = Independent          ▲ = Collaborative

**Infant or Child**

Anxiety; conduct problems; delayed cognitive development; depressive symptoms; difficulty establishing healthy intimate interpersonal relations; difficulty functioning socially; difficulty regulating emotion; extreme mood alterations; low academic performance; obesity; role reversal; somatic complaints; substance misuse

## Related Factors

Altered parental role; decreased emotion recognition abilities; depressive symptoms; difficulty managing complex treatment regimen; dysfunctional family processes; emotional vacillation; high use of internet-connected devices; inadequate knowledge about child development; inadequate knowledge about child health maintenance; inadequate parental role model; inadequate problem-solving skills; inadequate social support; inadequate transportation; inattentive to child's needs; increased anxiety symptoms; low self efficacy; marital conflict; nonrestorative sleep-wake cycle; perceived economic strain; social isolation; substance misuse; unaddressed intimate partner violence

## At-Risk Population

**Parent**

Adolescents; economically disadvantaged individuals; homeless individuals; individuals experiencing family substance misuse; individuals experiencing situational crisis; individuals with family history of post-traumatic shock; individuals with history of being abused; individuals with history of being abusive; individuals with history of being neglected; individuals with history of exposure to violence; individuals with history of inadequate prenatal care; individuals with history of prenatal stress; individuals with low educational level; sole parents

**Infant or Child**

Children experiencing prolonged separation from parent; children with difficult temperament; children with gender other than that desired by parent; children with history of hospitalization in neonatal intensive care; premature infants

## Associated Conditions

**Parent**

Depression; mental disorders

**Infant or Child**

Behavioral disorder; complex treatment regimen; emotional disorder; neurodevelopmental disabilities

## Client Outcomes

**Client Will (Specify Time Frame)**

- Initiate appropriate measures to develop a safe, nurturing environment

• = Independent        ▲ = Collaborative

- Acquire and display attentive, supportive parenting behaviors and child supervision
- Identify appropriate strategies to manage a child's inappropriate behaviors
- Identify strategies to protect child from harm and/or neglect and initiate action when indicated

## Nursing Interventions

- Use the Parenting Sense of Competence (PSOC) scale to measure parental self-efficacy.
- Determine parent/family sources of stress, using the Parental Stress Scale.
- Use family-centered care and role modeling for holistic care of families.
- Assess for the following signs of parental burnout: exhaustion in one's parental role, contrast with previous parental self, feelings of being fed up with one's parental role, and emotional distancing from one's children.
- ▲ Institute abuse/neglect protection measures if evidence exists of an inability to cope with family stressors or crises, signs of parental substance abuse are observed, or a significant level of social isolation is apparent.
- Evaluate the family's perceived strength of its social support system. Encourage the family to use social support.
- Support parents' competence in appraising their infant's behavior and responses and aim supportive interventions to minimize parents' experiences of strain or stress.
- ▲ Refer to parenting training programs.
- Refer to Readiness for Enhanced **Parenting** for additional interventions.

## Multicultural

- Acknowledge racial/ethnic differences at the onset of care.
- Assess for the influence of stigma related to parent help-seeking behaviors.
- Assess for the influence of cultural beliefs, norms, and values on the client's perceptions of the parental role.
- Acknowledge that value conflicts arising from acculturation stresses may contribute to increased anxiety and significant conflict with the parental role.
- Refer parents of young children in specific cultural communities to support programs.

• = Independent ▲ = Collaborative

**Home Care**

- The interventions previously described may be adapted for home care use.

**Client/Family Teaching and Discharge Planning**

- Encourage children and parent involvement in bereavement support groups, as an adjunct to grief therapy.
▲ Refer to a parenting program to facilitate learning of parenting skills.
- Teach the client about available community resources (e.g., therapists, ministers, counselors, self-help groups).
- Teach parents the importance of involvement with and monitoring of child/adolescent technology usage, social media presence, and online activities for digital safety.
- Promotion of better-quality relationships between parents and children is an effective strategy that can lead to enhanced learning. Good-quality parenting leads to improved cognitive and social skills for children.

# Readiness for Enhanced Parenting

**Domain 7** Role relationship    **Class 1** Caregiving roles

## NANDA-I Definition

A pattern of primary caregiver to nurture, protect, and promote optimal growth and development of the child, through a consistent, empathic exercise of authority and appropriate behavior in response to the child's needs, which can be strengthened.

## Defining Characteristics

Expresses desire to enhance acceptance of child; expresses desire to enhance attention quality; expresses desire to enhance child health maintenance; expresses desire to enhance childcare arrangements; expresses desire to enhance engagement with child; expresses desire to enhance home environmental safety; expresses desire to enhance mood stability; expresses desire to enhance parent-child relations; expresses desire to enhance patience; expresses desire to enhance positive communication; expresses desire to enhance positive parenting behaviors; expresses desire to enhance positive temperament; expresses desire to enhance response to infant behavioral cues

## Client Outcomes

**Client/Family Will (Specify Time Frame)**

- Affirm desire to improve parenting skills to further support growth and development of children
- Demonstrate loving relationship with children

• = Independent                    ▲ = Collaborative

- Provide a safe, nurturing environment
- Assess risks in home/environment and take steps to prevent possibility of harm to children
- Meet physical, psychosocial, and spiritual needs or seek appropriate assistance

## Nursing Interventions

- Use family-centered care and role modeling for holistic care of families.
- Use cell phone technology to enhance parenting interventions.
- Promote low-technology interventions, such as massage and multisensory interventions (maternal voice, eye-to-eye contact, and rocking) and music, to reduce maternal and infant stress and improve mother–infant relationship.
- Promote mindful parenting techniques such as being fully present during interactions, maintaining freedom from distractions or judgment, and responding with an open mind.
- Support skin-to-skin care for infants at risk at birth; maintain infants in an upright position during skin-to-skin contact.
- Encourage family meals and rituals.
- Refer to parenting training programs.
- Refer to the care plan for Impaired **Parenting** for additional interventions.

### Multicultural

- Understand and incorporate cultural differences into interventions to enhance the impact of interventions.
- Support programs for parents of young children in specific cultural communities.
- Acknowledge and praise parenting strengths noted.

### Home Care

- The nursing interventions previously described should be used in the home environment with adaptations as necessary.
- ▲ Refer to a parenting program to facilitate learning of parenting skills.

### Client/Family Teaching and Discharge Planning

- Refer to Client/Family Teaching and Discharge Planning for Impaired **Parenting** for suggestions that may be used with minor adaptations.
- Teach parents home safety: reduction of hot water temperature, proper poison storage, use of smoke alarms, and installation of safety gates for stairs.

P

• = Independent          ▲ = Collaborative

- Provide parent teaching about supportive emotion communication practices such as listening and connection, labeling feelings, and providing emotional support.
▲ Refer mothers of children with type 1 diabetes for community support in babysitting, child care, or respite.
▲ Refer parents of sexual minority adolescents to supportive parenting resources and programs.
- Teach parents the importance of involvement with and monitoring of child/adolescent technology usage, social media presence, and online activities for digital safety.
- Promotion of better-quality relationships between parents and children is an effective strategy that can lead to enhanced learning. Good-quality parenting leads to improved cognitive and social skills for children.

# Risk for Impaired Parenting

**Domain 7** Role relationship    **Class 1** Caregiving roles

**NANDA-I Definition**

Primary caregiver susceptible to a limitation to nurture, protect, and promote optimal growth and development of the child, through a consistent, empathic exercise of authority and appropriate behavior in response to the child's needs.

**Risk Factors**

Altered parental role; decreased emotion recognition abilities; depressive symptoms; difficulty managing complex treatment regimen; dysfunctional family processes; emotional vacillation; high use of Internet-connected devices; inadequate knowledge about child development; inadequate knowledge about child health maintenance; inadequate parental role model; inadequate problem-solving skills; inadequate social support; inadequate transportation; inattentive to child's needs; increased anxiety symptoms; low self efficacy; marital conflict; nonrestorative sleep-wake cycle; perceived economic strain; social isolation; substance misuse; unaddressed intimate partner violence

**At-Risk Population**

Parent

Adolescents; economically disadvantaged individuals; homeless individuals; individuals experiencing family substance misuse; individuals experiencing situational crisis; individuals with family history of post-traumatic shock; individuals with history of being abused; individuals with history of being abusive; individuals with history of being neglected; individuals with history of exposure to violence; individuals with history of inadequate prenatal care; individuals with history of prenatal stress; individuals with low educational level; sole parents

**Infant or Child**

Children experiencing prolonged separation from parent; children with difficult temperament; children with gender other than that desired by parent; children with history of hospitalization in neonatal intensive care; premature infants

## Associated Conditions

**Parent**

Depression; mental disorders

**Infant or Child**

Behavioral disorder; complex treatment regimen; emotional disorder; neurodevelopmental disabilities

## Client Outcomes, Nursing Interventions, and Client/Family Teaching and Discharge Planning

Refer to care plans for Readiness for Enhanced **Parenting** and Impaired **Parenting**.

**P**

# Risk for Perioperative Positioning Injury

**Domain 11** Safety/protection    **Class 2** Physical injury

## NANDA-I Definition

Susceptible to inadvertent anatomical and physical changes as a result of posture or positioning equipment used during an invasive/surgical procedure, which may compromise health.

## Risk Factors

Decreased muscle strength; dehydration; factors identified by standardized, validated screening tool; inadequate access to appropriate equipment; inadequate access to appropriate support surfaces; inadequate availability of equipment for individuals with obesity; malnutrition; obesity; prolonged non-anatomic positioning of limbs; rigid support surface

## At-Risk Population

Individuals at extremes of age; individuals in lateral position; individuals in lithotomy position; individuals in prone position; individuals in Trendelenburg position; individuals undergoing surgical procedure >1 hour

## Associated Conditions

Diabetes mellitus; edema; emaciation; general anesthesia; immobilization; neuropathy; sensoriperceptual disturbance from anesthesia; vascular diseases

• = Independent    ▲ = Collaborative

## Client Outcomes

### Client Will (Specify Time Frame)

- Demonstrate unchanged skin condition, with exception of the incision, throughout the perioperative experience
- Demonstrate resolution of redness of the skin at points of pressure within 30 minutes after pressure is eliminated
- Remain injury-free related to surgical positioning, including intact skin and absence of pain and/or numbness associated with surgical positioning
- Demonstrate unchanged or improved physical mobility from preoperative status
- Demonstrate unchanged or improved peripheral sensory integrity from preoperative status

## Nursing Interventions

### General Interventions for Any Surgical Client

▲ Positioning of the client during a surgical procedure is the responsibility of all members of the perioperative team, including registered nurse, surgical technologist, surgeon, and anesthesia professional (Spruce, 2018).
- Assess the client's skin integrity throughout the perioperative process to avoid skin breakdown during surgical/invasive procedures. Continuous evaluation of clinical changes in the client is necessary to assess outcomes and effects of nursing interventions for surgical positioning (Bjorkland-Lima et al, 2019).
- Recognize that surgery increases a client's risk for skin injury because of the time the client is immobile for the procedure (Park, Park, & Hwang, 2019).
- An operating room–related pressure injury is any pressure injury that develops within 48 to 72 hours intraoperatively, interoperatively, or postoperatively of a surgical procedure (Khong et al, 2020).

### Prevention of Pressure Injuries

- Complete a preoperative assessment to identify client factors that will increase a client's risk for pressure injuries. This includes physical alterations that may require additional precautions for procedure-specific positioning and to identify specific procedural positioning needs, type of anesthesia, and so on.
- Identify procedure risk factors such as length and type of surgery, potential for intraoperative hypotensive episodes, low core temperatures, and decreased mobility on postoperative day 1.

• = Independent            ▲ = Collaborative

- Recognize that all surgical clients should be considered at high risk for pressure ulcer development, because pressure ulcers can develop in as little as 20 minutes in the operating room.
- Remove all client jewelry and accessories.
- Protect the heels during surgery by elevating the heels completely.
- Use pressure-reducing devices and pressure-relieving mattresses as necessary to prevent pressure injury.
- Avoid using rolled sheets and towels as positioning devices because they tend to produce high and inconsistent pressures. Special positioning devices are available that redistribute pressure.
- Avoid covering positioning devices or placing extra blankets on top of a pressure-reducing surface.
- The nurse should demonstrate knowledge not only of the equipment but also of anatomy and the application of physiological principles to properly position the client.
- Monitor client position and pressure being applied to the client intraoperatively by staff, equipment, and/or instruments.
- Use additional pressure-redistributing padding on all bony prominences.
- Recognize that reddened areas or areas injured by pressure should not be massaged.
- Implement measures to prevent inadvertent hypothermia.
- Many surgical clients have medical devices placed as a part of the surgical procedure. Avoid positioning the client on the medical device and perform frequent assessments of the skin under and around the device (NPIAP & EPUAP, 2019; Cooper et al, 2020).

**Positioning the Perioperative Client**
- Ensure linens on the operating room table are free of wrinkles.
- Lock the operating room table, cart, or bed and stabilize the mattress before transferring/positioning the client. Monitor the client while on the operating room table at all times.
- Lift rather than pull or slide the client when positioning to reduce the incidence of skin injury from shearing and/or friction.
- Ensure that appropriate numbers of personnel are present to assist in positioning the client.
- Recognize that, optimally, clients (especially those with limited range of motion/mobility) should be asked to position themselves under the nurse's guidance before induction of anesthesia so that the nurse can verify that a position of comfort has been obtained.
- Ensure that nerves are protected by positioning extremities carefully.

• = Independent       ▲ = Collaborative

- Use slow and smooth movements during positioning to allow the circulatory system to readjust.
- Reassess the client after positioning and periodically during the procedure to maintain proper alignment and skin integrity.
- Frequently assess the eyes and/or monitor intraocular pressure, especially when client is in the prone, Trendelenburg, or knee-chest position.
- Position hips in proper alignment with knees flexed. Unaligned hips can cause pressure to the low back and hip joints.
- Position the arms extended on arm boards so that they do not extend beyond a 90-degree angle. The arms should be at the level of the bed and should not be allowed to hang off the bed. Do not position arms at sides unless surgically necessary.
- Protect the client's skin surfaces from injury by preventing pooling of preparative solutions, blood, irrigation, urine, and feces.
- Keep the client appropriately covered and limit traffic in the room during the procedure.
- When positioning the client prone, care should be taken to ensure the head and neck are properly positioned. In addition, 5- to 10-degree reverse Trendelenburg should be used, if possible, to reduce intraocular pressure and decrease facial edema.
- Recognize that clients positioned in the lithotomy position should be kept in this position for as short a time as possible.
- The lowest heel position should be used in the lithotomy position.
- Maintain normal body alignment.
- When applying body supports and restraint straps (safety belt), apply loosely and secure over waist or midthigh at least 2 inches above the knees, avoiding bony prominences by placing a blanket between the strap and the client.
- Assess the client's skin integrity immediately postoperatively.
- Ensure that complete, concise, accurate documentation of client assessment and use of positioning devices is in the client's medical record.

### Geriatric

- Common age-related diseases include cardiovascular, diabetes, lung, renal, musculoskeletal, and neurodegenerative diseases. Progression of these diseases can lead to impaired systems and organs, leading to complications including anemia, malnutrition, and recurrent infection (Jaul et al, 2018).
- The skin of older adults (i.e., ≥65 years) is fragile and prone to shear injuries as the skin is less elastic; the dermis is thin and has less

collagen, muscle, and adipose tissue than the skin of younger adults (Van Wicklin, 2019). These changes leave the older adult's skin more susceptible to pressure, bruising, skin tears, infection, impaired thermoregulation, and slow healing (Van Wicklin, 2019).

**Pediatric**

- Pressure injury sites in the pediatric client differ from those in the adult population due to differences in anatomic structure.
- Neonates are vulnerable to skin and pressure injuries because of an immature and underdeveloped epidermis and dermis (Broom, Dunk, & Mohamed, 2019).
- Neonates and children are at higher risk for nutritional deficiencies as a result of smaller appetites and dietary intake in combination with increased nutritional requirement necessary to meet growth needs (Van Wicklin, 2019).
- Use of pediatric- and neonatal-specific pressure injury risk assessment tools accounts for age-specific indicators.

**Client/Family Teaching and Discharge Planning**

- Teach the client/family signs and symptoms of pressure injury, extremity nerve damage, compartment syndrome, and ocular injury based on surgical positioning. Early detection and treatment is beneficial.

P

# Risk for Peripheral Neurovascular Dysfunction

**Domain 11** Safety/projection    **Class 2** Physical injury

## NANDA-I Definition

Susceptible to disruption in the circulation, sensation, and motion of an extremity, which may compromise health.

## Risk Factors

To be developed

## Associated Conditions

Bone fractures; burns; immobilization; mechanical compression; orthopedic surgery; trauma; vascular obstruction

## Client Outcomes

**Client Will (Specify Time Frame)**

- Maintain circulation, sensation, and movement of an extremity within client's own normal limits
- Explain signs of neurovascular compromise

• = Independent    ▲ = Collaborative

## Nursing Interventions

- Recognize the risk factors that may result in peripheral neurovascular dysfunction.
- Assess for the early onset of neurovascular dysfunction or compartment syndrome by performing the neurovascular assessment as ordered or as indicated by the client's condition, and report abnormal findings to the provider promptly.
  - Pain: Assess severity (using an appropriate pain scale), quality, radiation, and relief by medications.
  - Pulses: Assess the pulses distal to the injury and compare with the unaffected limb; use a 0-to-4 point scale (0 = absent and 4 = strong/bounding).
  - Pallor: Assess skin color and temperature changes below the injury site and compare with unaffected limb; assess capillary refill.
  - Paresthesia (change in sensation): Assess by lightly touching the skin proximal and distal to the injury; ask if the client has any unusual sensations such as hypersensitivity, tingling, prickling, decreased feeling, or numbness.
  - Paralysis: Ask the client to perform appropriate range-of-motion exercises in the unaffected and then the affected extremity.
  - In addition to the five Ps, assess for swelling or increase in compartment pressure by feeling the extremity; note new onset of firmness of the extremity. Intracompartmental pressures may also be measured with proprietary monitoring devices.
- Monitor appropriate application and function of corrective device (e.g., cast, splint, traction) as needed.
- For prevention of deep vein thrombosis (DVT), nursing care of DVT, and pulmonary embolism, refer to the interventions on DVT prevention and treatment in the care plan for Ineffective Peripheral **Tissue** Perfusion.

# Risk for Poisoning

**Domain 11** Safety/protection    **Class 4** Environmental hazards
### NANDA-I Definition

Susceptible to accidental exposure to, or ingestion of, drugs or dangerous products in sufficient doses, which may compromise health.

• = Independent      ▲ = Collaborative

## Risk Factors
### External
Access to dangerous product; access to illicit drugs potentially contaminated by poisonous additives; access to pharmaceutical preparations; occupational setting without adequate safeguards
### Internal
Excessive emotional disturbance; inadequate knowledge of pharmaceutical preparations; inadequate knowledge of poisoning prevention; inadequate precautions against poisoning; neurobehavioral manifestations; unaddressed inadequate vision

## Client Outcomes
### Client Will (Specify Time Frame)
- Prevent inadvertent ingestion of or exposure to toxins or poisonous substances
- Explain and undertake appropriate safety measures to prevent ingestion of or exposure to toxins or poisonous substances
- Verbalize appropriate response to apparent or suspected toxic ingestion or poisoning

## Nursing Interventions

- When a client presents with possible/actual poisoning, follow the ABCs (airway, breathing and circulation) and administer oxygen if needed.
- ▲ When a client presents with possible poisoning, call the poison control center.
- Obtain a thorough history of what was ingested, how much, and when, and ask to look at the containers. Note the client's age, weight, medications, medical conditions, and any history of vomiting, choking, coughing, or change in mental status. Also take note of any interventions performed before seeking treatment.
- ▲ Note results of toxicology screens, arterial blood gases, blood glucose levels, and other ordered laboratory tests.
- For suspected acetaminophen poisoning, obtain an accurate history of the time(s) of acetaminophen ingestion, the quantity, and the formulation of acetaminophen ingested.
- ▲ Initiate prescribed treatment for poisoning promptly. The poison control center will specify any treatment or medications that need to be administered.
- ▲ Ensure that recommendations from the poison control center are clearly documented and readily accessible in the client's chart.
- Follow the "five rights" as guidelines when administering medications.

• = Independent     ▲ = Collaborative

- Use a bar code scanning system for client identification whenever possible.
- Standardize use of abbreviations, acronyms, symbols, and dose designations and eliminate those that are prone to cause errors.
- Be aware of the medications that look/sound alike and ensure that the correct medication is ordered and administered.
- Identify all the client's current medications on admission to a health care facility and compare the list with the current ordered medications. Reconcile any differences in medications. Use the expertise of the pharmacy department if there is any uncertainty regarding the accuracy of the client's medications. Reconcile the list of medications if the client is transferred from one unit to another, when there is a handoff to the next provider of care, and when the client is discharged.
- Assess for possible interactions and adverse effects among prescribed medications and over-the-counter products with a computerized drug interaction checker.

**Pediatric**

▲ Evaluate lead exposure risk and consult the health care provider regarding lead screening measures as indicated (public/ambulatory health).
- Provide multifaceted medication teaching to parents that includes an easy-to-read dosing handout, a teaching session, a teach-back method, and a standardized dosing device for liquid medications.
- Provide guidance for parents and caregivers regarding age-related safety measures, including the following (Safe Kids Worldwide, 2021):
  ○ Store household products safely out of child's reach and sight to prevent poisoning.
  ○ Keep all household cleaning products in their original containers. Shop for child-resistant containers.
  ○ Read and follow product labels.
  ○ Check home for products such as cleaning supplies, liquid laundry packets, personal care products, plants, pesticides, alcohol, and medicine.
  ○ Post Poison Help number in phone and visibly at home: 1-800-222-1222.
- Advise families that syrup of ipecac is no longer recommended to be kept and used in the home.
- Advise families that over-the-counter cough and cold suppressant medications are not recommended and are no longer considered safe for children 2 or younger.

• = Independent     ▲ = Collaborative

- Recognize that some children may have been exposed to methamphetamines or the components used to make methamphetamines.
- Advise families to safely dispose of unused medications.

**Geriatric**

- Caution the client and family to avoid storing medications with similar appearances close to one another (e.g., nitroglycerin ointment near toothpaste or denture creams). Confusion and visual impairment can place the older person at risk of incorrectly identifying the contents. Place medications in a medication organizer that indicates when they are to be taken. Failing eyesight, the use of multiple drugs, and difficulty in remembering whether a medication was taken are among the causes of accidental poisoning in older persons.
- Perform medication reconciliation in all older clients entering the health care system and on discharge.
- Use the Screening Tool of Older People's Prescriptions (STOPP) and the Screening Tool to Alert Right Treatment (START) to promote safety, avoid omissions, and prevent inappropriateness in prescriptions.

**Home Care**

- The previous interventions may be adapted for home care use.
- Provide the client and/or family with information about the free poison control application webPOISONCONTROL.
- Identify poisonous substances in the immediate surroundings of the home, such as a garage or barn, including paints and thinners, fertilizers, rodent and bug control substances, animal medications, gasoline, and oil. Label with the name, a poison warning sign, and a poison control center number. Lock out of the reach of children.
- Identify the risk of toxicity from environmental activities such as spraying trees or roadside shrubs. Contact local departments of agriculture or transportation to obtain material safety data sheets or to prevent the activity in desired areas.
- To prevent carbon monoxide poisoning, instruct the client and family in the importance of using a carbon monoxide detector in the home and changing it every 6 months, having the home heating system serviced every year by a qualified technician, and ensuring proper installation and venting of all combustion equipment. Carbon monoxide results from fumes produced by portable generators, stoves, lanterns, gas ranges, running vehicles, or burning charcoal and wood, which can build up in enclosed or partially enclosed spaces and result in harm or death for people and animals exposed.

**P**

• = Independent      ▲ = Collaborative

**Multicultural**

- Prompt caregivers to take action to prevent lead poisoning.
- If children live in a high-lead environment, teach the need for handwashing before each meal, annual blood testing for lead levels, and avoidance of high-lead areas.

**Client/Family Teaching and Discharge Planning**

- The previous interventions may be adapted for teaching needs and discharge planning.
- Counsel the client and family members regarding the following points of medication safety:
  - Avoid sharing prescriptions.
  - Always use good light when preparing medication. Do not dispense medication during the night without a light on.
  - Read the label before you open the bottle, after you remove a dose, and again before you give it.
  - Always use child-resistant caps and lock all medications away from your child or confused older adult.
  - Give the correct dose. *Never* guess.
  - Do not increase or decrease the dose without calling the health care provider.
  - Always follow the weight and age recommendations on the label.
  - Avoid making conversions. If the label calls for 2 teaspoons and you have a dosing cup labeled only with ounces, do not use it.
  - Be sure the health care provider knows if you are taking more than one medication at a time.
  - Never let young children take medication by themselves.
  - Read and follow labeling instructions on all products; adjust dosage for age.
  - Avoid excessive amounts and/or frequency of doses. ("If a little does some good, a lot should do more.")

# Post-Trauma Syndrome

**Domain 9** Coping/stress tolerance   **Class 1** Post-trauma responses

## NANDA-I Definition

Sustained maladaptive response to a traumatic, overwhelming event.

## Defining Characteristics

Aggressive behaviors; alienation; altered attention; altered mood; anxiety (00146); avoidance behaviors; compulsive behavior; denial; depressive symptoms; dissociative amnesia; enuresis; exaggerated startle response; expresses anger; expresses numbness; expresses shame; fear (00148);

flashbacks; gastrointestinal irritation; headache; heart palpitations; hopelessness (00124); horror; hypervigilance; individuals with history of detachment; intrusive dreams; intrusive thoughts; irritable mood; neurosensory irritability; nightmares; panic attacks; rage; reports feeling guilty; repression; substance misuse

## Related Factors

Diminished ego strength: environment not conducive to needs; exaggerated sense of responsibility; inadequate social support; perceives event as traumatic; self-injurious behavior; survivor role

## At-Risk Population

Individuals displaced from home; individuals experiencing prolonged duration of traumatic event; individuals exposed to disaster; individuals exposed to epidemic; individuals exposed to event involving multiple deaths; Individuals exposed to event outside the range of usual human experience; individuals exposed to serious accident; individuals exposed to war; individuals in human service occupations; individuals suffering serious threat; individuals who witnessed mutilation; individuals who witnessed violent death; individuals whose loved ones suffered serious injuries; individuals whose loved ones suffered serious threats; individuals with destructed home; individuals with history of being a prisoner of war; individuals with history of being abused; individuals with history of criminal victimization; individuals with history of torture

## Associated Conditions

Depression

## Client Outcomes

### Client Will (Specify Time Frame)

- Return to pretrauma level of functioning as quickly as possible
- Acknowledge traumatic event and begin to work with the trauma by talking about the experience and expressing feelings of fear, anger, anxiety, guilt, and helplessness
- Identify support systems and available resources and be able to connect with them
- Return to and strengthen coping mechanisms used in previous traumatic event
- Acknowledge event and perceive it without distortions
- Assimilate event and move forward to set and pursue life goals

## Nursing Interventions

- Observe for a reaction to a traumatic event in all clients regardless of age or sex.
- Use a trauma-informed approach with survivors.

• = Independent ▲ = Collaborative

- After a traumatic event, assess for intrusive memories, avoidance and numbing, and hyperarousal.
- Use an open and nonthreatening body positioning and posture.
- Remain with the client and provide support during periods of overwhelming emotions.
- Help the individual to comprehend the trauma if possible.
- Use touch with the client's permission (e.g., a hand on the shoulder, holding a hand).
- Help the client regain previous sleeping and eating habits.
▲ Provide the client pain medication if he or she has physical pain.
▲ Assess the need for pharmacotherapy and refer as needed.
▲ Refer for appropriate psychotherapy: cognitive therapy, exposure therapy, eye movement desensitization and reprocessing (EMDR), and cognitive-behavioral therapy (CBT).
- Help the client use positive cognitive restructuring to reestablish feelings of self-worth.
- Provide the means for the client to express feelings through therapeutic drawing.
- Encourage the client to return to his or her normal routine as quickly as possible.
- Talk to and assess the client's social support after a traumatic event.

**Pediatric**
- Refer to nursing care plan Risk for **Post-Trauma** Syndrome.
▲ Carefully assess children exposed to disasters and trauma. Note behavior specific to developmental age. Refer for therapy as needed.

**Geriatric**
- Carefully screen older adults for signs of PTSD, especially after a disaster.
- Consider using the Impact of Event Scale—Revised (IES-R), which is an appropriate instrument to measure the subjective response to stress in the older population.
▲ Monitor the client for clinical signs of depression and anxiety; refer to a health care provider for medication if appropriate.
- Instill hope.

**Multicultural**
- Assess the influence of cultural beliefs, norms, and values on the client's ability to cope with a traumatic experience.
- Acknowledge racial and ethnic differences at the onset of care.
▲ Carefully assess refugees for PTSD and refer for treatment as appropriate.

• = Independent　　　　▲ = Collaborative

- Use a family-centered approach when working with Latin, Asian, African American, and Native American clients.
- When working with Asian American clients, provide opportunities by which the family can save face.
- Incorporate cultural traditions as appropriate.

**Home Care**

▲ Assess family support and the response to the client's coping mechanisms. Refer the family for medical social services or other counseling, as necessary.
- Assess the effect of the trauma on family and significant others and provide empathy and caring to them.

**Client/Family Teaching and Discharge Planning**

- Teach positive coping skills and avoidance of negative coping skills.
- Teach mindfulness strategies and encourage use when intrusive thoughts or flashbacks occur.
- Refer the client to peer support groups.
- Consider the use of complementary and alternative therapies.

# Risk for Post-Trauma Syndrome

**P**

**Domain 9** Coping/stress tolerance    **Class 1** Post-trauma responses

## NANDA-I Definition

Susceptible to sustained maladaptive response to a traumatic, overwhelming event, which may compromise health.

## Risk Factors

Diminished ego strength; environment not conducive to needs; exaggerated sense of responsibility; inadequate social support; perceives event as traumatic; self-injurious behavior; survivor role

## At-Risk Population

Individuals displaced from home; individuals experiencing prolonged duration of traumatic event; individuals exposed to disaster; individuals exposed to epidemic; individuals exposed to event involving multiple deaths; individuals exposed to event outside the range of usual human experience; individuals exposed to serious accident; individuals exposed to war; individuals in human service occupations; individuals suffering serious threat; individuals who witnessed mutilation; individuals who witnessed violent death; individuals whose loved ones suffered serious injuries; individuals whose loved ones suffered serious threats; individuals with destructed home; individuals with history of being a prisoner of war; individuals with history of being abused; individuals with history of criminal victimization; individuals with history of torture

• = Independent          ▲ = Collaborative

## Associated Conditions

Depression

## Client Outcomes

**Client Will (Specify Time Frame)**

- Identify symptoms associated with posttraumatic stress disorder (PTSD) and seek help
- Acknowledge event and perceive it without distortions
- Identify support systems and available resources and be able to connect with them
- State that he/she is not to blame for the event

## Nursing Interventions

- Assess for PTSD in a client who has chronic/critical illness, anxiety, or personality disorder; was a witness to severe injury or death; or experienced sexual molestation.
- Consider the use of a self-reported screening questionnaire.
- Assess for ongoing symptoms of posttraumatic stress such as dissociation, avoidance behavior, hypervigilance, and reexperiencing.
- Assess for past experiences with traumatic events.
- Consider screening for PTSD in a client who is a high user of medical care.
- ▲ Provide deployed combat veterans with previous history of low mental or physical health status before deployment with appropriate referral after deployment.
- Provide peer support to contact coworkers experiencing trauma to remind them that others in the organization are concerned about their welfare.
- Provide posttrauma debriefings. Effective posttrauma coping skills are taught, and each participant creates a plan for his or her recovery.
- Provide posttrauma counseling and debriefings.
- Consider exposure therapy for civilian trauma survivors after an assault or motor vehicle crash.
- ▲ Assess for a history of life-threatening illness such as cancer and provide appropriate counseling.
- Children with cancer should continue to be assessed for PTSD into adulthood.
- Provide protection for a child who has witnessed violence or who has had traumatic injuries. Help the child acknowledge the event and express grief over the event.
- Assess for a medical history of anxiety disorders.
- ▲ Assess children of deployed parents for PTSD and provide appropriate referrals.

• = Independent                    ▲ = Collaborative

- Consider implementation of a school-based program for children to decrease PTSD after catastrophic events.

**Geriatric and Multicultural**

- Refer to the care plan for **Post-Trauma** Syndrome.

**Home Care**

▲ Evaluate the client's response to a traumatic or critical event. If screening warrants, refer to a therapist for counseling/treatment.
- Refer to the care plan for **Post-Trauma** Syndrome.

**Client/Family Teaching and Discharge Planning**

- Provide education to explain that acute stress disorder symptoms may be common when preparing combatants for their role in deployment. Provide referrals if the symptoms persist.

# Readiness for Enhanced Power

**Domain 9** Coping/stress tolerance     **Class 2** Coping responses

## NANDA-I Definition

A pattern of participating knowingly in change for well-being, which can be strengthened.

## Defining Characteristics

Expresses desire to enhance awareness of possible changes; expresses desire to enhance decisions that could lead to changes; expresses desire to enhance independence by taking action for change; expresses desire to enhance involvement in change; expresses desire to enhance knowledge for participation in change; expresses desire to enhance participation in choices for daily living; expresses desire to enhance participation in choices for health; expresses desire to enhance power

## Client Outcomes

**Client Will (Specify Time Frame)**

- Describe power resources
- Identify realistic perceptions of control
- Develop a plan of action based on power resources
- Seek assistance as needed

## Nursing Interventions

- Assess the meaning of the event to the person.
- Establish a trusting relationship with the client.
- Assist and encourage the client to identify sources of emotional support.
- Provide support for client families to identify the balance between client care responsibilities and self-care.

• = Independent        ▲ = Collaborative

- Initiate and facilitate family health conversations between the client and their family.
- Provide the client with information and regular updates regarding their care.
- Refer client to an empowerment support group.

**Pediatric**

- Provide empowerment-based education for parents that includes a focus on caregiving knowledge, caring behaviors, self-efficacy, and indicators of the child's recovery.
- Initiate problem-solving opportunities, empowering discussions, and reflection to help families take action to manage their child's illness.
- Provide teaching so chronically ill children can learn about their illness, recommendations, identify their limitations, and adapt by changing their routines.

**Geriatric**

- The preceding interventions may be adapted for use with older adults.
- Provide health education for older individuals that is tailored, interactive, structured, and continuous and incorporates motivational and encouragement techniques.

**Multicultural**

- The preceding interventions may be adapted for use with diverse clients.
- Provide support and educational interventions that are culturally tailored.

**Home Care**

- The preceding interventions may be adapted for use in home care.
- Provide caregivers with support, listen to their concerns, and advocate for their needs.

# Powerlessness

**Domain 9** Coping/stress tolerance    **Class 2** Coping responses

## NANDA-I Definition

A state of actual or perceived loss of control or influence over factors or events that affect one's well-being, personal life, or the society (adapted from American Psychology Association).

## Defining Characteristics

Delayed recovery; depressive symptoms; expresses doubt about role performance; expresses frustration about inability to perform previous activities; expresses lack of purpose in life; expresses shame; fatigue; loss of independence; reports inadequate sense of control; social alienation

• = Independent        ▲ = Collaborative

## Related Factors

Anxiety; caregiver role strain; dysfunctional institutional environment; impaired physical mobility; inadequate interest in improving one's situation; inadequate interpersonal relations; inadequate knowledge to manage a situation; inadequate motivation to improve one's situation; inadequate participation in treatment regimen; inadequate social support; ineffective coping strategies; low self-esteem; pain; perceived complexity of treatment regimen; perceived social stigma; social marginalization

## At-Risk Population

Economically disadvantaged individuals; individuals exposed to traumatic events

## Associated Conditions

Cerebrovascular disorders; cognition disorders; critical illness; progressive illness; unpredictability of illness trajectory

## Client Outcomes

### Client Will (Specify Time Frame)

- State feelings of powerlessness and other feelings related to powerlessness (e.g., anger, sadness, hopelessness)
- Identify factors that are uncontrollable
- Participate in planning and implementing care; make decisions regarding care and treatment when possible
- Ask questions about care and treatment
- Verbalize hope for the future and sense of participation in planning and implementing care

## Nursing Interventions

Note: Before implementation of interventions in the face of client powerlessness, nurses should examine their own philosophies of care to ensure that control issues or lack of faith in client capabilities will not bias the ability to intervene sincerely and effectively.

- Assess powerlessness with tools that are available for general and specific client groups:
  - Measure of Powerlessness for Adult Patients (de Almeida Lopes Monteiro da Cruz & Braga, 2006)
  - Personal Progress Scale–Revised, tested with women (Johnson, Worell, & Chandler, 2005)
  - Life Situation Questionnaire–Powerlessness subscale, tested with stroke caregivers (Larson et al, 2005)
  - Making Decisions Scale, tested in clients with mental illness (Hansson & Björkman, 2005)
  - Family Empowerment Scale, tested on parents of children with emotional disorders (Koren, DeChillo, & Friesen, 1992)

• = Independent          ▲ = Collaborative

- Establish a trusting relationship with the client.
- Assist and encourage the client to identify sources of emotional support.
- Engage with clients using respectful listening and questioning to develop an awareness of clients' most important concerns.
- Provide clients with a collaborative decision-making process.
- Provide support for client families to identify the balance between client care responsibilities and self-care.
- Use a rehabilitative behavioral learning model that assists clients to understand how the mechanisms of habit and ritual work to reinforce powerlessness in their lives.
- Provide the client with information and regular updates regarding their care.
- Refer client to an empowerment support group.
- Refer to the care plans for **Hopelessness** and **Spiritual** Distress.

**Pediatric**
- Provided empowerment-based educational preparation for parents that includes a focus on caregiving knowledge, caring behaviors, self-efficacy, and indicators of the child's recovery.
- Initiate problem-solving opportunities, empowering discussions, and reflection to help families take action to manage their child's illness.
- Provide teaching so chronically ill children can learn about their illness, recommendations, identify their limitations, and adapt by changing their routines.

**Geriatric**
- The preceding interventions may be adapted for use with older adults.
- Initiate and facilitate family health conversations between older clients and their family.
- Provide health education for older individuals that is tailored, interactive, structured, and continuous and incorporates motivational and encouragement techniques.

**Multicultural**
- The preceding interventions may be adapted for use with diverse clients.
- Provide support and educational interventions that are culturally tailored.

**Home Care**
- The preceding interventions may be adapted for use in home care.
- Provide caregivers with support, listen to their concerns, and advocate for their needs.

• = Independent ▲ = Collaborative

**Client/Family Teaching and Discharge Planning**
- The preceding interventions may be adapted for teaching and discharge planning.

# Risk for Powerlessness

**Domain 9** Coping/stress tolerance    **Class 2** Coping responses

## NANDA-I Definition

Susceptible to a state of actual or perceived loss of control or influence over factors or events that affect one's well-being, personal life, or the society, which may compromise health (adapted from American Psychology Association).

## Risk Factors

Anxiety; caregiver role strain; dysfunctional institutional environment; impaired physical mobility; inadequate interest in improving one's situation; inadequate interpersonal relations; inadequate knowledge to manage a situation; inadequate motivation to improve one's situation; inadequate participation in treatment regimen; inadequate social support; ineffective coping strategies; low self-esteem; pain; perceived complexity of treatment regimen; perceived social stigma; social marginalization

## At-Risk Population

Economically disadvantaged; individuals exposed to traumatic events

## Associated Conditions

Cerebrovascular disorders, cognition disorders; critical illness; progressive illness; unpredictability of illness trajectory

## Client Outcomes, Nursing Interventions, and Client/Family Teaching and Discharge Planning

See the care plan for **Powerlessness.**

# Adult Pressure Injury

**Domain 11** Safety/protection    **Class 2** Physical injury

## NANDA-I Definition

Localized damage to the skin and/or underlying tissue of an adult, as a result of pressure, or pressure in combination with shear (European Pressure Ulcer Advisory Panel, 2019).

## Defining Characteristics

Blood-filled blister; erythema; full thickness tissue loss; full thickness tissue loss with exposed bone; full thickness tissue loss with exposed muscle; full thickness tissue loss with exposed tendon; localized heat in relation to surrounding tissue; pain at pressure points; partial thickness loss of dermis;

• = Independent      ▲ = Collaborative

purple localized area of discolored intact skin; ulcer is covered by eschar; ulcer is covered by slough

## Related Factors

### External Factors

Altered microclimate between skin and supporting surface; excessive moisture; inadequate access to appropriate equipment; inadequate access to appropriate health services; inadequate availability of equipment for individuals with obesity; inadequate caregiver knowledge of pressure injury prevention strategies; increased magnitude of mechanical load; pressure over bony prominence; shearing forces; surface friction; sustained mechanical load; use of linen with insufficient moisture wicking property

### Internal Factors

Decreased physical activity; decreased physical mobility; dehydration; dry skin; hyperthermia; inadequate adherence to incontinence treatment regimen; inadequate adherence to pressure injury prevention plan; inadequate knowledge of pressure injury prevention strategies; protein-energy malnutrition; smoking; substance misuse

### Other Factors

Factors identified by standardized, validated screening tool

## At-Risk Population

Individuals in aged care settings; individuals in intensive care units; individuals in palliative care settings; individuals in rehabilitation settings; individuals in transit to or between clinical care settings; individuals receiving home-based care; individuals with American Society of Anesthesiologists (ASA) Physical health status score ≥3; individuals with body mass index above normal range for age and gender; individuals with body mass index below normal range for age and gender; individuals with history of pressure injury; individuals with physical disability; older adults

## Associated Conditions

Anemia; cardiovascular diseases; chronic neurological conditions; critical illness; decreased serum albumin level; decreased tissue oxygenation; decreased tissue perfusion; diabetes mellitus; edema; elevated C-reactive protein; hemodynamic instability; hip fracture; immobilization; impaired circulation; intellectual disability; medical devices; peripheral neuropathy; pharmaceutical preparations; physical trauma; prolonged duration of surgical procedure; sensation disorders; spinal cord injuries

## Client Outcomes

### Client Will (Specify Time Frame)

- Report any altered sensation or pain at site of tissue impairment
- Skin, without redness over bony prominences and capillary refill of less than 6 seconds over areas of redness

• = Independent      ▲ = Collaborative

- Be repositioned off of bony prominences frequently if risk for pressure injuries is high (e.g., Braden Scale score ≤18)
- Demonstrate understanding of plan to reduce pressure injury risk
- Describe measures to protect the skin

## Nursing Interventions

▲ The National Pressure Ulcer Advisory Panel (NPUAP) redefined the definition of a pressure ulcer, which is now referred to as pressure injuries, during the NPUAP 2016 Staging Consensus Conference in 2016. The new definitions more accurately define alterations in tissue integrity from pressure. Classify pressure injuries (NPUAP & European Pressure Ulcer Advisory Panel [EPUAP], 2016) using national guidelines and definitions (see http://www.npuap.org/resources/educational-and-clinical-resources/npuap-pressure-injury-stages/).

   ○ **Pressure Injury:** A pressure injury is localized damage to the skin and underlying soft tissue usually over a bony prominence or related to a medical or other device. The injury can present as intact skin or an open ulcer and may be painful. The injury occurs as a result of intense and/or prolonged pressure or pressure in combination with shear. The tolerance of soft tissue for pressure and shear may also be affected by microclimate, nutrition, perfusion, comorbidities, and condition of the soft tissue (NPUAP & EPUAP, 2016).

   ○ **Stage 1 Pressure Injury:** Nonblanchable erythema of intact skin. Area of localized nonblanchable erythema that may appear differently in darkly pigmented skin, and changes in sensation, temperature, or firmness may precede visual changes. Color changes do not include purple or maroon discoloration, which is more likely to indicate deep tissue pressure injury (NPUAP & EPUAP, 2016).

   ○ **Stage 2 Pressure Injury:** Partial-thickness skin loss with exposed dermis. Partial-thickness skin loss with exposed dermis in which the wound bed is pink/red and moist and adipose (fat) and deeper tissues are not visible. Granulation tissue, slough, and eschar are not present. A stage 2 pressure injury may also present as an intact or ruptured blister. These injuries commonly result from adverse microclimate and shear in the skin over the pelvis and shear in the heel. This stage should not be used to describe moisture-associated skin damage (MASD) including incontinence-associated dermatitis (IAD), intertriginous dermatitis (ITD), medical

**P**

adhesive–related skin injury (MARSI), or traumatic wounds (skin tears, burns, and abrasions) (NPUAP & EPUAP, 2016).

○ **Stage 3 Pressure Injury:** Full-thickness skin loss. Full-thickness loss of skin, in which adipose is visible and granulation tissue and epibole (rolled wound edges) are often present and undermining/tunneling may occur. Slough and/or eschar may also be visible. Fascia, muscle, tendon, ligament, cartilage, and/or bone are not exposed. The depth of tissue damage varies by anatomical location, and areas of significant adiposity can develop deep wounds. If slough or eschar obscures the extent of tissue loss, this is an unstageable pressure injury (NPUAP & EPUAP, 2016).

○ **Stage 4 Pressure Injury:** Full-thickness skin and tissue loss. Full-thickness skin and tissue loss with exposed or directly palpable fascia, muscle, tendon, ligament, cartilage, or bone, and slough and/or eschar may be visible. Epibole, undermining, and/or tunneling often occur and depth varies by anatomical location. If slough or eschar obscures the extent of tissue loss, this is an unstageable pressure injury (NPUAP & EPUAP, 2016).

○ **Deep Tissue Pressure Injury:** Persistent nonblanchable deep red, maroon, or purple discoloration. Intact or nonintact skin with localized area of persistent nonblanchable deep red, maroon, or purple discoloration or epidermal separation revealing a dark wound bed or blood-filled blister. Pain and temperature change often precedes skin color changes. Discoloration may appear differently in darkly pigmented skin. This injury results from intense and/or prolonged pressure and shear forces at the bone–muscle interface. The wound may evolve rapidly to reveal the actual extent of tissue injury, or it may resolve without tissue loss. If necrotic tissue, subcutaneous tissue, granulation tissue, fascia, muscle, or other underlying structures are visible, this indicates a full-thickness pressure injury (unstageable, stage 3, or stage 4). Do not use deep tissue pressure injury to describe vascular, traumatic, neuropathic, or dermatological conditions (NPUAP & EPUAP, 2016).

○ **Unstageable Pressure Injury:** Obscured full-thickness skin and tissue loss. Full-thickness skin and tissue loss in which the extent of tissue damage within the ulcer cannot be confirmed because it is obscured by slough or eschar. If slough or eschar is removed, a stage 3 or stage 4 pressure injury will be revealed. Stable eschar (i.e., dry, adherent, intact without erythema or fluctuance) on the heel or ischemic limb should not be softened or removed (NPUAP & EPUAP, 2016).

• = Independent            ▲ = Collaborative

- Routinely assess clients for risk of pressure injuries using a valid and reliable risk assessment tool (National Pressure Injury Advisory Panel [NPIAP] & European Pressure Injury Advisory Panel [EPIAP], 2019). A validated risk-assessment tool such as the Norton scale or Braden scale should be used to identify clients at risk for pressure-related skin breakdown (NPIAP & EPIAP, 2019).
- Pressure injury risk assessment should be completed on admission, daily, and after procedures or changes in the client's condition (Baranoski & Ayello, 2016; NPIAP & EPIAP, 2019).
- Inspect the skin daily, especially bony prominences and dependent areas, for pallor, redness, and breakdown. In addition to assessing pressure injury risk, client-specific interventions should be implemented to prevent tissue injury. Implement the following interventions to prevent tissue breakdown:
  - Turn and reposition all individuals at risk for pressure injury, unless contraindicated because of medical condition or medical treatments.
  - Position client properly; use pressure-redistributing surfaces based on the individual's needs (e.g., pillows, gel or foam cushions, reactive/nonreactive foam mattresses, alternating pressure mattress, air-fluidized surface) if indicated. Continue to turn and reposition the individual regardless of the support surface in use. Establish turning frequency based on the characteristics of the support surface and the individual's response (NPIAP & EPIAP, 2019).
  - Lift and move client carefully using a turn sheet and adequate assistance; keep bed linens dry and wrinkle-free.
  - Perform actions to keep client from sliding down in bed (e.g., bend knees slightly when head of bed is elevated 30 degrees or higher) to reduce the risk of skin surface abrasion and shearing. Use the 30-degree tilted side-lying position (alternately, right side, back, left side). Maintain the head of the bed as flat as possible. Avoid extended use of prone positioning unless the individual can tolerate this and his or her medical condition allows (NPIAP & EPIAP, 2019).
  - Select a seated posture that is acceptable for the individual and minimizes the pressure and shear exerted on the skin and soft tissues. Limit time in seated position and encourage pressure relieving maneuvers (NPIAP & EPIAP, 2019).
  - Keep client's skin clean. Thoroughly dry skin after bathing and as often as needed, paying special attention to skinfolds and opposing skin surfaces (e.g., axillae, perineum, beneath breasts). Pat skin dry

rather than rub and use a mild soap for bathing. Avoid alkaline soaps and cleansers. Apply moisturizing lotion at least once a day (NPIAP & EPIAP, 2019).

○ Protect the skin from contact with urine and feces (e.g., keep perineal area clean and dry, apply a protective ointment or cream to perineal area).

○ Provide and encourage adequate daily fluid intake for hydration for an individual assessed to be at risk of or with a pressure injury (NPUAP & EPUAP, 2016). Adjust protein intake for individuals with or at risk for pressure injuries. This must be consistent with the individual's comorbid conditions and goals (NPIAP & EPIAP, 2019).

○ If the individual cannot be moved or is positioned with the head of the bed elevated over 30 degrees, place a polyurethane foam dressing on the sacrum (NPUAP & EPUAP, 2016). Use heel offloading device or polyurethane foam dressings on individuals at high risk for heel ulcers (NPUAP & EPUAP, 2016).

○ Consult with nutrition/dietary specialist to evaluate client's nutritional status.

○ Increase activity as allowed.

• Medical device–related pressure injuries (MDRPIs) result from the use of devices designed and applied for diagnostic or therapeutic purposes. The resultant pressure injury generally conforms to the pattern or shape of the device. The injury should be staged using the NPUAP pressure injury staging system and the etiology of the pressure injury noted to be caused by the device (NPUAP & EPUAP, 2016).

○ Assess the skin around and under medical devices routinely to identify signs of pressure-related injuries (NPIAP & EPIAP, 2019).

○ Common devices associated with pressure-related tissue injury include oxygen delivery and monitoring devices (e.g., face mask, nasal cannula, pulse oximetry, bilevel positive airway pressure [BiPAP] mask), feeding tubes (e.g., nasogastric, gastric, jejunal tubes), endotracheal devices (oral and/or nasal endotracheal tubes, tracheostomy tubes), urinary and bowel elimination equipment (indwelling urinary catheter, fecal containment catheter), and musculoskeletal appliances (cervical collar, splints, braces).

○ Assess and evaluate the purpose and function of the medical device. Remove medical devices as soon as medically feasible (NPIAP & EPIAP, 2019).

○ Assess proper fit of the medical device and securement to prevent

**P**

• = Independent          ▲ = Collaborative

tension, and assess the skin under the device regularly for pressure-related injury (NPIAP & EPIAP, 2019).

○ Protect the skin below and around the device to reduce pressure. Use a prophylactic dressing under the medical device to protect skin (NPIAP & EPIAP, 2019).

- **Mucosal Membrane Pressure Injury:** Mucosal membrane pressure injury is found on mucous membranes with a history of a medical device in use at the location of the injury. Due to the anatomy of the tissue these ulcers cannot be staged (NPUAP & EPUAP, 2016).
- Critically ill clients are at increased risk for pressure ulcers, often requiring frequent skin risk assessment and preventive interventions.
- Efforts must be taken to disseminate evidence-based guidelines and ensure that health care providers, in all settings, are making every effort to identify individuals who are at risk for pressure injuries and implement preventive and treatment interventions (Ratliff et al, 2017).
- A client at risk for skin, wound, and related complications can benefit from the expert knowledge and skill set of a certified wound, ostomy, continence nurse (Berke et al, 2019). See care plan for Impaired **Skin** Integrity for additional interventions if a pressure ulcer occurs.

**P**

### Geriatric

- Consider the older client's cognitive status when assessing the skin and in developing a comprehensive plan of care to prevent pressure injuries (NPUAP & EPUAP, 2016; NPIAP & EPIAP, 2019).
- Aging skin, medications (e.g., steroids), and moisture place the older client at increased risk for pressure-associated skin breakdown.
- Clients over age 65 years are at higher risk for pressure injuries because they have reduced subcutaneous fat and capillary blood flow, as well as physiological skin changes, including decreased cohesion of the dermis and epidermis and reduced sensory function (Podd, 2018).
- Use atraumatic wound dressings to prevent and treat pressure injuries (NPUAP & EPUAP, 2016) to reduce further injury to a frail older client's skin (NPIAP & EPIAP, 2019).
- For older clients with continence concerns, develop and implement an individualized continence management program (NPIAP & EPIAP, 2019).
- Regularly reposition the older client who is unable to reposition independently. Consider pressure redistribution support surface for clients assessed to be at high risk for pressure injuries (NPUAP & EPUAP, 2016; NPIAP & EPIAP, 2019).

### Home Care

- The interventions described previously may be adapted for home care use.

• = Independent      ▲ = Collaborative

- Instruct and assist the client and caregivers in how to assess the skin for excessive pressure. Provide written instructions for actions they can implement to reduce the risk of pressure injury development (NPUAP & EPUAP, 2016).
- Educate client and caregivers on proper nutrition and when to call the agency and/or health care provider with concerns.
▲ It may be beneficial to initiate a consultation in a case assignment with a wound, ostomy, continence nurse (or wounds specialist) to establish a comprehensive plan for pressure ulcer risk reduction for clients at high risk for skin breakdown.

## Risk for Adult Pressure Injury

**Domain 11** Safety/protection    **Class 2** Physical injury
### NANDA-I Definition

Adult susceptible to localized damage to the skin and/or underlying tissue, as a result of pressure, or pressure in combination with shear, which may compromise health (European Pressure Ulcer Advisory Panel, 2019).

### Risk Factors
#### External Factors

Altered microclimate between skin and supporting surface; excessive moisture; inadequate access to appropriate equipment; inadequate access to appropriate health services; inadequate availability of equipment for individuals with obesity; inadequate caregiver knowledge of pressure injury prevention strategies; increased magnitude of mechanical load; pressure over bony prominence; shearing forces; surface friction; sustained mechanical load; use of linen with insufficient moisture wicking property

#### Internal Factors

Decreased physical activity; decreased physical mobility; dehydration; dry skin; hyperthermia; inadequate adherence to incontinence treatment regimen; inadequate adherence to pressure injury prevention plan; inadequate knowledge of pressure injury prevention strategies; protein-energy malnutrition; smoking; substance misuse

#### Other Factors

Factors identified by standardized, validated screening tool

### At-Risk Population

Individuals in aged care settings; individuals in intensive care units; individuals in palliative care settings; individuals in rehabilitation settings; individuals in transit to or between clinical care settings; individuals receiving home-based care; individuals with American Society of Anesthesiologists

• = Independent        ▲ = Collaborative

(ASA) physical health status score ≥3; individuals with body mass index above normal range for age and gender; individuals with body mass index below normal range for age and gender; individuals with history of pressure injury; individuals with physical disability; older adults

## Associated Conditions

Anemia; cardiovascular diseases; chronic neurological conditions; critical illness; decreased serum albumin level; decreased tissue oxygenation; decreased tissue perfusion; diabetes mellitus; edema; elevated C-reactive protein; hemodynamic instability; hip fracture; immobilization; impaired circulation; intellectual disability; medical devices; peripheral neuropathy; pharmaceutical preparations; physical trauma; prolonged duration of surgical procedure; sensation disorders; spinal cord injuries

## Client Outcomes, Nursing Interventions, and Client/Family Teaching and Discharge Planning

See the care plan for Adult **Pressure** Injury.

# Child Pressure Injury

**Domain 11** Safety/protection    **Class 2** Physical injury

## NANDA-I Definition

Localized damage to the skin and/or underlying tissue of a child or adolescent, as a result of pressure, or pressure in combination with shear (European Pressure Ulcer Advisory Panel, 2019).

## Defining Characteristics

Blood-filled blister; erythema; full thickness tissue loss; full thickness tissue loss with exposed bone; full thickness tissue loss with exposed muscle; full thickness tissue loss with exposed tendon; localized heat in relation to surrounding tissue; pain at pressure points; partial thickness loss of dermis; purple localized area of discolored intact skin; ulcer is covered by eschar; ulcer is covered by slough

## Related Factors

### External Factors

Altered microclimate between skin and supporting surface; difficulty for caregiver to lift client completely off bed; excessive moisture; inadequate access to appropriate equipment; inadequate access to appropriate health services; inadequate access to appropriate supplies; inadequate access to equipment for children with obesity; inadequate caregiver knowledge of appropriate methods for removing adhesive materials; inadequate caregiver knowledge of appropriate methods for stabilizing devices; inadequate caregiver knowledge of modifiable factors; inadequate caregiver knowledge of pressure injury prevention strategies; increased magnitude of mechanical load; pressure over bony prominence; shearing forces; surface friction; sustained mechanical load; use of linen with insufficient moisture wicking property

**Internal Factors**

Decreased physical activity; decreased physical mobility; dehydration; difficulty assisting caregiver with moving self; difficulty maintaining position in bed; difficulty maintaining position in chair; dry skin; hyperthermia; inadequate adherence to incontinence treatment regimen; inadequate adherence to pressure injury prevention plan; inadequate knowledge of appropriate methods for removing adhesive materials; inadequate knowledge of appropriate methods for stabilizing devices; protein-energy malnutrition; water-electrolyte imbalance

**Other Factors**

Factors identified by standardized, validated screening tool

**At-Risk Population**

Children in intensive care units; children in long-term care facilities; children in palliative care settings; children in rehabilitation settings; children in transit to or between clinical care settings; children receiving home-based care; children with body mass index above normal range for age and gender; children with body mass index below normal range for age and gender; children with developmental issues; children with growth issues; children with large head circumference; children with large skin surface area

**Associated Conditions**

Alkaline skin pH; altered cutaneous structure; anemia; cardiovascular diseases; decreased level of consciousness; decreased serum albumin level; decreased tissue oxygenation; decreased tissue perfusion; diabetes mellitus; edema; elevated C-reactive protein; frequent invasive procedures; hemodynamic instability; immobilization; impaired circulation; intellectual disability; medical devices; pharmaceutical preparations; physical trauma; prolonged duration of surgical procedure; sensation disorders; spinal cord injuries

**Client Outcomes**

**Client Will (Specify Time Frame)**

• Report any altered sensation or pain at site of tissue impairment
• Skin, without redness over bony prominences and capillary refill of less than 6 seconds over areas of redness
• Be repositioned off of bony prominences frequently if risk for pressure injuries is high (e.g., Braden QD or Glamorgan scale score)
• Family/caregiver will demonstrate understanding of plan to reduce pressure injury risk
• Describe measures to protect the skin

• = Independent ▲ = Collaborative

## Nursing Interventions

- Consider the impact of skin maturity, perfusion, and oxygenation and medical devices related to risk for pressure injury development in neonates and children (National Pressure Injury Advisory Panel [NPIAP] & European Pressure Injury Advisory Panel [EPIAP], 2019).
- Perform an age-appropriate pressure injury (National Pressure Ulcer Advisory Panel [NPUAP] & European Pressure Ulcer Advisory Panel [EPUAP], 2016) risk assessment using a valid and reliable tool.
- Pressure injury risk assessment should be completed on admission, daily, and after procedures or changes in the client's condition (Baranoski & Ayello, 2016; Freundlich, 2017; NPIAP & EPIAP, 2019).
- ▲ NPUAP redefined the definition of a "pressure ulcer," which is now referred to as "pressure injuries," during the NPUAP 2016 Staging Consensus Conference in 2016. The new definitions more accurately define alterations in tissue integrity from pressure. Classify pressure injuries (NPUAP & EPUAP, 2016) using national guidelines and definitions (see http://www.npuap.org/resources/educational-and-clinical-resources/npuap-pressure-injury-stages/).
  - ○ **Pressure Injury:** A pressure injury is localized damage to the skin and underlying soft tissue usually over a bony prominence or related to a medical or other device. The injury can present as intact skin or an open ulcer and may be painful. The injury occurs as a result of intense and/or prolonged pressure or pressure in combination with shear. The tolerance of soft tissue for pressure and shear may also be affected by microclimate, nutrition, perfusion, comorbidities, and condition of the soft tissue (NPUAP & EPUAP, 2016).
  - ○ **Stage 1 Pressure Injury:** Nonblanchable erythema of intact skin. Area of localized nonblanchable erythema that may appear differently in darkly pigmented skin, and changes in sensation, temperature, or firmness may precede visual changes. Color changes do not include purple or maroon discoloration, which is more likely to indicate deep tissue pressure injury (NPUAP & EPUAP, 2016).
  - ○ **Stage 2 Pressure Injury:** Partial-thickness skin loss with exposed dermis. Partial-thickness skin loss with exposed dermis in which the wound bed is pink/red and moist and adipose (fat) and deeper tissues are not visible. Granulation tissue, slough, and eschar are

not present. A stage 2 pressure injury may also present as an intact or ruptured blister. These injuries commonly result from adverse microclimate and shear in the skin over the pelvis and shear in the heel. This stage should not be used to describe moisture-associated skin damage (MASD) including incontinence-associated dermatitis (IAD), intertriginous dermatitis (ITD), medical adhesive–related skin injury (MARSI), or traumatic wounds (skin tears, burns, and abrasions) (NPUAP & EPUAP, 2016).

○ **Stage 3 Pressure Injury:** Full-thickness skin loss. Full-thickness loss of skin, in which adipose is visible and granulation tissue and epibole (rolled wound edges) are often present and undermining/tunneling may occur. Slough and/or eschar may also be visible. Fascia, muscle, tendon, ligament, cartilage, and/or bone are not exposed. The depth of tissue damage varies by anatomical location, and areas of significant adiposity can develop deep wounds. If slough or eschar obscures the extent of tissue loss, this is an unstageable pressure injury (NPUAP & EPUAP, 2016).

○ **Stage 4 Pressure Injury:** Full-thickness skin and tissue loss. Full-thickness skin and tissue loss with exposed or directly palpable fascia, muscle, tendon, ligament, cartilage, or bone, and slough and/or eschar may be visible. Epibole, undermining, and/or tunneling often occur and depth varies by anatomical location. If slough or eschar obscures the extent of tissue loss, this is an unstageable pressure injury (NPUAP & EPUAP, 2016).

○ **Deep Tissue Pressure Injury:** Persistent nonblanchable deep red, maroon, or purple discoloration. Intact or nonintact skin with localized area of persistent nonblanchable deep red, maroon, or purple discoloration or epidermal separation revealing a dark wound bed or blood-filled blister. Pain and temperature change often precedes skin color changes. Discoloration may appear differently in darkly pigmented skin. This injury results from intense and/or prolonged pressure and shear forces at the bone–muscle interface. The wound may evolve rapidly to reveal the actual extent of tissue injury, or it may resolve without tissue loss. If necrotic tissue, subcutaneous tissue, granulation tissue, fascia, muscle, or other underlying structures are visible, this indicates a full-thickness pressure injury (unstageable, stage 3, or stage 4). Do not use deep tissue pressure injury to describe vascular, traumatic, neuropathic, or dermatological conditions (NPUAP & EPUAP, 2016).

○ **Unstageable Pressure Injury:** Obscured full-thickness skin and tissue loss. Full-thickness skin and tissue loss in which the extent of tissue damage within the ulcer cannot be confirmed because it is obscured by slough or eschar. If slough or eschar is removed, a stage 3 or stage 4 pressure injury will be revealed. Stable eschar (i.e., dry, adherent, intact without erythema or fluctuance) on the heel or ischemic limb should not be softened or removed (NPUAP & EPUAP, 2016).

- Routinely assess clients for risk of pressure injuries using a valid and reliable risk assessment tool (NPIAP & EPIAP, 2019). A validated risk-assessment tool such as the Norton Scale or Braden Scale should be used to identify clients at risk for pressure-related skin breakdown (NPIAP & EPIAP, 2019).

- Inspect the skin daily, especially bony prominences and dependent areas, for pallor, redness, and breakdown. In addition to assessing pressure injury risk, client specific interventions should be implemented to prevent tissue injury. Implement the following interventions to prevent tissue breakdown:
  - ○ Turn and reposition all individuals at risk for pressure injury, unless contraindicated because of medical condition or medical treatments.
  - ○ Position client properly; use pressure-redistributing surfaces based on the individual's needs (e.g., pillows, gel or foam cushions, reactive/nonreactive foam mattresses, alternating pressure mattress, air-fluidized surface) if indicated. Continue to turn and reposition the individual regardless of the support surface in use. Establish turning frequency based on the characteristics of the support surface and the individual's response (NPIAP & EPIAP, 2019).
  - ○ Lift and move client carefully using a turn sheet and adequate assistance; keep bed linens dry and wrinkle-free.
  - ○ Perform actions to keep client from sliding down in bed (e.g., bend knees slightly when head of bed is elevated 30 degrees or higher) to reduce the risk of skin surface abrasion and shearing. Use the 30-degree tilted side-lying position (alternately, right side, back, left side). Maintain the head of the bed as flat as possible (NPIAP & EPIAP, 2019).
  - ○ Select a seated posture that is acceptable for the individual and minimizes the pressure and shear exerted on the skin and soft tissues. Limit time in seated position and encourage pressure-relieving maneuvers (NPIAP & EPIAP, 2019).
  - ○ Keep client's skin clean and moisturized. Thoroughly dry skin after bathing and as often as needed, paying special attention to skinfolds and opposing skin surfaces (e.g., axillae, perineum). Pat

• = Independent          ▲ = Collaborative

skin dry rather than rub and use a mild soap for bathing. Avoid alkaline soaps and cleansers. Apply moisturizing lotion at least once a day (NPIAP & EPIAP, 2019).

○ Protect the skin from contact with urine and feces (e.g., keep perineal area clean and dry, apply a protective ointment or cream to perineal area). Avoid diapers when possible. Apply skin protectant cream with each episode of cleansing skin of urine and feces (NPIAP & EPIAP, 2019).

○ Provide and encourage adequate daily fluid intake for hydration for an individual assessed to be at risk of or with a pressure injury (NPUAP & EPUAP, 2016). Adjust protein intake for individuals with or at risk for pressure injuries. This must be consistent with the individual's comorbid conditions and goals (NPIAP & EPIAP, 2019).

○ If the individual cannot be moved or is positioned with the head of the bed elevated over 30 degrees, place a pressure reduction pillow under the occiput and if appropriate a polyurethane foam dressing on the sacrum (NPUAP & EPUAP, 2016).

○ Implement automated nutrition/dietary specialist consultations to evaluate client's nutritional status.

○ Increase activity as allowed.

- Evaluate high-risk areas for pressure injury. Changes in growth influences at risk areas of the body for pressure injury areas.

- Select an age-appropriate support surface for premature neonates and pediatric clients at high risk for pressure ulcers.

- Medical device–related pressure injuries (MDRPIs) result from the use of devices designed and applied for diagnostic or therapeutic purposes. The resultant pressure injury generally conforms to the pattern or shape of the device. The injury should be staged using the NPUAP pressure injury staging system and the etiology of the pressure injury noted to be caused by the device (NPUAP & EPUAP, 2016).

○ Assess the skin around and under medical devices routinely to identify signs of pressure-related injuries (NPIAP & EPIAP, 2019).

○ Common devices associated with pressure-related tissue injury include oxygen delivery and monitoring devices (e.g., face mask, nasal cannula, pulse oximetry), feeding tubes (e.g., nasogastric, gastric, jejunal tubes), endotracheal devices (oral and/or nasal endotracheal tubes, tracheostomy tubes), urinary and bowel elimination equipment (indwelling urinary catheter, fecal

• = Independent        ▲ = Collaborative

containment catheter), and musculoskeletal appliances (cervical collar, splints, braces).

- ○ Assess and evaluate the purpose and function of the medical device. Remove medical devices as soon as medically feasible (NPIAP & EPIAP, 2019).
- ○ Assess proper fit of the medical device and securement to prevent tension, and assess the skin under the device regularly for pressure-related injury (NPIAP & EPIAP, 2019).
- ○ Protect the skin below and around the device to reduce pressure. Use a prophylactic dressing under the medical device to protect skin (NPIAP & EPIAP, 2019).

- **Mucosal Membrane Pressure Injury:** Mucosal membrane pressure injury is found on mucous membranes with a history of a medical device in use at the location of the injury. Due to the anatomy of the tissue these ulcers cannot be staged (NPUAP & EPUAP, 2016).
- Critically ill children are at increased risk for pressure injury, often requiring frequent skin risk assessment and preventive interventions.
- Review evidence-based practice interventions to assess and implement nursing interventions to reduce pressure injury risk.
- Involve family/caregiver in education focused on reducing risks and management strategies for pressure injuries.
- Select an age-appropriate support surface for premature neonates and pediatric clients at high risk for pressure ulcers.
- Engage the client/family/legal guardian in the development of a client-specific plan of care to reduce pressure-related risk for skin breakdown (NPIAP & EPIAP, 2019).
- Document risk assessment and interventions implemented to reduce the client's risk for pressure injury development (NPUAP & EPUAP, 2016).

**Home Care**

- The interventions described previously may be adapted for home care use.
- Instruct and assist the client and caregivers in how to assess the skin for excessive pressure. Provide written instructions for actions they can implement to reduce the risk of pressure injury development (NPUAP & EPUAP, 2016).
- Educate family/caregivers and client (age-appropriate instruction) on proper nutrition and when to call the agency and/or health care provider with concerns.
- ▲ Initiate a consultation in a case assignment with a wound, ostomy, continence nurse (or wounds specialist) to establish a comprehensive

• = Independent          ▲ = Collaborative

plan for pressure ulcer risk reduction for clients at high risk for skin breakdown.

# Risk for Child Pressure Injury

**Domain 11** Safety/protection   **Class 2** Physical injury

## NANDA-I Definition

Child or adolescent susceptible to localized damage to the skin and/or underlying tissue, as a result of pressure, or pressure in combination with shear, which may compromise health (European Pressure Ulcer Advisory Panel, 2019).

## Risk Factors

### External Factors

Altered microclimate between skin and supporting surface; difficulty for caregiver to lift patient completely off bed; excessive moisture; inadequate access to appropriate equipment; inadequate access to appropriate health services; inadequate access to appropriate supplies; inadequate access to equipment for children with obesity; inadequate caregiver knowledge of appropriate methods for removing adhesive materials; inadequate caregiver knowledge of appropriate methods for stabilizing devices; inadequate caregiver knowledge of modifiable factors; inadequate caregiver knowledge of pressure injury prevention strategies; increased magnitude of mechanical load; pressure over bony prominence; shearing forces; surface friction; sustained mechanical load; use of linen with insufficient moisture wicking property

### Internal Factors

Decreased physical activity; decreased physical mobility; dehydration; difficulty assisting caregiver with moving self; difficulty maintaining position in bed; difficulty maintaining position in chair; dry skin; hyperthermia; inadequate adherence to incontinence treatment regimen; inadequate adherence to pressure injury prevention plan; inadequate knowledge of appropriate methods for removing adhesive materials; inadequate knowledge of appropriate methods for stabilizing devices; protein-energy malnutrition; water-electrolyte imbalance

### Other Factors

Factors identified by standardized, validated screening tool

## At-Risk Population

Children in intensive care units; children in long-term care facilities; children in palliative care settings; children in rehabilitation settings; children in transit to or between clinical care settings; children receiving home-based care; children with body mass index above normal range for age and gender; children with body mass index below normal range for age and gender;

children with developmental issues; children with growth issues; children with large head circumference; children with large skin surface area

## Associated Conditions

Alkaline skin pH; altered cutaneous structure; anemia; cardiovascular diseases; decreased level of consciousness; decreased serum albumin level; decreased tissue oxygenation; decreased tissue perfusion; diabetes mellitus; edema; elevated C-reactive protein; frequent invasive procedures; hemodynamic instability; immobilization; impaired circulation; intellectual disability; medical devices; pharmaceutical preparations; physical trauma; prolonged duration of surgical procedure; sensation disorders; spinal cord injuries

## Client Outcomes, Nursing Interventions, and Client/Family Teaching and Discharge Planning

See the care plan for Child **Pressure** Injury.

# Neonatal Pressure Injury

**Domain 11** Safety/protection　**Class 2** Physical injury

## NANDA-I Definition

Localized damage to the skin and/or underlying tissue of a neonate, as a result of pressure, or pressure in combination with shear (European Pressure Ulcer Advisory Panel, 2019).

## Defining Characteristics

Blood-filled blister; erythema; full thickness tissue loss; full thickness tissue loss with exposed bone; full thickness tissue loss with exposed muscle; full thickness tissue loss with exposed tendon; localized heat in relation to surrounding tissue; maroon localized area of discolored intact skin; partial thickness loss of dermis; purple localized area of discolored intact skin; skin ulceration; ulcer is covered by eschar; ulcer is covered by slough

## Related Factors

### External Factors

Altered microclimate between skin and supporting surface; excessive moisture; inadequate access to appropriate equipment; inadequate access to appropriate health services; inadequate access to appropriate supplies; inadequate caregiver knowledge of appropriate methods for removing adhesive materials; inadequate caregiver knowledge of appropriate methods for stabilizing devices; inadequate caregiver knowledge of modifiable factors; inadequate caregiver knowledge of pressure injury prevention strategies; increased magnitude of mechanical load; pressure over bony prominence; shearing forces; surface friction; sustained mechanical load; use of linen with insufficient moisture wicking property

• = Independent　　　▲ = Collaborative

**Internal Factors**

Decreased physical mobility; dehydration; dry skin; hyperthermia; water-electrolyte imbalance

**Other Factors**

Factors identified by standardized, validated screening tool

## At-Risk Population

Low birth weight neonates; neonates <32 weeks gestation; neonates experiencing prolonged intensive care unit stay; neonates in intensive care units

## Associated Conditions

Anemia; decreased serum albumin level; decreased tissue oxygenation; decreased tissue perfusion; edema; immature skin integrity; immature skin texture; immature stratum corneum; immobilization; medical devices; nutritional deficiencies related to prematurity; pharmaceutical preparations; prolonged duration of surgical procedure; significant comorbidity

## Client Outcomes

**Client Will (Specify Time Frame)**

- Intact skin; prevention of skin alterations
- Report any altered sensation or pain at site of tissue impairment
- Skin, without redness over bony prominences and capillary refill of less than 6 seconds over areas of redness
- Be repositioned off of bony prominences frequently if risk for pressure injuries is high
- Family/caregiver will demonstrate understanding of plan to reduce pressure injury risk
- Family/caregiver will describe measures to protect the skin

## Nursing Interventions

- Gestational age influences the development of the skin and its function as a barrier. Epidermal maturation is complete at 34 weeks of age. Prematurely or critically ill infants are at a higher risk of skin alterations related to intrinsic and extrinsic factors (Broom et al, 2019).
- Assess the presence of a medical device and pressure injury risk as well as illness severity and need for critical care in neonates and children (National Pressure Injury Advisory Panel [NPIAP] & European Pressure Injury Advisory Panel [EPIAP], 2019).
- Select medical devices that minimize tissue injury. Apply according to the manufacturer's recommendations, ensuring correct sizing and shape. Reposition devices regularly and remove as soon as they are no longer medically necessary. Apply prophylactic dressings under devices to reduce the risk of pressure injuries (NPIAP & EPIAP, 2019).

• = Independent        ▲ = Collaborative

- Protect neonates against toxicity due to topical agents, including iodine, isopropyl ethyl and methyl alcohol, infection, and injury until the stratum corneum has reached maturity (Delmore et al, 2019).
- Routine skin assessment is essential as a lower gestational age is at a higher risk for skin injury (Broom et al, 2019).
- Assess for excessive moisture, especially in between skinfolds and dependent areas.
- Risk assessment tools for high-risk neonates are limited; however, current best evidence has found the Braden QD and Glamorgan to be valid and reliable with assessing pressure injury risk in children and neonates. Clinicians should routinely perform an age-appropriate pressure injury (National Pressure Ulcer Advisory Panel [NPUAP] & European Pressure Ulcer Advisory Panel [EPUAP], 2016) risk assessment using a valid and reliable tool.
- Avoid daily bathing of the skin, which can disrupt normal barrier function.
- Avoid adhesives and products that increase adhesion, which may result in increased epidermal stripping (Delmore et al, 2019).
- Use support surfaces to alleviate poor tissue tolerance and shear and improve microclimate.
- Involve family/caregiver in education focused on reducing risks and management strategies for pressure injuries.

**Home Care**

- The interventions described previously may be adapted for home care use.
- Instruct and assist the client and caregivers in how to assess the skin for excessive pressure. Provide written instructions for actions they can implement to reduce the risk of pressure injury development (NPIAP & EPIAP, 2019).
- Educate client and caregivers on proper nutrition and when to call the agency and/or health care provider with concerns.
- ▲ Initiate a consultation in a case assignment with a wound, ostomy, continence nurse (or wound specialist) to establish a comprehensive plan for pressure ulcer risk reduction for clients at high risk for skin breakdown (Berke et al, 2019).
- ▲ Collaboration with health care professionals, including medical, nursing, nutrition, and industry stakeholders, is imperative to improve outcomes in pressure injury prevention (Delmore et al, 2019; NPIAP & EPIAP, 2019).

P

• = Independent          ▲ = Collaborative

# Risk for Neonatal Pressure Injury

**Domain 11** Safety/protection  **Class 2** Physical injury

## NANDA-I Definition

Neonate susceptible to localized damage to the skin and/or underlying tissue, as a result of pressure, or pressure in combination with shear, which may compromise health (European Pressure Ulcer Advisory Panel, 2019).

## Risk Factors

### External Factors

Altered microclimate between skin and supporting surface; excessive moisture; inadequate access to appropriate equipment; inadequate access to appropriate health services; inadequate access to appropriate supplies; inadequate caregiver knowledge of appropriate methods for removing adhesive materials; inadequate caregiver knowledge of appropriate methods for stabilizing devices; inadequate caregiver knowledge of modifiable factors; inadequate caregiver knowledge of pressure injury prevention strategies; increased magnitude of mechanical load; pressure over bony prominence; shearing forces; surface friction; sustained mechanical load; use of linen with insufficient moisture wicking property

### Internal Factors

Decreased physical mobility; dehydration; dry skin; hyperthermia; water-electrolyte imbalance

### Other Factors

Factors identified by standardized, validated screening tool

## At-Risk Population

Low birth weight neonates; neonates <32 weeks gestation; neonates experiencing prolonged intensive care unit stay; neonates in intensive care units

## Associated Conditions

Anemia; decreased serum albumin level; decreased tissue oxygenation; decreased tissue perfusion; edema; immature skin integrity; immature skin texture; immature stratum corneum; immobilization; medical devices; nutritional deficiencies related to prematurity; pharmaceutical preparations; prolonged duration of surgical procedure; significant comorbidity

## Client Outcomes, Nursing Interventions, and Client/Family Teaching and Discharge Planning

See the care plan for Neonatal **Pressure** Injury.

# Ineffective Protection

**Domain 1** Health promotion  **Class 2** Health management

• = Independent  ▲ = Collaborative

## NANDA-I Definition

Decrease in the ability to guard self from internal or external threats such as illness or injury.

## Defining Characteristics

Altered sweating; anorexia; chilling; coughing; disorientation; dyspnea; expresses itching, fatigue; impaired physical mobility; impaired tissue healing; insomnia; leukopenia; low serum hemoglobin level; maladaptive stress response; neurosensory impairment; pressure injury; psychomotor agitation; thrombocytopenia; weakness

## Related Factors

Depressive symptoms; difficulty managing complex treatment regimen; hopelessness; inadequate vaccination; ineffective health self-management; low self-efficacy; malnutrition; physical deconditioning; substance misuse

## Associated Conditions

Blood coagulation disorders; immune system diseases; neoplasms; pharmaceutical preparations; treatment regimen

## Client Outcomes

### Client Will (Specify Time Frame)

- Remain free of infection while in contact during contact with health care
- Remain free of any evidence of new bleeding as evident by stable vital signs
- Explain precautions to take to prevent infection including hand hygiene
- Explain precautions to take to prevent bleeding including fall prevention

## Nursing Interventions

- Take temperature, pulse, and blood pressure (e.g., every 1–4 hours).
- ▲ Observe nutritional status (e.g., weight, serum protein and albumin levels, muscle mass, and usual food intake). Work with the dietitian to improve nutritional status if needed.
- Observe the client's sleep pattern; if altered, see Nursing Interventions for Disturbed **Sleep** Pattern.
- Identify stressors in the client's life; stress can negatively affect the immune system. If stress is uncontrollable, see Nursing Interventions for Ineffective **Coping.**

### Prevention of Infection

- ▲ Monitor for and report any signs of infection (e.g., fever, chills, flushed skin, drainage, edema, redness, abnormal laboratory values, pain) and notify the health care provider promptly.

• = Independent          ▲ = Collaborative

- If white blood cell count is severely decreased (i.e., absolute neutrophil count of less than 1000/mm$^3$), initiate the following precautions:
  ○ Take vital signs every 2 to 4 hours.
  ○ Complete a head-to-toe assessment twice daily, including inspection of oral mucosa, invasive sites, wounds, urine, and stool; monitor for onset of new reports of pain.
▲ Avoid any invasive procedures, including catheterization, injections, or rectal or vaginal procedures, unless absolutely necessary.
  ○ Consider warming the client before elective surgery.
▲ Administer granulocyte growth factor as ordered.
  ○ Take meticulous care of all invasive sites; use chlorhexidine gluconate for cleansing.
  ○ Follow standard precautions, especially performing hand hygiene, to prevent health care–associated infections.
▲ Refer for appropriate prophylactic antifungal treatment and avoid pathogen exposure (through air filtration, regular hand hygiene, and avoidance of plants and flowers).
  ○ Have the client wear a mask when leaving the room.
  ○ Help the client bathe daily.
  ○ Practice food safety: a neutropenic diet may not be necessary.
  ○ Ensure that the client is well nourished. Provide food with protein and consider vitamin supplements. If appetite is suppressed, institute a dietary referral. Keep track of serum albumin levels and transferrin and prealbumin levels.
  ○ Help the client cough and practice deep breathing regularly. Maintain an appropriate activity level.
  ○ Obtain a private room for the client. Use high-energy particulate air filters if available and appropriate.
▲ Nurses play a pivotal role in the early identification and management of sepsis. Early identification is key to survival. Identifying abnormal vital signs is the first step in early sepsis recognition. If early signs of sepsis are identified, immediately notify the health care provider.
- Refer to care plan for Risk for **Infection.**
- Refer to care plan for Readiness for Enhanced **Nutrition** for additional interventions.

**Pediatric**
- Skin-to-skin contact (SSC) is the practice of placing a diapered infant onto the bare chest of the mother so that the mother and infant are in direct SSC contact with each other. In resource-rich countries, SSC has been motivated by a push to humanize a process that has

**•** = Independent          **▲** = Collaborative

become a medical experience. SSC has been a process to facilitate infant transition to extrauterine life.

- Assess postoperative fever in pediatric oncology clients promptly.

**Geriatric**

▲ If not contraindicated, encourage exercise to promote improved quality of life in older adults.

**Prevention of Bleeding**

▲ Immune thrombocytopenia (ITP), previously known as idiopathic thrombocytopenic purpura, is an autoimmune disorder characterized by a severe reduction in peripheral blood platelet count. Bleeding events are often unpredictable, and clients with ITP may not exhibit bleeding beyond bruising and petechiae. However, more serious mucosal bleeding may occur, including menorrhagia, epistaxis, gastrointestinal hemorrhage, hematuria, or intracranial hemorrhage (Khan et al, 2017; Neunert et al, 2019). Monitor the client's risk for bleeding; evaluate results of clotting studies and platelet counts.

- Watch for hematuria, melena, hematemesis, hemoptysis, epistaxis, bleeding from mucosa, petechiae, and ecchymoses.

▲ Give medications orally or intravenously only; avoid giving intramuscularly, subcutaneously, or rectally.

- Apply pressure for a longer time than usual to invasive sites, such as venipuncture or injection sites. Additional pressure is needed to stop bleeding of invasive sites in clients with bleeding disorders.
- Take vital signs often; watch for changes associated with fluid volume loss.
- Monitor menstrual flow if relevant; have the client use pads instead of tampons.
- Have the client use a moistened toothette or a very soft child's toothbrush instead of an adult toothbrush. Follow the dentist's recommendation for flossing and appropriate rinses to use. Control gum bleeding by applying pressure to gums with gauze pad soaked in ice water.

▲ To decrease risk of bleeding, avoid administering salicylates or nonsteroidal antiinflammatory drugs (NSAIDs) if possible.

**Home Care**

- Some of the interventions previously described may be adapted for home care use.

▲ The Patient-Centered Medical Home (PCMH) model facilitates a team-based approach to care, wherein providers coordinate care across all elements of the larger health care system (Frasso et al, 2017).

• = Independent ▲ = Collaborative

Consider using a nurse-led PCMH for monitoring high-need, high-cost clients (Breland et al, 2016).

- End-of-life (EOL) care is defined as care that helps those with advanced, progressive, incurable, and serious illness to live as well as possible until they die. EOL care in the United States is provided through palliative and hospice medicine. Both hospice and palliative care focus on ensuring the best possible quality of life for individuals with serious illness and their families by providing support, symptom management, and comfort care. Palliative care need depends on the psychosocial, spiritual, and physical necessities of each client rather than the diagnosis. Caution should be used when assessing need for palliative care; the diagnosis should not be the primary trigger but instead use of a provider tool consisting of three elements: nutritional decline, disease progression, and functional decline. Building trust and shared decision making among the health care team, client, and family are pivotal in all palliative care conversations. Seriously ill clients have a high symptom burden, depending on their diagnosis (Cruz-Oliver, 2017).

**P Client/Family Teaching and Discharge Planning**
**Depressed Immune Function**
- Discharge planning should start at admission. Key elements to focus on when providing discharge teaching to clients and their families to promote a successful transition from acute care to self-management at home are to develop health knowledge, provide resources, and promote self-efficacy. Identify clients' needs to provide tailored, individual support and education. Teach the client and family how and when to take the client's temperature and provide temperature parameters so the client/family knows when to call the provider (Pollack et al, 2016).
- Teach precautions to use to decrease the chance of infection. Teach/reinforce appropriate self-care, including good hand hygiene, personal hygiene, and ensuring a safe environment. Teach the client to avoid crowds and contact with persons who have infections. Teach the need for good nutrition, avoidance of stress, and adequate rest to maintain immune system function.

**Bleeding Disorder**
- Teach the client to wear a medical alert bracelet and to notify all health care personnel of the bleeding disorder.
- Teach the client and family the signs of bleeding, precautions to take to prevent bleeding, and action to take if bleeding begins. Caution the client to avoid taking over-the-counter medications without

• = Independent         ▲ = Collaborative

the permission of the health care provider. Medications containing salicylates can increase bleeding.

• Teach the client to wear loose-fitting clothes and avoid physical activity that might cause trauma.

# Rape-Trauma Syndrome

**Domain 9** Coping/stress tolerance     **Class 1** Post-trauma responses

## NANDA-I Definition

Sustained maladaptive response to a forced, violent, sexual penetration against the victim's will and consent.

## Defining Characteristics

Aggressive behaviors; altered interpersonal relations; anger behaviors; anxiety (00146); cardiogenic shock; confusion; denial, depressive symptoms; difficulty with decision-making; disordered thinking; expresses anger; expresses embarrassment; expresses shame; fear (00148); humiliation; hypervigilance; loss of independence; low self-esteem; mood variability; muscle spasm; muscle tension; nightmares; paranoia; perceived vulnerability; phobic disorders; physical trauma; powerlessness (00125); psychomotor agitation; reports altered sleep-wake cycle; reports feeling guilty; self-blame; sexual dysfunction (00059); substance misuse; thoughts of revenge

## Related Factors

To be developed

## At-Risk Population

Individuals who experienced rape; individuals with history of suicide attempt

## Associated Conditions

Depression; dissociative identity disorder

## Client Outcomes

**Client Will (Specify Time Frame)**

• Share feelings, concerns, and fears
• Recognize that the rape or attempt was not client's own fault
• State that, no matter what the situation, no one has the right to assault another
• Describe medical/legal treatment procedures and reasons for treatment
• Report absence of physical complications or pain
• Identify support resources and attend psychotherapy/group assistance in coping with the trauma and effects of the traumatic experience
• Function at same level as before crisis, including sexual functioning

• = Independent     ▲ = Collaborative

- Recognize that it is normal for full recovery to take a minimum of 1 year

## Nursing Interventions

- Use a trauma-informed approach with survivors of sexual assault.
- Introduce yourself and your role in all interactions.
- Escort the client to a treatment room immediately on arrival to the emergency department. Stay with the client and provide access to a community-based advocate.
- Assure the client of confidentiality.
- Provide a sexual assault response team (SART), if available, that includes a sexual assault nurse examiner (SANE), rape counseling advocate, and representative of law enforcement for best possible outcomes.
- Use an open and nonthreatening body positioning and posture.
- Use open-ended questions to document the client's chief complaint and request an event history of the sexual assault in his or her own words.
- Use the sexual assault evidence collection kits that have been reviewed by the SART members and provided by your state to collect adequate and accurate evidence for analysis by a forensic laboratory.
- Before proceeding with a medical forensic examination, consent for the medical evaluation and for evidence collection and release must be obtained from the sexual assault client.
- Ask permission before you touch the client.
- Provide anticipatory guidance by explaining every step of the physical examination and nursing care to the client before performing and check for understanding.
- Observe for signs of physical injury.
- Inform client of the risk of pregnancy and sexually transmitted infections (STIs) and offer available treatments.
- Assess sexual assault clients for health problems related to human sex trafficking: infectious diseases; noninfectious diseases (malnutrition, dental problems, and skin problems); reproductive health problems; substance abuse; mental health problems; and violence.
- Provide reassurance that the sexual violence was not the client's fault.
- Emphasize the client's resilience and strengths.
- Encourage the client to verbalize his or her feelings.
- Assess to determine whether physically abused women are also survivors of sexual assault.
- ▲ Encourage the client to report the sexual assault to a law enforcement agency.

• = Independent          ▲ = Collaborative

▲ Refer the client for cognitive behavioral therapy (CBT).
▲ Stress the necessity of follow-up care with counselors, mental health specialists, and medical subspecialists as appropriate.

**Male Rape**
- Some of the interventions described previously may be adapted for use with male clients.
- Assist male survivors of sexual assault to identify and verbalize their victimization experiences as rape.

**Geriatric**
- Some of the interventions described previously may be adapted for use with older clients.
- Build a trusting relationship with the client.
- All examinations should be done on older adults as they would be done on any adult client after sexual assault, with modifications for comfort if necessary.
- Assess for mobility limitations and cognitive impairment.
- Explain and encourage the client to report sexual abuse.
- Observe for psychosocial distress.

**Pediatric**
- Some of the interventions described previously may be adapted for use with child and adolescent populations.
- For minors, follow state-mandated reporting laws and report to Child Protective Services.
- Use language that is tailored to the age and abilities of the child or adolescent.
- Assess adolescent sexual assault clients for health problems related to human sex trafficking: infectious diseases; noninfectious diseases (malnutrition, dental problems, and skin problems); reproductive health problems; substance abuse; mental health problems; and violence.

**Multicultural**
- Some of the interventions described previously may be adapted for use with diverse clients.
- Assess how an individual's culture affects how they perceive trauma, safety, and privacy.
- Provide information and referrals for follow-up care that recognize and address the unique needs of sexual and gender minority clients.

**Home Care**
- Some of the interventions described previously may be adapted for home care use.

R

• = Independent          ▲ = Collaborative

- Assist the client with assessing the home setting for safety and/or selecting a safe living environment.
▲ Ensure that the client has systems in place for long-term support.
▲ Assess for other client vulnerabilities, such as mental health issues or addiction, and refer the client to social agencies for implementation of a therapeutic regimen.

**Client/Family Teaching and Discharge Planning**
- Provide teaching about the emotional and physical aftermath of sexual trauma.
- Screen the client for suicide risk and refer to appropriate services.

# Ineffective Relationship

**Domain 7** Role relationship    **Class 3** Role performance

## NANDA-I Definition

A pattern of mutual partnership that is insufficient to provide for each other's needs.

## Defining Characteristics

Delayed attainment of developmental goals appropriate for family life-cycle stage; expresses dissatisfaction with complementary interpersonal relations between partners; expresses dissatisfaction with emotional need fulfillment between partners; expresses dissatisfaction with idea sharing between partners; expresses dissatisfaction with information sharing between partners; expresses dissatisfaction with physical need fulfillment between partners; imbalance in autonomy between partners; imbalance in collaboration between partners; inadequate mutual respect between partners; inadequate mutual support in daily activities between partners; inadequate understanding of partner's compromised functioning; partner not identified as support person; reports unsatisfactory communication with partner

## Related Factors

Ineffective communication skills; stressors; substance misuse; unrealistic expectations

## At-Risk Population

Individuals experiencing developmental crisis; individuals with history of domestic violence; individuals with incarcerated intimate partner

## Associated Conditions

Cognitive dysfunction in one partner

## Client Outcomes

**Family/Client Will (Specify Time Frame)**
- Share thoughts and feelings with each other

• = Independent                    ▲ = Collaborative

- Communicate openly with each other
- Assist in performing family roles and tasks
- Provide support for each other
- Obtain appropriate assistance

## Nursing Interventions

- Assess communication patterns concerning role and satisfaction within the relationship, including elements associated with intimacy.
- Assess relationship quality using the Relationship Flourishing Scale.
- Focus on helping couples maintain or develop marital closeness, especially during times of extreme stress.
- Assess the presence of stressors; physical, emotional, and behavioral health; and physical health status of the couple.
- Explore the couple's perceptions of the impact of illness on the relationship.
- Assist couples to identify sources of their own perceived dyadic empathy in the relationship.
- Assist clients to identify sources of gratitude in their relationships.
- Encourage couples to engage in reappraisal of conflict in their relationship.
- Encourage the use of positive relational humor and humor evaluation between partners.
- Provide support resources to provide military members and their families with assistance in preparation for deployments and education about the importance of maintaining communication during deployment.
- Provide resources to military family members with posttraumatic stress disorder (PTSD).
- Encourage couples to participate together in leisure activities.
- Openly explore communication and satisfaction in the same-sex relationship without bias.
- Refer to care plans Readiness for Enhanced **Relationship**, Readiness for Enhanced **Family** Processes, and Readiness for Enhanced Family **Coping.**

### Geriatric

- Assess geriatric spousal caregivers for positive and negative consequences of providing medical care.
- Assess intimacy and sexuality of older adults.
- Facilitate and increase opportunities for social connectedness for older individuals through the use of technology training.

• = Independent          ▲ = Collaborative

**Multicultural**

- Assess relationship dynamics without bias as to race, gender identity, or ethnicity.
- Use culturally tailored cognitive behavioral techniques to promote communication, problem solving, self-disclosure, empathic response skills, and sexual education and counseling.

# Readiness for Enhanced Relationship

**Domain 7** Role relationship    **Class 3** Role performance

## NANDA-I Definition

A pattern of mutual partnership to provide for each other's needs, which can be strengthened.

## Defining Characteristics

Expresses desire to enhance autonomy between partners; expresses desire to enhance collaboration between partners; expresses desire to enhance communication between partners; expresses desire to enhance emotional need fulfillment for each partner; expresses desire to enhance mutual respect between partners; expresses desire to enhance satisfaction with complementary interpersonal relationship between partners; expresses desire to enhance satisfaction with emotional need fulfillment for each partner; expresses desire to enhance satisfaction with idea sharing between partners; expresses desire to enhance satisfaction with information sharing between partners; expresses desire to enhance satisfaction with physical need fulfillment for each partner; expresses desire to enhance understanding of partner's functional impairment

## Client Outcomes

**Family/Client Will (Specify Time Frame)**

- Share thoughts and feelings with each other
- Communicate openly with each other
- Assist in performing family roles and tasks
- Provide support for each other
- Obtain appropriate assistance

## Nursing Interventions

- Assess the ways in which the relationship has been altered (e.g., communication, sexuality, intimacy) from both partner's perspective.
- Assess relationship quality using the Relationship Flourishing Scale.
- Focus on helping couples maintain or develop marital closeness.
- Assist couples to identify sources of their own perceived dyadic empathy in the relationship.

• = Independent      ▲ = Collaborative

- Assist clients to identify sources of gratitude in their relationships.
- Encourage couples to engage in reappraisal of conflict in their relationship.
- Encourage the use of positive relational humor and humor evaluation between partners.
- Provide support resources to provide military members and their families with assistance in preparation for deployments and education about the importance of maintaining communication during deployment.
- Encourage couples to participate together in leisure activities such as dance.
- Refer to care plans Readiness for Enhanced **Family** Processes and Readiness for Enhanced Family **Coping.**

**Pediatric**
- Encourage guidance and information on communication for parents of seriously ill children.
- Encourage young children to express gratitude.

**Geriatric**
- Assess geriatric spousal caregivers for positive and negative consequences of providing medical care.
- Assess sexuality needs and support consensual sexual expression.
- Facilitate and increase opportunities for social connectedness for older individuals through the use of technology training.

**Multicultural**
- Provide a relationship-focused intervention to enhance communication for multicultural couples.
- Use culturally tailored cognitive behavioral techniques to promote communication, problem-solving, self-disclosure, empathic response skills, and sexual education and counseling.

# Risk for Ineffective Relationship

**Domain 7** Role relationship    **Class 3** Role performance

## NANDA-I Definition

Susceptible to developing a pattern that is insufficient for providing a mutual partnership to provide for each other's needs.

## Risk Factors

Inadequate communication skills; stressors; substance misuse; unrealistic expectations

## At-Risk Population

Individuals experiencing developmental crisis; individuals with history of domestic violence; individuals with incarcerated intimate partner

## Associated Conditions

Cognitive dysfunction in one partner

## Client Outcomes and Nursing Interventions

Refer to care plan for Ineffective **Relationship**.

# Impaired Religiosity

**Domain 10** Life Principles    **Class 3** Value/belief/action congruence

## NANDA-I Definition

Impaired ability to exercise reliance on beliefs and/or participate in rituals of a particular faith tradition.

## Defining Characteristics

Desires to reconnect with belief pattern; desires to reconnect with customs; difficulty adhering to prescribed religious beliefs; difficulty adhering to prescribed religious rituals; expresses distress about separation from faith community; questions religious beliefs; questions religious customs

## Related Factors

Anxiety; cultural barrier to practicing religion; depressive symptoms; environmental constraints; fear of death; inadequate social support; inadequate sociocultural interaction; inadequate transportation; ineffective caregiving; ineffective coping strategies; insecurity; pain; spiritual distress

## At-Risk Population

Hospitalized individuals; individuals experiencing end of life crisis; individuals experiencing life transition; individuals experiencing personal crisis; individuals experiencing spiritual crisis; individuals with history of religious manipulation; older adults

## Associated Conditions

Depression; impaired health status

## Client Outcomes

Client Will (Specify Time Frame)

- Express satisfaction with the ability to express religious practices
- Express satisfaction with access to religious materials and rituals
- Demonstrate balance between religious practices and healthy lifestyles
- Avoid high-risk, controlling religious relationships that inflict physical, sexual, or emotional harm and/or exploitation

## Nursing Interventions

**Adults**
- Recognize when clients integrate religious practices into their life.

• = Independent         ▲ = Collaborative

- Assist clients to work around or overcome barriers to participating in their usual religious rituals or practices that support coping.
- Encourage the use of prayer or meditation as appropriate.
- Promote family coping using religious practices to help cope with loss, as appropriate.
- Refer to a religious leader, professional counseling, or support group as needed.

**End-of-Life Care**
- Refer to a religious leader, professional counseling, or support group as needed.
- Implement QSEN competencies and evidence-based practice in providing end-of-life (EOL) care.

**Maternal–Child Health**
- Provide support for pregnant client's religiosity to promote health-seeking behaviors.

**Sexual Minority Individuals (Lesbian, Gay, Bisexual, Transgender, Queer)**
- Provide support using religiosity with caution.

**Pediatric**
- Provide spiritual care for children based on developmental level.
- **Parents:** Incorporate religious traditions and faith practices for parents with hospitalized and chronically ill children.

**Geriatric**
- Promote established religious practices in older adults.

**Multicultural**
Promote religious practices that are culturally appropriate:
- African American
- Hispanic
- Jordanian
- Muslim

**Multiprofessional**
- Refer to a religious leader, professional counseling, or support group as needed.

## Readiness for Enhanced Religiosity

**Domain 10** Life principles     **Class 3** Value/belief/action congruence
**NANDA-I Definition**

A pattern of reliance on religious beliefs and/or participation in rituals of a particular faith tradition, which can be strengthened.

• = Independent                    ▲ = Collaborative

## Defining Characteristics

Expresses desire to enhance connection with a religious leader; Expresses desire to enhance forgiveness; Expresses desire to enhance participation in religious experiences; Expresses desire to enhance participation in religious practices; Expresses desire to enhance religious options; Expresses desire to enhance use of religious material; Expresses desire to reestablish belief patterns; Expresses desire to reestablish religious customs

## Client Outcomes

### Client Will (Specify Time Frame)

- Express satisfaction with the ability to express religious practices
- Express satisfaction with access to religious materials and rituals
- Demonstrate balance between religious practices and healthy lifestyles
- Avoid high-risk, controlling religious relationships that inflict physical, sexual, or emotional harm and/or exploitation

## Nursing Interventions

### Adults
- Encourage centering prayer or other forms of meditation to promote mental and spiritual health.

### Disabled
- Use prayer as a coping mechanism for those with disabilities.

### Maternal–Child Health
- Provide support for pregnant client's religiosity to promote health-seeking behaviors.

### Sexual Minority Individuals (Lesbian, Gay, Bisexual, Transgender, Queer)
- Encourage the use of religion to decrease stigma and improve quality of life (QOL) for HIV-positive men.

### Uninsured/Low Income
- Explore the use of a faith community nurse to provide wellness services and care monitoring.

### Veterans
- Encourage the use of religion to help decrease sleep disturbances in veterans.

### End-of-Life Care
- Implement QSEN competencies and evidence-based practice in providing end-of-life (EOL) care.
- ▲ Refer to a religious leader, professional counseling, or support group as needed.

### Pediatric
- Provide spiritual care for children based on developmental level.

• = Independent          ▲ = Collaborative

- **Parents:** Incorporate religious traditions and faith practices for parents with hospitalized and chronically ill children.
- **School-Age Children:** Encourage faith community involvement and religious attendance with parent(s).
- **School-Age Children:** Encourage children to participate in faith community health programs.
- **African American Children:** Incorporate faith traditions in coping with chronic disease.
- **Latino Children:** Incorporate faith traditions among clients and families in pediatric settings.
- **Adolescents:** Encourage prayer, particularly within the African American community.
- **Adolescents/Young Adults:** Encourage religious coping in the adolescent/young adult population.

**Geriatric**
- Encourage listening to religious music.

**Multicultural**
- **African American:** Collaborate with faith communities to promote wellness. Also, incorporate faith traditions in coping with chronic disease.
- **Latino:** Incorporate faith traditions among clients and families in pediatric settings.
- **Thai:** Encourage both religious and spiritual coping strategies to help cope.

**Multiprofessional**
▲ Chaplain referral when individuals engage in religious coping mechanisms.

## Risk for Impaired Religiosity

**Domain 10** Life principles    **Class 3** Value/belief/action congruence
### NANDA-I Definition
Susceptible to an impaired ability to exercise reliance on religious beliefs and/or participate in rituals of a particular faith tradition, which may compromise health.
### Risk Factors
Anxiety; cultural barrier to practicing religion; depressive symptoms; environmental constraints; fear of death; inadequate social support; inadequate sociocultural interaction; inadequate transportation; ineffective caregiving; ineffective coping strategies; insecurity; pain; spiritual distress

• = Independent          ▲ = Collaborative

## At-Risk Population

Hospitalized individuals; individuals experiencing end of life crisis; individuals experiencing life transition; individuals experiencing personal crisis; individuals experiencing spiritual crisis; Individuals with history of religious manipulation; older adults

## Associated Conditions

Depression; impaired health status

## Client Outcomes and Nursing Interventions

Refer to care plan for Impaired **Religiosity.**

# Relocation Stress Syndrome

**Domain 9** Coping/stress tolerance   **Class 1** Post-trauma responses

## NANDA-I Definition

Physiological and/or psychosocial disturbance following transfer from one environment to another.

## Defining Characteristics

Anger behaviors; anxiety (00146); decreased self concept; depressive symptoms; expresses anger; expresses frustration; fear (00148); increased morbidity; increased physical symptoms; increased verbalization of needs; loss of identity; loss of independence; low self-esteem; pessimism; preoccupation; reports altered sleep-wake cycle; reports concern about relocation; reports feeling alone; reports feeling insecure; reports feeling lonely; social alienation; unwillingness to move

## Related Factors

Communication barriers; inadequate control over environment; inadequate predeparture counseling; inadequate social support; ineffective coping strategies; powerlessness; situational challenge to self-worth; social isolation

## At-Risk Population

Individuals facing unpredictability of experience; individuals who move from one environment to another; individuals with history of loss

## Associated Conditions

Depression; diminished mental competency; impaired health status; impaired psychosocial functioning

## Client Outcomes

**Client Will (Specify Time Frame)**

- Recognize and know the name of at least one staff member or new neighbor within 1 week of relocating
- Engage at least one staff member of new neighbor in a conversation within 2 weeks of relocating

• = Independent            ▲ = Collaborative

- Express concern about move when encouraged to do so during individual contacts within 24 hours of awareness of impending relocation
- Perform activities of daily living (ADLs) in safe manner
- Proactively ask for assistance with ADLs
- Maintain previous mental and physical health status (e.g., nutrition, elimination, sleep, social interaction, physical activity) within 2 months of relocating

## Nursing Interventions

- Orientation to the new environment is a proactive means that alleviates anxiety and increases confidence.
- Be aware that relocation to retirement communities may be a positive change.
- Begin relocation planning as early in the decision-making process as possible.
- Obtain a history, including the reason for the move, the client's usual coping mechanisms, history of losses, and family and financial support for the client.
- Identify to what extent the client can participate in the relocation decision-making process and advocate for this participation.
- Assess client's readiness to relocate and relocation self-efficacy.
- Consult an evidence-based practice guide for relocation.
- Assess family members' perceptions of client's ability to participate in relocation decisions. Particularly in incidences of neurocognitive impairment such as dementia, be attentive to health care workers' involvement in making the decision to relocate. They may need support and encouragement through the process.
- Consider the cultural and ethnic values of the client and family as much as possible when choosing roommates, foods, and other aspects of care.
- Promote clear communication between all participants involved in the relocation process.
- Observe the following procedures if the client is being transferred to an extended care or assisted living facility:
  - Facilitate the client's participation in decisions and choice of placement, and arrange a preadmission visit if possible.
  - If the client cannot visit the new facility, arrange for a visit or telephone call by a member of the staff to welcome the client and show a videotape or at least provide pictures of the new care facility.
  - Have a familiar person accompany the client to the new

• = Independent ▲ = Collaborative

facility. This lessens client and family anxiety, confusion, and dissatisfaction.

○ Encourage the resident and/or caregiver to write a journal regarding thoughts and feelings about the relocation.

○ Continue to assess caregiver psychological distress during a 6-month period after relocation. Caregivers experience guilt and distress because of the responsibility of moving their loved one.

- Identify previous routines for ADLs. Try to maintain as much continuity with the previous schedule as possible.
- Bring in familiar items from home (e.g., pictures, clocks, afghans).
- Establish the way the client would like to be addressed (Mr., Mrs., Miss, first name, or calling name/nickname).
- Thoroughly orient the client and the family to the new environment and routines; repeat directions as needed.
- Spend one-to-one time with the client. Allow the client to express feelings and convey acceptance of them; emphasize that the client's feelings are real and individual and that it is acceptable to be sad or angry about moving.
- Allocate an attentive staff member to help the client adjust to the move. Assign the same staff members to the client for care if the therapeutic relationship is compatible with client needs; maintain consistency in the staffing personnel with whom the client interacts on a daily basis.
- Encourage the client to verbalize one positive aspect of the new living situation each day. Helping the client to focus on the positive aspects of the move can facilitate adaptation and adjustment by reframing one's attitude in a positive fashion.
- Ask the client to verbalize one positive aspect of the new living situation each day.
- Monitor the client's well-being and provide appropriate interventions for problems with social interaction, nutrition, sleep, new onset of infection, or elimination problems.
- If the client is being transferred within a facility, have staff members from the new unit visit the client and the family, if possible, before transfer.
- Work with the caregivers and family members, helping them work with and adjust to the stages of "making the best of it," "making the move," and "making it better."
- If a client is being transferred from the intensive care unit (ICU), have previous staff make occasional visits until the client is

**•** = Independent        **▲** = Collaborative

comfortable in the new surroundings. Ensure that the family is told relevant information.

- Watch for coping problems (e.g., withdrawal, regression, angry behavior, impaired sleeping, refusal to eat, flat affect, anxiety) and intervene immediately.
- Encourage the client to express grief for the loss of former residence and of interpersonal relationships and explain that it is normal to feel sadness over change and loss.
- Assess the client's psychological needs along with physiological needs.
- Encourage clients to take a proactive role in their care as much as is possible inclusive of autonomous decision-making (e.g., arrangement of the furniture in the residence, choice of roommate, bathing routines).

## Pediatric

- Assess family history and contact information from children relocated to rescue shelters.
- Be aware that community relocation may be beneficial for children and assess community and academic resources of new location (Miller et al, 2019).
- Provide support for a child and family who must relocate to be near a higher acuity health care facility such as a transplant center (Søndergaard et al, 2016).
- In situations of familial discord such as divorce, recommend alternative dispute resolution versus traditional litigated settlement.
- Assess presence of allergies before and after relocation.
  - ○ If the client is an adolescent, try to avoid a move in the middle of the school year, find a newcomers' club for the adolescent to join, and refer for counseling if needed.
- Assess adolescents' perceptions of their acceptance by peers.
- Help parents recognize that relocation stress syndrome may persist for prolonged periods (e.g., 2 years), especially in adolescents.
- Be aware that adolescents may cope with the transition by exerting control in particular domains.
- The effects of frequent relocation may not manifest immediately and may have long-term effects on physical and mental health.

## Geriatric

- Monitor the need for transfer and relocate only when medically or psychologically necessary.
- Implement discharge planning early and engage the older adult in the planning and decision-making process about relocation.

• = Independent          ▲ = Collaborative

- Use technologies, such as sensing devices, to measure average in-home gait speed (AIGS) as a predictor of fall risk.
- Implement a registered nurse (RN) care coordination care planning model to restore older adults' health, maintain their independence, and reduce care costs.
- After the transfer, assess the client's mental status. Document and observe for any new onset of confusion. Confusion can follow relocation because of the overwhelming stress and sensory overload.
- Facilitate visits from companion animals.

**Client/Family Teaching and Discharge Planning**
- Teach family members about symptoms of relocation stress syndrome. Encourage them to monitor for signs of the syndrome.
- Help significant others learn how to support the client in the relocation process by setting up social engagements such as a schedule of visits, arranging for holidays, bringing familiar items from home, and establishing a system for contact when the client needs support.
- Assist family members and the relocating older adult to use Internet/webcam technology for interaction to supplement in-person visits.

# Risk for Relocation Stress Syndrome

**R**

**Domain 9** Coping/stress tolerance    **Class 1** Post-trauma responses

**NANDA-I Definition**

Susceptible to physiological and/or psychosocial disturbance following transfer from one environment to another, which may compromise health.

**Risk Factors**

Communication barriers; inadequate control over environment; inadequate predeparture counseling; inadequate social support; ineffective coping strategies; powerlessness; situational challenge to self-worth; social isolation

**At-Risk Population**

Individuals facing unpredictability of experience; individuals who move from one environment to another; individuals with history of loss

**Associated Conditions**

Diminished mental competency; impaired health status; impaired psychosocial functioning

**Client Outcomes, Nursing Interventions, and Client/Family Teaching and Discharge Planning**

Refer to care plan for **Relocation** Stress Syndrome.

• = Independent          ▲ = Collaborative

# Impaired Resilience

**Domain 9** Coping/stress tolerance     **Class 2** Coping responses

## NANDA-I Definition

Decreased ability to recover from perceived adverse or changing situations, through a dynamic process of adaptation.

## Defining Characteristics

Decreased interest in academic activities; decreased interest in vocational activities; depressive symptoms; expresses shame; impaired health status; inadequate sense of control; ineffective coping strategies; ineffective integration; low self-esteem; renewed elevation of distress; reports feeling guilty; social isolation

## Related Factors

Altered family relations; community violence; disrupted family rituals; disrupted family roles; dysfunctional family processes; inadequate health resources; inadequate social support; inconsistent parenting; ineffective family adaptation; multiple coexisting adverse situations; perceived vulnerability; substance misuse

## At-Risk Population

Economically disadvantaged individuals; individuals experiencing a new crisis; individuals experiencing chronic crisis; individuals exposed to violence; individuals who are members of an ethnic minority; individuals whose parents have mental disorders; individuals with history of exposure to violence; individuals with large families; mothers with low educational level; women

## Associated Conditions

Intellectual disability; psychological disorder

## Client Outcomes

**Client Will (Specify Time Frame)**
- Demonstrate reduced or cessation of drug and alcohol usage
- State effective life events on feelings about self
- Seek help when necessary
- Verbalize or demonstrate cessation of abuse
- Adapt to unexpected crises or challenges
- Verbalize positive outlook on illness, family, situation, and life
- Use available resources to meet coping needs
- Identify role models
- Identify available assets and resources
- Be able to verbalize meaning of one's life

## Nursing Interventions

- Encourage positive, health-seeking behaviors.
- Ensure access to biological, psychological, and spiritual resources.

• = Independent          ▲ = Collaborative

- Foster cognitive skills in decision-making.
- Assist client in cognitive restructuring of negative thought processes.
- Facilitate supportive family environments and communication.
- Promote engagement in positive social activities.
- Assist client to identify strengths and reinforce these.
- Help the client identify positive emotions during adverse situations.
- Build on supportive counseling and therapy.
- Identify protective factors such as assets and resources to enhance coping.
- Provide positive reinforcement and emotional support during the learning process.
- Encourage mindfulness, a conscious attention, and awareness of self.
- Educate and encourage the use of stress-reduction techniques.
- Enhance knowledge and use of self-care strategies.

**Pediatric**

- The preceding interventions may be adapted for the pediatric client.
- Promote nurturing, supportive relationships with family.
- Facilitate health and well-being opportunities.
- Promote the development of positive mentor relationships.
- ▲ Consider referral to appropriate community resource for children who have had adverse childhood experiences.

**R**

## Readiness for Enhanced Resilience

**Domain 9** Coping/stress tolerance    **Class 2** Coping responses

### NANDA-I Definition

A pattern of ability to recover from perceived adverse or changing situations, through a dynamic process of adaptation, which can be strengthened.

### Defining Characteristics

Expresses desire to enhance available resources; expresses desire to enhance communication skills; expresses desire to enhance environmental safety; expresses desire to enhance goal setting; expresses desire to enhance interpersonal relations; expresses desire to enhance involvement in activities; expresses desire to enhance own responsibility for action; expresses desire to enhance positive outlook; expresses desire to enhance progress toward goal; expresses desire to enhance psychological resilience; expresses desire to enhance self-esteem; expresses desire to enhance sense of control; expresses desire to enhance support system; expresses desire to enhance use of conflict management strategies; expresses desire to enhance use of coping skills; expresses desire to enhance use of resources

• = Independent      ▲ = Collaborative

## Client Outcomes

**Client Will (Specify Time Frame)**
- Adapt to adversities and challenges
- Communicate clearly and appropriately for age
- Take responsibility for own actions
- Make progress towards goals
- Use effective coping strategies
- Express emotions

## Nursing Interventions

- Listen to and encourage expressions of feelings and beliefs.
- Establish a therapeutic relationship based on trust and respect.
- Assist client in rating current level of resilience.
- Facilitate supportive family environments and communication.
- Assist client to identify and reinforce strengths.
- Enhance skills associated with social and executive functioning.
- Provide positive reinforcement and emotional support during implementation of nursing care.
▲ Facilitate the engagement with mentorship and volunteer opportunities.
- Determine how family behavior affects the client.
- Promote use of mindfulness and other stress-reduction techniques.

**Pediatric**
- The preceding interventions may be adapted for the pediatric client.
- Encourage the promotion of protective factors by fostering the seeking of opportunities to improve cognitive abilities, such as tutoring and other resources; the development of positive and supportive relations such as family, community members, or mentors; and the improvement of general health.

**Multicultural**
- Use teaching strategies that are culturally and age appropriate.

## Risk for Impaired Resilience

**Domain 9** Coping/stress tolerance     **Class 2** Coping responses

### NANDA-I Definition

Susceptible to decreased ability to recover from perceived adverse or changing situations, through a dynamic process of adaptation, which may compromise health.

### Risk Factors

Altered family relations; community violence; disrupted family rituals; disrupted family roles; dysfunctional family processes; inadequate health

• = Independent          ▲ = Collaborative

resources; inadequate social support; inconsistent parenting; ineffective family adaptation; multiple coexisting adverse situations; perceived vulnerability; substance misuse

## At-Risk Population

Economically disadvantaged individuals; individuals experiencing a new crisis; individuals experiencing chronic crisis; individuals exposed to violence; individuals who are members of an ethnic minority; individuals whose parents have mental disorders; individuals with history of exposure to violence; individuals with large families; mothers with low educational level; women

## Associated Conditions

Intellectual disability; psychological disorder

## Client Outcomes

### Client Will (Specify Time Frame)

- Identify available community resources
- Propose practical, constructive solutions for disputes
- Identify and access community resources for assistance
- Accept assistance with activities of daily living from family and friends
- Verbalize an enhanced sense of control
- Verbalize meaningfulness of one's life

## Nursing Interventions

- Determine how family behavior affects client.
- Help the client to identify personal rights, responsibilities, and conflicting norms.
- Encourage consideration of values underlying choices and consequences of the choice.
- Help the client practice conversational and social skills.
- Assist client to prioritize values.
- Foster an accepting, nonjudgmental atmosphere.
- Help to identify self-defeating thoughts.
- ▲ Refer to community resources/social services as appropriate.
- ▲ Help clarify problem areas in interpersonal relationships.
- ▲ Promote a sense of an individual's autonomy and control over choices to be made in one's environment.
- ▲ Identify and enroll high-risk families in follow-up programs.

# Parental Role Conflict

**Domain 7** Role relationship    **Class 3** Role performance
## NANDA-I Definition

Parental experience of role confusion and conflict in response to crisis.

• = Independent          ▲ = Collaborative

## Defining Characteristics

Anxiety; disrupted caregiver routines; expresses fear; expresses frustration; perceived inadequacy to provide for child's needs; perceived loss of control over decisions relating to child; reluctance to participate in usual caregiver activities; reports concern about change in parental role; reports concern about family; reports feeling guilty

## Related Factors

Interruptions in family life due to home treatment regimen; intimidated by invasive modalities; intimidation by restrictive modalities; parent–child separation

## At-Risk Population

Individuals living in nontraditional setting; individuals undergoing changes in marital status; parents with child requiring home care for special needs

## Client Outcomes

**Client Will (Specify Time Frame)**

- Express feelings and perceptions regarding effects of illness, disability, and/or hospitalization on parental role
- Participate in hospital and home care as much as able given the availability of resources and support systems
- Exhibit assertiveness and responsibility in active family decision-making regarding care of the child
- Describe and select available resources to support parental management of the needs of the child and family

## Nursing Interventions

- Assess and support parent's previous coping behaviors.
- Assess for the following signs of parental burnout: exhaustion in one's parental role, contrast with previous parental self, feelings of being fed up with one's parental role, and emotional distancing from one's children.
- Determine parent/family sources of stress, using the Parental Stress Scale.
- Evaluate the family's perceived strength of its social support system. Encourage the family to use social support.
- Determine the older childbearing woman's support systems and expectations for motherhood.
- Use family-centered care and role modeling for holistic care of families.
- ▲ Maintain parental involvement in shared decision-making regarding care by using the following steps: incorporate parents' information concerning the child's typical routines, behaviors, fears, likes, and dislikes; provide clear and direct firsthand information concerning

**R**

• = Independent        ▲ = Collaborative

the child's condition and progress; normalize the home/hospital environment as much as possible; and collaborate in care by providing choices when possible.

- Seek and support parental participation in care.
- ▲ Inform parents of financial resources, respite care, and home support to assist them in maintaining sufficient energy and personal resources to continue caregiving responsibilities.
- Provide family-centered care: allow parents to touch and talk to the child, and assist in the handling of medical equipment; offer open visiting hours; promote family presence at the bedside; promote open communication; provide for privacy.
- Refer parents to available telephone and/or Internet support groups.
- Involve new mother's partner or parents in clinical encounters and invite family members to discuss their expectations and parenting experiences.

## Multicultural

- Acknowledge racial/ethnic differences at the onset of care.
- Assess for the influence of cultural beliefs, norms, and values on the client's perceptions of the parental role.
- Acknowledge that value conflicts arising from acculturation stresses may contribute to increased anxiety and significant conflict with the parental role.
- ▲ Refer parents of young children in specific cultural communities to support programs.

## Home Care

- The interventions described previously may be adapted for home care use.
- Assess family preference for prenatal and postpartum visits; assist new parents to renegotiate parenting roles and responsibilities with coparenting.

## Client/Family Teaching and Discharge Planning

- Offer family-led education interventions to improve participants' knowledge about their condition and its treatment and decrease their information needs.
- Encourage children and parent involvement in bereavement support groups, as an adjunct to grief therapy.
- ▲ Refer to a parenting program to facilitate learning of parenting skills.
- Teach the client about available community resources (e.g., therapists, ministers, counselors, self-help groups).

# Ineffective Role Performance

**Domain 7** Role relationship    **Class 3** Role performance

## NANDA-I Definition

A pattern of behavior and self-expression that does not match the environmental context, norms, and expectations.

## Defining Characteristics

Altered pattern of responsibility; altered perception of role by others; altered role perception; altered role resumption; anxiety; depressive symptoms; domestic violence; harassment; inadequate confidence; inadequate external support for role enactment; inadequate knowledge of role requirements; inadequate motivation; inadequate opportunity for role enactment; inadequate self-management; inadequate skills; inappropriate developmental expectations; ineffective adaptation to change; ineffective coping strategies; ineffective role performance; perceived social discrimination; pessimism; powerlessness; reports social discrimination; role ambivalence; role denial; role dissatisfaction; system conflict; uncertainty

## Related Factors

Altered body image; conflict; fatigue; inadequate health resources; inadequate psychosocial support system; inadequate rewards; inadequate role models; inadequate role preparation; inadequate role socialization; inappropriate linkage with the health care system; low self-esteem; pain; role conflict; role confusion; role strain; stressors; substance misuse; unaddressed domestic violence; unrealistic role expectations

## At-Risk Population

Economically disadvantaged individuals; individuals with developmental level inappropriate for role expectation; individuals with high demand job role; individuals with low educational level

## Associated Conditions

Depression; neurological defect; personality disorders; physical illness; psychosis

## Client Outcomes

Client Will (Specify Time Frame)

- Identify realistic perception of role
- State personal strengths
- Acknowledge problems contributing to inability to perform usual role
- Accept physical limitations regarding role responsibility and consider ways to change lifestyle to accomplish goals associated with role performance
- Demonstrate knowledge of appropriate behaviors associated with new or changed role

• = Independent          ▲ = Collaborative

- State knowledge of change in responsibility and new behaviors associated with new responsibility
- Verbalize acceptance of new responsibility

## Nursing Interventions

- Assess the client's level of resilience and implement nursing actions that increase client resilience and sense of coherence.
- Assess the effect of uncertainty on the client's role and provide support and education.
- Assess the client's social support system.
- Assess for the presence of shame related to current health situation.
- Assess for the characteristics of role stress.
- Assess male military members for gender role stressors with the Male Gender Role Stressor Inventory (MGRSI).
- Ask the client what they need to feel prepared for the tasks and demands of their role.
- Support the client's spirituality practices.
- Refer to the care plans for Readiness for Enhanced Family **Coping,** Readiness for Enhanced **Decision-Making,** Ineffective **Home** Maintenance Behaviors, Impaired **Parenting,** Risk for **Loneliness,** Readiness for Enhanced Community **Coping,** Readiness for Enhanced **Self-Care,** and Ineffective **Sexuality** Pattern.

### Pediatric

- ▲ Provide parents of disabled children with information about and referrals to educational and social resources available to assist their child.
- Provide parents with information about mindfulness-based interventions (MBIs) to enhance coping when the role change is associated with a critically and chronically ill child.

### Geriatric

- Assess older adults' choices regarding their care and enable them to live as they wish and receive the help they want by carefully listening to their stories.
- Assess older adults for a sense of competence in their daily life.
- Provide support and practice for older adults to use technology.
- Support the client's spiritual beliefs and activities and provide appropriate spiritual support persons.

### Multicultural

- Assess for the influence of cultural beliefs, norms, values, and expectations on the individual's role.
- Negotiate with the client regarding the aspects of their role that can be modified and still honor cultural beliefs.

• = Independent      ▲ = Collaborative

- Identify perceived barriers to family to use support groups or other service programs to assist with role changes.
- The preceding interventions may be adapted for home care use.

**Client/Family Teaching and Discharge Planning**

▲ Refer client to comprehensive services to assist with transition needs at discharge.
- Provide educational materials to family members on client behavior management plus caregiver stress-coping management.
- Help the client identify resources for assistance in caring for a disabled or aging parent (e.g., adult day care, nursing home placement).

# Sedentary Lifestyle

**Domain 1** Health promotion   **Class 1** Health awareness

## NANDA-I Definition

An acquired mode of behavior that is characterized by waking hour activities that require low energy expenditure.

## Defining Characteristics

Average daily physical activity is less than recommended for age and gender; chooses a daily routine lacking physical exercise; does not exercise during leisure time; expresses preference for low physical activity; performs majority of tasks in a reclining posture; performs majority of tasks in a sitting posture; physical deconditioning

## Related Factors

Conflict between cultural beliefs and health practices; decreased activity tolerance; difficulty adapting areas for physical activity; exceeds screen time recommendations for age; impaired physical mobility; inadequate interest in physical activity; inadequate knowledge of consequences of sedentarism; inadequate knowledge of health benefits associated with physical activity; inadequate motivation for physical activity; inadequate resources for physical activity; inadequate role models; inadequate social support; inadequate time management skills; inadequate training for physical exercise; low self-efficacy; low self-esteem; negative affect toward physical activity; pain; parenting practices that inhibit child's physical activity; perceived physical disability; perceived safety risk

## At-Risk Population

Adolescents; individuals aged ≥60 years; individuals living in urban areas; individuals living with a partner; individuals with high educational level;

• = Independent   ▲ = Collaborative

individuals with high socioeconomic status; individuals with significant time constraints; married individuals; women

## Client Outcomes

### Client Will (Specify Time Frame)

- Engage in purposeful moderate-intensity cardiorespiratory (aerobic) exercise for 30 to 60 minutes/day on 5 or more days per week for a total of 2 hours and 30 minutes (150 minutes) per week
- Increase exercise to 20 minutes/day (>150 minutes/week); light to moderate intensity exercise may be beneficial in deconditioned persons
- Increase pedometer step counts by 1000 steps per day every 2 weeks to reach a daily step count of at least 7000 steps per day, with a daily goal for most healthy adults of 10,000 steps per day
- Perform resistance exercises that involve all major muscle groups (legs, hips, back, chest, abdomen, shoulders, and arms) performed 2 to 3 days/week
- Perform flexibility exercise (stretching) for each of the major muscle-tendon groups 2 days/week for 10 to 60 seconds to improve joint range of motion; greatest gains occur with daily exercise
- Engage in neuromotor exercise 20 to 30 minutes/day including motor skills (e.g., balance, agility, coordination, and gait), proprioceptive exercise training, and multifaceted activities (e.g., Tai chi and yoga) to improve and maintain physical function and reduce falls in those at risk for falling (older persons)

## Nursing Interventions

- Assess the client with the American College of Sports Medicine (ACSM, 2018) guidelines for exercise preparticipation health screening before implementing physical activity interventions.
- Observe the client for sedentary behaviors such as prolonged sitting, physical inactivity, and prolonged sleep.
- Recommend the client enter an exercise program with an active person who supports exercise behavior (e.g., friend or exercise buddy).
- Recommend the client use a mobile fitness application for customizing, cueing, tracking, and analyzing an exercise program.
- Encourage prescriptive resistance exercise of each major muscle group (hips, thighs, legs, back, chest, shoulders, and abdomen) using a variety of exercise equipment.
- Encourage gradual progression of greater resistance, more repetitions per set, and/or increasing frequency.
- Encourage pregnant clients to engage in regular physical activity.
- ▲ Assess the client for depression and refer for counseling and follow-up as appropriate.

• = Independent        ▲ = Collaborative

**Multicultural**

- Assess for reasons why the client would be unable to participate in regular physical activity; address reasons and refer to resources as needed.
- Assess for clients' perceptions of the neighborhood they reside in.
- Encourage and support spiritual practices.
- Encourage participation in group physical activity programs.

**Pediatric**

- Assess the child's current activity status using the Pediatric Inactivity Triad (Faigenbaum et al, 2018).
- Assess parent's perceptions of children's screen time and active play.
- Children and adolescents should participate in 60 minutes (1 hour) or more of physical activity daily.
  - Aerobic: Sixty or more minutes a day should be either moderate-intensity or vigorous-intensity aerobic physical activity and should include vigorous-intensity physical activity at least 3 days a week.
  - Muscle-strengthening: As part of daily physical activity, children and adolescents should include muscle-strengthening physical activity on at least 3 days of the week.
  - Bone-strengthening: As part of daily physical activity, children and adolescents should include bone-strengthening physical activity on at least 3 days of the week.
  - Providing activities that are age appropriate, are enjoyable, and offer variety will encourage young people to participate in physical activities (U.S. Department of Health and Human Services, 2018).
- Assist families to develop family-based interventions to increase child physical activity.
- Encourage parents and caregivers to adhere to the following American Academy of Pediatrics guidelines for children's media use (Chassiakos et al, 2016):
  - For children younger than 18 months, avoid use of screen media other than video-chatting.
  - Parents of children 18 to 24 months of age who want to introduce digital media should choose high-quality programming and watch it with their children to help them understand what they are seeing.
  - For children ages 2 to 5 years, limit screen use to 1 hour/day of high-quality programs. Parents should co-view media with children to help them understand what they are seeing and apply it to the world around them.
  - For children ages 6 and older, place consistent limits on the time

**S**

spent using media, and the types of media, and make sure media does not take the place of adequate sleep, physical activity, and other behaviors essential to health.

○ Designate media-free times together, such as dinner or driving, and media-free locations at home, such as bedrooms.

○ Have ongoing communication about online citizenship and safety, including treating others with respect online and off-line.

○ Encourage parents and caregivers to create their personalized family media plan (see https://www.healthychildren.org/English/media/Pages/default.aspx) (American Academy of Pediatrics, 2021).

**Geriatric**

• Use valid and reliable criterion-referenced standards for fitness testing (e.g., Senior Fitness Test) designed for older adults that can predict the level of capacity associated with maintaining physical independence into later years of life (e.g., get up and go test).

• Recommend the client begin a regular exercise program, even if generally active.

• Implement progressive resistance training plus balance exercise for older adults as indicated.

• Before surgery, refer clients to a personalized "prehabilitation" program that includes a warm-up followed by aerobic, strength, flexibility, neuromotor, and functional task work.

**Home Care**

• The preceding interventions may be adapted for home care use.

▲ Assess home environment for factors that create barriers to mobility. Refer to physical and occupational therapy services if needed to assist the client in restructuring home environment and daily living patterns.

**Client/Family Teaching and Discharge Planning**

• Provide teaching to clients and family to increase awareness of the health benefits of reducing sedentary behavior.

• Consider using motivational interviewing techniques when working with both children and adult clients to increase their activity.

# Readiness for Enhanced Self-Care

**Domain 4** Activity/rest   **Class 5** Self-care

**NANDA-I Definition**

A pattern of performing activities for oneself to meet health-related goals, which can be strengthened.

• = Independent         ▲ = Collaborative

## Defining Characteristics

Expresses desire to enhance independence with health; expresses desire to enhance independence with life; expresses desire to enhance independence with personal development; expresses desire to enhance independence with well-being; expresses desire to enhance knowledge of self-care strategies; expresses desire to enhance self-care

## Client Outcomes

### Client Will (Specify Time Frame)

- Evaluate current levels of self-care as optimum for abilities
- Express the need or desire to continue to enhance levels of self-care
- Seek health-related information as needed
- Identify strategies to enhance self-care
- Perform appropriate interventions as needed
- Monitor level of self-care
- Evaluate the effectiveness of self-care interventions at regular intervals

## Nursing Interventions

- For assessment of self-care, use a valid and reliable screening tool if available for specific characteristics of the person, such as arthritis, diabetes, stroke, heart failure (HF), or dementia.
- Support the person's awareness that enhanced self-care is an achievable, desirable, and positive life goal.
- Show respect for the person, regardless of characteristics and/or background.
- Promote trust and enhanced communication between the person and health care providers.
- Promote opportunities for spiritual care and growth.
- Promote social support through facilitation of family involvement.
- Provide opportunities for ongoing group support through establishment of self-help groups on the Internet.
- Help the person identify and reduce the barriers to self-care.
- Provide literacy-appropriate education for self-care activities.
- Facilitate self-efficacy by ensuring the adequacy of self-care education.
- Provide alternative mind–body therapies such as reiki, guided imagery, yoga, and self-hypnosis.
- Promote the person's hope to maintain self-care.

### Pediatric

- Assess and evaluate a child's level of self-care and adjust strategies as needed.
- Assist families to engage in and maintain social support networks.

• = Independent         ▲ = Collaborative

- Encourage activities that support or enhance spiritual care.

**Multicultural**

- Identify cultural beliefs, values, lifestyle practices, and problem-solving strategies when assessing the client's level of self-care.
- Recognize the effect of culture on SCBs.
- Provide culturally competent care.
- Support independent self-care activities.

**Home Care**

- The nursing interventions described previously may also be used in home care settings. Provide clients with information about digital resources and health applications.
- Assist individuals and families to identify self-care activities for prevention of exacerbations of chronic illness symptoms to avoid rehospitalization.
- Use educational guidelines for stroke survivors.
- Ensure appropriate multiprofessional communication to support client safety.
- For public safety, health care professionals and consumers should participate in decision-making when managing reflux-related symptoms in the self-care setting.
- Enhance individual and family coping with chronic illnesses.
- Encourage participation in a community care management program.

**Client/Family Teaching and Discharge Planning**

- Teach clients how to regularly assess their level of self-care.
- Instruct clients that a variety of interventions may be needed to enhance self-care.
- Help clients to understand that enhanced self-care is an achievable goal.
- Empower clients.
- Teach clients about the decision-making process and self-care activities needed to manage their illness state and promote well-being.
- Continuously stress that all self-care activities must be regularly evaluated to ensure that enhanced levels of self-care can be maintained.

# Bathing Self-Care Deficit

**Domain 4** Activity/rest    **Class 5** Self-care

**NANDA-I Definition**

Inability to independently complete cleansing activities.

• = Independent        ▲ = Collaborative

## Defining Characteristics

Difficulty accessing bathroom; difficulty accessing water; difficulty drying body; difficulty gathering bathing supplies; difficulty regulating bath water; difficulty washing body

## Related Factors

Anxiety; decreased motivation; environmental constraints; impaired physical mobility; neurobehavioral manifestations; pain; weakness

## At-Risk Population

Older adults

## Associated Conditions

Impaired ability to perceive body part; impaired ability to perceive spatial relationships; musculoskeletal diseases; neuromuscular diseases

## Client Outcomes

### Client Will (Specify Time Frame)

- Remain free of body odor and maintain intact skin
- State satisfaction with ability to use adaptive devices to bathe
- Maintain independency with bathing and hygiene
- Use methods to bathe safely and effectively with minimal difficulty
- Bathe with assistance of caregiver as needed and report satisfaction and dignity maintained during bathing experience
- Bathe with assistance of caregiver as needed without exhibiting defensive (aggressive) behaviors

## Nursing Interventions

- Ask clients about their bathing preferences, which can increase client privacy and satisfaction.
- Adjust room temperature above 20°C (68°F) and avoid hot water bathing, especially during cold seasons.
- Bathe critically ill clients or clients outside of critical care who have a central venous access device with a nonrinse chlorhexidine-impregnated wipe or chlorhexidine solution with rinsing.
- Avoid using a bath basin for bathing to avoid client exposure to multidrug-resistant pathogens from contaminated bath basins or hospital water supply.
- If a bath basin is used, use chlorhexidine gluconate solution for client bathing.
- Consider using a prepackaged bath for immobile clients who cannot shower.
- Avoid using high pressure during wiping. Monitor the client's skin and ask for feedback regarding sensation.
- Consider bathing for terminally ill cancer clients who have pain and anxiety to promote comfort.

• = Independent      ▲ = Collaborative

- Consider using music intervention in clients who have pain during bathing.
- Use person-centered bathing approach: plan for client's comfort and bathing preferences, show respect in communications by listening, critically think to solve issues that arise, and use a gentle approach.
▲ Provide pain relief measures, such as ice packs, heat, and analgesics for sore joints, 45 minutes before bathing; move extremities slowly and carefully; and inform the client before movements associated with pain occur (walking; transferring to a new location; moving joints; and washing genitals, face, and between toes and under arms). Have the client wash painful areas; recognize indicators of pain and apologize for any pain caused.
▲ Use a comfortable padded shower chair with foot support or adapt a chair: pad it with towels/washcloths, cover the cold back with dry towels, and cover the arms with foam pipe insulation.
- Ensure that bathing assistance preserves client dignity through use of privacy with a traffic-free bathing area and posted privacy signs, timeliness of personal care, and encourage client participation and involvement in the delivery of care.
- For cognitively impaired clients, avoid upsetting factors associated with bathing: instead of using the terms *bath, shower,* or *wash,* use comforting words, such as *warm, relaxing,* or *massage.* Start at the client's feet and bathe upward; bathe the face last after washing hands and using a clean cloth. Use a beautician/barber or wash hair at another time to avoid water dripping in the face.
- Use towel bathing to bathe client in bed, a bath blanket, and warm towels to keep the client covered the entire time. Warm and moisten towels/washcloths and place in plastic bags to keep them warm. Use the towels to massage large areas (front, back) and one washcloth for facial areas and another one for genital areas. No rinsing or drying is needed, as is commonly thought for bathing.
- For shower bathing use person-centered techniques, keep client covered with towels and cleanse under the towels, use no-rinse products, use favorite bathing items, and use a handheld shower with adjustable spray.
- Provide nighttime bathing or showering or a warm foot bath 1 to 2 hours before bedtime for at least 10 minutes to improve sleep.
▲ Request referral of client who has had a stroke to rehabilitation services.

**Geriatric**
▲ Advocate for the use of the Bathing Without a Battle educational program for clients with dementia.

• = Independent          ▲ = Collaborative

- Arrange the bathing environment to promote sensory comfort. Reduce noise of voices and water. Do not allow traffic into bathing room. Add fabric to absorb sound (three to four times the width of the opening for sound-absorbing folds). Play soft music.
- Design the bathing environment for comfort and safety. Use grab bars with nonslip grip and bathmats. Ensure that flooring is not slippery.
- Use music during shower for clients with dementia.
- Train caregivers bathing clients with dementia to avoid behaviors that can trigger assault: confrontational communication, invalidation of the resident's feelings, failure to prepare a resident for a task, initiating shower spray or touch during bathing without verbal prompts beforehand, washing the hair and face, speaking disrespectfully to the client, and hurrying the pace of the bath.
- Focus on the abilities of the client with dementia to obtain client's participation in bathing.

**Multicultural**

- Ask the client for input on bathing habits and cultural bathing preferences.

**Home Care**

- An individualized home-based caregiver training program can improve caregiver skills and competence with managing behavior issues with dementia clients during bathing.
- Provide home occupational therapy targeting self-bathing and environmental modifications for clients with bathing disabilities.
- Turn down temperature of water heater and recommend use of a water temperature-sensing shower valve to prevent scalding.
- Remove physical barriers in the home to maximize the client's ability to function independently and safely while bathing.

**Client/Family Teaching and Discharge Planning**

- Provide client/family education regarding chlorhexidine bathing for the reduction of common hospital-acquired infections.

## Dressing Self-Care Deficit

**Domain 4** Activity/Rest   **Class 5** Self-Care

**NANDA-I Definition**

Inability to independently put on or remove clothing.

**Defining Characteristics**

Difficulty choosing clothing; difficulty fastening clothing; difficulty gathering clothing; difficulty maintaining appearance; difficulty picking up clothing; difficulty putting clothing on lower body; difficulty putting clothing on upper body; difficulty putting on various items of clothing; difficulty removing clothing item; difficulty using assistive device; difficulty using zipper

## Related Factors

Anxiety; decreased motivation; discomfort; environmental constraints; fatigue; neurobehavioral manifestations; pain; weakness

## Associated Conditions

Musculoskeletal impairment; neuromuscular diseases

## Client Outcomes

### Client Will (Specify Time Frame)

- Dress and groom self to optimal potential
- Use assistive technology to dress and groom
- Explain and use methods to enhance strengths during dressing and grooming
- Dress and groom with assistance of caregiver as needed

## Nursing Interventions

▲ Assess independence in dressing and bathing skills after rehabilitation to determine the need for follow-up care.

▲ Assess the motor impairment and balance of all clients after stroke.

▲ Routinely assess functional impairment and report functional changes to the health care provider for hospitalized clients with advanced cancer.

▲ Refer clients with rehabilitation needs to physical and occupational therapy for functional rehabilitation with ADLs.

• For clients with spinal cord injury, encourage their self-efficacy and involve them in decision-making.

• Use adaptive dressing and grooming equipment as needed (e.g., button hooks, dressing stick, elastic shoelaces, long-handled shoehorn, reacher, sock application devices, Velcro clothing and shoes, zipper pull, long-handled brushes, soap-on-a-rope, suction holders). Use of adaptive clothing and devices for dressing and grooming can improve self-care ability and promote independence.

• Provide client analgesics before dressing as needed, sufficient time for dressing, and assist as needed. Analgesics, adequate time, and assistance if tiring can promote independence in dressing.

▲ For clients who are wheelchair dependent, consider the use of functional adaptive clothing.

## Geriatric

▲ Gather information on the client's personal clothing style and allow the client freedom to choose from a few selected outfits.

• = Independent          ▲ = Collaborative

▲ When dressing dementia clients, give short verbal instructions, provide encouragement, and provide positive reinforcement. Use gentle physical prompting when needed, never debate, and never argue.

▲ Provide training to nursing home direct care staff regarding how to assist dementia clients with dressing that maintains dignity and respect of choice.

**Multicultural**

• Consider use of assistive technology versus personal care assistance for Native Americans.

• Consider cultural differences in clothing choices for Latino/Hispanic clients and respect dressing norms.

**Home Care**

• Ensure the client is dressing in a safe area. The bathroom may increase risk for falls during dressing.

• Consider home occupational therapy for elderly frail clients living at home.

**Client/Family Teaching and Discharge Planning**

• Include caregiver's perceptions of client rehabilitation needs after stroke.

• Provide family caregiver training for assisting the client with dressing.

# Feeding Self-Care Deficit

**S**

**Domain 4** Activity/rest    **Class 5** Self-care

## NANDA-I Definition

Inability to eat independently.

## Defining Characteristics

Difficulty bringing food to mouth; difficulty chewing food; difficulty getting food onto utensils; difficulty handling utensils; difficulty manipulating food in mouth; difficulty opening containers, difficulty picking up cup, difficulty preparing food; difficulty self-feeding a complete meal; difficulty self-feeding in an acceptable manner; difficulty swallowing food; difficulty swallowing sufficient amount of food; difficulty using assistive device

## Related Factors

Anxiety; decreased motivation; discomfort; environmental constraints; fatigue; neurobehavioral manifestations; pain; weakness

## Associated Conditions

Musculoskeletal impairment; neuromuscular diseases

## Client Outcomes

**Client Will (Specify Time Frame)**

• Feed self safely and effectively

• = Independent          ▲ = Collaborative

- State satisfaction with ability to use adaptive devices for feeding
- Use assistance with feeding when necessary (caregiver)
- Maintain adequate nutritional intake

## Nursing Interventions

▲ Screen for oropharyngeal dysphagia and malnutrition in elderly and high-risk hospitalized clients.

▲ The Eating Assessment Tool-10 (EAT-10) may be used to screen for dysphagia.

▲ For critical care clients who receive prolonged endotracheal intubation (>48 hours), assess swallowing using a valid tool to avoid aspiration related to dysphagia.

▲ A formalized screening for dysphagia should be done in all stroke clients before any oral intake using the 3-ounce water swallow test by a trained clinician.

▲ The Edinburgh Feeding Evaluation in Dementia can be used to determine the presence of behaviors that lead to feeding or eating problems in late-stage dementia clients.

▲ Assess for fatigue, sedating medications, and frailty before meals. Supervision and eating assistance may be required to avoid aspiration.

▲ Individualize the feeding process to promote interdependence, especially for younger adults who need feeding assistance.

▲ Consider consultation with a speech and language pathologist for clients with dysphagia for diet modifications and swallowing exercise therapy.

▲ Assess the ability to self-feed and communicate which clients require feeding assistance to decrease missed meals and allow for adequate nutrition.

▲ Conduct repeat structured observations of clients at mealtime after a stroke to detect clients with eating difficulties to prevent possible social and functional consequences.

▲ Prioritize assisted feeding as important in a caregiver's assignment to allow adequate time for the client to eat.

▲ Consider using adaptive eating devices for clients with an upper limb motor impairment to assist with eating independently.

▲ Ensure oral care is provided to all clients using an American Dental Association–approved toothbrush and toothpaste after meals and at bedtime. Increase oral care frequency for clients who are on nothing-by-mouth (NPO) status.

## Geriatric

▲ Assess for absent teeth and ill-fitting dentures in older clients before feeding.

• = Independent          ▲ = Collaborative

▲ Establish a routine during mealtime and create a controlled stimulated environment with adequate lighting that simulates a home-like dining experience.

▲ Supervise the feeding of those with moderate dependency and provide physical assistance when needed.

▲ When eating assistance is needed, (1) position clients in an upright position; (2) do not provide too much food at one time (approximately $3/4$ spoonful); and (3) offer food slowly, allowing the food to be chewed completely. For visually impaired clients, press the food to the client's lips and provide encouragement.

▲ Consider implementing Montessori interventions for dementia clients who have eating problems, such as playing music for sensory stimulation and employing hand-eye coordination, scooping, pouring, and squeezing activities.

▲ Limit activities and avoid noise and interruptions during mealtimes.

▲ Use high-calorie oral nutritional supplements for clients with advanced dementia who cannot meet their nutrition requirements by food alone.

▲ Provide nutritional supplement drinks in a glass to older adults with cognitive impairment.

• Provide verbal cues and encouragement during mealtimes.

▲ Avoid changes or modifications to mealtime routines.

▲ Encourage family members to assist clients during mealtime for those who need eating assistance.

▲ Play familiar soothing music during meals for clients with dementia.

▲ Provide feeding training and education programs for caregivers.

**Multicultural**

▲ For those with impaired hand function who use chopsticks, suggest adapted chopsticks.

▲ Use the simplified Chinese Edinburgh Feeding Evaluation in Dementia scale to measure feeding problems in people with dementia from Mainland China and other Chinese cultural groups.

▲ The culturally adaptive Spanish version of the Edinburgh Feeding Evaluation in Dementia Scale is valid for measuring feeding difficulties in Spanish-speaking dementia clients.

**Home Care**

▲ For elderly home care clients with chronic diseases, assess nutritional status and chewing/swallowing ability.

▲ Provide multiprofessional nutritional support for home care clients by involving physical therapy, occupational therapy, and dietitians.

• = Independent          ▲ = Collaborative

S

**Client/Family Teaching and Discharge Planning**

▲ Educate family caregivers who are involved in the feeding of a family member by providing demonstration and hands-on training by a qualified trainer.

▲ Educate family members that neither insertion of a feeding tube nor timing of its insertion affects client survival for those with advanced dementia who have eating problems.

# Toileting Self-Care Deficit

**Domain 4** Activity/rest    **Class 5** Self-care

## NANDA-I Definition

Inability to independently perform tasks associated with bowel and bladder elimination.

## Defining Characteristics

Difficulty completing toilet hygiene; difficulty flushing toilet; difficulty manipulating clothing for toileting; difficulty reaching toilet; difficulty rising from toilet; difficulty sitting on toilet

## Related Factors

Anxiety; decreased motivation; environmental constraints; fatigue; impaired physical mobility; impaired transfer ability; neurobehavioral manifestation; pain; weakness

## Associated Conditions

Musculoskeletal impairment; neuromuscular diseases

## Client Outcomes

**Client Will (Specify Time Frame)**

• Remain free of incontinence and impaction with no urine or stool on skin

• State satisfaction with ability to use adaptive devices for toileting

• Explain and demonstrate use of methods to be safe and independent in toileting

## Nursing Interventions

• Assess clients for fall risk using established and valid fall risk assessment tools and implement fall prevention interventions for those at risk for falling.

• Implement purposeful hourly or 2-hourly rounding that targets toileting needs of the client.

• Perform a bladder scan for postvoid residual in neurological clients who are at high risk for neurogenic bladder and urinary retention.

• Use disposable underpads versus reusable washable underpads for hospitalized adult clients with urine or fecal incontinence.

• = Independent        ▲ = Collaborative

- In the acute care setting, use absorbent pads left open under the client for fecal and urine incontinence.
- Consider use of external urinary collection devices and avoid use of an indwelling urinary catheter for the purpose of incontinence.
- Perform intermittent straight catheterization for clients who are unable to empty their bladder and have urinary retention.
- Ensure a timely planned evacuation of bowel for spinal cord injury clients by implementing a low-fiber diet and digital stimulation.
- Assess bowel symptoms and self-management strategies of clients who have had sphincter-saving surgery. Develop client-specific interventions to continue to support and meet client needs.
- Consider use of a female urinal for female cancer clients who are receiving palliative care.
▲ Before use of a bedpan, discuss its use with clients.
- Promote use of assistive toileting equipment when needed for toileting transfer assistance.
- Avoid prolonged time sitting on a toilet, commode, or bedpan to reduce pressure-related skin injury risk. Use padded toilet cushions if needed.
- Consider use of toilet alarm systems for clients who are at risk for falling and not cognitively impaired.
- Close toilet lid before flushing toilet and teach client to do so.

**Geriatric**
- Assess residents without dementia for risk factors associated with toileting disability (such as rating health as fair or poor; living in a residence with four or less residents or that is for-profit; incontinence; physical, visual, or hearing impairment; and need for ADL or transferring assistance to guide prevention interventions).
- Promote a toileting pattern using timed voiding and verbal prompts to develop habits and promote continence in dementia clients.
- Assess the client's functional ability to manipulate clothing for toileting, and if necessary, modify clothing with Velcro fasteners, elastic waists, drop-front underwear, or slacks.
- Consider an exercise training of routine walking and pelvic floor exercises for frail incontinent women.

**Multicultural**
- Remove barriers to toileting, support client's cultural beliefs, and protect dignity during continence care.

**Home Care**
▲ Instruct client/family member or caregiver to develop a bladder diary to obtain a better understanding of incontinent patterns.

• = Independent          ▲ = Collaborative

▲ Involve the client's caregiver in developing a written plan for managing incontinence in dementia clients.

▲ Consider consultation with occupational therapy to evaluate home bathroom design, to evaluate assistive device needs, and to provide training for proper body mechanics for home caregivers.

• Consider the use of technology-assisted toilets with perineal washing ability.

**Client/Family Teaching and Discharge Planning**

• Instruct clients with mixed (stress and urge) urinary incontinence to perform pelvic floor exercises for at least 3 months and increase walking to build muscle strength.

• Instruct female clients not to use sanitary pads for urinary incontinence.

• Explain to family and caregivers of clients with dementia that toilet self-care activities decrease when self-awareness is lost.

• Educate male clients who perform self-straight catheterization on use of the coude tip catheter to avoid difficulties with insertion.

# Readiness for Enhanced Self-Concept

**Domain 6** Self-perception    **Class 1** Self-concept

**NANDA-I Definition**

A pattern of perceptions or ideas about the self, which can be strengthened.

**Defining Characteristics**

Expresses desire to enhance acceptance of limitations; expresses desire to enhance acceptance of strengths; expresses desire to enhance body image satisfaction; expresses desire to enhance confidence in abilities; expresses desire to enhance congruence between actions and words; expresses desire to enhance role performance; expresses desire to enhance satisfaction with personal identity; expresses desire to enhance satisfaction with sense of worth; expresses desire to enhance self-esteem

**Client Outcomes**

**Client Will (Specify Time Frame)**

• State willingness to enhance self-concept

• State satisfaction with thoughts about self, sense of worthiness, role performance, body image, and personal identity

• Demonstrate actions that are congruent with expressed feelings and thoughts

• State confidence in abilities

• Accept strengths and limitations

• = Independent          ▲ = Collaborative

## Nursing Interventions

- Encourage client to express feelings through songwriting.
- Refer to nutritional and exercise programs to support weight loss.
- Offer client complementary and alternative medicine (CAM) interventions such as acupressure, aromatherapy, compress, and massage.
- Support homeless individuals to identify and endorse a positive self-concept.
- Support unemployed individuals to cope with identity threats and support individual identity growth.
- Support establishing community-based partnerships to address health needs.
- For clients with a history of trauma, offer a mindfulness-based intervention of hatha yoga.

### Pediatric

- Facilitate healthy relationships with teachers, coaches, and other supportive adults in the adolescents' lives.
- Provide parents with information designed to promote body satisfaction, healthy eating, and weight management in early childhood.
- Promote the adoption of a recovery identity through online interactions and support groups for individuals with eating disorders.
- Provide activities to bolster physical self-concept.
- ▲ Provide overweight adolescents access to group-based weight control interventions.
- Provide an alternative school-based program for pregnant and parenting adolescents.

### Geriatric

- Encourage clients to consider online support programs when they are in a caregiving situation.
- Encourage activity and a strength, mobility, balance, and endurance training program.
- Support meaning and purpose in the lives of older adults through a focus on everyday well-being and facilitation of personally treasured activities.
- Use an approach that reduces the emphasis put on ageist self-concept attributions when working with older clients.

### Multicultural

- Refer to the care plans Disturbed **Body Image,** Readiness for Enhanced **Coping,** Chronic Low **Self-Esteem,** and Readiness for Enhanced **Spiritual** Well-Being.

• = Independent          ▲ = Collaborative

Home Care
- Previously discussed interventions may be used in the home care setting.

# Chronic Low Self-Esteem

**Domain 6** Self-perception    **Class 2** Self-esteem
## NANDA-I Definition

Long-standing negative perception of self-worth, self-acceptance, self-respect, competence, and attitude toward self.

## Defining Characteristics

Dependent on others' opinions; depressive symptoms; excessive guilt; excessive seeking of reassurance; expresses loneliness; hopelessness; insomnia; loneliness; nonassertive behavior; overly conforming behaviors; reduced eye contact; rejects positive feedback; reports repeated failures; rumination; self-negating verbalizations; shame; suicidal ideation; underestimates ability to deal with situation

## Related Factors

Decreased mindful acceptance; difficulty managing finances; disturbed body image; fatigue; fear of rejection; impaired religiosity; inadequate affection received; inadequate attachment behavior; inadequate family cohesiveness; inadequate group membership; inadequate respect from others; inadequate sense of belonging; inadequate social support; ineffective communication skills; insufficient approval from others; low self efficacy; maladaptive grieving; negative resignation; repeated negative reinforcement; spiritual incongruence; stigmatization; stressors; values incongruent with cultural norms

## At-Risk Population

Economically disadvantaged individuals; individuals experiencing repeated failure; individuals exposed to traumatic situation; individuals with difficult developmental transition; individuals with history of being abandoned; individuals with history of being abused; individuals with history of being neglected; individuals with history of loss

## Associated Conditions

Depression; functional impairment; mental disorders; physical illness

## Client Outcomes

Client Will (Specify Time Frame)
- Demonstrate improved ability to interact with others (e.g., maintains eye contact, engages in conversation, expresses thoughts/feelings)
- Verbalize increased self-acceptance through positive self-statements about self

• = Independent            ▲ = Collaborative

- Identify personal strengths, accomplishments, and values
- Identify and work on small, achievable goals
- Improve independent decision-making and problem-solving skills

## Nursing Interventions

- Assess existing strengths and coping abilities, and provide opportunities for their expression and recognition.
- Assess the client's self-esteem using valid and established tools such as the Rosenberg Self-Esteem Scale.
- Assess the client for addictive use of social media.
- Reinforce the personal strengths and positive self-perceptions that a client identifies.
- Encourage self-affirmations by reflecting on values and strengths, in response to daily threats.
- Identify client's negative self-assessments.
- Assess individuals with low self-esteem for nonsuicidal self-injury (NSSI).
- Assess individuals with low self-esteem for symptoms of depression.
- Encourage realistic and achievable goal setting and resources and identify impediments to achievement.
- Assist client in challenging negative perceptions of self and performance.
- Encourage the client's usual religious or spiritual practices.
- Promote maintaining a level of functioning in the community and a sense of community feeling.

### Pediatric

- Assess children/adolescents with chronic illness for evidence of reduced self-esteem and make needed referrals.
- Encourage parents to use active listening to foster respectful relationships with children and adolescents.
- Monitor young adolescents during the transition to middle school for changes in self-concept.
- Encourage mothers of premature infants to use skin-to-skin care for at least 30 minutes/day.
- Implement interventions that promote and maintain positive peer relations for adolescent clients.
- Encourage attendance at social support groups.
- Encourage parents to praise children in ways that are not overly positive or inflated.
- Provide parents with information designed to promote body satisfaction, healthy eating, and weight management in early childhood.

• = Independent          ▲ = Collaborative

- Assess children/adolescents that express a body image of self-perceived underweight, self-perceived overweight, and/or frustration with appearance for evidence of bullying.
▲ Provide bully prevention programs and include information on cyberbullying.

**Geriatric**
- Support client in identifying and adapting to functional changes.
- Implement reminiscence therapy.
- Encourage older adult clients to participate in flexibility, toning, and balance exercise.
- Encourage regular physical activity with prerecorded workouts.
- Encourage participation in intergenerational social activities.
- Encourage activities in which a client can volunteer to support/help others.
- Encourage home and community gardening activities.

**Multicultural**
- Assess for the influence of cultural beliefs, norms, and values on the client's sense of self-esteem.
- Assess individuals with low self-esteem for symptoms of depression.
- Validate the client's feelings regarding ethnic or racial identity.

**Home Care**
- Assess a client's immediate support system/family for relationship patterns and content of communication.
▲ Refer to continuous support and help from medical social services to assist the family in care of the client and support the caregiver's well-being.
▲ If a client is involved in counseling or self-help groups, monitor and encourage attendance. Help the client identify the value of group participation after each group encounter. Discussion about group participation clarifies and reinforces group feedback and support.

**Client/Family Teaching and Discharge Planning**
- Encourage clients to consider online support programs when they are in a caregiving situation.
▲ Refer to community agencies for psychotherapeutic counseling.

## Situational Low Self-Esteem

**Domain 6** Self-perception   **Class 2** Self-esteem
**NANDA-I Definition**

Change from positive to negative perception of self-worth, self-acceptance, self-respect, competence, and attitude toward self in response to a current situation.

• = Independent          ▲ = Collaborative

## Defining Characteristics

Depressive symptoms; expresses loneliness; helplessness; indecisive behavior; insomnia; loneliness; nonassertive behavior; purposelessness; rumination; self-negating verbalizations; underestimates ability to deal with situation

## Related Factors

Behavior incongruent with values; decrease in environmental control; decreased mindful acceptance; difficulty accepting alteration in social role; difficulty managing finances; disturbed body image; fatigue; fear of rejection; impaired religiosity inadequate attachment behavior; inadequate family cohesiveness; inadequate respect from others; inadequate social support; ineffective communication skills; low self efficacy; maladaptive perfectionism; negative resignation; powerlessness; stigmatization; stressors; unrealistic self-expectations; values incongruent with cultural norms

## At-Risk Population

Individuals experiencing a change in living environment; individuals experiencing alteration in body image; individuals experiencing alteration in economic status; individuals experiencing alteration in role function; individuals experiencing death of a significant other; individuals experiencing divorce; individuals experiencing new additions to the family; individuals experiencing repeated failure; individuals experiencing unplanned pregnancy; individuals with difficult developmental transition; individuals with history of being abandoned; individuals with history of being abused; individuals with history of being neglected; individuals with history of loss; individuals with history of rejection

## Associated Conditions

Depression; functional impairment; mental disorders; physical illness

## Client Outcomes

### Client Will (Specify Time Frame)

- State effect of life events on feelings about self
- State personal strengths
- Acknowledge presence of guilt and not blame self if an action was related to another person's appraisal
- Seek help when necessary
- Demonstrate self-perceptions are accurate given physical capabilities
- Demonstrate separation of self-perceptions from societal stigmas

## Nursing Interventions

▲ Assess the client for signs and symptoms of depression and potential for suicide and/or violence. If present, immediately notify the appropriate personnel of symptoms. See care plans for Risk for Other-Directed **Violence** and Risk for **Suicidal Behavior.**

• = Independent      ▲ = Collaborative

- Assess the client's environmental and everyday stressors, including evidence of abusive relationships.
- Assess the client's self-esteem using valid and established tools such as the Rosenberg Self-Esteem Scale.
- Encourage expressions of gratitude through a gratitude journal or kind acts.
- Use a cognitive approach such as problem-solving education (PSE) to assist in the identification of problems and situational factors that contribute to problems and offer options for resolution.
- Encourage self-affirmations by reflecting on values and strengths, in response to daily threats.
- Accept client's own pace in working through grief or crisis situations.
- Encourage the client to accept their own defenses, feelings, and urges in dealing with the crisis.
- Teach the client mindfulness techniques to cope more effectively with strong emotional responses.
- Encourage objective appraisal of self and life events and challenge negative or perfectionist expectations of self.
- Acknowledge the presence of societal stigma. Teach management tools.
- Validate the effect of negative past experiences on self-esteem and work on corrective measures.

**Pediatric, Geriatric, and Multicultural**
- See care plan for Chronic Low **Self-Esteem**.

**Home Care**
- Establish an emergency plan and contract with the client for its use. Having an emergency plan is reassuring to the client. Establishing a contract validates the worth of the client and provides a caring link between the client and society.
- Access supplies that support a client's success at independent living.
- See care plan for Chronic Low **Self-Esteem**.

**Client/Family Teaching and Discharge Planning**
- Previously discussed interventions may be used in the home care setting.
▲ Refer to appropriate community resources or crisis intervention centers.
▲ Refer to resources for handicap and/or disability services.
- See care plan for Chronic Low **Self-Esteem**.

• = Independent       ▲ = Collaborative

# Risk for Chronic Low Self-Esteem

**Domain 6** Self-perception   **Class 2** Self-esteem

## NANDA-I Definition

Susceptible to long-standing negative perception of self-worth, self-acceptance, self-respect, competence, and attitude toward self, which may compromise health.

## Risk Factors

Decreased mindful acceptance; difficulty managing finances; disturbed body image; fatigue; fear of rejection; impaired religiosity; inadequate affection received; inadequate attachment behavior; inadequate family cohesiveness; inadequate group membership; inadequate respect from others; inadequate sense of belonging; inadequate social support; ineffective communication skills; insufficient approval from others; low self-efficacy; maladaptive grieving; negative resignation; repeated negative reinforcement; spiritual incongruence; stigmatization; stressors; values incongruent with cultural norms

## At-Risk Population

Economically disadvantaged individuals; individuals experiencing repeated failure; individuals exposed to traumatic situation; individuals with difficult developmental transition; individuals with history of being abandoned; individuals with history of being abused; individuals with history of being neglected; individuals with history of loss

## Associated Conditions

Depression; functional impairment; mental disorders; physical illness

## Client Outcomes and Nursing Interventions

Refer to care plan for Chronic Low **Self-Esteem.**

# Risk for Situational Low Self-Esteem

**Domain 6** Self-perception   **Class 2** Self-esteem

## NANDA-I Definition

Susceptible to change from positive to negative perception of self-worth, self-acceptance, self-respect, competence, and attitude toward self in response to a current situation, which may compromise health.

## Risk Factors

Behavior incongruent with values; decrease in environmental control; decreased mindful acceptance; difficulty accepting alteration in social role; difficulty managing finances; disturbed body image; fatigue; fear of rejection; impaired religiosity; inadequate attachment behavior; inadequate family cohesiveness; inadequate respect from others; inadequate social support; individuals experiencing repeated failure; ineffective communication skills; low self efficacy; maladaptive perfectionism; negative resignation; powerlessness; stigmatization; stressors; unrealistic self-expectations; values incongruent with cultural norms

## At-Risk Population

Individuals experiencing a change in living environment; individuals experiencing alteration in body image; individuals experiencing alteration in economic status; individuals experiencing alteration in role function; individuals experiencing death of a significant other; individuals experiencing divorce; individuals experiencing new additions to the family; individuals experiencing unplanned pregnancy; individuals with difficult developmental transition; individuals with history of being abandoned; individuals with history of being abused; individuals with history of being neglected; individuals with history of loss; individuals with history of rejection

## Associated Conditions

Depression; functional impairment; mental disorders; physical illness

## Client Outcomes

### Client Will (Specify Time Frame)

- State accurate self-appraisal
- Demonstrate the ability to self-validate
- Demonstrate the ability to make decisions independent of primary peer group
- Express effects of media on self-appraisal
- Express influence of substances on self-esteem
- Identify strengths and healthy coping skills
- State life events and change as influencing self-esteem

## Nursing Interventions

- Assist client to challenge negative perceptions of self and performance.
- Assess the client's self-esteem using valid and established tools such as the Rosenberg Self-Esteem Scale.
- Encourage client to maintain highest level of community functioning.
- Encourage self-affirmations by reflecting on values and strengths, in response to daily threats.
- Encourage realistic and achievable goal setting and resources and identify impediments to achievement.
- ▲ Assess the client for symptoms of depression and anxiety. Refer to specialist as needed. Prompt and effective treatment can prevent exacerbation of symptoms or safety risks.
- See care plans for Disturbed Personal **Identity,** Situational Low **Self-Esteem,** and Chronic Low **Self-Esteem.**

• = Independent        ▲ = Collaborative

## Pediatric

- Assess children/adolescents who are either a victim or an offender of cyberbullying for low self-esteem.
- Encourage attendance at social support groups.
- ▲ Encourage a combination of extracurricular activity for adolescents in a safe, supportive, and empowering environment.

## Geriatric

- Support humor as a coping mechanism.
- Support client in identifying and adapting to functional changes.
- Encourage participation in intergenerational social activities.
- Support meaning and purpose in the lives of older adults through a focus on everyday well-being and facilitation of personally treasured activities.
- Use an approach that reduces the emphasis put on ageist self-concept attributions when working with older clients.
- See care plans for Situational Low **Self-Esteem** and Chronic Low **Self-Esteem**.

## Home Care

- Previously discussed interventions may be used in the home care setting.
- See care plans for Situational Low **Self-Esteem** and Chronic Low **Self-Esteem**.

## Client/Family Teaching and Discharge Planning

- ▲ Refer the client to community agencies that offer support and environmental resources. Make referrals as needed.
- See care plans for Situational Low **Self-Esteem** and Chronic Low **Self-Esteem**.

**S**

# Self-Mutilation

**Domain 11** Safety/protection    **Class 3** Violence

## NANDA-I Definition

Deliberate self-injurious behavior causing tissue damage with the intent of causing nonfatal injury to attain relief of tension.

## Defining Characteristics

Abrading skin; biting; constricting a body part; cuts on body; hitting; ingested harmful substance; inhaled harmful substance; insertion of object into body orifice; picking at wound; scratches on body; self-inflicted burn; severing of a body part

## Related Factors

Absence of family confidant; altered body image; dissociation; disturbed interpersonal relations; eating disorder; excessive emotional disturbance;

• = Independent        ▲ = Collaborative

feeling threatened with loss of significant interpersonal relations; impaired self-esteem; inability to express tension verbally; ineffective communication between parent and adolescent; ineffective coping strategies; irresistible urge for self-directed violence; irresistible urge to cut self; labile behavior; loss of control over problem-solving situation; low self-esteem; mounting tension that is intolerable; negative feelings; pattern of inability to plan solutions; pattern of inability to see long term consequences; perfectionism; requires rapid stress reduction; social isolation; substance misuse; use of manipulation to obtain nurturing interpersonal relations with others

## At-Risk Population

Adolescents; battered children; incarcerated individuals; individuals experiencing family divorce; individuals experiencing family substance misuse; individuals experiencing loss of significant interpersonal relations; individuals experiencing sexual identity crisis; individuals living in nontraditional setting; individuals whose peers self-mutilate; individuals with family history of self-destructive behavior; individuals with history of childhood abuse; individuals with history of childhood illness; individuals with history of childhood surgery; individuals with history of self-directed violence; individuals witnessing violence between parental figures

## Associated Conditions

Autism; borderline personality disorder; character disorder; depersonalization; developmental disabilities; psychotic disorders

## Client Outcomes

### Client Will (Specify Time Frame)

- Have injuries treated
- Refrain from further self-injury
- State appropriate ways to cope with increased psychological or physiological tension
- Express feelings
- Seek help when having urges to self-mutilate
- Maintain self-control without supervision
- Use appropriate community agencies when caregivers are unable to attend to emotional needs

## Nursing Interventions

- Before implementing interventions for nonsuicidal self-injury (NSSI), nurses should examine their own knowledge base and emotional responses to incidents of self-harm.
- Assess clients with a diagnosis of borderline personality disorder or an eating disorder for NSSI.
- Assess veterans seeking treatment for posttraumatic stress disorder (PTSD) for NSSI behaviors.

• = Independent          ▲ = Collaborative

- A nonjudgmental approach to clients is critical.
- Consider using a measure of self-harm risk that is available for clients.
▲ Provide medical treatment for injuries. Use aseptic technique when caring for wounds. Care for the wounds in a matter-of-fact manner.
- Assess for risk of suicide or other self-damaging behaviors.
- Assess for the presence of hallucinations. Ask specific questions: "Do you hear voices that other people do not hear?" "Are they telling you to hurt yourself?"
- Monitor the client's behavior closely, using engagement and support as elements of safety checks while avoiding intrusive overstimulation.
- Focus on understanding the function that self-harm serves for the client and on managing the client's distress.
- Establish trust, listen to client, convey safety, and assist in developing positive goals for the future.
▲ Refer for Treatment for Self-Injurious Behaviors (T-SIB) therapy.

**Pediatric**
- Assess children and adolescents placed in psychiatric settings for NSSI.
- Assess adolescents with a diagnosis of borderline personality disorder or an eating disorder for NSSI.
- Assess children and adolescents for experiences of bullying or rejection by peers.
- Ask adolescent clients directly if they use social media to post communication about or share images of wounds related to self-injury.
▲ Refer adolescents who self-harm to cognitive behavioral therapy (CBT) treatments.
▲ Refer self-injuring students for psychological or psychiatric treatment. Treatment includes starting therapy and medications, increasing coping skills, facilitating decision-making, encouraging positive relationships, and fostering self-esteem.

**Home Care and Client/Family Teaching and Discharge Planning**
- Provide family teaching about NSSI and treatments.
▲ Refer family and client to outpatient family-focused cognitive behavioral treatment (F-CBT).
▲ Refer family and client to dialectical behavior therapy (DBT).

• = Independent ▲ = Collaborative

**S**

# Risk for Self-Mutilation

**Domain 11** Safety/protection    **Class 3** Violence
## NANDA-I Definition

Susceptible to deliberate self-injurious behavior causing tissue damage with the intent of causing nonfatal injury to attain relief of tension.
## Risk Factors

Absence of family confidant; altered body image; dissociation; disturbed interpersonal relations; eating disorder; excessive emotional disturbance; feeling threatened with loss of significant interpersonal relations; impaired self-esteem; inability to express tension verbally; ineffective communication between parent and adolescent; ineffective coping strategies; irresistible urge for self-directed violence; irresistible urge to cut self; labile behavior; loss of control over problem-solving situation; low self-esteem; mounting tension that is intolerable; negative feelings; pattern of inability to plan solutions; pattern of inability to see long-term consequences; perfectionism; requires rapid stress reduction; social isolation; substance misuse; use of manipulation to obtain nurturing interpersonal relations with others
## At-Risk Population

Adolescents; battered children; incarcerated individuals; individuals experiencing family divorce; individuals experiencing family substance misuse; individuals experiencing loss of significant interpersonal relations; individuals experiencing sexual identity crisis; individuals living in nontraditional setting; individuals whose peers self-mutilate; individuals with family history of self-destructive behavior; individuals with history of childhood abuse; individuals with history of childhood illness; individuals with history of childhood surgery; individuals with history of self-directed violence; individuals witnessing violence between parental figures
## Associated Conditions

Autism; borderline personality disorder; character disorder; depersonalization; developmental disabilities; psychotic disorders
## Client Outcomes, Nursing Interventions, and Client/Family Teaching

Refer to care plan for **Self-Mutilation.**

# Self-Neglect

**Domain 4** Activity/rest    **Class 5** Self-care
## NANDA-I Definition

A constellation of culturally framed behaviors involving one or more self-care activities in which there is a failure to maintain a socially accepted standard of health and well-being (Gibbons, Lauder, & Ludwick, 2006).

• = Independent      ▲ = Collaborative

## Defining Characteristics

Inadequate environmental hygiene; inadequate personal hygiene; nonadherence to health activity

## Related Factors

Fear of institutionalization; impaired executive function; inability to maintain control; lifestyle choice; neurobehavioral manifestations; stressors; substance misuse

## Associated Conditions

Capgras syndrome; frontal lobe dysfunction; functional impairment; learning disability; malingering; mental disorders; psychotic disorders

## Client Outcomes

### Client Will (Specify Time Frame)

- Reveal improvement in cognition (e.g., if reversible and treatable)
- Show improvement in mental health problems (e.g., depression)
- Show improvement in chronic medical problems
- Demonstrate improvement in functional status (e.g., basic and IADLs)
- Demonstrate adherence to health activities (e.g., medications and medical appointments)
- Exhibit improved personal hygiene
- Exhibit improved environmental hygiene
- Have fewer hospitalizations and emergency room visits
- Increase safety of client
- Increase safety of community in which client lives
- Agree to necessary personal and environmental changes that eliminate risk/endangerment to self or others (e.g., neighbors)
- Improve social networks and social engagement
- Identify eligibility for public services and other benefits

Note: Because self-neglect is present along a continuum of severity and includes an array of behavioral and environmental issues, a change in a client's status must occur in such a way that it balances obligation for protection and respects individual rights (e.g., autonomy and self-determination) while ensuring individual health and well-being. This is accomplished through a client–provider partnership that keeps the door open, even though the client may initially decline help. Building a relationship with the client will improve trust and assist in developing an individually tailored care plan to address problems contributing to self-neglect. Multiprofessional collaboration and teamwork, and in some instances assistance of next of kin and/or adult protective services (APS) may be needed (e.g., a state agency or local social services program).

• = Independent        ▲ = Collaborative

## Nursing Interventions

- Monitor individuals with acute or chronic mental and physical illness for defining characteristics for self-neglect.
- Assist individuals with complex mental and physical health issues to adopt positive health behaviors so that they may maintain their health status in the community.
- Assist individuals with reconnecting with family, friends, communities, and other social networks available.
- Assist individuals whose self-care is failing with managing their medication regimen.
- Assist persons with self-care deficits caused by impairments in activities of daily living (ADLs) or instrumental ADLs (IADLs).
- Assess persons with failing self-care for changes in cognitive function (e.g., dementia or delirium).
- ▲ Refer persons with failing self-care to appropriate specialists (e.g., psychologist, psychiatrist, social worker) and therapists (e.g., physical therapy, occupational therapy).
- ▲ Responding to clients with self-neglect requires that plan of care be person centered and outcome focused and clarify how real and potential risks will be addressed, by whom, and within what timeframe. Professional judgment and complexity of cases and situations can present an exceptionally fine line in making decisions and judgments.
- Use behavioral modification as appropriate (describing all options and consequences of refusing care or treatment) to bring about client changes that lead to improvement in personal hygiene, environmental hygiene, and adherence to medical regimen.
- Monitor persons with substance abuse disorders (i.e., drugs, alcohol, smoking) and depression for adequate health and safety.
- ▲ Refer persons with failing self-care who are significantly impaired cognitively (e.g., executive function, dementia) or functionally and/or who are suspected victims of abuse to APS.

## Geriatric

- ▲ Assess client's socioeconomic status and refer for appropriate support.
- ▲ Refer persons demonstrating a significant decline in self-care abilities (e.g., posing a threat to themselves or to their community) for formal evaluation of capacity and executive function.

## Multicultural

- Deliver health care that is sensitive to the culture and philosophy of individuals whose self-care appears inadequate.

• = Independent          ▲ = Collaborative

# Sexual Dysfunction

**Domain 8** Sexuality    **Class 2** Sexual function

## NANDA-I Definition

A state in which an individual experiences a change in sexual function during the sexual response phases of desire, arousal, and/or orgasm, which is viewed as unsatisfying, unrewarding, or inadequate.

## Defining Characteristics

Altered interest in others; altered self-interest; altered sexual activity; altered sexual excitation; altered sexual role; altered sexual satisfaction; decreased sexual desire; perceived sexual limitation; seeks confirmation of desirability; undesired alteration in sexual function

## Related Factors

Inaccurate information about sexual function; inadequate knowledge about sexual function; inadequate role models; insufficient privacy; perceived vulnerability; unaddressed abuse; value conflict

## At-Risk Population

Individuals without a significant other

## Associated Conditions

Altered body function; altered body structure

## Client Outcomes

**Client Will (Specify Time Frame)**

- Identify individual cause of sexual dysfunction
- Identify stressors that contribute to dysfunction
- Discuss alternative, satisfying, and acceptable sexual practices for self and partner
- Identify the degree of sexual interest by the client and partner
- Adapt sexual technique as needed to cope with sexual problems
- Discuss with partner concerns about body image and sex role

## Nursing Interventions

- Gather the client's sexual history, noting normal patterns of functioning and the client's vocabulary, and encouraging clients to ask questions or discuss sexual problems experienced.
- Gather a sexual history for transgender clients, including their view and importance of sexuality and the presence of coexisting sexual dysfunctions such as low desire, inability to achieve orgasm, disturbance in body image, or experiencing pain with sexual intercourse.
- ▲ Assess duration and risk factors for sexual dysfunction and explore potential causes such as medications, medical problems, aging process, or psychosocial issues.

• = Independent          ▲ = Collaborative

▲ Assess for history of sexual abuse.

▲ Assess and provide treatment for sexual dysfunction, involving the person's partner in the process, and evaluating pharmacological and nonpharmacological interventions.

• Assess risk factors for sexual dysfunction, especially with varying sexual partners.

• Observe for stress and anxiety as possible causes of dysfunction.

▲ Assess for depression as a possible cause of sexual dysfunction and institute appropriate treatment.

• Observe for grief-related loss (e.g., amputation, mastectomy, ostomy) because a change in body image often precedes sexual dysfunction. See care plan for Disturbed **Body** Image.

▲ Explore physical causes of sexual dysfunction such as diabetes, cardiovascular disease, arthritis, or BPH.

▲ Consider that ED may indicate the presence of cardiovascular disease, and screening and referral of men is recommended.

• Certain chronic diseases such as cancer often have significant effects on sexual function, and both the disease process and treatment can contribute to sexual dysfunction.

• Consider that neurological diseases can affect sexual function directly, with secondary effects caused by disability related to the illness and social and emotional effects.

• Explore behavioral or other causes of sexual dysfunction, such as smoking, dietary factors, or obesity.

▲ Consider medications as a cause of sexual dysfunction.

▲ Refer to appropriate medical providers for consideration of medication for premature ejaculation, ED, or orgasmic problems.

• Refer to the care plan Ineffective **Sexuality** Pattern for additional interventions.

**Geriatric**

▲ Carefully assess the sexuality needs and sexual dysfunction of older adults and refer for counseling if needed.

• Teach about normal changes that occur with aging that may be perceived as sexual dysfunction, such as reduction in vaginal lubrication and reduction in duration and resolution of orgasm for women; for men these changes include increased time required for erection and for subsequent erections, erection without ejaculation, less firm erection, and decreased volume of seminal fluid.

• If prescribed, instruct clients with chronic pain to take pain medication before sexual activity.

• See care plan for Ineffective **Sexuality** Pattern.

• = Independent            ▲ = Collaborative

**Multicultural**

- Evaluate culturally influenced risk factors for sexual function and dysfunction.
- Validate client feelings and emotions regarding the changes in sexual behavior by letting the client know that the nurse heard and understands what was said, promoting the nurse–client relationship.

**Home Care**

- Previously discussed interventions may be adapted for home care use.
- ▲ Identify specific sources of concern about sexual dysfunction and provide reassurance and instruction on appropriate expectations as indicated.
- ▲ Confirm that physical reasons for dysfunction have been addressed, and refer for therapy and/or support groups if appropriate.
- See care plan for Ineffective **Sexuality** Pattern.

**Client/Family Teaching and Discharge Planning**

- Provide accurate information for clients regarding interventions for sexual dysfunction.
- Include the partner/family in discharge instructions because partner concerns are often overlooked regarding sexual issues.
- Teach the client and partner about condom use, for those at risk.
- ▲ Refer to appropriate community resources, such as a clinical specialist, family counselor, or cardiac rehabilitation, including the partner if appropriate; for complex issues, a referral to a sex counselor, urologist, gynecologist, or other specialist may be needed.
- ▲ Refer for medical advice when ED lasts longer than 2 months or is recurring.
- Teach the following interventions to decrease the likelihood of ED: limit or avoid the use of alcohol, stop smoking, exercise regularly, reduce stress, get enough sleep, deal with anxiety or depression, and see a health care provider for regular checkups and medical screening tests.
- See care plan for Ineffective **Sexuality** Pattern.

## Ineffective Sexuality Pattern

**Domain 8** Sexuality    **Class 2** Sexual function

### NANDA-I Definition

Expressions of concern regarding own sexuality.

### Defining Characteristics

Altered sexual activity; altered sexual behavior; altered sexual partner relations; altered sexual role; difficulty with sexual activity; difficulty with sexual behavior; value conflict

• = Independent          ▲ = Collaborative

## Related Factors

Conflict about sexual orientation; conflict about variant preference; fear of pregnancy; fear of sexually transmitted infection; impaired sexual partner relations; inadequate alternative sexual strategies; inadequate role models; insufficient privacy

## At-Risk Population

Individuals without a significant other

## Client Outcomes

### Client Will (Specify Time Frame)

- State knowledge of difficulties, limitations, or changes in sexual behaviors or activities
- State knowledge of sexual anatomy and functioning
- State acceptance of altered body structure or functioning
- Describe acceptable alternative sexual practices
- Identify importance of discussing sexual issues with significant other
- Describe practice of safe sex with regard to pregnancy and avoidance of sexually transmitted infections (STIs)

## Nursing Interventions

- After establishing rapport or therapeutic relationship, give the client permission to discuss issues dealing with sexuality, for example, "Have you been or are you concerned about functioning sexually because of your health status?"
- Use assessment questions and standardized instruments to assess sexual problems, where possible.
- ▲ Assess any risks associated with sexual activity, particularly coronary risks.
- Assess knowledge about sexual functioning and return to sexual activity after experiencing a health problem with both clients and partners.
- Encourage the client to discuss concerns with his or her partner.
- Explore attitudes about sexual intimacy and changes in sexuality patterns.
- Assess psychosocial function such as anxiety, fear, depression, and low self-esteem.
- Discuss alternative sexual expressions for altered body functioning or structure, including closeness and sexual and nonsexual touching as other forms of expression.
- Assess the client's sexual orientation and usual pattern of sexual activities, and discuss prevention of illnesses for which the client may be at increased risk (e.g., anorectal cancer), asking specific questions about sexual orientation, for example, "Do you have sexual relationships with men, women, or both?" Assess use of safer

• = Independent     ▲ = Collaborative

sex practices (e.g., condom use); the frequency of anal intercourse; number of sexual partners in the last year; last HIV screening/results; and use of medications, alcohol, and illicit drugs.

- Specific guidelines for sexual activity for clients who have had total hip arthroplasty (THA) include the following: sexual activity can be generally resumed 1 to 2 months after surgery, and positioning to avoid hip dislocation, for example, a supine position ("missionary") at maximum abduction in extension, or the man and woman standing, with the woman's legs slightly bent and the man approaching the woman from behind (Issa et al, 2017).
- Specific guidelines for those who have had a myocardial infarction (MI) include the following: sexual activity can generally be resumed 1 week after MI unless complications are experienced, such as arrhythmias or cardiac arrest, if the client does not have cardiac symptoms during mild to moderate physical activity; begin with activities that require less exertion, such as fondling or kissing, building confidence in tolerance for sexual activity before sexual intercourse; engage in sexual activity in familiar surroundings with the usual partner; have a comfortable room temperature, and be well rested to minimize cardiac stress; avoid heavy meals or alcohol for 2 to 3 hours before sexual activity; and choose a position of comfort to minimize stress of the cardiac client (Steinke et al, 2016).
- Specific guidelines include that those who have had complete coronary revascularization, in addition to those mentioned with MI, including those with successful percutaneous cardiovascular revascularization without complication, can resume sex within a few days, and those who have had standard coronary artery bypass grafting or noncoronary open heart surgery may resume sex in 6 to 8 weeks. Incisional pain with sexual activity can be managed by premedicating with a mild pain reliever, and reassurance should be provided to the partner that sexual activity will not harm the sternum as long as direct pressure is avoided (Jelavić et al, 2018).
- Specific guidelines for those with an implantable cardioverter defibrillator (ICD) include returning to sexual activity is generally safe after ICD implantation if moderate physical activity does not precipitate arrhythmias; avoid strain on the incision at the implant site; assure the client and partner that fears about being shocked during sexual activity are normal; if the ICD discharges with sexual activity, the client should stop, rest, and later notify the health care provider that the device fired so that a determination can be made if

**S**

this was an appropriate shock or not; and report any dyspnea, chest pain, or dizziness with sexual activity (Steinke et al, 2016).

• Specific guidelines for those with chronic lung disease include planning for sexual activity when energy level is highest; use of controlled breathing techniques; avoiding physical exertion before sexual activity; using positions that minimize shortness of breath, such as a semireclining position; engaging in sexual activity when medications are at peak effectiveness; use of an oxygen cannula, if prescribed, to provide oxygen before, during, or after sex; and use of continuous positive airway pressure (CPAP) therapy, if prescribed (Steinke et al, 2016).

• Specific guidelines for those with MS include treatment of symptoms with prescribed medications, assessing changes in body image, and supportive therapies to assist with a more satisfying sexual experience, including treatment of neuropathic pain, sexual positions that are most supportive, discussing changes in sensation and stimulation with the partner, use of stretching exercise for tight muscles before sexual activity, and avoiding a distended bowel or bladder that may cause discomfort.

• Refer to the care plan **Sexual** Dysfunction for additional interventions.

**Pediatric**

• Initiate discussions regarding sexual health, attitudes, and knowledge about sexual behavior and sexual abstinence, providing information that is age appropriate and accurate regarding sexual activity and risky sexual behaviors.

• Provide age-appropriate information for adolescents regarding HIV/AIDS and sexual behavior, and discuss STIs, particularly human papillomavirus, including the risks of perinatal transmission and methods to reduce risks among adolescents with HIV.

• Provide age-appropriate information regarding potential for sexual abuse.

**Geriatric**

• Carefully assess the sexuality needs of the older client and refer for counseling as needed.

▲ Explore possible changes in sexuality related to health status, menopause, medications, and sexual risk, and make appropriate referrals.

• Allow the client to verbalize feelings regarding loss of sexual partner, and acknowledge problems such as disapproving children, lack of available partner for women, and environmental variables that make forming new relationships difficult.

• = Independent          ▲ = Collaborative

▲ Provide a milieu that allows for discussion of sexual issues and a higher level of sexual satisfaction, including allowing couples to room together and the provision of privacy.

• See care plan for **Sexual** Dysfunction.

**Multicultural**

• Assess for the influence of cultural beliefs, norms, and values on client's perceptions of sexual behavior.

**Home Care**

• Previously discussed interventions may be adapted for home care use. Also see care plan for **Sexual** Dysfunction.

• Help the client and significant other identify a place and time in the home and daily living for privacy in sharing sexual or relationship activity, and, if necessary, help the client communicate the need for privacy to family members.

• Confirm that physical reasons for dysfunction have been addressed, and provide support for coping behaviors, including participation in support groups or therapy if appropriate.

**Client/Family Teaching and Discharge Planning**

▲ Refer to appropriate community agencies (e.g., certified sex counselor, Reach to Recovery, Ostomy Association, American Association of Sex Educators, Counselors, and Therapists).

▲ Sexuality education is important to all populations, whether hearing or deaf, sighted or blind, disabled or not disabled; discuss contraceptive choices as appropriate, safer sexual practices, and refer to a health professional (e.g., gynecologist, urologist, nurse practitioner).

**S**

## Risk for Shock

**Domain 11** Safety/protection    **Class 2** Physical injury

### NANDA-I Definition

Susceptible to an inadequate blood flow to tissues that may lead to cellular dysfunction, which may compromise health.

### Risk Factors

Bleeding; deficient fluid volume; factors identified by standardized, validated screening tool; hyperthermia; hypothermia; hypoxemia; hypoxia; inadequate knowledge of bleeding management strategies; inadequate knowledge of infection management strategies; inadequate knowledge of modifiable factors; ineffective medication self-management; nonhemorrhagic fluid losses; smoking; unstable blood pressure

• = Independent          ▲ = Collaborative

## At-Risk Population

Individuals admitted to the emergency care unit; individuals at extremes of age; individuals with history of myocardial infarction

## Associated Conditions

Artificial respiration; burns; chemotherapy; diabetes mellitus; embolism; heart diseases; hypersensitivity; immunosuppression; infections; lactate levels ≥2 mmol/L; liver diseases; medical devices; neoplasms; nervous system diseases; pancreatitis; radiotherapy; sepsis; sequential organ failure assessment (SOFA) score ≥3; simplified acute physiology score (SAPS III >70); spinal cord injuries; surgical procedures; systemic inflammatory response syndrome (SIRS); trauma

## Client Outcomes

### Client Will (Specify Time Frame)

- Discuss precautions to prevent complications of disease
- Maintain adherence to agreed-on medication regimens
- Maintain adequate hydration
- Monitor for infection signs and symptoms
- Maintain a mean arterial pressure (MAP) above 65 mm Hg
- Maintain a heart rate between 60 and 100 with a normal rhythm
- Maintain urine output greater than 0.5 mL/kg/hr
- Maintain warm, dry skin

## Nursing Interventions

- Review data pertaining to client risk status including age, primary diseases, immunosuppression, antibiotic use, and presence of hemodynamic alterations such as tachycardia, tachypnea, and decrease in blood pressure (BP).
- Review client's medical and surgical history, noting conditions that place the client at higher risk for shock, including trauma, myocardial infarction, pulmonary embolism, head injury, dehydration, infection, endocrine problems, certain medications, and pregnancy.
- Complete a full nursing physical examination.
- Monitor circulatory status (e.g., BP, MAP, skin color, skin temperature, heart sounds, heart rate and rhythm, presence and quality of peripheral pulses, pulse oximetry, and end-tidal carbon dioxide monitoring [EtCO$_2$]). Anticipate additional studies that will evaluate dynamic changes in cardiac tissue such as ultrasonography.
- Maintain intravenous (IV) access and provide isotonic IV fluids such as 0.9% normal saline or Ringer's lactate as ordered; these fluids are commonly used in the prevention and treatment of shock.
- Monitor for inadequate tissue oxygenation (e.g., apprehension, increased anxiety, altered mental status, agitation, oliguria,

• = Independent        ▲ = Collaborative

cool/mottled periphery) and determinants of tissue oxygen delivery (e.g., Pao$_2$, SpO$_2$, ScvO$_2$/SvO$_2$, MAP, hemoglobin levels, lactate levels, CO).

▲ Maintain vital signs (BP, pulse, respirations, and temperature) and pulse oximetry within normal parameters.

▲ Administer oxygen immediately to maintain SpO$_2$ greater than 90%, and antibiotics and other medications as prescribed to any client presenting with symptoms of early shock.

▲ Monitor trends in noninvasive hemodynamic parameters (e.g., MAP) as appropriate.

▲ Monitor serum lactate levels and interpret them within the context of each client.

**Critical Care**

▲ Prepare the client for the placement of an additional IV line, a central line, and/or a pulmonary artery catheter as prescribed. Adequate IV and central line access may be required for fluid resuscitation and medication delivery. Maintaining more than one IV access ensures rapid IV medication and fluid delivery in a cri-sis situation. Large amounts of fluid can be delivered more efficiently through centrally placed vascular access sites. Most vasoactive agents, especially vasopressors, should be delivered only through central lines because of risk of tissue sloughing.

▲ Monitor trends in hemodynamic parameters (e.g., central venous pressure [CVP], CO, cardiac index [CI], systemic vascular resistance [SVR], pulmonary artery pressure [PAP], MAP) as appropriate.

▲ Monitor electrocardiography. Myocardial ischemia can present as ST segment changes, which can be seen before a decrease in BP as a compensatory mechanism.

▲ Monitor arterial blood gases, coagulation, blood chemistries, blood glucose, cardiac enzymes, blood cultures, and hematology laboratory test results.

▲ Administer vasopressor agents as prescribed.

• If the client is in shock, refer to the following care plans: Risk for Ineffective **Renal** Perfusion, Risk for Ineffective **Gastrointestinal** Perfusion, Impaired **Gas** Exchange, and Decreased **Cardiac** Output.

**Client/Family Teaching and Discharge Planning**

▲ Teach client and family or significant others about any medications prescribed. Instruct the client to report any adverse side effects to his or her health care provider. Medication teaching includes the drug name, purpose, administration instructions (e.g., with or without food), and any side effects.

• = Independent          ▲ = Collaborative

- Instruct the client and family on disease process and rationale for care.
- Instruct clients and their family members on the signs and symptoms of low BP to report to their health care provider (dizziness, lightheadedness, fainting, dehydration and unusual thirst, lack of concentration, blurred vision, nausea, cold, clammy, pale skin, rapid and shallow breathing, fatigue, and depression).
- Promote a culture of client safety and individual accountability.

# Impaired Sitting

**Domain 4** Activity/rest    **Class 2** Activity/exercise
## NANDA-I Definition

Limitation of ability to independently and purposefully attain and/or maintain a rest position that is supported by the buttocks and thighs, in which the torso is upright.

## Defining Characteristics

Difficulty adjusting position of one or both lower limbs on uneven surface; difficulty attaining postural balance; difficulty flexing or moving both hips; difficulty flexing or moving both knees; difficulty maintaining postural balance; difficulty stressing torso with body weight

## Related Factors

Insufficient energy; insufficient muscle strength; malnutrition; neurobehavioral manifestations; pain; self-imposed relief posture

## Associated Conditions

Impaired metabolism; mental disorders; neurological disorder; orthopedic surgery; prescribed posture; sarcopenia

## Client Outcomes

### Client Will (Specify Time Frame)

- Verbalize importance of being able to sit as a method to engage in activities of daily living
- Understand somatic physiology of posture control
- Choose health care options that enhance ability to sit
- Engage in physical conditioning exercises to enhance sitting ability
- Understand relationship of posture and emotions
- Control pain to increase ability to sit

## Nursing Interventions

- Acknowledge the importance of being able to sit as a method to engage in activities of daily living.
- Understand the somatic physiology of posture control.
- Encourage engagement in physical conditioning exercises to enhance proper sitting ability.

- Understand the relationship of posture and emotions.
- Maintain pain levels below 3 to 4 on a 0-to-10 scale to increase ability to sit.

**Pediatric**
- Promote proper sitting ability to increase cognitive and physical functioning.

**Geriatric**
- Promote proper sitting ability to increase cognitive and physical functioning.

**Multicultural**
- Understand the importance of unimpaired sitting to different populations.

**Home Care**
- Encourage proper sitting posture in the home environment to promote health.

# Impaired Skin Integrity

**Domain 11** Safety/protection    **Class 2** Physical injury

## NANDA-I Definition

Altered epidermis and/or dermis.

## Defining Characteristics

Abscess; acute pain; altered skin color; altered turgor; bleeding; blister; desquamation; disrupted skin surface; dry skin; excoriation; foreign matter piercing skin; hematoma; localized area hot to touch; macerated skin; peeling; pruritus

## Related Factors

### External Factors

Excessive moisture; excretions; humidity; hyperthermia; hypothermia; inadequate caregiver knowledge about maintaining tissue integrity; inadequate caregiver knowledge about protecting tissue integrity; inadequate use of chemical agent; pressure over bony prominence; psychomotor agitation; secretions; shearing forces; surface friction; use of linen with insufficient moisture wicking property

### Internal Factors

Body mass index above normal range for age and gender; body mass index below normal range for age and gender; decreased physical activity; decreased physical mobility; edema; inadequate adherence to incontinence treatment regimen; inadequate knowledge about maintaining tissue integrity; inadequate knowledge about protecting tissue integrity; malnutrition;

• = Independent          ▲ = Collaborative

psychogenic factor; self mutilation; smoking; substance misuse; water-electrolyte imbalance

## At-Risk Population

Individuals at extremes of age; individuals in intensive care units; individuals in long-term care facilities; individuals in palliative care settings; individuals receiving home-based care

## Associated Conditions

Altered pigmentation; anemia; cardiovascular diseases; decreased level of consciousness; decreased tissue oxygenation; decreased tissue perfusion; diabetes mellitus; hormonal change; immobilization; immunodeficiency; impaired metabolism; infections; medical devices; neoplasms; peripheral neuropathy; pharmaceutical preparations; punctures; sensation disorders

## Client Outcomes

**Client Will (Specify Time Frame)**

- Regain integrity of skin surface
- Report any altered sensation or pain at site of skin impairment
- Demonstrate understanding of plan to heal skin and prevent reinjury or complications
- Describe measures to protect and heal the skin and to care for any skin lesion

## Nursing Interventions

- NPUAP redefined the definition of a pressure ulcer, now referred to as pressure injuries, during the NPUAP 2016 Staging Consensus Conference. The new definitions more accurately define alterations in tissue integrity from pressure as the following: A pressure injury is localized damage to the skin and underlying soft tissue usually over a bony prominence or related to a medical or other device. The injury can present as intact skin or an open ulcer and may be painful. The injury occurs as a result of intense and/or prolonged pressure or pressure in combination with shear. The tolerance of soft tissue for pressure and shear may also be affected by microclimate, nutrition, perfusion, comorbidities, and condition of the soft tissue (NPUAP, 2016).
- Pressure ulcer is no longer a current clinical term; rather, pressure injury is used to describe an alteration in tissue integrity from pressure (NPUAP, 2016). Similarly, hospital-acquired pressure ulcers (HAPUs) are currently referred to as hospital-acquired pressure injuries (HAPIs).
- Assess site of skin impairment and determine cause or type of wound (e.g., acute or chronic wound, burn, dermatological lesion, pressure injury, skin tear).

• = Independent ▲ = Collaborative

- Use a risk assessment tool to systematically assess client risk factors for skin breakdown caused by pressure.
- Determine the extent of the skin impairment caused by pressure using the revised classification system and definition for pressure injuries (NPUAP, 2016).
  - ○ **Stage 1 Pressure Injury:** Nonblanchable erythema of intact skin. Area of localized nonblanchable erythema that may appear differently in darkly pigmented skin and changes in sensation, temperature, or firmness may precede visual changes. Color changes do not include purple or maroon discoloration, which is more likely to indicate deep tissue pressure injury (NPUAP, 2016).
  - ○ **Stage 2 Pressure Injury:** Partial-thickness skin loss with exposed dermis. Partial-thickness skin loss with exposed dermis in which the wound bed is pink/red and moist and adipose (fat) and deeper tissues are not visible. Granulation tissue, slough, and eschar are not present. A stage 2 pressure injury may also present as an intact or ruptured blister. These injuries commonly result from adverse microclimate and shear in the skin over the pelvis and shear in the heel. This stage should not be used to describe moisture-associated skin damage (MASD) including incontinence-associated dermatitis (IAD), intertriginous dermatitis (ITD), medical adhesive–related skin injury (MARSI), or traumatic wounds (skin tears, burns, and abrasions) (NPUAP, 2016).
  - ○ **Stage 3 Pressure Injury:** Full-thickness skin loss. Full-thickness loss of skin, in which adipose is visible and granulation tissue and epibole (rolled wound edges) are often present and undermining/tunneling may occur. Slough and/or eschar may also be visible. Fascia, muscle, tendon, ligament, cartilage, and/or bone are not exposed. The depth of tissue damage varies by anatomical location, and areas of significant adiposity can develop deep wounds. If slough or eschar obscures the extent of tissue loss, this is an unstageable pressure injury (NPUAP, 2016).
  - ○ **Stage 4 Pressure Injury:** Full-thickness skin and tissue loss. Full-thickness skin and tissue loss with exposed or directly palpable fascia, muscle, tendon, ligament, cartilage or bone, and slough and/or eschar may be visible. Epibole, undermining, and/or tunneling often occur, and depth varies by anatomical location. If slough or eschar obscures the extent of tissue loss, this is an unstageable pressure injury (NPUAP, 2016).
  - ○ **Deep Tissue Pressure Injury:** Persistent nonblanchable deep red, maroon, or purple discoloration. Intact or nonintact skin

**S**

with localized area of persistent nonblanchable deep red, maroon, or purple discoloration or epidermal separation revealing a dark wound bed or blood-filled blister. Pain and temperature change often precede skin color changes. Discoloration may appear differently in darkly pigmented skin. This injury results from intense and/or prolonged pressure and shear forces at the bone–muscle interface. The wound may evolve rapidly to reveal the actual extent of tissue injury, or it may resolve without tissue loss. If necrotic tissue, subcutaneous tissue, granulation tissue, fascia, muscle, or other underlying structures are visible, this indicates a full-thickness pressure injury (unstageable, stage 3, or stage 4). Do not use the term deep tissue pressure injury to describe vascular, traumatic, neuropathic, or dermatological conditions (NPUAP, 2016).

○ **Unstageable Pressure Injury:** Obscured full-thickness skin and tissue loss. Full-thickness skin and tissue loss in which the extent of tissue damage within the ulcer cannot be confirmed because it is obscured by slough or eschar. If slough or eschar is removed, a stage 3 or stage 4 pressure injury will be revealed. Stable eschar (i.e., dry, adherent, intact without erythema or fluctuance) on the heel or ischemic limb should not be softened or removed (NPUAP, 2016).

○ **Mechanical Device–Related Pressure Injury:** Used to describe alterations in tissue integrity caused by pressure from mechanical devices used in the care of clients (e.g., indwelling urinary catheters, endotracheal tubes, nasogastric tubes, drains). The pressure injury typically conforms to the shape of the device (NPUAP, 2016).

○ **Mucosal Membrane Pressure Injury:** Mucosal membrane pressure injury is found on mucous membranes with a history of a medical device in use at the location of the injury. Because of the anatomy of the tissue, these ulcers cannot be staged (NPUAP, 2016).

• Inspect and monitor site of skin impairment at least once a day for color changes, erythema, edema, warmth, pain, changes in sensation, moisture, or other signs of infection.

• Monitor the client's skin care practices, noting type of soap or other cleansing agents used, temperature of water, and frequency of skin cleansing.

• Consider using physiologically compatible cleansers with each wound dressing change.

- Maintain good skin hygiene, using mild nondetergent soap, drying gently, and lubricating with lotion or emollient to reduce the risk of dermal trauma; improve circulation; and promote comfort.
- Urinary and fecal incontinence can cause skin breakdown.
- For clients with limited mobility and activity, use a risk assessment tool to systematically assess immobility and activity-related risk factors.
- Do not position the client on site of skin impairment. If consistent with overall client management goals, reposition the client as determined by individualized tissue tolerance and overall condition. Reposition and transfer the client with care to protect against the adverse effects of external mechanical forces such as pressure, friction, and shear. Maintain the head of the bed as flat as possible. Use a 30-degree lateral positioning (NPIAP, EPIAP, & PPPIA, 2019).
- Evaluate for use of support surfaces (specialty mattresses, beds), chair cushions, or devices as appropriate. Maintain the head of the bed at the lowest possible degree of elevation to reduce shear and friction, and use lift devices, pillows, foam wedges, and pressure-reducing devices in the bed (Brienza et al, 2016; NPIAP, EPIAP, & PPPIA, 2019).
- Implement a written treatment plan for topical treatment of the site of skin impairment.
- Select a topical treatment that will maintain a moist wound-healing environment (stage 2) that is balanced with the need to absorb exudate. Stage 1 pressure injuries may be managed by keeping the client off of the area and using a protective dressing (Baranoski & Ayello, 2016).
- Avoid massaging around the site of skin impairment and over bony prominences.
- Assess the client's nutritional status. Refer for a nutritional consultation and/or institute dietary supplements as necessary.
- Identify the client's phase of wound healing (inflammation, proliferation, or maturation) and stage of injury.

**Home Care**

- The interventions described previously may be adapted for home care use.
- Instruct and assist the client and caregivers in how to change dressings and maintain a clean environment. Provide written instructions and observe the client completing the dressing change before hospital discharge and in the home setting.
- Educate client and caregivers on proper nutrition, signs and symptoms of infection, and when to call the agency and/or health care provider with concerns.

• = Independent ▲ = Collaborative

▲ Treating wounds requires a multiprofessional approach with the frontline nurse an essential member (Cox, 2019).

**Client/Family Teaching and Discharge Planning**

• Teach skin and wound assessment and ways to monitor for signs and symptoms of infection, complications, and healing. Early assessment and intervention help prevent serious problems from developing.

• Teach the client why a topical treatment has been selected.

• If consistent with overall client management goals, teach how to reposition as client condition warrants.

• Teach the client to use pillows, foam wedges, chair cushions, and pressure-redistribution devices to prevent pressure injury (Brienza et al, 2016).

# Risk for Impaired Skin Integrity

**Domain 11** Safety/protection    **Class 2** Physical injury

**NANDA-I Definition**

Susceptible to alteration in epidermis and/or dermis, which may compromise health.

**Risk Factors**

**External Factors**

Excessive moisture; excretions; humidity; hyperthermia; hypothermia; inadequate caregiver knowledge about maintaining tissue integrity; inadequate caregiver knowledge about protecting tissue integrity; inadequate use of chemical agent; pressure over bony prominence; psychomotor agitation; secretions; shearing forces; surface friction; use of linen with insufficient moisture wicking property

**Internal Factors**

Body mass index above normal range for age and gender; body mass index below normal range for age and gender; decreased physical activity; decreased physical mobility; edema; inadequate adherence to incontinence treatment regimen; inadequate knowledge about maintaining skin integrity; inadequate knowledge about protecting skin integrity; malnutrition; psychogenic factor; self mutilation; smoking; substance misuse; water-electrolyte imbalance

**At-Risk Population**

Individuals at extremes of age; individuals in intensive care units; individuals in long-term care facilities; individuals in palliative care settings; individuals receiving home-based care

• = Independent                    ▲ = Collaborative

## Associated Conditions

Altered pigmentation; anemia; cardiovascular diseases; decreased level of consciousness; decreased tissue oxygenation; decreased tissue perfusion; diabetes mellitus; hormonal change; immobilization; immunodeficiency; impaired metabolism; infections; medical devices; neoplasms; peripheral neuropathy; pharmaceutical preparations; punctures; sensation disorders

## Client Outcomes

**Client Will (Specify Time Frame)**

- Report altered sensation or pain at risk areas as soon as noted
- Demonstrate understanding of personal risk factors for impaired skin integrity
- Verbalize a personal plan for preventing impaired skin integrity

## Nursing Interventions

- The NPUAP redefined the definition of a pressure ulcer, which is now referred to as a pressure injury, during the NPUAP 2016 Staging Consensus Conference in 2016. The new definition more accurately defines alterations in tissue integrity from pressure as the following: A pressure injury is localized damage to the skin and underlying soft tissue, usually over a bony prominence or related to a medical or other device. The injury can present as intact skin or an open ulcer and may be painful. The injury occurs as a result of intense and/or prolonged pressure or pressure in combinations with shear. The tolerance of soft tissue for pressure and shear may also be affected by microclimate, nutrition, perfusion, comorbidities, and conditions of the soft tissue (NPUAP, 2016).
- Identify clients at risk for impaired skin integrity as a result of immobility, chronological age, malnutrition, incontinence, compromised perfusion, immunocompromised status, or chronic medical condition, such as diabetes mellitus, spinal cord injury, or renal failure.
- Inspect and monitor skin condition at least once a day for color or texture changes, redness, localized heat, edema or induration, pressure damage, dermatological conditions, or lesions and any incontinence-associated dermatitis. Determine whether the client is experiencing loss of sensation or pain.
- Monitor the client's skin care practices, noting type of soap or other cleansing agents used, temperature of water, and frequency of skin cleansing.
- Keep skin clean and dry. Cleanse the skin gently with pH-balanced cleansers, avoiding alkaline soaps and cleansers.
- ▲ Develop and implement an individualized continence management plan. Cleanse the skin promptly after episodes of incontinence. Use incontinence skin barriers including creams, ointments, pastes, or

S

film-forming skin protectants as needed to protect skin and maintain intact skin (Wound, Ostomy and Continence Nurses Society–Wound Guidelines Task Force, 2017). Use highly absorbent incontinence products (NPIAP, EPIAP, & PPPIA, 2019).

- For clients with limited mobility, inspect and monitor condition of skin covering bony prominences.
- Implement and communicate a client-specific prevention plan.
- At-risk clients should be frequently repositioned.
- Evaluate for use of specialty mattresses, beds, or devices as appropriate.
▲ Assess the client's nutritional status; refer for a nutritional consultation, and/or institute dietary supplements.

### Geriatric

- Limit the number of complete baths to two or three per week, and alternate them with partial baths. Use a tepid water temperature (between 90°F [32.2°C] and 105°F [40.5°C]) for bathing or use a no-rinse alternative product.
- Use lotions and moisturizers to prevent skin from drying out, especially in the winter.
- Increase fluid intake within cardiac and renal limits to a minimum of 1500 mL/day.
- Increase humidity in the environment, especially during the winter, by using a humidifier or placing a container of water on a warm object. Increasing the moisture in the air helps keep moisture in the skin.

### Home Care

- Assess client and caregiver ability to recognize potential risk for skin breakdown. Provide resources for client/caregiver to contact health care provider with questions/concerns related to skin and incontinence care as needed. Engage family, caregivers, or legal guardian when establishing goals of care and validate their understanding of these goals. Educate the individual and his or her caregiver regarding skin changes in aging and at end of life.
- See the care plan for Impaired **Skin** Integrity.

### Client/Family Teaching and Discharge Planning

- Teach the client skin assessment and ways to monitor for impending skin breakdown. Early assessment and intervention help prevent the development of serious problems.
- If consistent with overall client management goals, teach how to turn and reposition the client.
- Teach the client and/or caregivers to use pillows, foam wedges, and pressure-reducing devices to prevent pressure injury (NPIAP, EPIAP, & PPPIA, 2019).

• = Independent          ▲ = Collaborative

# Sleep Deprivation

**Domain 4** Activity/rest    **Class 1** Sleep/rest
## NANDA-I Definition

Prolonged periods of time without sustained natural, periodic suspension of relative consciousness that provides rest.

## Defining Characteristics

Altered attention; anxiety; apathy; combativeness; confusion; decreased functional ability; drowsiness; expresses distress; fatigue; fleeting nystagmus; hallucinations; heightened sensitivity to pain; irritable mood; lethargy; prolonged reaction time; psychomotor agitation; transient paranoia; tremors

## Related Factors

Age-related sleep stage shifts; average daily physical activity is less than recommended for age and gender; discomfort; environmental disturbances; environmental overstimulation; late day confusion; nonrestorative sleep-wake cycle; sleep terror; sleep walking; sustained circadian asynchrony; sustained inadequate sleep hygiene

## At-Risk Population

Individuals with familial sleep paralysis

## Associated Conditions

Conditions with periodic limb movement; idiopathic central nervous system hypersomnolence; narcolepsy; neurocognitive disorders; nightmares; sleep apnea; sleep-related enuresis; sleep-related painful erections; treatment regimen

## Client Outcomes

**Client Will (Specify Time Frame)**

- Verbalize plan that provides adequate time for sleep
- Identify actions that can be taken to ensure adequate sleep time
- Awaken refreshed once adequate time is spent sleeping
- Be less sleepy during the day once adequate time is spent sleeping

## Nursing Interventions

- Minimize care-environmental factors that may lead to sleep deprivation if they persist. See Nursing Interventions for Disturbed **Sleep** Pattern.
- Address personal client factors that may lead to sleep deprivation if they persist. See Nursing Interventions for **Insomnia.**
- Assess for hypersensitivity to pain in sleep-deprived clients.
- Assess the amount of sleep obtained each night compared with the amount of sleep needed given the client's age, medical diagnoses, and personal preferences.

• = Independent        ▲ = Collaborative

- Assess the extent to which clients can be provided 3 to 4 consecutive hours of sleep time that is free from disturbance.
- If sleep-disrupting environmental factors that are inherent in hospitalization cannot be reduced adequately to prevent sleep deprivation, schedule specific times for rest and sleep during the day.
- If personal sleep-disrupting factors that are inherent in insomnia cannot be reduced adequately to prevent the client's sleep deprivation, consider scheduling a specific time for rest and sleep during the day.
- If caffeine is used by the client to alleviate daytime drowsiness, monitor amounts and time of use.
- If naps are inadequate for preventing excessive daytime sleepiness due to sleep deprivation, consider and carefully evaluate use of unstudied, but commonly used, countermeasures for fighting drowsiness.
- ▲ If daytime drowsiness occurs despite adequate periods of undisturbed nighttime sleep and supplemental daytime naps, consider undiagnosed sleep apnea as a possible cause.

**Pediatric**

- Assess the amount of sleep obtained every 24 hours compared with the amount of sleep needed for the child given age, medical diagnoses, and individual differences.
- Encourage daily schedules that allow for late awakening times for adolescents.
- Encourage an age-appropriate nap schedule that adequately supplements the child's nighttime sleep duration.
- See the Pediatric section of Nursing Interventions for Disturbed **Sleep** Pattern.

**Geriatric**

- Assess the amount of sleep obtained each night compared with the amount of sleep needed for an older adult given advancing age, medical diagnoses, and individual differences.
- ▲ If an older adult has daytime sleepiness despite adequate nighttime sleep, consider a referral to a sleep laboratory to rule out sleep apnea.
- Assess how much time the older adult spends in bed unable to sleep and their comfort with low sleep efficiency.
- If a client is obtaining less sleep than required for optimal daytime function, explore if daytime napping will supplement, rather than replace, nighttime sleep.
- See the Geriatric section of Nursing Interventions for Disturbed **Sleep** Pattern and **Insomnia**.

**Multicultural**

- Be aware of racial and ethnic disparities in sleep deprivation.

• = Independent        ▲ = Collaborative

**Home Care**

- Assessments and interventions discussed previously can all be adapted for use in home care.
▲ If daytime drowsiness occurs despite adequate periods of undisturbed nighttime sleep and supplemental daytime naps, consider sleep apnea as a possible cause.
- Teach family members about the prevalence and long-term consequences of inadequate amounts of sleep for both clients and family caregivers.
▲ If sleep is deprived due to insomnia, refer client to a nurse practitioner or other sleep specialist trained in cognitive behavioral therapies for insomnia (CBT-I).
- Teach client/family caregivers about the need for those with medical conditions to avoid schedules and commitments that interfere with obtaining adequate amounts of sleep.
- Promote adoption of behaviors that ensure adequate amounts of sleep for all family members.
- Teach family members ways to avoid chronic sleep loss.
- Advise against chronic use of caffeinated drinks to overcome daytime fatigue and drowsiness while focusing on elimination of factors that lead to chronic sleep loss.

**S**

# Readiness for Enhanced Sleep

**Domain 4** Activity/rest    **Class 1** Sleep/rest

## NANDA-I Definition

A pattern of natural, periodic suspension of relative consciousness to provide rest and sustain a desired lifestyle, which can be strengthened.

## Defining Characteristics

Expresses desire to enhance sleep-wake cycle

## Client Outcomes

**Client Will (Specify Time Frame)**

- Verbalize a current interest in what constitutes normal sleep
- Reflect on own experiences and beliefs about sleep
- Verbalize an interest in nonpharmacological approaches to sleep promotion
- Take concrete steps to establish an environment conducive to sleep initiation and maintenance

## Nursing Interventions

- Assess client's current knowledge and beliefs about sleep need and factors affecting sleep quantity and quality.

• = Independent        ▲ = Collaborative

- Whenever there is a lack of knowledge or false beliefs about sleep requirements, provide information regarding sleep need and encourage clients to identify their personal sleep requirements.
- Based on your assessment, focus on one or more of the following sleep hygiene strategies, choosing the most relevant for the client:
  - ○ Regular scheduling of the nighttime sleep period, daytime exposure to light, exercise, napping, and mealtimes characterized by (1) exercise during the day, (2) avoidance of long periods of daytime sleep (unless a night-shift worker), (3) avoidance of large meals before bed, and (4) arising at the same time each day even if sleep was poor during the previous night.
  - ○ Use of a relaxing bedtime routine that includes (1) activities that calm the mind (e.g., mindfulness or other types of meditation, listening to music, prayer) and (2) activities that relax the body (e.g., warm baths, massage, progressive muscle relaxation).
  - ○ Use of essential oils.
  - ○ Creation of an environment conducive to sleep, including (1) comfortable sleepwear, sleep surface, and room temperature; (2) low or masked levels of light and noise; and (3) a sleep space as free as possible from interruptions from others.
  - ○ Management of any sources of pain as needed before sleep. (See further Nursing Interventions for Acute **Pain** and Chronic **Pain**.)
  - ○ Avoidance of late-day electronic device use.
  - ○ Monitoring of late-day intake of caffeine from all sources, including energy drinks, coffee, colas, teas, and chocolate.
  - ○ Avoidance of alcoholic beverages to induce sleep.
  - ○ Avoidance of nicotine.
  - ○ Avoidance of a sedentary lifestyle.

**Geriatric**
- Interventions discussed previously can all be adapted for use with geriatric clients.
- Counsel the older client regarding normal age-related sleep changes.
- Elicit the older client's beliefs about sleep and correct any misconceptions, which may manifest as undue concern for some elders, but too little concern for others.
- Review older clients' prescription medications; use of over-the-counter (OTC) medications; and use of caffeine, tobacco, and alcohol.
- Assess and refer as appropriate whenever coexisting conditions may be affecting older clients' sleep.
- Expand older clients' awareness of sleep hygiene behaviors for improving sleep.

• = Independent          ▲ = Collaborative

- Encourage the older client to walk and engage in other exercise outside unless contraindicated.

**Home Care**

- All interventions discussed previously can be adapted for home care use.
- Assess family caregivers' readiness for enhancing sleep.
- Assess the conduciveness of the home environment for promoting sleep and the resources needed to improve the sleep environment.

# Disturbed Sleep Pattern

**Domain 4** Activity/rest   **Class 1** Sleep/rest

## NANDA-I Definition

Time-limited awakenings due to external factors.

## Defining Characteristics

Difficulty in daily functioning; difficulty initiating sleep; difficulty maintaining sleep state; expresses dissatisfaction with sleep; expresses tiredness; nonrestorative sleep-wake cycle; unintentional awakening

## Related Factors

Disruption caused by sleep partner; environmental disturbances; insufficient privacy

## Associated Conditions

Immobilization

## Client Outcomes

**Client Will (Specify Time Frame)**

- Verbalize plan to implement sleep promotion routines
- Maintain a regular schedule of sleep and waking
- Fall asleep without difficulty
- Remain asleep throughout the night
- Awaken naturally, feeling refreshed and is not fatigued during day

## Nursing Interventions

- Assess the client's sleep environment to determine its adequacy for providing undisturbed sleep.
- Obtain a sleep history to identify the following: (1) the client's perception of smells, noise, and light levels in the sleep environment; (2) the client's preferred bedding; (3) client activities occurring in the sleep environment during hours of sleep, including use of handheld technology; (4) number of times the client typically awakens during the sleep period; and (5) when, during the sleep period, time is available for undisturbed sleep.
- Keep environment as quiet as possible during sleep periods.

• = Independent        ▲ = Collaborative

- Consider masking hospital noise that cannot be eliminated.
- Offer earplugs when feasible.
- Dim the lights during sleep periods.
- Offer eye covers when lighting cannot be dimmed.
- Be aware that use of eye covers in intubated clients may lead to sensory deprivation and anxiety.
- Negotiate use of handheld technology whenever clients have access to electronic devices in the care setting.
- Consolidate essential care to provide the opportunity for uninterrupted sleep the first 3 to 4 hours of the sleep period. Follow with periods of 90 to 110 minutes between interruptions.
- If the client must be disturbed during the first 3 to 4 hours of the sleep period, attempt to protect 90- to 110-minute blocks of time between awakenings.
- When feasible, schedule newly ordered medications to avoid the need to wake the client the first few hours of the night.
- Combine the previously mentioned interventions as feasible to create a sleep-promotion care bundle.
- Assess for medications and other stimulants that fragment sleep. Use caution when administering sleep medications. See Nursing Interventions for **Insomnia.**

**Pediatric**
- Adapt interventions described above with caution because of limited empirical evidence regarding the effects of their use for pediatric clients.
- Assess use of evening and nighttime texting and consider limiting as needed to protect sleep.

**Geriatric**
- Most interventions discussed above can all be adapted for use with geriatric clients.
- Use of earplugs and eye covers with ataxic clients and clients with dementia may contribute to disorientation.

**Multicultural**
- Be aware that cultural sleep practices may alter the kinds of environmental sleep disruptors that require management.

**Home Care**
- Consider the unique characteristics of each home sleep environment when addressing sleep disruption.
- In addition, see the Home Care section of Nursing Interventions for Readiness for Enhanced **Sleep.**

• = Independent            ▲ = Collaborative

# Impaired Social Interaction

**Domain 7** Role relationship **Class 3** Role performance

## NANDA-I Definition

Insufficient or excessive quantity or ineffective quality of social exchange.

## Defining Characteristics

Anxiety during social interaction; dysfunctional interaction with others; expresses difficulty establishing satisfactory reciprocal interpersonal relations; expresses difficulty functioning socially; expresses difficulty performing social roles; expresses discomfort in social situations; expresses dissatisfaction with social connection; family reports altered interaction; inadequate psychosocial support system; inadequate use of social status toward others; low levels of social activities; minimal interaction with others; reports unsatisfactory social engagement; unhealthy competitive focus; unwillingness to cooperate with others

## Related Factors

Altered self-concept; depressive symptoms; disturbed thought processes; environmental constraints; impaired physical mobility; inadequate communication skills; inadequate knowledge about how to enhance mutuality; inadequate personal hygiene; inadequate social skills; inadequate social support; maladaptive grieving; neurobehavioral manifestations; sociocultural dissonance

## At-Risk Population

Individuals without a significant other

## Associated Conditions

Halitosis; mental diseases; neurodevelopmental disorders; therapeutic isolation

## Client Outcomes

Client Will (Specify Time Frame)

- Identify barriers that cause impaired social interactions
- Discuss feelings that accompany impaired and successful social interactions
- Use available opportunities to practice interactions
- Use successful social interaction behaviors
- Report increased comfort in social situations
- Communicate, state feelings of belonging, demonstrate caring and interest in others
- Report effective interactions with others

## Nursing Interventions

- Encourage the client to keep a gratitude journal.
- Encourage dancing with Parkinson's programs for individuals with Parkinson's disease.

• = Independent ▲ = Collaborative

- Consider use of social cognition and interaction training (SCIT) to improve social functioning.
- Consider use of animal-assisted therapy (AAT).
- Encourage visually challenged clients to use text-based computer-mediated communications to facilitate social interaction.
- Provide management strategies to individuals experiencing auditory hallucinations.
- Refer to care plans for Risk for **Loneliness** and **Social** Isolation for additional interventions.

**Pediatric**

- Assess children with social impairments for experiences of bullying or victimization.
- For adolescent clients, consider use of a peer network intervention to increase social interactions.
- Provide supervised interaction opportunities for children of chronically ill parents.
- Encourage family style dining (FSD) for preschool children to promote social interactions during mealtimes.
- Use peer-mediated interaction (PMI) to increase social interactions of children on the autistic spectrum.
- Consider Social Story with self-modeling for children with autism spectrum disorder.
- Encourage a responsive parenting style for parents of children with autism spectrum disorder.
- ▲ Refer children with autism spectrum disorder to "Play Time/Social Time" (PT/ST) and "I Can Problem Solve" (ICPS) programs.

**Geriatric**

- Assess older clients for hearing loss and refer for hearing aids as needed.
- Encourage socialization through physical activity and meaningful activities incorporated into normal daily care practices.
- Provide live concert music for clients with dementia.
- ▲ Refer depressed clients to services for cognitive-behavioral therapy (CBT).
- Refer to care plans for **Frail** Elderly Syndrome, Risk for **Loneliness,** and **Social** Isolation for additional interventions.

**Multicultural**

- Approach individuals of color with respect, warmth, and professional courtesy.
- Use professional interpreters as needed.
- Refer to care plan for **Social** Isolation for additional interventions.

• = Independent          ▲ = Collaborative

**Home Care**
- Previously discussed interventions may be adapted for home care use.

**Client/Family Teaching and Discharge Planning**
- Previously discussed interventions may be adapted for client/family teaching and discharge planning.

## Social Isolation

**Domain 12** Comfort **Class 3** Social comfort

### NANDA-I Definition

A state in which the individual lacks a sense of relatedness connected to positive, lasting, and significant interpersonal relationships.

### Defining Characteristics

Expresses dissatisfaction with respect from others; expresses dissatisfaction with social connection; expresses dissatisfaction with social support; expresses loneliness; flat affect; hostility; impaired ability to meet expectations of others; low levels of social activities; minimal interaction with others; preoccupation with own thoughts; purposelessness; reduced eye contact; reports feeling different from others; reports feeling insecure in public; sad affect; seclusion imposed by others; sense of alienation; social behavior incongruent with cultural norms; social withdrawal

### Related Factors

Difficulty establishing satisfactory reciprocal interpersonal relations; difficulty performing activities of daily living; difficulty sharing personal life expectations; fear of crime; fear of traffic; impaired physical mobility; inadequate psychosocial support system; inadequate social skills; inadequate social support; inadequate transportation; low self-esteem; negative perception of support system; neurobehavioral manifestations; values incongruent with cultural norms

### At-Risk Population

Economically disadvantaged individuals; immigrants; individuals living alone; individuals living far from significant others; individuals moving to unfamiliar locations; individuals with history of rejection; individuals experiencing altered social role; individuals experiencing loss of significant other; individuals with history of traumatic event; individuals with ill family member; individuals with no children; institutionalized individuals; older adults; widowed individuals

### Associated Conditions

Altered physical appearance; chronic disease; cognitive disorders

## Client Outcomes

**Client Will (Specify Time Frame)**
- Identify feelings of isolation
- Practice social and communication skills needed to interact with others
- Initiate interactions with others; set and meet goals
- Participate in activities and programs at level of ability and desire
- Describe feelings of self-worth

## Nursing Interventions

- Assess the client's feelings regarding social isolation.
- Assess individuals in quarantine or other socially isolating situations for the negative psychological effects of social isolation.
- For individuals who require quarantine, provide clear rationale for quarantine and information about protocols, and ensure sufficient supplies are provided. Tell people what is happening and why, explain how long it will continue, provide meaningful activities for them to do while in quarantine, provide clear communication, ensure basic supplies (such as food, water, and medical supplies) are available, and reinforce a sense of altruism.
- Provide the client with social skills training.
- Encourage limits on social media use.
- Recommend involvement in organizations and other activities that encourage socialization.
- See the care plan for Risk for **Loneliness.**

**Pediatric**
- Assess for experiences of bullying and/or cyberbullying.
- Encourage limits on technology and social media use for children and adolescents.
- Provide positive social support and assist the child to identify supportive adults in their lives.
- Promote adequate sleep time.
- ▲ Refer children and adolescents to mental health treatment as necessary.
- ▲ Refer parents of disabled or seriously ill children to support groups.

**Geriatric**
- The interventions described previously may be adapted for use with older clients.
- Assess for risks and experiences associated with social isolation.
- Identify social engagement activities such as volunteering, engaging in social activities, and growing spirituality that are acceptable to the client.
- ▲ Refer client to pet therapy or consider pet ownership if feasible.

• = Independent        ▲ = Collaborative

- Consider telephone outreach for isolated older individuals.
- Consider use of technology such as computers, video conferencing, Internet, or apps to alleviate or reduce loneliness or social isolation among older adults.
- Implement fall precautions for clients experiencing social isolation.

**Multicultural**
- The interventions described previously may be adapted for use with diverse clients.
- Assess for experiences of interpersonal and institutional racism.

**Home Care**
- The interventions described previously may be adapted for home care use.
- Assist clients to interact and engage with neighbors when they move to a supported housing community.

**Client/Family Teaching and Discharge Planning**
- See the care plan for **Caregiver** Role Strain and Risk for **Loneliness.**

# Chronic Sorrow

**Domain 9** Coping/stress tolerance    **Class 2** Coping responses

**NANDA-I Definition**

Cyclical, recurring, and potentially progressive pattern of pervasive sadness experienced (by a parent, caregiver, individual with chronic illness or disability) in response to continual loss, throughout the trajectory of an illness or disability.

**Defining Characteristics**

Expresses feeling that interferes with well-being; overwhelming negative feelings; sadness

**Related Factors**

Disability management crisis; illness management crisis; missed milestones; missed opportunities

**At-Risk Population**

Individuals experiencing developmental crisis; individuals experiencing loss of significant other; individuals working in caregiver role for prolonged period of time

**Associated Conditions**

Chronic disability; chronic disease

**Client Outcomes**

**Client Will (Specify Time Frame)**
- Express appropriate feelings of guilt, fear, anger, or sadness
- Identify problems associated with sorrow (e.g., changes in appetite, insomnia, nightmares, loss of libido, decreased energy, alteration in activity levels)

• = Independent          ▲ = Collaborative

- Seek help in dealing with grief-associated problems
- Plan for the future one day at a time
- Function at normal developmental level

**Nursing Interventions**

- Determine the client's degree of sorrow.
- Assess for the four discrete stages of grieving in clients with chronic disease.
- Provide coping strategies for caregivers who may experience chronic sorrow.
- Develop a trusting relationship to care for clients with chronic sorrow.
- Provide information about support groups and counseling.
- Encourage use of positive coping techniques:
- ▲ Refer the client for mental health services as needed.
- ▲ Refer clients for financial assistance as needed.

**Pediatric**

- Encourage the parents of children with uncommon diseases to use online resources to manage their chronic sorrow.
- Educate parents that an increase in chronic sorrow can occur after stressful events.
- Nurses should assess for chronic sorrow and discuss coping strategies for parents of children who have been in the neonatal intensive care unit (NICU).
- Educate parents that children may grieve differently than adults.
- ▲ Refer grieving children to peer support groups.
- Encourage children experiencing grief to participate in bereavement activities and camps.
- Encourage children who are grieving to participate in other forms of therapy, in addition to individual counseling and psychotherapy.
- Help the adolescent with chronic sorrow determine sources of support and refer for counseling if needed.
- Provide family-centered care to parents of children with disabilities, and encourage parents to attend support groups.
- Encourage parents with chronic sorrow to participate in an online support group and learn coping strategies.
- Parents of children with chronic illnesses may experience chronic sorrow.
- Provide information to parents who are experiencing chronic sorrow.
- Respite care can be beneficial for parents of children with chronic illnesses.
- Recognize that mothers who have a miscarriage or lose an infant often grieve and experience sorrow.

• = Independent        ▲ = Collaborative

**Geriatric**
- Identify previous losses and assess the client for depression.
- Evaluate the social support system of the older client and refer for bereavement counseling if needed.

**Home Care**
- In-home bereavement follow-up by nurses should be considered if available.
- Assess the client for depression and refer for mental health services if appropriate.
- Provide empathetic communication for family/caregivers.
- The interventions described previously may be adapted for home care use.
- See care plans for Chronic Low **Self-Esteem**, Risk for **Loneliness**, and **Hopelessness**.

## Spiritual Distress

**Domain 10** Life principles     **Class 3** Value/belief/action congruence

### NANDA-I Definition

A state of suffering related to the impaired ability to integrate meaning and purpose in life through connections with self, others, the world, or a superior being.

### Defining Characteristics

Anger behaviors; crying; decreased expression of creativity; disinterested in nature; dysomnias; excessive guilt; expresses alienation; expresses anger; expresses anger toward power greater than self; expresses concern about beliefs; expresses concern about the future; expresses concern about values system; expresses concerns about family; expresses feeling abandoned by power greater than self; expresses feeling of emptiness; expresses feeling unloved; expresses feeling worthless; expresses insufficient courage; expresses loss of confidence; expresses loss of control; expresses loss of hope; expresses loss of serenity; expresses need for forgiveness; expresses regret; expresses suffering; fatigue; fear; impaired ability for introspection; inability to experience transcendence; maladaptive grieving; perceived loss of meaning in life; questions identity; questions meaning of life; questions meaning of suffering; questions own dignity; refuses to interact with others

### Related Factors

Altered religious ritual; altered spiritual practice; anxiety; barrier to experiencing love; cultural conflict; depressive symptoms; difficulty accepting the aging process; inadequate environmental control; inadequate interpersonal relations; loneliness; loss of independence; low self-esteem; pain;

perception of having unfinished business; self-alienation; separation from support system; social alienation; sociocultural deprivation; stressors; substance misuse

## At-Risk Population

Individuals experiencing birth of a child; individuals experiencing death of a significant other; individuals experiencing infertility; individuals experiencing life transition; individuals experiencing racial conflict; individuals experiencing unexpected life event; individuals exposed to death; individuals exposed to natural disaster; individuals exposed to traumatic events; individuals receiving bad news; individuals receiving terminal care; individuals with low educational level

## Associated Conditions

Chronic disease; depression; loss of body part; loss of function of a body part; treatment regimen

## Client Outcomes

### Client Will (Specify Time Frame)

- Express meaning and purpose in life
- Express sense of hope in the future
- Express sense of connectedness with self
- Express sense of connectedness with family/friends
- Express ability to forgive
- Express acceptance of health status
- Find meaning in relationships with others
- Find meaning in relationship with a higher power
- Find meaning in personal and health care treatment choices

## Nursing Interventions

- Observe clients for cues indicating difficulties in finding meaning, purpose, or hope in life.
- Observe seriously ill clients with poor prognosis or life-changing conditions for loss of meaning, purpose, and hope in life.
- Promote a sense of love, caring, and compassion in nursing encounters.
- Be physically present and actively listen to the client.
- Assist clients to participate in their usual religious rituals or practices that support coping with cancer and its treatment.
- Help the client find a reason for living, be available for support, and promote hope.
- Respect the client's beliefs; avoid imposing your own spiritual beliefs on the client. Be aware of your own belief systems and accept the client's spirituality.
- Monitor and promote supportive social contacts and spiritual and religious practices.

• = Independent        ▲ = Collaborative

- Integrate and assist family in searching for meaning in the client's health care situation.
- Offer spiritual support to family and caregivers.
- Screen for spiritual needs and if a need arises, offer chaplain referral.
- Support mind–body interventions (e.g., meditation, guided imagery, relaxation, massage). Support outdoor activities.
- Encourage journaling.
- Provide privacy or a "sacred space."
- Integrate spiritual care in multiprofessional palliative care teams.
- Encourage life review at end of life, including recalling, evaluating, and integrating life experiences.

**Geriatric**
- Offer opportunities to practice one's religion.

**Pediatric**
- Offer adolescents with cancer opportunities for reflection to express their spirituality and spiritual needs to enhance efficient coping strategies.
- Foster spiritual activities among adolescents.

**Multicultural**
- Recognize the importance of spirituality and provide culturally competent spiritual care to specific populations:
  - African American
  - Latino/Hispanic
  - Muslim
  - Veterans of armed services. Recognize the unique spiritual needs of veterans and provide spiritual support or appropriate referrals.

**Home Care**
- All the nursing interventions described previously apply in the home setting.

## Risk for Spiritual Distress

**Domain 10** Life principles    **Class 3** Value/belief/action congruence
### NANDA-I Definition

Susceptible to an impaired ability to integrate meaning and purpose in life through connectedness within self, literature, nature, and/or a power greater than oneself, which may compromise health.

### Risk Factors

Altered religious ritual; altered spiritual practice; anxiety; barrier to experiencing love; cultural conflict; depressive symptoms; difficulty accepting the aging process; inadequate environmental control; inadequate interpersonal relations; loneliness; loss of independence; low self-esteem; pain; perception of having unfinished business; self-alienation; separation from support system; social alienation; sociocultural deprivation; stressors; substance misuse

## At-Risk Population

Individuals experiencing birth of a child; individuals experiencing death of significant other; individuals experiencing infertility; individuals experiencing life transition; individuals experiencing racial conflict; individuals experiencing unexpected life event; individuals exposed to death; individuals exposed to natural disaster; individuals exposed to traumatic events; individuals receiving bad news; individuals receiving terminal care; individuals with low educational level

## Associated Conditions

Chronic disease, depression; loss of a body part; loss of function of a body part; treatment regimen

## Client Outcomes and Nursing Interventions

Refer to care plan for **Spiritual** Distress.

# Readiness for Enhanced Spiritual Well-Being

**S** **Domain 10** Life principles    **Class 2** Beliefs

## NANDA-I Definition

A pattern of integrating meaning and purpose in life through connectedness with self, others, art, music, literature, nature, and/or a power greater than oneself which can be strengthened.

## Defining Characteristics

Expresses desire to enhance acceptance; expresses desire to enhance capacity to self-comfort; expresses desire to enhance comfort in one's faith; expresses desire to enhance connection with nature; expresses desire to enhance connection with power greater than self; expresses desire to enhance coping; expresses desire to enhance courage; expresses desire to enhance creative energy; expresses desire to enhance forgiveness from others; expresses desire to enhance harmony in the environment; expresses desire to enhance hope; expresses desire to enhance inner peace; expresses desire to enhance interaction with significant other; expresses desire to enhance joy; expresses desire to enhance love; expresses desire to enhance love of others; expresses desire to enhance meditative practice; expresses desire to enhance mystical experiences; expresses desire to enhance oneness with nature; expresses desire to enhance oneness with power greater than self; expresses desire to enhance participation in religious practices; expresses desire to enhance peace with power greater than self; expresses desire to enhance prayerfulness; expresses desire to enhance reverence; expresses desire to enhance satisfaction with life; expresses desire to enhance self-awareness; expresses desire to enhance self-forgiveness; expresses desire to enhance sense of awe; expresses desire to enhance sense of harmony within oneself; expresses desire to enhance sense of identity; expresses desire to enhance sense of magic in the environment; expresses desire to enhance serenity; expresses desire to enhance service to others; expresses desire to enhance strength in one's faith; expresses desire to enhance surrender

## Client Outcomes

### Client Will (Specify Time Frame)

- Express hope
- Express sense of meaning and purpose in life
- Express peace and serenity
- Express love
- Express acceptance
- Express surrender
- Express forgiveness of self and others
- Express satisfaction with philosophy of life
- Express joy
- Express courage
- Describe being able to cope
- Describe use of spiritual practices
- Describe providing service to others
- Describe interaction with spiritual leaders, friends, and family
- Describe appreciation for art, music, literature, and nature

**S**

## Nursing Interventions

- ▲ Perform a spiritual assessment that includes the client's relationship with God, meaning and purpose in life, religious affiliation, and any other significant beliefs.
- Be present and actively listen to the client.
- Encourage the client to engage in other spiritual meditative or mind–body practices.
- Coordinate or encourage nurses to participate in spiritual care education courses and simulation.
- Perform actions to address spiritual need.
- Encourage clients to reflect on what is meaningful to them in life.
- Offer spiritual support to family and caregivers.
- Offer opportunities to facilitate religious or spiritual practices, including reflection, prayer, and relaxation techniques with deep breathing and listening to scripture verses.

• = Independent          ▲ = Collaborative

- Support spiritual practices, including meditation, guided imagery, journaling, relaxation, and involvement in art, music, or poetry.
- Encourage expressions of spirituality.
- Encourage integration of spirituality in healthy lifestyle choices.

**Geriatric**

▲ Offer opportunities to practice one's religion.
- Encourage social relationships and connections with family for institutionalized older adults.
- For those with chronic disease, encourage individual spiritual practices that promote meaning and peace.
▲ For those with terminal illness, encourage clients to attend meaning-centered psychotherapy, spiritual therapy intervention, life review, dignity therapy, yoga, meditation, and mind-body stress reduction if appropriate.
- During bereavement, encourage bereavement life review to promote spiritual well-being and alleviate depression.

**Pediatric**

- Offer adolescents with cancer opportunities for reflection and storytelling to express their spirituality and spiritual needs to enhance efficient coping strategies.
- Foster spiritual activities among adolescents.

**Multicultural**

- Recognize the importance of spirituality and provide culturally competent spiritual care to specific populations:
  ○ African American
  ○ Armed forces
  ○ Chinese
  ○ Homeless
  ○ Indonesian
  ○ Latino/Hispanic
  ○ Thai

**Home Care**

- All the nursing interventions described previously apply in the home setting.

# Impaired Standing

**Domain 4** Activity/rest     **Class 2** Activity/exercise
**NANDA-I Definition**

Limitation of ability to independently and purposefully attain and/or maintain the body in an upright position from feet to head.

• = Independent          ▲ = Collaborative

## Defining Characteristics

Difficulty adjusting position of one or both lower limbs on uneven surface; difficulty attaining postural balance; difficulty extending one or both hips; difficulty extending one or both knees; difficulty flexing one or both hips; difficulty flexing one or both knees; difficulty maintaining postural balance; difficulty moving one or both hips; difficulty moving one or both knees; difficulty stressing torso with body weight

## Related Factors

Excessive emotional disturbance; insufficient energy; insufficient muscle strength; insufficient physical endurance; malnutrition; obesity; pain; self-imposed relief posture

## Associated Conditions

Circulatory perfusion disorder; impaired metabolism; injury to lower extremity; neurological disorder; prescribed posture; sarcopenia, surgical procedures

## Client Outcomes

### Client Will (Specify Time Frame)

- Demonstrate optimal independence and safety when standing
- Demonstrate the proper use of assistive devices
- State benefits of standing

## Nursing Interventions

- Encourage clients to stand at intervals throughout the day.
- Advise clients of the physical and psychological benefits of being upright and active.
- Educate clients about the health risks of sitting.
- Geriatric
- Advise older clients who have difficulty standing to use assistive devices.
- Encourage the use of trunk exercises along with walking and balance exercises in older adults.
- Encourage clients who are unable to stand to consider chair exercises.
- Encourage poststroke clients to participate in rehabilitation interventions that promote standing.
- Mechanical sit-stand lifts can be used with clients who require assistance with transfers.
- Educate older adults who have fallen about the need for balance and muscle training of the ankle joint.
- Educate adults older than age 80 years on the need for vitamin D.
- Assess for risk of falls among older adults with difficulty standing.
- Advise older clients who are at risk for falls to avoid doing multiple tasks at one time while standing.

S

• = Independent　　▲ = Collaborative

**Client/Family Teaching and Discharge Planning**

- Educate clients that standing can be beneficial for their health.
- Teach clients about the need to take frequent breaks when standing for long periods.
- Instruct clients about the use of yoga for individuals who have difficulty with standing balance.

## Stress Overload

**Domain 9** Coping/stress tolerance    **Class 2** Coping responses

### NANDA-I Definition

Excessive amounts and types of demands that require action.

### Defining Characteristics

Difficulty with decision-making; expresses feeling pressured; expresses increased anger; expresses tension; impaired functioning; increased impatience; negative impact from stress

### Related Factors

Inadequate resources; repeated stressors; stressors

### Client Outcomes

**Client Will (Specify Time Frame)**

- Review the amounts and types of stressors in daily living
- Identify stressors that can be modified or eliminated
- Mobilize social supports to facilitate lower stress levels
- Reduce stress levels through use of health promoting behaviors and other strategies

### Nursing Interventions

- Assist client in identification of stress overload during vulnerable life events.
- Listen actively to descriptions of stressors and the stress response.
- In younger adult women, assess interpersonal stressors.
- Categorize stressors as modifiable or nonmodifiable.
- Help clients modify or mitigate stressors identified as modifiable.
- Help clients distinguish among short-term, chronic, and secondary stressors.
- Provide information as needed to reduce stress responses to acute and chronic illnesses.
- ▲ Explore possible therapeutic approaches such as cognitive-behavioral therapy, biofeedback, neurofeedback, acupuncture, pharmacological agents, and complementary and alternative therapies.
- Help the client to reframe his or her perceptions of some of the stressors.

• = Independent        ▲ = Collaborative

- Assist the client to mobilize social supports for dealing with recent stressors.

**Pediatric**

- With children, nurses should work with parents to help them reduce children's stressors.
- Help children to manage their feelings related to self-concept.
- Help children to deal with bullies and other sources of violence in schools and neighborhoods.
- Help children to manage the complexities of chronic illnesses.

**Geriatric**

- Assess for chronic stress with older adults and provide a variety of stress relief techniques.
- ▲ Encourage older adults to seek appropriate counseling.

**Multicultural**

- Review cultural beliefs and acculturation level in relation to perceived stressors.

**Home Care**

- The preceding interventions may be adapted for home care use.
- Develop community-based programs for stress management as needed for groups with increased risk of stress overload (e.g., firefighters, policemen, military personnel, nurses).
- Support and encourage neighborhood stability.

**Client/Family Teaching and Discharge Planning**

- Diagnose the possibility of stress overload before teaching.
- Establish readiness for learning.
- Provide manageable amounts of information at the appropriate educational level.
- Evaluate the need for additional teaching and learning experiences.

# Acute Substance Withdrawal Syndrome

**Domain 9** Coping/stress tolerance    **Class 3** Neurobehavioral stress

## NANDA-I Definition

Serious, multifactorial sequelae following abrupt cessation of an addictive compound.

## Defining Characteristics

Acute confusion (00128); anxiety (00146); disturbed sleep pattern (00198); nausea (00134); risk for electrolyte imbalance (00195); risk for injury (00035)

• = Independent    ▲ = Collaborative

## Related Factors

Developed dependence to addictive substances; excessive use of an addictive substance over time; malnutrition; sudden cessation of an addictive substance

## At-Risk Population

Individuals with history of withdrawal symptoms; older adults

## Associated Conditions

Significant comorbidity

## Client Outcomes

### Client Will (Specify Time Frame)

- Stabilize and remain free from physical injury
- Verbalize effects of substances on body
- Maintain vital signs and laboratory values within normal range
- Verbalize importance of adequate nutrition

## Nursing Interventions

### Alcohol-Induced Withdrawal Syndrome

- Assess for the client's pattern of alcohol use, last drink, and current blood alcohol levels.
- Implement seizure precautions.
- Rule out other causes of symptoms.
- Monitor vital signs.
- Assess for progression of withdrawal symptoms such as insomnia, anxiety, nausea/vomiting, tremulousness, headache, diaphoresis, palpitations, increased body temperature, tachycardia, and hypertension.
- Monitor severity of withdrawal symptoms with the Clinical Institute Withdrawal Assessment (CIWA-Ar).
- Evaluate the client for progression to delirium tremens (DTs).
- Assess nutritional status for risk of malnutrition. Assess for thiamine (B$_1$) deficiency, which is associated with chronic alcohol abuse, folate deficiency, and vitamin D deficiency associated with a history of inadequate exposure to sunlight. Consult with health care provider as needed for supplement order.
- Address hydration needs.
- Determine hepatic and renal functioning before administration of medications.

### Opioid-Induced Withdrawal Syndrome

- Assess for the client's opioid of choice, last use, and current withdrawal symptoms.
- Monitor severity of withdrawal symptoms with the Clinical Opiate Withdrawal Scale (COWS).

• = Independent        ▲ = Collaborative

- Nurses should wait to administer the first dose of buprenorphine to opioid-dependent clients until clients are experiencing mild to moderate opioid withdrawal symptoms.
- Assess and manage early opioid withdrawal symptoms (agitation, anxiety, insomnia, muscle aches, increased lacrimation, rhinorrhea, sweating, and yawning) and late opioid withdrawal symptoms (abdominal cramping, diarrhea, pupillary dilation, nausea, vomiting, and piloerection).
- Monitor vital signs.
- Teach the client about the anticipated withdrawal symptoms and opioid cravings while offering support and encouragement.
▲ Monitor laboratory reports and report to health care provider.
▲ Refer client for buprenorphine, methadone, or naltrexone treatment.

**Benzodiazepine-Induced Withdrawal Syndrome**
- Assess for the client's last benzodiazepine use and current withdrawal symptoms.
- Implement seizure precautions.
- Rule out delirium from other causes or other withdrawal syndromes.
▲ Anticipate use of the same treatment protocols as for alcohol withdrawal and use of a long-acting benzodiazepine in tapering doses over time.

**Cocaine/Methamphetamine-Induced Withdrawal Syndrome**
- Assess for the client's last stimulant use and current withdrawal symptoms.

**Cannabis-Induced Withdrawal Syndrome**
- Assess for the client's last cannabis use and current withdrawal symptoms.
- Direct nursing actions to address anxiety, irritability, sleep disturbances, and decreased appetite.

**Nicotine-Induced Withdrawal Syndrome**
- Assess for the client's last nicotine use and current withdrawal symptoms.
- Rule out nicotine withdrawal as the cause of delirium in critically ill clients.

**All Withdrawal Syndromes**
- Obtain a drug and/or alcohol history using a tool such as the AUDIT-C or the DAST-10.
- Implement and follow institutional withdrawal protocols.
- Assess for signs of recent trauma or head injury.
- Assess the client's level of consciousness, monitor for changes in behavior, and orient to reality as needed.
- Assess vital signs and monitor for existing medical conditions and current medications.

• = Independent          ▲ = Collaborative

- Assess and monitor for expression of psychological distress.
- Collect urine/serum samples for laboratory tests.
- Address craving for substances with mindfulness-based techniques.
- Respond to agitated behavior with deescalation techniques.
- Administer as-needed (PRN) medications for agitation and symptom control as ordered.
- Provide a quiet room without dark shadows, noises, or other excessive stimuli.
- Provide suicide precautions and 1:1 staffing for clients who are delirious or who may present a danger to themselves or others.

**Client/Family Teaching and Discharge Planning**

▲ After withdrawal symptoms have subsided, refer the client to substance use treatment and long-term management.

▲ Refer for smoking cessation services that target nicotine craving.

# Risk for Acute Substance Withdrawal Syndrome

**Domain 9** Coping/stress tolerance     **Class 3** Neurobehavioral stress

**NANDA-I Definition**

Susceptible to serious, multifactorial sequelae following abrupt cessation of an addictive compound, which may compromise health.

**Risk Factors**

Developed dependence to addictive substance; excessive use of an addictive substance over time; malnutrition; sudden cessation of an addictive substance

**At-Risk Population**

Individuals with history of withdrawal symptoms; older adults

**Associated Conditions**

Significant comorbidity

**Client Outcomes**

**Client Will (Specify Time Frame)**

- Stabilize and remain free from physical injury
- Verbalize effects of substances on body
- Maintain vital signs and laboratory values within normal range
- Verbalize importance of adequate nutrition

**Nursing Interventions**

**Risk for Alcohol-Induced Withdrawal Syndrome**

- Assess for the client's pattern of alcohol use, last drink, and current blood alcohol levels.
- Implement seizure precautions.

• = Independent          ▲ = Collaborative

- Rule out other causes of symptoms.
- Monitor vital signs.
- Assess for progression of withdrawal symptoms such as insomnia, anxiety, nausea/vomiting, tremulousness, headache, diaphoresis, palpitations, increased body temperature, tachycardia, and hypertension.
- Monitor severity of withdrawal symptoms with the Clinical Institute Withdrawal Assessment (CIWA-Ar).
- Evaluate the client for progression to delirium tremens (DTs).
- Assess nutritional status for risk of malnutrition, thiamine ($B_1$) deficiency associated with chronic alcohol abuse, folate deficiency, and vitamin D deficiency–associated history of inadequate exposure to sunlight. Consult with health care provider as needed for supplement order.
- Address hydration needs.
- Determine hepatic and renal functioning before administration of medications.

**Risk for Opioid-Induced Withdrawal Syndrome**
- Assess for the client's opioid of choice, last use, and current withdrawal symptoms.
- Monitor severity of withdrawal symptoms with the Clinical Opiate Withdrawal Scale (COWS).
- Assess and manage early opioid withdrawal symptoms (agitation, anxiety, insomnia, muscle aches, increased lacrimation, rhinorrhea, sweating, and yawning) and late opioid withdrawal symptoms (abdominal cramping, diarrhea, pupillary dilation, nausea, vomiting, and piloerection).
- Monitor vital signs.
- Clients should be taught about risk of relapse and other safety concerns from using opioid withdrawal management as stand-alone treatment for opioid use disorder.
- Teach the client about the anticipated withdrawal symptoms and opioid cravings, while offering support and encouragement.
- ▲ Monitor laboratory reports and report to health care provider.
- ▲ Refer client for buprenorphine or methadone treatment.

**Risk for Benzodiazepine-Induced Withdrawal Syndrome**
- Assess for the client's last benzodiazepine use and current withdrawal symptoms.
- Implement seizure precautions.
- Rule out delirium from other causes or other withdrawal syndromes.

• = Independent          ▲ = Collaborative

▲ Anticipate use of the same treatment protocols as for alcohol withdrawal and use of a long-acting benzodiazepine in tapering doses over time.

**Risk for Cocaine/Methamphetamine-Induced Withdrawal Syndrome**

• Assess for the client's last stimulant use and current withdrawal symptoms.

**Risk for Cannabis-Induced Withdrawal Syndrome**

• Assess for the client's last cannabis use and current withdrawal symptoms.
• Direct nursing actions to address anxiety, irritability, sleep disturbances, and decreased appetite.

**Risk for Nicotine-Induced Withdrawal Syndrome**

• Assess for the client's last nicotine use and current withdrawal symptoms.
• Rule out nicotine withdrawal as the cause of delirium in critically ill clients.

**All Withdrawal Syndromes**

• Obtain a drug and/or alcohol history using a tool such as the AUDIT-C or the DAST-10.
• Implement and follow institutional withdrawal protocols.
• Assess for signs of recent trauma or head injury.
• Assess the client's level of consciousness, monitor for changes in behavior, and orient to reality as needed.
• Assess vital signs and monitor for existing medical conditions and current medications.
• Assess and monitor for expression of psychological distress.
• Collect urine/serum samples for laboratory tests.
• Address craving for substances with mindfulness-based techniques.
• Respond to agitated behavior with deescalation techniques.
• Administer as-needed (PRN) medications for agitation and symptom control as ordered.
• Provide a quiet room without dark shadows, noises, or other excessive stimuli.
• Provide suicide precautions and 1:1 staffing for clients who are delirious or who may present a danger to themselves or others.

**Client/Family Teaching and Discharge Planning**

▲ After withdrawal symptoms have subsided, refer client to substance use treatment.
▲ Refer for smoking cessation services that target nicotine craving.

• = Independent          ▲ = Collaborative

# Ineffective Infant Suck-Swallow Response

**Domain 2** Nutrition    **Class 1** Ingestion

## NANDA-I Definition

Impaired ability of an infant to suck or to coordinate the suck-swallow response.

## Defining Characteristics

Arrhythmia; bradycardic events; choking; circumoral cyanosis; excessive coughing; finger splaying; flaccidity; gagging; hiccups; hyperextension of extremities; impaired ability to initiate an effective suck; impaired ability to sustain an effective suck; impaired motor tone; inability to coordinate sucking, swallowing, and breathing; irritability; nasal flaring; oxygen desaturation; pallor; subcostal retraction; time-out signals; use of accessory muscles of respiration

## Related Factors

Hypoglycemia; hypothermia; hypotonia; inappropriate positioning; unsatisfactory sucking behavior

## At-Risk Population

Infants born to mothers with substance misuse; infants delivered using obstetrical forceps; infants delivered using obstetrical vacuum extraction; infants experiencing prolonged hospitalization; premature infants

## Associated Conditions

Convulsive episodes; gastroesophageal reflux; high flow oxygen by nasal cannula; lacerations during delivery; low Appearance, Pulse, Grimace, Activity, & Respiration (APGAR) scores; neurological delay; neurological impairment; oral hypersensitivity; oropharyngeal deformity; prolonged enteral nutrition

## Client Outcomes

**Infant Will (Specify Time Frame)**

- Consume adequate calories that will result in appropriate weight gain and optimal growth and development
- Have opportunities for skin-to-skin experiences
- Have opportunities for "trophic" (i.e., small volume of breast milk/ formula) enteral feedings prior to full oral feedings
- Progress to stable, neurobehavioral organization (e.g., motor, state, self-regulation, attention-interaction)
- Demonstrate presence of mature oral reflexes that are necessary for safe feeding
- Progress to safe, self-regulated oral feedings
- Coordinate the suck-swallow-breathe sequence while nippling

• = Independent          ▲ = Collaborative

**S**

- Display clear behavioral cues related to hunger and satiety
- Display approach/engagement cues, with minimal avoidance/disengagement cues
- Have opportunities to pace own feeding, taking breaks as needed
- Display evidence of being in the "quiet-alert" state while nippling
- Progress to and engage in mutually positive parent/caregiver–infant/child interactions during feedings

**Parent/Family Will (Specify Time Frame)**

- Recognize necessity of adequate calories for appropriate weight gain and optimal growth and development
- Learn to read and respond contingently to infant's behavioral cues (e.g., hunger, satiety, approach/engagement, stress/avoidance/disengagement)
- Learn strategies that promote organized infant behavior
- Learn appropriate positioning and handling techniques
- Learn effective ways to relieve stress behaviors during nippling
- Learn ways to help infant coordinate suck-swallow-breathe sequence (i.e., external pacing techniques)
- Engage in mutually positive interactions with infant during feeding
- Recognize ways to facilitate effective feedings: feed in quiet-alert state; keep length of feeding appropriate; burp; prepare/structure environment; recognize signs of sensory overload; encourage self-regulation; respect need for breaks and breathing pauses; avoid pulling and twisting nipple during pauses; allow infant to resume sucking when ready; provide oral support (cheek and/or jaw) as needed; use appropriate nipple hole size and flow rate

**Nursing Interventions**

- Refer to care plans for Disorganized **Infant** Behavior, Ineffective **Breastfeeding**, Interrupted **Breastfeeding**, Insufficient **Breast Milk Production**, Ineffective Infant **Feeding** Dynamics as needed.

**Mother–Baby Dyad Interventions**

- Assess for any factors that may disrupt successful breastfeeding after birth.
- Provide opportunities for skin-to-skin care.
- Allow the stable newborn to breastfeed within the first 30 to 60 minutes after birth.
- Encourage rooming-in.
- Assess and document the effectiveness of mixed breastfeeding and bottle-feeding.
- Position infant in semiupright position, with head, shoulders, and hips in a straight line facing the mother with the infant's nose level with the mother's nipple.

• = Independent        ▲ = Collaborative

▲ Refer to a multiprofessional team (e.g., neonatal/pediatric nutritionist, physical or occupational therapist, speech pathologist, lactation specialist) as needed.

**Maternal Interventions**
• Assess for any maternal issues related to breastfeeding.
• Support the mother's confidence in her ability to breastfeed.
• Educate mothers to recognize and respond to their infant's cues for feeding.
• Assess for proper latch at the breast.
• Determine the reason for the poor latch, including inverted nipples, flat nipples, ankyloglossia, small mandible, or nipple confusion, and offer alternatives to mothers for unsuccessful latch.
• Council mothers on various feeding positions to encourage successful latch.

**Infant Interventions**
• Observe coordination of infant's suck, swallow, and gag reflex.
• Assess for neonatal signs of inadequate milk supply/intake.

**Premature Infants/Infants Requiring Specialty/Intensive Care**
• Provide developmentally supportive neonatal intensive care for preterm infants.
• Foster direct breastfeeding as early as possible and enable the first oral feed to be at the breast in the neonatal intensive care unit (NICU).
• Before the infant is ready for oral feedings, implement gavage feedings (or other alternative) as ordered, using expressed breast milk whenever possible.
• Provide a naturalistic environment for tube feedings (naso-orogastric, gavage, or other) that approximates a pleasurable oral feeding experience: hold infant in semiupright/flexed position; offer nonnutritive sucking; pace feedings; allow for semidemand feedings contingent with infant cues; offer rest breaks; burp, as appropriate.
• Continue to provide support for the mother discharged before the infant by encouraging skin-to-skin technique and regular breastfeeding.

**Home Care**
• The previously mentioned appropriate interventions may be adapted for home care use.
• Provide breastfeeding mothers instruction on the technique of expressing milk by hand or pump.
▲ Provide lists of various local peer support groups and services (e.g., mother-to-mother support groups such as La Leche League; hospital/clinic-based support groups; and governmental supported groups such as Special Supplemental Nutrition Program for Women,

**S**

Infants, and Children [WIC] in the United States, with phone numbers, contact names, and addresses).

**Client/Family Teaching and Discharge Planning**

- Before discharge, anticipation of breastfeeding problems should be assessed based on maternal and/or infant risk factors.
- Include mothers and appropriate others (e.g., fathers, partners, grandmothers, support persons) in teaching of anticipatory guidance for key discharge issues.

# Risk for Sudden Infant Death

**Domain 11** Safety/protection    **Class 2** Physical injury

## NANDA-I Definition

Infant susceptible to unpredicted death.

## Risk Factors

Delayed prenatal care; inadequate prenatal care; inattentive to second-hand smoke; infant < 4 months placed in sitting devices for routine sleep; infant overheating; infant overwrapping; infant placed in prone position to sleep; infant placed in side-lying position to sleep; soft sleep surface; soft, loose objects placed near infant

## At-Risk Population

Boys; infants aged 2-4 months; infants exposed to alcohol in utero; infants exposed to cold climates; infants exposed to illicit drug in utero; infants fed with expressed breast milk; infants not breastfed exclusively; infants of African descent; infants whose mothers smoked during pregnancy; infants with postnatal exposure to alcohol; infants with postnatal exposure to illicit drug; low birth weight infants; Native American infants; premature infants

## Client Outcomes

**Client Will (Specify Time Frame)**

- Explain appropriate measures to prevent sudden infant death syndrome (SIDS)
- Demonstrate correct techniques for positioning and blanketing the infant, protecting the infant from harm

## Nursing Interventions

- Position the infant supine to sleep during naps and night; do not position in the prone position or side-lying position.
- Avoid overbundling, overheating, and swaddling the infant. The infant should not feel hot to touch.

**Home Care**

- Most of the interventions and client teaching information are relevant to home care.

• = Independent        ▲ = Collaborative

- Evaluate home for potential safety hazards, such as inappropriate cribs, cradles, or strollers.
- Determine where and how the child sleeps, and provide instructions on safe sleeping positions and environments as needed.

**Multicultural**

- Safe to Sleep recommendations should be tailored to include the mother's culture and experience, provided to all members of the family, and reviewed frequently.
- Provide teaching to African American mothers on how pacifier use reduces SIDS risk.
- Recommend to African American and Hispanic mothers the need to abstain from smoking during the prenatal period.

**Client/Family Teaching and Discharge Planning**

- Teach the safety guidelines for infant care in the previous interventions.
- Teach parents and caregivers the following measures for a Safe Infant Sleeping Environment recommended by the American Academy of Pediatrics (AAP) Task Force on Sudden Infant Death Syndrome (2016):
  - Place infant in supine positioning.
  - Use a firm sleep surface.
  - Room-sharing without bed-sharing.
  - Avoidance of soft bedding.
  - Avoid overheating.
  - Offer infant a pacifier.
  - Avoid smoke exposure during pregnancy and after birth.
  - Avoid alcohol and illicit drug use during pregnancy and after birth.
  - Infants should be immunized in accordance with AAP and Centers for Disease Control and Prevention (CDC) recommendations.
  - Do not use home cardiorespiratory monitors as a strategy to reduce the risk of SIDS.
  - Breastfeeding is a protective factor.
- Provide parents of both term and preterm infants with verbal and written education about SIDS and ways to reduce the risk of SIDS before discharge to home.
- Recommend breastfeeding.
- Teach the need to stop smoking during pregnancy and to not smoke around the infant. Do not allow the infant to be exposed to any secondhand smoke.

**S**

• = Independent          ▲ = Collaborative

# Risk for Suffocation

**Domain 11** Safety/protection     **Class 2** Physical injury

## NANDA-I Definition

Susceptible to inadequate air availability for inhalation, which may compromise health.

## Risk Factors

Access to empty refrigerator/freezer; eating large mouthfuls of food; excessive emotional disturbance; gas leak; inadequate knowledge of safety precautions; low-strung clothesline; pacifier around infant's neck; playing with plastic bag; propped bottle placed in infant's crib; small object in airway; smoking in bed; soft sleep surface; unattended in water; unvented fuel-burning heater; vehicle running in closed garage

## Associated Conditions

Altered olfactory function; face/neck disease; face/neck injury; impaired motor functioning

## Client Outcomes

**Client Will (Specify Time Frame)**

- Undertake appropriate measures to prevent suffocation
- Demonstrate correct techniques for emergency rescue maneuvers (e.g., Heimlich maneuver, rescue breathing, cardiopulmonary resuscitation [CPR]) and describe situations that require them

## Nursing Interventions

- Identify hospitalized clients at particular risk for suffocation, including the following:
  - Clients with altered levels of consciousness
  - Infants or young children
  - Clients with developmental delays
  - Clients with mental illness, especially schizophrenia
  - Clients who have been physically or chemically restrained
- Practice caution with physical restraints and follow all institutional policies and procedures as restraint use has been associated with mortality.
- Institute safety measures such as proper positioning and feeding precautions. See the care plans for Risk for **Aspiration** and Impaired **Swallowing** for additional interventions.
- Vigilance and special protective measures are necessary for clients at greater risk for suffocation.

### Pediatric

- Provide families with education about interventions and modifiable risk factors to prevent infant suffocation:
  - Use a firm sleep surface with a fitted sheet.

• = Independent          ▲ = Collaborative

○ Do not place infants in adult beds, on couches, or in armchairs to sleep.

○ Do not overbundle the infant.

○ Avoid soft bedding and do not have loose bedding in crib with infant.

○ Use caution with infant head coverings and keep blanket end at infant chest.

○ Do not practice bed sharing or co-sleeping with infants.

• Conduct risk factor identification, noting special circumstances in which preventive or protective measures are indicated. Note the presence of environmental hazards, including plastic bags; cribs with slats wider than 2 inches; ill-fitting crib mattresses that can allow the infant to become wedged between the mattress and crib; pillows/loose bedding in cribs; placement of crib near windows with blinds or cords; co-sleeping; abandoned large appliances such as refrigerators, dishwashers, or freezers; clothing with cords or hoods that can become entangled; bibs; pacifiers on a string; necklaces in infants and children; drapery cords; and pull-toy strings.

• Counsel families to evaluate household furniture for safety, including large dressers, televisions, bookshelves, and appliances, which may need to be anchored to the wall to prevent the child from climbing on the furniture and it falling forward and suffocating the child.

• Counsel families about items that are most associated with choking in children.

• Counsel families to keep the following items away from the sight and reach of infants and toddlers: buttons, beads, jewelry, pins, nails, marbles, coins, stones, magnets, and balloons. Choose age-appropriate toys and games for children and check for any small parts that may be a choking hazard because children have the need to put everyday objects in their mouths.

• Stress water and pool safety and stress including vigilant, uninterrupted parental supervision.

• Underscore the necessity of not allowing children to play with or near electric garage doors and of keeping garage door openers out of the reach of young children.

• For adolescents, watch for signs of depression that could result in suicide by suffocation.

**Geriatric**

• Monitor client during feeding for coughing or choking when eating and drinking, being unable to chew food properly, and losing food and drink from the front of the mouth.

• = Independent          ▲ = Collaborative

- A swallowing assessment by a speech-language pathologist is recommended in clients with suspected or confirmed dysphagia to ensure the appropriate type and consistency of diet to mitigate choking and aspiration risk.
- Ensure proper positioning during and after feeding to decrease the risk of aspiration.
- Recognize that older adults in depression may use hanging, strangulation, and suffocation as a means of suicide.

**Home Care**
- Assess the home for potential safety hazards and refer as needed to community resources.
- Assist the family to develop an emergency preparedness plan for potential escape routes from the home in the event of detectors going off, fire, or other emergencies.

**Client/Family Teaching and Discharge Planning**
- Recommend that families who are seeking day care or in-home care for children, geriatric family members, or at-risk family members with developmental or functional disabilities inspect the environment for hazards and examine the first aid preparation and vigilance of providers.
- Ensure family members learn and practice rescue techniques, including treatment of choking and lack of breathing, as well as CPR.

**S**

# Risk for Suicidal Behavior

**Domain 11** Safety/protection    **Class 3** Violence
## NANDA-I Definition
Susceptible to self-injurious acts associated with some intent to die.
## Related Factors
### Behavioral
Apathy; difficulty asking for help; difficulty coping with unsatisfactory performance; difficulty expressing feelings; ineffective chronic pain self-management; self-injurious behavior; self-negligence; stockpiling of medication; substance misuse
### Psychological
Anxiety; depressive symptoms; hostility; expresses deep sadness; expresses frustration; expresses loneliness; low self-esteem; maladaptive grieving; perceived dishonor; perceived failure; reports excessive guilt; reports helplessness; reports hopelessness; reports unhappiness; suicidal ideation
### Situational
Easy access to weapon; loss of independence; loss of personal autonomy

• = Independent        ▲ = Collaborative

## Social

Dysfunctional family processes; inadequate social support; inappropriate peer pressure; legal difficulty; social deprivation; social devaluation; social isolation; unaddressed violence by others

## At-Risk Population

Adolescents; adolescents living in foster care; economically disadvantaged individuals; individuals changing a will; individuals experiencing situational crisis; individuals facing discrimination; individuals giving away possessions; individuals living alone; individuals obtaining potentially lethal materials; individuals preparing a will; individuals who frequently seek care for vague symptomatology; individuals with disciplinary problems; individuals with family history of suicide; individuals with history of suicide attempt; individuals with history of violence; individuals with sudden euphoric recovery from major depression; institutionalized individuals; men; Native American individuals; older adults

## Associated Conditions

Depression; mental disorders; physical illness; terminal illness

## Client Outcomes

### Client Will (Specify Time Frame)

- Not harm self
- Maintain connectedness in relationships
- Disclose and discuss suicidal ideas and plan if present; seek help
- Express decreased anxiety and control of impulses
- Talk about feelings; express anger appropriately
- Identify a safety plan
- Identify protective factors
- Refrain from using mood-altering substances
- Obtain no access to harmful objects
- Yield access to harmful objects
- Maintain self-control without supervision

## Nursing Interventions

The American Psychiatric Nurses Association (APNA, 2015) has adapted a set of essential competencies for psychiatric nurses, all of which can be useful for generalist nurses. These competencies have been incorporated in the following sections.

- Assess using suicide risk measures that are available for nurses.
- Before implementing interventions in the face of suicidal behavior, nurses should examine their own emotional responses to incidents of suicide to ensure that interventions will not be based on countertransference reactions.

• = Independent ▲ = Collaborative

- Pursue an understanding of suicide as a phenomenon at all levels of nursing practice.
- Assess for suicidal ideation when the history reveals the following: depression; substance abuse; bipolar disorder; schizophrenia; anxiety disorders, posttraumatic stress disorder, dissociative disorder, eating disorders, substance use disorders, or antisocial or other personality disorders; attempted suicide, current or past; recent stressful life events (divorce and/or separation, relocation, problems with children); recent unemployment; recent bereavement; adult or childhood physical or sexual abuse; LGBTQ+ identities, family history of suicide; and history of chronic trauma.
- Assess all medical clients and clients with chronic illnesses, traumatic injuries, or pain for their perception of health status and suicidal ideation.
- Be alert for the following warning signs of suicide: making statements such as, "I can't go on," "Nothing matters anymore," "I wish I were dead"; becoming depressed or withdrawn; behaving recklessly; getting affairs in order and giving away valued possessions; showing a marked change in behavior, attitudes, or appearance; abusing drugs or alcohol; and suffering a major loss or life change.
- Take suicide notes seriously and ask if a note was left in any previous suicide attempts. Consider themes of notes in determining appropriate interventions.
- Question family members regarding the preparatory actions mentioned.
- Determine the presence and degree of suicidal risk. A number of questions will elicit the necessary information: "Have you been thinking about hurting or killing yourself?" "How often do you have these thoughts and how long do they last?" "Do you have a plan?" "What is it?" "Do you have access to the means to carry out that plan?" "How likely is it that you could carry out the plan?" "Are there people or things that could prevent you from hurting yourself?" "What do you see in your future a year from now?" "Five years from now?" "What do you expect would happen if you died?" "What has kept you alive up to now?"
- Observe, record, and report any changes in mood or behavior that may signify increasing suicide risk and document results of regular surveillance checks.
- Develop a positive therapeutic relationship with the client; do not make promises that may not be kept. Clarify with the clients that anything they share will be communicated only to other staff involved in their care.

- Express desire to help client. Provide education about suicide and the effectiveness of intervention. Validate the client's experience of psychological pain while maintaining a safe environment for the client.
▲ Refer for mental health counseling and possible hospitalization if evidence of suicidal intent exists, which may include evidence of preparatory actions (e.g., obtaining a weapon, making a plan, putting affairs in order, giving away prized possessions, preparing a suicide note).
- Perform risk assessment for possible suicidality on admission to the hospital and thereafter during hospitalization. Alert treatment team to level of risk.
- Determine client's need for supervision and assign a hospitalized client to a room located near the nursing station.
- Search the newly hospitalized client and the client's personal belongings for weapons or potential weapons and hoarded medications during the inpatient admission procedure, as appropriate. Remove dangerous items.
- Monitor the client during the use of potential weapons (e.g., razor, scissors) and limit access to windows and exits unless locked and shatterproof, as appropriate.
- Increase surveillance of a hospitalized client at times when staffing is predictably low (e.g., staff meetings, change of shift report, periods of unit disruption).
- Ensure that all oncoming staff members have adequate information to assist the client, using the acronym SBARR.
▲ If imminent suicide is suspected or an attempt has occurred, call for assistance and do not leave the client alone. Client and staff safety will be served by assistance in the response. The client may attempt additional self-harm if left alone.
- Place the client in the least restrictive, safe, and monitored environment that allows for the necessary level of observation. Assess suicidal risk at least daily and more frequently as warranted.
▲ Refer for treatment and participate in the management of any mental illness or symptoms that may be contributing to the client's suicidal ideation or behavior.
▲ Verify that the client has taken medications as ordered (e.g., conduct mouth checks after medication administration).
▲ Maintain increased surveillance of the client whenever use of an antidepressant has been initiated or the dose increased.
- Involve the client in treatment planning and self-care management of psychiatric disorders.

• = Independent          ▲ = Collaborative

- Explore with the client all circumstances and motivations related to the suicidality. Listen to the client's own views on his or her problems.
- Explore with the client reasons to live and sources of hope.
- Keep discussions oriented to the present and future.
- ▲ Document client behavior in detail to support involuntary commitment or an overnight psychiatric observation program for an actively suicidal client.
- Use cognitive-behavioral techniques that help the client to modify thinking styles that promote depression, hopelessness, and a belief that suicide is a valid means of escaping the current situation.
- Engage the client in group interventions that can be useful to address recurrent suicide attempts.
- See the care plans for Risk for Self-Directed **Violence, Hopelessness,** and Risk for **Self-Mutilation.**

**Pediatric**

- The previously discussed interventions may be appropriate for pediatric clients.
- Assess specifically for bullying and cyberbullying.
- Assess for exposure to trauma and other adverse childhood experiences.
- Assess for exposure to suicide of a significant other.
- Assess for the presence of school victimization around lesbian, gay, bisexual, and transgender (LGBT) issues and be prepared to advocate for the client.
- Evaluate for the presence of self-mutilation and related risk factors. Refer to care plan for Risk for **Self-Mutilation** for additional information.
- Support the implementation of school-based suicide prevention programs.

**Geriatric**

- Evaluate the older client's perceived mental and physical health status and financial stressors.
- Explore with the client perceived pressures about being a burden or being burdensome.
- Conduct a thorough assessment of clients' medications.
- When assessing suicide risk factors, note a higher degree of risk for older men and for some older adults who have lost a loved one in the previous year.
- An older adult who shows self-destructive behaviors should be evaluated to rule out a diagnosis of dementia.
- ▲ Refer older adults in primary care settings for integrated care management.
- Consider telephone contacts as an effective intervention for suicidal older adults.

• = Independent          ▲ = Collaborative

**Multicultural**
- Assess for the influence of cultural beliefs, norms, and values on the client's perceptions of suicide and on the nurse's perception and approach to suicide.
- Validate the individual's feelings regarding concerns about the current crisis and family functioning.

**Home Care**
- Communicate the degree of risk to family and caregivers; assess the family and caregiving situation for the ability to protect the client and to understand the client's suicidal behavior.
- Assess access to lethal means in the home.
- Assist the client and family to develop a suicide safety plan that includes lethal means reduction, brief problem solving and coping skills, increasing social support, and identifying emergency contacts to use during a suicide crisis.

**Client/Family Teaching and Discharge Planning**
- Involve the family in discharge planning (e.g., illness/medication teaching, recognition of increasing suicidal risk, client's plan for dealing with recurring suicidal thoughts, community resources).
- Teach cognitive-behavioral activities to the client and family, such as active problem-solving, reframing (reappraising the situation from a different perspective), or thought stopping (in response to a negative thought, picturing a large stop sign and replacing the image with a prearranged positive alternative). Teach the client to confront his or her own negative thought patterns (or cognitive distortions), such as catastrophizing (expecting the very worst), dichotomous thinking (perceiving events in only one of two opposite categories), or magnification (placing distorted emphasis on a single event).
- ▲ Refer family members and friends to local mental health agencies and crisis intervention centers if the client has suicidal ideation or a suspicion of suicidal thoughts exists.
- ▲ In the event of successful suicide, refer the family to a therapy group for survivors of suicide.

## Delayed Surgical Recovery

**Domain 11** Safety/protection    **Class 2** Physical injury
**NANDA-I Definition**

Extension of the number of postoperative days required to initiate and perform activities that maintain life, health, and well-being.

• = Independent          ▲ = Collaborative

## Defining Characteristics

Anorexia; difficulty in moving about; difficulty resuming employment; excessive time required for recuperation; expresses discomfort; fatigue; interrupted surgical area healing; perceived need for more time to recover; postpones resumption of work; requires assistance for self-care

## Related Factors

Delirium; impaired physical mobility; increased blood glucose level; malnutrition; negative emotional response to surgical outcome; obesity; persistent nausea; persistent pain; persistent vomiting; smoking

## At-Risk Population

Individuals aged ≥80 years; individuals experiencing intraoperative hypothermia; individuals requiring emergency surgery; individuals requiring perioperative blood transfusion; individuals with American Society of Anesthesiologists (ASA) Physical Status Classification score ≥3; individuals with history of myocardial infarction; individuals with low functional capacity; individuals with preoperative weight loss >5%

## Associated Conditions

Anemia; diabetes mellitus; extensive surgical procedures; pharmaceutical preparations; prolonged duration of perioperative surgical wound infection; psychological disorder in postoperative period; surgical wound infection

## Client Outcomes

**Client Will (Specify Time Frame)**

- Have surgical area that shows evidence of healing: no redness, induration, draining, dehiscence, or immobility
- State that appetite is regained
- State that no nausea is present
- Demonstrate ability to move about
- Demonstrate ability to complete self-care activities
- State that no fatigue is present
- State that surgical pain is controlled or relieved
- Resume employment activities/ADLs
- State no depression or anxiety related to surgical procedure

## Nursing Interventions

- Encourage smoking cessation before surgery.
- Perform a thorough preoperative assessment of the client's health literacy level.
- Assess for the presence of medical conditions and treat appropriately before surgery.
- Carefully assess the client's use of herbal and dietary supplements such as feverfew, fish oil, ginkgo biloba, garlic, ginseng, ginger, valerian, kava, St. John's wort, ephedra (Ma huang or metabolite), and

• = Independent      ▲ = Collaborative

echinacea. It is recommended that all dietary supplements are stopped at least 1 week before major surgical or diagnostic procedures.
- Assess and treat for depression and anxiety in a client before surgery and postoperatively.
- Play music of the client's choice preoperatively, intraoperatively, and postoperatively.
- Consider using healing touch and other mind-body-spirit interventions such as stress control, therapeutic massage, and imagery.
- Maintain perioperative normothermia. Use reflective blankets to reduce heat loss during surgery.
- Postoperatively, discuss vital sign parameters with the surgeon, as well as signs and symptoms that could indicate early postoperative infection.
- Use careful aseptic technique when caring for wounds.
- Clients should bathe before surgery.
- Clients should be allowed to shower after surgery to maintain cleanliness, if not contraindicated because of the presence of pacemaker wires or other contraindications.
- Optimize the client's preoperative, intraoperative, and postoperative condition to minimize client stress and retain homeostasis.
- Carefully assess functional status of the client postoperatively using a fall-risk stratification tool, such as the Morse Fall Scale, to identify clients at high risk for fall.
- See care plans for **Anxiety**, Acute **Pain, Fatigue**, Risk for Perioperative **Positioning** Injury, Impaired Physical **Mobility,** and **Nausea.**

**Pediatric**
- Provide age-appropriate procedural information and postoperative expectations, including pain, function, and emotional care needs.
- Teach imagery and encourage distraction for children for postsurgical pain relief.

**Geriatric**
- Clients over age 65 should undergo a comprehensive geriatric assessment before surgery.
- The condition of the client' skin should be noted and fully documented.
- Routinely assess pain using a pain scale appropriate for clients with impaired cognition or inability to verbalize.
- Serially evaluate the client's vital signs, including temperature. Check baseline vital signs and monitor trends.

• = Independent ▲ = Collaborative

- The older client should be evaluated for signs and symptoms of delirium. Ensure that hearing aids and glasses are also available as needed.
- Offer spiritual support.

**Home Care**

- The preceding interventions may be adapted for the home setting.
- Provide supportive telephone calls from nurse to client as a means of decreasing anxiety and providing the psychosocial support necessary for recovery from surgery.

**Client/Family Teaching and Discharge Planning**

- Provide discharge planning and teaching in a language that is appropriate to the client and caregiver's education and literacy level.
- Create a discharge plan that includes measurable functional goals, expectations for recovery, and signs and symptoms of postoperative complications.

# Risk for Delayed Surgical Recovery

**Domain 11** Safety/protection    **Class 2** Physical injury

## NANDA-I Definition

Susceptible to an extension of the number of postoperative days required to initiate and perform activities that maintain life, health, and well-being, which may compromise health.

## Risk Factors

Delirium; impaired physical mobility; increased blood glucose level; malnutrition; negative emotional response to surgical outcome; obesity; persistent nausea; persistent pain; persistent vomiting; smoking

## At-Risk Population

Individuals aged ≥ 80 years; individuals experiencing intraoperative hypothermia; individuals requiring emergency surgery; individuals requiring perioperative blood transfusion; individuals with American Society of Anesthesiologists (ASA) Physical Status classification score ≥ 3; individuals with history of myocardial infarction; individuals with low functional capacity; individuals with preoperative weight loss > 5%

## Associated Conditions

Anemia; diabetes mellitus; extensive surgical procedures; pharmaceutical preparations; prolonged duration of perioperative surgical wound infection; psychological disorder in postoperative period; surgical wound infection

## Client Outcomes, Nursing Interventions, and Client/Family Teaching and Discharge Planning

See the care plan for Delayed **Surgical** Recovery.

• = Independent      ▲ = Collaborative

# Impaired Swallowing

**Domain 2** Nutrition    **Class 1** Ingestion
**NANDA-I Definition**

Abnormal functioning of the swallowing mechanism associated with deficits in oral, pharyngeal, or esophageal structure or function.

## Defining Characteristics
### First Stage: Oral

Abnormal oral phase of swallow study; bruxism; choking prior to swallowing; choking when swallowing cold water; coughing prior to swallowing; drooling; food falls from mouth; food pushed out of mouth; gagging prior to swallowing; impaired ability to clear oral cavity; inadequate consumption during prolonged meal time; inadequate lip closure; inadequate mastication; incidence of wet hoarseness twice within 30 seconds; inefficient nippling; inefficient suck; nasal reflux; piecemeal deglutition; pooling of bolus in lateral sulci; premature entry of bolus; prolonged bolus formation; tongue action ineffective in forming bolus

### Second Stage: Pharyngeal

Abnormal pharyngeal phase of swallow study; altered head position; choking; coughing; delayed swallowing; fevers of unknown etiology; food refusal; gagging sensation; gurgly voice quality; inadequate laryngeal elevation; nasal reflux; recurrent pulmonary infection; repetitive swallowing

### Third Stage: Esophageal

Abnormal esophageal phase of swallow study; acidic-smelling breath; difficulty swallowing; epigastric pain; food refusal; heartburn; hematemesis; hyperextension of head; nighttime awakening; nighttime coughing; odynophagia; regurgitation; repetitive swallowing; reports "something stuck"; unexplained irritability surrounding mealtimes; volume limiting; vomiting; vomitus on pillow

## Related Factors

Altered attention; behavioral feeding problem; protein-energy malnutrition; self-injurious behavior

## At-Risk Population

Individuals with history of enteral nutrition; older adults; premature infants

## Associated Conditions

Acquired anatomic defects; brain injuries; cerebral palsy; conditions with significant muscle hypotonia; congenital heart disease; cranial nerve involvement; developmental disabilities; esophageal achalasia; gastroesophageal reflux disease; laryngeal diseases; mechanical obstruction; nasal defect; nasopharyngeal cavity defect; neurological problems; neuromuscular diseases; oropharynx abnormality; pharmaceutical preparations;

• = Independent    ▲ = Collaborative

prolonged intubation; respiratory condition; tracheal defect; trauma; upper airway anomaly; vocal cord dysfunction

## Client Outcomes

### Client Will (Specify Time Frame)

- Demonstrate effective swallowing without signs of aspiration (see the section Defining Characteristics)
- Remain free from aspiration (e.g., lungs clear, temperature within normal range)

## Nursing Interventions

- Assess for risk factors associated with impaired swallowing.
- Complete swallow screen per facility protocol.
- ▲ Do not feed clients with impaired swallowing orally until an appropriate diagnostic workup is completed.
- ▲ Ensure proper nutrition by consulting with a health care provider regarding alternative nutrition and hydration when oral nutrition is not safe/adequate.
- ▲ Refer to a speech-language pathologist for evaluation and diagnostic evaluation of swallowing to determine swallowing problems and solutions as soon as oral and/or pharyngeal dysphagia is suspected.
- ▲ To manage impaired swallowing, use a multiprofessional dysphagia team composed of a speech pathologist, dietitian, nursing, health care provider, and medical staff. A comprehensive assessment from a multiprofessional dysphagia team can lead to personalized therapeutic interventions that can help the client learn to swallow safely and maintain a good nutritional status.
- ▲ Observe the following feeding guidelines:
  - ○ Before giving oral feedings, determine the client's readiness to eat (e.g., alert, able to hold head erect, follow instructions, move tongue in mouth, and manage oral secretions). If one of these elements is missing, it may be advisable to withhold oral feeding and use enteral feeding for nourishment.
  - ○ Monitor client during oral feedings and provide cueing as needed to ensure client follows swallowing guidelines/aspiration precautions recommended by speech-language pathologist or dysphagia specialist. Note: General aspiration precautions include the following: sit at 90 degrees for all oral feedings; take small bites/sips; eat at a slow rate; if client is being fed, position the feeder at eye level with the client; and no straws. However, client-specific strategies will be determined via bedside and/or instrumental swallowing evaluation performed by dysphagia specialist.
  - ○ Keep bolus size to 5 mL or smaller.

• = Independent ▲ = Collaborative

- ○ During feeding, adapt environment to decrease noise and distractions.
- ○ If the client is older or has gastroesophageal reflux disease, ensure the client is kept in an upright posture for an hour after eating.
- Monitor client during feeding for coughing or choking when eating and drinking, being unable to chew food properly, and losing food and drink from the front of the mouth.
- Use standardized diet and fluid descriptors such as the International Dysphagia Diet Standardisation Initiative (IDDSI) for diet and fluid modification.
- During meals and all oral intake, observe for wet voice, dysarthria (slurred speech), drooling, inability to cough on command, and an absent gag reflex as an indication of silent aspiration.
- ▲ If signs of aspiration or pneumonia are present, auscultate lung sounds after feeding. Note new onset of crackles or wheezing, or elevated temperature.
- ▲ Assess for signs of malnutrition and dehydration and keep a record of food intake.
- ▲ Evaluate nutritional status daily. Weigh the client weekly to help evaluate nutritional status. If the client is not adequately nourished, work with the dysphagia team to determine whether the client needs therapeutic feeding only or needs enteral feedings until the client can swallow adequately.
- ▲ Assist client in following dysphagia specialist's recommendations and provide open, accurate, and effective communication with dysphagia team regarding client's diet tolerance.
- ▲ Document and notify the provider and dysphagia team of changes in medical, nutritional, or swallowing status.
- ▲ Work with the client on swallowing exercises prescribed by the dysphagia team.
- ▲ Recognize that the client can aspirate oral feedings, even if there are no symptoms of coughing or distress. This phenomenon is called silent aspiration and is common.
- ▲ Ensure oral hygiene is maintained.
- ▲ For clients receiving mechanical ventilation with a tracheostomy tube or after postextubation, request a referral to a speech-language pathologist or dysphagia specialist for an instrumental swallowing evaluation before beginning oral diet.

**Pediatric**
- ▲ Refer children and infants who have difficulty swallowing, difficulty manipulating food, or delayed swallowing to a speech-language pathologist or dysphagia specialist for further assessment and testing.

• = Independent          ▲ = Collaborative

▲ Consult with occupational therapy to evaluate positioning for pediatric clients related to feeding.

▲ For at-risk infants, consult with a feeding specialist regarding nipple selection to address sucking and swallowing coordination before bottle feeding.

• For at-risk infants, provide external pacing by lowering the bottle to remove milk from the nipple or removing the nipple from the mouth entirely.

• For a preterm infant, provide opportunities for patterned nonnutritive sucking (NNS) or oral stimulation.

**Geriatric**

▲ Recognize that age-related changes can affect swallowing and these changes have a more pronounced effect when superimposed on neurological disease and other chronic problems.

• Assess for difficulty swallowing medications and modify medication administration as needed.

▲ Evaluate the medications the client is taking and collaborate with pharmacists and other appropriate professionals for assistance with modifications, correct dosages, and drug interactions.

**Home Care**

▲ Refer to speech therapy. Speech-language pathologists can work with clients to enhance swallowing ability and teach compensatory strategies.

**Client/Family Teaching and Discharge Planning**

▲ Teach the client and family restorative and rehabilitative techniques prescribed by the dysphagia team.

• Teach the client, family, and caregivers about standardized diet and fluid descriptors such as the International Dysphagia Diet Standardisation Initiative (IDDSI) for diet and fluid modification.

• Teach the family and caregivers how to monitor the client to prevent and detect aspiration during eating.

# Risk for Thermal Injury

**Domain 11** Safety/protection    **Class 2** Physical injury
## NANDA-I Definition

Susceptible to extreme temperature damage to skin and mucous membranes, which may compromise health.

## Risk Factors

Fatigue; inadequate caregiver knowledge of safety precautions; inadequate knowledge of safety precautions; inadequate protective clothing; inadequate supervision; inattentiveness; smoking; unsafe environment

• = Independent        ▲ = Collaborative

## At-Risk Population

Individuals exposed to environmental temperature extremes

## Associated Conditions

Alcoholic intoxication; drug intoxication; neuromuscular diseases; neuropathy; treatment regimen

## Client Outcomes

### Client Will (Specify Time Frame)

- Be free of thermal injury to skin or tissue
- Explain actions can take to protect self and others from thermal injury

## Nursing Interventions

- Teach the following interventions to prevent fires in the home, to handle any possible fire, and to have a readily available exit from the home:
  - Avoid plugging several appliance cords into the same electrical socket.
  - Do not use open candles or allow smoking in the home.
  - Keep a fire extinguisher within reach in case a fire should occur.
  - Install smoke alarms on every level of the home and in every sleeping area.
  - Keep furniture and other heavy objects out of the way of doors and windows.
  - Develop a fire escape plan that includes two ways out of every room and an outside meeting place. Practice the escape plan at least twice a year.
- Teach clients about home fire safety to prevent thermal injury and prevention.
- Apply sunscreen as directed on the container when out in the sun. Also use sun-blocking clothing, and stay in the shade if possible.
- Teach clients safety measures to prevent fires in the home in which medical oxygen is in use:
  - **Never smoke** in a home in which medical oxygen is in use. "No smoking" signs should be posted inside and outside the home.
  - Do not wear oxygen near an ignition source (e.g., open flame, gas stove, fireplace, candles, cigarettes, matches, lighters) (Fields, Whitney, & Bell, 2020). Note that petroleum jelly, lip balm, skin lotion, or the like will **not** spontaneously combust in the presence of supplemental oxygen without an ignition source (e.g., flame or spark) and are safe to use on the face and in bed in the presence of oxygen (Winslow & Jacobsen, 1998).
  - Homes with medical oxygen must have working smoke alarms that are tested monthly (Fields, Whitney, & Bell, 2020).

• = Independent          ▲ = Collaborative

- ○ Test fire extinguishers every 3 to 6 months. Keep a fire extinguisher within reach. If a fire occurs, turn off the oxygen, leave the home, and summon the fire department (NFPA, 2021).
- ○ Develop a fire escape plan that includes two ways out of every room and an outside meeting place. Practice the escape plan at least twice a year (NFPA, 2021).
- Be aware that thermal injury also includes injury from cold materials and environmental conditions, including freezing injury, nonfreezing injury, and hypothermia.
- Provide adequate environmental temperatures. Older clients and others at risk for temperature dysregulation can easily become hypothermic in air-conditioned environments (e.g., a surgical suite), with inadequate clothing, inhaling cold gases, or when exposed to room temperature or chilled fluids (e.g., intravenous, gastric lavage, bowel prep, continuous renal replacement therapy [CRRT], dialysis).
- Be aware that fine motor coordination decreases as a very early sign of hypothermia. Preventing progression of thermal injury is critical to client outcomes. Shivering is the body's attempt to generate heat through muscle activity; it consumes considerable metabolic energy, and is a **late** sign of hypothermia.
- Monitor temperature in vulnerable clients. Core temperature is the best measure to assess for hypothermia. If a pulmonary artery catheter is not available, use a thermometer calibrated for lower body temperature such as a distal esophageal, rectal, temporal artery, or bladder temperature probe.
- Use active warming measures to help clients maintain body temperature (e.g., warming blankets, warmed fluids, forced warm air warming devices, foil wraps, radiant warmers) as indicated. Be aware that passive devices (e.g., clothing items or blankets) do not add heat to body tissues.
- Ensure that exposed skin is protected from cold:
- ○ From environment, with adequate clothing
- ○ From cold topical applications (e.g., ice packs or circulating cold water therapy systems), with padding
- Monitor for developing cold thermal injury by checking skin color, peripheral circulation, temperature, and sensation. Be aware that fine motor coordination decreases as a very early sign of hypothermia. Shivering, the body's attempt to generate heat through muscle activity, is a late sign of hypothermia.
- Check the temperature of all equipment and other materials before allowing them to contact client skin, especially if client has increased risk factors for thermal injury.

• = Independent          ▲ = Collaborative

**Pediatric**
- Teach the following activities to clients with young children:
  - ○ Lock up matches and lighters out of sight and reach.
  - ○ Never leave a hot stove unattended.
  - ○ Do not allow small children to use the microwave until they are at least 7 or 8 years of age.
  - ○ Keep all portable heaters out of children's reach and at least 3 feet away from anything that can burn.
  - ○ Teach fire prevention and safety to older children.
- Install thermostatic mixer valves in a hot water system to prevent extreme hot water causing scalding burns.

# Ineffective Thermoregulation

**Domain 11** Safety/protection     **Class 6** Thermoregulation

## NANDA-I Definition

Temperature fluctuation between hypothermia and hyperthermia.

## Defining Characteristics

Cyanotic nail beds; flushed skin; hypertension; increased body temperature above normal range; increased respiratory rate; mild shivering; moderate pallor; piloerection; reduction in body temperature below normal range; seizure; skin cool to touch; skin warm to touch; slow capillary refill; tachycardia

## Related Factors

Dehydration; environmental temperature fluctuations; inactivity; inappropriate clothing for environmental temperature; increased oxygen demand; vigorous activity

## At-Risk Population

Individuals at extremes of weight; individuals exposed to environmental temperature extremes; individuals with inadequate supply of subcutaneous fat; individuals with increased body surface area to weight ratio

## Associated Conditions

Altered metabolic rate; brain injury; condition affecting temperature regulation; decreased sweat response; impaired health status; inefficient nonshivering thermogenesis; pharmaceutical preparations; sedation; sepsis; trauma

## Client Outcomes

**Client Will (Specify Time Frame)**
- Maintain temperature within normal range
- Explain measures needed to maintain normal temperature
- Describe two to four symptoms of hypothermia or hyperthermia
- List two or three self-care measures to treat hypothermia or hyperthermia

• = Independent          ▲ = Collaborative

## Nursing Interventions

### Temperature Measurement

- Measure and record the client's temperature using a consistent method of temperature measurement every 1 to 4 hours depending on the severity of the situation or whenever a change in condition occurs (e.g., chills, change in mental status).
- Select core, near core, or peripheral temperature monitoring mode based on ability to obtain an accurate temperature from that site and clinical situation, dictating the need for mode of temperature monitoring required for clinical treatment decisions.
- Caution should be taken in interpreting extreme values of temperature (less than 35°C [95 \°F] or greater than 39°C [102.2°F]) from a near core temperature site device.
- Evaluate the significance of a decreased or increased temperature.
- ▲ Notify the health care provider of temperature according to institutional standards or written orders, or when temperature reaches 100.5°F (38.3°C) and above; use a lower threshold for immunocompromised clients who will be less likely to exhibit a fever when seriously ill (Niven & Laupland, 2016). Also notify the health care provider of the presence of a change in mental status and temperature greater than 100.5°F (38.3°C) or less than 96.8°F (36°C).

### Fever (Pyrexia)

- Recognize that fever is characterized as a temporary elevation in internal body temperature 1°C to 2°C higher than the client's normal body temperature.
- Recognize that fever is a normal physiological response to a perceived threat by the body, frequently in response to an infection.
- ▲ Review client history, including current medical diagnosis, medications, recent procedures/interventions, recent travel, environmental exposure to infectious agents, recent blood product administration, and review of laboratory analysis for cause of ineffective thermoregulation.
- Recognize that fever may be low grade (96.8°F–100.4°F [36°C–38°C]) in response to an inflammatory process such as infection, allergy, trauma, illness, or surgery; moderate to high-grade fever (100.4°F–104°F [38°C–40°C]) indicates a more concerted inflammatory response from a systemic infection; hyperpyrexia (40°C and higher) occurs as a result of damage of the hypothalamus, bacteremia, or an extremely overheated room (Niven & Laupland, 2016; Walter et al, 2016).

• = Independent          ▲ = Collaborative

▲ Monitor and intervene to provide comfort during a fever by:
  ○ Obtaining vital signs and accurate intake and output
  ○ Checking laboratory analysis trends of white blood cell counts and other markers of infection
  ○ Providing blankets when the client complains of being cold but removing surplus of blankets when the client is too warm
  ○ Encouraging fluid and nutrition
  ○ Limiting activity to conserve energy
  ○ Providing frequent oral care
  ○ Adjusting room temperature for client comfort

## Hypothermia

- Take vital signs frequently, noting changes associated with hypothermia, such as increased blood pressure, pulse, and respirations, that then advance to decreased values as hypothermia progresses.
- Monitor the client for signs of hypothermia (e.g., shivering, cool skin, piloerection, pallor, slow capillary refill, cyanotic nail beds, decreased mentation, dysrhythmias) (Paal et al, 2016; Zafren, 2017).
- See the care plan for **Hypothermia** as appropriate.

## Hyperthermia

- Recognize that hyperthermia is a different etiology than fever, so the cause of the elevated body temperature should be explored for definitive treatment.
- Note changes in vital signs associated with hyperthermia, such as rapid, bounding pulse; increased respiratory rate; and decreased blood pressure, accompanied by orthostatic hypotension; and signs and symptoms of dehydration (Niven & Laupland, 2016; Gaudio & Grissom, 2016).
- Monitor the client for signs of hyperthermia (e.g., headache, nausea and vomiting, weakness, extreme fatigue, delirium, coma).
- Adjust clothing to facilitate passive warming or cooling as appropriate.
- See the care plan for **Hyperthermia** as appropriate.

## Pediatric

- For routine measurement of temperature, use an electronic thermometer in the axilla in infants younger than 4 weeks; for a child up to 5 years of age, use an electronic thermometer in the axilla or an infrared temporal artery thermometer.
- Recognize that pediatric clients have a decreased ability to adapt to temperature extremes. Take the following actions to maintain body temperature in the infant/child:
  ○ Keep the head covered.

• = Independent          ▲ = Collaborative

○ Use blankets to keep the client warm.
○ Keep the client covered during procedures, transport, and diagnostic testing.
○ Keep the room temperature at 72°F (22.2°C).
- Recognize that the infant and small child are both vulnerable to developing heat stroke in hot weather; ensure that they receive sufficient fluids and are protected from hot environments.
- Antipyretic treatments typically are not indicated unless the child's temperature is higher than 38.3°C [100.4°F] and may be given to provide comfort.

**Geriatric**
- Do not allow an older client to become chilled; keep the client covered when giving a bath and offer socks to wear in bed; be aware of factors such as room temperature (heating/air conditioning), clothing (layered/loose), and fluid intake.
- Recognize that the older client may have an infection without a significant rise in body temperature.
- Fever from infection in older adults does not confer a higher mortality risk; thus, fever should not be treated with antipyretic agents or other cooling methods unless the client is demonstrating limited cardiorespiratory reserves (Young et al, 2019).
- Ensure that older clients receive sufficient fluids during hot days and stay out of the sun.
- Assess the medication profile for the potential risk of drug-related altered body temperature.

**Home Care**
**Treating Fever**
- Instruct client/parents on the physiological benefits of fever and provide interventions to treat fever symptoms, avoiding antipyretic agents and external cooling interventions.
- Ensure that client/parents know when to contact a health care provider for fever-related concerns.

**Client/Family Teaching and Discharge Planning**
- Teach the client and family the signs of fever, hypothermia, and hyperthermia and appropriate actions to take if either condition develops.
- Teach the client and family an age-appropriate method for taking the temperature.
- Teach the client to avoid alcohol and medications that depress cerebral function.

• = Independent          ▲ = Collaborative

# Risk for Ineffective Thermoregulation

**Domain 11** Safety/protection    **Class 6** Thermoregulation

### NANDA-I Definition

Susceptible to temperature fluctuation between hypothermia and hyperthermia, which may compromise health.

### Risk Factors

Dehydration; environmental temperature fluctuations; inactivity; inappropriate clothing for environmental temperature; increased oxygen demand; vigorous activity

### At-Risk Population

Individuals at extremes of weight; individuals exposed to environmental temperature extremes; individuals with inadequate supply of subcutaneous fat; individuals with increased body surface area to weight ratio

### Associated Conditions

Altered metabolic rate; brain injuries; condition affecting temperature regulation; decreased sweat response; impaired health status; inefficient nonshivering thermogenesis; pharmaceutical preparations; sedation; sepsis; trauma

### Client Outcomes, Nursing Interventions, and Client/Family Teaching and Discharge Planning

Refer to care plans for Ineffective **Thermoregulation, Hyperthermia,** or **Hypothermia.**

**T**

# Risk for Thrombosis

**Domain 4** Activity/rest    **Class 4** Cardiovascular/pulmonary responses

### NANDA-I Definition

Susceptible to obstruction of a blood vessel by a thrombus that can break off and lodge in another vessel, which may compromise health.

### Risk Factors

Atherogenic diet; dehydration; excessive stress; impaired physical mobility; inadequate knowledge of modifiable factors; ineffective management of preventive measures; ineffective medication self-management; obesity; sedentary lifestyle; smoking

### At-Risk Population

Economically disadvantaged individuals; individuals aged ≥60 years; individuals with family history of thrombotic disease; individuals with history of thrombotic disease; pregnant women; women <6 weeks postpartum

• = Independent    ▲ = Collaborative

## Associated Conditions

Atherosclerosis; autoimmune diseases; blood coagulation disorders; chronic inflammation; critical illness; diabetes mellitus; dyslipidemias; endovascular procedures; heart diseases; hematologic diseases; high acuity illness; hormonal therapy; hyperhomocysteinemia; infections; kidney diseases; medical devices; metabolic syndrome; neoplasms; surgical procedures; trauma; vascular diseases

## Client Outcomes

### Client Will (Specify Time Frame)

- Not develop a thromboembolism during hospitalization
- State the relevant risk factors associated with the development of a thrombosis
- Engage in behaviors or lifestyle changes to reduce risk of developing a thrombosis

## Nursing Interventions

- It is estimated that 40% of clients with a deep vein thrombosis (DVT) will progress to postthrombotic syndrome (PTS); therefore, prevention of DVT is a key component.
- Assess client's risk factors to develop venous thromboembolism (VTE).
  - Venous stasis as a result of dehydration, immobility, heart failure, or venous compressions from a tumor
  - Hypercoagulable states from disease, obesity, and trauma
  - Immobilization from prolonged bed rest or limb casting
  - Surgery and trauma, especially hip, pelvic, and spinal surgery and leg amputation; several burns also predispose clients to DVT
  - Pregnancy results in a hypercoagulable state placing these clients at risk; although fatal events are rare
  - Oral contraceptives and estrogen replacement may place clients at risk, which is proportional to the estrogen content; postmenopausal women on hormone replacement therapy are considered at risk
  - In malignancy cases 17% of clients with VTE have a neoplasm with the most frequent occurrence in clients with pancreatic cancer
- Use a VTE risk assessment tool to determine individual susceptibility to thrombosis.
- ▲ Implement evidence-based prevention methods, both chemical (pharmacological) and/or mechanical.
- ▲ Chemical thromboprophylaxis should be anticipated in the postoperative care of critically ill clients.
- Implement mechanical prophylaxis through use of intermittent pneumatic compression (IPC) devices (Ho & Harahsheh, 2016).

• = Independent          ▲ = Collaborative

- Ensure proper fit and application of the device.
- Implement progressive mobility and early ambulation as the client tolerates to reduce risk of VTE.
- Provide education to the client and family about the importance of continued use of IPC after the client is ambulatory. Ensure that IPC is reapplied after ambulation (Hanison & Corbett, 2016; Dunn & Ramos, 2017).
- Perform a skin inspection during bathing.
- IPC should be applied even when the client is sitting in a chair (Dunn & Ramos, 2017).
- Provide appropriate education or referral to a smoking cessation program. Smoking is a well-established risk factor for atherosclerotic disease that increases the client's risk for VTE (McLendon et al, 2021).
- Obesity is an independent risk for VTE.
- Clients with cancer are at an increased risk of developing DVT mainly because of the release of certain chemicals from the tumor and spread of the tumor into blood vessels. Generally, bloodstream cancers such as leukemia carry the highest risk for development of DVT, followed by solid tumors of the pancreas, stomach, lungs, ovaries, uterus, bladder, and brain (Udoh, 2016).

**Pediatric**

- The nurse should be alert to certain diagnoses that increase the pediatric client's risk for VTE.
- The most frequent diagnosis associated with VTE in the pediatric population is trauma (Yen et al, 2016).
- Incidence of VTE in children is low; however, the rate of VTE in hospitalized children is much higher (Austin, Jenkins, & Hines, 2017).
- Risk factors for pediatric development of VTE include use of central venous access devices (Simmons, 2017).
- Neonatal and adolescent age groups are at higher risk for VTE compared with other pediatric age groups (Monagle et al, 2012). Additional studies are needed to further understand the risks and interventions for this population.

**Geriatric**

- The risk of VTE increases with age, increasing 90% between the ages of 15 and 80.
- It is well established that older clients are at a greater risk of developing atrial fibrillation (Heeringa et al, 2006).

**Home Care**

- Provide client education on the importance of continued use of compression stockings as directed.

• = Independent ▲ = Collaborative

- Provide education to the client and/or family caregiver about the continued use of anticoagulant pharmacological therapy as directed. The client and/or family caregiver may need instruction on proper injection technique if the client is not discharged on an oral anticoagulant.
- Clients who take the anticoagulant warfarin should have dietary education. Warfarin's effects may be decreased with a diet rich in vitamin K.
- The newer anticoagulants, such as rivaroxaban, apixaban, and edoxaban, do not have the same medication–food interactions as warfarin.

# Disturbed Thought Process

**Domain 5** Perception/cognition    **Class 4** Cognition

## NANDA-I Definition

Disruption in cognitive functioning that affects the mental processes involved in developing concepts and categories, reasoning, and problem solving.

## Defining Characteristics

Difficulty communicating verbally; difficulty performing instrumental activities of daily living; disorganized thought sequence; expresses unreal thoughts; impaired interpretation of events; impaired judgment; inadequate emotional response to situations; limited ability to find solutions to everyday situations; limited ability to make decisions; limited ability to perform expected social roles; limited ability to plan activities; limited impulse control ability; obsessions; phobic disorders; suspicions

## Related Factors

Acute confusion; anxiety; disorientation; fear; grieving; non-psychotic depressive symptoms; pain; stressors; substance misuse; unaddressed trauma

## At-Risk Population

Economically disadvantaged individuals; individuals in the early postoperative period; older adults; pregnant women

## Associated Conditions

Brain injuries; critical illness; hallucinations; mental disorders; neurodegenerative disorders; pharmaceutical preparations

## Client Outcomes

**Client Will (Specify Time Frame)**

- Recognize and verbalize that delusions are occurring
- Verbalize reality based thoughts and ideas

• = Independent      ▲ = Collaborative

- Differentiate between delusions and reality
- Refrain from acting on delusional ideation
- Remain free from injury

## Nursing Interventions

- Assess client for the presence of delusions with an established tool such as the Positive and Negative Syndrome Scale (PANSS).
- Assess and monitor the client for suicidal ideation.
- Assess and monitor how the client copes with delusions and impaired reality testing.
- Assess and monitor clients for side effects associated with antipsychotic medications.
- Use active listening to identify the meaning attributed to delusional thoughts.
- Respond to delusional statements with advanced empathy response techniques. Advanced empathy responses include the following:
  - Acknowledge what the person said with a "You say" statement. "You say you have microchips in your brain." Frame the question as exploratory to gain clarification.
  - Acknowledge your understanding with a statement. "I can't see any microchips and the test results do not show microchips in your brain." State your perceptions, what you have seen, heard, or been told.
  - Acknowledge how you imagine the other person feels with a perspective-taking statement such as, "I don't know what it would feel like to have microchips in my brain, but I imagine it might feel scary." Express genuine interest in the client's feelings and ask open-ended questions about their experience.
  - Explore the client's feelings and methods of coping.
- Use nursing presence to provide support to clients who experience grandiose or persecutory delusions.
- Use asynchronous email as a method to promote engagement with clients who experience psychosis.
- Assist the client to identify how daily stress can contribute to impaired thinking and cognitive symptoms.
- Provide the client with psychoeducation that includes information about their illness, treatment, disease management, problem-solving, coping skills, and how to access community mental health care services.
- ▲ Refer the client for cognitive behavioral therapy (CBT).
- ▲ Refer the client for metacognitive training (MCT). MCT is available in a module format, with modules that target common cognitive errors and problem-solving biases.
- ▲ Refer the client for art therapy group or services.

• = Independent ▲ = Collaborative

Geriatric
- The previous interventions can be adapted for use with geriatric clients.

Multicultural
- The previous interventions can be adapted for use with multicultural clients.
- Assess for the impact of socioenvironmental risk factors, such as discrimination, on cognitions.

Home Care
- The previous interventions can be adapted for use with home care clients.

Client/Family Teaching and Discharge Planning
- Assess family reactions to the client's illness.
- Provide family and caregivers information about delusions.
- Teach family members how to respond to delusions or expressions of impaired thinking.

# Impaired Tissue Integrity

**Domain 11** Safety/protection    **Class 2** Physical injury

## NANDA-I Definition

Damage to the mucous membrane, cornea, integumentary system, muscular fascia, muscle, tendon, bone, cartilage, joint capsule, and/or ligament.

## Defining Characteristics

Abscess; acute pain; bleeding, decreased muscle strength; decreased range of motion; difficulty bearing weight; dry eye; hematoma, impaired skin integrity; localized area hot to touch, localized deformity; localized loss of hair; localized numbness; localized swelling; muscle spasms; reports lack of balance; reports tingling sensation; stiffness; tissue exposure below the epidermis redness, tissue damage

## Related Factors

### External Factors

Excretions; humidity; hyperthermia; hypothermia; inadequate caregiver knowledge about maintaining tissue integrity; inadequate caregiver knowledge about protecting tissue integrity; inadequate use of chemical agent; pressure over bony prominence; psychomotor agitation; secretions; shearing forces; surface friction; use of linen with insufficient moisture wicking property

### Internal Factors

Body mass index above normal range for age and gender; body mass index below normal range for age and gender; decreased blinking frequency; decreased physical activity; fluid imbalance; impaired physical mobility;

impaired postural balance; inadequate adherence to incontinence treatment regimen; inadequate blood glucose level management; inadequate knowledge about maintaining tissue integrity; inadequate knowledge about restoring tissue integrity; inadequate ostomy care; malnutrition; psychogenic factor; self mutilation; smoking; substance misuse

## At-Risk Population

Homeless individuals; individuals at extremes of age; individuals exposed to environmental temperature extremes; individuals exposed to high-voltage power supply; individuals participating in contact sports; individuals participating in winter sports; individuals with family history of bone fracture; individuals with history of bone fracture

## Associated Conditions

Anemia; autism spectrum disorder; cardiovascular diseases; chronic neurological conditions; critical illness; decreased level of consciousness; decreased serum albumin level; decreased tissue oxygenation; decreased tissue perfusion; hemodynamic instability; immobilization; intellectual disability; medical devices; metabolic diseases; peripheral neuropathy; pharmaceutical preparations; sensation disorders; surgical procedures

## Client Outcomes

### Client Will (Specify Time Frame)

- Report any altered sensation or pain at site of tissue impairment
- Demonstrate understanding of plan to heal tissue and prevent reinjury
- Describe measures to protect and heal the tissue, including wound care
- Experience a wound that decreases in size and has increased granulation tissue

## Nursing Interventions

- The National Pressure Ulcer Advisory Panel (NPUAP) redefined the definition of a pressure ulcer, which is now referred to as a pressure injury, during the NPUAP 2016 Staging Consensus Conference. The new definitions more accurately define alterations in tissue integrity from pressure as follows: A pressure injury is localized damage to the skin and underlying soft tissue usually over a bony prominence or related to a medical device or other device. The injury can present as intact skin or an open ulcer and may be painful. The injury occurs as a result of intense and/or prolonged pressure or pressure in combination with shear. The tolerance of soft tissue for pressure and shear may also be affected by microclimate, nutrition, perfusion, comorbidities, and condition of the soft tissue (NPUAP, 2016).
- The first step is to identify etiological factors or what is causing the impairment.
- Determine the size (length, width) and depth of the wound.

▲ Classify pressure injuries (NPUAP, 2016) using national guidelines and definitions (see http://www.npuap.org/resources/educational-and-clinical-resources/npuap-pressure-injury-stages/).

○ **Pressure Injury:** A pressure injury is localized damage to the skin and underlying soft tissue usually over a bony prominence or related to a medical or other device. The injury can present as intact skin or an open ulcer and may be painful. The injury occurs as a result of intense and/or prolonged pressure or pressure in combination with shear. The tolerance of soft tissue for pressure and shear may also be affected by microclimate, nutrition, perfusion, comorbidities, and condition of the soft tissue (NPUAP, 2016).

○ **Stage 1 Pressure Injury:** Nonblanchable erythema of intact skin. Area of localized nonblanchable erythema that may appear differently in darkly pigmented skin, and changes in sensation, temperature, or firmness may precede visual changes. Color changes do not include purple or maroon discoloration, which is more likely to indicate deep tissue pressure injury (NPUAP, 2016).

○ **Stage 2 Pressure Injury:** Partial-thickness skin loss with exposed dermis. Partial-thickness skin loss with exposed dermis in which the wound bed is pink/red and moist and adipose (fat) and deeper tissues are not visible. Granulation tissue, slough, and eschar are not present. A stage 2 pressure injury may also present as an intact or ruptured blister. These injuries commonly result from adverse microclimate and shear in the skin over the pelvis and shear in the heel. This stage should not be used to describe MASD, including incontinence-associated dermatitis (IAD), intertriginous dermatitis (ITD), medical adhesive–related skin injury (MARSI), or traumatic wounds (skin tears, burns, and abrasions) (NPUAP, 2016).

○ **Stage 3 Pressure Injury:** Full-thickness skin loss. Full-thickness loss of skin, in which adipose is visible and granulation tissue and epibole (rolled wound edges) are often present, and undermining/tunneling may occur. Slough and/or eschar may also be visible. Fascia, muscle, tendon, ligament, cartilage, and/or bone are not exposed. The depth of tissue damage varies by anatomical location, and areas of significant adiposity can develop deep wounds. If slough or eschar obscures the extent of tissue loss, this is an unstageable pressure injury (NPUAP, 2016).

○ **Stage 4 Pressure Injury:** Full-thickness skin and tissue loss. Full-thickness skin and tissue loss with exposed or directly palpable

• = Independent                    ▲ = Collaborative

fascia, muscle, tendon, ligament, cartilage, or bone and slough and/ or eschar may be visible. Epibole, undermining, and/or tunneling often occur and depth varies by anatomical location. If slough or eschar obscures the extent of tissue loss, this is an unstageable pressure injury (NPUAP, 2016).

○ **Deep Tissue Pressure Injury:** Persistent nonblanchable deep red, maroon, or purple discoloration. Intact or nonintact skin with localized area of persistent nonblanchable deep red, maroon, or purple discoloration or epidermal separation revealing a dark wound bed or blood-filled blister. Pain and temperature change often precede skin color changes. Discoloration may appear differently in darkly pigmented skin. This injury results from intense and/or prolonged pressure and shear forces at the bone–muscle interface. The wound may evolve rapidly to reveal the actual extent of tissue injury, or it may resolve without tissue loss. If necrotic tissue, subcutaneous tissue, granulation tissue, fascia, muscle, or other underlying structures are visible, this indicates a full-thickness pressure injury (unstageable, stage 3, or stage 4). Do not use deep tissue pressure injury to describe vascular, traumatic, neuropathic, or dermatological conditions (NPUAP, 2016).

○ **Unstageable Pressure Injury:** Obscured full-thickness skin and tissue loss. Full-thickness skin and tissue loss in which the extent of tissue damage within the ulcer cannot be confirmed because it is obscured by slough or eschar. If slough or eschar is removed, a stage 3 or stage 4 pressure injury will be revealed. Stable eschar (i.e., dry, adherent, intact without erythema or fluctuance) on the heel or ischemic limb should not be softened or removed (NPUAP, 2016).

○ **Medical Device–Related Pressure Injury:** This describes an etiology. Medical device–related pressure injuries result from the use of devices designed and applied for diagnostic or therapeutic purposes. The resultant pressure injury generally conforms to the pattern or shape of the device. The injury should be staged using the staging system (NPUAP, 2016).

○ **Mucosal Membrane Pressure Injury:** Mucosal membrane pressure injury is found on mucous membranes with a history of a medical device in use at the location of the injury. Due to the anatomy of the tissue, these ulcers cannot be staged (NPUAP, 2016).

• Inspect and monitor the site of impaired tissue integrity at least once daily for color changes, redness, swelling, warmth, pain, or other signs of infection or per facility/agency policy. Monitor the status of the skin around the wound. Pay special attention to all high-risk areas such as bony prominences, skinfolds, sacrum, and heels. There is evidence that stage 1 pressure injuries are underdetected in individuals with darkly pigmented skin because areas of redness are not easily identified.

- Determine whether the client is experiencing changes in sensation or pain.
- Individualizing plans for bathing frequency, pH-balanced soaps, and applying moisturizing products while skin is still damp can help improve skin integrity (Murphree, 2017).
- Assess for incontinence and implement an individualized plan for management.
- Monitor for correct placement of tubes, catheters, and other devices. Assess the skin and tissue affected by the pressure of the devices and tape used to secure these devices.
- Medical device–related pressure injury describes an etiology.
- Assess frequently for correct placement of foot boards, restraints, traction, casts, or other devices, and assess skin and tissue integrity.
- ▲ Implement and communicate a comprehensive treatment plan for the topical treatment of the skin impairment site.
- ▲ Identify a plan for debridement if necrotic tissue (eschar or slough) is present and if consistent with overall client management goals (i.e., curative versus palliative care).
- Select a topical treatment that maintains a moist, wound-healing environment and also allows absorption of exudate and filling of dead space.
- Avoid positioning the client on the site of impaired tissue integrity.
- Select a support surface that meets the needs of the individual based on the level of immobility/activity, size and weight, need for microclimate management, and history of pressure injuries (NPIAP, EPIAP, & PPPIA, 2019).
- If the goal of care is to keep the client comfortable (e.g., for a terminally ill client), repositioning may not be appropriate.
- ▲ Assess the client's nutritional status. Refer for a nutritional consultation and/or institute dietary supplements as necessary.
- ▲ Review client nutrition plan evaluating for the intake of 1.25 to 1.5 g of protein per kilogram body weight daily, unless medically contraindicated, for adults at risk of a pressure injury or with existing pressure injuries. Offer 1 mL of fluid intake per kilocalorie per day, unless medically contraindicated (Wound, Ostomy and Continence

Nurses Society–Wound Guidelines Task Force, 2017). Reassess as condition changes (NPIAP, EPIAP, & PPPIA, 2019).
▲ Develop a comprehensive plan of care that includes a thorough wound assessment, treatment interventions, support surfaces, nutritional products, adjunctive therapies, and evaluation of the outcome of care.

**Home Care**
• Some of the interventions previously described may be adapted for home care use.
▲ Assess the client's current phase of wound healing (inflammation, proliferation, or maturation) and stage of injury; initiate appropriate wound management.
• Instruct and assist the client and caregivers in understanding how to change dressings and in the importance of maintaining a clean environment. Provide written instructions and observe them completing the dressing change.
▲ Initiate a consultation in a case assignment with a wound specialist or wound, ostomy, and continence nurse to establish a comprehensive plan as soon as possible. Plan case conferencing to promote optimal wound care.
▲ Consult with other health care disciplines to provide a thorough, comprehensive assessment.

**Client/Family Teaching and Discharge Planning**
• Teach skin and wound assessment and ways to monitor for signs and symptoms of infection, complications, and healing.
• Teach the client why a topical treatment has been selected. Explain wound bed changes that the caregiver can expect to see. Instruct on when the dressing needs to be changed. Assess pressure injuries with each wound dressing change and confirm the appropriateness of the current dressing regimen (NPIAP, EPIAP, & PPPIA, 2019).
▲ Teach the use of pillows, foam wedges, and pressure-reducing devices on beds and chairs to prevent pressure injury.

## Risk for Impaired Tissue Integrity

**Domain 11** Safety/protection    **Class 2** Physical injury
**NANDA-I Definition**

Susceptible to damage to the mucous membrane, cornea, integumentary system, muscular fascia, muscle, tendon, bone, cartilage, joint capsule, and/or ligament, which may compromise health.

• = Independent          ▲ = Collaborative

## Risk Factors

### External Factors

Excretions; humidity; hyperthermia; hypothermia; inadequate caregiver knowledge about maintaining tissue integrity; inadequate caregiver knowledge about protecting tissue integrity; inadequate use of chemical agent; pressure over bony prominence; psychomotor agitation; secretions; shearing forces; surface friction; use of linen with insufficient moisture wicking property

### Internal Factors

Body mass index above normal range for age and gender; body mass index below normal range for age and gender; decreased blinking frequency; decreased physical activity; fluid imbalance; impaired physical mobility; impaired postural balance; inadequate adherence to incontinence treatment regimen; inadequate blood glucose level management; inadequate knowledge about maintaining tissue integrity; inadequate knowledge about restoring tissue integrity; inadequate ostomy care; malnutrition; psychogenic factor; self mutilation; smoking; substance misuse

### At-Risk Population

Homeless individuals; individuals at extremes of age; individuals exposed to environmental temperature extremes; individuals exposed to high-voltage power supply; individuals participating in contact sports; individuals participating in winter sports; individuals with family history of bone fracture; individuals with history of bone fracture

### Associated Conditions

Anemia; autism spectrum disorder; cardiovascular diseases; chronic neurological conditions; critical illness; decreased level of consciousness; decreased serum albumin level; decreased tissue oxygenation; decreased tissue perfusion; hemodynamic instability; immobilization; intellectual disability; medical devices; metabolic diseases; peripheral neuropathy; pharmaceutical preparations; sensation disorders; surgical procedures

### Client Outcomes, Nursing Interventions, and Client/Family Teaching and Discharge Planning

Refer to care plan for Impaired **Tissue** Integrity.

# Ineffective Peripheral Tissue Perfusion

**Domain 4** Activity/rest    **Class 4** Cardiovascular/pulmonary responses

## NANDA-I Definition

Decrease in blood circulation to the periphery, which may compromise health.

• = Independent        ▲ = Collaborative

## Defining Characteristics

Absence of peripheral pulses; altered motor function; altered skin characteristics; ankle-brachial index <0.90; capillary refill time >3 seconds; color does not return to lowered limb after 1 minute of leg elevation; decreased blood pressure in extremities; decreased pain-free distances during a 6-minute walk test; decreased peripheral pulses; delayed peripheral wound healing; distance in the 6-minute walk test below normal range; edema; extremity pain; femoral bruit; intermittent claudication; paresthesia; skin color pales with limb elevation

## Related Factors

Excessive sodium intake; inadequate knowledge of disease process; inadequate knowledge of modifiable factors; sedentary lifestyle; smoking

## Associated Conditions

Diabetes mellitus; endovascular procedure; hypertension; trauma

## Client Outcomes

### Client Will (Specify Time Frame)

- Demonstrate adequate tissue perfusion as evidenced by palpable peripheral pulses, relief of pain, increased exercise tolerance, warm and dry skin, adequate urine output, and absence of respiratory distress
- Verbalize knowledge of treatment regimen, including appropriate exercise and medications and their actions and possible side effects
- Identify changes in lifestyle needed to increase tissue perfusion

## Nursing Interventions

▲ Assess the brachial, radial, dorsalis pedis, posterior tibial, and popliteal pulses bilaterally. If unable to palpate them, use a handheld Doppler device and notify the health care provider immediately with a decrease in pulse quality or new onset of absence of pulses along with a cold extremity.

- Note skin color; assess skin temperature, sensation and movement, and capillary refill.

- Assess for pain in the extremities, noting severity, quality, timing, and exacerbating and alleviating factors. Differentiate venous from arterial disease.

- Note skin texture and the presence of hair, ulcers, or gangrenous areas on the legs or feet.

- Assess for the presence of edema in the extremities and rate severity on a four-point scale. Measure the circumference of the ankle and calf at the same time each day in the early morning (Busti, 2016).

▲ Prepare for vascular laboratory tests.

▲ Prepare for revascularization procedures.

• = Independent          ▲ = Collaborative

**Arterial Insufficiency**

▲ Monitor peripheral pulses. If there is new onset of loss of pulses with bluish, purple, or black areas and extreme pain, notify the health care provider immediately.

▲ Measure ankle-brachial index (ABI) via Doppler imaging.

• Avoid elevating the legs above the level of the heart. With arterial insufficiency, leg elevation decreases arterial blood supply to the legs.

▲ In clients with intermittent claudication, exercise programs are recommended, such as walking or riding an exercise bicycle from 30 to 45 minutes per day, three times a week as ordered by the health care provider.

• Keep the client warm and have the client wear clean all-cotton or all-wool socks and rounded-toe shoes or sheepskin-lined slippers when mobile. Clients with arterial insufficiency report being cold; keep extremities warm to maintain vasodilation and blood supply. Do not apply heat. Heat application can easily damage ischemic tissues.

▲ Pay careful attention to foot care. Refer to a podiatrist if the client has thick, overgrown nails or calluses. Ischemic feet are vulnerable to injury; meticulous foot care can prevent further injury.

• If the client has ischemic arterial ulcers, refer to the care plan for Impaired **Tissue** Integrity.

▲ If the client smokes, recommend the client stop smoking and offer specific smoking cessation interventions. Refer to the health care provider for medications to support nicotine withdrawal.

▲ If the client has diabetes, good glycemic control is recommended.

• Educate the client on the use and safety of antiplatelet medications. Encourage the client to wear a medical alert bracelet.

**Venous Insufficiency**

• Elevate edematous legs as ordered and ensure no pressure under the knee and heels to prevent pressure ulcers.

▲ Apply graduated compression stockings as ordered. Ensure proper fit by measuring accurately. Remove the stockings at least twice a day, in the morning with the bath and in the evening, to assess the condition of the extremity, then reapply. Knee length is preferred rather than thigh length.

• Encourage the client to walk with compression stockings on and perform toe-up and point-flex exercises.

• If the client is overweight, encourage weight loss to decrease venous disease.

• If the client has venous leg ulcers, encourage the client to avoid prolonged sitting, standing, and elevation of the involved leg.

• = Independent        ▲ = Collaborative

Encourage proper use of compression stockings. Pain may prevent compliance.

▲ If the client is mostly immobile, consult with the health care provider regarding use of a calf-high intermittent pneumatic compression device for prevention of deep venous thrombosis (DVT).

• Assess for signs of DVT, including pain, tenderness, dilated superficial veins, a palpable cord indicating a thrombosed vein, swelling in the calf and thigh, and warmth and erythema in the involved extremity. Obtain serial leg measurements of the thigh and calf circumferences. In some clients a tender venous cord can be felt in the popliteal fossa. Do not rely on Homan's sign.

▲ Note the results of a D-dimer test and ultrasounds.

• If DVT is present, observe for symptoms of a pulmonary embolism (PE).

• Educate on use and safety of anticoagulant and antiplatelet medications.

**Geriatric**

• Complete a thorough lower extremity assessment, documenting the slightest change from previous assessment, and implement a plan immediately.

• Recognize that older adults have an increased risk for development of DVT and PE.

**Home Care**

• The interventions previously described may be adapted for home care use.

• If arterial disease is present and the client smokes, encourage smoking cessation using motivational interviewing techniques and evidence-based clinical practice guidelines (AHRQ, 2008; AHA, 2021; CDC, n.d.).

• Examine the feet carefully at frequent intervals for changes and new ulcerations. Encourage the client to perform regular assessment of the feet.

▲ Assess the client's nutritional status, paying special attention to obesity, hyperlipidemia, and malnutrition. Refer to a dietitian if appropriate.

• Monitor for development of gangrene, venous ulceration, and symptoms of cellulitis (redness, pain, and increased swelling in an extremity).

**Client/Family Teaching and Discharge Planning**

• Explain the importance of good foot care. Teach the client and family to wash daily with mild soap and tepid water. Teach the client and

• = Independent            ▲ = Collaborative

family to inspect the feet daily. Recommend that the diabetic client wear properly fitting shoes to prevent the formation of blisters and calluses. Clients with diabetes should be instructed to never walk barefoot (Berti-Hearn & Elliott, 2018).

▲ Teach diabetic clients that they should have a comprehensive foot examination at least annually. The examination should include sensory assessments. If good sensation is not present, refer to a footwear professional for fitting of therapeutic shoes and inserts, the cost of which may be covered by insurance and/ or Medicare.

• For arterial disease, stress the importance of not smoking, following a weight loss program (if the client is obese), carefully controlling a diabetic condition, controlling hyperlipidemia, managing hypertension, maintaining intake of antiplatelet therapy, and reducing stress.

• Encourage clients to walk or engage in other forms of physical activity.

• Teach the client to avoid exposure to cold; limit exposure to brief periods if going out in cold weather and wear warm clothing.

• For venous disease, stress the importance of not smoking, and teach the importance of wearing compression stockings as ordered, elevating the legs at intervals (30 minutes, three to four times a day), weight loss if overweight, regular exercise such as walking, and watching for skin breakdown on the legs.

• Educate clients about any medications prescribed to treat their venous disease.

• Educate clients about the importance of taking prescribed medications to achieve therapeutic anticoagulation (Roberts & Lawrence, 2017).

• Teach clients to avoid crossing legs when sitting or standing for prolonged periods (Berti-Hearn & Elliott, 2019).

• Teach client to avoid long periods of sitting or standing to reduce the pooling of blood (D'Alesandro, 2016).

• Teach the client to recognize the signs and symptoms that should be reported to a health care provider (e.g., change in skin temperature, color, or sensation, or the presence of a new lesion on the foot).

• Provide clear, simple instructions about plan of care.

• Instruct and provide emotional support for clients undergoing hyperoxygenation treatment.

• = Independent          ▲ = Collaborative

# Risk for Ineffective Peripheral Tissue Perfusion

**Domain 4** Activity/rest    **Class 4** Cardiovascular/pulmonary responses

**NANDA-I Definition**

Susceptible to a decrease in blood circulation to the periphery, which may compromise health.

**Risk Factors**

Excessive sodium intake; inadequate knowledge of disease process; inadequate knowledge of modifiable factors; sedentary lifestyle; smoking

**Associated Conditions**

Diabetes mellitus; endovascular procedures; hypertension; trauma

**Client Outcomes, Nursing Interventions, and Client/Family Teaching and Discharge Planning**

Refer to care plan for Ineffective Peripheral **Tissue** Perfusion.

# Impaired Transfer Ability

**Domain 4** Activity/rest    **Class 2** Activity/exercise

**NANDA-I Definition**

Limitation of independent movement between two nearby surfaces.

**Defining Characteristics**

Difficulty transferring between bed and chair; difficulty transferring between bed and standing position; difficulty transferring between car and chair; difficulty transferring between chair and floor; difficulty transferring between chair and standing position; difficulty transferring between floor and standing position; difficulty transferring between uneven levels; difficulty transferring in or out of bath tub; difficulty transferring in or out of shower stall; difficulty transferring on or off a bedside commode; difficulty transferring on or off a toilet

**Related Factors**

Environmental constraints; impaired postural balance; inadequate knowledge of transfer techniques; insufficient muscle strength; neurobehavioral manifestation; obesity; pain; physical deconditioning

**Associated Conditions**

Musculoskeletal impairment; neuromuscular diseases; vision disorders

**Client Outcomes**

Client Will (Specify Time Frame)

- Transfer from bed to chair and back successfully
- Transfer from chair to chair successfully
- Transfer from wheelchair to toilet and back successfully

• = Independent                    ▲ = Collaborative

- Transfer from wheelchair to car and back successfully

**Nursing Interventions**

- Specify level of independence using a standardized functional scale.
- Assess level of client ability to perform specific tasks before transfer of client.
- Assess client's dependence, weight, strength, balance, tolerance to position change, cooperation, fatigue level, and cognition plus available equipment and staff ratio/experience to decide whether to do a manual or device-assisted transfer because devices can reduce staff injury (American Nurses Association [ANA], 2015; Riccoboni et al, 2021).
▲ Complications associated with immobility and resultant muscle loss begin within 48 hours of onset of injury and are greatest during the first 2 to 3 weeks (Cameron et al, 2015). Request a consultation for a physical therapist (PT) and/or occupational therapist (OT) to develop a plan of care for safe client handling and mobility.
▲ Obtain a consultation for a PT, OT, or orthotist to evaluate and fit clients with proper orthoses, braces, collars, and walking aids before helping them stand.
▲ Help client put on/take off collars, braces, prostheses in bed, and put on/take off antiembolism stockings and abdominal binders. If applying antiembolism stockings is prescribed to reduce the risk of DVT, apply while the client is in bed for ease of application.
▲ Collaborate with PT and OT to use algorithms to identify technological aids to handle and transfer dependent and obese clients. Use assistive mobility devices such as gait belts, lifts, and transport devices to move obese clients to avoid harm to both client and health care professional (Choi & Brings, 2015).
- Implement and document type of transfer (e.g., slide board, pivot), weight-bearing status (non–weight-bearing, partial), equipment (walker, sling lift), and level of assistance (standby, moderate) on care plan, white board in room, and/or electronic medical record.
- Apply a gait belt with handles before transferring clients with partial weight-bearing abilities; keep the belt and client close to provider during the transfer.
- Help clients when wearing shoes with nonskid soles and socks/hose.
- Remove or swivel wheelchair armrests, leg rests, and footplates to the side, especially with squat or slide board transfers. This gives clients and nurses feet space in which to maneuver and provides fewer obstacles to trip over.

• = Independent          ▲ = Collaborative

- Adjust transfer surfaces so that they are similar in height. For example, lower a hospital bed to about an inch higher than commode height.
- Place wheelchair and commode at a slight angle toward the surface onto which the client will transfer.
- Teach client to consistently lock brakes on wheelchair/commode/ shower chair before transferring.
- Give clear, simple instructions, allow client time to process information, and let him or her do as much of the transfer as possible.
▲ Remind clients to comply with weight-bearing restrictions ordered by their health care provider. Weight-bearing may retard healing in fractured bones.
- Place client in set position before standing him or her, for example, sitting on edge of surface with bilateral weight bearing on buttocks and hips, with knees flexed, balls of feet aligned under knees, and head in midline.
- Support and stabilize client's weak knees by placing one or both of your knees next to or encircling client's knees, rather than blocking them. This allows client to flex his or her knees and lean forward to stand and transfer.
   ○ Squat transfer: client leans well forward, slightly raises flexed hips off the surface, pivots, and sits down on new surface.
   ○ Standing pivot transfer: client leans forward with hips flexed and pushes up with hands from seat surface (or arms of chair), then stands erect, pivots, and sits down on new surface.
   ○ Slide board transfer: client should have on pants or have a pillowcase over the board. Remove arm and leg rest from wheelchair on one side, then slightly angle chair toward new surface. Help client lean sideways, shifting his or her weight so the transfer board can be placed well under the upper thigh of the leg next to new surface. Make sure the board is safely angled across both surfaces. Help client to sit upright and place one hand on the board and the other hand on the surface. Remind and help client perform a series of pushups with arms while leaning slightly forward and lifting (not sliding) hips in small increments across the board with each pushup.
- Position walking aids appropriately so a standing client can grasp and use them once he or she is upright.
- Reinforce to clients who use walkers to place one hand on walker and push with opposite hand against chair arm or surface from which

**T**

• = Independent          ▲ = Collaborative

they are arising to stand up. Placing both hands on the walker may cause it to tip and the client to lose balance and fall.

- Use ceiling-mounted or bedside mechanical bariatric lifts to transfer dependent bariatric (extremely obese) clients.
- Use bariatric devices and use available safe client handling equipment for lifting, transferring, positioning, and sliding client as an effective tool to reduce risk of injury from client handling (Choi & Brings, 2015; Lee & Lee, 2017).
- Place a mechanical lift sling in the wheelchair preventively. Place two transfer sheets or a slide board under the bariatric client.
- Perform initial and subsequent fall risk assessment. Use standardized tools for fall risk assessment and multiprofessional multifactorial interventions to reduce falls and risk of falling in hospitals.
▲ Collaborate with PT, OT, and pharmacist for individualized preventive/postfall plans; for example, scheduled toileting, balance and strength training, removal of hazards, chair alarms, call system/phone in reach, and review of medications.
- Coordinate a follow-up encounter within 30 days of discharge from any inpatient facility with a licensed provider to perform a medication reconciliation, including all medications the client has been taking or receiving before the outpatient visit to provide quality care and improve quality of communication related to medications.
- Encourage an exercise component such as Tai chi, physical therapy, or another exercise for balance, gait, and strength training in group programs or at home.
- Integrate structured, progressive exercise protocols into a client's plan of care and innovative partnerships with other providers to create longer-duration interventions for clients at risk of falling.
- Modify the environment for safety; recommend vision assessment and consideration for cataract removal.
- To reduce the risk of falling, assess the physical environment (e.g., poor lighting, high bed position, improper equipment).
- Recommend polypharmacy assessment with special consideration to sedatives, antidepressants, and drugs affecting the central nervous system; recommend evaluation for orthostatic hypotension and irregular heartbeats; and recommend vitamin D supplementation 800 international units/day (National Committee for Quality Assurance, 2015b).

**Home Care**

▲ Obtain referral for OT and PT to teach home exercises and balance and fall prevention and recovery. They also evaluate for potential

• = Independent          ▲ = Collaborative

modifications such as an entry ramp, elevated toilet seat/toilevator (raised base under toilet), tub seat or shower chair, need for shower stall with built-in seat or wheel-in shower stall without a curb/threshold, handheld flexible shower head, lever-type facets, pull-out drawers with loop handles versus cupboards, and standing lift.

- Develop a multifactorial/multicomponent interventions risk strategy to reduce the risk for falls that includes adaptation or modification of the home environment; withdrawal or minimization of psychoactive medications; withdrawal or minimization of other medications; management of postural hypotension; management of foot problems and footwear; and exercise, particularly balance, strength, and gait training (National Committee for Quality Assurance, 2015a).
- Assess for adequate lighting and hazards such as throw/area rugs, clutter, cords, and unfitted bedspreads. Suggest safe floor surfaces, such as use of adhesive nonslip strips in tubs, thresholds, and areas in which floor height changes; removal of wax from slippery floors; and installing low-pile carpet or nonglazed or nonglossy tiles, wood, or linoleum coverings. Encourage relocating commonly used items to shelves/drawers in reach; applying remote controls to appliances; and optimizing furniture placement for function, maneuverability, and stability.
- Assess clients for impairment of vision because this can result in a loss of function in activities of daily living and, consequently, result in impaired functional capacity and is an important risk factor for falls.
- Nurses can provide further safety assessments by suggesting installing hand rails in bathrooms and by stairs, using slip-resistant floor surfaces, ensuring client's slippers and clothes fit properly, and recommending repairing or discarding broken equipment in the home (Keall et al, 2015; E et al, 2020).
- ▲ Involve social worker or case manager to educate clients about potential assistive technology, financial cost and benefits, regulations of payers, and local resources.
- ▲ Implement approaches for home care staff and family to safely handle and transfer clients.
- For further information, refer to care plans for Impaired Physical **Mobility** and Impaired **Walking**.

**Client/Family Teaching and Discharge Planning**
- Assess for readiness to learn and use teaching modalities conducive to personal learning styles, including written instructions for home use.

• = Independent      ▲ = Collaborative

- Supervise practice sessions in which client and family apply items such as gait belts, braces, and orthoses. Check skin once aids are removed.
- Teach and monitor client/family for consistent use of safety precautions for transfers (e.g., nonskid shoes, correctly placed equipment/chairs, locked brakes, leg rests swiveled away) and for correct performance of transfer or use of lifts/slings.
- Teach client/family how to check brakes on chairs to ensure they engage and how to check tires for adequate air pressure; advise routine inspection and annual tune-up of devices.
- Offer information on safe use of shower and commode chairs to prevent discomfort, pressure, and falls during transfer, transport, care, and hygiene.
- For further information, refer to the care plans for Impaired Physical **Mobility,** Impaired **Walking,** and Impaired Wheelchair **Mobility.**

# Risk for Physical Trauma

**Domain 11** Safety/protection    **Class 2** Physical injury
## NANDA-I Definition

Vulnerable to accidental tissue injury (e.g., wound, burn, fracture), which may compromise health.
## Risk Factors
### External

Absence of call for aid device; absence of stairway gate; absence of window guard; access to weapon; bathing in very hot water; bed in high position; children riding in front seat of car; defective appliance; delay in ignition of gas appliance; dysfunctional call for aid device; electrical hazard (e.g., faulty plug, frayed wire, overloaded outlet/fuse box); exposure to corrosive product; exposure to dangerous machinery; exposure to radiation; exposure to toxic chemical; extremes of environmental temperature; flammable object (e.g., clothing, toys); gas leak; grease on stove; high-crime neighborhood; icicles hanging from roof; inadequate stair rails; inadequately stored combustible (e.g., matches, oily rags); inadequately stored corrosive (e.g., lye); insufficient lighting; insufficient protection from heat source; misuse of headgear (e.g., hard hat, motorcycle helmet); misuse of seat restraint; insufficient antislip material in bathroom; nonuse of seat restraints; obstructed passageway; playing with dangerous object; playing with explosive; pot handle facing front of stove; proximity to vehicle pathway (e.g., driveway, railroad track); slippery floor; smoking in bed; smoking near oxygen; struggling with restraints; unanchored electric wires; unsafe operation of heavy equipment (e.g., excessive speed while intoxicated with required eyewear); unsafe road; unsafe walkway; use of cracked dishware; use of throw rugs; use of unstable chair; use of unstable ladder; wearing loose clothing around open flame

**Internal**

Alteration in cognitive functioning; alteration in sensation (e.g., resulting from spinal cord injury, diabetes mellitus); decrease in eye–hand coordination; decrease in muscle coordination; economically disadvantaged; emotional disturbance; history of trauma (e.g., physical, psychological, sexual); impaired balance; insufficient knowledge of safety precautions; insufficient vision; weakness

## Client Outcomes

### Client Will (Specify Time Frame)

- Remain free from trauma
- Explain actions that can be taken to prevent trauma

## Nursing Interventions

- Provide vision aids for visually impaired clients.
- Assist the client with ambulation. Encourage the client to use assistive devices in activities of daily living (ADLs) as needed.
- Evaluate client's risk for burn injury.
- Assess the client for causes of impaired cognition.
- Provide assistive devices in the home.
- ▲ Question the client concerning his or her sense of safety.
- ▲ Assess for a substance abuse problem and refer to appropriate resources for drug and alcohol education.
- Review drug profile for potential side effects that may inhibit performance of ADLs.
- See care plans for Risk for **Aspiration,** Risk for **Falls,** Impaired **Home** Maintenance, Risk for **Injury,** Risk for **Poisoning,** and Risk for **Suffocation.**

### Pediatric

- Assess the client's socioeconomic status.
- Never leave young children unsupervised.
- Keep flammable and potentially flammable articles out of reach of young children.
- Lock up harmful objects such as guns.

### Geriatric

- Assess the geriatric client's cognitive level of functioning.
- Assess for routine eye examinations.
- Perform a home safety assessment and recommend the following preventive measures: keep electrical cords out of the flow of traffic;

remove small rugs or make sure they are slip resistant; increase lighting in hallways and other dark areas; place a light in the bathroom; keep towels, curtains, and other items that might catch fire away from the stove; store harmful products away from food products; provide at least one grab bar in tubs and showers; check prescribed medications for appropriate labels; store medications in original containers or in a dispenser of some type (e.g., egg carton, 7-day plastic dispenser). If the client cannot administer medications according to directions, secure someone to administer medications. Mark stove knobs with bright colors (yellow or red) and outline the borders of steps.
- Discourage driving at night.
- Encourage the client to participate in resistance and impact exercise programs as tolerated.

**Client/Family Teaching and Discharge Planning**
- Educate the family regarding age-appropriate child safety precautions, environmental safety precautions, and intervention in an emergency.
- Teach the family to assess the child care provider's knowledge regarding child safety.
- Educate the client and family regarding helmet use during recreation and sports activities.
- Encourage the proper use of car seats and safety belts.
- Teach parents to restrict driving for teens.
- Teach parents the importance of monitoring children after school.
- Teach firearm safety.
- For further information, refer to care plans for Risk for **Aspiration,** Risk for **Falls,** Impaired **Home** Maintenance, Risk for **Injury,** Risk for **Poisoning,** and Risk for **Suffocation.**

## Unilateral Neglect

**Domain 5** Perception/cognition **Class 1** Attention
**NANDA-I Definition**

Impairment in sensory and motor response, mental representation, and spatial attention of the body, and the corresponding environment, characterized by inattention to one side and overattention to the opposite side. Left-side neglect is more severe and persistent than right-side neglect.

**Defining Characteristics**

Altered safety behavior on neglected side; disturbed sound lateralization; failure to dress neglected side; failure to eat food from portion of plate on neglected side; failure to groom neglected side; failure to move eyes in the

• = Independent ▲ = Collaborative

neglected hemisphere; failure to move head in the neglected hemisphere; failure to move limbs in the neglected hemisphere; failure to move trunk in the neglected hemisphere; failure to notice people approaching from the neglected side; hemianopsia; impaired performance on line bisection tests; impaired performance on line cancellation tests; impaired performance on target cancellation tests; left hemiplegia from cerebrovascular accident; marked deviation of the eyes to stimuli on the non-neglected side; marked deviation of the trunk to stimuli on the non-neglected side; omission of drawing on the neglected side; perseveration; representational neglect; substitution of letters to form alternative words when reading; transfer of pain sensation to the non-neglected side; unaware of positioning of neglected limb; unilateral visuospatial neglect; uses vertical half of page only when writing

## Related Factors

To be developed

## Associated Conditions

Brain injuries

## Client Outcomes

**Client Will (Specify Time Frame)**

- Use techniques that can be used to minimize unilateral neglect (UN)
- Care for both sides of the body appropriately and keep affected side free from harm
- Return to the highest functioning level possible based on personal goals and abilities
- Remain free from injury

## Nursing Interventions

▲ Assess the client for signs of UN (e.g., not washing, shaving, or dressing one side of the body; sitting or lying inappropriately on affected arm or leg; failing to respond to environmental stimuli contralateral to the side of lesion; eating food on only one side of plate; reading words on one side of the page; or failing to look to one side of the body).

▲ Collaborate with health care provider for referral to a rehabilitation team (including, but not limited to, rehabilitation clinical nurse specialist, physical medicine and rehabilitation health care provider, neuropsychologist, occupational therapist, physical therapist, and speech and language pathologist) for continued help in dealing with UN.

- Use the principles of rehabilitation to progressively increase the client's ability to compensate for UN by using assistive devices, feedback, and support.

U

• = Independent          ▲ = Collaborative

- Teach the client to be aware of the problem and modify behavior and environment.
- Set up the environment so that essential activity is on the unaffected side:
  - ○ Place the client's personal items within view and on the unaffected side.
  - ○ Position the bed so that client is approached from the unaffected side.
  - ○ Monitor and assist the client to achieve adequate food and fluid intake.
- Implement fall prevention interventions as clients with right hemisphere brain damage are twice as likely to fall as those with left hemisphere damage.
- Position affected extremity in a safe and functional manner.
- ▲ Collaborate closely with rehabilitation professionals to identify and reinforce therapies aimed at reducing neglect symptoms.

**Home Care**

- Many of the previously listed interventions may be adapted for use in the home care setting.
- Position bed at home so that client gets out of bed on unaffected side.

**Client/Family Teaching and Discharge Planning**

- Engage discharge planning specialists for comprehensive assessment and planning early in the client's stay.
- Encourage family participation in care to promote safety.
- Explain pathology and symptoms of UN to both the client and family. Family members may not understand that inattention is a complication of the neurological injury.
- Teach the client how to scan regularly to check the position of body parts and to regularly turn head from side to side for safety when ambulating, using a wheelchair, or doing self-care tasks.
- Teach caregivers to cue the client to the environment.

# Impaired Urinary Elimination

**Domain 3** Elimination and exchange    **Class 1** Urinary function

## NANDA-I Definition

Dysfunction in urine elimination.

## Defining Characteristics

Dysuria; frequent voiding; nocturia; urinary hesitancy; urinary incontinence; urinary retention; urinary urgency

     • = Independent          ▲ = Collaborative

## Related Factors

Alcohol consumption; altered environmental factor; caffeine consumption; environmental constraints; fecal impaction; improper toileting posture; ineffective toileting habits; insufficient privacy; involuntary sphincter relaxation; obesity; pelvic organ prolapse; smoking; use of aspartame; weakened bladder muscle; weakened supportive pelvic structure

## At-Risk Population

Older adults; women

## Associated Conditions

Anatomic obstruction; diabetes mellitus; sensory motor impairment; urinary tract infection

## Client Outcomes

**Client Will (Specify Time Frame)**

- State absence of pain or excessive urgency during urination
- Demonstrate voiding frequency no more than every 2 hours

## Nursing Interventions

- Ask the client about urinary elimination patterns and concerns.
- Question the client regarding the following:
  - ○ Presence of symptoms such as incontinence, dribbling, frequency, urgency, dysuria, and nocturia
  - ○ Presence of pain in the area of the bladder
  - ○ Pattern of urination and approximate amount
  - ○ Possible aggravating and alleviating factors for urinary problems
- Ask the client to keep a bladder diary/bladder log.
- For interventions on urinary incontinence, refer to the following nursing diagnosis care plans as appropriate: Stress Urinary **Incontinence,** Urge Urinary **Incontinence,** Mixed Urinary **Incontinence, Urinary Retention,** or Disability-Associated Urinary **Incontinence.**
- ▲ Perform a focused physical assessment including inspecting the perineal skin integrity, percussion, and palpation of the lower abdomen looking for obvious bladder distention or an enlarged kidney.
- ▲ If signs of urinary obstruction are present, refer client to a urologist.
- Check for costovertebral tenderness.
- ▲ Review results of urinalysis for the presence of urinary infection such as white blood cells, red blood cells, bacteria, and positive nitrites.
- ▲ If blood or protein is present in the urine, recognize that both hematuria and proteinuria are serious symptoms, and the client should be referred to a urologist to receive a workup to rule out pathology.

• = Independent ▲ = Collaborative

- Inquire about the client's history of smoking.

**Urinary Tract Infection**

▲ Consult the provider for culture and sensitivity testing and antibiotic treatment in the individual with evidence of a symptomatic UTI.

▲ Teach the client to recognize symptoms of UTI, such as dysuria that crescendos as the bladder nears complete evacuation; urgency to urinate followed by micturition of only a few drops; suprapubic aching discomfort; malaise; voiding frequency; and sudden exacerbation of urinary incontinence with or without fever, chills, and flank pain. Recognize that cloudy or malodorous urine, in the absence of other lower urinary tract symptoms, may not indicate the presence of a UTI and that asymptomatic bacteriuria in the older adult does not justify a course of antibiotics.

▲ Refer the individual with chronic lower urinary tract pain to a urologist or specialist in the management of pelvic pain.

**Pediatric**

- Initial management of childhood urinary incontinence: (1) thorough history and physical examination; (2) bladder diary; (3) urinalysis; (4) urinary tract ultrasound; (5) screening for behavioral problems (Maternik, Krzeminska, & Zurowska, 2015).

- Standard practice recommendations when caring for pediatric clients include an aggressive bowel regimen, timed voiding, and escalating urotherapy with biofeedback. Medications may be considered as a secondary measure (Arlen, 2017).

- Encourage children to void on a timed schedule every 2 hours, void two times with every void, drink two bottles of water during and after school, stop drinking 2 hours before bed, and void two times before bed.

**Geriatric**

- Evidence for behavioral interventions include the following: (1) Prompted voiding is suitable for older adult clients, with or without cognitive impairment, who have a consistent caregiver; (2) prompted voiding is unsuccessful in clients who require more than one person for transfers, are not able to follow one-step commands, and a successful toileting rate of less than 66% after a 3-day prompted voiding trial; and (3) a key factor in the success of prompted voiding is caregiver education (Newman, 2019).

- Encourage older women to consume one to two servings of fresh blueberries and consider drinking at least 10 ounces of cranberry juice daily or supplement the diet with cranberry concentrate capsules as ordered.

• = Independent                    ▲ = Collaborative

- ▲ Refer the older woman with recurrent UTIs to her health care provider for possible use of topical estrogen creams for treatment of atrophic vaginal mucosa from decreased hormonal stimulation, which can predispose to UTIs (Nicolle & Norrby, 2016).
- Postresidual volumes (PRVs) should be assessed in older women with overactive bladder (OAB). A volume of greater than 200 mL is significant.
- ▲ Recognize that UTIs in older men are typically associated with prostatic hyperplasia or strictures of the urethra. Refer the client to a urologist (Nicolle & Norrby, 2016).
- Analysis of urinary elimination patterns of clients could help in clinical follow-up of elderly postoperative clients and in the selection of best nursing interventions.
- Frailty, not age, should guide urinary elimination treatment decisions.
- Managing incontinence-associated dermatitis in the geriatric population involves regular, ongoing skin assessments to identify damaged skin as well as areas for potential skin damage.

**Client/Family Teaching and Discharge Planning**
- Teach the client/family methods to keep the urinary tract healthy. Refer to Client/Family Teaching in the care plan for Readiness for Enhanced **Urinary** Elimination.
- Teach the following measures to women to decrease the incidence of UTIs:
  - Urinate at appropriate intervals. Do not ignore need to void, which can result in stasis of urine.
  - Drink plenty of liquids, especially water.
  - Wipe from front to back. This helps prevent bacteria in the anal region from spreading to the vagina and urethra.
  - Wear underpants that have a cotton crotch. This allows air to circulate in the area and decreases moisture in the area, which predisposes to infection.
  - Avoid potentially irritating feminine products.
- Teach the sexually active woman with recurrent UTIs prevention measures:
  - Void after intercourse to flush bacteria out of the urethra and bladder.
  - Use a lubricating agent as needed during intercourse to protect the vagina from trauma and decrease the incidence of vaginitis.
  - Watch for signs of vaginitis and seek treatment as needed.
  - Avoid use of diaphragms with spermicide.

• = Independent     ▲ = Collaborative

- Teach clients with spinal cord injury and neurogenic bladder dysfunction to consider adding cranberry extract tablets or cranberry juice or fruits containing D-mannose (e.g., apples, oranges, peaches, blueberries) on a daily basis and to monitor fluid intake. The client is encouraged to discuss the use of probiotics and antibiotic therapy with the provider for frequent recurrent symptomatic UTIs.
- Teach all persons to recognize hematuria and to promptly seek care if this symptom occurs.

# Urinary Retention

**Domain 3** Elimination and exchange    **Class 1** Urinary function

## NANDA-I Definition

Incomplete emptying of the bladder.

## Defining Characteristics

Absence of urinary output; bladder distention; dysuria; increased daytime urinary frequency; minimal void volume; overflow incontinence; reports sensation of bladder fullness; reports sensation of residual urine; weak urine stream

## Related Factors

Environmental constraints; fecal impaction; improper toileting posture; inadequate relaxation of pelvic floor muscles; insufficient privacy; pelvic organ prolapse; weakened bladder muscle

## At-Risk Population

Puerperal women

## Associated Conditions

Benign prostatic hyperplasia; diabetes mellitus; nervous system diseases; pharmaceutical preparations; urinary tract obstruction

## Client Outcomes

**Client Will (Specify Time Frame)**

- Demonstrate consistent ability to urinate when desire to void is perceived
- Have measured urinary residual volume of less than 300 mL
- Experience correction or relief from dysuria, nocturia, postvoid dribbling, and voiding frequently
- Be free of a urinary tract infection

## Nursing Interventions

- Obtain a focused urinary history including questioning the client about episodes of acute urinary retention (UR; complete inability to void) or chronic retention (documented elevated postvoid residual volumes), as well as symptoms such as dysuria, nocturia, postvoid dribbling, and voiding frequently.

- Question the client concerning specific risk factors for UR:
  - ○ Medications, including antispasmodics/parasympatholytics, alpha-adrenergic agonists, antidepressants, sedatives, narcotics, psychotropic medications, illicit drugs
  - ○ Vaginal delivery within the past 48 hours
  - ○ Bowel elimination patterns, history of fecal impaction, encopresis
  - ○ Metabolic disorders such as diabetes mellitus, chronic alcoholism, and related conditions associated with polyuria and peripheral polyneuropathies
  - ○ Spinal cord injuries
  - ○ Ischemic stroke
  - ○ Herpetic infection
  - ○ Heavy-metal poisoning (lead, mercury) causing peripheral polyneuropathies
  - ○ Advanced stage HIV infection
  - ○ Recent surgery requiring general or spinal anesthesia
  - ○ Recent surgical procedures
  - ○ Recent prostatic biopsy
- Complete a pain assessment including pain intensity using a self-report pain tool, such as the 0 to 10 numerical pain rating scale. Also determine location, quality, onset/duration, intensity, aggravating/ alleviating factors, and effects of pain on function and quality of life.
- Perform a focused physical assessment including perineal skin integrity and inspection, percussion, and palpation of the lower abdomen, looking for obvious bladder distention or an enlarged kidney.
- Recognize that unrelieved obstruction of urine can result in kidney damage and, if severe, kidney failure. UR can be a medical emergency and should be reported to the primary provider as soon as possible.
- Review laboratory test results, including serum electrolytes, blood urea nitrogen (BUN), and creatinine, along with calcium, phosphate, magnesium, uric acid, and albumin.
- Monitor for signs of dehydration, peripheral edema, elevated blood pressure, and heart failure.
- Ask the client to complete a bladder diary including patterns of urine elimination, urine loss (if present), nocturia, and volume and type of fluids consumed for a period of 3 to 7 days.
- ▲ Consult with the health care provider concerning eliminating or altering medications suspected of producing or exacerbating UR.

| U |

• = Independent        ▲ = Collaborative

- Both men and women may develop UR from obstruction of the bladder outlet and abnormalities in detrusor contractility.
- In clients treated with an indwelling urethral catheter (IUC), complications such as catheter-associated urinary tract infections are common, whereas underuse of IUC may cause harmful UR.
- Advise the male client with UR related to benign prostatic hyperplasia (BPH) to avoid risk factors associated with acute UR:
  - ○ Avoid over-the-counter (OTC) cold remedies containing a decongestant (alpha-adrenergic agonist) or antihistamine, such as diphenhydramine, which has anticholinergic effects.
  - ○ Avoid taking OTC dietary medications (frequently contain alpha-adrenergic agonists).
  - ○ Discuss voiding problems with a health care provider before beginning new prescription medications.
  - ○ After prolonged exposure to cool weather, warm the body before attempting to urinate.
  - ○ Avoid overfilling the bladder by regular urination patterns and refrain from excessive intake of alcohol.
- Advise the client who is unable to void of specific strategies to manage this potential medical emergency as follows:
  - ○ Attempt urination in complete privacy.
  - ○ Place the feet solidly on the floor.
  - ○ If unable to void using these strategies, take a warm sitz bath or shower and void (if possible) while still in the tub or shower.
  - ○ Drink a warm cup of caffeinated coffee or tea to stimulate the bladder, which may promote voiding.
  - ○ If unable to void within 6 hours or if bladder distention is producing significant pain, seek urgent or emergency care.
- Perform sterile (in acute care) or clean intermittent catheterization at home as ordered for clients with UR. Refer to care plan for Mixed Urinary **Incontinence** for more information about intermittent catheterization.
- ▲ Insert an indwelling catheter only as ordered by a health care provider. Understand the indication for the urinary catheter to be placed as part of client management. Catheter-associated urinary tract infections (CAUTIs) are among the most common health care–associated infections and result in unnecessary health care costs. A CAUTI also increases the risk of a bloodstream infection.
- Nurse-led and computer-based reminders are both successful in reducing how long urinary catheters remain in place (Timmons et al, 2017).

• = Independent          ▲ = Collaborative

- Nurse-driven practice recommendations to reduce CAUTI risk include securing catheters; maintaining drainage bags lower than level of bladder; emptying drainage bags every 8 hours, when two-thirds full, and before any transfer; daily evaluation of catheter indication/need to promote removal; and use of bladder scanner to prevent reinsertion.
- Current practice recommendations support aseptic catheter insertions, whereas the use of hydrophilic-coated catheters for clean intermittent catheters can reduce the rate of CAUTIs. Suprapubic catheterization is not more effective than urethral catheterization in reducing the incidence of catheter-related bacteremia.
- For the individual with UR who is not a suitable candidate for intermittent catheterization, recognize that the catheter can be a significant cause of harm to the client through development of a CAUTI or through genitourinary trauma when the catheter is pulled.
- Advise clients with indwelling catheters that bacteria in the urine is an almost universal finding after the catheter has remained in place for more than 1 week and that only symptomatic infections warrant treatment.
- Use the following strategies to reduce the risk for CAUTI whenever feasible:
  ○ Insert the indwelling catheter with sterile technique, only when insertion is indicated.
  ○ Remove the indwelling catheter as soon as possible; acute care facilities should institute a policy for regular review of the necessity of an indwelling catheter.
  ○ Maintain a closed drainage system whenever feasible.
  ○ Maintain unobstructed urine flow, avoiding kinks in the tubing and keeping the collecting bag below the level of the bladder at all times.
  ○ Regularly cleanse the urethral meatus with a gentle cleanser to remove apparent soiling.
  ○ Change the long-term catheter every 4 weeks; more frequent catheter changes should be reserved for clients who experience catheter encrustation and blockage.
- Educate staff about the risks for CAUTI development and specific strategies to reduce these risks.

**Postoperative Urinary Retention**
- UR is a common complication of surgery, anesthesia, and advancing age. If conservative measures do not help the client pass urine, the bladder needs to be drained using either an intermittent catheter or

U

IUC, which places the client at risk for development of CAUTI (Lee et al, 2017).

- Remove the IUC at midnight in the hospitalized postoperative client to reduce the risk for acute UR.
- Perform a bladder scan before considering inserting a catheter to determine PVR volume after surgery.
- Spinal anesthesia is a risk factor associated with postoperative urinary retention (Bjerregaard et al, 2015).

**Geriatric**

- Aggressively assess older clients, particularly those with dribbling urinary incontinence, urinary tract infection, and related conditions, for UR.
- Assess older clients for impaction when UR is documented or suspected; monitor older male clients for retention related to BPH or prostate cancer. Prostate enlargement in older men increases the risk for acute and chronic UR.

**Home Care**

- Encourage the client to report any inability to void.
- Maintain an up-to-date medication list; evaluate side-effect profiles for risk of UR. New medications or changes in dose may cause UR.
- ▲ Refer the client for health care provider evaluation if UR occurs. Identification of cause is important. Left untreated, UR may lead to urinary tract infection or kidney failure.

**Client/Family Teaching and Discharge Planning**

- Teach the client with mild to moderate obstructive symptoms to double void by urinating, resting in the bathroom for 3 to 5 minutes, and then trying again to urinate.
- Teach the client with UR and infrequent voiding to urinate by the clock.
- Teach the client with an indwelling catheter to assess the tube for patency, maintain the drainage system below the level of the symphysis pubis, and routinely cleanse the bedside bag as directed.
- Teach the client with an indwelling catheter or undergoing intermittent catheterization the symptoms of a significant urinary infection, including hematuria, acute-onset incontinence, dysuria, flank pain, fever, or acute confusion.

# Risk for Urinary Retention

**Domain 3** Elimination and exchange     **Class 1** Urinary function

## NANDA-I Definition

Susceptible to incomplete emptying of the bladder.

## Related Factors

Environmental constraints; fecal impaction; improper toileting posture; inadequate relaxation of pelvic floor muscles; insufficient privacy; pelvic organ prolapse; weakened bladder muscle

## At-Risk Population

Puerperal women

## Associated Conditions

Benign prostatic hyperplasia; diabetes mellitus; nervous system diseases; pharmaceutical preparations; urinary tract obstruction

## Client Outcomes, Nursing Interventions, and Client/Family Teaching and Discharge Planning

Refer to care plan for **Urinary Retention.**

# Risk for Vascular Trauma

**Domain 11** Safety/projection     **Class 2** Physical injury

## NANDA-I Definition

Susceptible to damage to vein and its surrounding tissues related to the presence of a catheter and/or infusion solutions, which may compromise health.

## Risk Factors

Inadequate available insertion site; prolonged period of time catheter is in place

## Associated Conditions

Irritating solution; rapid infusion rate

## Client Outcomes

**Client Will (Specify Time Frame)**

- Remain free from vascular trauma
- Remain free from signs and symptoms that indicate vascular trauma
- Remain free of signs and symptoms of vascular inflammation or infection
- Remain free from impaired tissue and/or skin
- Maintain skin integrity, tissue perfusion, usual tissue temperature, color, and pigment
- Report any altered sensation or pain
- State site is comfortable

• = Independent     ▲ = Collaborative

## Nursing Interventions

### Client Preparation

▲ Verify objective and estimate duration of treatment. Check health care provider's order.

• Assess client's clinical situation when venous infusion is indicated.

• Assess if client is prepared for an intravenous (IV) procedure. Explain the procedure if necessary, to decrease stress.

• Provide privacy and make the client comfortable during the IV insertion.

• Teach the client what symptoms of possible vascular trauma he or she should be alert to and to immediately inform staff if any of these symptoms are noticed.

### Insertion

• Wash hands before and after touching the client, as well as when inserting, replacing, accessing, repairing, or dressing an intravascular catheter (O'Grady et al, 2011; Infusion Nurses Society [INS], 2016; Kaur, 2019).

• Maintain aseptic technique for the insertion and care of intravascular catheters.

• In preparation, assess the client's medical history for disease processes such as diabetes and hypertension, frequent venipuncture, variations in skin color, skin alteration, age, obesity, fluid volume deficit, and IV drug use; these factors may lead to difficult vascular visualization (INS, 2016).

• When vascular visualization is difficult, consider the use of visible light devices that provide transillumination of the peripheral veins or ultrasonography (INS, 2016). Ultrasonography reduces the number of venipuncture attempts and procedure time.

• Avoid areas of joint flexion or bony prominences.

• Avoid the use of the antecubital area, which has high failure rates, and do not use lower extremities unless necessary because of the risk of tissue damage, thrombophlebitis, and ulceration (INS, 2016).

▲ Avoid the dorsal hand, radial wrist, and the volar (inner) wrist, if possible.

▲ Consider topical anesthetic before IV cannula insertion to reduce pain (Kaur, 2019).

• Choose an appropriate vascular access device (VAD) based on the types and characteristics of the devices and insertion site. Consider the following:

  ○ Peripheral cannulae: these are short devices that are placed into a peripheral vein. They can be straight, winged, or ported and winged.

  ○ Midline catheters or peripherally inserted central catheters (PICCs) that range from 7.5 to 20 cm.

  ○ Central venous access devices (CVADs) are terminated in the central venous circulation and are available in a range of gauge sizes; they can be nontunneled catheters, skin-tunneled catheters, implantable injection ports, or PICCs.

- ○ Polyurethane venous devices and silicone rubber may cause less friction and, consequently, may reduce the risk of mechanical phlebitis (Phillips, 2014).
- ▲ Choose a device with consideration of the nature, volume, and flow of prescribed solution.
- • If possible, choose the venous access site considering the client's preference. Engaging the client in choosing the venous access site, when possible, may facilitate line patency.
- • Select the gauge of the venous device according to the duration of treatment, purpose of the procedure, and size of the vein.
- • Verify whether the client is allergic to fixation or device material.
- • Disinfect the venipuncture site. Assess that skin is dry before puncturing to achieve maximal benefit of the disinfection agent.
- • Provide a comfortable, safe, hypoallergenic, easily removable stabilization dressing, allowing for visualization of the access site.
- • Use sterile, transparent, semipermeable dressing to cover catheter site. Replace dressing with catheter change, or at a minimum every 7 days for transparent dressings (INS, 2016).
- • Document insertion date, site, type of VAD, number of punctures performed, other occurrences, and measures/arrangements.
- • Always decontaminate the device before infusing medication or manipulating IV equipment.
- ▲ Verify the sequence of drugs to be administrated.

**Monitoring Infusion**
- • Monitor permeability and flow rate at regular intervals.
- • Monitor catheter–skin junction and surrounding tissues at regular intervals, observing possible appearance of burning, pain, erythema, altered local temperature, infiltration, extravasation, edema, secretion, tenderness, or induration. Remove promptly.
- ▲ Replace device according to institution protocol.
- ▲ Flush vascular access according to organizational policies and procedures and as recommended by the manufacturer.
- • When locking a catheter, use enough fluid to fill the entire catheter and use a positive pressure technique when disconnecting the syringe (Porritt, 2016).
- • Remove catheter on suspected contamination, if the client develops signs of phlebitis or infection, the catheter is malfunctioning, or when the catheter is no longer required.

**V**

• = Independent         ▲ = Collaborative

- Encourage clients to report any discomfort such as pain, burning, swelling, or bleeding (Kaur, 2019).

**Pediatric**

- The preceding interventions may be adapted for the pediatric client.
- Inform the client and family about the IV procedure; obtain permissions, maintain client's comfort, and perform appropriate assessment before venipuncture. Assess the client for any allergies or sensitivities to tape, antiseptics, or latex.
- Consider using a two-dimensional ultrasound for venous cannulation.
- The use of an appropriate device to obtain blood samples reduces discomfort in the pediatric client.
- Avoid areas of joint flexion or bony prominences.
- For insertion in pediatric clients, use upper extremities, lower extremities, or the scalp in neonates or young infants (O'Grady et al, 2011).
- ▲ Consider whether sedation or the use of local anesthetic is suitable for insertion of a catheter, taking into consideration the age of the pediatric client.
- ▲ Use diversion while performing the procedure.

**Geriatric**

- The preceding interventions may be adapted for the geriatric client.
- Consider the physical, emotional, and cognitive changes related to older adults.
- Use strict aseptic technique for venipuncture of older clients.

**Home Care**

- Some devices may remain after discharge. Provide device-specific education to the client and family members about care of the selected device.
- Help in the choice of actions that support self-care. The nurse can provide valuable information that can be used to guide decision-making to maximize the self-care abilities of clients receiving home infusion therapy.
- Select, with the client, the insertion site most compatible with the development of activities of daily living (ADLs).
- Minimize the use of continuous IV therapy whenever possible.

# Impaired Spontaneous Ventilation

**Domain 4** Activity/rest    **Class 4** Cardiovascular/pulmonary responses

## NANDA-I Definition

Inability to initiate and/or maintain independent breathing that is adequate to support life.

• = Independent          ▲ = Collaborative

## Defining Characteristics

Apprehensiveness; decreased arterial oxygen saturation; decreased cooperation; decreased partial pressure of oxygen; decreased tidal volume; increased accessory muscle use; increased heart rate; increased metabolic rate; increased partial pressure of carbon dioxide ($PCO_2$); psychomotor agitation

## Related Factors

Respiratory muscle fatigue

## Associated Conditions

Impaired metabolism

## Client Outcomes

**Client Will (Specify Time Frame)**

- Maintain arterial blood gases within safe parameters
- Remain free of dyspnea or restlessness
- Effectively maintain airway
- Effectively mobilize secretions

## Nursing Interventions

▲ Collaborate with the client, family, and provider regarding possible intubation and ventilation. Ask whether the client has advance directives and, if so, integrate them into the plan of care with clinical data regarding overall health and reversibility of the medical condition.

• Assess and respond to changes in the client's respiratory status. Monitor the client for dyspnea, increase in respiratory rate, use of accessory muscles, retraction of intercostal muscles, flaring of nostrils, decrease in $O_2$ saturation, cyanosis, and subjective complaints (Gallagher, 2017; Loscalzo, 2018).

• Have the client use a numerical scale (0–10) or visual analog scale to self-report dyspnea before and after interventions.

• Assess for history of chronic respiratory disorders when administering oxygen.

▲ Collaborate with the health care provider and respiratory therapists in determining the appropriateness of noninvasive positive pressure ventilation/noninvasive ventilation (NPPV/NIV) for the decompensated client with respiratory diseases (including COPD). Ventilatory support during an exacerbation can be provided by either noninvasive or invasive ventilation (GOLD, 2020). NIV improves respiratory acidosis and decreases respiratory rate, severity of breathlessness, incidence of ventilator-associated pneumonia (VAP), and hospital length of stay (American Association of Critical Care Nurses, 2017a; GOLD, 2020).

**V**

▲ Assist with implementation, client support, and monitoring if NPPV/NIV is used.

• If the client has apnea, respiratory muscle fatigue, somnolence, hypoxemia, and/or acute respiratory acidosis, prepare the client for possible intubation and mechanical ventilation.

• If a client with acute respiratory failure (ARF) has a Rapid Shallow Breathing Index (RSBI) >105, endotracheal intubation is likely needed with invasive mechanical ventilation. A client with ARF with an RSBI of <105 may require only noninvasive ventilation (Karthika et al, 2016).

**Ventilator Support**

▲ Explain the endotracheal intubation and mechanical ventilation process to the client and family as appropriate, and during intubation administer sedation for client comfort according to the health care provider's orders.

• Secure the endotracheal tube in place using either tape or a commercially available device, auscultate bilateral breath sounds, use a $CO_2$ detector, and obtain a chest radiograph to confirm endotracheal tube placement.

▲ Review ventilator settings with the health care provider and respiratory therapy to ensure support is appropriate to meet the client's minute ventilation requirements (Chacko et al, 2015).

▲ Suction as needed and hyperoxygenate according to facility policy.

• Check that monitor alarms are set appropriately at the start of each shift.

• Respond to ventilator alarms promptly. If unable to immediately locate the source/cause of an alarm, use a manual self-inflating resuscitation bag to ventilate the client while waiting for assistance.

• Prevent unplanned extubation by maintaining stability of endotracheal tube (Goodrich, 2017).

• Drain collected fluid from condensation out of ventilator tubing as needed.

• Note ventilator settings of flow of inspired oxygen, peak inspiratory pressure, tidal volume, and alarm activation at intervals and when removing the client from the ventilator for any reason.

▲ Administer analgesics and sedatives as needed to facilitate client comfort and rest. Use behavioral and sedation scales for nonverbal clients to provide a consistent way of monitoring pain and sedation levels and ensuring that therapeutic outcomes are being met.

- Tools such as the Riker Sedation-Agitation Scale, the Motor Activity Assessment Scale, the Ramsey Scale, or the Richmond Agitation-Sedation Scale may be useful in monitoring levels of sedation.
- Alternatives to medications for decreasing anxiety should be attempted, such as music therapy with selections of the client's choice played on headphones at intervals.
- Analyze and respond to arterial blood gas results, end-tidal $CO_2$ levels, and pulse oximetry values. Ventilatory support must be closely monitored to ensure adequate oxygenation and acid-base balance.
- Use an effective means of verbal and nonverbal communication with the client. Barriers to communication include endotracheal tubes, sedation, and general weakness associated with a critical illness.
- Move the endotracheal tube from side to side at least every 24 hours, and tape it or secure it with a commercially available device. Assess and document client's skin condition, and ensure correct tube placement at lip line (Vollman et al, 2017).
- Implement steps to prevent ventilator-associated events (VAEs), such as ventilator-associated pneumonia (VAP), including continuous removal of subglottic secretions, elevation of the head of bed to 30 to 45 degrees (Hospital Quality Institute, 2015; American Association of Critical Care Nurses, 2017a) unless medically contraindicated, change of the ventilator circuit no more than every 48 hours, and handwashing before and after contact with each client.
- The accumulation of contaminated oropharyngeal secretions above the endotracheal tube may contribute to the risk of aspiration.
- Position the client in a semirecumbent position with the head of the bed at a 30- to 45-degree angle to decrease the aspiration of gastric, oral, and nasal secretions (Hospital Quality Institute, 2015; American Association of Critical Care Nurses, 2017a; Vollman et al, 2017).
- Consider use of kinetic therapy, using a kinetic bed that slowly moves the client with 40-degree turns.
- Perform handwashing using both soap and water and alcohol based solution before and after all mechanically ventilated client contact to prevent spread of infections (Centers for Disease Control and Prevention, 2019e).
- Provide routine oral care using tooth brushing and oral rinsing with an antimicrobial agent if needed (American Association of Critical Care Nurses, 2017a, 2017b; Vollman et al, 2017).
- Maintain proper cuff inflation for both endotracheal tubes and cuffed tracheostomy tubes with minimal leak volume or minimal occlusion

V

volume to decrease risk of aspiration and reduce incidence of VAP (American Association of Critical Care Nurses, 2016; Johnson, 2017).

- Reposition the client as needed. Use rotational bed or kinetic bed therapy in clients for whom side-to-side turning is contraindicated or difficult.
▲ Clients mechanically ventilated for more than 24 hours can benefit from protocolized rehabilitation directed toward early mobilization (Schmidt et al, 2017).
- Assess bilateral anterior and posterior breath sounds every 2 to 4 hours and as needed; respond to any relevant changes (Gallagher, 2017).
- Assess responsiveness to ventilator support; monitor for subjective complaints and sensation of dyspnea (Gallagher, 2017).
▲ Collaborate with the multiprofessional team in treating clients with acute respiratory failure. Collaborate with the health care team to meet the client's ventilator care needs and avoid complications.
- Document assessments and interventions according to policy.

**Geriatric**
- Recognize that critically ill older adults have a high rate of morbidity when mechanically ventilated.
▲ NPPV may be used during acute treatment of older clients with impaired ventilation.

**Home Care**
▲ Some of the interventions listed previously may be adapted for home care use. Begin discharge planning as soon as possible with the case manager or social worker to assess the need for home support systems, assistive devices, and community or home health services.
▲ With help from a medical social worker, assist the client and family to determine the fiscal effect of care in the home versus an extended care facility.
- Assess the home setting during the discharge process to ensure the home can safely accommodate ventilator support (e.g., adequate space and electricity).
- Have the family contact the electric company and place the client residence on a high-risk list in case of a power outage. Some home-based care requires special conditions for safe home administration.
- Assess the caregivers for commitment to supporting a ventilator-dependent client in the home.
- Be sure that the client and family or caregivers are familiar with operation of all ventilation devices, know how to suction secretions if needed, are competent in doing tracheostomy care, and know schedules for cleaning equipment. Have the designated caregiver or

• = Independent          ▲ = Collaborative

caregivers demonstrate care before discharge. Some home-based care involves specialized technology and requires specific skills for safe and appropriate care.
- Assess client and caregiver knowledge of the disease, client needs, and medications to be administered via ventilation-assistive devices. Avoid analgesics. Assess knowledge of how to use equipment. Teach as necessary.
- A client receiving ventilation support may not be able to articulate needs. Respiratory medications can have side effects that change the client's respiration or level of consciousness.
- Establish an emergency plan and criteria for use. Identify emergency procedures to be used until medical assistance arrives. Teach and role-play emergency care. A prepared emergency plan reassures the client and family and ensures client safety.

**Client/Family Teaching and Discharge Planning**
- Explain to the client the potential sensations that will be experienced, including relief of dyspnea, the feeling of lung inflations, the noise of the ventilator, and the reality of alarms.
- Explain to the client and family about being unable to speak, and work out an alternative system of communication. See previously mentioned interventions (Gallagher, 2017).
- Demonstrate to the family how to perform simple procedures, such as suctioning secretions in the mouth with a tonsil-tip catheter, providing range-of-motion exercises, and reconnecting the ventilator immediately if it becomes disconnected.
- Offer both the client and family explanations of how the ventilator works and answer any questions.

# Dysfunctional Adult Ventilatory Weaning Response

**Domain 4** Activity/rest    **Class 4** Cardiovascular/pulmonary responses
### NANDA-I Definition
Inability of individuals >18 years of age, who have required mechanical ventilation at least 24 hours, to successfully transition to spontaneous ventilation.
### Defining Characteristics
Early Response (30 minutes)
Adventitious breath sounds; audible airway secretions; decreased blood pressure (<90 mm Hg or >20% reduction from baseline); decreased heart rate (>20% reduction from baseline); decreased oxygen saturation (<90%

• = Independent                    ▲ = Collaborative

when fraction of inspired oxygen ratio >40%); expresses apprehensiveness; expresses distress; expresses fear of machine malfunction; expresses feeling warm; hyperfocused on activities; increased blood pressure (systolic pressure >180 mm Hg or >20% from baseline); increased in heart rate (>140 bpm or >20% from baseline); increased respiratory rate (>35 rpm or >50% over baseline); nasal flaring; panting; paradoxical abdominal breathing; perceived need for increased oxygen; psychomotor agitation; shallow breathing; uses significant respiratory accessory muscles; wide-eyed appearance

### Intermediate Response (30-90 minutes)

Decreased pH (<7.32 or >0.07 reduction from baseline); diaphoresis; difficulty cooperating with instructions; hypercapnia (>50 mm Hg increase in partial pressure of carbon dioxide or >8 mm Hg increase from baseline); hypoxemia (partial pressure of oxygen 50% or oxygen >6 L/min)

### Late Response (>90 minutes)

Cardiorespiratory arrest; cyanosis; fatigue; recent onset arrhythmias

### Related Factors

Altered sleep-wake cycle; excessive airway secretions; ineffective cough; malnutrition

### At-Risk Population

Individuals with history of failed weaning attempt; individuals with history of lung diseases; individuals with history of prolonged dependence on ventilator; individuals with history of unplanned extubation; individuals with unfavorable pre-extubation indexes; older adults

### Associated Conditions

Acid-base imbalance; anemia; cardiogenic shock; decreased level of consciousness; diaphragm dysfunction acquired in the intensive care unit; endocrine system diseases; heart diseases; high acuity illness; hyperthermia; hypoxemia; infections; neuromuscular diseases; pharmaceutical preparations; water-electrolyte imbalance

### Client Outcomes

**Client Will (Specify Time Frame)**

- Wean from ventilator with adequate arterial blood gases
- Remain free of unresolved dyspnea or restlessness
- Effectively clear secretions

### Nursing Interventions

▲ Assess client's readiness for weaning as evidenced by the following:
  ○ Physiological and psychological readiness.
  ○ Resolution of initial medical problem that led to ventilator dependence.
  ○ Hemodynamic stability.

• = Independent ▲ = Collaborative

- ○ Normal hemoglobin levels.
- ○ Absence of fever.
- ○ Normal state of consciousness.
- ○ Metabolic, fluid, and electrolyte balance.
- ○ Adequate nutritional status with serum albumin levels >2.5 g/dL.
- ○ Adequate sleep.
- ○ Adequate pain management and minimal sedation.
- ▲ Evaluate serum electrolytes, complete blood count, and nutritional status as a measure of client readiness to wean.
- ▲ Assess arterial blood gas analysis as part of weaning interventions. Monitor pulse oximetry and not correlation of pulse oximeter reading with arterial blood gas results.
- ▲ If the client has a central venous catheter, monitor changes in values during weaning as a symptom of hemodynamic stability along with changes in blood pressure and heart rate.
- ▲ Monitor respiratory parameters for weaning and extubation determination. Review and collaborate with respiratory therapists and providers to note improvements in NIF.
- ▲ Monitor respiratory rate and volume of independent breaths while on mechanical ventilation. Supporting independent breathing strengthens the diaphragm.
- ▲ Collaborate with respiratory therapy and provider tests to evaluate diaphragm strength for readiness to wean.
- ▲ Assess the presence and strength of the client's gag reflexes.
- ▲ Collaborate with respiratory therapy and providers to review client readiness to wean using a standardized checklist. Checklist may be referred to as mechanical ventilator liberation protocols or spontaneous awakening trails with spontaneous breathing trials (SAT/SBT) protocols.
- ▲ Use evidence-based weaning and extubation protocols as appropriate.
- ▲ A client may require noninvasive ventilation (NIV) or bilevel positive airway pressure (BiPAP) once extubated from mechanical ventilation to reduce the risk of reintubation.
- ▲ An early mobility and walking program can promote weaning from a ventilator support as a client's overall strength and endurance improve. Collaborate with respiratory therapy and physical therapy to implement early mobility programs for clients on mechanical ventilation.
- ▲ Evaluate client nutritional status as a critical element for successful weaning and ability to be successful with rehabilitation program.

• = Independent        ▲ = Collaborative

▲ Provide adequate nutrition to ventilated clients, using enteral feeding when possible.

• Identify reasons for previous unsuccessful weaning attempts, and include that information in development of the weaning plan.

▲ Collaborate with respiratory therapy and provide for optimal oxygen delivery plan once the client is successfully weaned from mechanical ventilation.

▲ Clients with neurological diseases may need special considerations to successfully wean from mechanical ventilation.

▲ Collaborate with a multiprofessional team (provider, nurse, respiratory therapist, physical therapist, and dietitian) to develop a weaning plan with a timeline and goals; revise this plan throughout the weaning period.

• Assist client to identify personal strategies that result in relaxation and comfort (e.g., music, visualization, relaxation techniques, reading, television, family visits). Support implementation of these strategies.

• Provide a safe and comfortable environment. Orient the client to the call light button. Ensure that the call light button is readily available, and assure the client that needs will be met responsively.

▲ Coordinate pain and sedation medications to minimize sedative effects while optimizing analgesia needs.

• Administer analgesics and sedatives as needed to facilitate client comfort and rest. Use behavioral and sedation scales for nonverbal clients to provide a consistent way of monitoring pain and sedation levels and ensuring that therapeutic outcomes are being met.

• Tools such as the Riker Sedation-Agitation Scale, the Motor Activity Assessment Scale, the Ramsey Scale, or the Richmond Agitation-Sedation Scale may be useful in monitoring levels of sedation (Devlin et al, 2018).

• Schedule weaning periods for the time of day when the client is most rested. Cluster care activities to promote successful weaning. Avoid other procedures during weaning: keep the environment quiet and promote restful activities between weaning periods.

• Promote a normal sleep-wake cycle, allowing uninterrupted periods of nighttime sleep.

• During weaning, monitor the client's physiological and psychological responses; acknowledge and respond to fears and subjective complaints. Validate the client's efforts during the weaning process.

• Involve the client and family in the weaning plan. Inform them of the weaning plan and possible client responses to the weaning process

• = Independent          ▲ = Collaborative

(e.g., potential feelings of dyspnea). Foster a partnership between clients and nurses in care planning for weaning.

- Coach the client through episodes of increased anxiety. Remain with the client or place a supportive and calm significant other in this role. Give positive reinforcement, and with permission use touch to communicate support and concern.

- Terminate weaning when the client demonstrates predetermined criteria or when the following signs of weaning intolerance occur:
  - ○ Tachypnea, dyspnea, or chest and abdominal asynchrony
  - ○ Agitation or mental status changes
  - ○ Decreased oxygen saturation: $SaO_2$ <90%
  - ○ Increased $PaCO_2$ or end-tidal $CO_2$ ($EtCO_2$)
  - ○ Change in pulse rate or blood pressure or onset of new dysrhythmias

▲ If the dysfunctional weaning response is severe, consider slowing weaning to brief periods. Continue to collaborate with the team to determine whether an untreated physiological cause for the dysfunctional weaning pattern remains. Consult with health care provider regarding use of noninvasive ventilation immediately after discontinuing ventilation. Consider an alternative care setting (subacute, rehabilitation facility, home) for clients with prolonged ventilator dependence as a strategy that can positively affect outcomes.

**Geriatric**

- Recognize that older clients may require longer periods to wean.
▲ NPPV may be used during acute treatment of older clients with impaired ventilation.
- Explore the client's wishes, if possible, before requiring mechanical ventilation support. Collaborate with the client, family, and provider regarding possible intubation and ventilation. Ask whether the client has advance directives and, if so, integrate them into the plan of care with clinical data regarding overall health and reversibility of the medical condition.

**Home Care**

- Weaning from a ventilator at home should be based on client stability and comfort of the client and caregivers under an intermittent care plan. Generally the client will be safer weaning in a hospital environment.

**V**

# Dysfunctional Ventilatory Weaning Response

**Domain 4** Activity/rest **Class 4** Cardiovascular/pulmonary responses
**NANDA-I Definition**

Inability to adjust to lowered levels of mechanical ventilator support that interrupts and prolongs the weaning process

**Defining Characteristics**

**Mild**

Breathing discomfort; expresses feeling warm; fatigue; fear of machine malfunction; increased focus on breathing; mildly increased respiratory rate over baseline; perceived need for increased oxygen; psychomotor agitation

**Moderate**

Abnormal skin color; apprehensiveness; blood pressure increased from baseline (<20 mm Hg); decreased air entry on auscultation; diaphoresis; difficulty cooperating; difficulty responding to coaching; facial expression of fear; heart rate increased from baseline (<20 beats/min); hyperfocused on activities; minimal use of respiratory accessory muscles; moderately increased respiratory rate over baseline

**Severe**

Adventitious breath sounds; agitation; asynchronized breathing with the ventilator; blood pressure increased from baseline (≥20 mm Hg); deterioration in arterial blood gases from baseline; gasping breaths; heart rate increased from baseline (≥20 beats/min); paradoxical abdominal breathing; profuse diaphoresis; shallow breathing; significantly increased respiratory rate above baseline; use of significant respiratory accessory muscles

**Related Factors**

**Physiological Factors**

Altered sleep-wake cycle; ineffective airway clearance; malnutrition; pain

**Psychological Factors**

Anxiety; decreased motivation; fear; hopelessness; inadequate knowledge of weaning process; inadequate trust in health care professional; low self-esteem; powerlessness; uncertainty about ability to wean

**Situational**

Environmental disturbances; inappropriate pace of weaning process; uncontrolled episodic energy demands

**At-Risk Population**

Individuals with history of unsuccessful weaning attempt; individuals with history of ventilator dependence >4 days

• = Independent　　　▲ = Collaborative

## Associated Conditions

Decreased level of consciousness

## Client Outcomes, Nursing Interventions, and Client/Family Teaching and Discharge Planning

Refer to care plan for Dysfunctional Adult **Ventilatory** Weaning Response.

# Risk for Other-Directed Violence

**Domain 11** Safety/protection    **Class 3** Violence

## NANDA-I Definition

Susceptible to behaviors in which an individual demonstrates that he or she can be physically, emotionally, and/or sexually harmful to others.

## Risk Factors

Easy access to weapon; negative body language; pattern of aggressive anti social behavior; pattern of indirect violence; pattern of other-directed violence; pattern of threatening violence; suicidal behavior

## At-Risk Population

Individuals with history of childhood abuse; individuals with history of cruelty to animals; individuals with history of fire-setting; individuals with history of motor vehicle offense; individuals with history of substance misuse; individuals with history of witnessing family violence

## Associated Conditions

Neurological impairment; pathological intoxication; perinatal complications; prenatal complications; psychotic disorders

## Client Outcomes

### Client Will (Specify Time Frame)

- Stop all forms of abuse (physical, emotional, sexual; neglect; financial exploitation)
- Display no aggressive activity
- Refrain from verbal outbursts
- Refrain from violating others' personal space
- Refrain from antisocial behaviors
- Maintain relaxed body language and decreased motor activity
- Identify factors contributing to abusive/aggressive behavior
- Demonstrate impulse control or state feelings of control
- Identify impulsive behaviors
- Identify and talk about feelings; express anger appropriately
- Displace anger to meaningful activities
- Communicate needs appropriately
- Identify responsibility to maintain control
- Express empathy for victim

• = Independent         ▲ = Collaborative

- Obtain no access or yield access to harmful objects
- Use alternative coping mechanisms for stress
- Obtain and follow through with counseling

**Victim (and Children if Applicable) Will (Specify Time Frame)**

- Have safe plan for leaving situation or avoiding abuse
- Resolve depression or traumatic response

**Parent Will (Specify Time Frame)**

- Monitor social/play contacts
- Provide supervision and nurturing environment
- Intervene to prevent high-risk social behaviors

**Nursing Interventions**

- Aggressive/violent behavior may be impulsive, but more commonly it evolves in reaction to the environment (internal or external). In either case, nursing staff must go through specialized training to be prepared for a quick response.
- Monitor the environment, evaluate situations that could become violent, and intervene early to deescalate the situation. Know and follow institutional policies and procedures concerning violence. Consider that family members or other staff may initiate violence in all settings. Enlist support from other staff rather than attempting to handle situations alone.
- Assessment with tools that measure violence may be useful in predicting or tracking behavior and serving as outcome measures.
- Identify clients with interpersonal hostile-dominance personality characteristics.

- Assess for the presence of command hallucinations.
- Apply verbal deescalation techniques when clients show increased irritability, hostility, or aggression.
- Apply **STAMPEDAR** as an acronym for assessing the immediate potential for violence.
- Determine the presence and degree of homicidal or suicidal risk. Refer to the care plan for Risk for **Suicidal** Behavior.
- Establish trust, listen to client, convey safety, and assist in developing positive goals for the future.
- Review state laws and mental health codes to determine local mandates for threat reporting by specific health care professionals. Many mental health providers are required to report harm or threats of harm to another person, referred to as the "duty to warn."
- Place the client on the appropriate precaution monitoring and observation protocol.

• = Independent  ▲ = Collaborative

- Monitor the client's behavior closely, using engagement and support as elements of safety checks while avoiding intrusive overstimulation.
- Offer information about treatment, unit rules, and procedures.
- Implement recovery-focused care interventions.
▲ After a violent event on a unit, debriefing and support of both staff and clients should be made available.
▲ Initiate and promote staff attendance at aggression management training programs.

**Pediatric**
- Assess for predictors of anger that can lead to violent behavior.
▲ In the case of child abuse or neglect, refer to child protective services.
▲ Refer the adolescent client to a violence prevention program.

**Geriatric**
- Assess for aggressive behavior in clients with a diagnosis of dementia or severe mental illness.
- For clients with dementia, provide music therapy.
- Document and record suspected elder abuse according to mandated reporter regulations.

**Multicultural**
- Exercise caution when using violence risk instruments for populations that have not been included in the testing of the instrument.

**Home Care**
- Be alert to the potential for violent behavior in the home setting. Respond to verbal aggression with interventions to deescalate negative emotional states. Violence is a process that can be recognized early. Deescalation involves reducing client stressors, responding to the client with respect, acknowledging the client's feeling state, and assisting the client to regain control. If deescalation does not work, the nurse should leave the home.
- Assess family members or caregivers for their ability to protect the client and themselves. The safety of the client between home visits is a nursing priority. Caregivers often need assistance with recognizing or admitting fear of or danger from a loved one.
- Assess access to lethal means risk factors in the home.
▲ For situations of suspected neglect or abuse, assist the client to develop an emergency plan with access to a cell phone.
- Encourage safe storage of firearms.

**Client/Family Teaching and Discharge Planning**
- Teach relaxation and exercise as ways to release anger and deal with stress.

**V**

• = Independent      ▲ = Collaborative

- Teach cognitive-behavioral activities, such as active problem-solving, reframing (reappraising the situation from a different perspective), or thought stopping (in response to a negative thought, picture a large stop sign and replace the image with a prearranged positive alternative). Teach the client to confront his or her own negative thought patterns (or cognitive distortions), such as catastrophizing (expecting the very worst), dichotomous thinking (perceiving events in only one of two opposite categories), magnification (placing distorted emphasis on a single event), or unrealistic expectations (e.g., "should get what I want when I want it").
▲ Refer perpetrators of violence to acceptance and commitment therapy.
- Teach clients and families the use of appropriate community resources in emergency situations (e.g., hotline, economic resources access, community mental health agency, ED, 911 in most places in the United States, the toll-free National Domestic Violence Hotline [1-800-799-SAFE]). Virtual resources are increasing and should be made available to clients.

# Risk for Self-Directed Violence

**Domain 11** Safety/protection    **Class 3** Violence
## NANDA-I Definition
Susceptible to behaviors in which an individual demonstrates that he or she can be physically, emotionally, and/or sexually harmful to self.
## Risk Factors
Behavioral cues of suicidal intent; conflict about sexual orientation; conflict in interpersonal relations; employment concern; engagement in autoerotic sexual acts; inadequate personal resources; social isolation; suicidal ideation; suicidal plan; verbal cues of suicidal intent
## At-Risk Population
Individuals aged 15-19 years; individuals aged ≥45 years; individuals in occupations with high suicide risk; individuals with history of multiple suicide attempts; individuals with pattern of difficulties in family background
## Associated Conditions
Mental health issues; physical health issues; psychological disorder
## Client Outcomes
Client Will (Specify Time Frame)
- Stop all forms of abuse/violence to self (physical, self-injurious emotional, sexual; neglect)
- Refrain from self-deprecation
- Identify factors contributing to abusive/self-injurious behavior

• = Independent        ▲ = Collaborative

- Demonstrate impulse control or state feelings of control
- Identify impulsive behaviors
- Identify precursors to impulsive actions
- Identify consequences of impulsive actions to self
- Avoid high-risk environments and situations
- Identify and talk about feelings; express anger appropriately
- Communicate needs appropriately
- Demonstrate self control
- Use alternative coping mechanisms for stress
- Obtain and follow through with counseling

**Client (and Children if Applicable) Will**

- Have safe plan for leaving situation
- Resolve depression or traumatic response

**Parent/Caregiver Will**

- Monitor social/play contacts
- Provide supervision and nurturing environment
- Intervene to prevent high-risk social behaviors

## Nursing Interventions

- Assess with suicide-screening tools as a part of a comprehensive clinical practice. Such tools can be helpful predictors of future self-harm.
- Screen clients for adverse childhood experiences (ACEs) and refer to ACE-informed services.
- Assess the client's use of substances such as cigarettes, alcohol, and other drugs, and suggest monitoring and/or decreasing usage.
- Assess parental mental health history and recommend treatment for parents who suffer from psychiatric disease. Parental history of mental illness is a risk factor for self-harming behaviors, equally for males and females.
- Place the client on the appropriate precaution monitoring and observation protocol.
- ▲ Refer the client to dialectical behavior therapy (DBT).
- ▲ Refer the client to an emergency department for monitoring and/or surveillance.

**Pediatric**

- Assess levels of violence in the home environment, and, if necessary, take steps to decrease aggression in the family.
- Discuss the client's experience in school, as students who feel unconnected to school, are unhappy at school, or feel that teachers are unfair may be more likely to self-harm in the future.

• = Independent          ▲ = Collaborative

- Review the client's experience online, because victims—and also, but to a lesser extent, perpetrators—of cyberbullying have a greater incidence of self-harm.
- Investigate the use of cell phone applications to address and monitor self-harming tendencies.

### Geriatric
- Conduct a comprehensive assessment, reviewing previous mental and physical disease diagnoses.
- Closely monitor medication prescribing and dosage in this population. Provide medication education and discuss alternatives to avoid potential adverse situations.

### Client/Family Teaching and Discharge Planning
- Teach clients about healthy sleep patterns.
- Involve family members in the care of geriatric clients, whose incidents of self-harm may indicate distress that cannot easily be expressed in words.

## Impaired Walking

**Domain 4** Activity/rest    **Class 2** Activity/exercise
### NANDA-I Definition
Limitation of independent movement within the environment on foot.
### Defining Characteristics
Difficulty ambulating on decline; difficulty ambulating on incline; difficulty ambulating on uneven surface; difficulty ambulating required distance; difficulty climbing stairs; difficulty navigating curbs

### Related Factors
Altered mood; environmental constraints; fear of falling; inadequate knowledge of mobility strategies; insufficient muscle strength; insufficient physical endurance; neurobehavioral manifestations; obesity; pain; physical deconditioning

### Associated Conditions
Cerebrovascular disorders; impaired postural balance; musculoskeletal impairment; neuromuscular diseases; vision disorders

### Client Outcomes/Goals
Client Will (Specify Time Frame)
- Demonstrate optimal independence and safety in walking
- Demonstrate the ability to direct others on how to assist with walking
- Demonstrate the ability to use and care for assistive walking devices properly and safely

• = Independent          ▲ = Collaborative

## Nursing Interventions

- Progressive mobilization as tolerated (gradually raising head of bed [HOB], sitting in reclined chair, standing, with assistance). Progressing mobility gradually from bed rest to increased sit-to-stand times to short-distance walking and timed testing can result in shorter admission stays and time to recovery (Snow, 2019). See also the care plan for Impaired Physical **Mobility.**
- Consider and monitor for side effects of prescribed hydration and medications; medical diagnosis, physical condition; length of immobility contributing to orthostatic hypotension; and/or if lightheadedness, dizziness, syncope, or unexplained falls occur.
- ▲ Assess for orthostatic hypotension if systolic pressure falls 15 mm Hg or diastolic pressure falls 7 mm Hg from sitting to standing within 3 minutes. If this occurs, replace client in bed and notify prescriber. Evaluation of change in heart rate can be useful to determine if orthostatic hypotension could be neurogenic.
- Apply thromboembolic deterrent (TED) stockings and/or elastic leg wraps as prescribed; raise HOB slowly in small increments to sitting, have client move feet/legs up and down, and then stand slowly; avoid prolonged standing. Movement enhances venous return, improving cardiac output and decreasing syncope.
- Assess for cognitive, neuromuscular, and sensory deficits that will affect safety when walking (e.g., stroke, diabetic neuropathy, history of falls).
- ▲ Take pulse rate/rhythm, respiratory rate, and pulse oximetry before walking clients, and reassess within 5 minutes of walking, then ongoing as needed. If abnormal, have the client sit for 5 minutes, then remeasure. If still abnormal, walk clients more slowly and with more help or for a shorter time, or notify physician. If uncontrolled diabetes/angina/arrhythmias/tachycardia (100 beats per minute or more) or resting systolic blood pressure at or above 200 mm Hg or diastolic blood pressure at or above 110 mm Hg occurs, do not initiate walking exercise. Refer to the care plan Decreased **Activity** Tolerance.
- Assist clients to apply orthosis, immobilizers, splints, braces, and compression stockings as prescribed before walking.
- Eat frequent small, low-carbohydrate meals. Low-carbohydrate meals help prevent postprandial hypotension.
- Reinforce correct use of prescribed mobility devices, and remind clients of weight-bearing restrictions.

• = Independent          ▲ = Collaborative

- Emphasize the importance of wearing properly fitting, low-heeled shoes with nonskid soles and socks/hose and of seeking medical care for foot pain or problems with abnormal toenails, corns, calluses, or diabetes. Refer to podiatric consultation if indicated.

▲ Use a snug gait belt with handles and assistive devices while walking clients, as recommended by the physical therapist.

- Walk clients frequently with an appropriate number of people; have one team member state short, simple motor instructions.

- Cue and manually guide clients with neglect as they walk.

- Document the number of helpers, level of assistance (e.g., maximum, standby), type of assistance, and devices needed in communication tools (e.g., plan of care, client room signage, verbal report).

**Special Considerations: Lower Extremity Amputation**

▲ Consult with physical therapist for best practices for postoperative mobilization for the individual case. In most cases, a prosthesis will not be fitted until wound healing occurs.

- Recognize that ambulation with a prosthesis is more labor-intensive than with a native limb.

- Teach clients the importance of avoiding prolonged hip and knee flexion. If contractures occur, they will affect prosthesis fit and function and ability to achieve a more normal gait.

**Geriatric**

▲ Assess for swaying, poor balance, weakness, and fear of falling while elders stand/walk using an objective fall-risk tool if possible. If present, implement fall protection precautions and refer for physical therapy evaluation and recommendations (Thiamwong et al, 2020).

▲ Review medications for polypharmacy (more than five drugs) and medications that increase the risk of falls, including sedatives, antidepressants, and drugs affecting the central nervous system.

- Encourage tai chi, physical therapy, or another exercise for balance, gait, and strength training in group programs or at home.

- Recommend vision assessment and consideration for cataract removal if needed.

**Home Care**

- Establish a support system for emergency and contingency care (e.g., wearable medical alert alarm, Internet-connected smart speaker; notify local emergency medical services [EMS] of potential need). Impaired walking may be life-threatening during a crisis (e.g., fall, fire, orthostatic episode).

- Assess for and modify any barriers to walking in the home environment.

• = Independent     ▲ = Collaborative

▲ Use a standardized tool to assess need for referral for occupational therapist (OT) or physical therapist (PT). If indicated, refer to OT/ PT for home assessment and evaluation for home assessment for barriers, individualized strength, balance retraining, an exercise plan, and environmental modifications for safety (Tan et al, 2021).

▲ Refer to home health services for support and assistance with activities of daily living (ADLs).

**Client/Family Teaching and Discharge Planning**

• Teach clients to check ambulation devices weekly for cracks, loose nuts, or worn tips and to clean dust and dirt on tips.

• Teach diabetics that they are at risk for foot ulcers and teach them preventive interventions. See care plan for Risk for Ineffective Peripheral **Tissue Perfusion.**

▲ Instruct clients at risk for osteoporosis or hip fracture to bear weight, walk, engage in resistance exercise (with appropriate adjustments for conditions), ensure good nutrition (especially adequate intake of calcium and vitamin D), drink milk, stop smoking, monitor alcohol intake, and consult a physician for appropriate medications.

## Wandering

**Domain 4** Activity/rest    **Class 3** Energy balance

**NANDA-I Definition**

Meandering, aimless, or repetitive locomotion that exposes the individual to harm; frequently incongruent with boundaries, limits, or obstacles.

**Defining Characteristics**

Eloping behavior; frequent movement from place to place; fretful locomotion; haphazard locomotion; hyperactivity; locomotion interspersed with nonlocomotion; locomotion into unauthorized spaces; locomotion resulting in getting lost; locomotion that cannot be easily dissuaded; long periods of locomotion without an apparent destination; pacing; periods of locomotion interspersed with periods of nonlocomotion; persistent locomotion in search of something; scanning behavior; searching behavior; shadowing a caregiver's locomotion; trespassing

**Related Factors**

Altered sleep-wake cycle; desire to go home; environmental overstimulation; neurobehavioral manifestations; physiological state; separation from familiar environment

**At-Risk Population**

Individuals with premorbid behavior

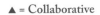

• = Independent                    ▲ = Collaborative

## Associated Conditions

Cortical atrophy; psychological disorder; sedation

## Client Outcomes

### Client Will (Specify Time Frame)

- Remain safe and free from falls
- Maintain psychological well-being and reduce need to wander
- Reduce episodes of wandering in restricted areas/getting lost/ elopement
- Maintain appropriate body weight
- Maintain physical activity and remain comfortable and free of pain

### Caregiver Will (Specify Time Frame)

- Be able to explain interventions they can use to provide a safe environment for a care receiver who displays wandering behavior
- Develop strategies to reduce caregiver stress levels

## Nursing Interventions

- Provide safe and secure surroundings that deter and detect accidental elopements, using perimeter control devices (door alarms) or electronic tracking systems (including radiofrequency identification [RFID] tags, global positioning system [GPS] locator, smart watch, or cell phone application).
- Assess for physical distress or unmet needs (e.g., hunger, thirst, pain/ discomfort, elimination needs).
- Assess for emotional or psychological distress, such as anxiety, fear, or feeling lost, considering the situated experience of the client.
- Assess and document the pattern, rhythm, and frequency of wandering over time.
- Obtain a psychosocial history from caregivers, including stress-coping behaviors.
- Observe the location and environmental conditions in which wandering is occurring and modify those that appear to provoke boundary transgression or unsafe wandering.
  - Assess the person's environment and advocate for appropriate modifications using a survey such as the Wayfinding Evidence-Based Checklist and Rating (WEBCAR) instrument (Benbow, 2013).
  - Use a full-length mirror in front of exit doors to deter elopement.
  - Use camouflage (a cloth panel, painted mural, or wall hanging) to cover doorknobs or locks (check fire safety code/policy and never obscure an emergency red EXIT sign).
  - Change the floor pattern in front of door that should not be opened to create a visual, subjective barrier (e.g., illusion of a step, black hole, or pit).

• = Independent    ▲ = Collaborative

- Increase social interaction and offer structured activity and stress-reducing approaches, such as walking, exercise, music, massage, rocking chair, and activities using household methods and a prepared environment (e.g., watering plants, flower arranging, gardening, preparing meals, shining shoes, setting table, wrapping boxes, watercolor painting, sewing buttons, sorting objects, folding laundry, matching socks, stereognostic/mystery bags, doll therapy, puzzles, games, and crafts).
- When using electronic tracking technologies, an approach emphasizing relationships, respect, and the individual needs of the person and caretaker is best suited to finding solutions that both protect and empower.
- Role model person-centered care and provide appropriate supervision, support, and education of direct-care staff.
- Help older adults find their rooms by placing signs with their names and portraits of themselves at a younger age next to the doorways.
- Provide a regularly scheduled and supervised exercise or walking program, particularly if wandering occurs excessively during the night or at times that are dangerous.
- Refer to the care plan for **Caregiver** Role Strain. For clients with dementia, also see care plan for Chronic **Confusion.**

**Multicultural**

- Assess preferences for use of social services and family caregiver availability and willingness to provide care.

**Client/Family Teaching and Discharge Planning**

- Teach caregivers about missing person resources such AMBER and Silver Alert public safety systems, MedicAlert Safe Return/Safely Home, Project Lifesaver, and related resources from the Alzheimer's Association and National Autism Association; for example, the Autism Wandering Awareness Alerts Response and Education (AWAARE) Collaboration's Big Red Safety Box and Digital Toolkits for Caregivers (available in English and Spanish), First Responders, and Teachers.

**Home Care**

- The previously mentioned interventions may be adapted for home care use.
- Help the caregiver set up a plan to reduce and manage wandering behavior, including a plan of action to use if the client elopes or is missing:
  - Assist the family to set up a plan of exercise for the client, including safe walking within appropriate geographic boundaries.

• = Independent          ▲ = Collaborative

- Assess the home environment for modifications that will protect the client and prevent elopement.
- Refer to supportive community and social services, such as an Area Office on Aging, the Alzheimer's Association, National Autism Association, home health care (psychiatric/geriatric nurse, occupational therapist, medical social worker), and companion or respite care to assist with the impact of caregiving for the wandering client.
- Provide information about therapy dog/assistance dog resources.

# Nursing Care Plans for Hearing Loss and Vision Loss

## Hearing Loss

### Definition

A condition where there is the inability to detect some or all frequencies of sound and may involve complete or partial impairment of the ability to hear. *Note:* **Hearing Loss** is not a NANDA-I accepted diagnosis, but it is included here because of the frequency of occurrence of hearing loss, especially in the geriatric population.

### Defining Characteristics

Inability to hear in noisy environments; difficulty following conversations with more than one person; change in speech; change in usual response to stimuli; disorientation; impaired communication; irritability; poor concentration; restlessness; sensory distortions

### Related Factors

Altered sensory integration; altered sensory reception; altered sensory transmission; biochemical imbalance; electrolyte imbalance; excessive noise exposure; psychological stress

### Client Outcomes

Client Will (Specify Time Frame)

- Demonstrate understanding by a verbal, written, or signed response
- Demonstrate relaxed body movements and facial expressions
- Explain plan to modify lifestyle to accommodate hearing impairment
- Demonstrate familiarity with hearing assistive devices

### Nursing Interventions

- Observe for signs of hearing loss, especially in people exposed to loud noise and people older than 60 years of age.
- Use the National Institutes of Health (NIH) Toolbox to test hearing as available.
- Recognize that certain populations are especially vulnerable to noise-induced hearing loss, including farmers, industrial workers, firefighters, construction workers, musicians, and music lovers using personal listening devices.

• = Independent ▲ = Collaborative

▲ Refer client to otolaryngologist and/or audiologist.

• Keep background noise to a minimum. Turn off the television and radio when communicating with the client. If in a noisy environment, take the client to a private room and shut the door.

• Stand or sit directly in front of the client when communicating. Make sure adequate light is on the nurse's face, avoid chewing gum or covering mouth or face with hands while speaking, establish eye contact, and use nonverbal gestures.

• Speak clearly in lower voice tones if possible. Do not over-enunciate or shout at the client.

• Verify that the client understands critical information by asking the client to repeat the information.

• If necessary, provide a communication board, personnel who know sign language, or any method helpful to increase understanding for the hearing-impaired client. Health care institutions are required to provide and pay for qualified interpreters under the Americans with Disabilities Act.

• Prepare pictures or diagrams depicting tests or procedures; have books with relevant pictures available for more detailed discussions. The use of visual aids can improve communication when hearing is impaired.

• Watch for signs of depression such as withdrawal, impaired sleep, and flat affect, and refer for treatment if needed.

• Encourage the client to wear a hearing aid if available.

• Recognize that clients with a hearing aid may choose to wear a hearing aid intermittently because hearing aids can create distortion of speech and extraneous noise that is bothersome (Shah & Lotke, 2019).

• Review the client's nutritional status and suggest a diet diary to evaluate nutritional habits.

• Ask the client about smoking. Refer the client to a smoking cessation program if indicated.

• Review the client's environmental risk factors for hearing loss, including occupational noise.

**Critical Care**

• Develop a communication cart to foster communication with hearing-impaired clients. Contents can include spiral notebooks, felt-tip markers, clipboards, communication boards (picture, word, entire phrases, and alphabet), hearing aid batteries, and electronic speech generators.

• Develop good communication skills to interact with hearing-impaired clients. It is unfair to expect critically ill older adults to understand what is being said to them only through auditory means.

• = Independent         ▲ = Collaborative

**Pediatric**

▲ Refer infants or children for hearing tests as indicated so that treatment/therapy begins early as needed.

• In the child, recommend that parents watch for signs of hearing loss, including worsening speech or school performance, withdrawal from social activities, playing alone, and playing the television and music increasingly loud (Shah & Lotke, 2019).

• Refer the child to an audiologist to explore the use of computer-based auditory training programs.

• Recognize that children who are deaf or hard of hearing are particularly vulnerable to abuse, both by parents/caregivers and by sexual predators.

• Recommend that teenagers avoid use of personal listening devices, or try to keep the volume down.

**Geriatric**

▲ Routinely screen geriatric clients for presence of hearing loss.

▲ Inspect the ear canal for wax buildup in the ears.

• Work with the client to ensure contact with others and maintenance of meaningful activities to strengthen the social network and maintain cognitive abilities.

**Home Care**

• The previously listed interventions are applicable in the home care setting.

• Recommend that the client change the home environment if needed for better acoustics. Avoid glossy walls, high and reflective ceilings, reflective glass counters, and tiled floors. Use acoustic paneling if needed. The goal is to reduce noise reverberating off the walls, floors, and surfaces of the home.

• Suggest installation of devices such as strobe lights for the telephone, alarm clock, fire alarms, and doorbell; sensors that detect an infant's cry; alarm clocks that vibrate the bed; and closed caption decoders for television sets. Other helpful devices include telephone amplifiers, speakerphones, cell phones with text messaging or instant messaging, pocket talker personal listening systems, and FM and infrared amplification systems that connect directly to a television or audio output jack. Also available is a telecommunication device, which is a typewriter keyboard with an alphanumeric display that allows the hearing-impaired person to send typed messages over the telephone line. Use of hearing ear dogs (dogs specially trained to alert their owners to specific sounds) may also be helpful.

• = Independent          ▲ = Collaborative

### Client/Family Needs and Discharge Planning

- Teach the client to avoid excessive noise at work or at home and to wear hearing protection when necessary.
- Teach the client to avoid inserting objects such as cotton-tipped swabs or bobby pins into the ears.

# Vision Loss

## Definition

Decreased or absence of vision when it existed previously; vision loss can be either acute in onset or occur as a slow progressive chronic visual loss. *Note:* **Vision Loss** is not a NANDA-I nursing diagnosis. The authors have identified this health problem because vision loss is commonly seen in nursing practice.

## Defining Characteristics

Change in behavior pattern; change in problem-solving abilities; disorientation; decreased visual acuity; loss of vision; visual hallucinations

## Related Factors

Aging; diabetes mellitus; exposure to ultraviolet (UV) light; impaired visual function; impaired visual integration; impaired visual reception; impaired visual transmission; nutritional deficiency (Adapted from the work of NANDA-I.)

## Client Outcomes

**Client Will (Specify Time Frame)**

- Demonstrate relaxed body movements and facial expressions
- Remain as independent as possible
- Explain plan to modify lifestyle to accommodate visual impairment
- Incorporate use of lighting to maximize visual abilities
- Demonstrate familiarity with vision assistive devices
- Remain free of physical harm resulting from loss of vision

## Nursing Interventions

- When providing sensitive care, post visual impairment signage for interprofessional team service support (Luckowski & Luckowski, 2015).
- Knock before entering and address client by name. Introduce yourself and title. If you want to shake hands, verbalize intent first, and in a normal, natural tone of voice, explain exactly what you are going to do. Check the call bell to ensure it is in place and usable. Place other items such as the phone and bedside table within reach and let the client know where they are located. Describe the bedrail controls and room layout, including the bathroom. Keep area clean and free from

clutter. Indicate when a conversation is over and when you are leaving the room (Luckowski & Luckowski, 2015).

- When handing an item, place it directly in the client's hand or place the client's hand on top of the item. Use the sight-guided technique to assist ambulation. Offer the back of your arm just above the elbow and walk one step ahead. Inform the client of stairs or turns. When sitting, guide the client's hand to the back of the chair or place to sit on the bed (Luckowski & Luckowski, 2015).
- Use the clock's coordinates to describe the location of food on the plate. Open containers as requested. Encourage utilization of talking clocks and watches, books, radio, and service dogs. Read education and discharge information to the client and refer for social support services as required (Luckowski & Luckowski, 2015).
- Provide environmental predictability. Consistently remind staff, family members, and visitors to tell the client when something is added or removed from the environment.
- Evaluate the environment for effective and adequate light sources.
- Make doorframes and light switches a contrasting color to the walls.
- Ensure access to eyeglasses or magnifying devices as needed.
- Encourage expression of feelings and expect grieving behavior if onset of vision loss and/or blindness is new. People grieve the loss of vision and experience a loss of identity and control over their lives.
- Recommend that clients have vision evaluated by an optometrist or ophthalmologist as appropriate to determine whether an improvement in visual acuity is possible.
- Question the client regarding the presence of visual hallucinations (Charles Bonnet syndrome).
- Take protective measures to prevent falls. Refer to the care plans for Risk for Adult **Falls** and Risk for Child **Falls.**
- Explore and enhance available support systems to ensure a safe discharge. Caregivers and/or family may not have the ability to assist the client after discharge.
- Assess the client's visual and other sensory loss using valid and reliable tools such as the Snellen eye chart (visual acuity) or Amsler grid (central vision loss with macular degeneration).
- Annual dilated eye examinations for clients with diabetes are recommended.
- Use valid and reliable tools to identify visual impairments of clients.
- Encourage the client to implement lifestyle strategies that promote avoidance of cardiovascular disease and diabetes to prevent vision loss.

• = Independent          ▲ = Collaborative

- Nursing actions that create a sense of good nursing care in clients with wet age-related macular degeneration identified two main areas of focus. The first theme was related to being perceived as an individual, specifically being respected, and answering questions politely and focusing on them as individuals and being engaged. The second theme was client empowerment through encouragement of participation to create confidence. Creating trust by building partnerships and shared decision-making is best (Emsfors, Christensson, & Elgán, 2017).

**Geriatric**
- Low vision is defined as central acuity of 20/70 or worse corrected. Legal blindness is defined as 20/200 or worse. Determination of legal blindness may qualify people for Social Security and Disability benefits. Driving contraindications must be heeded for safety (Pelletier, Rojas-Roldan, & Coffin, 2016).
- Sight loss is linked to increasing age and can have a profound effect on quality of life.
▲ Important implications for practice include the following: (1) untreatable vision loss is not an inevitable consequence of aging, and any vision loss should be investigated; (2) cataract extraction is a common procedure that results in visual rehabilitation; and (3) eye drops are often-prescribed medications, and missed doses can cause untreatable vision loss (Marsden, 2017).
- Older people with sight loss are more prone to falls and the risk of injury, including hip fractures, which double in older clients.
- Evidence supports daily age-related eye disease study (AREDS) vitamin supplementation to delay vision loss with age-related macular degeneration. Intravitreal injections of vascular endothelial growth factor stabilize vision in clients with neovascular macular degeneration or diabetic edema (Pelletier, Rojas-Roldan, & Coffin, 2016).
- Low vision rehabilitation to promote independence while reducing risk for injury must incorporate aging adults' perspective on risk and analysis of environmental factors (Laliberte Rudman et al, 2016).
- Keep the environment quiet, soothing, and familiar. Use consistent caregivers. These measures are comforting to older adults with a sensory loss and help decrease confusion (Nyman, Innes, & Heward, 2017).
▲ The leading causes of sight loss in older people are uncorrected refractive error (treatable with prescriptions), cataracts (treatable with surgery), glaucoma (preventable), diabetic retinopathy (preventable with good glycemic control), and age-related macular degeneration (sometimes treatable) (Marsden, 2017).

• = Independent          ▲ = Collaborative

- Cataracts are the leading cause of reversible vision impairment and may increase the risk for falls in older adults.
- Hearing and vision rehabilitation services need to screen for dual sensory impairment.
▲ Refer to a comprehensive vision rehabilitation center early in the disease process of macular degeneration to prevent some of the negative consequences of vision loss (Pondorfer et al, 2020).
- Teach the client methods to preserve remaining vision as much as possible, including avoiding smoking or breathing secondhand smoke, protecting the eyes from sunlight, and including fish and leafy green vegetables in the diet (Young, 2015).
- Vision impairment is independently associated with malnutrition.
- Monitor for signs of new onset of increased vision loss, such as not recognizing familiar people, difficulty seeing in bright light or low light, new problems with reading, and complaints of tired eyes and/ or vision problems with current glasses facilitating effective vision (Ventocilla & Wicker, 2016).
- Age-related visual problems can also occur with stroke.
- Watch for signs of depression such as decreased appetite, withdrawal from usual life activities, flat affect, excessive time in bed, and somatization.
- For the client with both vision loss and dementia, provide the following nursing care:
  ○ Recognize that vision loss can increase problems for the client with dementia, including decreased orientation, decreased recognition of others, less recall, impaired judgment, and possibly aggression (Young, 2015).
  ○ Use one-to-one conversations to maintain socialization.
  ○ Obtain and use visual aids to help maintain orientation and contact with the environment, including such things as talking clocks, speaking Freeview digital boxes to give an auditory version of what is on the television, and use of memory photo dial pads so that clients can use the telephone to maintain contact with others (Abraha et al, 2017; Young, 2015).

**Multicultural**
- Consider race/ethnicity as a possible related factor to vision loss.

**Home Care**
- Most of the listed interventions are applicable in the home care setting.
- Monitor home care clients for recent visual loss and resulting decrease in social activity.

• = Independent ▲ = Collaborative

- Enable the visually impaired client to do things for himself or herself to maintain independence as long as possible (Nihata et al, 2018).

**Client/Family Teaching and Discharge Planning**

- Use contrast to increase visibility of items; for example, place a dark background around the light switch so that it can be located more easily.
- Place red, yellow, or orange identifiers on important items that need to be seen, such as a red strip at the edge of steps, a red marker behind a light switch, or a red dot on a stove or washing machine to indicate how far to turn the knob, or use a dial marker that will offer a tactile cue to the client to turn on ovens, stoves, and washing machines. Color cues can improve the legibility of the environment and increase the ability to target objects quickly.
- Use a watch or clock that verbally tells time and a phone with large numerals and emergency numbers programmed into it (Ventocilla & Wicker, 2016).
- Teach blind clients how to feed themselves; associate food on the plate with hours on a clock so that the client can identify the location of food.
- Use low vision aids, including magnifying devices for near vision and telescopes for seeing objects at a distance, a closed-circuit television that magnifies print, and guides for writing checks and envelopes.
- Teach the client with vision loss to do the following:
  - Use a magnifying mirror to shave or apply makeup; use an electric razor only.
  - Put personal care products in brightly colored pump containers (red, yellow, or orange) for identification.
  - Use tactile clues such as safety pins or buttons placed in hems to help client match clothing, or place matching outfits of clothing in separate plastic bags.
  - Use a prefilled medication organizer with large lettering or three-dimensional (3D) markers.
- ▲ Increase lighting in the home to help vision in the following ways:
  - Ensure adequate illumination of the entire home, adding light fixtures and increasing wattage of existing bulbs as needed.
  - Decrease glare; where light reflects on shiny surfaces, move or cover objects.
  - Use nonglare wax on the floor.
  - Use motion lights that turn on automatically when a person enters the room for nighttime use.
  - Add indoor strip or "runway"-type lighting to baseboards.

• = Independent                    ▲ = Collaborative

▲ Refer the client to an occupational therapist for assistance in dealing with vision loss and learning how to meet personal needs to maintain maximum independence.

• Consider referral to a psychologist due to the risk of depression in clients with vision impairment (Brunes & Heir, 2020).

• Encourage the client to wear a hat and sunglasses when out in the sun.

• Work with the client to find rewarding recreational pursuits.

• Arrange transportation sources because driving is contraindicated.

• = Independent          ▲ = Collaborative

# BIBLIOGRAPHY

Abraha, I., Rimland, J. M., Trotta, F. M., et al. (2017). Systematic review of systematic reviews of non-pharmacological interventions to treat behavioural disturbances in older patients with dementia. The SENATOR-OnTop series. *BMJ Open*, *7*(3), e012759. https://doi.org/10.1136/bmjopen-2016-012759.

ACOG Committee Opinion Committee on Obstetric Practice. (2020). Obstetric management of patients with spinal cord injuries. *Obstetrics & Gynecology*, *135*(5), e230–e236. https://doi.org/10.1097/AOG.0000000000003842.

Adalja, A., Toner, E., & Inglesby, T. V. (2015). Clinical management of bioterrorism-related conditions. *New England Journal of Medicine*, *372*(10), 954–962. https://doi.org/10.1056/NEJMra1409755.

Agency for Healthcare Research and Quality. (2017). *Early mobility guide for reducing ventilator-associated events in mechanically ventilated patients*. Retrieved from https://www.ahrq.gov/sites/default/files/wysiwyg/professional s/quality-patient-safety/hais/tools/mvp/modules/technical/early-mobility-mvpguide.pdf. Accessed 25 June 2021.

Agency for Healthcare Research and Quality (AHRQ). (2015). *Toolkit for reducing catheter-associated urinary tract infections in hospital units: Implementation guide*. AHRQ Pub No. 15-0013-2-EF. Retrieved from https://www.ahrq.gov/hai/cauti-tools/impl-guide/index.html. Accessed 12 July 2021.

Agency for Healthcare Research and Quality (AHRQ). (2008). *Treating tobacco use and dependence: 2008 update—clinical practice guideline*. Washington, D.C.: AHRQ. Retrieved from https://www.ahrq.gov/prevention/guidelines/tobacc o/clinicians/update/index.html. Accessed 2 August 2021.

Agiostratidou, G., Anhalt, H., Ball, D., et al. (2017). Standardizing clinically meaningful outcome measures beyond $HbA_{1c}$ for type 1 diabetes: a consensus report of the American Association of Clinical Endocrinologists, the American Association of Diabetes Educators, the American Diabetes Association, the Endocrine Society, JDRF International, The Leona M. and Harry B. Helmsley Charitable Trust, the Pediatric Endocrine Society, and the T1D Exchange. *Diabetes Care*, *40*(12), 1622–1630. https://doi.org/10.2337/dc17-1624.

Allen, L. A., Stevenson, L. W., Grady, K. L., et al. (2012). Decision making in advanced heart failure: A scientific statement from the American Heart Association. *Circulation*, *125*(15), 1928–1952. https://doi.org/10.1161/CIR.0b013e31824f2173.

American Academy of Audiology. (2021). *How's your hearing?*. Retrieved from https://www.audiology.org/consumers-0. Accessed 10 June 2021.

American Academy of Oral Medicine (AAOM). (2016). AAOM clinical practice statement: Subject: Clinical management of cancer therapy-induced salivary gland hypofunction and xerostomia. *Oral Surgery Oral Medicine Oral Pathology Oral Radiology*, *122*(3), 310–312. https://doi.org/10.1016/j.oooo.2016.04.015.

American Academy of Pediatrics. (2021). *Family media plan*. Healthychildren.org. Retrieved from https://www.healthychildren.org/English/media/Pages/default.aspx. Accessed July 26, 2021.

American Academy of Pediatrics Task Force on Sudden Infant Death Syndrome. (2016). SIDS and other sleep-related infant deaths: Updated 2016 recommendations for a safe infant sleeping environment. *Pediatrics, 138*(5), e20162938. https://doi.org/10.1542/peds.2016-2938.

American Association of Critical Care Nurses. (2017a). AACN practice alert: Prevention of ventilator-associated pneumonia in adults. *Critical Care Nurse, 37*(3), e22–e25. Retrieved from https://www.aacn.org/~/media/aacn-website/clincial-resources/practice-alerts/preventingvapinadults2017.pdf. Accessed 4 August 2021.

American Association of Critical Care Nurses. (2017b). AACN practice alert: Oral care for acutely and critically ill patients. *Critical Care Nurse, 37*(3), e19–e21. Retrieved from https://www.aacn.org/~/media/aacn-website/clincial-resources/practice-alerts/oralcarepractalert2017.pdf. Accessed 4 August 2021.

American Association of Critical Care Nurses. (2016). AACN practice alert: Prevention of aspiration in adults. *Critical Care Nurse, 36*(1), e20–e24. Retrieved from https://www.aacn.org/~/media/aacn-website/clincial-resources/practice-alerts/preventionaspirationpracticealert.pdf. Accessed 7 June 2021.

American College of Nurse-Midwives (ACNM). (2020). Coping with labor pain. *Journal of Midwifery and Women's Health, 65*(3), 435–436. https://doi.org/10.1111/jmwh.13127.

American College of Radiology. (2021). *ACR manual on contrast media.* Retrieved from https://www.acr.org/-/media/ACR/files/clinical-resources/contrast_media.pdf. Accessed 14 June 2021.

American College of Sports Medicine (ACSM). (2018). *American College of Sports Medicine's guidelines for exercise testing and prescription* (10th ed.). Philadelphia: Lippincott Williams & Wilkins.

American Dental Association (ADA). (2020). *Home oral care.* Retrieved from https://www.ada.org/en/member-center/oral-health-topics/home-care. Accessed 19 July 2021.

American Diabetes Association (ADA). (2021). Standards of medical care in diabetes—2021. *Diabetes Care, 44*(Suppl 1), S15–S33. https://doi.org/10.2337/dc21-S002.

American Geriatrics Society. (2015). American Geriatrics Society 2015 Updated Beers criteria for potentially inappropriate medication use in older adults. *Journal of the American Geriatrics Society, 63*(11), 2227–2246. https://doi.org/10.1111/jgs.13702.

American Geriatrics Society (AGS). (2011). *2010 AGS/BGS clinical practice guideline: Prevention of falls in older persons: Summary of recommendations.* Retrieved from https://hsctc.org/wp-content/uploads/2017/07/2010-American-Geriatrics-Society-Guideline_-Prevention-of-Falls-in-Older-Persons.pdf. Accessed 25 June 2021.

American Heart Association (AHA). (2021). *PAD toolkit for health care professionals.* Retrieved from https://www.heart.org/en/health-topics/peripheral-artery-disease/pad-toolkit. Accessed 2 August 2021.

American Nurses Association (ANA). (2015). *Safe patient handling and mobility: Understanding the benefits of a comprehensive SPHM program.* Retrieved from https://www.nursingworld.org/~498de8/globalassets/practiceandpolicy/work-environment/health—safety/ana-sphmcover__finalapproved.pdf Accessed 2 August 2021.

American Psychiatric Nurses Association (APNA). (2015). *Psychiatric-mental health nurse essential competencies for assessment and management of individuals at risk for suicide.* Retrieved from http://www.apna.org/i4a/pages/index.cfm ?pageid=5684. Accessed 30 July 2021.

American Society of Anesthesiologists Committee. (2011). Practice guidelines for preoperative fasting and the use of pharmacologic agents to reduce the risk of pulmonary aspiration: Application to healthy patients undergoing elective procedures: An updated report by the American Society of Anesthesiologists Committee on Standards and Practice Parameters. *Anesthesiology, 114*(3), 495–511. https://doi.org/10.1097/ALN.0b013e3181fcbfd9.

American Society of PeriAnesthesia Nurses (ASPAN). (2021). Normothermia clinical guideline. In *2021-2022 Perianesthesia nursing standards: Practice recommendations and interpretive statements.* Cherry Hill, NJ: ASPAN.

Americans with Disabilities Act. (n.d.). (ADA requirements and technical assistance. Retrieved from https://www.ada.gov/ada_req_ta.htm. Accessed 12 July 2021.

Amsterdam, E. A., Wenger, N. K., Brindis, R. G., et al. (2014). 2014 AHA/ACC guideline for the management of patients with non-ST elevation acute coronary syndromes: A report of the American College of Cardiology/American Heart Association Task Force on Practice Guidelines. *Circulation, 130*(25), e344–e426. https://doi.org/10.1161/CIR.0000000000000134.

Anderson, K., Ewen, H., & Miles, E. (2010). The grief support in healthcare scale: Development and testing. *Nursing Research, 59*(6), 372–379. https://doi.org/10.1097/NNR.0b013e3181fca9de.

Anderson, P. A., Savage, J. W., Vaccaro, A. R., et al. (2017). Prevention of surgical site infection in spine surgery. *Neurosurgery, 80*(3S), S114–S123. https://doi.org/10.1093/neuros/nyw066.

Andreucci, M., Faga, T., Pisani, A., Perticone, M., & Michael, A. (2017). The ischemic/nephrotoxic acute kidney injury and the use of renal biomarkers in clinical practice. *European Journal of Internal Medicine, 39*, 1–8. https://doi.org/10.1016/j.ejim.2016.12.001.

Appleton, R. T., Kinsella, J., & Quasim, T. (2015). The incidence of intensive care unit-acquired weakness syndromes: A systematic review. *Journal of the Intensive Care Society, 16*(2), 126–136. https://doi.org/10.1177/1751143714563016.

Arlen, A. M. (2017). Dysfunctional voiders—Medication versus urotherapy? *Current Urology Reports, 18*(2), 14. https://doi.org/10.1007/s11934-017-0656-0.

Arnett, D. K., Blumenthal, R. S., Albert, M. A., et al. (2019). 2019 ACC/AHA guideline on the primary prevention of cardiovascular disease: A report of the American College of Cardiology/American Heart Association Task Force on Clinical Practice Guidelines. *Circulation, 140*(11), e596–e646. https://doi.org/10.1161/CIR.0000000000000678.

Asl, B. M. H., Vatanchi, A., Golmakani, N., & Najafi, A. (2018). Relationship between behavioral indices of pain during labor pain with pain intensity and duration of delivery. *Electronic Physician, 10*(1), 6240–6248. https://doi.org/10.19082/6240.

Austin, P., Jenkins, S., & Hines, A. (2017). Thromboembolic events in PICU: A descriptive study. *Pediatric Nursing, 43*(3), 132–137.

Baer, A.N., & Sankar, V. (2020). Treatment of dry mouth and other non-ocular sicca symptoms in Sjögren's syndrome. Fox, R., & Romain, P.L., (Eds), *UpToDate,* Waltham, MA. Retrieved from https://www.uptodate.com/contents/treatment-of-dry-mouth-and-other-non-ocular-sicca-symptoms-in-sjogrens-syndrome. Accessed 19 July 2021.

Baldwin, J., & Cox, J. (2016). Treating dyspnea: Is oxygen therapy the best option for all patients? *Medical Clinics of North America*, *100*(5), 1123–1130. https://doi.org/10.1016/j.mcna.2016.04.018.

Ban, K. A., Minei, J. P., Laronga, C., et al. (2017). American College of Surgeons and Surgical Infection Society: Surgical site infection guidelines, 2016 update. *Journal of the American College of Surgeons*, *224*(1), 59–74. https://doi.org/10.1016/j.jamcollsurg.2016.10.029.

Baranoski, S., & Ayello, E. A. (Eds.). (2016). *Wound care essentials: Practice principles* (4th ed.) Ambler, PA: Lippincott Williams & Wilkins.

Barton, G., Vanderspank-Wright, B., & Shea, J. (2016). Optimizing oxygenation in the mechanically ventilated patient: Nursing practice implications. *Critical Care Nursing Clinics of North America*, *28*(4), 425–435. https://doi.org/10.1016/j.cnc.2016.07.003.

Beeckman, D. (2017). A decade of research on Incontinence-Associated Dermatitis (IAD): Evidence, knowledge gaps and next steps. *Journal of Tissue Viability*, *26*(1), 47–56. https://doi.org/10.1016/j.jtv.2016.02.004.

Benbow, W. (2013). Evidence-based checklist for wayfinding design in dementia care facilities. *Canadian Nursing Home*, *24*(1), 4–10. Retrieved from http://wabenbow.com/wp-content/uploads/2014/02/Wayfinding-Compressed.pdf. Accessed 5 August 2021.

Berke, C., Conley, M. J., Netsch, D., et al. (2019). Role of the wound, ostomy and continence nurse in continence care: 2018 update. *Journal of Wound Ostomy and Continence Nursing*, *46*(3), 221–225. https://doi.org/10.1097/WON.0000000000000529.

Berríos-Torres, S. I., Umscheid, C. A., Bratzler, D. W., et al. (2017). Centers for Disease Control and Prevention guideline for the prevention of surgical site infection, 2017. *JAMA Surgery*, *152*(8), 784–791. https://doi.org/10.1001/jamasurg.2017.0904.

Berti-Hearn, L., & Elliott, B. (2019). Chronic venous insufficiency: A review for nurses. *Nursing2019*, *49*(12), 24–30. https://doi.org/10.1097/01.NURSE.0000604688.03299.aa.

Berti-Hearn, L., & Elliott, B. (2018). A closer look at lower extremity peripheral arterial disease. *Nursing2018*, *48*(1), 34–41. https://doi.org/10.1097/01.NURSE.0000527596.79097.9a.

Bickley, L. S., Szilagyi, P., Hoffman, R. M., & Soriano, R. P. (2020a). Foundations of health assessment. In L. S. Bickley, et al. (Ed.), *Bate's guide to physical examination and history taking* (13th ed.) (pp. 1–210). Philadelphia: Wolters Kluwer.

Bickley, L. S., Szilagyi, P., Hoffman, R. M., & Soriano, R. P. (2020b). Thorax and lungs. In L. S. Bickley, et al. (Ed.), *Bates' guide to physical examination and history taking* (13th ed.) (pp. 441–487). Philadelphia: Wolters Kluwer.

Bjerregaard, L. S., Bogø, S., Raaschou, S., et al. (2015). Incidence of and risk factors for postoperative urinary retention in fast-track hip and knee arthroplasty. *Acta Orthopaedica*, *86*(2), 183–188. https://doi.org/10.3109/17453674.2014.972262.

Bjorkland-Lima, L., Müller-Staub, M., Cardoso e Cardozo, M., de Souza Bernardes, D., & Rabelo-Silva, E. R. (2019). Clinical indicators of nursing outcomes classification for patient with risk for perioperative positioning injury: A cohort study. *Journal of Clinical Nursing*, *28*(23-24), 4367–4378. https://doi.org/10.1111/jocn.15019.

Blekken, L. E., Vinsnes, A. G., Gjeilo, K. H., & Bliss, D. Z. (2018). Management of fecal incontinence in older adults in long-term care. In D. Z. Bliss

(Ed.), *Management of fecal incontinence for the advanced practice nurse* (pp. 149–169). New York: Springer.

Bliss, D. Z., Funk, T., Jacobson, M., & Savik, K. (2015). Incidence and characteristics of incontinence-associated dermatitis in community-dwelling persons with fecal incontinence. *Journal of Wound Ostomy and Continence Nursing, 42*(5), 525–530. https://doi.org/10.1097/WON.0000000000000159.

Blodgett, T. J., Gardner, S. E., Blodgett, N. P., Peterson, L. V., & Pietraszak, M. (2015). A tool to assess the signs and symptoms of catheter associated urinary tract infection: Development and reliability. *Clinical Nursing Research, 24*(4), 341–356. https://doi.org/10.1177/1054773814550506.

Boettler, T., Newsome, P. N., Mondelli, M. U., et al. (2020). Care of patients with liver disease during the COVID-19 pandemic: EASL-ESCMID position paper. *JHEP Reports, 2*(3), 100113. https://doi.org/10.1016/j.jhep.2020.100113.

Bolen, B. B. (2020). *What to eat when you have diarrhea.* Verywell Health [website]. Retrieved from https://www.verywellhealth.com/what-to-eat-for-diarrhea-1944822. Accessed 30 June 2021.

Bounds, M., Kram, S., Speroni, K. G., et al. (2016). Effect of ABCDE bundle implementation on prevalence of delirium in intensive care unit patients. *American Journal of Critical Care, 25*(6), 535–544. https://doi.org/10.4037/ajcc2016209.

Boyd, K. (2018). *Remedies to reduce dry eye symptoms.* American Academy of Ophthalmology [website]. Retrieved from https://www.aao.org/eye-health/tips-prevention/dry-eye-tips. Accessed 25 June 2021.

Boynton, T., Kelly, L., Perez, A., Miller, M., An, Y., & Trudgen, C. (2014). Banner mobility assessment tool for nurses: Instrument validation. *American Journal of Safe Patient Handling & Movement, 4*(3), 86–92.

Bozkurt, B., Aguilar, D., Deswal, A., et al. (2016). Contributory risk and management of comorbidities of hypertension, obesity, diabetes mellitus, hyperlipidemia, and metabolic syndrome in chronic heart failure: A scientific statement from the American Heart Association. *Circulation, 134*(23), e535–e578. https://doi.org/10.1161/CIR.0000000000000450.

Breland, J. Y., Asch, S. M., Slightam, C., Wong, A., & Zulman, D. M. (2016). Key ingredients for implementing intensive outpatient programs within patient-centered medical homes: A literature review and qualitative analysis. *Healthcare (Amsterdam Netherlands), 4*(1), 22–29. https://doi.org/10.1016/j.hjdsi.2015.12.005.

Brienza, D. M., Zulkowski, K., Sprigle, S., & Geyer, M. J. (2016). Pressure redistribution: Seating, positioning, and support surfaces. In S. Baranoski, & E. A. Ayello (Eds.), *Wound care essentials: Practice principles* (4th ed.). Philadelphia, PA: Wolters Kluwer.

Brodshaug, I., Tettum, B., & Raeder, J. (2019). Thermal suit or forced air warming in prevention of perioperative hypothermia: A randomized controlled trial. *Journal of PeriAnesthesia Nursing, 34*(5), 1006–1015. org/10.1016/j.jopan.2019.03.002.

Broom, M., Dunk, A. M., & Mohamed, A. L. E. (2019). Predicting neonatal skin injury: The first step to reducing skin injuries in neonates. *Health Services Insights, 12*, 1178632919845630. https://doi.org/10.1177/1178632919845630.

Brown, H. W., Dyer, K. Y., & Rogers, R. G. (2020). Management of fecal incontinence. *Obstetrics & Gynecology, 136*(4), 811–822. https://doi.org/10.1097/AOG.0000000000004054.

Brunes, A., & Heir, T. (2020). Visual impairment and depression: Age-specific prevalence, associations with vision loss, and relation to life satisfaction. *World Journal of Psychiatry*, *10*(6), 139–149. https://doi.org/10.5498/wjp.v10.i6.139.

Bu, N., Zhao, E., Gao, Y., et al. (2019). Association between perioperative hypothermia and surgical site infection. A meta-analysis. *Medicine*, *98*(6):e14392. https://doi.org/10.1097/MD.0000000000014392.

Bureau of Labor Statistics. (2008). More seniors working fulltime. *TED: The Economics Daily*. Retrieved from https://www.bls.gov/opub/ted/2008/aug/wk1/art03.htm. Accessed 12 July 2021.

Busti, A. J. (2016). *Pitting edema assessment*. Evidence-Based Medicine Consult [website]. Retrieved from https://www.ebmconsult.com/articles/pitting-edema-assessment. Accessed 2 August 2021.

Çalış, A. S., Kaya, E., Mehmetaj, L., et al. (2019). Abdominal palpation and percussion maneuvers do not affect bowel sounds. *Turkish Journal of Surgery*, *35*(4), 309–313. https://doi.org/10.5578/turkjsurg.4291.

Cameron, S., Ball, I., Cepinskas, G., et al. (2015). Early mobilization in the critical care unit: A review of adult and pediatric literature. *Journal of Critical Care*, *30*(4), 664–672. https://doi.org/10.1016/j.jcrc.2015.03.032.

Campbell, M. L. (2017). Dyspnea. *Critical Care Nursing Clinics of North America*, *29*(4), 461–470. https://doi.org/10.1016/j.cnc.2017.08.006.

Carson, R. A., Mudd, S. S., & Madati, P. J. (2017). Evaluation of a nurse-initiated acute gastroenteritis pathway in the pediatric emergency department. *Journal of Emergency Nursing*, *43*(5), 406–412. https://doi.org/10.1016/j.jen.2017.01.001.

Cassard, A. M., Gérard, P., & Perlemuter, G. (2017). Microbiota, liver diseases, and alcohol. *Microbiology Spectrum*, *5*(4). https://doi.org/10.1128/microbiolspec.BAD-0007-2016.

Caughey, A.B., & Tilden, E. (2021). Nonpharmacologic approaches to management of labor pain. C.J. Lockwood, & K. Eckler (Eds), *UpToDate*, Waltham, MA. Retrieved from https://www.uptodate.com/contents/nonpharmacologic-approaches-to-management-of-labor-pain. Accessed 22 July 2021.

Centers for Disease Control and Prevention (CDC). (2021a). Older adult fall prevention. Retrieved from https://www.cdc.gov/falls. Accessed 25 June 2021.

Centers for Disease Control and Prevention (CDC). (2021b). Violence prevention: Risks and protective factors. Retrieved from https://www.cdc.gov/violenceprevention/childabuseandneglect/riskprotectivefactors.html. Accessed 25 June 2021.

Centers for Disease Control and Prevention (CDC). (2021c). *Pneumococcal ACIP vaccine recommendations*. Retrieved from https://www.cdc.gov/vaccines/hcp/acip-recs/vacc-specific/pneumo.html. Accessed 15 December 2021.

Centers for Disease Control and Prevention (CDC). (2021d). *Prevent seasonal flu*. Retrieved from www.CDC.gov/flu/protect/vaccine. Accessed 8 July 2021.

Centers for Disease Control and Prevention (CDC). (2021e). *Traumatic occupational injuries*. Retrieved from https://www.cdc.gov/niosh/injury/fastfacts.html. Accessed 29 September 2021.

Centers for Disease Control and Prevention. (2020a). *Adult immunization schedules for ages 19 years or older, United States, 2020*. Retrieved from http://www.cdc.gov/vaccines/schedules/hcp/imz/adult.html. Accessed 9 June 2021.

Centers for Disease Control and Prevention. (2020b). *Hand hygiene guidance.* Retrieved from https://www.cdc.gov/handhygiene/providers/guideline.ht ml. Accessed 14 June 2021.

Centers for Disease Control and Prevention. (2020c). *Optimizing personal protective equipment (PPE) supplies.* Retrieved from https://www.cdc.gov/ coronavirus/2019-ncov/hcp/ppe-strategy/index.html. Accessed 14 June 2021.

Centers for Disease Control and Prevention, National Center for Injury Prevention and Control. (2020d). *STEADI Program—Older adult fall prevention.* Retrieved from https://www.cdc.gov/steadi/materials.html. Accessed 25 June 2021.

Centers for Disease Control and Prevention (CDC). (2020e). *Heat stress. NI-OSH workplace safety and health tips.* Retrieved from https://www.cdc.gov/n iosh/topics/heatstress/. Accessed 6 July 2021.

Centers for Disease Control and Prevention (CDC). (2020f). *Surgical site infection event.* Retrieved from https://www.cdc.gov/nhsn/PDFs/pscManual/9p scSSIcurrent.pdf. Accessed 6 July 2021.

Centers for Disease Control and Prevention (CDC). (2020g). *Health effects of cigarette smoking.* Retrieved from https://www.cdc.gov/tobacco/data_statis tics/fact_sheets/health_effects/effects_cig_smoking/index.htm. Accessed 8 July 2021.

Centers for Disease Control and Prevention (CDC). (2020h). *The ABCs of hepatitis.* Retrieved from https://www.cdc.gov/hepatitis/resources/professi onals/pdfs/abctable.pdf. Accessed 13 July 2021.

Centers for Disease Control and Prevention (CDC). (2020i). *Body mass index (BMI).* Retrieved from https://www.cdc.gov/healthyweight/assessing/bmi/ index.html. Accessed 19 July 2021.

Centers for Disease Control and Prevention. (2019a). *International adoption.* Retrieved from https://www.cdc.gov/nceh/lead/prevention/adoption.htm. Accessed 14 June 2021.

Centers for Disease Control and Prevention (CDC). (2019b). *Protect the ones you love: Child injuries are preventable.* Retrieved from https://www.cdc.gov /safechild/falls/. Accessed 25 June 2021.

Centers for Disease Control and Prevention (CDC). (2019c). *Core elements of hospital antibiotic stewardship programs.* Retrieved from https://www.cdc.gov/antibiotic-use/healthcare/pdfs/hospital-core-ele ments-H.pdf. Accessed 30 September 2021.

Centers for Disease Control and Prevention (CDC). (2019d). *Vaccine Information Statement (VIS): Influenza.* Retrieved from https://www.cdc.gov/vaccin es/hcp/vis/. Accessed 8 July 2021.

Centers for Disease Control and Prevention (CDC). (2019e). *Hand hygiene in healthcare settings.* Retrieved from http://www.cdc.gov/handhygiene/Basics .html. Accessed 4 August 2021.

Centers for Disease Control and Prevention (CDC). (2016). *National Center for Health Statistics: Resources for the general public.* Atlanta, GA: CDC. Available at: https://www.cdc.gov/nchs/nchs_for_you/general_public.htm. Accessed 28 June 2021.

Centers for Disease Control and Prevention (CDC). (n.d.). *A practical guide to help your patients quit using tobacco.* Retrieved from https://www.cdc.gov/t obacco/patient-care/pdfs/hcp-conversation-guide.pdf. Accessed 4 January 2022.

Chacko, B., Peter, J. V., Tharyan, P., John, G., & Jeyaseelan, L. (2015). Pressure-controlled versus volume-controlled ventilation for acute respiratory failure due to acute lung injury (ALI) or acute respiratory distress syndrome (ARDS). *Cochrane Database of Systematic Reviews*, *1*, CD008807. https://doi.org/10.1002/14651858.CD008807.pub2.

Chalmers, J. D., Aliberti, S., & Blasi, F. (2015). Management of bronchiectasis in adults. *European Respiratory Journal*, *45*(5), 1446–1462. https://doi.org/10.1183/09031936.00119114.

Chassiakos, Y. L. R., Radesky, J., Christakis, D., Moreno, M. A., Cross, C., & Council on Communications and Media. (2016). Children and adolescents and digital media. *Pediatrics*, *138*(5), e20162593. https://doi.org/10.1542/peds.2016-2593.

Chaudhary, S., Figueroa, J., Shaikh, S., et al. (2018). Pediatric falls ages 0-4: Understanding demographics, mechanisms, and injury severities. *Injury Epidemiology*, *5*(Suppl. 1), 7. https://doi.org/10.1186/s40621-018-0147-x.

Choi, S. D., & Brings, K. (2015). Work-related musculoskeletal risks associated with nurses and nursing assistants handling overweight and obese patients: A literature review. *Work*, *53*(2), 439–448. https://doi.org/10.3233/WOR-152222.

Cieniewicz, A., Trzebicki, J., Mayzner-Zawadzka, E., Kostera-Pruszczyk, A., & Owczuk, R. (2019). Malignant hyperthermia - What do we know in 2019? *Anaesthesiology Intensive Therapy*, *51*(3), 169–177. https://doi.org/10.5114/ait.2019.87646.

Cooper, K. D., McQueen, K. M., Halm, M. A., & Flayter, R. (2020). Prevention and treatment of device-related hospital-acquired pressure injuries. *American Journal of Critical Care*, *29*(2), 150–154. https://doi.org/10.4037/ajcc2020167.

Corbitt, N., Harrington, J., Kendall, T., et al. (2019). *Prevention of bleeding*. Oncology Nursing Society [website]. Retrieved from https://www.ons.org/pep/prevention-bleeding. Accessed 8 June 2021.

Coutts, A. (2019). Nursing management of irritable bowel syndrome. *Nursing Standard (Royal College of Nursing (Great Britain): 1987)*, *34*(5), 76–81. https://doi.org/10.7748/ns.2019.e11363.

Cox, J. (2019). Wound care 101. *Nursing 2019*, *49*(10), 33–39. https://doi.org/10.1097/01.NURSE.0000580632.58318.08.

Coyer, F., Gardner, A., & Doubrovsky, A. (2017). An interventional skin care protocol (InSPiRE) to reduce incontinence-associated dermatitis in critically ill patients in the intensive care unit: A before and after study. *Intensive and Critical Care Nursing*, *40*, 1–10. https://doi.org/10.1016/j.iccn.2016.12.001.

Cruz-Oliver, D. M. (2017). Palliative care: An update. *Missouri Medicine*, *114*(2), 110–115.

D'Alesandro, M. A. (2016). Focusing on lower extremity DVT. *Nursing2016*, *46*(4), 28–36. https://doi.org/10.1097/01.NURSE.0000481417.73469.00.

Damluji, A. A., Forman, D. E., van Diepen, S., et al. (2019). Older adults in the cardiac intensive care unit: Factoring geriatric syndromes in the management, prognosis, and process of care: A scientific statement from the American Heart Association. *Circulation*, *141*(2), e6–e32. https://doi.org/10.1161/CIR.0000000000000741.

Danzl, D. F. (2018). Hypothermia and peripheral cold injuries. In J. L. Jameson, A. S. Fauci, D. L. Kasper, S. L. Hauser, D. L. Longo, & J. Loscalzo (Eds.), *Harrison's principles of internal medicine* (20th ed.). New York: McGraw-Hill.

Da Silva, G., & Sirany, A. (2019). Recent advances in managing fecal incontinence [online]. *F1000Research*. https://doi.org/10.12688/f1000research.15270.2. 8, F1000 Faculty Rev-1291.

de Almeida Lopes Monteiro da Cruz, D., & Braga, C. G. (2006). Construction and validation of an instrument to assess powerlessness [Abstract]. *International Journal of Nursing Terminologies and Classifications*, 17(1), 67.

Dean, E. (2020). Acute kidney injury: Who is at risk and how to care for patients. *Nursing Standard*, 35(5), 67–68. https://doi.org/10.7748/ns.35.5.67.s23.

Delmore, B., Deppisch, M., Sylvia, C., Luna-Anderson, C., & Nie, A. M. (2019). Pressure injuries in the pediatric population: A National Pressure Ulcer Advisory Panel white paper. *Advances in Skin and Wound Care*, 32(9), 394–408. https://doi.org/10.1097/01.ASW.0000577124.58253.66.

Devlin, J. W., Skrobik, Y., Gélinas, C., et al. (2018). Clinical practice guidelines for the prevention and management of pain, agitation/sedation, delirium, immobility, and sleep disruption in adult patients in the ICU. *Critical Care Medicine*, 46(9), e825–e873. https://doi.org/10.1097/CCM.0000000000003299.

Dikmen, H. A., & Terzioglu, F. (2019). Effects of reflexology and progressive muscle relaxation on pain, fatigue, and quality of life during chemotherapy in gynecologic cancer patients. *Pain Management Nursing*, 20(1), 47–53. https://doi.org/10.1016/j.pmn.2018.03.001.

DiGerolamo, K., & Davis, K. F. (2017). An integrative review of pediatric fall risk assessment tools. *Journal of Pediatric Nursing*, 34, 23–28. https://doi.org/10.1016/j.pedn.2017.02.036.

Dirkes, S. M., & Kozlowski, C. (2019). Early mobility in the intensive care unit: Evidence, barriers, and future directions. *Critical Care Nurse*, 39(3), 33–42. https://doi.org/10.4037/ccn2019654.

Dirks, J. (2017). Continuous venous oxygen saturation monitoring. In D. L. Wiegand (Ed.), *AACN procedure manual for high acuity, progressive, and critical care* (7th ed.) (pp. 116–122). Philadelphia: Elsevier.

Doenges, M. E., Moorhouse, M. F., & Murr, A. C. (2016). *A nurse's pocket guide: Diagnoses, prioritized interventions and rationales* (14th ed.). Philadelphia, PA: FA Davis.

Douglas, M. K., Rosenkoetter, M., Pacquiao, D. F., et al. (2014). Guidelines for implementing culturally competent nursing care. *Journal of Transcultural Nursing*, 25(2), 109–121. https://doi.org/10.1177/1043659614520998.

Dow, J., Giesbrecht, G. G., Danzl, D. F., et al. (2019). Wilderness Medical Society clinical practice guidelines for the out-of-hospital evaluation and treatment of accidental hypothermia: 2019 update. *Wilderness & Environmental Medicine*, 30(4S), S47–S69. https://doi.org/10.1016/j.wem.2019.10.002.

Drake, M. G. (2018). High-flow nasal cannula oxygen in adults: An evidence-based assessment. *Annals of the American Thoracic Society*, 15(2), 145–155. https://doi.org/10.1513/AnnalsATS.201707-548FR.

Dunn, N., & Ramos, R. (2017). Preventing venous thromboembolism: The role of nursing with intermittent pneumatic compression. *American Journal of Critical Care*, 26(2), 164–167. https://doi.org/10.4037/ajcc2017504.

Dykes, P. C. (2020). Using fall risk assessment tools in care planning. *Center for Patient Safety Research and Practice*. Center for Nursing Excellence, Brigham and Women's Hospital. Retrieved from https://www.ahrq.gov/sites/

default/files/wysiwyg/professionals/systems/hospital/fallprevention-training/webinars/webinar4_falls_usingriskassttools.pdf. Accessed 15 July 2021.

E, J. Y., Li, T., Mcinally, L., et al. (2020). Environmental and behavioural interventions for reducing physical activity limitation and preventing falls in older people with visual impairment. *Cochrane Database of Systematic Reviews, 9*, CD009233. https://doi.org/10.1002/14651858.CD009233.pub3.

Eamudomkarn, N., Kietpeerakool, C., Kaewrudee, S., Jampathong, N., Ngamjarus, C., & Lumbiganon, P. (2018). Effect of postoperative coffee consumption on gastrointestinal function after abdominal surgery: A systematic review and meta-analysis of randomized controlled trials. *Scientific Reports, 8*(1), 17349. https://doi.org/10.1038/s41598-018-35752-2.

Eman, S. M., & Lohrmann, C. (2015). Prevalence of fecal and double fecal and urinary incontinence in hospitalized patients. *Journal of Wound Ostomy & Continence Nursing, 42*(1), 89–93. https://doi.org/10.1097/WON.0000000000000082.

Emsfors, Å., Christensson, L., & Elgán, C. (2017). Nursing actions that create a sense of good nursing care in patients with wet age-related macular degeneration. *Journal of Clinical Nursing, 26*(17-18), 2680–2688. https://doi.org/10.1111/jocn.13749.

Ergin, E., Sagkal Midilli, T., & Baysal, E. (2018). The effect of music on dyspnea severity, anxiety, and hemodynamic parameters in patients with dyspnea. *Journal of Hospice and Palliative Nursing, 20*(1), 81–87. https://doi.org/10.1097/NJH.0000000000000403.

Ersan, T., & Schwer, W. A. (2021). *Perioperative management of the geriatric patient.* Medscape [website]. Retrieved from https://emedicine.medscape.com/article/285433-overview#a2. Accessed 8 July 2021.

Fabrellas, N. (2017). Research about nursing care for persons with liver disease: A step in the right direction. *Nursing Research, 66*(6), 419–420. https://doi.org/10.1097/NNR.0000000000000233.

Faigenbaum, A. D., Rebullido, T. R., & MacDonald, J. P. (2018). Pediatric inactivity triad: A risky PIT. *Current Sports Medicine Reports, 17*(2), 45–47. https://doi.org/10.1249/JSR.0000000000000450.

Fairchild, E., Roberts, L., Zelman, K., Michelli, S., & Hastings-Tolsma, M. (2017). Implementation of Robert's Coping with Labor Algorithm© in a large tertiary care facility. *Midwifery, 50*, 208–218. https://doi.org/10.1016/j.midw.2017.03.008.

Fields, B. E., Whitney, R. L., & Bell, J. F. (2020). Home oxygen therapy. *American Journal of Nursing, 120*(11), 51–57. https://doi.org/10.1097/01.NAJ.0000721940.02042.99.

Franjoine, M. R., Gunther, J. S., & Taylor, M. J. (2003). Pediatric balance scale: A modified version of the berg balance scale for the school-age child with mild to moderate motor impairment. *Pediatric Physical Therapy, 15*(2), 114–128. https://doi.org/10.1097/01.PEP.0000068117.48023.18.

Frasso, R., Golinkoff, A., Klusaritz, H., et al. (2017). How nurse-led practices perceive implementation of the patient-centered medical home. *Applied Nursing Research, 34*, 34–39. https://doi.org/10.1016/j.apnr.2017.02.005.

Freundlich, K. (2017). Pressure injuries in medically complex children: A review. *Children (Basel Switzerland), 4*(4), 25. https://doi.org/10.3390/children4040025.

Fusco, N., Stead, T. G., Lebowitz, D., & Ganti, L. (2019). Traumatic corneal abrasion. *Cureus, 11*(4), e4396. https://doi.org/10.7759/cureus.4396.

Gallagher, J. (2017). Invasive mechanical ventilation (through an artificial airway): Volume and pressure modes. In D. L. Wiegand (Ed.), *AACN procedure manual for high acuity, progressive, and critical care* (7th ed.) (pp. 227–248). Philadelphia: Elsevier.

Gaudio, F. G., & Grissom, C. K. (2016). Cooling methods in heat stroke. *Journal of Emergency Medicine, 50*(4), 607–616. https://doi.org/10.1016/j.jemermed.2015.09.014.

Gbinigie, O. A., Ordóñez-Mena, J. M., Fanshawe, T. R., Plüddemann, A., & Heneghan, C. (2018). Diagnostic value of symptoms and signs for identifying urinary tract infection in older adult outpatients: Systematic review and meta-analysis. *Journal of Infection, 77*(5), 379–390. https://doi.org/10.1016/j.jinf.2018.06.012.

Gibbons, S., Lauder, W., & Ludwick, R. (2006). Self-neglect: A proposed new NANDA diagnosis. *International Journal of Nursing Terminologies and Classifications, 17*(1), 10–18. https://doi.org/10.1111/j.1744-618X.2006.00018.x.

Global Initiative for Chronic Obstructive Lung Disease (GOLD). (2020). Global strategy for the diagnosis, management, and prevention of COPD (revised 2020). *Global Initiative for Chronic Obstructive Lung Disease.* Retrieved from https://goldcopd.org/wp-content/uploads/2019/12/GOLD-2020-FINAL-ver1.2-03Dec19_WMV.pdf. Accessed 8 June 2021.

Gok Metin, Z., Karadas, C., Izgu, N., Ozdemir, L., & Demirci, U. (2019). Effects of progressive muscle relaxation and mindfulness meditation on fatigue, coping styles, and quality of life in early breast cancer patients: An assessor blinded, three-arm, randomized controlled trial. *European Journal of Oncology Nursing, 42*, 116–125. https://doi.org/10.1016/j.ejon.2019.09.003.

Goldberg, T. E., Chen, C., Wang, Y., et al. (2020). Association of delirium with long-term cognitive decline: A meta-analysis. *JAMA Neurology, 77*(11), 1373–1381. https://doi.org/10.1001/jamaneurol.2020.2273.

Goldner, D., & Lavine, J. E. (2020). Nonalcoholic fatty liver disease in children: Unique considerations and challenges. *Gastroenterology, 158*(7), 1967–1983. e1. https://doi.org/10.1053/j.gastro.2020.01.048.

Goodrich, C. (2017). Endotracheal intubation (perform). In D. L. Wiegand (Ed.), *AACN procedure manual for high acuity, progressive, and critical care* (7th ed.) (pp. 8–22). Philadelphia: Elsevier.

Goodwin, V. A., Abbott, R. A., Whear, R., et al. (2014). Multiple component interventions for preventing falls and fall related injuries among older people: Systematic review and meta-analysis. *BMC Geriatrics, 14*, 15–21. https://doi.org/10.1186/1471-2318-14-15.

Goodwin Veenema, T. (2019). *Disaster nursing and emergency preparedness for chemical, biological, radiological terrorism and other hazards* (4th ed.). New York: Springer.

Gotekar, R. B. (2017). A clinical study of accidental fingernail injuries to the cornea in Alquwayiah General Hospital, Ridyadh Region, KSA. *Journal of Evolution of Medical and Dental Sciences, 6*(62), 4526. https://doi.org/10.14260/jemds/2017/979.

Gould, C. V., Umscheid, C. A., Agarwal, R. K., Kuntz, G., Pegues, D. A., & Healthcare Infection Control Practices Advisory Committee. (2019). *Guideline for prevention of catheter-associated urinary tract infections 2009.*

Retrieved from https://www.cdc.gov/infectioncontrol/guidelines/cauti/. Accessed 12 July 2021.

Grabiner, M. D. (2014). Exercise-based fall prevention programmes decrease fall-related injuries. *Evidence-Based Nursing, 17*(4), 125. https://doi.org/10.1136/eb-2013-101703.

Granum, M. N., Kaasby, K., Skou, S. T., & Grønkjaer, M. (2019). Preventing inadvertent hypothermia in patients undergoing major spinal surgery: A non-randomized controlled study of two different methods of preoperative and intraoperative warming. *Journal of PeriAnesthesia Nursing, 34*(5), 999–1005. https://doi.org/10.1016/j.jopan.2019.03.004.

Gray, M., McNickol, L., & Nix, D. (2016). Incontinence-associated dermatitis progress, promises, and ongoing challenges. *Journal of Wound Ostomy and Continence Nursing, 43*(2), 188–192. https://doi.org/10.1097/WON.0000000000000217.

Gray-Miceli, D., & Quigley, P. A. (2021). Assessing, managing, and preventing falls in acute care. In M. Boltz, E. Capezuti, D. Zwicker, & T. Fulmer (Eds.), *Evidence-based geriatric nursing protocols for best practice* (6th ed.). New York: Springer.

Green, M., Marzano, V., Leditschke, I. A., Mitchell, I., & Bissett, B. (2016). Mobilization of intensive care patients: A multidisciplinary practical guide for clinicians. *Journal of Multidisciplinary Healthcare, 9*, 247–256. https://doi.org/10.2147/JMDH.S99811.

Greenberg, S. A. (2019). *Try This:® Best practices in nursing care to older adults. Assessment of fear of falling in older adults: The Falls Efficacy Scale-International (FES-I).* New York: Hartford Institute for Geriatric Nursing. Retrieved from https://hign.org/consultgeri/try-this-series/assessment-fear-falling-older-adults-falls-efficacy-scale-international. Accessed 25 June 2021.

Greenberg, S. A., Sullivan-Marx, E., Sommers, M. L. S., Chittams, J., & Cacchione, P. Z. (2016). Measuring fear of falling among high-risk, urban, community-dwelling older adults. *Geriatric Nursing, 37*(6), 489–495. https://doi.org/10.1016/j.gerinurse.2016.08.018.

Greenberg, S. A. (2012). Analysis of measurement tools of fear of falling among high-risk, community-dwelling older adults. *Clinical Nursing Research, 21*(1), 113–130. https://doi.org/10.1177/1054773811433824.

Grover, M., Farrugia, G., & Stanghellini, V. (2019). Gastroparesis: A turning point in understanding and treatment. *Gut, 68*(12), 2238–2250. https://doi.org/10.1136/gutjnl-2019-318712.

Guandalini, S., Frye, R. E., & Tamer, M. A. (2020). *Diarrhea.* Medscape [website]. Retrieved from https://emedicine.medscape.com/article/928598-overview. Accessed 30 June 2021.

Gupta, N. M., Lindenauer, P. K., Yu, P. C., Imrey, P. B., Haessler, S., Deshpande, A., & et al (2019). Association between alcohol use disorders and outcomes of patients hospitalized with community-acquired pneumonia. *JAMA Network Open, 2*(6), e195172. https://doi.org/10.1001/jamanetworkopen.2019.5172.

Gupta, R. (2016). Diarrhea. In R. Wyllie, J. S. Hyams, & M. Kay (Eds.), *Pediatric gastrointestinal and liver disease* (5th ed.) (pp. 104–114). Philadelphia: Elsevier.

Hamilton, L. A., Collins-Yoder, A., & Collins, R. E. (2016). Drug-induced liver injury. *AACN Critical Care*, *27*(4), 430–440. https://doi.org/10.4037/aacnacc2016953.

Hanison, E., & Corbett, K. (2016). Non-pharmacological interventions for the prevention of venous thromboembolism: A literature review. *Nursing Standard*, *31*(8), 48–57. https://doi.org/10.7748/ns.2016.e10473.

Hansson, L., & Björkman, T. (2005). Empowerment in people with a mental illness: Reliability and validity of the Swedish version of an empowerment scale. *Scandinavian Journal of Caring Sciences*, *19*(1), 32–38. https://doi.org/10.1111/j.1471-6712.2004.00310.x.

Hedrick, T. L., McEvoy, M. D., Mythen, M. M. G., et al. (2018). American Society for Enhanced Recovery and Perioperative Quality Initiative joint consensus statement on postoperative gastrointestinal dysfunction within an enhanced recovery pathway for elective colorectal surgery. *Anesthesia and Analgesia*, *126*(6), 1896–1907. https://doi.org/10.1213/ANE.0000000000002742.

Heeringa, J., van der Kuip, D. A. M., Hofman, A., et al. (2006). Prevalence, incidence and lifetime risk of atrial fibrillation: The Rotterdam study. *European Heart Journal*, *27*(8), 949–953. https://doi.org/10.1093/eurheartj/ehi825.

Helmerhorst, H. J. F., Schultz, M. J., van der Voort, P. H. J., de Jong, E., & van Westerloo, D. J. (2015). Bench-to bedside review: The effects of hyperoxia during critical illness. *Critical Care (London England)*, *19*(1), 284. https://doi.org/10.1186/s13054-015-0996-4.

Hendrich, A. (2013). *Try This:® Best practices in nursing care to older adults. Fall risk assessment for older adults: The Hendrich II Fall Risk Model^(TM)*. New York: Hartford Institute for Geriatric Nursing. Retrieved from http://www.wsha.org/wp-content/uploads/Hendrich-II-Fall-Risk.pdf. Accessed 18 September 2021.

Hjorth, M., Sjöberg, D., Svanberg, A., Kaminsky, E., Langenskiöld, S., & Rorsman, F. (2018). Nurse-led clinic for patients with liver cirrhosis—effects on health-related quality of life: Study protocol of a pragmatic multicentre randomized controlled trial. *BMJ Open*, *8*(10), e023064. https://doi.org/10.1136/bmjopen-2018-023064.

Ho, K. M., & Harahsheh, Y. (2016). Intermittent pneumatic compression is effective in reducing proximal DVT. *Evidence-Based Nursing*, *19*(2), 47. https://doi.org/10.1136/eb-2015-102265.

Hockenberry, M. J., Wilson, D., & Rodgers, C. C. (Eds.). (2019). *Wong's nursing care of infants and children* (11th ed.) St. Louis: Elsevier.

Hodgson, C. L., Needham, D., Haines, K., et al. (2014). Feasibility and inter-rater reliability of the ICU Mobility Scale. *Heart and Lung*, *43*(1), 19–24. https://doi.org/10.1016/j.hrtlng.2013.11.003.

Hoffman, A. J., Brintnall, R. A., Given, B. A., von Eye, A., Jones, L. W., & Brown, J. K. (2017). Using perceived self-efficacy to improve fatigue and fatigability in postsurgical lung cancer patients: A pilot randomized controlled trial. *Cancer Nursing*, *40*(1), 1–12. https://doi.org/10.1097/NCC.0000000000000378.

Hogan, N. S., Worden, J. W., & Schmidt, L. A. (2004). An empirical study of the proposed complicated grief disorder criteria. *Omega*, *48*(3), 263–277. https://doi.org/10.2190/GX7H-H05N-A4DN-RLU9.

Hospital Quality Institute. (2015). *Eliminating ventilator-associated events (VAP) and ventilator-associated pneumonia (VAP/VAE). HQI toolkit.* Retrieved from http://www.hqinstitute.org/hqi-toolkit/eliminating-vapvae. Accessed 4 August 2021.

Houston, A., & Fuldauer, P. (2017). Enteral feeding: Indications, complications, and nursing care. *American Nurse Today*, *12*(1), 20–25.

Hutzler, L., & Williams, J. (2017). Decreasing the incidence of surgical site infections following joint replacement surgery. *Bulletin of the Hospital for Joint Diseases*, *75*(4), 268–273.

Imam, S. S., Shinkar, D. M., Mohamed, N. A., & Mansour, H. E. (2019). Effect of right lateral position with head elevation on tracheal aspirate pepsin in ventilated preterm neonates: Randomized controlled trial. *Journal of Maternal-Fetal & Neonatal Medicine*, *32*(22), 3741–3746. https://doi.org/10.1080/14767058.2018.1471674.

Infusion Nurses Society (INS). (2016). Infusion therapy standards of practice. *Journal of Infusion Nursing*, *39*(Suppl. 1), 1–169. Retrieved from https://source.yiboshi.com/20170417/1492425631944540325.pdf. Accessed 4 August 2021.

Institute for Healthcare Improvement. (2020). *Age-friendly health systems: Guide to using the 4Ms in the care of older adults.* Massachusetts: Institute for Healthcare Improvement. Retrieved from http://www.ihi.org/Engage/Initiatives/Age-Friendly-Health-Systems/Documents/IHIAgeFriendlyHealthSystems_GuidetoUsing4MsCare.pdf. Accessed 5 January 2022.

International Foundation for Functional Gastrointestinal Disorders. (2019). *Diet strategies for managing chronic diarrhea.* Retrieved from https://www.iffgd.org/lower-gi-disorders/diarrhea/nutrition-strategies.html. Accessed 14 June 2021.

Islam, S. (2015). Gastroparesis in children. *Current Opinion in Pediatrics*, *27*(3), 377–382. https://doi.org/10.1097/MOP.0000000000000216.

Issa, K., Pierce, T. P., Brothers, A., Festa, A., Scillia, A. J., & Mont, M. A. (2017). Sexual activity after total hip arthroplasty: A systematic review of outcomes. *Journal of Arthroplasty*, *32*(1), 336–340. https://doi.org/10.1016/j.arth.2016.07.052.

Jacobs, D.S. (2021). Corneal abrasions and corneal foreign bodies: Management. M.F. Gardiner, R.G. Bachur, J. F. Wiley (Eds.). *UpToDate*, Waltham, MA. Retrieved from http://www.uptodate.com/contents/corneal-abrasions-and-corneal-foreign-bodies-management?source=see_link. Accessed 8 July 2021.

Jain, Y., Srivatsan, R., Kollannur, A., & Zachariah, A. (2018). Heatstroke: Causes, consequences and clinical guidelines. *National Medical Journal of India*, *31*(4), 224–227. https://doi.org/10.4103/0970-258X.258224.

Jauch, E. C., Saver, J. L., Adams, H. P., Jr., et al. (2013). Guidelines for the early management of patients with acute ischemic stroke: A guideline for healthcare professionals from the American Heart Association/American Stroke Association. *Stroke*, *44*(3), 870–947. https://doi.org/10.1161/STR.0b013e318284056a.

Jaul, E., Barron, J., Rosenweig, J. P., & Menczel, J. (2018). An overview of comorbidities and the development of pressure ulcers among older adults. *BMC Geriatrics*, *18*(1), 305. https://doi.org/10.1186/s12877-018-0997-7.

Jeffs, L., Law, M. P., Zahradnik, M., et al. (2018). Engaging nurses in optimizing antimicrobial use in ICUs: A qualitative study. *Journal of Nursing Care Quality*, *33*(2), 173–179. https://doi.org/10.1097/NCQ.0000000000000281.

Jelavić, M. M., Krstačić, G., Perenčević, A., & Pintarić, H. (2018). Sexual activity in patients with cardiac disease. *Acta Clinical Croatica*, *57*(1), 141–148. https://doi.org/10.20471/acc.2018.57.01.18.

Johnson, D. M., Worell, J., & Chandler, R. K. (2005). Assessing psychological health and empowerment in women: The personal progress scale revised. *Women and Health*, *41*(1), 109–129. https://doi.org/10.1300/J013v41n01_07.

Johnson, R. (2017). Tracheostomy cuff and tube care. In D. L. Wiegand (Ed.), *AACN procedure manual for high acuity, progressive, and critical care* (7th ed.) (pp. 89–102). Philadelphia: Elsevier.

Jordan, A. H., & Litz, B. T. (2014). Prolonged grief disorder: Diagnostic, assessment, and treatment considerations. *Professional Psychology Research and Practice*, *45*(3), 180–187. https://doi.org/10.1037/a0036836.

Karthika, M., Al Enezi, F. A., Pillai, L. V., & Arabi, Y. M. (2016). Rapid shallow breathing index. *Annals of Thoracic Medicine*, *11*(3), 167–176. https://doi.org/10.4103/1817-1737.176876.

Kaur, A. (2019). *Peripheral Intravenous Cannula (PIVC): Insertion*. Joanna Briggs Institute EBP Database, JBI140045.

Kaye, A. D., Renschler, J. S., Cramer, K. D., et al. (2019). Postoperative management of corneal abrasions and clinical implications: A comprehensive review. *Current Pain and Headache Reports*, *23*(7), 48. https://doi.org/10.1007/s11916-019-0784-y.

Keall, M. D., Pierse, N., Howden-Chapman, P., et al. (2015). Home modifications to reduce injuries from falls in the home injury prevention intervention (HIPI) study: A cluster-randomised controlled trial. *Lancet*, *385*(9964), 231–238. https://doi.org/10.1016/S0140-6736(14)61006-0.

Kear, T. M. (2017). Fluid and electrolyte management across the age continuum. *Nephrology Nursing Journal*, *44*(6), 491–496.

Khan, F. U., Khan, Z., Ahmed, N., & Rehman, A. U. (2020). A general overview of incidence, associated risk factors, and treatment outcomes of surgical site infections. *Indian Journal of Surgery*, *82*(4), 449–459. https://doi.org/10.1007/s12262-020-02071-8.

Khan, A. M., Mydra, H., & Nevarez, A. (2017). Clinical practice updates in the management of immune thrombocytopenia. *P & T*, *42*(12), 756–763.

Khan, M. H., Kunselman, A. R., Leuenberger, U. A., et al. (2002). Attenuated sympathetic nerve responses after 24 hours of bed rest. *American Journal of Physiology Heart and Circulatory Physiology*, *282*(6), H2210–H2215. https://doi.org/10.1152/ajpheart.00862.2001.

Khong, B. P. C., Goh, B. C., Phang, L. Y., & David, T. (2020). Operating room nurses' self-reported knowledge and attitude on perioperative pressure injury. *International Wound Journal*, *17*(2), 455–465. https://doi.org/10.1111/iwj.13295.

Klompas, M., Branson, R., Eichenwald, E., et al. (2014). Strategies to prevent ventilator-associated pneumonia in acute care hospitals: 2014 update. *Infection Control and Hospital Epidemiology*, *35*(8), 915–936. https://doi.org/10.1086/677144.

Knapik, J. J., & Epstein, Y. (2019). Exertional heat stroke: Pathophysiology, epidemiology, diagnosis, treatment, and prevention. *Journal of Special Operations Medicine, 19*(2), 108–116.

Kolanowski, A., Boltz, M., Galik, E., et al. (2017). Determinants of behavioral and psychological symptoms of dementia: A scoping review of the evidence. *Nursing Outlook, 65*(5), 515–529. https://doi.org/10.1016/j.outlook.2017.06.006.

Kolb, H., Snowden, A., & Stevens, E. (2018). Systematic review and narrative summary: Treatments for and risk factors associated with respiratory tract secretions (death rattle) in the dying adult. *Journal of Advanced Nursing, 74*(7), 1446–1462. https://doi.org/10.1111/jan.13557.

Kollmann-Camaiora, A., Alsina, E., Domínguez, A., et al. (2017). Clinical protocol for the management of malignant hyperthermia. *Revista Espanola de Anestesiologia y Reanimacion, 64*(1), 32–40. https://doi.org/10.1016/j.redar.2016.06.004.

Koren, P. E., DeChillo, N., & Friesen, B. J. (1992). Measuring empowerment in families whose children have emotional disabilities: A brief questionnaire. *Rehabilitation Psychology, 37*(4), 305–321. https://doi.org/10.1037/h0079106.

Kranz, J., Schmidt, S., Wagenlehner, F., & Schneidewind, L. (2020). Catheter associated urinary tract infections in adult patients. *Deutsches Arzteblatt International, 117*(6), 83–88. https://doi.org/10.3238/arztebl.2020.0083.

Laliberte Rudman, D., Egan, M. Y., McGrath, C. E., et al. (2016). Low vision rehabilitation, age-related vision loss, and risk: A critical interpretive synthesis. *Gerontologist, 56*(3), e32–e45. https://doi.org/10.1093/geront/gnv685.

Lambert, P., Chaisson, K., Horton, S., et al. (2017). Reducing acute kidney injury due to contrast material: How nurses can improve patient safety. *Critical Care Nurse, 37*(1), 13–26. https://doi.org/10.4037/ccn2017178.

Larson, J., Franzén-Dahlin, A., Billing, E., Murray, V., & Wredling, R. (2005). Spouse's life situation after partner's stroke: Psychometric testing of a questionnaire. *Journal of Advanced Nursing, 52*(3), 300–306. https://doi.org/10.1111/j.1365-2648.2005.03590.x.

Lawton, S., & Shepherd, E. (2019). The underlying principles and procedure for bed bathing patients. *Nursing Times [online], 115*(5), 45–47. https://www.nursingtimes.net/roles/hospital-nurses/the-underlying-principles-and-procedure-for-bed-bathing-patients-25-04-2019/.

Lee, K. S., Koo, K. C., & Chung, B. H. (2017). Risk and management of postoperative urinary retention following spinal surgery. *International Neurology Journal, 21*(4), 320–328. https://doi.org/10.5213/inj.1734994.497.

Lee, S. J., & Lee, J. H. (2017). Safe patient handling behaviors and lift use among hospital nurses: A cross-sectional study. *International Journal of Nursing Studies, 74*, 53–60. https://doi.org/10.1016/j.ijnurstu.2017.06.002.

Lešnik, A., Piko, N., Železnik, D., & Bevc, S. (2017). Dehydration of older patients in institutional care and the home environment. *Research in Gerontological Nursing, 10*(6), 260–266. https://doi.org/10.3928/19404921-20171013-03.

Leyk, D., Hoitz, J., Becker, C., Glitz, K. J., Nestler, K., & Piekarski, C. (2019). Health risks and interventions in exertional heat stress. *Deutsches Arzteblatt International, 116*(31-32), 537–544. https://doi.org/10.3238/arztebl.2019.0537.

Lindahl, S. B. (2020). Intraoperative irrigation: Fluid administration and management amidst conflicting evidence. *AORN Journal, 111*(5), 495–507. https://doi.org/10.1002/aorn.13010.

Link, T. (2020). Guidelines in practice: Hypothermia prevention. *AORN Journal, 111*(6), 653–666. https://doi.org/10.1002/aorn.13038.

Lipman, G. S., Gaudio, F. G., Eifling, K. P., Ellis, M. A., Otten, E. M., & Grissom, C. K. (2019). Wilderness Medical Society Clinical Practice Guidelines for the prevention and treatment of heat illness: 2019 update. *Wilderness & Environmental Medicine, 30*(4S), S33–S46. https://doi.org/10.1016/j.wem.2018.10.004.

Loscalzo, J. (2018). Hypoxia and cyanosis. In J. L. Jameson, A. S. Fauci, D. L. Kasper, S. L. Hauser, D. L. Longo, & J. Loscalzo (Eds.), *Harrison's principles of internal medicine* (20th ed.). New York: McGraw-Hill.

Lough, M. E., Berger, S. J., Larsen, A., & Sandoval, C. P. (2022). Cardiovascular diagnostic procedures. In L. D. Urden, K. M. Stacy, & M. E. Lough (Eds.), *Critical care nursing diagnosis and management* (8th ed.) (pp. 206–297). St. Louis: Elsevier.

Lu, Y., Li, Y.-W., Wang, L., et al. (2019). Promoting sleep and circadian health may prevent postoperative delirium: A systematic review and meta-analysis of randomized clinical trials. *Sleep Medicine Reviews, 48*, 101207. https://doi.org/10.1016/j.smrv.2019.08.001.

Luckowski, A., & Luckowski, M. (2015). Caring for a patient with vision loss. *Nursing2015, 45*(11), 55–58. https://doi.org/10.1097/01.NURSE.0000471416.42130.35.

Maddock, K., & Connor, K. (2020). Drug fever: A patient case scenario and review of the evidence. *AACN Advanced Critical Care, 31*(3), 233–238. https://doi.org/10.4037/aacnacc2020311.

Mahler, D. A. (2017). Evaluation of dyspnea in the elderly. *Clinics in Geriatric Medicine, 33*(4), 503–521. https://doi.org/10.1016/j.cger.2017.06.004.

Malafa, M. M., Coleman, J. E., Bowman, R. W., & Rohrich, R. J. (2016). Perioperative corneal abrasion: Updated guidelines for prevention and management. *Plastic and Reconstructive Surgery, 137*(5), 790e–798e. https://doi.org/10.1097/PRS.0000000000002108.

Malignant Hyperthermia Association of the United States (MHAUS). (2020). *Website*. Retrieved from http://www.mhaus.org/. Accessed 6 July 2021.

Manworren, R. C. B., & Stinson, J. (2016). Pediatric pain measurement, assessment, and evaluation. *Seminars in Pediatric Neurology, 23*(3), 189–200. https://doi.org/10.1016/j.spen.2016.10.001.

Marcott, S., Dewan, K., Kwan, M., Baik, F., Lee, Y. J., & Sirjani, D. (2020). Where dysphagia begins: Polypharmacy and xerostomia. *Federal Practitioner, 37*(5), 234–241.

Marsden, J. (2017). Preserving vision and promoting visual health in older people. *Nursing Older People, 29*(6), 22–26. https://doi.org/10.7748/nop.2017.e935.

Marx, W., Kiss, N., McCarthy, A. L., McKavanagh, D., & Isenring, L. (2016). Chemotherapy-induced nausea and vomiting: A narrative review to inform dietetics practice. *Journal of the Academy of Nutrition & Dietetics, 116*(5), 819–827. https://doi.org/10.1016/j.jand.2015.10.020.

Maternik, M., Krzeminska, K., & Zurowska, A. (2015). The management of childhood urinary incontinence. *Pediatric Nephrology, 30*(1), 41–50. https://doi.org/10.1007/s00467-014-2791-x.

Matura, L. A., Malone, S., Jaime-Lara, R., & Riegel, B. (2018). A systematic review of biological mechanisms of fatigue in chronic illness. *Biological Research For Nursing, 20*(4), 410–421. https://doi.org/10.1177/1099800418764326.

McClurg, D., & Norton, C. (2016). What is the best way to manage neurogenic bowel dysfunction? *BMJ (Clinical research ed.), 354*, i3931. https://doi.org/10.1136/bmj.i3931.

McDonald, L. C., Gerding, D. N., Johnson, S., et al. (2018). Clinical practice guidelines for Clostridium difficile infection in adults and children: 2017 Update by the Infectious Diseases Society of America (IDSA) and Society for Healthcare Epidemiology of America (SHEA). *Clinical Infectious Disease, 66*(7), 987–994. https://doi.org/10.1093/cid/ciy149.

McLendon, K., Goyal, A., Bansal, P., & Attia, M. (2021). Deep venous thrombosis risk factors. In *StatPearls [Internet]*. Treasure Island, FL: StatPearls Publishing.

McIlwaine, M., Button, B., & Nevitt, S. J. (2019). Positive expiratory pressure physiotherapy for airway clearance in people with cystic fibrosis. *Cochrane Database of Systematic Reviews, 11*, CD003147. https://doi.org/10.1002/14651858.CD003147.pub5.

Meddings, J., Saint, S., Fowler, K. E., et al. (2015). The Ann Arbor criteria for appropriate urinary catheter use in hospitalized medical patients: Results obtained by using the RAND/UCLA Appropriateness Method. *Annals of Internal Medicine, 162*(Suppl. 9), S1–S34. https://doi.org/10.7326/M14-1304.

Mekonen, C. (2019). Graded motor imagery to address pain and motor dysfunction from phantom limb pain, complex regional pain syndrome, chronic musculoskeletal pain, and stroke. *Journal of Nurse Life Care Planning, 19*(3), 45–51.

Menees, S. B., Almario, C. V., Spiegel, B. M., & Chey, W. D. (2018). Prevalence of and factors associated with fecal incontinence: Results from a population-based survey. *Gastroenterology, 154*(6), 1672–1681.e3. https://doi.org/10.1053/j.gastro.2018.01.062.

Miller, K. K., Brown, C. R., Shramko, M., & Svetaz, M. V. (2019). Applying trauma – informed practices to the care of refugee and immigrant youth: 10 clinical pearls. *Children, 6*(8), 94. https://doi.org/10.3390/children6080094.

Milrad, S. F., Hall, D. L., Jutagir, D. R., et al. (2018). Depression, evening salivary cortisol and inflammation in chronic fatigue syndrome: A psychoneuroendocrinological structural regression model. *International Journal of Psychophysiology, 131*, 124–130. https://doi.org/10.1016/j.ijpsycho.2017.09.009.

Mody, L., Greene, M. T., Meddings, J., et al. (2017). A national implementation project to prevent catheter-associated urinary tract infection in nursing home residents. *JAMA Internal Medicine, 177*(8), 1154–1162. https://doi.org/10.1001/jamainternmed.2017.1689.

Molinari, L., Sakhuja, A., & Kellum, J. A. (2020). Perioperative renoprotection: General mechanisms and treatment approaches. *Anesthesia & Analgesia, 131*(6), 1679–1692. https://doi.org/10.1213/ANE.0000000000005107.

Momani, T. G., & Berry, D. L. (2017). Integrative therapeutic approaches for the management and control of nausea in children undergoing cancer treatment: A systematic review. *Journal of Pediatric Oncology Nursing, 34*(3), 173–184. https://doi.org/10.1177/1043454216688638.

Monagle, P., Chan, A., Goldenberg, N. A., Ichord, R. N., Journeycake, J. M., Nowak-Göttl, U., et al. (2012). Antithrombotic therapy in neonates and children: antithrombotic therapy and prevention of thrombosis, 9th ed. American College of Chest Physicians Evidence-Based Clinical Practice Guidelines. *Chest*, *141*(Suppl. 2), e737S–e801S. https://doi.org/10.1378/chest.11-2308.

Monsees, E., Lee, B., Wirtz, A., & Goldman, J. (2020). Implementation of a nurse-driven antibiotic engagement tool in 3 hospitals. *American Journal of Infection Control*, *48*(12), 1415–1421. https://doi.org/10.1016/j.ajic.2020.07.002.

Morse, J. M., Tylko, S. J., & Dixon, H. A. (1987). Characteristics of the fall-prone patient. *Gerontologist*, *27*(4), 516–522. https://doi.org/10.1093/geront/27.4.516.

Mukamal, R. (2020). *12 treatments for dry eyes: What patients should know.* American Academy of Ophthalmology [website]. Retrieved from https://www.aao.org/eye-health/tips-prevention/how-to-treat-dry-eye-devices. Accessed 25 June 2021.

Murphree, R. W. (2017). Impairments in skin integrity. *Nursing Clinics of North America*, *52*(3), 405–417. https://doi.org/10.1016/j.cnur.2017.04.008.

Musa, M. K., Saga, S., Blekken, L. E., Harris, R., Goodman, C., & Norton, C. (2019). The prevalence, incidence, and correlates of fecal incontinence among older people residing in care homes: A systematic review. *Journal of the American Medical Directors Association*, *20*(8), 956–962.e8. https://doi.org/10.1016/j.jamda.2019.03.033.

Myles, P. S., Andrews, S., Nicholson, J., Lobo, D. N., & Mythen, M. (2017). Contemporary approaches to perioperative IV fluid therapy. *World Journal of Surgery*, *41*(10), 2457–2463. https://doi.org/10.1007/s00268-017-4055-y.

Nagarwala, J., Dev, S., & Markin, A. (2016). The vomiting patient: Small bowel obstruction, cyclic vomiting, and gastroparesis. *Emergency Medical Clinics of North America*, *34*(2), 271–291. https://doi.org/10.1016/j.emc.2015.12.005.

Nahar, D. (2017). Prophylactic management of contrast-induced kidney injury in high-risk patients. *Nephrology Nursing Journal*, *43*(3), 244–249.

Naik, S., Lucerne, C., Kevorkova, Y., et al. (2019). Significant reduction of non-ventilator hospital acquired pneumonia (HAP) with a prevention bundle and clinical and leadership feedback in a large integrated healthcare system. *Open Forum Infectious Diseases*, *6*(Suppl. 2), S423. https://doi.org/10.1093/ofid/ofz360.1044.

National Center for Public Policy and Higher Education. (2005). *Income of U.S. workforce projected to decline if education doesn't improve.* Retrieved from http://www.highereducation.org/reports/pa_decline/index.shtml. Accessed 12 July 2021.

National Committee for Quality Assurance–Health Care Accreditation Organization. (2015a). *Geriatrics: Percentage of patients aged 65 and older with a history of falls who had a plan of care for falls documented within 12 months.* National Quality Measures Clearinghouse [website]. Retrieved from https://www.guidelinecentral.com/share/quality-measures/49449#h2_measure-domain. Accessed 27 November 2021.

National Committee for Quality Assurance–Health Care Accreditation Organization. (2015b). *Geriatrics: Percentage of patients aged 65 and older discharged from any inpatient facility (e.g., hospital, skilled nursing facility, or rehabilitation facility) and seen within 30 days of discharge in the office by the physician, prescribing practitioner, registered nurse, or clinical pharmacist who had reconciliation of the discharge medications with the current medication list in the outpatient medical record documented.* National Quality Measures Clearinghouse [website]. Retrieved from https://www.guidelinecentral.com/share/quality-measures/49444#h2_measure-domain. Accessed 27 November 2021.

National Comprehensive Cancer Network. (2021). *NCCN clinical practice guidelines in oncology cancer–related fatigue, version 1. 2021.* Retrieved from https://www.nccn.org/professionals/physician_gls/pdf/fatigue.pdf.

National Consensus Project for Quality Palliative Care. (2018). *Clinical practice guidelines for quality palliative care* (4th ed.). Retrieved from. https://www.nationalcoalitionhpc.org/ncp/. Accessed 9 June 2021.

National Council on Aging. (2021). *About the Falls Free® Initiative.* Retrieved from https://www.ncoa.org/article/about-the-falls-free-initiative. Accessed 5 January 2022.

National Fire Protection Association (NFPA). (2021). *Public education* [multiple resources]. Retrieved from https://www.nfpa.org/Public-Education. Accessed 30 July 2021.

National Institute for Health and Care Excellence. (2020). *Constipation. Clinical Knowledge summaries.* Retrieved from https://www.nice.org.uk/guidance/conditions-and-diseases/digestive-tract-conditions/constipation. Accessed 2 November 2020.

National Health Service (NHS). (2018). *Dry eyes.* Retrieved from http://www.nhs.uk/Conditions/Dry-eye-syndrome/Pages/Prevention.aspx. Accessed 25 June 2021.

National Kidney Foundation. (2021). *Aging and kidney disease.* Retrieved from https://www.kidney.org/news/monthly/wkd_aging. Accessed 30 June 2021.

National Pressure Injury Advisory Panel (NPIAP) and European Pressure Ulcer Advisory Panel (EPUAP). (2019). In E. Haesler (Ed.), *Prevention and Treatment of Pressure Ulcers.* Perth, Australia: Cambridge Media.

National Pressure Injury Advisory Panel (NPIAP), European Pressure Injury Advisory Panel (EPIAP), and Pan Pacific Pressure Injury Alliance (PPPIA). (2019). In E. Haesler (Ed.), *Prevention and treatment of pressure ulcers: Quick reference guide.* Osborne Park, Australia: Cambridge Media.

National Pressure Ulcer Advisory Panel (NPUAP) and European Pressure Ulcer Advisory Panel (EPUAP). (2016). *Pressure injury stages.* Retrieved from http://www.npuap.org/resources/educational-and-clinical-resources/npuap-pressure-injury-stages/. Accessed 16 November 2020.

National Pressure Ulcer Advisory Panel (NPUAP). (2016). *Pressure injury stages.* Retrieved from https://npiap.com/page/PressureInjuryStages. Accessed 29 July 2021.

Neunert, C., Terrel, D. R., Arnold, D. M., et al. (2019). American Society of Hematology 2019 guidelines for immune thrombocytopenia. *Blood Advances, 3*(23), 3829–3866. https://doi.org/10.1182/bloodadvances.2019000966.

Newman, D. K. (2019). Evidence-based practice guideline: Prompted voiding for individuals with urinary incontinence. *Journal of Gerontological Nursing, 45*(2), 14–26. https://doi.org/10.3928/00989134-20190111-03.

Nicolle, L. E., & Norrby, S. R. (2016). Approach to the patient with urinary tract infection. In L. Goldman, & A. Schafer (Eds.), *Goldman's Cecil medicine* (25th ed.) (pp. 1872–1876). Philadelphia: Elsevier.

Nihata, K., Fukuma, S., Hiratsuka, Y., et al. (2018). Association between vision-specific quality of life and falls in community-dwelling older adults: LOHAS. *PLoS One, 13*(4), e0195806. https://doi.org/10.1371/journal. pone.0195806.

Niven, D. J., & Laupland, K. B. (2016). Pyrexia: Aetiology in the ICU. *Critical Care, 20*(1), 247. https://doi.org/10.1186/s13054-016-1406-2.

Nordgren, M., Herborg, O., Hamberg, Sandström, E., Larsson, G., & Söderström, L. (2020). The effectiveness of four intervention methods for preventing inadvertent perioperative hypothermia during total knee or total hip arthroplasty. *AORN Journal, 111*(3), 303–312. https://doi.org/10.1002/aorn.12961.

Nyman, S. R., Innes, A., & Heward, M. (2017). Social care and support needs of community-dwelling people with dementia and concurrent visual impairment. *Aging & Mental Health, 21*(9), 961–967. https://doi.org/10.1080/13 607863.2016.1186151.

Oates, L. L., & Price, C. I. (2017). Clinical assessments and care interventions to promote oral hydration amongst older patients: A narrative systematic review. *BMC Nursing, 16*, 4. https://doi.org/10.1186/s12912-016-0195-x.

O'Donnell, K. F. (2020). Fecal incontinence: A stepwise approach to primary care management. *Journal for Nurse Practitioners, 16*(8), 586–589. https:// doi.org/10.1016/j.nurpra.2020.05.006.

Ofei, S. Y., & Fuchs, G. J., 3rd. (2019). Principles and practice of oral rehydration. *Current Gastroenterology Reports, 21*(12), 67. https://doi.org/10.1007/ s11894-019-0734-1.

O'Grady, N. P., Alexander, M., Burns, L. A., et al. (2011). Guidelines for the prevention of intravascular catheter-related infections. *American Journal of Infection Control, 39*(4 Suppl. 1), S1–S34. https://doi.org/10.1016/j. ajic.2011.01.003.

Olans, R. D., Olans, R. N., & Witt, D. J. (2017). Good nursing is good antibiotic stewardship. *American Journal of Nursing, 117*(8), 58–63. https://doi. org/10.1097/01.NAJ.0000521974.76835.e0.

Olinsky, C., & Norton, C. E. (2017). Implementation of a safe patient handling program in a multihospital health system from inception to sustainability: Successes over 8 years and ongoing challenges. *Workplace Health and Safety, 65*(11), 546–559. https://doi.org/10.1177/2165079917704670.

Onyimba, F. U., & Clarke, J. O. (2019). Helping patients with gastroparesis. *Medical Clinics of North America, 103*(1), 71–87. https://doi.org/10.1016/j. mcna.2018.08.013.

Osborn, K. S., Wraa, C. E., Watson, A. S., et al. (2013). *Nutrition. Medical-surgical nursing, preparation for practice* (2nd ed.). Upper Saddle River, NJ: Pearson.

Özdemir, I. A., Comba, C., Demirayak, G., et al. (2019). Impact of pre-operative walking on post-operative bowel function in patients with gynecologic cancer. *International Journal of Gynecological Cancer, 29*(8), 1311–1316. https:// doi.org/10.1136/ijgc-2019-000633.

Paal, P., Gordon, L., Strapazzon, G., et al. (2016). Accidental hypothermia— An update. *Scandinavian Journal of Trauma Resuscitation and Emergency Medicine, 24*(1), 111. https://doi.org/10.1186/s13049-016-0303-7.

Paquette, I. M., Varma, M. G., Kaiser, A. M., Steele, S. R., & Rafferty, J. F. (2017). The American Society of Colon and Rectal Surgeons' clinical practice guideline for the treatment of fecal incontinence. *Diseases of the Colon and Rectum, 58*(7), 623–636. https://doi.org/10.1097/DCR.0000000000000397.

Park, S., Park, H., & Hwang, H. (2019). Development and comparison of predictive models for pressure injuries in surgical patients. *Journal of Wound Ostomy & Continence Nursing*, *46*(4), 291–297. https://doi.org/10.1097/WON.0000000000000544.

Pedersen, C. M., Rosendahl-Nielsen, M., Hjermind, J., et al. (2009). Endotracheal suctioning of the adult intubated patient—what is the evidence? *Intensive and Critical Care Nursing*, *25*(1), 21–30. https://doi.org/10.1016/j.iccn.2008.05.004.

Pelletier, A. L., Rojas-Roldan, L., & Coffin, J. (2016). Vision loss in older adult. *American Family Physician*, *94*(3), 219–226.

Pender, N. J., Murdaugh, C. L., & Parsons, M. A. (2015). *Health promotion in nursing practice* (7th Ed.). Upper Saddle River, NJ: Prentice Hall.

Perkins, A. (2020). Spinal cord injury: A lifelong condition. *Nursing Made Incredibly Easy!*, *18*(5), 34–43. Retrieved from https://journals.lww.com/nursingmadeincrediblyeasy/Fulltext/2020/09000/Spinal_cord_injury__A_lifelong_condition.7.aspx. Accessed 7 June 2021.

Phillips, D., Griffin, D., Przybylski, T., et al. (2018). Development and validation of a modified performance-oriented mobility assessment tool for assessing mobility in children with hypophosphatasia. *Journal of Pediatric Rehabilitation Medicine*, *11*(3), 187–192. https://doi.org/10.3233/PRM-170523.

Phillips, L. D. (2014). *Manual of IV therapeutics: Evidence-based practice for infusion therapy* (6th ed.). Philadelphia: F.A. Davis.

Pileggi, D. J., & Cook, A. M. (2016). Neuroleptic malignant syndrome: Focus on treatment and rechallenge. *Annals of Pharmacotherapy*, *50*(11), 973–981. https://doi.org/10.1177/1060028016657553.

Pitchika, V., Pink, C., Völzke, H., Welk, A., Kocher, T., & Holtfreter, B. (2019). Long-term impact of powered toothbrush on oral health: 11-year cohort study. *Journal of Clinical Periodontology*, *46*(7), 713–722. https://doi.org/10.1111/jcpe.13126.

Pitta, M. R., Campos, F. M., Monteiro, A. G., Cunha, A. F., Porto, J. D., & Gomes, R. R. (2019). Tutorial on diarrhea and enteral nutrition: A comprehensive step-by-step approach. *Journal of Parenteral and Enteral Nutrition*, *43*(8), 1008–1019. https://doi.org/10.1002/jpen.1674.

Plemons, J. M., Al-Hashimi, I., & Marek, C. L. (2014). Managing xerostomia and salivary gland hypofunction: Executive summary of a report from the American Dental Association Council on Scientific Affairs. *Journal of the American Dental Association*, *145*(8), 867–873. https://doi.org/10.14219/jada.2014.44.

Podd, D. (2018). Beyond skin deep, managing pressure injuries. *JAAPA*, *31*(4), 10–17. https://doi.org/10.1097/01.JAA.0000531043.87845.9e.

Podsiadlo, D., & Richardson, S. (1991). The timed "Up & Go": A test of basic functional mobility for frail elderly persons. *Journal of the American Geriatrics Society*, *39*(2), 142–148. https://doi.org/10.1111/j.1532-5415.1991.tb01616.x.

Pollack, A. H., Backonja, U., Miller, A. D., et al. (2016). Closing the gap: supporting patients' transition to self-management after hospitalization. Proceedings of the SIGCHI Conference on Human Factors in Computing Systems. *CHI Conference*, *2016*, 5324–5336. https://doi.org/10.1145/2858036.2858240.

Pondorfer, S. G., Heinemann, M., Wintergerst, M. W. M., et al. (2020). Detecting vision loss in intermediate age-related macular degeneration: A comparison of visual function tests. *PLoS One*, *15*(4), e0231748. https://doi.org/10.1371/journal.pone.0231748.

Porritt, K. (2016). *Intravascular therapy: Maintaining catheter lumen patency.* Joanna Briggs Institute EBP Database, JBI14448.

Pozuelo-Carrascosa, D. P., Herráiz-Adillo, Á., Alvarez-Bueno, C., Añón, J. M., Martínez-Vizcaíno, V., & Cavero-Redondo, I. (2020). Subglottic secretion drainage for preventing ventilator-associated pneumonia: An overview of systematic reviews and an updated meta-analysis. *European Respiratory Review*, *29*(155), 190107. https://doi.org/10.1183/16000617.0107-2019.

Preas, M. A., O'Hara, L., & Thom, K. (2017). 2017 HICPAC-CDC guideline for prevention of surgical site infection: What the IP needs to know. Prevention Strategist. *Fall 2017*, 69–72. Retrieved from https://apic.org/Resource_/TinyMceFileManager/Periodical_images/SSI_2017_Fall_PS.pdf. Accessed 8 July 2021.

Raghu Ram, S. S. R. (2019). Halitosis-bad breath: Etiology, diagnosis, treatment. *Indian Journal of Public Health Research & Development*, *10*(11), 917–920.

Rathjen, N. A., Shahbodaghi, S. D., & Brown, J. A. (2019). Hypothermia and cold weather injuries. *American Family Physician*, *100*(11), 680–686.

Ratliff, C. R., Droste, L. R., Bonham, P., Wound, Ostomy and Continence Nurses Society-Wound Guidelines Task Force, et al. (2017). WOCN 2016 guideline for prevention and management of pressure injuries (ulcers). An executive summary. *Journal of Wound Ostomy and Continence Nursing*, *44*(3), 241–246. https://doi.org/10.1097/WON.0000000000000321.

Raynor, H. A., & Champagne, C. M. (2016). Position of the academy of nutrition and dietetics: Interventions for the treatment of overweight and obesity in adults. *Journal of the Academy of Nutrition and Dietetics*, *116*(1), 129–147. https://doi.org/10.1016/j.jand.2015.10.031.

Rhodes, A., Evans, L. E., Alhazzani, W., et al. (2017). Surviving sepsis campaign: International guidelines for management of sepsis and septic shock: 2016. *Critical Care Medicine*, *45*(3), 486–552. https://doi.org/10.1097/CCM.0000000000002255.

Riazi, S., Kraeva, N., & Hopkins, P. M. (2018). Updated guide for the management of malignant hyperthermia. *Canadian Journal of Anaesthesia*, *65*(6), 709–721. https://doi.org/10.1007/s12630-018-1108-0.

Riccoboni, J. B., Monnet, T., Eon, A., Lacouture, P., Gazeau, J. P., & Campone, M. (2021). Biomechanical comparison between manual and motorless device assisted patient handling: Sitting to and from standing position. *Applied Ergonomics*, *90*, 103284. https://doi.org/10.1016/j.apergo.2020.103284.

Richardson, M. G., Raymond, B. L., Baysinger, C. L., Kook, B. T., & Chestnut, D. H. (2019). A qualitative analysis of parturients' experiences using nitrous oxide for labor analgesia: It is not just about pain relief. *Birth*, *46*(1), 97–104. https://doi.org/10.1111/birt.12374.

Rischall, M. L., & Rowland-Fisher, A. (2016). Evidence-based management of accidental hypothermia in the emergency department. *Emergency Medicine Practice*, *18*(1), 1–18.

Roberts, S. H., & Lawrence, S. M. (2017). Venous thromboembolism: Updated management guidelines. *American Journal of Nursing*, *117*(5), 38–47. https://doi.org/10.1097/01.NAJ.0000516249.54064.53.

Rose, O., Schaffert, C., Czarnecki, K., et al. (2015). Effect evaluation of an interprofessional medication therapy management approach for multimorbid patients in primary care: A cluster-randomized controlled trial in community care (WestGem study protocol). *BMC Family Practice, 16*, 84. https://doi.org/10.1186/s12875-015-0305-y.

Rose, T. A., Jr., & Choi, J. W. (2015). Intravenous imaging contrast media complications: The basics that every clinician needs to know. *American Journal of Medicine, 128*(9), 943–949. https://doi.org/10.1016/j.amjmed.2015.02.018.

Safe Kids Worldwide. (2021). *Poison*. Retrieved from https://www.safekids.org/poisonsafety. Accessed 22 July 2021.

Saint, S., Greene, M. T., Krein, S. L., et al. (2016). A program to prevent catheter-associated urinary tract infection in acute care. *New England Journal of Medicine, 374*(22), 2111–2119. https://doi.org/10.1056/NEJMoa1504906.

Şanci, E., Coşkun, F. E., & Bayram, B. (2020). Impact of high-flow nasal cannula on arterial blood gas parameters in the emergency department. *Cureus, 12*(9), e10516. https://doi.org/10.7759/cureus.10516.

Sanders, M., Jones, S., Löwenstein, O., Jansen, J.-P., Miles, H., & Simpson, K. (2015). New formulation of sustained released naloxone can reverse opioid induced constipation without compromising the desired opioid effects. *Pain Medicine, 16*(8), 1540–1550. https://doi.org/10.1111/pme.12775.

Sauls, J. L. (2021). Acute respiratory failure. In M. Sole, D. Klein, M. Moseley, et al. (Eds.), *Introduction to critical care nursing* (pp. 375–403). St. Louis, MO: Elsevier.

Schallom, M., Dykeman, B., Metheny, N., Kirby, J., & Pierce, J. (2015). Head-of-bed elevation and early outcomes of gastric reflux, aspiration, and pressure ulcers: A feasibility study. *American Journal of Critical Care, 24*(1), 57–66. https://doi.org/10.4037/ajcc2015781.

Schiller, L. R., Pardi, D. S., & Sellin, J. H. (2017). Chronic diarrhea: Diagnosis and management. *Clinical Gastroenterology and Hepatology, 15*(2), 182–193. https://doi.org/10.1016/j.cgh.2016.07.028. e3.

Schmidt, G. A., Girard, T. D., Kress, J. P., et al. (2017). Official executive summary of an American Thoracic Society/American College of Chest Physicians clinical practice guideline: Liberation from mechanical ventilation in critically ill adults. *American Journal of Respiratory and Critical Care Medicine, 195*(1), 115–119. https://doi.org/10.1164/rccm.201610-2076ST.

Seckel, M. (2017). Suctioning: Endotracheal tube or tracheostomy tube. In D. L. Wiegland (Ed.), *AACN procedure manual for critical care* (7th ed.). Philadelphia: Elsevier.

Sgro, M., Campbell, D. M., & Gandhi, N. (2016). Nontherapeutic neonatal hypothermia. *Paediatrics and Child Health, 21*(4), 178–180. https://doi.org/10.1093/pch/21.4.178.

Shah, A., & Madhok, M. (2019). Management of pediatric hypothermia and peripheral cold injuries in the emergency department. *Pediatric Emergency Medicine Practice, 16*(1), 1–16.

Shah, R. K., & Lotke, M. (2019). *Hearing impairment*. Medscape [website]. Retrieved from https://emedicine.medscape.com/article/994159-overview. Accessed 9 August 2021.

Shah, S. M. (2019). *Indwelling catheter care*. Medline Plus [website]. Retrieved from https://medlineplus.gov/ency/patientinstructions/000140.htm. Accessed 12 July 2021.

Shahoei, R., Shahghebi, S., Rezaei, M., & Naqshbandi, S. (2017). The effect of transcutaneous electrical nerve stimulation on the severity of labor pain among nulliparous women: A clinical trial. *Complementary Therapies in Clinical Practice, 28*, 176–180. https://doi.org/10.1016/j.ctcp.2017.05.004.

Shane, A. L., Mody, R. K., Crump, J. A., et al. (2017). 2017 Infectious diseases society of America clinical practice guidelines for the diagnosis and management of infectious diarrhea. *Clinical Infectious Diseases, 65*(12), e45–e80. https://doi.org/10.1093/cid/cix669.

Shaw-Battista, J. (2017). Systemic review of hydrotherapy research: Does a warm bath in labor promote normal physiologic childbirth? *Journal of Perinatal & Neonatal Nursing, 31*(4), 303–316. https://doi.org/10.1097/JPN.0000000000000260.

Shen, S., Xu, J., Lamm, V., Vachaparambil, C. T., Chen, H., & Cai, Q. (2019). Diabetic gastroparesis and nondiabetic gastroparesis. *Gastrointestinal Endoscopy Clinics of North America, 29*(1), 15–25. https://doi.org/10.1016/j.giec.2018.08.002.

Sherani, F., Boston, C., & Mba, N. (2019). Latest update on prevention of acute chemotherapy-induced nausea and vomiting in pediatric cancer patients. *Current Oncology Reports, 21*(10), 88–89. https://doi.org/10.1007/s11912-019-0840-0.

Shrimanker, I., & Bhattarai, S. (2020). *Electrolytes. StatPearls [Internet].* Treasure Island, FL: StatPearls Publishing.

Sidebottom, A., Vacquier, M., Simon, K., et al. (2020). Maternal and neonatal outcomes in hospital-based deliveries with water immersion. *Obstetrics & Gynecology, 136*(4), 707–715. https://doi.org/10.1097/AOG.0000000000003956.

Siegel, J. D., Rhinehart, E., Jackson, M., Chiarello, L., & Health Care Infection Control Practices Advisory Committee. (2007). Guideline for isolation precautions: Preventing transmission of infectious agents in health care settings. *American Journal of Infection Control, 35*(10 Suppl. 2), S65–S164. https://doi.org/10.1016/j.ajic.2007.10.007.

Siela, D. (2010). Evaluation standards for management of artificial airways. *Critical Care Nurse, 30*(4), 76–78. https://doi.org/10.4037/ccn2010306.

Siela, D., & Kidd, M. (2017). Oxygen requirements for acutely and critically ill patients. *Critical Care Nurse, 37*(4), 58–70. https://doi.org/10.4037/ccn2017627.

Simmons, K. (2017). Sequential compression devices in the pediatric patient population. *AORN Journal, 106*(2), 13–14. https://doi.org/10.1016/S0001-2092(17)30658-0.

Singer, M. (2016). The new sepsis consensus definitions (Sepsis-3): The good, the not-so-bad, and the actually-quite-pretty. *Intensive Care Medicine, 42*(12), 2027–2029. https://doi.org/10.1007/s00134-016-4600-4.

Snow, T. M. (2019). *The use of a progressive mobility protocol to enhance patient outcomes [Dissertation].* Newark, Delaware: University of Delaware, School of Nursing.

Solà-Miravete, E., López, C., Martínez-Segura, E., Adell-Lleixà, M., Juvé-Udina, M. E., & Lleixà-Fortuño, M. (2018). Nursing assessment as an effective tool for the identification of delirium risk in older in-patients: A case-control study. *Journal of Clinical Nursing, 27*(1-2), 345–354. https://doi.org/10.1111/jocn.13921.

Sommers, J., Engelbert, R. H., Dettling-Ihnenfeldt, D., et al. (2015). Physiotherapy in the intensive care unit: An evidence-based, expert driven, practical statement and rehabilitation recommendations. *Clinical Rehabilitation, 29*(11), 1051–1063. https://doi.org/10.1177/0269215514567156.

Søndergaard, S., Robertson, K., Silfversten, E., et al. (2016). *Families support to transition: A systematic review of the evidence.* Santa Monica, CA: RAND Corporation. Retrieved from https://www.rand.org/pubs/research_reports /RR1511.html. Accessed 26 July 2021.

Spruce, L. (2018). Back to basics: Orthopedic positioning. *AORN Journal, 107*(3), 355–367. https://doi.org/10.1002/aorn.12071.

St. Clair, J., & MacDermott, J. (2017). Continuous lateral rotation therapy. In D. L. Wiegand (Ed.), *AACN procedure manual for high acuity, progressive, and critical care* (7th ed.) (pp. 111–115). Philadelphia: Elsevier.

Steinke, E. E., Johansen, P. P., Fridlund, B., & Broström, A. (2016). Determinants of sexual dysfunction and interventions for patients with obstructive sleep apnoea: A systematic review. *International Journal of Clinical Practice, 70*(1), 5–19. https://doi.org/10.1111/ijcp.12751.

Sullivan, A., Temperley, L., & Ruban, A. (2020). Pathophysiology, aetiology and treatment of gastroparesis. *Digestive Diseases and Sciences, 65*(6), 1615–1631. https://doi.org/10.1007/s10620-020-06287-2.

Suzman, D. L., Pelosof, L., Rosenberg, A., & Avigan, M. I. (2018). Hepatotoxicity of immune checkpoint inhibitors: An evolving picture of risk associated with a vital class of immunotherapy agents. *Liver International, 38*(6), 976–987. https://doi.org/10.1111/liv.13746.

Tablan, O. C., Anderson, L. J., Besser, R., et al. (2004). Guidelines for preventing health-care–associated pneumonia, 2003: Recommendations of CDC and the Healthcare Infection Control Practices Advisory Committee. *Morbidity and Mortality Weekly Report: Recommendations and Reports, 53*(RR-3), 1–36 (Reviewed 2015).

Tan, E. S. Z., Mackenzie, L., Travassaros, K., & Yeo, M. (2021). A pilot study to investigate the feasibility of the Modified Blaylock Tool for Occupational Therapy Referral (MBTOTR) for use by nurses in acute care. *Disability and Rehabilitation, 43*(3), 414–422. https://doi.org/10.1080/09638288.2019.1624840.

Tanasiewicz, M., Hildebrandt, T., & Obersztyn, I. (2016). Xerostomia of various etiologies: A review of the literature. *Advanced Clinical Exploratory Medicine, 25*(1), 199–206. https://doi.org/10.17219/acem/29375.

Tatsumi, H. (2019). Enteral tolerance in critically ill patients. *Journal of Intensive Care, 7*, 30. https://doi.org/10.1186/s40560-019-0378-0.

Taurchini, M., Del Naja, C., & Tancredi, A. (2018). Enhanced recovery after surgery: A patient centered process. *Journal of Visualized Surgery, 4*, 40. https://doi.org/10.21037/jovs.2018.01.20.

The Joint Commission. (2021). *Hospital National Patient Safety Goals.* Retrieved from https://www.jointcommission.org/-/media/tjc/documents/standards/ national-patient-safety-goals/2021/simplified-2021-hap-npsg-goals-final-11420.pdf. Accessed 8 July 2021.

The Joint Commission. (2020). *Home care. 2020 National Patient Safety Goals. Goal 9. Reduce the risk of patient harm resulting from falls.* Retrieved from https://www.jointcommission.org/-/media/tjc/documents/standards/nati onal-patient-safety-goals/2020/npsg_chapter_ome_jul2020.pdf. Accessed 25 June 2021.

Thiamwong, L., Sole, M. L., Ng, B. P., Welch, G. F., Huang, H. J., & Stout, J. R. (2020). Assessing fall risk appraisal through combined physiological and perceived fall risk measures using innovative technology. *Journal* of Gerontological Nursing, 2020, 46(4), 41–47. https://doi.org/10.3928/00989134-20200302-01.

Thiel, B., Sarau, A., & Ng, D. (2017). Efficacy of topical analgesics in pain control for corneal abrasions: A systematic review. Cureus, 9(3), e1121. https://doi.org/10.7759/cureus.1121.

Thompson, M. C., & Wachs, J. E. (2012). Occupational health nursing in the United States. Workplace Health and Safety, 60(3), 127–133. https://doi.org/10.1177/216507991206000308.

Timmons, B., Vess, J., & Conner, B. (2017). Nurse-driven protocol to reduce indwelling catheter time: A health care improvement initiative. Journal of Nursing Care Quality, 32(2), 104–107. https://doi.org/10.1097/NCQ.0000000000000221.

Torossian, A., Van Gerven, E., Geertsen, K., Horn, B., Van de Velde, M., & Raeder, J. (2016). Active perioperative patient warming using a self-warming blanket (BARRIER EasyWarm) is superior to passive thermal insulation: A multinational, multicenter, randomized trial. Journal of Clinical Anesthesia, 34, 547–554. https://doi.org/10.1016/j.jclinane.2016.06.030.

Tsantes, A. G., Papadopoulos, D. V., Lytras, T., et al. (2020). Association of malnutrition with surgical site infection following spinal surgery: Systematic review and meta-analysis. Journal of Hospital Infection, 104(1), 111–119. https://doi.org/10.1016/j.jhin.2019.09.015.

UCSF Department of Radiology and Biomedical Imaging. (2020a). Vascular access and use of central lines and ports in adults. University of California San Francisco. Retrieved from https://radiology.ucsf.edu/patient-care/patient-safety/contrast/iodinated/vascular-access-adults. Accessed 14 June 2021.

UCSF Department of Radiology and Biomedical Imaging. (2020b). Vascular access and use of central lines and ports in pediatrics. University of California San Francisco. Retrieved from https://radiology.ucsf.edu/patient-care/patient-safety/contrast/iodinated/vacular-access-pediatrics. Accessed 14 June 2021.

Udoh, I. (2016). Understanding venous thromboembolism in patients with cancer. Journal for Nurse Practitioners, 12(1), 53–59. https://doi.org/10.1016/j.nurpra.2015.10.015.

U.S. Army Medical Research Institute of Infectious Diseases. (2014). USAMRIID's medical management of biological casualties handbook (8th ed.). Frederick, MD: USAMRIID. Retrieved from. https://www.usamriid.army.mil/education/bluebookpdf/USAMRIID%20BlueBook%208th%20Edition%20-%20Sep%202014.pdf. Accessed 14 June 2021.

U.S. Department of Health and Human Services. (2019). People at risk: Children under five. FoodSafety.gov [website]. Retrieved from https://www.foodsafety.gov/people-at-risk/children-under-five. Accessed 24 June 2021.

U.S. Department of Health and Human Services. (2018). Physical activity guidelines for Americans (2nd ed). Washington, DC: US Department of Health and Human Services. Retrieved from. https://health.gov/our-work/physical-activity/current-guidelines. Accessed 15 July 2021.

U.S. Department of Justice, Civil Rights Division. (2020). A Guide to Disability Rights Laws. Retrieved from https://www.ada.gov/cguide.htm. Accessed 15 July 2021.

Van der Gucht, N., & Lewis, K. (2015). Women's experience of coping with pain during childbirth: A critical review of qualitative research. Midwifery, 31(3), 349–358. https://doi.org/10.1016/j.midw.2014.12.005.

Van Horn, L., Carson, J. S., Appel, L. J., et al. (2016). Recommended dietary pattern to achieve adherence to the American Heart Association/American College of Cardiology (AHA/ACC) guidelines: A scientific statement from the American Heart Association. *Circulation, 134*(22), e505–e529. https://doi.org/10.1161/CIR.0000000000000462.

van Rensburg, R., & Decloedt, E. H. (2019). An approach to the pharmacotherapy of neuroleptic malignant syndrome. *Psychopharmacology Bulletin, 49*(1), 84–91.

Van Wicklin, S. A. (2019). *Guideline for positioning the patient.* Retrieved from http://aornguidelines.org/guidelines/content?sectionid=173734066&view=book#173734066. Accessed 28 September 2020.

Vavricka, S. R., & Greuter, T. (2019). Gastroparesis and dumping syndrome: Current concepts and management. *Journal of Clinical Medicine, 8*(8), 1127. https://doi.org/10.3390/jcm8081127.

Venara, A., Neunlist, M., Slim, K., et al. (2016). Postoperative ileus: Pathophysiology, incidence, and prevention. *Journal of Visceral Surgery, 153*(6), 439–446. https://doi.org/10.1016/j.jviscsurg.2016.08.010.

Ventocilla, M., & Wicker, D. (2016). Low vision therapy. *Medscape.* Retrieved from http://emedicine.medscape.com/article/1832033-overview. Accessed 9 August 2021.

Vizioli, L. H., Winckler, F. D., da Luz, L. C., Marques, G. K., Callegari-Jacques, S. M., & Fornari, F. (2020). Abdominal palpation does not modify the number of bowel sounds in healthy volunteers and gastrointestinal outpatients. *American Journal of the Medical Sciences, 360*(4), 378–382. https://doi.org/10.1016/j.amjms.2020.05.041.

Vollman, K., Sole, M., & Quinn, B. (2017). Endotracheal tube care and oral care practices for ventilated and non-ventilated patients. In D. L. Wiegand (Ed.), *AACN procedure manual for high acuity, progressive, and critical care* (7th ed.) (pp. 32–39). Philadelphia: Elsevier.

Wakai, A., Lawrenson, J. G., Lawrenson, A. L., et al. (2017). Topical non-steroidal anti-inflammatory drugs for analgesia in traumatic corneal abrasions. *Cochrane Database of Systematic Reviews, 5*, CD009781. https://doi.org/10.1002/14651858.CD009781.pub2.

Walsh-Irwin, C. (2021). Cardiovascular alterations. In M. L. Sole, D. G. Klein, M. J. Moseley, M. B. F. Makic, & L. T. Morata (Eds.), *Introduction to critical care nursing* (8th ed.) (pp. 282–330). St. Louis: Elsevier.

Walter, E. J., Hanna-Jumma, S., Carraretto, M., & Forni, L. (2016). The pathophysiological basis and consequences of fever. *Critical Care (London England), 20*(1), 200. https://doi.org/10.1186/s13054-016-1375-5.

Wangen, T., Hatlevig, J., Pifer, G., & Vitale, K. (2019). Preventing aspiration complications, implementing a swallow screening tool. *Clinical Nurse Specialist, 33*(5), 237–243. https://doi.org/10.1097/NUR.0000000000000471.

Ware, M. R., Feller, D. B., & Hall, K. L. (2018). Neuroleptic malignant syndrome: Diagnosis and management. *Primary Care Companion for CNS Disorders, 20*(1), 17r02185. https://doi.org/10.4088/PCC.17r02185.

Waszak, D. L., Mitchell, A. M., Ren, D., & Fennimore, L. A. (2018). A quality improvement project to improve education provided by nurses to ED patients prescribed opioid analgesics at discharge. *Journal of Emergency Nursing, 44*(4), 336–344. https://doi.org/10.1016/j.jen.2017.09.010.

Wattchow, K. A., McDonnell, M. N., & Hillier, S. L. (2018). Rehabilitation interventions for upper limb function in the first four weeks following stroke:

A systematic review and meta-analysis of the evidence. *Archives of Physical Medicine and Rehabilitation*, *99*(2), 367–382. https://doi.org/10.1016/j.apmr.2017.06.014.

West, G. F., Rose, T., & Throop, M. D. (2018). Assessing nursing interventions to reduce patient falls. *Nursing2018*, *48*(8), 59–60. https://doi.org/10.1097/01.NURSE.0000541404.79920.4e.

Whelton, P. K., Carey, R. M., Aronow, W. S., et al. (2018). 2017 ACC/AHA/AAPA/ABC/ACPM/AGS/APhA/ASH/ASPC/NMA/PCNA guideline for the prevention, detection, evaluation, and management of high blood pressure in adults; executive summary: A report of the American College of Cardiology/American Heart Association Task Force on Clinical Practice Guidelines. *Hypertension*, *71*(6), 1269–1324. https://doi.org/10.1161/HYP.0000000000000066.

Whelton, P. K., Carey, R. M., Aronow, W. S., et al. (2017). ACC/AHA/AAPA/ABC/ACPM/AGS/APha/ASH/ASPC/NMA/PCNA guidelines for the prevention, detection, evaluation, and management of high blood pressure in adults: A report of the American College of Cardiology/American Heart Association Task Forces on Clinical Practice Guidelines. *Journal of the American College of Cardiology*, *71*, e127–e248. https://doi.org/10.1016/j.jacc.2017.11.006.

Whitehead, W. E., Palsson, O. S., & Simren, M. (2016). Treating fecal incontinence: An unmet need in primary care medicine. *North Carolina Medical Journal*, *77*(3), 211–215. https://doi.org/10.18043/ncm.77.3.211.

Wilson, J. E., Mart, M. F., Cunningham, C., et al. (2020). Delirium. *Nature Reviews Disease Primers*, *6*(1), 90. https://doi.org/10.1038/s41572-020-00223-4.

Winslow, E. H., & Jacobson, A. F. (1998). Dispelling the petroleum jelly myth. *American Journal of Nursing*, *98*(11), 16RR.

Witt, D. M., Clark, N. P., Kaatz, S., Schnurr, T., & Ansell, J. E. (2016). Guidance for the practical management of warfarin therapy in the treatment of venous thromboembolism. *Journal of Thrombosis and Thrombolysis*, *41*(1), 187–205. https://doi.org/10.1007/s11239-015-1319-y.

World Health Organization (WHO). (2018). *Global guidelines for the prevention of surgical site infection*. Geneva, Switzerland: WHO Press. Retrieved from https://www.who.int/publications/i/item/global-guidelines-for-the-prevention-of-surgical-site-infection-2nd-ed. Accessed 11 November 2021.

Wound, Ostomy and Continence Nurses Society–Wound Guidelines Task Force. (2017). WOCN 2016 Guideline for prevention and management of pressure injuries (ulcers). *Journal of Wound Ostomy and Continence Nursing*, *44*(3), 241–246. https://doi.org/10.1097/WON.0000000000000321.

Yancy, C. W., Jessup, M., Bozkurt, B., et al. (2017). 2017 ACCF/AHA/HFSA focused update of the 2013 ACCF/AHA guideline for the management of heart failure: A report of the American College of Cardiology Foundation/American Heart Association Task Force on Clinical Practice Guidelines and the Heart Failure Society of America. *Circulation*, *136*(6), e137–e161. https://doi.org/10.1161/CIR.0000000000000509.

Yancy, C. W., Jessup, M., Bozkurt, B., et al. (2013). 2013 ACCF/AHA guideline for the management of heart failure: A report of the American College of Cardiology Foundation/American Heart Association Task Force on Practice Guidelines. *Circulation*, *128*(16), e240–e327. https://doi.org/10.1161/CIR.0b013e31829e8776.

Yardley, L., Beyer, N., Hauer, K., Kempen, G., Piot-Ziegler, C., & Todd, C. (2005). Development and initial validation of the Falls Efficacy Scale-International (FES-I). *Age and Ageing, 34*(6), 614–619. https://doi.org/10.1093/ageing/afi196.

Yen, J., Van Arendonk, K. J., Streiff, M. B., et al. (2016). Risk factors for venous thromboembolism in pediatric trauma patients and validation of a novel scoring system: the risk of clots in kids with trauma score. *Pediatric Critical Care Medicine, 17*(5), 391–399. https://doi.org/10.1097/PCC.0000000000000699.

Young, C. J., Zahid, A., Koh, C. E., & Young, J. M. (2017). Hypothesized summative anal physiology score correlates but poorly predicts incontinence severity. *World Journal of Gastroenterology, 23*(31), 5732–5738. https://doi.org/10.3748/wjg.v23.i31.5732.

Young, J. S. (2015). Age-related eye diseases and recommendations for low-vision AIDS. *Home Healthcare Now, 33*(1), 10–19. https://doi.org/10.1097/NHH.0000000000000177.

Young, P. J., Bellomo, R., Bernard, G. R., et al. (2019). Fever control in critically ill adults. An individual patient data meta-analysis of randomised controlled trials. *Intensive Care Medicine, 45*(4), 468–476. https://doi.org/10.1007/s00134-019-05553-w.

Zafren, K. (2017). Out-of-hospital evaluation and treatment of accidental hypothermia. *Emergency Medicine Clinics of North America, 35*(2), 261–279. https://doi.org/10.1016/j.emc.2017.01.003.

Zhao, Y. L., Bott, M., He, J., Kim, H., Park, S. H., & Dunton, N. (2019). Evidence on fall and injurious fall prevention in acute care hospitals. *Journal of Nursing Administration, 49*(2), 86–92. https://doi.org/10.1097/NNA.0000000000000715.

Zimmerman, D. R., Shneor, E., Millodot, M., & Gordon-Shaag, A. (2019). Corneal and conjunctival injury seen in urgent care centres in Israel. *Ophthalmic and Physiological Optics, 39*(1), 46–52. https://doi.org/10.1111/opo.12600.

# INDEX

## A

Abdominal distention, 3
Abdominal hysterectomy, 3
Abdominal pain, 3
Abdominal surgery, 3
Abdominal trauma, 3
Ablation, radiofrequency catheter, 3
Abortion
  induced, 3
  spontaneous, 4
Abruptio placentae, 4
Abscess formation, 4
Absorbent underpads, in impaired
    wheelchair mobility, 556
Abuse
  in child, 4
  laxative, 83
  in parent, 4–5
  physical, 114
  protection, in impaired parenting, 611
  in significant other, 4–5
  in spouse, 4–5
Accessory muscle use, to breathe, 5
Accident prone, 5
Accidental hypothermia, nursing inter-
    ventions for, 452–454
Acculturation stresses, in impaired
    parenting, 611
Achalasia, 5
Acid base imbalances, 5
Acidosis
  lactic, 82
  metabolic, 5, 92
  respiratory, 5, 128
Acne, 5
Acquired immunodeficiency syndrome
    (AIDS), 9–10
  in child, 10
  dementia, 10
  in ineffective sexuality pattern, 716
Acromegaly, 5
Active warming measures, 776
Activities of daily living (ADLs),
    fatigue and, 369
Activity intolerance, potential to
  develop, 6

Activity planning, ineffective, 164–166
  client outcomes of, 165
  defining characteristics of, 165
  nursing interventions, 165–166
  related factors, 165
  risk for, 166–167
  at risk population, 165
Activity tolerance, decreased, 159–164
  associated condition, 159
  client outcomes of, 159
  client/family teaching and discharge
      planning for, 163–164
  defining characteristics of, 159
  nursing interventions, 159
  related factors, 159
  risk for, 164
  at risk population, 159
Acupoint pressure, for PONV, 569
Acute abdominal pain, 6
Acute alcohol intoxication, 6
Acute back pain, 6
Acute confusion, 6, 246–251
  risk for, 255
Acute coronary syndrome, 6
Acute kidney injury, signs of,
    279–280
Acute lymphocytic leukemia (ALL),
    6
Acute pain, 595–600
Acute renal failure, 6
Acute respiratory distress syndrome
    (ARDS), 6, 17
  in impaired gas exchange, 398
Acute stress disorder, in combatants, 629
Acute stroke, HOB elevation for, 547
Acute substance withdrawal syndrome,
    6–7, 749–752
  associated conditions, 750
  at-risk population, 750
  client outcomes, 750
  defining characteristics, 749
  nursing interventions, 750–752
  related factors, 750
  risk for, 752–754
Acute traveler's diarrhea, 324
Adams-Stokes syndrome, 7

Adaptive capacity, decreased intracra-
nial, 547
Addiction, 7
Addiction, nicotine, 103
Addiction, opioid, 106
Addiction, technology, 146
Addison's disease, 7
Adenoidectomy, 7
    tonsillectomy and, 145–146, 149
Adhesions, lysis of, 7
Adjustment disorder, 7
Adjustment impairment, 7
Adolescents
    enhanced religiosity in, 667
    exposure to community violence, 290
    ineffective eating dynamics of,
        332–334
    loneliness in, 533
    maturational issues, 90
    pregnant, 7–8
    terminally ill, 147
Adoption, giving child up for, 8
Adrenocortical insufficiency, 8
Adult
    enhanced religiosity in, 666
    obesity in, 584
    older, 105
    terminally ill, 147
Adult falls, risk for, 351–358
Adult pressure injury, 633–640
    risk for, 640–641
Adult Protective Services (APS), 709
Advance directives, 8
Adverse childhood experiences (ACEs),
    833
Aerobic exercise
    moderate-intensity, for impaired
        physical mobility, 552
    for readiness for enhanced exercise
        engagement, 346
    for sedentary lifestyle, 683
Affective disorders, 8
African American, enhanced religiosity
    in, 667
Afterload, altered, in decreased cardiac
    output, 210–211
Age, compromised host defenses and,
    500
Age-Friendly Health System's Model
    of Care, 355

Age-related growth charts, 335, 377
Age-related macular degeneration, 8
Age-related safety measures, 622
Aggressive behavior, 8
Aging, 9
Agitation, 9
Agnosia, compensatory strategies for,
    557
Agoraphobia, 9
Agranulocytosis, 9
AIDS. *See* Acquired immunodeficiency
    syndrome
Airborne-transmitted microorganisms,
    precautions for, 496–497
Airway clearance, ineffective, 167–172
    associated condition, 167
    client outcomes of, 167–172
    defining characteristics of, 167
    nursing interventions, 167–172
    related factors, 167
    at risk population, 167
Airway obstruction/secretions, 10
Alcohol
    defensive coping and, 284
    use
        in disturbed maternal-fetal
            dyad, 540
        during pregnancy, 232
    withdrawal from, 155
Alcohol-based hand rub, 496
Alcohol-induced withdrawal syndrome,
    750–752
    risk for, 752–754
Alcohol intoxication, acute, 6
Alcohol withdrawal, 10–11
Alcoholic ketoacidosis, 79
Alcoholism, 11
    dysfunctional family processes, 11, 364
Alkalosis, 11
Alkalosis, metabolic, 92
ALL. *See* Acute lymphocytic leukemia
All withdrawal syndromes, 751–752
    risk of, 754
Allergic reaction
    to contrast media, 280–281
    latex, 83
    risk for, 172–175
        causes of, 173–175
        client outcomes of, 172
        first aid, 173

Allergic reaction *(Continued)*
  nursing interventions, 172–175
  prevention of, 174–175
  risk factors, 172
  at risk population, 172
  severe, 173–174
  symptoms, 173
Allergies, 11
  dry eyes and, 349
  impaired oral mucous membrane
      integrity and, 579, 584
Alopecia, 11
ALS. *See* Amyotrophic lateral sclerosis
Altered afterload, risk for decreased
      cardiac output, 218
Altered contractility, risk for decreased
      cardiac output, 218
Altered health status, interrupted fam-
      ily processes and, 364
Altered heart rate, in decreased cardiac
      output, 218
Altered heart rhythm, in decreased
      cardiac output, 218
Altered mental status, 11
Altered preload, risk for decreased
      cardiac output, 218
Altered role performance, 130
Altered water source, dysfunctional gas-
      trointestinal motility and, 400, 405
Alternative mind-body therapies, 685
Alveolar-capillary membrane changes,
      impaired gas exchange and, 395
Alvimopan, for postoperative ileus, 403
Alzheimer's disease, 11–12
Ambulation, in labor pain, 608
AMD. *See* Age-related macular
      degeneration
Amenorrhea, 12
American College of Obstetricians and
      Gynecologists (ACOG), 568
American Psychiatric Nurses Associa-
      tion (APNA), 763–766
AMI (acute myocardial infarction). *See*
      Myocardial infarction
Amnesia, 12
Amniocentesis, 12
Amnionitis, 12
Amniotic membrane rupture, 12
Amputation, 12–13
Amyotrophic lateral sclerosis (ALS), 13

Anal fistula, 13
Analgesia, patient-controlled, 111
Analgesics, for pain
  around the clock, 597
  delivery methods, 597
  before painful procedures, 598
  response to, 596
  route of administration of, 597
Anaphylactic shock, 13
Anaphylaxis prevention, 13
Anasarca, 13
Anemia, 13
  aplastic, 17
  delayed surgical recovery and,
      768
  fatigue and, 369, 372
  impaired skin integrity and, 722
  maternal, delayed infant motor
      development and, 317
  pernicious, 113
  in pregnancy, 13
  risk for adult falls and, 352
  sickle cell, 13, 136–137
Anencephaly, 13, 101–102
Aneurysm
  abdominal aortic repair surgery, 13–14
  cerebral, 14
Anger, 14
Angina, 14
Angiocardiography, 14
Angioplasty, coronary, 14
Animal-assisted therapy, 736
  for decreased diversional activity
      engagement, 331
Anomaly, fetal/newborn, 14–15
Anorectal abscess, 15
Anorexia, 15
  frail elderly syndrome and, 393, 395
Anorexia nervosa, 15
Anosmia, 15
Antenatal education, 232–233
Antepartum care, in ineffective child-
      bearing process, 231–232
Antepartum period, 15
Anterior repair, anterior colporrhaphy,
      16
Antibiotic stewardship, for diarrhea,
      322
Anticipatory grieving interventions,
      415–418

Anticipatory guidance, for decision making, 303–304

Anticoagulant therapy, 16
  administration, safety guidelines for, 193–194

Antidepressants, for suicidal behavior, 765

Antidiarrheals, for deficient fluid volume, 385

Antiemetics
  for deficient fluid volume, 385
  nausea and, 567–569

Antifungal agents, for dry mouth, 565

Antifungal treatment, prophylactic, 654

Antipsychotic medications
  for delirium, 249
  in metabolic imbalance syndrome, 544

Antipyretic treatments, 780

Antisocial personality disorder, 16

Anuria, 16

Anxiety, 16, 175–178, 769
  assessment of, 252
  associated condition, 176
  for chronic insomnia, 521
  client outcomes of, 176–178
  death, 178–180
    associated condition, 178
    client outcomes of, 178–179
    defining characteristics of, 178
    nursing interventions, 179–180
    related factors, 178
    at risk population, 178
  defining characteristics of, 175–176
  dysfunctional gastrointestinal motility and, 400, 405
  frail elderly syndrome and, 393, 395
  high attachment, maladaptive grieving and, 412, 414
  in ineffective sexuality pattern, 714
  maladaptive grieving and, 414
  nausea and, in pregnancy, 569
  nursing interventions, 176–178
  in post-trauma syndrome, 626
  related factors, 176
  at risk population, 176
  separation, 135

Anxiety disorder, 16

Aortic valvular stenosis, 16

APGAR scores, ineffective infant suck-swallow response, 755

Aphasia, 16–17

Aplastic anemia, 17

Apnea
  in infancy, 17
  obstructive sleep, 104
  sleep, 138

Apneustic respirations, 17

Appendectomy, 17

Appendicitis, 17

Apprehension, 17

Aprepitant, for nausea, 570

ARDS. *See* Acute respiratory distress syndrome

Arrhythmia, 17

Arterial blood gases, monitor, in risk for shock, 719

Arterial insufficiency, 17
  in ineffective peripheral tissue perfusion, 794–796

Arteriolar nephrosclerosis, 88

Arthritis, 17
  fatigue and, 372
  rheumatoid, 125

Arthrocentesis, 17

Arthroplasty, 17–18

Arthroscopy, 18

Artificial respiration, dry eye and, 351

Ascites, 18

Asian American clients, post-trauma syndrome in, 627

Asperger's syndrome, 18

Asphyxia, birth, 18

Aspiration
  danger of, 18
  meconium, 91, 129
  risk for, 180–185
    associated condition, 181
    client outcomes of, 181
    nursing interventions, 181–185
    related factors, 181
    at risk population, 181
  signs of, 773

Assault victim, 18

Assaultive client, 18

Assisted living facility, for relocation stress syndrome, 669–670

Assistive devices
  for disuse syndrome, 328
  for impaired physical mobility, 552
  for walking
    risk for adult falls and, 352
    risk for child falls and, 359

Assistive technology, for impaired memory, 542–543
Asthma, 18–19
  impaired gas exchange and, 395
Ataxia, 19
Atelectasis, 19
Atherosclerosis, 19
  risk for ineffective cerebral tissue perfusion, 228–229
Athlete's foot, 19
ATN. *See* Tubular necrosis, kidney, acute
Atresia, tricuspid, 151
Atrial fibrillation, 19
  risk for ineffective cerebral tissue perfusion, 228–229
Atrial myxoma, risk for ineffective cerebral tissue perfusion, 228–229
Atrial septal defect, 19
Atrophic vaginal changes, 486
Atrophy, muscular, 97
Attachment, parent, 110
Attention deficit disorder, 19
Attentional fatigue, 371–372
Attention-interaction system, of disorganized infant behavior, 489
Audiologist, for impaired verbal communication, 244
Audiology consultation, for hearing loss, 244
Autism, 19–20
  in risk for self-mutilation, 708
  self-mutilation and, 706
Autism spectrum disorder
  risk for elopement attempt and, 339
  screening, for delayed child development, 315
Autoimmune diseases, dry eyes and, 349, 351
Autonomic dysreflexia, 20, 188–190
  associated condition, 188
  client outcomes of, 189
  defining characteristics of, 188
  nursing interventions, 189–190
  related factors, 188
  risk for, 191
  at risk population, 188
Autonomic hyperreflexia, 20
Autosomal disorder, impaired oral mucous membrane integrity and, 579, 584

Awakening and Breathing Coordination, Delirium Monitoring and Management, and Early Mobility (ABCDE) ICU, 250

**B**

Baby care, 20
Back pain, acute, 6
Bacteremia, 20
Balanced energy field, 20
Bariatric equipment, in impaired bed mobility, 549
Barrel chest, 20
Bathing
  assistance, 687
  for cognitively impaired clients, 688
  problems, 20
  towel, 688
Battered child syndrome, 20
Battered person, 20
Bed mobility, impaired, 20, 94, 545–550
Bed positioning, in impaired bed mobility, 548–549
Bed rails, for impaired bed mobility, 547
Bed rest, prolonged, 20–21
Bedbugs, infestation, 20
Bedpan, for toileting self-care deficit, 695
Bedside commode, for constipation, 260
Bedside Mobility Assessment Tool 2.0 (BMAT 2.0), 352–353
Bedsores, 21
Bedwetting, 21
Behavior
  in acute confusion, 247
  of anxiety, 175
  decreased cardiac output and, 211
  health, risk-prone, 420–422
  of ineffective lymphedema self-management, 534–535
  infant, enhanced organized, readiness for, 493
  maladaptive, 88
  manipulative, 89
  in sedentary interventions, 684
  smoking, 138
  violent, 154
  wellness-seeking, 155

Behavioral causes, in sexual dysfunction, 712

Behavioral disorder, impaired oral mucous membrane integrity and, 579, 584

Behavioral modification, in self-neglect, 710

Behavioral screening and intervention (BSI), 363

Bell's palsy, 21

Benign prostatic hypertrophy (BPH), 21, 24
  urinary retention and, 812

Bent-leg sit-ups, for constipation, 260

Benzodiazepine-induced withdrawal syndrome, 751
  risk for, 753–754

Bereaved person, interacting with, activities when, 416–417

Bereavement, 21

Bethanechol HCL saliva stimulant, in dry mouth, 566

Biliary atresia, 21

Biliary calculus, 21

Biliary obstruction, 21

Bilingual members, outside of traditional health care system, 525

Bilirubin elevation in neonate, 21

Biofeedback therapy, for chronic functional constipation, 267

Biofield therapy, for enhancing comfort, 240

Biological exposure, contamination and, 269

Biopsy, 21
  breast, 25
  liver, 85

Bioterrorism, 21

Bipolar disorder, 21–22

Bipolar disorder I, manic disorder, 89

Birth
  ineffective childbearing process during, 231
  readiness for enhanced childbearing process after, 234

Birth asphyxia, 22

Birth control, 22

Bladder
  cancer, 22
  neurogenic, 102

Bladder diary
  for disability-associated urinary incontinence, 475
  for stress urinary incontinence, 482
  for toileting self-care deficit, 695–696
  for urge urinary incontinence, 485–486

Bladder distention, 22

Bladder function, in acute confusion, 249

Bladder habits
  in disability-associated urinary incontinence, 474–475
  in stress urinary incontinence, 481
  in urge urinary incontinence, 485

Bladder log, 481

Bladder temperature, in perioperative hypothermia, 462

Bladder training, 22
  in child, 22

Bladder training program, 487

Bleeding
  prevention of, 655
  risk for, 192–194
    associated condition, 192
    client outcomes of, 192
    nursing interventions, 192–194
    risk factors, 192
    at risk population, 192
  uterine, 153

Bleeding disorder
  client/family teaching and discharge planning for, 656–657
  platelet count and, 582

Bleeding tendency, 22

Blepharitis, symptoms of, 349

Blepharoplasty, 22

Blindness, 22

Blood coagulation disorders, frail elderly syndrome and, 393, 395

Blood disorder, 22

Blood glucose
  control, 22
  low, 86

Blood pressure, low, 86

Blood pressure alteration, 22

Blood transfusion, 23

Blurred vision, dry eyes and, 348

Board transfer, slide, in impaired transfer ability, 798

Body dysmorphic disorder, 23

Body image
  change, 23
  disturbed, 197–200
Body mass index (BMI)
  impaired skin integrity and, 721–722
  in nutrition, 572–573
  in obesity, 584–586
  in overweight, 587, 589–590,
    593
Body requirements, less than, 574–578
Body temperature, altered, 23
Bone fractures
  chronic pain and, 601
  peripheral neurovascular dysfunction
    and, 619
Bone marrow biopsy, 23
Bone strengthening, 683
  for readiness for enhanced exercise
    engagement, 346
Border-defining pillow/mattress, adult
  falls and, 354
Borderline personality disorder, 23
  self-mutilation and, 706
Boredom, 23
Botulism, 23
Bowel continence, impaired, 273–278
  associated condition, 274
  client outcomes of, 274
  defining characteristics of, 273–274
  nursing interventions, 274–278
  related factors, 274
  at risk population, 274
Bowel function, in acute confusion, 249
Bowel habits
  in chronic functional constipation,
    265–266
  in constipation, 256
  in perceived constipation, 262
  7-day diary of, 257, 262, 266
Bowel incontinence, 23
Bowel movements, 86
  monitor frequency of, 598
Bowel obstruction, 23, 104
Bowel program, for constipation, 260
Bowel resection, 23
Bowel sounds
  absent/diminished, 24
  hyperactive, 24
Bowel training, 24
  in child, 24

Bracelet, medical alert, 656
Braden scale score, 635
Bradycardia, 24
Bradypnea, 24
Brain injury, 24
  impaired swallowing and, 771–772
  labile emotional control and, 341
  risk for ineffective cerebral tissue
    perfusion, 228–229
Brain neoplasm, risk for ineffective
    cerebral tissue perfusion, 228–229
Brain surgery, 24
Brain tumor, 24
Braxton Hicks contraction, 24–25
Breast
  lumps, 25
  painful
    due to engorgement, 108
    due to sore nipples, 108
Breast cancer, 25
  compromised family coping and, 295
Breast examination, self, 25
Breast milk production, insufficient, 25
Breast pumping, 25
Breastfeeding
  effective, 25
  ineffective, 25, 201–203
    associated condition, 202
    client outcomes of, 202
    defining characteristics of, 201
    nursing interventions, 202–203
    related factors, 201–202
    at risk population, 202
  interrupted, 25, 203–205
  with pregnant client, 235
  readiness for enhanced, 205–206
  sore nipples and, 139
Breath sounds, decreased/absent, 25
Breathing
  mouth, in dry mouth, 563
  pattern
    alteration, 25
    ineffective, 206–210
Breech birth, 25
Bristol Stool Scale, 257
Bronchitis, 25–26
Bronchopulmonary dysplasia, 26
Bronchoscopy and, 26
Bruits, carotid, 26
Bruxism, impaired dentition and, 308

Bryant's traction, 26
Buck's traction, 26
Buerger's disease, 26
Bulimia, 26
Bullying, 26
Bunion, 26
Bunionectomy, 26
Burning eyes, dry eyes and, 348
Burns, 27
   peripheral neurovascular dysfunction
      and, 619
   risk, 27
Bursitis, 27
Bypass graft, 27
   coronary artery, 40
   femoral popliteal, 56

## C

CABG. *See* Coronary artery bypass
     grafting
Cachexia, 27
Caffeine
   intake, in sleep deprivation, 730
   to lower urinary tract symptoms,
     487
Calcium alteration, 27
Calibrated thermometer, 776
Calming activities, for insomnia, 521
Cancer, 27–28
   fatigue with, 371–372
   liver, 85
   lung, 86
   pancreatic, 109
   skin, 137
Candidiasis, oral, 28
Cannabis-induced withdrawal syn-
     drome, 751
   risk for, 754
Capgras syndrome, self-neglect and,
     709
Capillary refill time, prolonged, 28
Carbon monoxide poisoning, 28,
     623
Carcinoma, ovarian, 107–108
Cardiac arrest, 28
Cardiac catheterization, 28–29
Cardiac disease, fatigue with,
     371–372
Cardiac disorders, in pregnancy, 29
Cardiac dysrhythmia, 29

Cardiac output, decreased, 29, 210–217
   associated condition, 211
   client outcomes of, 211
   defining characteristics of, 210–211
   nursing interventions, 211–217
   related factors, 211
   risk for, 218
Cardiac tamponade, 29
   risk for decreased cardiac tissue
     perfusion, 218
Cardiac tissue perfusion, decreased, risk
     for, 218–222
Cardiogenic shock, 29, 136
   unstable blood glucose level and,
     406
Cardiometabolic abnormalities, screen-
     ing for, in metabolic imbalance
     syndrome, 545
Cardiorespiratory (aerobic) exercise,
     moderate-intensity, for impaired
     physical mobility, 552
Cardiovascular disease
   decreased activity tolerance due to,
     162
   impaired skin integrity and, 722
Care receiver, role strain, 225
Care staff, communication among,
     effectiveness of, 505
Caregiver
   care situation and, 225
   in factors of disorganized infant
     behavior, 490
   health literacy of, 523
   health status of, 223–224
   role strain, 29, 223–227
     associated condition, 225
     client outcomes of, 225
     defining characteristics of,
       223–224
     nursing interventions, 225–227
     related factors, 224–225
     risk of, 227–228
     at risk population, 225
Caregiver-care receiver relationship, 224
   defining characteristics of, 224
   risk for caregiver role strain and, 227
Caregiving activities
   defining characteristics of, 223
   related factors (r/t) in, 224
   risk for caregiver role strain and, 228

Care-resistant behavior, in dementia or delirium, 583
Caring, for trauma, 627
Carious teeth, 29
Carotid endarterectomy, 29–30
Carotid stenosis, risk for ineffective cerebral tissue perfusion, 228–229
Carpal tunnel syndrome, 30
Casts, 30
    traction and, 150–151
Cataract extraction, 30
Catatonic schizophrenia, 30
Catheter
    condom, 479–480
    indwelling urinary
        in disability-associated urinary incontinence, 477
        in risk for urinary tract injury, 517
    peripheral, 497
    urinary, 152–153
        proper placement, 518
Catheter- associated urinary tract infections (CAUTIs), 812
Catheterization
    left heart, 84
    urinary, 30
Causative factors, in nausea, 567–568
Cavities in teeth, 30
Celiac disease, 30
Cellulitis, 30–31
    periorbital, 31
Centers for Disease Control and Prevention's Stopping Elderly Accidents, Deaths, & Injuries (STEADI) initiative, 356
Central line insertion, 31
Central nervous system sensitization, chronic pain and, 601
Cerebral aneurysm, 31
    risk for ineffective cerebral tissue perfusion, 228–229
Cerebral palsy, 31
    impaired swallowing and, 771–772
Cerebral perfusion, 31
Cerebral perfusion pressure (CPP), reducing risk of, 230
Cerebral tissue perfusion, ineffective, risk for, 228–230

Cerebrovascular accident (CVA), 31, 41–42
    impaired physical mobility and, 553
Cervical dilation, labor pain and, 607
Cervicitis, 31
Cervix, incompetent, 120
Cesarean delivery, 31–32
Cevimeline, for dry mouth, 564
Chairs, for impaired physical mobility, 553
Character disorder, self-mutilation and, 706
Chemical dependence, 32
Chemical exposure
    contamination and, 268–269
    corneal injury and, 511
Chemosis, dry eyes and, 348
Chemotherapy, 32
    client receiving, 581–583
    dry eyes and, 349, 351
    fatigue and, 369, 372
    impaired oral mucous membrane integrity and, 579, 584
    nausea after, 569
Chemotherapy-induced diarrhea (CID), 324
Chest pain, 32
Chest tubes, 32
Chewing gum, for postoperative ileus, 402
Cheyne-Stokes respiration, 32
Chickenpox, 32
    communicable diseases, childhood as, 37
Child
    abuse, 32
    with chronic condition, 33–34
    delayed development, 314–316
    eating dynamics of, ineffective, 334–337
    exposed to methamphetamines, 623
    falls, risk for, 358–361
    in impaired parenting
        associated condition, 610, 615
        characteristics of, 610
        related factors for, 610
        at risk population, 610, 615
    in ineffective breastfeeding, 201
    neglect, 33
    nursing interventions for, impaired dentition in, 312

Child *(Continued)*
   pressure injury, 641–649
      risk for, 648
   risk factors for, falls in, 358–361
   sepsis, 135
   terminally ill, 147
Childbearing problems, 33
Childbearing process
   ineffective, 230–233
      client outcomes of, 231–232
      defining characteristics of, 231
      nursing interventions, 232–233
      related factors, 231
      risk for, 236
      at risk population, 231
   readiness for enhanced, 233–236
      client outcomes of, 234
      defining characteristics of, 233–234
      nursing Interventions, 235–236
Childbirth, 34
Childhood obesity, 34
Chills, 34
Chlamydia infection, 34
Chloasma, 34
Chlorhexidine gluconate
   for cleansing, 654
   mouthwash, for VAE and VAP, 582
Choking or coughing with eating, 34
Cholecystectomy, 34
   laparoscopic laser, 82
Cholelithiasis, 34
Chorioamnionitis, 34
Chromosomal disorders, ineffective
      infant feeding dynamics and, 376
Chronic confusion, 34, 251–255
   adult falls and, 354
Chronic disability, chronic sorrow and,
      739
Chronic disease
   chronic sorrow and, 739
   fatigue and, 369
   frail elderly syndrome and, 393, 395
   ineffective family health self-
      management and, 427
   ineffective health maintenance
      behaviors and, 429
   in sexual dysfunction, 712
   social isolation and, 737
   spiritual distress and, 742

Chronic disease-related malnutrition,
      575–576
Chronic fatigue syndrome, 370
Chronic functional constipation, 34,
      264–267
   associated condition, 265
   defining characteristics of, 264
   related factors, 264
   at risk population, 265
Chronic heart failure, 389
Chronic inflammation, fatigue and, 369
Chronic insomnia, 521
Chronic low self-esteem, 698–700
   associated conditions, 698
   at-risk population, 698
   client outcomes, 698–699
   defining characteristics, 698
   nursing interventions, 699–700
   related factors, 698
   risk for, 703
Chronic lung disease, in ineffective
      sexuality pattern, 716
Chronic lymphocytic leukemia, 34
Chronic musculo-skeletal diseases,
      chronic pain and, 601
Chronic obstructive pulmonary disease
      (COPD), 34
Chronic pain, 34, 600–606
Chronic pain syndrome, 606
Chronic renal failure, 34
Chronic sorrow, 739–741
   associated conditions, 739
   at-risk population, 739
   client outcomes, 739–740
   defining characteristics, 739
   nursing interventions, 740–741
   related factors, 739
Chronic vomiting, impaired dentition
      and, 308
Chvostek's sign, 35
Circumcision, 35
Cirrhosis, 35
Cleaners, household, eye injury and, 510
Cleft lip/cleft palate, 35
   ineffective infant feeding dynamics
      and, 376
Client
   health literacy of, 523
   identification of, accuracy of, 505
   perioperative, positioning, 617–618

Client *(Continued)*
  receiving chemotherapy/radiation,
    581–583
  surgical
    general interventions for,
      616–619
    risk for pressure ulcer, 617
  on ventilator, 582
Client/network interventions, for im-
    paired mood regulation, 559–560
Client outcomes
  in acute confusion, 246–247
  in acute pain, 595–596
  in acute substance withdrawal
    syndrome, 750
  in adult pressure injury, 634–635, 641
  in anxiety, 176–178
  in autonomic dysreflexia, 189
  in child pressure injury, 642, 649
  in chronic confusion, 252
  in chronic functional constipation,
    265
  in chronic low self-esteem, 698–699
  in chronic pain, 601–602
  in chronic pain syndrome, 606
  in chronic sorrow, 739–740
  in compromised family coping, 292
  in compromised human dignity, 439
  in constipation, 256
  in contamination, 270
  in death anxiety, 178–179
  in decision making, 299, 302, 304–305
  in decisional conflict, 300–301
  in decreased activity tolerance, 159
  in decreased cardiac output, 211
  in decreased diversional activity
    engagement, 330
  in defensive coping, 283
  in deficient community health, 418
  in deficient fluid volume, 384
  in deficient knowledge, 523
  in delayed child development, 314
  in delayed infant motor develop-
    ment, 318
  in delayed surgical recovery, 768
  in diarrhea, 320
  in disability-associated urinary
    incontinence, 474
  in disabled family coping, 296
  in disorganized infant behavior,
    490–491

Client outcomes *(Continued)*
  in disturbed body image, 198
  in disturbed family identity syn-
    drome, 465
  in disturbed personal identity, 467
  in disturbed thought process,
    784–785
  in disuse syndrome, 326
  in dry eyes, 351
  in dysfunctional adult ventilatory
    weaning response, 824
  in dysfunctional family processes,
    362–363
  in dysfunctional gastrointestinal
    motility, 400–401, 405
  in dysfunctional ventilatory weaning
    response, 824
  in electrolyte imbalance, 337
  in enhanced nutrition, 572
  in enhanced parenting, 612–613
  in enhanced power, 629
  in enhanced relationship, 662
  in enhanced religiosity, 666
  in enhanced resilience, 675
  in excess fluid volume, 389
  in family processes, 367
  in fatigue, 369–373
  in fear, 374
  in female genital mutilation, 378
  in frail elderly syndrome, 393, 395
  in hope, 433, 435
  in hopelessness, 437
  in hyperthermia, 446
  in hypothermia, 451–452, 458, 461
  in imbalanced fluid volume, 380–381
  in imbalanced nutrition, 575
  in impaired bowel continence, 274
  in impaired comfort, 237
  in impaired dentition, 309
  in impaired gas exchange, 396
  in impaired oral mucous membrane,
    579, 584
  in impaired parenting, 610–611, 615
  in impaired physical mobility,
    551–552
  in impaired religiosity, 664
  in impaired resilience, 673
  in impaired skin integrity, 722
  in impaired social interaction, 735
  in impaired spontaneous ventila-
    tion, 819

Client outcomes *(Continued)*
  in impaired standing, 747
  in impaired swallowing, 772
  in impaired transfer ability, 797–798
  in impaired urinary elimination, 807
  in impaired verbal communication, 243
  in impaired walking, 834
  in impaired wheelchair mobility, 556
  in ineffective activity planning, 165
  in ineffective adolescent eating dynamics, 333
  in ineffective airway clearance, 167–172
  in ineffective breastfeeding, 202
  in ineffective breathing pattern, 207
  in ineffective child eating dynamics, 335
  in ineffective childbearing process, 231–232
  in ineffective coping, 285
  in ineffective denial, 306
  in ineffective dry eye self-management, 349
  in ineffective family health self-management, 427
  in ineffective health maintenance behaviors, 429
  in ineffective health self-management, 423
  in ineffective home maintenance behaviors, 431, 434
  in ineffective impulse control, 472
  in ineffective infant feeding dynamics, 377
  in ineffective infant suck-swallow response, 755–756
  in ineffective lymphedema self-management, 535
  in ineffective peripheral tissue perfusion, 793
  in ineffective protection, 653
  in ineffective relationship, 660–661
  in ineffective role performance, 679–680
  in ineffective sexuality pattern, 714
  in ineffective thermoregulation, 777
  in insomnia, 520
  in insufficient breast milk production, 200

Client outcomes *(Continued)*
  in interrupted family processes, 365
  in labile emotional control, 341
  in labor pain, 607
  in maladaptive grieving, 412
  in mixed urinary incontinence, 478
  in nausea, 567
  in neonatal abstinence syndrome, 571
  in neonatal hyperbilirubinemia, 441
  in neonatal hypothermia, 459
  in neonatal pressure injury, 650, 652
  in nipple-areolar complex injury, 515
  in obesity, 585
  in overweight, 589, 592
  in parental role conflict, 677
  in perceived constipation, 261
  in perioperative positioning injury, 616
  in peripheral neurovascular dysfunction, 619
  in post-trauma syndrome, 625, 628
  in powerlessness, 631, 633
  in rape-trauma syndrome, 657–658
  in readiness for enhanced childbearing process, 234
  in readiness for enhanced comfort, 239
  in readiness for enhanced coping, 287–288
  in readiness for enhanced exercise engagement, 345
  in readiness for enhanced family coping, 297–298
  in readiness for enhanced grieving, 415
  in readiness for enhanced health literacy, 528
  in readiness for enhanced health self-management, 425
  in readiness for enhanced knowledge, 524
  in readiness for enhancing communication, 241
  in relocation stress syndrome, 668–669
  in risk for adult falls, 352
  in risk for aspiration, 181
  in risk for autonomic dysreflexia, 191
  in risk for bleeding, 192
  in risk for child falls, 359
  in risk for complicated immigration transition, 470

Client outcomes *(Continued)*
  in risk for corneal injury, 508
  in risk for decreased activity toler-
      ance, 164
  in risk for deficient fluid volume, 392
  in risk for delayed infant motor
      development, 320
  in risk for disturbed maternal-fetal
      dyad, 539
  in risk for dry mouth, 562–563
  in risk for elopement attempt, 339
  in risk for impaired attachment, 185
  in risk for impaired liver function,
      529
  in risk for ineffective activity plan-
      ning, 167
  in risk for ineffective cerebral tissue
      perfusion, 229
  in risk for infection, 494–495
  in risk for injury, 505
  in risk for iodinated contrast media,
      adverse reaction to, 279
  in risk for latex allergy reaction, 526
  in risk for loneliness, 532–533
  in risk for maladaptive grieving, 414
  in risk for metabolic syndrome,
      543–544
  in risk for neonatal hyperbilirubine-
      mia, 444
  in risk for occupational injury, 511
  in risk for other-directed violence,
      829
  in risk for poisoning, 621
  in risk for suffocation, 760
  in risk for suicidal behavior, 763
  in risk for surgical site infection, 499
  in risk for thermal injury, 775
  in risk for unstable blood pressure,
      195
  in risk for urinary tract injury, 517
  in risk for vascular trauma, 815
  in risk-prone health behavior, 420
  in sedentary lifestyle, 682
  in self-mutilation, 706
  in self-neglect, 709
  in sexual dysfunction, 711
  in situational low self-esteem, 701
  in sleep deprivation, 729
  in social isolation, 738
  in spiritual distress, 742
  in stress urinary incontinence, 481

Client outcomes *(Continued)*
  in unilateral neglect, 805
  in unstable blood glucose level,
      406–407
  in urge urinary incontinence, 484
  in urinary retention, 810
  in wandering, 838
Client/family teaching
  for acute confusion, 251
  for acute pain, 599–600
  for acute substance withdrawal
      syndrome, 752
  for adult pressure injury, 641
  for anxiety, 177–178
  for anxiety in, 177–178
  for autonomic dysreflexia, 190
  for bathing self-care deficit, 689
  for caregiver role strain, 227
  for child pressure injury, 649
  for chronic confusion, 254–255
  for chronic low self-esteem, 700
  for chronic pain, 605–606
  for chronic pain syndrome, 606
  for compromised family coping, 295
  for compromised human dignity, 440
  for constipation, 260
  for contamination, 272
  for death anxiety, 180
  for decision making, 300
  for decisional conflict, 301
  for decreased activity tolerance,
      163–164
  for decreased cardiac output, 217
  for decreased diversional activity
      engagement, 332
  for defensive coping, 284
  for deficient community health, 420
  for deficient fluid volume, 388
  for delayed child development, 316
  for delayed surgical recovery, 770
  for diarrhea, 326
  for disabled family coping, 297
  for disorganized infant behavior, 492
  for disturbed body image, 200
  for disturbed family identity syn-
      drome, 466
  for disturbed personal identity, 469
  for disturbed thought process, 786
  for disuse syndrome, 330
  for dressing self-care deficit, 691
  for dry eyes, 351

Client outcomes *(Continued)*
  for dysfunctional family processes, 364
  for dysfunctional gastrointestinal motility, 405
  for electrolyte imbalance, 338
  for enhanced nutrition, 574
  for enhanced parenting, 613–614
  for excess fluid volume, 391–392
  for family processes, 368
  for fatigue, 373
  for fear, 376
  for feeding self-care deficit, 694
  for frail elderly syndrome, 394
  for hope, 434, 436
  for hopelessness, 438
  for hyperthermia, 451
  for hypothermia, 457–458, 464
  for imbalanced energy field, 344
  for imbalanced nutrition, 578
  for impaired bed mobility, 550
  for impaired comfort, 238
  for impaired dentition, 313
  for impaired gas exchange, 399–400
  for impaired memory, 542–543
  for impaired oral mucous membrane, 583–584
  for impaired parenting, 612, 615
  for impaired physical mobility, 554
  for impaired skin integrity, 726
  for impaired social interaction, 737
  for impaired spontaneous ventilation, 823
  for impaired standing, 748
  for impaired swallowing, 774
  for impaired tissue integrity, 791
  for impaired transfer ability, 801–802
  for impaired urinary elimination, 809–810
  for impaired verbal communication, 246
  for impaired walking, 837
  for impaired wheelchair mobility, 559–560
  for ineffective adolescent eating dynamics, 334
  for ineffective airway clearance, 171–172
  for ineffective breastfeeding, 203
  for ineffective breathing pattern, 210

Client outcomes *(Continued)*
  for ineffective child eating dynamics, 336–337
  for ineffective coping, 286–287
  for ineffective denial, 308
  for ineffective dry eye self-management, 350
  for ineffective family health self-management, 428
  for ineffective health maintenance behaviors, 430
  for ineffective health self-management, 424
  for ineffective home maintenance behaviors, 432–434
  for ineffective impulse control, 473
  for ineffective infant feeding dynamics, 378
  for ineffective infant suck-swallow response, 758
  for ineffective lymphedema self-management, 537–538
  for ineffective peripheral tissue perfusion, 795–796
  for ineffective protection, 656
  for ineffective role performance, 681
  for ineffective sexuality pattern, 717
  for ineffective thermoregulation, 780
  for insomnia, 522
  for interrupted breastfeeding, 205
  for interrupted family processes, 366
  for labile emotional control, 342–343
  for metabolic imbalance syndrome, 545
  for nausea, 570
  for neonatal abstinence syndrome, 572
  for neonatal hyperbilirubinemia, 443
  for neonatal pressure injury, 652
  for obesity, 588
  for overweight, 591, 595
  for parental role conflict, 678
  for perceived constipation, 263–264
  for perioperative positioning injury, 619
  for post-trauma syndrome, 627, 629
  for powerlessness, 633
  for rape-trauma syndrome, 660
  for readiness for enhanced breastfeeding, 206

Client outcomes *(Continued)*
 for readiness for enhanced childbearing process, 235
 for readiness for enhanced comfort, 241
 for readiness for enhanced coping, 289
 for readiness for enhanced exercise engagement, 347
 for readiness for enhanced health literacy, 528
 for readiness for enhanced health self-management, 426
 for readiness for enhancing communication, 242
 for readiness for self-care, 686
 for relocation stress syndrome, 672
 for risk for acute substance withdrawal syndrome, 754
 for risk for adult falls, 358
 for risk for aspiration, 184–185
 for risk for autonomic dysreflexia, 191
 for risk for bleeding, 194
 for risk for child falls, 361
 for risk for corneal injury, 509–510
 for risk for decreased activity tolerance, 164
 for risk for decreased cardiac tissue perfusion, 221–222
 for risk for deficient fluid volume, 392
 for risk for delayed infant motor development, 320
 for risk for elopement attempt, 340
 for risk for impaired liver function, 532
 for risk for impaired skin integrity, 728
 for risk for ineffective activity planning, 167
 for risk for infection, 498, 507
 for risk for injury, 507
 for risk for iodinated contrast media, adverse reaction to, 281
 for risk for latex allergy reaction, 527
 for risk for loneliness, 534
 for risk for maladaptive grieving, 414
 for risk for neonatal hyperbilirubinemia, 445

Client outcomes *(Continued)*
 for risk for other-directed violence, 831–832
 for risk for physical trauma, 804
 for risk for poisoning, 624
 for risk for self-directed violence, 834
 for risk for shock, 719–720
 for risk for situational low self-esteem, 705
 for risk for sudden infant death, 759
 for risk for suffocation, 762
 for risk for suicidal behavior, 767
 for risk for unstable blood pressure, 197
 for risk for urinary tract injury, 519
 for risk-prone health behavior, 422
 with safety risks, 506
 for sedentary lifestyle, 684
 for self-mutilation, 707
 for sexual dysfunction, 713
 for situational low self-esteem, 702
 for social isolation, 739
 for stress overload, 749
 for toileting self-care deficit, 696
 for unilateral neglect, 806
 for unstable blood glucose level, 410–411
 for urinary retention, 814
 for wandering, 839
Clinical Opiate Withdrawal Scale (COWS), 750
Closeness, physical, for disorganized infant behavior, 491
*Clostridium difficile*, diarrhea and, 321
Clotting disorder, 35
Coagulopathy
 risk for ineffective cerebral tissue perfusion, 228–229
 signs and symptoms of, hypothermia and, 453
Cocaine baby, 35
Cocaine/methamphetamine-induced withdrawal syndrome, 751
 risk for, 754
Codependency, 35–36
Cognition, in acute confusion, 247
Cognition impairment, in imbalanced nutrition, 577
Cognitive-behavioral activities, 767

Cognitive disorders
  memory techniques for, 541
  social isolation and, 737
Cognitive factors, of anxiety, 176
Cognitive function, in self-neglect, 710
Cognitive stimulation
  for acute confusion, 249
  for chronic confusion, 249
Cognitive-behavioral therapy (CBT),
    736, 766
  in enhanced relationship, 663
  family-focused, 707
  for fatigue, 371
  for fear, 375
  for labile emotional control, 342
Cold, viral, 36
Cold suppressant medications, 622
Cold thermal injury, 776
Colectomy, 36
Colitis, 36
  ulcerative, 152
Collagen disease, 36
Colon, spastic, 139
Colostomy, 36
Colporrhaphy, anterior, 36
Coma, 36–37
Comfort
  enhanced, readiness for, 239–241
  impaired, 236–238
  loss of, 37
Comfortable padded shower chair,
    688
Comfort-function goal, 595, 599–600,
    602, 605
Communicable diseases, childhood, 37
Communication, 37
  among care staff, effectiveness of, 505
  for enhancing comfort, 239
  nature of, 523
  for person and provider, 685
  problems, 37
  specialists, for impaired verbal com-
    munication, 244
  verbal, impaired, 242–246
Community
  church settings, for ineffective com-
    munity coping, 291
  coping, 37
  enhanced, readiness for,
    281–283
  ineffective, 289–291

Community (Continued)
  health, deficient, 418–420
  health problems, 37
Community-based prevention educa-
    tion, in metabolic imbalance
    syndrome, 545
Companion animal, 37
Compartment syndrome, 37, 620
Complementary and alternative medi-
    cine (CAM), 697
Complementary healing modalities,
    for ineffective health maintenance
    behaviors, 429–430
Complicated immigration transition,
    risk for, 470–472
Complimentary health approaches,
    guidelines in, for imbalanced
    energy field, 344
Comprehensive nursing assessment,
    for impaired verbal communica-
    tion, 243
Compromised family coping,
    291–295
Compromised host defenses,
    500–504
Compromised human dignity, risk for,
    439–440
Compromised regulatory mechanism,
    electrolyte imbalance and, 337
Compulsion, 37
Condom catheter, 479–480
Conduction disorders, 37
Conflict
  decisional, 300–301
  parental role, 110–111
  value system, 153
Confusion
  acute, 37, 246–251
    risk for, 255
  chronic, 37, 251–255
    adult falls and, 354
Congenital heart disease
  cardiac anomalies, 38
  impaired swallowing and, 771–772
  ineffective infant feeding dynamics
    and, 376
Congestive heart failure (CHF), 38
  fatigue and, 372
Conjunctival hyperemia, dry eyes and,
    348
Conjunctivitis, 38

Consciousness, altered level of, 38
Consent, for assessment, 481
Constipation, 38, 255–260
  associated condition, 256
  chronic functional, 38, 264–267
    associated condition, 265
    defining characteristics of, 264
    related factors, 264
    risk for, 267–268
    at risk population, 265
  client outcomes of, 256
  defining characteristics of, 255
  nursing interventions, 256–260
  perceived, 38, 261–264
  related factors, 255–256
  risk for, 38, 260–261
  at risk population, 256
Contact-transmitted microorganisms,
    precautions for, 497
Contamination, 38–39, 268–272
  associated condition, 269
  client outcomes of, 270
  defining characteristics of, 268
  nursing interventions, 270–272
  pesticide, 114
  related factors, 269
  risk for, 273
  at risk population, 269
Continence, in impaired wheelchair
    mobility, 556
Continent ileostomy (Kock pouch), 39
Continuity of care, for acute confusion,
    249
Continuous positive airway pressure
    (CPAP) therapy, 716
Continuous renal replacement therapy
    (CRRT), for excess fluid volume,
    391
Contraceptive method, 39
Contractility, altered, in decreased
    cardiac output, 211
Contrast-induced nephropathy (CIN),
    279–281
Contrast media, allergic reaction to,
    280–281
Control, impulse, ineffective, 472–473
Contusion, chronic pain and, 601
Convulsion, 39
COPD. See Chronic obstructive pul-
    monary disease

Coping, 39
  community
    enhanced, readiness for,
      281–283
    ineffective, 289–291
  defensive, 283–284
  family
    compromised, 291–295
    disabled, 295–297
    enhanced, readiness for,
      297–298
  ineffective, 284–287
  problems, 39–40
    in relocation stress syndrome,
      671
  skills, age-related deterioration in, 296
Core temperature, 776
Corneal abrasion, 508–509
Corneal injury, 40
  risk for, 508–510
Corneal reflex, absent, 40
Corneal surgery, nearsightedness, 99
Corneal transplant, 40
Coronary artery bypass grafting
    (CABG), 40
  in ineffective sexuality pattern, 715
Coronary artery stent, 141
Coronary risks, in ineffective sexuality
    pattern, 714
Coronary syndrome, acute, 6
Corrective device, monitor of, 620
Costovertebral angle tenderness, 40
Cough
  ineffective, 40
  over-the-counter, medications, 622
  stress test, 482
  whooping, 113–114
Coughing, 771
Counseling
  for disabled family coping, 296
  posttrauma, 628
  in readiness for enhanced family
    coping, 298
COVID-19, fatigue and, 372
Crackles in lungs, coarse, 40
Crackles in lungs, fine, 40
Craniectomy/craniotomy, 40
Crepitation, subcutaneous, 40
Crisis, 40–41
  midlife, 93

Critical care
  in acute confusion, 250–251
  for client on a ventilator, 582
  for imbalanced nutrition, 577–578
  of ineffective airway clearance,
    168–169
  nursing interventions
    in disuse syndrome, 328–330
    in impaired gas exchange,
      398–400
    for ineffective dry eye self-
      management, 349–350
  in risk for aspiration, 183
  in risk for shock, 719–720
  in risk for unstable blood pressure,
    196–197
Critically ill, nursing interventions for
  in decreased cardiac output, 214–217
  in deficient fluid volume, 385–388
  in excess fluid volume, 390–392
Crohn's disease, 41
Cross contamination, prevention of, 270
Croup, 41
Crush syndrome, chronic pain and, 601
Cryosurgery, for retinal detachment, 41
Crystalloids, fluid challenge of, for
  deficient fluid volume, 386
Cuing strategies, for impaired memory,
  542
Cultural assessment, in ineffective
  childbearing process, 233
Cultural values, in relocation stress
  syndrome, 669
Culturally tailored cognitive behavioral
  techniques, in enhanced
  relationship, 663
Cushing's syndrome, 41
Cuts (wounds), 41
CVA. *See* Cerebrovascular accident
Cyanosis
  central, 42
  of nail beds, 42
  of oral mucous membrane, 42
  peripheral, 42
  symptoms of, in deficient fluid
    volume, 384
Cystic fibrosis, 42
Cystitis, 42
Cystocele, 42
Cystoscopy, 42–43

# D

Daytime drowsiness, 730
Deafness, 43
Death, 43
  anxiety, 178–180
    associated condition, 178
    client outcomes of, 178–179
    defining characteristics of,
      178
    nursing interventions, 179–180
    related factors, 178
    at risk population, 178
  oncoming, 43
Debridement, of wound, 155
Decisional conflict, 300–301
Decision-making
  impaired emancipated, 302–303
    risk for, 305–306
  readiness for, enhanced, 299–300
  readiness for, enhanced emancipated,
    303–304
  shared, 677–678
Decisions, difficulty making, 43
Decreased activity tolerance, 159–164
  Addison's disease and, 7
  associated condition, 159
  client outcomes of, 159
  client/family teaching and discharge
    planning for, 163–164
  defining characteristics of, 159
  nursing interventions, 159
  related factors, 159
  at risk population, 159
Decreased cardiac output, 210–217
  associated condition, 211
  client outcomes of, 211
  defining characteristics of, 210–211
  nursing interventions, 211–217
  related factors, 211
  risk for, 218
  in risk for shock, 719
Decreased cardiac tissue perfusion, risk
  for, 218–222
  associated condition, 218
  client outcomes of, 218–219
  nursing interventions, 219–222
  risk factors, 218
  at risk population, 218
Decreased diversional activity engagement, 330–332

Decreased intracranial adaptive capacity, 547
Decreased level of consciousness, 84
Decreased sodium, 138
Decreased temperature, 146
Decubitus ulcer, 43
Deep tissue injury, in impaired tissue integrity, 789
Deep tissue pressure injury, 636, 644, 723–724
  in impaired tissue integrity, 789
Deep vein thrombosis (DVT), 43, 795
  prevention of, 620
  signs of, 328
Defecation
  pattern of, 321
  posture for, 258, 267
  privacy for, 258
  straining with, 141
  usual pattern of, 256, 262, 265
Defensive behavior, 43
Defensive coping, 283–284
Deficient community health, 418–420
Deficient fluid volume, 383–388
  risk for, 392
Deficient knowledge, 522–524
  associated condition, 523
  client outcomes of, 523
  defining characteristics of, 522
  kidney transplantation recipient and, 81
  nursing interventions, 523–524
  related factors in, 522
  at risk population, 523
Deficit
  memory, 91
  pulse, 124
  self-care
    bathing, 686–689
    dressing, 689–691
    feeding, 691–694
    toileting, 694–696
Degeneration, macular, 87
Dehiscence
  abdominal, 43
  of wound, 156
Dehydration, 43–44, 386
  assessment for, diarrhea and, 322–323
  early signs of, 338
  mild or moderate signs of, 324

Dehydration Risk Appraisal Checklist, 386
Delayed child development, 314–316
  risk for, 316
Delayed infant motor development, 316–319
  risk for, 319–320
Delayed surgical recovery, 144, 767–770
Delirium, 44, 247
  care-resistant behavior in, 583
  predisposing factors of, 248
  risk factors or causes of, 248
  types of, 247
Delirium tremens (DT), 44
Delivery, 44
  ineffective childbearing process during, 231
  readiness for enhanced childbearing process during, 234
Delusions, 44
Dementia, 44
  care-resistant behavior in, 583
  delirium and, 248, 250
  fatigue and, 369
  multi-infarct, 96, 153
  in relocation stress syndrome, 669
  senile, 134–135
  vascular, 153
Denial
  for defensive coping, 284
  of health status, 44
  ineffective, 306–308
Dental caries, 44
  in dry mouth, 563
Dental prosthesis, in dry mouth, 565
Dentition, impaired, 308–313
Depersonalization, self-mutilation and, 706
Depressed immune function, client/ family teaching and discharge planning for, 656
Depression, 44–45
  assessment of, in disturbed maternal-fetal dyad, 539
  chronic low self-esteem and, 698
  chronic pain and, in older clients, 605
  delayed child development and, 314, 316
  dysfunctional family processes and, 362

Depression *(Continued)*
  fatigue and, 372
  frail elderly syndrome and, 393, 395
  impaired oral mucous membrane
    integrity and, 579, 584
  in impaired physical mobility, 554
  ineffective adolescent eating dynamics
    and, 333
  ineffective child eating dynamics
    and, 335
  ineffective home maintenance
    behaviors and, 431, 434
  in ineffective sexuality pattern, 714
  labor pain and, 607
  maladaptive grieving and, 414
  postpartum, 118
  post-trauma syndrome and, 625, 628
  during pregnancy, 232
  risk for adult falls and, 352
  screening, in ineffective childbearing
    process, 232
  signs of, 252, 329
  situational low self-esteem and, 701
  spiritual distress and, 742
Depressive disorder, major, 87
Dermatitis, 45
Despondency, 45
Destructive behavior, toward others, 45
Detachment, retinal, 129
Development
  delayed child, 314–316
  delayed infant motor, risk for,
    319–320
Developmental concerns, 45
Developmental disabilities
  dry eyes and, 349
  dysfunctional family processes and,
    362
  impaired swallowing and, 771–772
  ineffective health maintenance
    behaviors and, 429
  ineffective health self-management
    and, 423
  risk for elopement attempt and,
    339
  self-mutilation and, 706
Dexamethasone, for nausea, 570
Diabetes, in pregnancy, 45. *See also*
    Gestational diabetes.
Diabetes insipidus, 45

Diabetes mellitus, 45–46
  compromised host defenses and,
    500–501
  delayed surgical recovery and, 768
  dysfunctional gastrointestinal motil-
    ity and, 400, 405
  impaired skin integrity and, 722
  juvenile, 46
  perioperative positioning injury
    and, 615
  risk for decreased cardiac tissue
    perfusion, 218
  unstable blood glucose level and, 406
Diabetic coma, 46
Diabetic ketoacidosis, 46, 79–80
Diabetic neuropathy, 46
Diabetic retinopathy, 46, 129
Dialectical behavior therapy (DBT)
    group, for labile emotional control,
    342
Dialysis, 46
  peritoneal, 113
Diapers, in impaired wheelchair mobil-
    ity, 556
Diaphragmatic hernia, 46, 129
Diarrhea, 46, 320–326
  chemotherapy-induced, 324
  definition of, 321
  radiation-induced, 324
  traveler's, 146, 151
Diary
  bladder
    in disability-associated urinary
      incontinence, 475
    for stress urinary incontinence,
      482
    for urge urinary incontinence,
      485–486
  of pain, 603
DIC. *See* Disseminated intravascular
    coagulation
Dietary measures, in nausea, 567
Dietary modifications, for nausea, in
    pregnancy, 568
Dietary referral, 654
Dietary supplements, for overweight,
    590, 594
Digital resources, in disturbed
    maternal-fetal dyad, 540
Digitalis toxicity, 47

Dignity
  human, compromised, risk for,
    439–440
  loss of, 47
Dilated cardiomyopathy, risk for inef-
    fective cerebral tissue perfusion,
    228–229
Dilation and curettage (D&C), 47
Dilemmas, moral/ethical, 95
Dirty body, for prolonged period,
    47
Disabilities, pregnant woman with,
    in disturbed maternal-fetal dyad,
    539
Disability-associated urinary inconti-
    nence, 473–477
  associated condition, 474
  client outcomes of, 474
  defining characteristics of, 474
  nursing interventions, 474–477
  related factors in, 474
  at risk population, 474
Disabled family coping, 295–297
Discharge planning, 47
  for acute confusion, 251
  for acute pain, 599–600
  for acute substance withdrawal
    syndrome, 752
  for adult pressure injury, 641
  for anxiety, 177–178
  for bathing self-care deficit, 689
  for caregiver role strain, 227
  for child pressure injury, 649
  for chronic confusion, 254–255
  for chronic low self-esteem, 700
  for chronic pain, 605–606
  for chronic pain syndrome, 606
  for compromised family coping, 295
  for compromised human dignity, 440
  for constipation, 260
  for contamination, 272
  for death anxiety, 180
  for decision making, 300
  for decisional conflict, 301
  for decreased activity tolerance,
    163–164
  for decreased cardiac output, 217
  for decreased diversional activity
    engagement, 332
  for defensive coping, 284

Discharge planning (Continued)
  for deficient community health, 420
  for deficient fluid volume, 388
  for delayed surgical recovery, 770
  for diarrhea, 326
  for disabled family coping, 297
  for disorganized infant behavior, 492
  for disturbed body image, 200
  for disturbed family identity syn-
    drome, 466
  for disturbed personal identity,
    469
  for disturbed thought process, 786
  for disuse syndrome, 330
  for dressing self-care deficit, 691
  for dry eyes, 351
  for dysfunctional family processes,
    364
  for dysfunctional gastrointestinal
    motility, 405
  for electrolyte imbalance, 338
  for enhanced nutrition, 574
  for enhanced parenting, 613–614
  for excess fluid volume, 391–392
  for family processes, 368
  for fatigue, 373
  for fear, 376
  for feeding self-care deficit, 694
  for hope, 434, 436
  for hopelessness, 438
  for hyperthermia, 451
  for hypothermia, 457–458, 464
  for imbalanced energy field, 344
  for imbalanced nutrition, 578
  for impaired bed mobility, 550
  for impaired comfort, 238
  for impaired dentition, 313
  for impaired gas exchange, 399–400
  for impaired memory, 542–543
  for impaired oral mucous membrane,
    583
  for impaired parenting, 612, 615
  for impaired physical mobility, 554
  for impaired skin integrity, 726
  for impaired social interaction, 737
  for impaired spontaneous ventilation,
    823
  for impaired standing, 748
  for impaired swallowing, 774
  for impaired tissue integrity, 791

Discharge planning *(Continued)*
  for impaired transfer ability, 801–802
  for impaired urinary elimination, 809–810
  for impaired verbal communication, 246
  for impaired walking, 837
  for impaired wheelchair mobility, 559–560
  for ineffective adolescent eating dynamics, 334
  for ineffective airway clearance, 171–172
  for ineffective breastfeeding, 203
  for ineffective breathing pattern, 210
  for ineffective child eating dynamics, 336–337
  for ineffective coping, 286–287
  for ineffective denial, 308
  for ineffective dry eye self-management, 350
  for ineffective family health self-management, 428
  for ineffective health maintenance behaviors, 430
  for ineffective health self-management, 424
  for ineffective home maintenance behaviors, 432–434
  for ineffective impulse control, 473
  for ineffective infant feeding dynamics, 378
  for ineffective infant suck-swallow response, 758
  for ineffective lymphedema self-management, 537–538
  for ineffective peripheral tissue perfusion, 795–796
  for ineffective protection, 656
  for ineffective role performance, 681
  for ineffective sexuality pattern, 717
  for ineffective thermoregulation, 780
  for insomnia, 522
  for interrupted breastfeeding, 205
  for interrupted family processes, 366
  for labile emotional control, 342–343
  for metabolic imbalance syndrome, 545
  for nausea, 570
  for neonatal abstinence syndrome, 572
  for neonatal hyperbilirubinemia, 443

Discharge planning *(Continued)*
  for neonatal pressure injury, 652
  for obesity, 588
  for overweight, 591, 595
  for parental role conflict, 678
  for perceived constipation, 263–264
  for perioperative positioning injury, 619
  for postoperative interventions, 502–503
  for post-trauma syndrome, 627, 629
  for powerlessness, 633
  for rape-trauma syndrome, 660
  for readiness for enhanced breast-feeding, 206
  for readiness for enhanced childbearing process, 235
  for readiness for enhanced comfort, 241
  for readiness for enhanced coping, 289
  for readiness for enhanced exercise engagement, 347
  for readiness for enhanced health literacy, 528
  for readiness for enhanced health self-management, 426
  for readiness for enhancing communication, 242
  for readiness for self-care, 686
  for relocation stress syndrome, 672
  for risk for acute substance withdrawal syndrome, 754
  for risk for adult falls, 358
  for risk for aspiration, 184–185
  for risk for autonomic dysreflexia, 191
  for risk for bleeding, 194
  for risk for child falls, 361
  for risk for corneal injury, 509–510
  for risk for decreased activity tolerance, 164
  for risk for decreased cardiac tissue perfusion, 221–222
  for risk for elopement attempt, 340
  for risk for impaired liver function, 532
  for risk for impaired skin integrity, 728
  for risk for ineffective activity planning, 167

Discharge planning *(Continued)*
  for risk for infection, 498, 507
  for risk for injury, 507
  for risk for iodinated contrast media,
    adverse reaction to, 281
  for risk for latex allergy reaction, 527
  for risk for loneliness, 534
  for risk for maladaptive grieving, 414
  for risk for neonatal hyperbilirubine-
    mia, 445
  for risk for other-directed violence,
    831–832
  for risk for physical trauma, 804
  for risk for poisoning, 624
  for risk for self-directed violence, 834
  for risk for shock, 719–720
  for risk for situational low self-
    esteem, 705
  for risk for sudden infant death, 759
  for risk for suffocation, 762
  for risk for suicide, 767
  for risk for unstable blood pressure,
    197
  for risk for urinary tract injury, 519
  for risk-prone health behavior, 422
  for sedentary lifestyle, 684
  for self-mutilation, 707
  for sexual dysfunction, 713
  for situational low self-esteem, 702
  for social isolation, 739
  for stress overload, 749
  for suffocation, 762
  for toileting self-care deficit, 696
  for unilateral neglect, 806
  for unstable blood glucose level,
    410–411
  for urinary retention, 814
  for wandering, 839
Discomforts, of pregnancy, 47
Disk, ruptured, 131
Dislocation, of joint, 47
Disorganized infant behavior, 489–493
  risk for, 493–494
Dissecting aneurysm, 47
Dissection, radical neck, 126
Disseminated intravascular coagulation
  (DIC), 46–47
Dissociative identity disorder, 47–48, 96
Distention, bladder, 22
Distention, neck vein, 99

Distraction techniques, for fear, 375
Distress, 48
  moral, 561–562
  spiritual, 741–743
    associated conditions, 742
    at-risk population, 742
    client outcomes, 742
    defining characteristics, 741
    nursing interventions, 742–743
    related factors, 741–742
    risk for, 743–744
Disturbed body image, 197–200
  associated condition, 198
  client outcomes of, 198
  defining characteristics of, 197
  nursing interventions, 198–200
  related factors, 197
  at risk population, 198
Disturbed family identity syndrome,
  464–466
  client outcomes, 465
  defining characteristics of, 464
  nursing interventions, 465–466
  related factors in, 464
  risk for, 466–467
  at risk population, 464–465
Disturbed maternal-fetal dyad, risk for,
  539–540
Disturbed personal identity, 467–469
  risk for, 469–470
Disturbed sleep pattern, 733–734
Disturbed thought process, 784–786
  associated conditions, 784
  at-risk population, 784
  client outcomes, 784–785
  defining characteristics, 784
  nursing interventions, 785–786
  related factors, 784
Disuse syndrome
  potential to develop, 48
  risk of, 326–330
Diuretics, for excess fluid volume, 390
Diverse analgesic delivery methods, for
  pain, 597
Diversion, urinary, 153
Diversional activity engagement, lack
  of, 48
Diverticulitis, 48
Dizziness, 48
Doll therapy, for impaired comfort, 238

Domestic violence, 48
  during pregnancy, 232
Door hardware, for impaired wheel-
    chair mobility, 559
Dopamine agonists, ineffective impulse
    control and, 473
Down syndrome, 48
Doxylamine, for nausea, in pregnancy,
    568
Dress self, inability to, 48
Dribbling, of urine, 48
Driving, restrictions to, 510
Drooling, 49
Droplet-transmitted microorganisms,
    precautions for, 497
Dropout, from school, 49
Drowning, near, 99
Drug abuse, 49
Drug fever, nursing interventions for,
    449
Drug therapy, 270–271
Drug withdrawal, 49
Dry eye, 49
  risk for, 350–351
  self-management, ineffective,
      347–350
  signs of, 348
  symptoms of, 348
Dry eye syndrome, 79
Dry mouth, 49
  in impaired oral mucous membrane,
      581
  risk for, 562–566
Dry stool, 141
DT. *See* Delirium tremens
Duodenal ulcer, 152
DVT. *See* Deep vein thrombosis
Dyad, maternal-fetal, disturbed, 539–540
Dying client, 49
Dysfunction
  erectile, 52, 54
  neurovascular, peripheral, risk for,
      619–620
  sexual, 135, 711–713
    associated conditions, 711
    at-risk population, 711
    client outcomes, 711
    defining characteristics, 711
    nursing interventions, 711–713
    related factors, 711

Dysfunctional adult ventilatory wean-
    ing response, 823–827
  associated conditions, 824
  at-risk population, 824
  client outcomes, 824
  defining characteristics, 823–824
  nursing interventions, 824–827
  related factors, 824
Dysfunctional eating pattern, 49
Dysfunctional family processes,
    361–364
Dysfunctional family unit, 49
Dysfunctional gastrointestinal motility,
    400–405
  risk for, 405
Dysfunctional ventilatory weaning, 49
  response, 823–827
    associated condition, 824
    client outcomes, 824
    defining characteristics,
        823–824
    nursing interventions, 824–827
    related factors, 824
Dysmenorrhea, 49
Dyspareunia, 49
Dyspepsia, 49–50
Dysphagia, 50, 773
  in impaired bed mobility, 547
Dysphasia, 50
Dyspnea, 50
  nocturnal paroxysmal, 104
Dysreflexia
  autonomic, 20, 188–190
    associated condition, 188
    client outcomes of, 189
    defining characteristics of, 188
    nursing interventions, 189–190
    related factors, 188
    risk for, 191
    at risk population, 188
  spinal injury and, 479
Dysrhythmia, 50
Dysthymic disorder, 50
Dystocia, 50
Dystrophy, muscular, 97–98
Dysuria, 50

E
Ear surgery, 51
Earache, 51

Early dumping syndrome, signs and symptoms of, 403
Eating Assessment Tool- 10 (EAT-10), 692
Eating disorder, 263, 359
Eating dynamics
  adolescent, 51
  child, 51
  ineffective
    adolescent, 332–334
    child, 334–337
  infant, 51
Eating habit
  dysfunctional gastrointestinal motility and, 400, 405
  ineffective child eating dynamics and, 334
Eclampsia, 51
ECMO. *See* Extracorporeal membrane oxygenator
ECT. *See* Electroconvulsive therapy
Ectopic pregnancy, 51–52
Eczema, 52
ED. *See* Erectile dysfunction
Edema, 52
  extent of, 389
  location of, 389
  perioperative positioning injury and, 615
  pulmonary, 124
Edinburgh Feeding Evaluation in Dementia, 692
Edmonton Frail Scale, 393
Education
  in disabled family coping, 296
  patient, 111
Elasticity, change in, in skin turgor, 137
Elder abuse, 52
Elderly, 52
Elective surgery, in impaired physical mobility, 553
Electric/power mobility devices, drivers of, safety rules for, 557
Electroconvulsive therapy (ECT), 51–52
Electrolyte imbalance, 52
  risk for, 337–338
Electronic thermometer, 779
Elevated waist circumference, in metabolic imbalance syndrome, 544

Elopement attempt, risk for, 339–340
Emaciated person, 52
Emaciation, perioperative positioning injury and, 615
Emancipated decision-making, impaired, 52
Embolectomy, 52
Emboli, 52
Embolism
  in leg or arm, 52
  risk for ineffective cerebral tissue perfusion, 228–229
Emergency department visits, for corneal injury, 508–510
Emesis, 52
Emotion
  of anxiety, 175
  decreased cardiac output and, 211
Emotional control, labile, 340–343
Emotional influences
  in chronic functional constipation, 266
  in constipation, 257
  in perceived constipation, 262
Emotional problems, 52
Emotional status, of caregiver, 224
Empathy, 52–53
  for trauma, 627
Emphysema, 53
Emptiness, 53
Encephalitis, 53, 91
Endocardial cushion defect, 53
Endocarditis, 53
Endocrine system diseases
  diarrhea and, 320
  risk for adult falls and, 352
Endometriosis, 53
Endometritis, 53
Enemas
  for chronic functional constipation, 267
  for constipation, 259–260
  for perceived constipation, 263
Energy, decreased, frail elderly syndrome and, 393, 395
Energy conservation, for fatigue, 373
Energy field, imbalanced, 343–344
Energy therapy, for enhancing comfort, 240

Enhanced readiness
  for childbearing process, 233–236
  for comfort, 239–241
  for communication, 239
  for coping, 297–298
    community, 281–283
    family, 297–298
  for decision-making, 299–300
  for emancipated decision-making, 303–304
  for exercise engagement, 344–347
  for family processes, 366–368
  for grieving, 415–418
  for health self-management, 425–426
  for hope, 433–436
  for infant behavior, organized, 493
  for knowledge, 524–525
  for nutrition, 572–574
  for parenting, 612–614
  for power, 629–630
  for relationship, 662–663
  for religiosity, 665–667
  for resilience, 674–675
  for self-care, 684–686
  for self-concept, 696–698
  for sleep, 731–733
  for spiritual well-being, 744–746
Enteral feedings, 182–185
Enteral nutrition
  diarrhea and, 320
  dysfunctional gastrointestinal motility and, 400, 405
  prolonged
    ineffective infant feeding dynamics and, 376
    ineffective infant suck-swallow response, 755
Enterocolitis, necrotizing, 99–100
Enuresis, 53
Environmental exposure to pathogens, increased, 497
Environmental factors
  adult falls and, 351
  child falls and, 359
  ineffective child eating dynamics and, 334
Environmental interpretation problems, 53

Environmental risk factors, for occupational injury, 510
Environmental stressors, 272
Environmental temperatures, 776
Epidermal necrolysis, toxic, 147
Epididymitis, 53
Epiglottitis, 53
Epilepsy, 53–54, 134
Epiphora, dry eyes and, 348
Episiotomy, 54
Epistaxis, 54
Epstein-Barr virus, 54
Equianalgesic dosing charts, 598
Erectile dysfunction (ED), 52, 54
Erythema multiforme, 150
Escherichia coli infection, 54
Esophageal achalasia, impaired swallowing and, 771–772
Esophageal varices, 54
Esophagitis, 54
Ethical dilemmas, 95
Ethnic values, in relocation stress syndrome, 669
Evisceration, 54
  of wound, 156
Excess fluid volume, 388–392
Exercise
  for impaired bed mobility, 548–550
  for impaired physical mobility, 548–550
  for sleep, 522
Exhaustion, 54
  frail elderly syndrome and, 393, 395
Experiential avoidance, for labile emotional control, 341
Exposure
  to hot or cold environment, 54
  to pathogens, environmental, increased, 494
Extended care facility, for relocation stress syndrome, 669–670
External abdominal massage
  for chronic functional constipation, 267
  for constipation, 258
  for perceived constipation, 263
External fixation, 54
External risk factors, for poisoning, 621
Extracorporeal membrane oxygenator (ECMO), 51

Extraoral examination, for dry mouth, 563
Extremities
  pallor of, 108
  rubor of, 131
Eye
  discomfort, 54
  dry, 49
    risk for, 350–351
    self-management, ineffective, 347–350
    signs of, 348
    symptoms of, 348
  pink, 115
Eye drops, 349
Eye fatigue, dry eyes and, 348
Eye surgery, 54–55

F
Face, moon, 95
Facilitator role *vs.* authority role, 524
Failure to thrive
  child, 55
  delayed infant motor development and, 317
  risk for delayed infant motor development and, 320
Fallot, tetralogy of, 148
Falls
  assessment of, in impaired bed mobility, 547
  risk for, 55, 506
  toileting self-care deficit and, 694
Falls Free Initiative, 352
Family-centered approach, 523
  in post-trauma syndrome, 627
Family-centered care, 613
Family coping
  compromised, 291–295
  disabled, 295–297
  enhanced, readiness for, 297–298
Family decision-makers, psychosocial support services for, 297
Family health self-management, ineffective, 426–428
Family identity syndrome, disturbed, 464–466
  client outcomes, 465
  defining characteristics of, 464
  nursing interventions, 465–466

Family identity syndrome, disturbed *(Continued)*
  related factors in, 464
  risk for, 466–467
  at risk population, 464–465
Family outcomes, in readiness for enhanced grieving, 415
Family problems, 55
Family processes, 55
  defining characteristics of, 224
  dysfunctional, 361–364
  enhanced, readiness for, 366–368
  ineffective child eating dynamics and, 334
  interrupted, 364–366
  related factors (r/t) in, 224
  risk for caregiver role strain and, 228
Family style dining, 736
Family teaching
  in acute pain, 599–600
  in acute substance withdrawal syndrome, 752
  in adult pressure injury, 641
  in anxiety, 177–178
  in autonomic dysreflexia, 190
  in bathing self-care deficit, 689
  in caregiver role strain, 227
  in child pressure injury, 649
  in chronic low self-esteem, 700
  in chronic pain, 605–606
  in chronic pain syndrome, 606
  in compromised family coping, 295
  in compromised human dignity, 440
  in constipation, 260
  in contamination, 272
  in death anxiety, 180
  in decision making, 300
  in decisional conflict, 301
  in decreased activity tolerance, 163–164
  in decreased cardiac output, 217
  in decreased diversional activity engagement, 332
  in defensive coping, 284
  in deficient community health, 420
  in deficient fluid volume, 388
  in delayed child development, 316
  in delayed surgical recovery, 770
  in diarrhea, 326
  in disabled family coping, 297

Family teaching *(Continued)*
  in disorganized infant behavior, 492
  in disturbed body image, 200
  in disturbed family identity syndrome, 466
  in disturbed personal identity, 469
  in disturbed thought process, 786
  in disuse syndrome, 330
  in dressing self-care deficit, 691
  in dry eyes, 351
  in dysfunctional family processes, 364
  in dysfunctional gastrointestinal motility, 405
  in electrolyte imbalance, 338
  in enhanced nutrition, 574
  in enhanced parenting, 613–614
  in excess fluid volume, 391–392
  in family processes, 368
  in fatigue, 373
  in fear, 376
  in feeding self-care deficit, 694
  in frail elderly syndrome, 394
  in hope, 434, 436
  in hopelessness, 438
  in hyperthermia, 451
  in hypothermia, 457–458, 464
  in imbalanced energy field, 344
  in imbalanced nutrition, 578
  in impaired bed mobility, 550
  in impaired dentition, 313
  in impaired gas exchange, 399–400
  in impaired memory, 542–543
  in impaired oral mucous membrane, 583–584
  in impaired parenting, 612, 615
  in impaired physical mobility, 554
  in impaired skin integrity, 726
  in impaired social interaction, 737
  in impaired spontaneous ventilation, 823
  in impaired standing, 748
  in impaired swallowing, 774
  in impaired tissue integrity, 791
  in impaired transfer ability, 801–802
  in impaired urinary elimination, 809–810
  in impaired walking, 837
  in impaired wheelchair mobility, 559–560

Family teaching *(Continued)*
  in ineffective adolescent eating dynamics, 334
  in ineffective airway clearance, 171–172
  in ineffective breastfeeding, 203
  in ineffective breathing pattern, 210
  in ineffective child eating dynamics, 336–337
  in ineffective coping, 286–287
  in ineffective denial, 308
  in ineffective dry eye self-management, 350
  in ineffective family health self-management, 428
  in ineffective health maintenance behaviors, 430
  in ineffective health self-management, 424
  in ineffective home maintenance behaviors, 432–434
  in ineffective impulse control, 473
  in ineffective infant feeding dynamics, 378
  in ineffective infant suck-swallow response, 758
  in ineffective lymphedema self-management, 537–538
  in ineffective peripheral tissue perfusion, 795–796
  in ineffective protection, 656
  in ineffective role performance, 681
  in ineffective sexuality pattern, 717
  in ineffective thermoregulation, 780
  in insomnia, 522
  in interrupted breastfeeding, 205
  in interrupted family processes, 366
  in labile emotional control, 342–343
  in metabolic imbalance syndrome, 545
  in nausea, 570
  in neonatal abstinence syndrome, 572
  in neonatal hyperbilirubinemia, 443
  in neonatal pressure injury, 652
  in obesity, 588
  in overweight, 591, 595
  in parental role conflict, 678
  in perioperative positioning injury, 619
  in post-trauma syndrome, 627, 629

Family teaching *(Continued)*
in powerlessness, 633
in rape-trauma syndrome, 660
in readiness for enhanced breastfeeding, 206
in readiness for enhanced childbearing process, 235
in readiness for enhanced comfort,
241
in readiness for enhanced exercise
engagement, 347
in readiness for enhanced health
literacy, 528
in readiness for enhanced health self-
management, 426
in readiness for enhancing communication, 242
in readiness for self-care, 686
in relocation stress syndrome, 672
in risk for acute substance withdrawal syndrome, 754
in risk for adult falls, 358
in risk for aspiration, 184–185
in risk for autonomic dysreflexia, 191
in risk for bleeding, 194
in risk for child falls, 361
in risk for corneal injury, 509–510
in risk for decreased activity tolerance, 164
in risk for decreased cardiac tissue
perfusion, 221–222
in risk for deficient fluid volume, 392
in risk for delayed infant motor
development, 320
in risk for elopement attempt, 340
in risk for impaired liver function,
532
in risk for impaired skin integrity,
728
in risk for ineffective activity planning, 167
in risk for infection, 498
in risk for injury, 507
in risk for iodinated contrast media,
adverse reaction to, 281
in risk for latex allergy reaction, 527
in risk for loneliness, 534
in risk for maladaptive grieving, 414
in risk for neonatal hyperbilirubinemia, 445

Family teaching *(Continued)*
in risk for other-directed violence,
831–832
in risk for physical trauma, 804
in risk for poisoning, 624
in risk for self-directed violence, 834
in risk for shock, 719–720
in risk for situational low self-
esteem, 705
in risk for sudden infant death, 759
in risk for suffocation, 762
in risk for suicidal behavior, 767
in risk for unstable blood pressure,
197
in risk for urinary tract injury, 519
in risk-prone health behavior, 422
in sedentary lifestyle, 684
in self-mutilation, 707
in sexual dysfunction, 713
in situational low self-esteem, 702
in social isolation, 739
in stress overload, 749
in toileting self-care deficit, 696
in unilateral neglect, 806
in unstable blood glucose level,
410–411
in urinary retention, 814
in wandering, 839
Family-centered theory, 367
Fatigue, 55, 368–373, 769
Fear, 55, 373–376
in breast biopsy, 25
of falling, frail elderly syndrome and,
393, 395
Febrile seizures, 55, 134
Fecal impaction, 55, 325
Fecal incontinence, 55. *See also* Bowel
incontinence.
Feeding
assistance, for acute confusion, 250
physical challenge with
ineffective adolescent eating
dynamics and, 333
ineffective child eating dynamics
and, 335
ineffective infant feeding dynamics and, 376
self-care deficit, 691–694
Feeding disorders, risk for child falls
and, 359

Feeding dynamics, infant, 56
    ineffective, 376–378
Feeding problems, newborn, 56
Feeding protocol, in imbalanced nutri-
    tion, 576
Feelings, in dysfunctional family
    processes, 362
Female genital mutilation, 56
    risk for, 378–380
Femoral popliteal bypass, 56
Fetal alcohol syndrome, 56
Fetal distress, 56
Fetal expulsion, labor pain and, 607
Fever (pyrexia), 57
    in ineffective thermoregulation,
        778–779
    postoperative, 655
    treating, in ineffective thermoregula-
        tion, 780
Fiber intake
    for chronic functional constipation,
        266
    for constipation, 258
    for perceived constipation, 263
Fibrillation, ventricular, 154
Fibrocystic breast disease, 57
Fibromyalgia, fatigue and, 369
Filamentary keratitis, dry eyes and, 348
Filthy home environment, 57
Financial crisis, in the home environ-
    ment, 57
Fingernail, in corneal abrasions, 509
Fire escape, 775
First aid, risk for allergy reaction, 173
Fistula, tracheoesophageal, 150
Fistulectomy, 57
5-foot turning space, in impaired
    wheelchair mobility, 559
"Five Ps," of assessment, 620
5 Minute Appearance, Pulse, Grimace,
    Activity, & Respiration (APGAR)
    score
    delayed infant motor development
        and, 317
    risk for delayed infant motor devel-
        opment and, 320
Fixation, internal, open reduction of
    fracture with, 106
Flail chest, 57
Flashbacks, 57
Flat affect, 57

Flexibility exercise (stretching), 345, 682
    for impaired physical mobility, 551
Floor clutter, in impaired wheelchair
    mobility, 557
Fluid volume, 769
    deficient, 383–388
        risk for, 392
    deficit, 57
    excess, 57, 388–392
    imbalance, risk for, 57, 380–383
Foam sticks, in impaired oral mucous
    membrane, 580
Food
    allergies, 57
    consumed, in nutrition, 572
    contamination of, 273
    intolerance, 57
Food intolerance, dysfunctional gastro-
    intestinal motility and, 400, 405
Food safety, 654
Foodborne illness, 57
Foreign body aspiration, 58
Formalized screening tool, for impaired
    bed mobility, 548
Formula feeding, of infant, 58
Fracture, 58
    hip, 58
    rib, 130
Frail elderly clients
    acute confusion and, 251
    in ineffective coping, 287
Frail elderly syndrome, 58, 392–394
    confusion and, acute, 37
    risk for, 394–395
Frailty Index, 393
Frequency, of urination, 58
Friendship, 58
Frontal lobe dysfunction, self-neglect
    and, 709
Frostbite, 58
Frothy sputum, 58–59
Full medication profile, for acute pain,
    599
Full-thickness skin loss, 788
Functional constipation, chronic,
    264–267
    associated condition, 265
    defining characteristics of, 264
    related factors, 264
    risk for, 267–268
    at risk population, 265

Functional impairment
  chronic low self-esteem and, 698
  labile emotional control and, 341
  self-neglect and, 709
  situational low self-esteem and, 701
Fusion, lumbar, 59

## G

Gag reflex, depressed or absent, 59
Gallop rhythm, 59
Gallstones, 59
Gang member, 59
Gangrene, 59
Gas exchange, impaired, 59, 395–400
  in risk for shock, 719
Gastric ulcer, 59, 152
Gastritis, 59
Gastroenteritis, 59
  child, 59
  viral, 154–155
Gastroesophageal reflux disease
    (GERD), 59–60
  child, 60
  dysfunctional gastrointestinal motil-
    ity and, 400, 405
  impaired swallowing and, 771–772
Gastrointestinal (GI) bleeding, 60–61
  lower, 86
Gastrointestinal circulation, decreased,
    dysfunctional gastrointestinal
    motility and, 400, 405
Gastrointestinal diseases, diarrhea
    and, 320
Gastrointestinal hemorrhage, 60
Gastrointestinal motility
  dysfunctional, 400–405
    risk for, 405
  increased, nursing interventions for,
    403–404
Gastrointestinal perfusion, in risk for
    shock, 719
Gastrointestinal stimuli, autonomic
    dysreflexia and, 188, 191
Gastrointestinal surgery, 60
Gastroschisis, 60
Gastrostomy, 60
Gender dysphoria, 60
General anesthesia
  impaired gas exchange and, 395
  perioperative positioning injury and,
    615

General interventions, for surgical cli-
    ent, 616–619
Genetic counseling, in disturbed
    maternal-fetal dyad, 540
Genital herpes, 60
Genital warts, 60
GERD. *See* Gastroesophageal reflux
    disease
Geriatric client
  acute confusion in, 250–251
  acute pain in, 599
  adult pressure injury in, 639–640
  anxiety in, 177
  caregiver role strain in, 226–227
  chronic confusion in, 254–255
  chronic low self-esteem in, 700
  chronic pain in, 604–605
  chronic sorrow in, 741
  compromised family coping in, 293
  compromised human dignity in, 440
  constipation in, 259–260
  contamination in, 272
  death anxiety in, 179–180
  decision making in, 299–300, 303
  decisional conflict in, 301
  decreased activity tolerance in, 162
  decreased cardiac output in, 215–216
  decreased diversional activity en-
    gagement in, 331–332
  defensive coping in, 284
  deficient community health in, 419
  deficient fluid volume in, 386–387
  deficient knowledge in, 524
  delayed surgical recovery in, 769–770
  diarrhea in, 324–325
  disabled family coping in, 296
  disturbed body image in, 199
  disturbed family identity syndrome
    in, 465
  disturbed personal identity in, 468
  disturbed sleep pattern in, 734
  disturbed thought process in, 786
  disuse syndrome in, 329
  dressing self-care deficit in, 690–691
  dysfunctional adult ventilatory wean-
    ing response in, 827
  dysfunctional family processes in,
    363
  dysfunctional gastrointestinal motil-
    ity in, 405
  electrolyte imbalance in, 338

Geriatric client *(Continued)*
  enhanced nutrition in, 574
  enhanced power in, 630
  enhanced relationship in, 663
  enhanced religiosity in, 667
  excess fluid volume in, 391
  family processes in, 368
  fatigue in, 372
  fear in, 375
  feeding self-care deficit in, 692–694
  hope in, 433–434
  hopelessness in, 438
  hyperthermia in, 450
  hypothermia in, 456–457
  imbalanced energy field in, 344
  imbalanced fluid volume in, 383
  imbalanced nutrition in, 577–578
  impaired bed mobility in, 549
  impaired bowel continence in, 278
  impaired comfort in, 238
  impaired dentition in, 312–313
  impaired gas exchange in, 398
  impaired memory in, 542–543
  impaired oral mucous membrane in,
    582–583
  impaired physical mobility in,
    553–554
  impaired religiosity in, 665
  impaired sitting in, 721
  impaired social interaction in, 736
  impaired spontaneous ventilation
    in, 822
  impaired swallowing in, 774
  impaired urinary elimination in,
    808–809
  impaired verbal communication
    in, 245
  impaired walking in, 836
  impaired wheelchair mobility in,
    558
  ineffective activity planning in, 166
  ineffective airway clearance in, 170
  ineffective breathing pattern in, 209
  ineffective coping in, 286
  ineffective denial in, 307–308
  ineffective dry eye self-management
    in, 349
  ineffective family health self-
    management in, 428
  ineffective health maintenance
    behaviors in, 430

Geriatric client *(Continued)*
  ineffective health self-management
    in, 424
  ineffective home maintenance
    behaviors in, 432–433
  ineffective impulse control in, 473
  ineffective peripheral tissue perfusion
    in, 795
  ineffective protection in, 655
  ineffective relationship in, 661–662
  ineffective role performance in, 680
  ineffective sexuality pattern in,
    716–717
  ineffective thermoregulation in, 780
  insomnia in, 521–522
  interrupted family processes in, 366
  labile emotional control in, 342
  maladaptive grieving in, 413–414
  metabolic imbalance syndrome in,
    545
  nausea in, 569
  obesity in, 587
  overweight in, 589, 594
  perioperative positioning injury in,
    618–619
  post-trauma syndrome in, 626, 629
  powerlessness in, 632
  rape-trauma syndrome in, 659
  readiness for enhanced comfort in,
    240–241
  readiness for enhanced coping in,
    288
  readiness for enhanced exercise
    engagement in, 347
  readiness for enhanced family coping
    in, 298
  readiness for enhanced grieving in,
    417
  readiness for enhanced health
    literacy in, 528
  readiness for enhanced knowledge
    in, 525
  readiness for enhanced sleep in,
    732–733
  readiness for enhanced spiritual well-
    being in, 746
  readiness for enhancing communica-
    tion in, 242
  readiness for self-concept in, 697
  relocation stress syndrome in,
    671–672

Geriatric client *(Continued)*
  risk for adult falls in, 354–358
  risk for aspiration in, 183–184
  risk for decreased cardiac tissue
    perfusion in, 221–222
  risk for dry mouth in, 566
  risk for elopement attempt in, 340
  risk for impaired skin integrity in, 728
  risk for infection in, 498
  risk for injury in, 507
  risk for iodinated contrast media,
    adverse reaction to, 281
  risk for loneliness in, 533
  risk for occupational injury in, 513–514
  risk for other-directed violence in, 831
  risk for physical trauma in, 803–804
  risk for poisoning in, 623
  risk for self-directed violence in, 834
  risk for situational low self esteem
    in, 705
  risk for suffocation in, 761–762
  risk for suicide in, 766
  risk for surgical site infection in,
    503–504
  risk for unstable blood pressure in, 197
  risk for vascular trauma in, 818
  risk-prone health behavior in, 421
  sedentary lifestyle in, 684
  self-neglect in, 710
  sexual dysfunction in, 712–713
  situational low self-esteem in, 702
  sleep deprivation in, 732–733
  social isolation in, 738–739
  spiritual distress in, 743
  spousal caregivers, in enhanced
    relationship, 663
  stress overload in, 749
  toileting self-care deficit in, 695–696
  unstable blood glucose level in,
    409–411
  urinary retention in, 814
  violence in, 831
Gestational diabetes, 61
Gestations, multiple, 96
Gestures, in impaired physical mobility,
  553
Gingiva, in impaired oral mucous
  membrane, 580
Gingival recession, in dry mouth, 563
Gingivitis, 61

Glaucoma, 61
Glomerulonephritis, 61
Glucose level, blood, unstable, risk for,
  406–411
Gluten allergy, 61
Gonorrhea, 61
Good quality parenting, in impaired
  parenting, 612
Gout, 61
Graduated compression stockings, for
  disuse syndrome, 328
Graft *versus* host disease, dry eyes and,
  349
Grand mal seizure, 61
Grandiosity, 61
Grandparents, raising grandchildren,
  61–62
Granulocyte growth factor, 654
Graves' disease, 62
Great vessels, transposition of, 151
Grief, in compromised family coping,
  295
Grieving
  maladaptive, 62, 412–414
  risk for, 414
Groom self, inability to, 62
Growth
  chart, in imbalanced nutrition, 577
  development lag and, 62
  of readiness for self-care, 685
Guided imagery
  for impaired comfort, 238
  for labile emotional control, 342
Guillain-Barré syndrome, 62
Guilt, 62
Gum bleeding, control of, 655

## H

Habits, bladder
  in disability-associated urinary
    incontinence, 474–475
  in stress urinary incontinence, 481
  in urge urinary incontinence, 485
Hair loss, 62
Halitosis, 62
  in impaired oral mucous membrane,
    581
  impaired social interaction and,
    735
Hallucinations, 62

Hand hygiene, regimens, for chronic functional constipation, 266

Hand massage, for impaired comfort, 238

Hand rub, alcohol-based, 496

Hand washing
   for constipation, 256
   for contamination, 271
   for perceived constipation, 262

Hands, trembling of, 151

Hard stool, 141

Head injury, 63

Headache, 63
   migraine, 93

Head-to-toe assessment, 654

Healing modalities, complementary, for ineffective health maintenance behaviors, 429–430

Healing touch, for impaired comfort, 237

Health, community, deficient, 418–420

Health behavior, risk-prone, 63, 420–422

Health care-acquired pneumonia, 496
   geriatric, 498

Health care-associated infections (HAIs), 495

Health coach, internet-based, for disturbed personal identity, 469

"Health coaching", 525

Health education, 632

Health information technology (HIT), for enhancing comfort, 240

Health literacy
   of clients and caregivers, 523
   readiness for enhanced, 527–528

Health maintenance behaviors, ineffective, 428–430

Health maintenance problems, 63

Health promotion education, pediatric, 525

Health self-management
   enhanced, readiness for, 425–426
   ineffective, 422–424
      family, 426–428

Health-seeking person, 63

Hearing impairment, 63

audiology consultation for, 244

Heart attack, 63

Heart diseases, impaired gas exchange and, 395

Heart failure, 63

Heart palpitations, 108

Heart rate, altered, in decreased cardiac output, 210

Heart surgery, 63

Heartburn, 63

Heat stroke, 63
   nursing interventions for, 446–448

Heels, during surgery, 617

Hematemesis, 64

Hematuria, 64

Hemianopia, 64

Hemiplegia, 64

Hemiplegic shoulder, in impaired bed mobility, 549

Hemodialysis, 64
   for excess fluid volume, 392

Hemodynamic monitoring, 64

Hemodynamic parameters, noninvasive, in risk for shock, 719

Hemolytic uremic syndrome, 64

Hemophilia, 64–65

Hemoptysis, 65

Hemorrhage, 65
   subarachnoid, 142

Hemorrhoidectomy, 65

Hemorrhoids, 65

Hemothorax, 65

Hendrich II Model, 352

Hepatitis, 65

Hernia, 65
   diaphragmatic, 46, 129
   hiatal, 66

Herniated disk, 65

Herniorrhaphy, 65

Herpes
   genital. *See* Herpes simplex II
   in pregnancy, 65

Herpes simplex I, 65

Herpes simplex II, 65–66

Herpes zoster, 66

HHNS. *See* Hyperosmolar hyperglycemic nonketotic syndrome

Hiatal hernia, 66

Hierarchy of Pain Measures, 596

High acuity illness, ineffective health self-management and, 423

High attachment anxiety, maladaptive grieving and, 412, 414

High-energy particulate air filters, 654

High-risk pregnancy, fear related to, in disturbed maternal-fetal dyad, 539

High sitting position, for impaired bed mobility, 547

Hip fracture, 66

Hip replacement, 66

Hirschsprung's disease, 66

Hirsutism, 66

History
life, for disturbed personal identity, 468
of life-threatening illness, 628
medical
in disability-associated urinary incontinence, 475
in risk factors for stress incontinence, 481
for poisoning, 621
in relocation stress syndrome, 669
travel, 495

Hitting behavior, 66–67

HIV. *See* Human immunodeficiency virus

Hodgkin's disease, 67

Holistic assessment, for compromised family coping, 293

Home
rats in, 126
roaches, invasion of, 130
rodents in, 126

Home care
for acute confusion, 251
for acute pain, 599
for adult pressure injury, 639–640
for anxiety, 177
for autonomic dysreflexia, 190
for bathing self-care deficit, 689
for caregiver role strain, 227
for child pressure injury, 647–648
for chronic confusion, 254
for chronic low self-esteem, 700
for chronic pain, 605
for chronic sorrow, 741
for compromised family coping, 294
for compromised human dignity, 440
for constipation, 259–260
for contamination, 272
for death anxiety, 180
for decision making, 300, 303–304
for decisional conflict, 301

Home care *(Continued)*
for decreased activity tolerance, 162–163
for decreased cardiac output, 216
for decreased diversional activity engagement, 332
for defensive coping, 284
for deficient community health, 420
for deficient fluid volume, 387–388
for deficient knowledge, 524
for delayed surgical recovery, 770
for diarrhea, 325
for disabled family coping, 297
for disorganized infant behavior, 492
for disturbed body image, 199–200
for disturbed family identity syndrome, 466
for disturbed personal identity, 469
for disturbed sleep pattern, 734
for disturbed thought process, 786
for disuse syndrome, 329–330
for dressing self-care deficit, 691
for dry mouth, 566
for dysfunctional adult ventilatory weaning response, 827
for dysfunctional family processes, 364
for enhanced parenting, 613
for enhanced power, 630
for excess fluid volume, 391
for family processes, 368
for fatigue, 372–373
for fear, 376
for feeding self-care deficit, 693
for frail elderly syndrome, 394
for hope, 434, 436
for hopelessness, 438
for hyperthermia, 450–451
for hypothermia, 457, 463–464
for imbalanced energy field, 344
for imbalanced nutrition, 578
for impaired bed mobility, 549–550
for impaired bowel continence, 278
for impaired dentition, 313
for impaired gas exchange, 398–399
for impaired memory, 542
for impaired oral mucous membrane, 583
for impaired parenting, 612
for impaired physical mobility, 554

Home care *(Continued)*
for impaired sitting, 721
for impaired skin integrity, 725–726
for impaired social interaction, 737
for impaired spontaneous ventilation, 822–823
for impaired swallowing, 774
for impaired tissue integrity, 791
for impaired transfer ability, 800–802
for impaired verbal communication, 246
for impaired walking, 836–837
for impaired wheelchair mobility, 559
for ineffective activity planning, 166
for ineffective adolescent eating dynamics, 333–334
for ineffective airway clearance, 170–171
for ineffective breastfeeding, 203
for ineffective breathing pattern, 209–210
for ineffective child eating dynamics, 336
for ineffective coping, 286–287
for ineffective denial, 307–308
for ineffective health maintenance behaviors, 430
for ineffective health self-management, 424
for ineffective home maintenance behaviors, 432
for ineffective infant feeding dynamics, 377–378
for ineffective infant suck-swallow response, 757–758
for ineffective peripheral tissue perfusion, 795
for ineffective protection, 655–656
for ineffective sexuality pattern, 717
for insomnia, 522
for interrupted breastfeeding, 205
for interrupted family processes, 366
for labile emotional control, 342
for maladaptive grieving, 414
for metabolic imbalance syndrome, 545
for moral distress, 562
for nausea, 570
for neonatal abstinence syndrome, 572

Home care *(Continued)*
for neonatal pressure injury, 651
for nipple-areolar complex injury, 515
for parental role conflict, 678
for post-trauma syndrome, 627, 629
for powerlessness, 632
for rape-trauma syndrome, 659–660
for readiness for enhanced breastfeeding, 206
for readiness for enhanced childbearing process, 235
for readiness for enhanced comfort, 240–241
for readiness for enhanced coping, 288–289
for readiness for enhanced exercise engagement, 347
for readiness for enhanced grieving, 417–418
for readiness for enhanced sleep, 733
for readiness for enhanced spiritual well-being, 746
for readiness for enhancing communication, 242
for readiness for self-care, 686
for readiness for self-concept, 698
for risk for adult falls, 356–358
for risk for aspiration, 184
for risk for child falls, 360–361
for risk for complicated immigration transition, 472
for risk for elopement attempt, 340
for risk for impaired attachment, 187
for risk for impaired liver function, 531
for risk for infection, 498
for risk for injury, 507
for risk for latex allergy reaction, 527
for risk for loneliness, 534
for risk for other-directed violence, 831
for risk for poisoning, 623
for risk for situational low self-esteem, 705
for risk for sudden infant death, 758–759
for risk for suicide, 767
for risk for surgical site infection in, 504
for risk for urinary tract injury, 519

Home care *(Continued)*
for risk for vascular trauma, 818
for risk-prone health behavior, 422
for sedentary lifestyle, 684
for self-mutilation, 707
for sexual dysfunction, 713
for situational low self-esteem, 702
for sleep deprivation, 728
for social interaction, 739
for spiritual distress, 743
for stress overload, 749
for swallowing, 774
for tissue integrity, 791
for toileting self-care deficit, 695–696
for unilateral neglect, 806
for unstable blood glucose level, 410
for urinary retention, 814
for violence, 831
for wandering, 839–840
Home maintenance
behaviors, ineffective, 431–433
problems, 67
Home safety, in risk for child falls, 359
Home-based exercise-training program,
for frail elderly syndrome, 394
Homelessness, 67
Hope, 67
enhanced, readiness for, 433–436
Hopelessness, 67, 436–438, 766
Hospitalization, for corneal injury, 509
Hospitalized child, 67
Hostile behavior, 67
Household cleaners, eye injury and, 510
HTN. *See* Hypertension
Human dignity, compromised, risk for,
439–440
Human energy field, 68
Human immunodeficiency virus
(HIV), 67
in ineffective sexuality pattern, 716
Human milk, for pain, 599
Human papillomavirus, in sexual
dysfunction, 716
Humidified oxygen, administration of,
in impaired gas exchange, 397
Humiliating experience, 68
Huntington's disease, 68
Hydration
for acute confusion, 250
for stress urinary incontinence, 483

Hydrocele, 68
Hydrocephalus, 68
Hydrotherapy, in labor pain, 608
Hygiene
inability to provide own, 68
problems, 20
Hyperactive delirium, 247
Hyperactive syndrome, 68
Hyperbilirubinemia, neonatal, 69, 101
Hypercalcemia, 69
Hypercapnia, 69
Hypercholesterolemia, risk for inef-
fective cerebral tissue perfusion,
228–229
Hyperemesis gravidarum, 69
Hyperemia, conjunctival, dry eyes and,
348
Hyperglycemia, 69
signs and symptoms of, unstable
blood glucose level, 409
Hyperkalemia, 69
Hyperlipidemia, risk for decreased
cardiac tissue perfusion, 218
Hypernatremia, 69
Hyperosmolar hyperglycemic nonke-
totic syndrome (HHNS), 66
Hyperphosphatemia, 70
Hyperpyrexia, in ineffective thermoreg-
ulation, 778
Hypersensitivity, to slight criticism, 70
Hypertension, 67–68, 195
malignant, 88
risk for decreased cardiac tissue
perfusion, 218
risk for ineffective cerebral tissue
perfusion, 228–229
Hyperthermia, 70, 445–451
in ineffective thermoregulation, 779
malignant, 88
Hyperthyroidism, 70
Hypertrophy, prostatic, 123
Hyperventilation, 70
Hypervolemia, intraoperative, signs of,
in imbalanced fluid volume, 382
Hypoactive delirium, 247
Hypocalcemia, 70
Hypoglycemia, 70
signs and symptoms of, unstable
blood glucose level, 408
Hypokalemia, 70

Hypomagnesemia, 70
Hypomania, 70
Hyponatremia, 70–71
    monitoring of, in imbalanced fluid
        volume, 382
Hypoplastic left lung, 71
Hypotension, 71
    orthostatic, 107
Hypothalamus-pituitary-adrenal axis
        dysregulation, fatigue and, 369
Hypothermia, 71, 382, 451–458
    inadvertent, prevention of, 617
    in ineffective thermoregulation, 779
    perioperative, 112
        risk for, 461–464
        unintentional, nursing interven-
            tions for, 462–463
    risk for, 458
Hypothyroidism, 71
Hypotonia, impaired swallowing and,
        771–772
Hypovolemia
    intraoperative, signs of, in imbal-
        anced fluid volume, 382
    risk for decreased cardiac tissue
        perfusion, 218
    signs of, 384
Hypovolemic shock, 71, 136
Hypoxemia, risk for decreased cardiac
        tissue perfusion, 218
Hypoxia, 71
    risk for decreased cardiac tissue
        perfusion, 218
Hysterectomy, 71
    vaginal, 153
Hysteroscopic procedures, monitoring
        of, in imbalanced fluid volume,
        382

I

IBS. See Irritable bowel syndrome
ICD. See Implantable cardioverter/
        defibrillator
IDDM (insulin-dependent diabetes
        mellitus). See Diabetes mellitus
Identification, client, accuracy of, 505
Identity, disturbed, 72, 467–469
    risk for, 469–470
Idiopathic thrombocytopenic purpura
        (ITP), 72
Ileal conduit, 72

Ileostomy, 72
Ileus, 72
    paralytic, 110
    postoperative, nursing interventions
        for, 402–403
Illness, mental, 92
Imbalance
    acid-base, 5
    body temperature, risk for, 776
    electrolyte, 52
        risk for, 337–338
    energy field, 343–344
    fluid volume, risk for, 380–383
    nutrition, 574–578
Immigration transition, risk for compli-
        cated, 72
Immobility, 73
Immobilization
    disturbed sleep pattern and, 733
    impaired skin integrity and, 722
    perioperative positioning injury
        and, 615
    peripheral neurovascular dysfunction
        and, 619
    risk for disuse syndrome and, 326
Immune system diseases
    chronic pain and, 601
    impaired oral mucous membrane
        integrity and, 579, 584
Immunization, 73
Immunodeficiency, impaired skin
        integrity and, 722
Immunosuppression, 73
    compromised host defenses and, 500
    diarrhea and, 320
    impaired oral mucous membrane
        integrity and, 579, 584
Impaction
    constipation and, 257
    fecal, 55, 325
    of stool, 73
Impaired attachment, risk for,
        185–187
    client outcomes of, 185
    nursing interventions, 186–187
    related factors, 185
    at risk population, 185
    special considerations, 187
Impaired bed mobility, 545–550
Impaired cardiovascular function, risk
        for, 222–223

Impaired comfort, 236–238
  associated condition, 237
  client outcomes of, 237
  defining characteristics of, 237
  nursing interventions, 237–238
  related factors, 237
Impaired communication, verbal,
    242–246
  associated condition, 243
  defining characteristics of, 242–243
  related factors, 243
  at risk population, 243
Impaired dentition, 308–313
Impaired emancipated decision-
    making, 302–303
  risk for, 305–306
Impaired gas exchange, 395–400
  in risk for shock, 719
Impaired health status, imbalanced
    energy field and, 343
Impaired liver function, risk for,
    528–532
Impaired memory, 540–543
Impaired mobility
  bathing problems and, 20
  bed, 94, 545–550
  hygiene problems and, 20
  physical, 550–554, 769
  wheelchair, 555–560
Impaired mood regulation, 560–561
Impaired oral mucous membrane
    integrity, 96, 579–583
  risk for, 584
Impaired parenting, 609–612
  risk for, 111, 614–615
Impaired physical mobility, 550–554,
    769
  associated condition, 551
  client outcomes of, 551–552
  defining characteristics of,
    550–551
  dysfunctional gastrointestinal motil-
    ity and, 400, 405
  nursing interventions of, 552–554
  related factors, 551
  risk for, 94
Impaired postural balance, frail elderly
    syndrome and, 393, 395
Impaired religiosity, 664–665
  risk for, 667–668

Impaired resilience, 673–674
  risk for, 675–676
Impaired sitting, 73, 720–721
Impaired skin integrity, 721–726
  associated conditions, 722
  at-risk population, 722
  client outcomes, 722
  defining characteristics, 721
  nursing interventions, 722–726
  related factors, 721–722
  risk for, 726–728
Impaired social interaction, 138,
    735–737
  associated conditions, 735
  at-risk population, 735
  client outcomes, 735
  defining characteristics, 735
  nursing interventions, 735–737
  related factors, 735
Impaired spontaneous ventilation,
    818–823
  associated conditions, 819
  client outcomes, 819
  defining characteristics, 819
  nursing interventions, 819–823
  related factors, 819
Impaired standing, 73, 746–748
  associated conditions, 747
  client outcomes, 747
  defining characteristics, 747
  nursing interventions, 747–748
  related factors, 747
Impaired swallowing, 771–774
  associated conditions, 771–772
  at-risk population, 771
  client outcomes, 772
  defining characteristics, 771
  nursing interventions, 772–774
  related factors, 771
Impaired temperature regulation, 146
Impaired tissue integrity, 786–791
Impaired transfer ability, 797–802
  associated conditions, 797
  client outcomes, 797–798
  defining characteristics, 797
  nursing interventions, 798–802
  related factors, 797
Impaired urinary elimination, 153,
    806–810
  associated conditions, 807

Impaired urinary elimination
   *(Continued)*
   at-risk population, 807
   client outcomes, 807
   defining characteristics, 806
   nursing interventions, 807–810
   related factors, 807
Impaired walking, 155, 834–837
   associated condition, 834
   client outcomes/goals, 834
   defining characteristics, 834
   nursing interventions, 835–837
   related factors, 834
   special considerations, 836–837
Impaired wheelchair mobility, 94,
      555–560
   associated condition, 555
   client outcomes of, 556
   defining characteristics of, 555
   nursing interventions of, 556–560
   related factors, 555
   at risk population, 555
Imperforate anus, 73
Impetigo, 73
Implant, lens, 84
Implantable cardioverter/defibrillator
      (ICD), 72
   in ineffective sexuality pattern,
      715–716
Impotence, 73
Impulse control, ineffective, 472–473
Impulsiveness, 73
Inactivity, 73–74
Inadequate support system, 143
Inadequate tissue oxygenation, in risk
      for shock, 718–719
Inborn genetic diseases
   chronic pain and, 601
   delayed child development and,
      314, 316
   ineffective infant feeding dynamics
      and, 376
   obesity and, 585
   overweight and, 589, 592
Incompatibility, Rh factor, 130
Incompetent cervix, 74, 120
Incontinence
   reflex, 127
   of stool, 74
   urinary, 153

Incontinence *(Continued)*
   disability-associated, 473–477
   mixed, 477–480
   stress, 480–484
   urge, 484–488
   of urine, 74
Increased sodium, 138
Indigestion, 74
Individual, risk factors, for occupational
      injury, 510
Induction, of labor, 74, 81
Indwelling urinary catheter
   in deficient fluid volume, 385
   in disability-associated urinary
      incontinence, 477
   in excess fluid volume, 390–391
   in risk for urinary tract injury, 517
Ineffective activity planning, 164–166
   client outcomes of, 165
   defining characteristics of, 165
   nursing interventions, 165–166
   related factors, 165
   risk for, 166–167
   at risk population, 165
Ineffective adolescent eating dynamics,
      332–334
Ineffective airway clearance, 167–172
   associated condition, 167
   client outcomes of, 167–172
   defining characteristics of, 167
   nursing interventions, 167–172
   related factors, 167
   at risk population, 167
Ineffective breathing pattern, 206–210
   associated condition, 207
   client outcomes of, 207
   defining characteristics of, 206–207
   nursing interventions, 207–210
   related factors, 207
   at risk population, 207
Ineffective child eating dynamics,
      334–337
Ineffective childbearing process,
      230–233
   risk for, 236
Ineffective community coping, 289–291
Ineffective coping, 284–287
Ineffective denial, 306–308
Ineffective dry eye self-management,
      347–350

Ineffective health maintenance behaviors, 428–430
Ineffective health self-management, 422–424
    family, 426–428
Ineffective home maintenance behaviors, 431–433
    risk for, 434
Ineffective impulse control, 472–473
Ineffective infant feeding dynamics, 376–378
Ineffective infant suck-swallow response, 755–758
    associated conditions, 755
    at-risk population, 755
    client outcomes, 755–756
    defining characteristics, 755
    nursing interventions, 756–758
    related factors, 755
Ineffective lymphedema self-management, 534–538
    risk for, 538
Ineffective peripheral tissue perfusion, 792–796
    associated conditions, 793
    client outcomes, 793
    defining characteristics, 793
    nursing interventions, 793–796
    related factors, 793
    risk for, 797
Ineffective protection, 652–657
Ineffective relationship, 660–662
    risk for, 663–664
Ineffective role performance, 679–681
Ineffective sexuality pattern, 136, 713–717
    at-risk population, 714
    client outcomes, 714
    defining characteristics, 713
    nursing interventions, 714–717
    related factors, 714
Ineffective thermoregulation, 148, 777–780
    associated conditions, 777
    at-risk population, 777
    client outcomes, 777
    defining characteristics, 777
    nursing interventions, 778–780
    related factors, 777
    risk for, 781

Infant
    apnea, 74
    behavior, 74
        disorganized, 489–493
        enhanced organized, readiness for, 493
    behavioral communication cues in, 245
    care, 74
    delivery of, in labor pain, 608
    of diabetic mother, 75
    disorganized infant behavior in, 490
    feeding dynamics, ineffective, 74, 376–378
    impaired parenting in
        associated condition, 610, 615
        characteristics of, 610
        related factors for, 610
        at risk population, 610, 615
    in ineffective breastfeeding, 201
    in interrupted breastfeeding, 204
    motor development, delayed, 316–319
    nursing interventions in
        for delayed child development, 315
        for delayed infant motor development, 318–319
    impaired dentition in, 311
    requiring specialty, 186–187
    of substance-abusing mother, 75
    terminally ill, 147
Infantile polyarteritis, 75
Infantile spasms, 134
Infection
    control, in risk for injury, 506
    diarrhea and, 320
    dysfunctional gastrointestinal motility and, 400, 405
    impaired oral mucous membrane integrity and, 579, 584
    impaired skin integrity and, 722
    maternal, 90
    opportunistic, 106
    potential for, 75
    prevention of, 653–657
    respiratory, acute childhood, 129
    risk for, 494–498
    in surgical site, 144
    unstable blood glucose level and, 406
    in upper respiratory, 152

Infection *(Continued)*
    urinary tract, symptomatic, 479
    of wound, 156
Infectious processes, 75
Infertility, 75
    male, 88
Inflammatory bowel disease, child and
        adult, 75
Influenza, 75
    vaccines, contamination and, 271
Information, presentation of, 523
Infusion of diuretic drips, 391
Ingestion, of poison, 620
Inguinal hernia repair, 75–76
Inhalation, of smoke, 138
Injury, 76
    corneal, risk for, 508–510
    occupational, 105
        risk for, 510–514
    perioperative positioning, risk for,
        615–619
    pressure, 122, 635, 643
    risk for, 505–507
    spinal cord, 139–140
    thermal
        cold, 776
        risk for, 774–777
    urinary tract, risk for, 516–519
Injury-related malnutrition, 575–576
Insomnia, 76, 519–522, 730–731
    associated condition, 520
    chronic, 521
    client outcomes of, 520
    defining characteristics of, 519
    fatigue and, 372
    nursing interventions, 520–522
    related factors, 519–520
    at risk population, 520
    short-term, 520–522
Insufficient breast milk production,
        200–201
Insulin shock, 76
Integrative therapies, for nausea, 570
Integrity, skin, impaired, 721–726
    associated conditions, 722
    at-risk population, 722
    client outcomes, 722
    defining characteristics, 721
    nursing interventions, 722–726
    related factors, 721–722
    risk for, 726–728

Integumentary stimuli
    autonomic dysreflexia and, 188
    risk for autonomic dysreflexia, 191
Intellectual disability, 76
Intensive care, 186–187
Intensive care unit (ICU), for reloca-
        tion stress syndrome, 670–671
Intermittent claudication, 76
Intermittent self-catheterization,
        479–480
Internal body temperature, 778
Internal cardioverter/defibrillator
        (ICD). *See* Implantable cardio-
        verter/defibrillator
Internal factors, contamination and, 269
Internal fixation, 76
    open reduction of fracture with, 106
Internal risk factors, for poisoning, 621
International Dysphagia Diet Stand-
        ardisation Initiative (IDDSI), 773
Internet
    for compromised family coping, 294
    for impaired comfort, 238
Internet-based health coach, for dis-
        turbed personal identity, 469
Interrupted family processes, 364–366
Interstitial cystitis, 76–77
Interventions, general, for surgical cli-
        ent, 616–619
Interviewing techniques, motivational,
        525
Intestinal obstruction, 77
Intestinal perforation, 77
Intimacy, sexual, in ineffective sexuality
        pattern, 714
Intimacy dysfunction, dysfunctional
        family processes and, 362
Intolerance
    lactose, 82
    milk, 94
Intoxication, 77
Intraaortic balloon counterpulsation, 77
Intracranial adaptive capacity, de-
        creased, 547
Intracranial pressure, increased, 77
Intraoperative hypervolemia, signs of,
        in imbalanced fluid volume, 382
Intraoperative hypovolemia, signs of, in
        imbalanced fluid volume, 382
Intraoral examination, for dry mouth,
        563

Intrauterine growth retardation, 77
Intravenous (IV) fluids, in risk for shock, 718
Intravenous therapy, 77
Intubation
    endotracheal or nasogastric, 77–78
    prolonged, impaired swallowing and, 771–772
Invasive procedures, in prevention of infection, 654
Invertebral disk excision, 77
Iodinated contrast media, adverse reaction to, risk for, 278–281
Iodine reaction with diagnostic testing, 78
Ipecac, 622
Irregular pulse, 78
Irritable bowel syndrome (IBS), 71, 78
Ischemia, chronic pain and, 601
Ischemic attack, transient, 149, 151
Isolation, 78
    social, 138, 737–739
Isotonic IV solutions, for deficient fluid volume, 385
Itching, 78
ITP. *See* Idiopathic thrombocytopenic purpura

## J

Jaundice, 78
    neonatal, 78
Jaw pain, heart attacks and, 78
Jaw surgery, 78
Jittery, 78
Jock itch, 78
Joint dislocation, 78
Joint pain, 78
Joint replacement, 78–79
JRA. *See* Juvenile rheumatoid arthritis
Juvenile rheumatoid arthritis (JRA), 79

## K

Kangaroo care, for disorganized infant behavior, 491
Kaposi's sarcoma, 79
Kawasaki disease, 79
Keloids, 79
Keratoconjunctival staining, with fluorescein, dry eyes and, 348
Keratoconjunctivitis sicca, 79
Keratoplasty, 79

Ketoacidosis
    alcoholic, 79
    diabetic, 79–80
Keyhole heart surgery, 80
Kidney
    disease screening for, 80
    failure, 80
        acute, child, 80
        chronic, child, 80
        nonoliguric, 80
    stone, 80
    transplant, 80
    transplantation
        donor, 80
        recipient, 80–81
    tubular, necrosis, 99
    tumor, 81
Kissing disease, 81
Knee replacement, 81
Knowledge, 81
    deficient, 81, 522–524
    enhanced, readiness for, 524–525
    of nurse, to positioning, 617
Kock pouch, 81
Korsakoff's syndrome, 81

## L

Labile emotional control, 340–343
Labor
    induction of, 81
    ineffective childbearing process during, 231
    normal, 81–82
    preterm, 122–123
    readiness for enhanced childbearing process during, 234
    suppression of, 143
    uterine atony in, 153
Labor pain, 82, 606–609
Labyrinthitis, 82
Lacerations, 82
    ineffective infant suck-swallow response, 755
Lactation, 82
Lactic acidosis, 82
Lactose intolerance, 82
Laminectomy, 82
Language barriers, impaired verbal communication and, 245
Language impairment, 82
Laparoscopic laser cholecystectomy, 82

Laparoscopic procedures, monitoring of, in imbalanced fluid volume, 382

Laparoscopy, 83

Laparotomy, 83

Large bowel resection, 83

Laryngeal diseases, impaired swallowing and, 771–772

Laryngectomy, 83

Laser-assisted in situ keratomileusis, 83

Laser surgery, 83

Lasik eye surgery, 83

Latex allergic reaction, 83
 risk for, 525–527

Latino, enhanced religiosity in, 667

Laxatives
 abuse, 83
 for chronic functional constipation, 267
 for constipation, 258
 for perceived constipation, 263

Lead, in drinking water, 272

Lead poisoning, 84, 624

Learning, reinforcement of, 523

Learning disability, self-neglect and, 709

Left heart catheterization, 84

Legionnaires' disease, 84

Lens implant, 84

Lesbian, gay, bisexual, or transgender (LGBTQ) youth, 364
 in interrupted family processes, 366

Lesions, of mouth, 95

Lethargy, 84

Leukemia, 84

Leukocytosis, dry eyes and, 349, 351

Leukopenia, 84

Level of attention, in acute confusion, 247

Level of consciousness
 in acute confusion, 247
 decreased, 84
  dry eye and, 351
  impaired skin integrity and, 722
  risk for disuse syndrome and, 326

Level of psychomotor behavior, in acute confusion, 247

Lice, 84
 childhood communicable diseases, 37

"Life history," for disturbed personal identity, 468

Lifestyle
 assessment
  in chronic functional constipation, 265–266
  in constipation, 256
  in perceived constipation, 262
  in stress urinary incontinence, 482
 modifications, for nausea, in pregnancy, 568
 sedentary, 84, 133, 681–684

Ligation, tubal, 152

Light, insomnia and, 522

Lightheadedness, 84

Limb reattachment procedures, 84–85

Liposuction, 85

Lips, lubricate, in dry mouth, 565

Listlessness, 84

Lithotripsy, 85

Liver
 biopsy, 85
 cancer, 85
 disease, 85
 function, 85
  impaired, risk for, 528–532
 transplant, 85

Living conditions, unsanitary, 152

Living will, 85

Lobectomy, 85

Loneliness, 86
 risk for, 532–534

Loose-fitting clothes
 for bleeding disorder, 657
 in disability-associated urinary incontinence, 476

Loose stools, 86

Loss
 of ability to smell, 138
 of bladder control, 86
 of bowel control, 86

Lou Gehrig's disease, 86

Low attachment avoidance, maladaptive grieving and, 412, 414

Low back pain, 86

Low self-esteem
  chronic, 134, 698–700
    associated conditions, 698
    at-risk population, 698
    client outcomes, 698–699
    defining characteristics, 698
    low, risk for, 703
    nursing interventions, 699–700
    related factors, 698
    risk for, 703
  in ineffective sexuality pattern, 714
  situational, 700–702
    associated conditions, 701
    at-risk population, 701
    client outcomes, 701
    defining characteristics, 701
    nursing interventions, 701–702
    related factors, 701
    risk for, 703–705
Low-technology interventions, for
    enhanced parenting, 613
Lower back pain, fear of, 375
Lower extremity amputation,
    836–837
Lower gastrointestinal (GI) bleed-
    ing, 86
Lower limb prosthesis, risk for adult
    falls and, 352
Lumbar puncture, 86
Lump, rectal, 127
Lumpectomy, 86
Lung cancer, 86
Lung disease, chronic, in ineffective
    sexuality pattern, 716
Lung surgery, 86
Lupus erythematosus, 86–87
    systemic, 145
Lyme disease, 87
Lymph nodes, in dry mouth, 563
Lymphedema, 87
    of ineffective lymphedema self-
        management
        signs, 534
        symptoms, 534
Lymphoma, 87

# M

Macular degeneration, 87
Magnetic resonance imaging (MRI),
    87, 95

Maintenance behaviors
  health, ineffective, 428–430
  home, ineffective, 431–433
    risk for, 434
Major depressive disorder, 87
Malabsorption syndrome, 87–88
Maladaptive behavior, 88
Maladaptive grieving, 180, 412–414
    risk for, 414
Malaise, 88
Malaria, 88
Male infertility, 88
Malignancy, 88
Malignant hypertension, 88
Malignant hyperthermia, 88
    nursing interventions for, 448
Malignant syndrome, neuroleptic, nurs-
    ing interventions for, 448–449
Malingering, self-neglect and, 709
Malnutrition, 88–89, 575–577
    dysfunctional gastrointestinal motil-
        ity and, 400, 405
    frail elderly syndrome and, 393, 395
Malnutrition Universal Screening Tool
    (MUST), 394
Mammography, 89
Manic disorder, bipolar I, 89
Manipulative behavior, 89
Marfan syndrome, 89
Massage, for impaired comfort, 237
Mastectomy, 89–90
    modified radical, 94
Mastitis, 90
Maternal anemia
    delayed infant motor development
        and, 317
    risk for delayed infant motor devel-
        opment and, 320
Maternal breastfeeding, in interrupted
    breastfeeding, 204
Maternal-fetal dyad, disturbed, risk for,
    539–540
Maternal infection, 90
Maternal mental disorders
    delayed child development and,
        314, 316
    delayed infant motor development
        and, 317
    risk for delayed infant motor devel-
        opment and, 320

Maternal/parental interventions, 186

Maternal physical illnesses, delayed child development and, 314, 316

Maternal prepregnancy obesity
delayed infant motor development and, 317
risk for delayed infant motor development and, 320

Matter-of-fact manner, in constipation, 259

Maturational issues, adolescent, 90

MAZE III procedure, 90

MD. *See* Muscular dystrophy

Measles, 91
childhood communicable diseases, 37

Measurement, temperature, nursing interventions for
hyperthermia in, 446–451
hypothermia in, 452–458, 461–464

Mechanical compression, peripheral neurovascular dysfunction and, 619

Mechanical device-related pressure injury, 724

Mechanical obstruction, impaired swallowing and, 771–772

Mechanical prosthetic valve, risk for ineffective cerebral tissue perfusion, 228–229

Meconium
aspiration, 91, 129
delayed, 91

Medical alert bracelet, for bleeding disorder, 656

Medical device-related pressure injury, 638–639, 646–647, 789

Medical devices, impaired skin integrity and, 722

Medical history
in chronic functional constipation, 266
compromised host defenses and, 500
in constipation, 257
in disability-associated urinary incontinence, 475
in perceived constipation, 262
in risk factors for stress incontinence, 481

Medical marijuana, 91

Medical mistrust, 307

Medical oxygen, 775–776

Medical professional, risk for allergy reaction, 174

Medical social services, for compromised family coping, 294

Medication reconciliation, 623

Medication safety, 505–506, 624

Medications
for acute confusion, 248
postoperative interventions and, 503
sexual dysfunction and, 712

Melanoma, 91

Melena, 91

Membranes, premature rupture of, 121

Memory, impaired, 540–543

Memory deficit, 91

Memory techniques, for cognitive disorders, 541

Ménière's disease, 91

Meningitis, 91

Meningocele, 91, 101–102

Menopause, 91–92

Menorrhagia, 92

Menstrual flow, 655

Mental activities, for ineffective coping, 285

Mental disorders
chronic low self-esteem and, 698
frail elderly syndrome and, 393, 395
impaired social interaction and, 735
ineffective family health self-management and, 427
ineffective health maintenance behaviors and, 429
ineffective home maintenance behaviors and, 431, 434
labile emotional control and, 341
maternal
delayed child development and, 314, 316
delayed infant motor development and, 317
risk for delayed infant motor development and, 320
risk for adult falls and, 352
risk for elopement attempt and, 339
self-neglect and, 709
situational low self-esteem and, 701

Mental health care, contamination and, 270

Mental health counseling, 765

Mental illness, 92

Mental status examination, in acute confusion, 247–248

Mentoring strategies, for ineffective community coping, 291

Metabolic acidosis, 92

Metabolic alkalosis, 92

Metabolic diseases, dry eyes and, 349, 351

Metabolic imbalance syndrome, 92

Metabolic syndrome, risk for, 543–545

Metabolism, impaired
  chronic pain and, 601
  impaired sitting and, 720
  impaired skin integrity and, 722
  impaired standing and, 747

Metacognitive training (MCT), 785

Metastasis, 92

Methamphetamines, exposed to, in children, 623

Methicillin-resistant *Staphylococcus aureus* (MRSA), 92, 95

MI. *See* Myocardial infarction

MIDCAB. *See* Minimally invasive direct coronary artery bypass

Midlife crisis, 93

Migraine headache, 93

Military families, personnel, 93–94

Military members, in enhanced relationship, 663

Milk, intolerance, 94

Mindfulness
  for enhancing comfort, 240
  meditation, 473

Mindfulness-based interventions
  in enhanced nutrition, 573
  for obesity, 586
  for overweight, 590, 593

Mindfulness-based stress reduction (MBSR) program, for interrupted family processes, 366

Mindfulness-based training program, for fear, 374

Minimally invasive direct coronary artery bypass (MIDCAB), 93–94

Mirror-mirror technique, for impaired dentition, 312

Miscarriage, 94

Mistrust, medical, 307

Mitral stenosis, 94
  risk for ineffective cerebral tissue perfusion, 228–229

Mitral valve prolapse, 94

Mixed delirium, 247

Mixed urinary incontinence, 477–480
  associated condition, 477
  client outcomes of, 478
  defining characteristics of, 477
  nursing interventions, 478–480
  related factors in, 477
  at risk population, 477

Mobility, impaired
  bed, 94, 545–550
  physical, 94, 550–554
  wheelchair, 94, 555–560
    associated condition, 555
    client outcomes of, 556
    defining characteristics of, 555
    nursing interventions of, 556–560
    related factors, 555
    at risk population, 555

Mobility skills, in impaired physical mobility, 552

Moderate- to vigorous-intensity physical activity, for obesity, 586

Moderate-intensity cardiorespiratory (aerobic) exercise, 345, 682
  for impaired physical mobility, 552

Moderate-intensity physical activity, for overweight, 589, 593

Modified radical mastectomy, 94

Mononucleosis, 94

Montessori interventions, for dementia clients, 693

Montreal Cognitive Assessment, in impaired memory, 541

Mood disorders, 95
  labile emotional control and, 341

Mood regulation, impaired, 560–561

Moon face, 95

Moral distress, 561–562

Moral/ethical dilemmas, 95

Morning sickness, 95

Morse Fall Scale, for falls, 547

Mother, in ineffective breastfeeding, 201

Mother-Baby Dyad interventions, 186–187

Motion sickness, 95

Motivational interviewing techniques, 525
 for obesity, 585
 for overweight, 589, 592

Motive-oriented therapeutic relationship (MOTR), for labile emotional control, 342

Motor system, of disorganized infant behavior, 489

Motor vehicle crash (MVC), 98

Mottling of peripheral skin, 95

Mourning, 95

Mouth, dry, risk for, 562–566

Mouth breathing, in dry mouth, 563

Mouth lesions, 95

Movement restrictions, prescribed
 decreased diversional activity engagement and, 330
 risk for disuse syndrome and, 326

MRI. *See* Magnetic resonance imaging

MRSA. *See* Methicillin-resistant *Staphylococcus aureus*

MS. *See* Multiple sclerosis

Mucocutaneous lymph node syndrome, 96

Mucosal membrane pressure injury, 639, 647, 724
 in impaired tissue integrity, 789

Mucositis, treatment of, 582

Mucous membrane, impaired oral integrity, 96, 579–583
 risk for, 584

Mucous plaques, dry eyes and, 348

Multicomponent cognitive rehabilitation program, for impaired memory, 542

Multicultural
 in acute pain, 599
 in anxiety, 177
 in bathing self-care deficit, 689
 in caregiver role strain, 226
 in chronic confusion, 254
 in chronic low self-esteem, 700
 in chronic pain, 605
 in compromised family coping, 293–294
 in compromised human dignity, 440
 in contamination, 272
 in death anxiety, 180

Multicultural *(Continued)*
 in decision making, 299, 303–304
 in decisional conflict, 301
 in defensive coping, 284
 in deficient community health, 419
 in deficient knowledge, 524
 in disabled family coping, 297
 in disorganized infant behavior, 492–493
 in disturbed body image, 199
 in disturbed family identity syndrome, 466
 in disturbed personal identity, 469
 in disturbed sleep pattern, 734
 in disturbed thought process, 786
 in dressing self-care deficit, 691
 in dysfunctional family processes, 364
 in enhanced nutrition, 574
 in enhanced parenting, 613–614
 in enhanced power, 630
 in enhanced relationship, 663
 in enhanced religiosity, 667
 in enhanced resilience, 675
 in family processes, 368
 in fear, 375–376
 in feeding self-care deficit, 693
 in frail elderly syndrome, 394
 in hope, 434
 in hopelessness, 438
 in imbalanced energy field, 344
 in impaired comfort, 238
 in impaired dentition, 313
 in impaired memory, 542–543
 in impaired parenting, 611–612
 in impaired religiosity, 665
 in impaired sitting, 721
 in impaired social interaction, 736
 in impaired verbal communication, 245–246
 in ineffective activity planning, 166
 in ineffective adolescent eating dynamics, 333–334
 in ineffective breastfeeding, 203
 in ineffective child eating dynamics, 336–337
 in ineffective childbearing process, 233
 in ineffective community coping, 290–291
 in ineffective coping, 286
 in ineffective denial, 307

Multicultural *(Continued)*
in ineffective family health self-management, 428
in ineffective health maintenance behaviors, 430
in ineffective health self-management, 424
in ineffective home maintenance behaviors, 432
in ineffective infant feeding dynamics, 377–378
in ineffective lymphedema self-management, 537
in ineffective relationship, 662
in ineffective role performance, 680–681
in ineffective sexuality pattern, 717
in insufficient breast milk production, 201
in interrupted breastfeeding, 205
in interrupted family processes, 366
in labile emotional control, 342
in maladaptive grieving, 414
in metabolic imbalance syndrome, 545
in neonatal abstinence syndrome, 572
in neonatal hyperbilirubinemia, 443
in neonatal hypothermia, 460
in obesity, 587–588
in overweight, 591, 595
in parental role conflict, 678
in post-trauma syndrome, 626–627, 629
in powerlessness, 632
in rape-trauma syndrome, 659
in readiness for enhanced breastfeeding, 206
in readiness for enhanced comfort, 240
in readiness for enhanced community coping, 282–283
in readiness for enhanced coping, 288
in readiness for enhanced exercise engagement, 347
in readiness for enhanced family coping, 298
in readiness for enhanced grieving, 417

Multicultural *(Continued)*
in readiness for enhanced health literacy, 528
in readiness for enhanced health self-management, 426
in readiness for enhanced knowledge in, 525
in readiness for enhanced spiritual well-being, 746
in readiness for enhancing communication, 242
in readiness for self-care, 686
in readiness for self-concept, 697
in risk for
dry mouth, 566
elopement attempt, 340
impaired attachment, 187
injury in, 507
loneliness, 533–534
occupational injury in, 513–514
other-directed violence, 831
poisoning, 624
sudden infant death, 759
suicide, 767
surgical site infection in, 504
in risk-prone health behavior, 421–422
in sedentary lifestyle, 683–684
in self-neglect, 710
in sexual dysfunction, 713
in situational low self-esteem, 702
in sleep deprivation, 730
in social isolation, 739
in spiritual distress, 743
in stress overload, 749
in toileting self-care deficit, 695
in unstable blood glucose level, 410
in violence, 831
in wandering, 839–840
Multidrug-resistant organism (MDRO), 495
Multi-infarct dementia, 96, 153
Multimicronutrient supplements, for pregnant clients, 233
Multiple gestations, 96
Multiple personality disorder, 96
Multiple sclerosis (MS), 96–97
fatigue and, 372
Mumps, 97
childhood communicable diseases, 37

Murmurs, 97
Muscle strength
  decreased, frail elderly syndrome and,
    393, 395
  in impaired physical mobility, 552
  insufficient, impaired sitting and, 720
Muscle-strengthening, 683
  for readiness for enhanced exercise
    engagement, 346
Muscular atrophy, 97
Muscular dystrophy (MD), 90, 97–98
Musculoskeletal diseases
  bathing self-care deficit and, 687
  dressing self-care deficit and, 690
  feeding self-care deficit and, 691
  risk for adult falls and, 352
  risk for child falls and, 359
  toileting self-care deficit and, 694
Musculoskeletal impairment, labile
    emotional control and, 341
Musculoskeletal-neurological stimuli
  autonomic dysreflexia and, 188
  risk for autonomic dysreflexia, 191
Music therapy, for impaired comfort,
    238
Mutilation, self, 705–707
MVC. *See* Motor vehicle crash
Myasthenia gravis, 98
  fatigue and, 369
Mycoplasma pneumonia, 98
Myelocele, 98
Myelomeningocele, 98, 101–102
Myocardial infarction (MI), 12, 93, 98
  ineffective sexuality pattern and, 715
Myocarditis, 98
Myringotomy, 98
Myxedema, 98

N
NANDA-I, definition
  of acute confusion, 246
  of anxiety, 175
  of autonomic dysreflexia, 188
  of caregiver role strain, 223
  of chronic confusion, 254–255
  of chronic functional constipation,
    264
  of compromised family coping, 291
  of constipation, 255
  of contamination, 268
  of death anxiety, 178

NANDA-I, definition *(Continued)*
  of decreased activity tolerance,
    159–164
  of decreased cardiac output, 210
  of defensive coping, 283
  of deficient knowledge, 522
  of disability-associated urinary
    incontinence, 473
  of disabled family coping, 295
  of disorganized infant behavior, 489
  of disturbed body image, 197
  of disturbed family identity syn-
    drome, 464–466
  of enhanced nutrition, 572
  of imbalanced nutrition, 574
  of impaired bed mobility, 545
  of impaired bowel continence, 273
  of impaired comfort, 237
  of impaired memory, 540
  of impaired physical mobility, 550
  of impaired verbal communication,
    242
  of impaired wheelchair mobility,
    555
  of ineffective activity planning, 164
  of ineffective airway clearance, 167
  of ineffective breastfeeding, 201
  of ineffective breathing pattern, 206
  of ineffective childbearing process,
    230
  of ineffective community coping, 289
  of ineffective coping, 284
  of ineffective impulse control, 472
  of ineffective lymphedema self-
    management, 534
  of insomnia, 519
  of mixed urinary incontinence, 477
  of nausea, 566
  of nipple-areolar complex injury, 514
  of perceived constipation, 261
  of readiness for enhanced breastfeed-
    ing, 205
  of readiness for enhanced childbear-
    ing process, 233
  of readiness for enhanced comfort,
    239
  of readiness for enhanced commu-
    nity coping, 281
  of readiness for enhanced coping, 287
  of readiness for enhanced family
    coping, 297

NANDA-I, definition *(Continued)*
  of readiness for enhanced health
    literacy, 527
  of readiness for enhanced home
    maintenance behaviors, 433
  of readiness for enhanced hope, 435
  of readiness for enhanced knowledge,
    524
  of readiness for enhanced organized
    infant behavior, 493
  of readiness for enhancing commu-
    nication, 241
  risk for
    allergy reaction, 172
    aspiration, 180–185
    autonomic dysreflexia, 191
    bleeding, 192
    caregiver role strain, 227
    complicated immigration transi-
      tion, 470
    corneal injury, 508
    decreased activity tolerance, 164
    decreased cardiac output, 218
    decreased cardiac tissue perfu-
      sion, 218
    disorganized infant behavior,
      493
    disturbed family identity syn-
      drome, 466
    disturbed maternal-fetal dyad,
      539
    disturbed personal identity, 469
    dry mouth, 562
    impaired, 185
    impaired cardiovascular func-
      tion, 222–223
    impaired liver function, 528
    ineffective activity planning, 166
    ineffective childbearing process,
      236
    ineffective home maintenance
      behaviors, 434
    ineffective lymphedema self-
      management, 538
    infection, 494
    injury, 505–507
    iodinated contrast media, ad-
      verse reaction to, 278–281
    latex allergy reaction, 525
    loneliness, 532

NANDA-I, definition *(Continued)*
    metabolic syndrome, 543
    nipple–areolar complex injury, 516
    occupational injury, 510
    surgical site infection, 499
    unstable blood pressure, 194
    urge urinary incontinence, 488
    urinary tract injury, 516
  of stress urinary incontinence, 480
Narcissistic personality disorder, 98–99
Narcolepsy, 99
  sleep deprivation and, 729
Narcotic use, 99
Nasal defect, impaired swallowing and,
    771–772
Nasal turbinates, in dry mouth, 563
Nasogastric suction, 99
Nasopharyngeal cavity defect, impaired
    swallowing and, 771–772
National Patient Safety Goals, 505
National Pressure Ulcer Advisory Panel
    (NPUAP), 787
Nausea, 99, 566–570, 769
  after chemotherapy, 569
  after surgery, 569
  in pregnancy, 568–569
  and vomiting, postoperative, 569
Near-drowning, 99
Nearsightedness, 99
  corneal surgery, 99
Neck vein distention, 99
Necrolysis, toxic epidermal, 147
Necrosis, tubular, kidney, acute, 99
Necrotizing enterocolitis, 99–100
Negative feelings, about self, 100
Neglect
  protection, in impaired parenting, 611
  self-, 708–710
  unilateral, 100, 804–806
    client outcomes, 805
    defining characteristics,
      804–805
    nursing interventions, 805–806
Neglectful care, of family member, 100
Neonatal abstinence syndrome, 100,
    570–572
  delayed infant motor development
    and, 317
  risk for delayed infant motor devel-
    opment and, 320

Neonatal hyperbilirubinemia, 101, 440–443
  risk for, 444–445
Neonatal hypothermia, 458–460
  risk for, 460
Neonatal intensive care unit (NICU), 740
Neonatal pressure injury, 649–651
  risk for, 652
Neonate, 101
  nursing intervention in
    for delayed child development, 315
    for delayed infant motor development, 318–319
  pain in, 599
  respiratory conditions of, 129
Neoplasms, 101
  chronic pain and, 601
  fatigue and, 369
  impaired skin integrity and, 722
  ineffective home maintenance behaviors and, 431, 434
Nephrectomy, 101
Nephropathy, contrast-induced, 279–281
Nephrostomy, percutaneous, 101
Nephrotic syndrome, 101
Nerve compression syndromes, chronic pain and, 601
Nervous system diseases, chronic pain and, 601
Neural tube defects, 101–102
  ineffective infant feeding dynamics and, 376
Neuralgia, 102
  trigeminal, 151
Neuritis, 102
Neurocognitive disorders
  ineffective family health self-management and, 427
  ineffective health self-management and, 423
  ineffective home maintenance behaviors and, 431, 434
  risk for adult falls and, 352
  risk for child falls and, 359
  sleep deprivation and, 729
Neurodevelopmental disorders
  delayed infant motor development and, 317

Neurodevelopmental disorders *(Continued)*
  impaired social interaction and, 735
  risk for delayed infant motor development and, 320
Neurogenic bladder, 102
Neurogenic bowel dysfunction, constipation and, 257
Neuroleptic malignant syndrome, nursing interventions for, 448–449
Neurological delay, ineffective infant suck-swallow response, 755
Neurological disorders, 102
  impaired sitting and, 720
  impaired standing and, 747
  in sexual dysfunction, 712
Neurological impairment, ineffective infant suck-swallow response, 755
Neurological injury, dry eyes and
  with motor reflex loss, 349, 351
  with sensory reflex loss, 349, 351
Neurological problems, impaired swallowing and, 771–772
Neuromotor exercise, 682
  for impaired physical mobility, 551–552
Neuromuscular blockade, dry eyes and, 351
Neuromuscular diseases
  bathing self-care deficit and, 687
  dressing self-care deficit and, 690
  feeding self-care deficit and, 691
  impaired swallowing and, 771–772
  toileting self-care deficit and, 694
Neuropathic component, of chronic pain, 603
Neuropathy
  perioperative positioning injury and, 615
  peripheral, 102, 112
Neurosurgery, 102
Neurovascular dysfunction, peripheral, risk for, 619–620
Newborn
  normal, 103
  postmature, 103
  small for gestational age, 103
Nicotine addiction, 103
Nicotine-induced withdrawal syndrome, 751
  risk for, 754

NIDDM. *See* Non-insulin-dependent diabetes mellitus
Nightmares, 103
  sleep deprivation and, 729
Nipple soreness, 103
Nipple-areolar complex injury, 514–515
  risk for, 515–516
Nitrous oxide, in labor pain, 609
Nocturia, 103–104
Nocturnal myoclonus, 104
Nocturnal paroxysmal dyspnea, 104
Noise, insomnia and, 522
Noncoronary open heart surgery, in ineffective sexuality pattern, 715
Non-insulin-dependent diabetes mellitus (NIDDM), 103–104
Noninvasive hemodynamic parameters, in risk for shock, 719
Nonopioid analgesic
  for acute pain, 597
  for chronic pain, 603
Nonpharmacological interventions, in nausea, 568
Nonpharmacological methods
  for acute pain, 598, 600
  for chronic pain, 605–606
Nonpharmacological pain relief, 608
Nonreassuring fetal heart rate pattern, 56
Non-ST-elevation myocardial infarction (NSTEMI), 104
Nonsteroidal antiinflammatory drugs (NSAIDs), 195, 655
Nonsuicidal self-injury (NSSI), 699, 706
Nonverbal cues, in impaired physical mobility, 553
Nonverbal therapeutic communication
  for ineffective coping, 285
  for labile emotional control, 343
Normal bed mobility, components of, 546
Normal labor, 81–82
Normal pressure hydrocephalus (NPH), 104
Nothing per mouth (NPO), 381
NPH. *See* Normal pressure hydrocephalus
NSTEMI. *See* Non-ST-elevation myocardial infarction

Nursing, 104
Nursing home care, decision making in, 304
Nursing interventions
  in acute confusion, 247–251
  in acute pain, 596–600
  in acute substance withdrawal syndrome, 750–752
  in adult pressure injury, 635–641
  in anxiety, 176–178
  in autonomic dysreflexia, 189–190
  in child pressure injury, 643–649
  in chronic confusion, 252–255
  in chronic functional constipation, 265–267
  in chronic low self-esteem, 699–700
  in chronic pain, 602–606
  in chronic pain syndrome, 606
  in chronic sorrow, 740–741
  in compromised family coping, 292–295
  in compromised human dignity, 439–440
  in constipation, 256–260
  in contamination, 270–272
  in death anxiety, 179–180
  in decision making, 299–300, 303–306
  in decisional conflict, 301
  in decreased activity tolerance, 159–164
  in decreased diversional activity engagement, 330–332
  in defensive coping, 283–284
  in deficient community health, 418–420
  in deficient fluid volume, 384–388
  in deficient knowledge, 523–524
  in delayed child development, 314–316
  in delayed infant motor development, 318–319
  in delayed surgical recovery, 768–770
  in diarrhea, 321–326
  in disability-associated urinary incontinence, 474–477
  in disabled family coping, 296–297
  in disorganized infant behavior, 491–493
  in disturbed body image, 198–200

Nursing interventions *(Continued)*
  in disturbed personal identity, 467–469
  in disturbed thought process, 785–786
  in disuse syndrome, 326–330
  in dry eyes, 351
  in dysfunctional adult ventilatory weaning response, 824–827
  in dysfunctional family processes, 363–364
  in dysfunctional gastrointestinal motility, 401–405
  in dysfunctional ventilatory weaning response, 824–827
  in electrolyte imbalance, 337–338
  in enhanced nutrition, 572–574
  in enhanced parenting, 613–614
  in enhanced power, 629–630
  in enhanced relationship, 662–663
  in enhanced religiosity, 666–667
  in enhanced resilience, 675
  in excess fluid volume, 389–392
  in family processes, 367–368
  in fatigue, 369–373
  in fear, 374–376
  in female genital mutilation, 378–380
  in frail elderly syndrome, 393–395
  in hope, 433–436
  in hopelessness, 437–438
  in hyperthermia, 446–451
  in hypothermia, 452–458, 461–464
  in imbalanced energy field, 343–344
  in imbalanced fluid volume, 381–383
  in imbalanced nutrition, 575–578
  in impaired bowel continence, 274–278
  in impaired comfort, 237–238
  in impaired dentition, 309–313
  in impaired gas exchange, 396–400
  in impaired oral mucous membrane, 580–584
  in impaired parenting, 611–612, 615
  in impaired physical mobility, 552–554
  in impaired religiosity, 664–665
  in impaired resilience, 673–674
  in impaired skin integrity, 722–726
  in impaired social interaction, 735–737

Nursing interventions *(Continued)*
  in impaired spontaneous ventilation, 819–823
  in impaired standing, 747–748
  in impaired swallowing, 772–774
  in impaired transfer ability, 798–802
  in impaired urinary elimination, 807–810
  in impaired verbal communication, 243–246
  in impaired walking, 835–837
  in impaired wheelchair mobility, 556–560
  in ineffective activity planning, 165–166
  in ineffective adolescent eating dynamics, 333–334
  in ineffective airway clearance, 167–172
  in ineffective breastfeeding, 202–203
  in ineffective breathing pattern, 207–210
  in ineffective child eating dynamics, 335–337
  in ineffective childbearing process, 232–233
  in ineffective community coping, 290–291
  in ineffective coping, 285–287
  in ineffective denial, 307–308
  in ineffective dry eye self-management, 349–350
  in ineffective family health self-management, 427–428
  in ineffective health maintenance behaviors, 429–430
  in ineffective health self-management, 423–424
  in ineffective home maintenance behaviors, 431–434
  in ineffective impulse control, 472–473
  in ineffective infant feeding dynamics, 377–378
  in ineffective infant suck-swallow response, 756–758
  in ineffective lymphedema self-management, 535–538
  in ineffective peripheral tissue perfusion, 793–796
  in ineffective protection, 653–657
  in ineffective relationship, 661–662

Nursing interventions *(Continued)*
  in ineffective role performance,
    680–681
  in ineffective sexuality pattern,
    714–717
  in ineffective thermoregulation,
    778–780
  in insomnia, 520–522
  in insufficient breast milk produc-
    tion, 200–201
  in interrupted breastfeeding,
    204–205
  in interrupted family processes,
    365–366
  in labile emotional control, 341–343
  in labor pain, 607–609
  in maladaptive grieving, 412–414
  in metabolic imbalance syndrome,
    544–545
  in mixed urinary incontinence,
    478–480
  in nausea, 567–570
  in neonatal abstinence syndrome,
    571–572
  in neonatal hyperbilirubinemia,
    441–443
  in neonatal hypothermia, 459–460
  in neonatal pressure injury, 650–652
  in nipple-areolar complex injury,
    515
  in obesity, 585–588
  in overweight, 589–595
  in parental role conflict, 677–678
  in perceived constipation, 262–264
  in perioperative positioning injury,
    616–619
  in peripheral neurovascular dysfunc-
    tion, 620
  in post-trauma syndrome, 625–629
  in powerlessness, 631–633
  in rape-trauma syndrome, 658–660
  in readiness for enhanced breastfeed-
    ing, 205–206
  in readiness for enhanced childbear-
    ing process, 235–236
  in readiness for enhanced comfort,
    239–241
  in readiness for enhanced commu-
    nity coping, 282–283
  in readiness for enhanced coping,
    288–289

Nursing interventions *(Continued)*
  in readiness for enhanced exercise
    engagement, 345–347
  in readiness for enhanced family
    coping, 298
  in readiness for enhanced grieving,
    415–418
  in readiness for enhanced health
    literacy, 528
  in readiness for enhanced health self-
    management, 425–426
  in readiness for enhanced knowledge,
    524–525
  in readiness for enhancing commu-
    nication, 241–242
  in relocation stress syndrome,
    669–672
  in risk for
    adult falls, 352–358
    allergic reaction, 172–175
    aspiration, 181–185
    autonomic dysreflexia, 191
    bleeding, 192–194
    child falls, 359–361
    complicated immigration transi-
      tion, 470–472
    corneal injury, 508–510
    decreased activity tolerance, 164
    decreased cardiac tissue perfu-
      sion, 219–222
    deficient fluid volume, 392
    delayed infant motor develop-
      ment, 320
    disturbed maternal-fetal dyad,
      539–540
    dry mouth, 563–566
    elopement attempt, 339–340
    impaired attachment, 186–187
    impaired liver function, 529–532
    ineffective activity planning, 167
    ineffective cerebral tissue perfu-
      sion, 229–230
    infection, 495–498
    injury, 505–507
    iodinated contrast media, ad-
      verse reaction to, 279–281
    latex allergy reaction, 526–527
    loneliness, 533–534
    maladaptive grieving, 414
    neonatal hyperbilirubinemia,
      445

Nursing interventions *(Continued)*
    occupational injury, 511–514
    other-directed violence, 830–832
    poisoning, 621–624
    suffocation, 760–762
    suicidal behavior, 763–767
    surgical site infection, 499–504
    thermal injury, 775–777
    unstable blood pressure,
        195–197
    urinary tract injury, 517–519
    vascular trauma, 816–818
    in risk-prone health behavior,
        420–422
    in sedentary lifestyle, 682–684
    in self-mutilation, 706–707
    in self-neglect, 710
    in sexual dysfunction, 711–713
    in situational low self-esteem,
        701–702
    in sleep deprivation, 729–731
    in social isolation, 738–739
    in spiritual distress, 742–743
    in stress urinary incontinence,
        481–484
    in unilateral neglect, 805–806
    in unstable blood glucose level,
        407–411
    in urge urinary incontinence,
        484–488
    in urinary retention, 810–814
    in wandering, 838–840
Nursing staff, for impaired verbal com-
        munication, 244
Nutrition, 104
    enhanced, readiness for, 572–574
    imbalanced, 104, 574–578
Nutrition follow-up, postoperative
        interventions and, 503
Nutritional intake, during pregnancy,
        233
Nutritional screening tool, for imbal-
        anced nutrition, 577
Nutritional status
    evaluation of, 773
    in ineffective protection, 653
Nutritional supplements, in imbalanced
        nutrition, 576
Nutritional teaching, in metabolic
        imbalance syndrome, 544

# O

Obesity, 104, 584–588
    fatigue and, 372
    frail elderly syndrome and, 393, 395
    in metabolic imbalance syndrome,
        544
    obstructive sleep apnea and, 104
OBS. *See* Organic brain syndrome
Obsessive-compulsive disorder (OCD),
        104–105
Obstruction, bowel, 104
Obstructive sleep apnea, 104
Occupational injury, 105
    risk for, 510–514
Occupational therapy services, in im-
        paired physical mobility, 554
OCD. *See* Obsessive-compulsive
        disorder
Ocular dryness, dry eyes and, 348
Ocular foreign body, dry eyes and, 348
Ocular itching, dry eyes and, 348
ODD. *See* Oppositional defiant
        disorder
Office of Minority Health of the U.S.
        Department of Health and Hu-
        man Services standards, impaired
        verbal communication and, 246
Off-pump coronary artery bypass
        (OPCAB), 105
Older adult, 105
Older children, nursing interventions
        for, impaired dentition in, 312
Oliguria, 105
Omphalocele, 60, 105
Onychomycosis, 149
Oophorectomy, 105
OPCAB. *See* Off-pump coronary artery
        bypass
Open heart surgery, 106
    noncoronary, in ineffective sexuality
        pattern, 715
Open reduction of fracture with inter-
        nal fixation, 106
Open wound, 156
Opioid addiction, 106
Opioid-induced withdrawal syndrome,
        750–751
    risk for, 753
Opioid use, 106
Opioid use disorder, 597, 603–604

Opioids
    for acute pain, 598
    for chronic pain, 602, 605
    constipation and
        causing, 257–259
        side effect of, 257–258, 266
    converting, 598
    for moderate to severe acute pain,
        597
    in multimodal analgesic plan, 598
Opportunistic infection, 106
Opportunities, of readiness for self-
    care, 685
Oppositional defiant disorder (ODD),
    105–106
Oral care, for vomits, 568
Oral cavity, in impaired oral mucous
    membrane, 580
Oral hygiene
    for dry mouth, 564–565
    for impaired dentition, 313
    for impaired oral mucous membrane,
        580
    infant, nursing interventions for,
        impaired dentition in, 311
Oral hypersensitivity, ineffective infant
    suck-swallow response, 755
Oral intake, in imbalanced nutrition,
    578
Oral Mucositis Assessment Scale, 581
Oral mucous membrane, impaired
    integrity, 106, 579–583
    risk for, 584
Oral nutritional supplements, in imbal-
    anced nutrition, 576
Oral rehydration solution, for diarrhea,
    323
Oral replacement therapy, for deficient
    fluid volume, 385
Oral screening, in dry mouth, 564
Oral temperature sensitivity, impaired
    dentition and, 308
Oral thrush, 106
Oral trauma, impaired oral mucous
    membrane integrity and, 579, 584
Orchitis, 106
Organic brain syndrome (OBS), 104
Organic mental disorders, 106
Organized infant behavior, enhanced,
    readiness for, 493

Oropharyngeal deformity, ineffective
    infant suck-swallow response, 755
Orthopedic surgery
    impaired sitting and, 720
    peripheral neurovascular dysfunction
        and, 619
Orthopedic traction, 106–107
Orthopnea, 107
Orthostatic hypotension, 107
    assessment for, 507
    risk for adult falls and, 352
Osteoarthritis, 107
    impaired physical mobility and, 553
Osteomyelitis, 107
Osteoporosis, 107
Ostomy, 107
Otitis media, 107
Outdoor relaxation, for fatigue, 373
Output, decreased cardiac, 210–217
    associated condition, 211
    client outcomes of, 211
    defining characteristics of, 210–211
    nursing interventions, 211–217
    related factors, 211
    risk for, 218
Ovarian carcinoma, 107–108
Overload, stress, 748–749
Over the counter mouthwashes, for
    impaired oral mucous mem-
    brane, 580
Over-the-counter cough medications,
    622
Overweight, 588–591
    risk for, 591–595
Oximetry, pulse, 125
Oxygen
    humidified, administration of, in
        impaired gas exchange, 397
    medical, 775–776
Oxygen therapy, dry eyes and, 349,
    351

**P**

P6 acupoint stimulation, for PONV,
    569
Pacemaker, 108
Paget's disease, 108
Pain, 769
    acute, 595–600
    in acute confusion, 249

Pain *(Continued)*
  back, low, 86
  chronic, 600–606
    syndrome, 606
  in corneal injury, 510
  diary of, 603
  due to constipation, 257–258
  labor, 606–609
  neurovascular assessment for, 620
Pain flow sheet, 597
Pain intensity, level of, assessment for, 596
Pain level, reassess, in impaired bed mobility, 548
Pain management
  acute, 108
  approach, explain to the client, 597, 603
  chronic, 108
  interventions, 596–597
  IV medications for, 609
  in labor pain, 608
"Pain medicine," use the term, 599, 605
Pain relief measures, 688
Pain scale, for pediatric, 598, 604
Palliative care, opioids for, 257–258
Pallor
  of extremities, 108
  neurovascular assessment for, 620
Palpitations, heart, 108
Pancreatic cancer, 109
Pancreatic diseases, unstable blood glucose level and, 406
Pancreatitis, 109
Panic attacks, 109
Panic disorders, 109
Papillomavirus, human, in sexual dysfunction, 716
Paralysis, 109–110
  neurovascular assessment for, 620
  risk for disuse syndrome and, 326
Paralytic ileus, 110
Paranoid personality disorder, 110
Paraplegia, 110
Parathyroidectomy, 110
Parent
  attachment, 110
  disorganized infant behavior in, 490–491
  enhanced religiosity in, 667

Parent *(Continued)*
  in impaired parenting
    associated condition, 610, 615
    characteristics of, 609
    related factors for, 610
    at risk population, 610, 614–615
  nursing interventions for
    maladaptive grieving in, 413–414
    in readiness for enhanced grieving, 417
  physical health issue of
    ineffective adolescent eating dynamics and, 333
    ineffective child eating dynamics and, 335
    ineffective infant feeding dynamics and, 376
  psychological health issue of
    ineffective adolescent eating dynamics and, 333
    ineffective child eating dynamics and, 335
    ineffective infant feeding dynamics and, 376
  terminally ill, 147–148
Parental factors, ineffective child eating dynamics and, 334
Parental presence, for enhancing comfort, 240
Parental psychiatric disorder
  ineffective adolescent eating dynamics and, 333
  ineffective child eating dynamics and, 335
  ineffective infant feeding dynamics and, 376
Parental role conflict, 110–111, 676–678
Parenteral nutrition, total, 150
Parenting, 111
  impaired, 111, 609–612
    risk for, 614–615
  readiness for enhanced, 612–614
  risk for, impaired, 111
  stress, 613
Parents' competence, in impaired parenting, 611
Paresthesia, 111
  neurovascular assessment for, 620
Parkinson's disease, 111
  fatigue and, 372

Paroxysmal nocturnal dyspnea (PND), 104, 111, 117
Passive ROM exercises, in impaired physical mobility, 548
Patent ductus arteriosus (PDA), 111
Pathogen
  environmental exposure to, increased, 494
  exposure of, 654
Patient-controlled analgesia (PCA), 111
Patient education, 111
Pattern
  disturbed sleep, 733–734
  ineffective sexuality, 713–717
PCA. *See* Patient-controlled analgesia
PDA. *See* Patent ductus arteriosus
PE. *See* Pulmonary embolism
Pectus excavatum, 111
Pediatric(s)
  in anxiety, 177
  in caregiver role strain, 226
  in chronic low self-esteem, 699–700
  in chronic sorrow, 740–741
  in compromised family coping, 292–295
  in contamination, 272
  in decreased activity tolerance, 162
  in delayed surgical recovery, 769–770
  in disabled family coping, 296–297
  in disturbed body image, 199–200
  in disturbed sleep pattern, 734
  in impaired sitting, 721
  in impaired social interaction, 736–737
  in impaired swallowing, 773–774
  in impaired urinary elimination, 808
  in impaired verbal communication, 245–246
  in ineffective activity planning, 165–166
  in ineffective airway clearance, 170
  in ineffective community coping, 290–291
  in ineffective coping, 286–287
  in ineffective sexuality pattern, 716–717
  in ineffective thermoregulation, 779–780
  in insufficient breast milk production, 201

Parent *(Continued)*
  in readiness for enhanced comfort, 240
  in readiness for enhanced community coping, 282–283
  in readiness for enhanced coping, 288–289
  in readiness for enhanced family coping, 298
  in readiness for enhanced spiritual well-being, 746
  in readiness for enhancing communication, 242
  in readiness for self-care, 685–686
  in readiness for self-concept, 697–698
  in risk for
    allergy reaction, 175
    bleeding, 194
    impaired attachment, 187
    iodinated contrast media, adverse reaction to, 281
    other-directed violence, 831–832
    physical trauma, 803–804
    self-directed violence, 833–834
    self-mutilation, 707
    situational low self-esteem, 705
    suffocation, 760–762
    suicide, 766–767
    thermal injury, 777
    trauma, 803–804
    unstable blood pressure, 196–197
    vascular trauma, 818
  in sedentary lifestyle, 683–684
  in self-mutilation, 707
  in sleep deprivation, 730–731
  in social isolation, 738–739
  in spiritual distress, 743
  in stress overload, 749
  thermal injury in, 777
  in violence, 831–832
Pediatric clients, nursing interventions for
  in acute pain, 598–600
  in chronic pain, 604–606
  in decision making, 303–304, 306
  in decreased diversional activity engagement, 331–332
  deficient community health in, 419–420

Pediatric clients, nursing interventions for *(Continued)*
  in deficient fluid volume, 386
  deficient knowledge in, 523–524
  in diarrhea, 324–326
  disturbed family identity syndrome in, 465–466
  disturbed personal identity in, 468–469
  in dysfunctional family processes, 363–364
  in dysfunctional gastrointestinal motility, 404
  for enhanced nutrition, 573–574
  in enhanced power, 630
  in enhanced relationship, 663
  in enhanced religiosity, 666–667
  in enhanced resilience, 675
  in family processes, 367–368
  in fear, 375–376
  in female genital mutilation, 380
  in hyperthermia, 449
  in hypothermia, 456, 463
  in imbalanced energy field, 344
  in imbalanced fluid volume, 383
  in imbalanced nutrition, 577
  in impaired religiosity, 665
  in impaired resilience, 674
  in impaired wheelchair mobility, 558–560
  ineffective family health self-management in, 428
  ineffective impulse control in, 473
  in ineffective lymphedema self-management, 537–538
  in ineffective protection, 654–655
  in ineffective role performance, 680–681
  in interrupted family processes, 365–366
  in labile emotional control, 342–343
  in maladaptive grieving, 413–414
  in metabolic imbalance syndrome, 545
  in nausea, 570
  in obesity, 587–588
  in overweight, 591, 594–595
  in perioperative positioning injury, 619

Pediatric clients, nursing interventions for *(Continued)*
  in post-trauma syndrome, 626–627
  in powerlessness, 632–633
  in rape-trauma syndrome, 659
  in readiness for enhanced exercise engagement, 346–347
  in readiness for enhanced grieving, 417
  readiness for enhanced knowledge in, 525
  in relocation stress syndrome, 671–672
  in risk for
    complicated immigration transition, 471–472
    elopement attempt, 340
    impaired liver function in, 531–532
    infection in, 497–498
    injury in, 507
    loneliness, 533–534
    poisoning, 622–624
    surgical site infection in, 503
  risk-prone health behavior in, 421–422
  in unstable blood glucose level, 410
Pediatric Inactivity Triad, for readiness for enhanced exercise engagement, 346
Pediculosis, 111
Pedometer, 682
Pedometer step counts, 551
Peer-mediated interaction, 736
PEG. *See* Percutaneous endoscopic gastrostomy
Pelvic floor training program, for urge urinary incontinence, 486–488
Pelvic inflammatory disease (PID), 112, 114–115
Pelvic organ prolapse, female, 483
Penile prosthesis, 112
Peptic ulcer, 112, 152
Perceived constipation, 261–264
Percutaneous endoscopic gastrostomy (PEG), 111
Percutaneous nephrostomy, 101
Percutaneous transluminal coronary angioplasty (PTCA), 112, 124
Perfusion, tissue, ineffective peripheral, 792–796

Perfusion disorder, circulatory, impaired standing and, 747
Pericardial friction rub, 112
Pericarditis, 112
Periodic limb movement, sleep deprivation and, 729
Periodontal disease, 112
Perioperative care surgery, 144
Perioperative client, positioning of, 617–618
Perioperative hypothermia
　risk for, 112, 461–464
　unintentional, nursing interventions for, 462–463
Perioperative positioning
　injury, 769
　　risk for, 615–619
　risk for, 112
Peripheral catheter, 497
Peripheral neuropathy, 102, 112
　impaired skin integrity and, 722
Peripheral neurovascular dysfunction, risk for, 112, 619–620
Peripheral pulses, absent or diminished, 125
Peripheral skin, mottling of, 95
Peripheral tissue perfusion, 149
　ineffective, 792–796
　　associated conditions, 793
　　client outcomes, 793
　　defining characteristics, 793
　　nursing interventions, 793–796
　　related factors, 793
　　risk for, 797
Peripheral vascular disease (PVD), 112
Peritoneal dialysis, 113
Peritonitis, 113
Pernicious anemia, 113
Persistent fetal circulation, 113
Person-centered approaches, 523
Personal identity
　disturbed, 467–469
　　risk for, 469–470
　problems, 113
Personality disorder, 113
　narcissistic, 98–99
Pertussis, 113–114
Pesticide contamination, 114, 268
Petechiae, 114
Petit mal seizure, 114

Pharmaceutical preparations
　deficient fluid volume and, 384
　diarrhea and, 320
　dry eyes and, 349, 351
　dysfunctional gastrointestinal motility and, 400, 405
　excess fluid volume and, 389
　imbalanced fluid volume and, 380
　impaired dentition and, 308
　labile emotional control and, 341
　risk for adult falls and, 352
　risk for child falls and, 359
　risk for deficient fluid volume and, 392
　unstable blood glucose level and, 406
Pharyngitis, 114
Phenylketonuria (PKU), 114–115
Pheochromocytoma, 114
Phlebitis, 114
Phobia, specific, 114
Photosensitivity, 114
Physical abuse, 114
Physical activity
　for chronic functional constipation, 267
　for constipation, 258
　for enhanced nutrition, 572–573
　for metabolic imbalance syndrome, 544
　for obesity, 586
　for overweight, 589, 593
　for perceived constipation, 263
　for postpartum women, 236
Physical appearance, altered, social isolation and, 737
Physical assessment, focused, for urge urinary incontinence, 485
Physical closeness, for disorganized infant behavior, 491
Physical disability, labile emotional control and, 341
Physical examination, of constipation, 257
Physical illness
　chronic low self-esteem and, 698
　maternal, delayed child development and, 314, 316
　situational low self-esteem and, 701

Physical mobility, impaired, 550–554, 769
  associated condition, 551
  client outcomes of, 551–552
  defining characteristics of, 550–551
  nursing interventions of, 552–554
  related factors, 551
Physical Self-Description Questionnaire short form (PSDQ-s), for readiness for enhanced exercise engagement, 346
Physical therapist (PT), for disuse syndrome, 327
Physical therapy
  for adult falls, 354
  for child falls, 360
  for impaired physical mobility, 554
  postoperative interventions and, 503
Physical trauma, risk for, 151
Physiological alterations
  in acute confusion, 248
  in ineffective coping, 286
Physiological dyspnea, 208–209
Physiological factors
  adult falls and, 351
  of anxiety, 175
  child falls and, 358
  fear and, 373
Physiological status, of caregiver, 223
Physiological system, of disorganized infant behavior, 489
Pica, 114
PID. See Pelvic inflammatory disease
Pigmentation, altered, impaired skin integrity and, 722
PIH. See Pregnancy-induced hypertension
Pilates, for fear, 375
Pillow, for impaired bed mobility, 549
Pilocarpine, for dry mouth, 564
Piloerection, 115
Pink eye, 115
Pinworms, 115
Pituitary tumor, benign, 115
Pivot transfer, standing, in impaired transfer ability, 799
PKU. See Phenylketonuria
Placenta abruptio, 115–116
Placenta previa, 116
Plantar fasciitis, 116

Platelet count, bleeding disorder and, 582
Play therapy, for fear, 375
Playground safety, in risk for child falls, 359–360
Pleural effusion, 116
Pleural friction rub, 116
Pleural tap, 116
Pleurisy, 116
PMS. See Premenstrual syndrome
PND. See Paroxysmal nocturnal dyspnea
Pneumonectomy, 117
Pneumonia, 117, 773
  health care-acquired, 496
    geriatric, 498
  HOB elevation for, 547
  mycoplasma, 98
  ventilator-associated, 582
Pneumothorax, 117
Poison control center, 621
Poisoning
  lead, 84
  risk for, 117, 620–624
Poliomyelitis, 117
Pollution, contamination and, 269
POLST form, for decisional conflict, 301
Polycystic ovary syndrome, unstable blood glucose level and, 406
Polydipsia, 117
Polyethylene glycol 3350 (PEG- 3350), for constipation, 260
Polyphagia, 117
Polypharmacy, ineffective health self-management and, 423
Polyuria, 118
Positioning
  devices, covering, 617
  for impaired bed mobility, 546, 548–549
  of perioperative client, 112, 617–618
Positive and Negative Syndrome Scale (PANSS), 785
Positive therapeutic relationship, 764
Postnatal infection
  delayed infant motor development and, 317
  risk for delayed infant motor development and, 320

Postoperative care, 118

Postoperative care, surgery, 144

Postoperative ileus, nursing interventions for, 402–403

Postoperative interventions, risk for, surgical site infection, 502–503

Postoperative nausea and vomiting, 569

Postoperative urinary retention, 813–814

Postpartum, uterine atony in, 153

Postpartum care
  in ineffective childbearing process, 232
  normal, 118–119

Postpartum depression (PPD), 118
  screening for, 292

Postpartum hemorrhage, 118

Posttrauma counseling, 628

Posttrauma debriefings, 628

Post-trauma related condition, chronic pain and, 601

Post-trauma syndrome, 119, 624–627
  risk for, 119, 627–629

Posttraumatic stress disorder (PTSD), 119, 124
  assessment for, 628
  in geriatric, 626
  in refugees, 626

Postural balance, impaired, frail elderly syndrome and, 393, 395

Posture, prescribed
  impaired sitting and, 720
  impaired standing and, 747

Potassium, increase/decrease in, 119

Power, 119
  enhanced, readiness for, 629–630
  rotation-oscillation toothbrush, for impaired oral mucous membrane, 580

Powerlessness, 119, 630–633
  factors of, 631
  measure of, 631
  risk for, 633

Practical Interventions to Achieve Therapeutic Lifestyle Changes (TLC), for disuse syndrome, 328

Preadolescent, terminally ill, 147

Preconception, nursing intervention in
  delayed child development in, 314–316
  delayed infant motor development in, 318–319

Preeclampsia, 115, 119
  unstable blood glucose level and, 406

Pregnancy
  cardiac disorders in, 119
  ineffective childbearing process during, 231
  loss, 119–120
  nausea in, 568–570
  normal, 120
  nursing interventions in
    delayed child development in, 314–316
    delayed infant motor development in, 318–319
    impaired dentition in, 311–313
    readiness for enhanced childbearing process during, 233
  trauma in, 151

Pregnancy-induced hypertension (PIH), 115, 119
  unstable blood glucose level and, 406

Preload, altered, in decreased cardiac output, 210

Premature dilation, of cervix, 120

Premature infant
  child, 120–121
  parent, 121
  requiring specialty, 186–187

Premature rupture, of membranes, 121

Premenstrual syndrome (PMS), 116–117

Premenstrual tension syndrome (PMS), 121

Prenatal care, normal, 122

Prenatal substance misuse, delayed child development and, 314, 316

Prenatal testing, 122

Preoperative care surgery, 144

Preoperative teaching, 122

Preoperative walking program, for postoperative ileus, 403

Preschool child, terminally ill, 147

Preschooler, nursing intervention in, for delayed child development, 315–316

Prescribed mobility restriction, labor pain and, 607

Pressure, for bleeding, prevention of, 655

Pressure injuries, 122, 635, 643
  deep tissue, 636, 644
  in impaired tissue integrity, 788–789
  prevention of, 616–617
  stage 1, 635, 643
  stage 2, 635–636, 643–644
  stage 3, 636, 644
  stage 4, 636, 644
  unstageable, 636, 644–645

Pressure-related skin breakdown, 637, 645

Pressure ulcer
  defined, 727
  prevention of, in impaired bed mobility, 548
  risk for, 617

Preterm labor, 122–123

Prevention
  of bleeding, 655
  of deep vein thrombosis, 620
  of inadvertent hypothermia, 617
  of infection, 653–657

Primary care office visit, for corneal injury, 508–510

Probiotics, for diarrhea, 322

Problem-solving dysfunction, 123

Problem-solving education (PSE), 702

Procedure-related risk factors, exogenous, risk for, surgical site infection, 501–503

Processed foods, in metabolic imbalance syndrome, 545

Progressive muscle relaxation (PMR) exercise, for labile emotional control, 342

Projection, 123

Prolapse, mitral valve, 94

Prolapsed umbilical cord, 123

Prone positioning, for impaired bed mobility, 547

Prophylactic antifungal treatment, 654

Proptosis, dry eyes and, 349, 351

Prostate cancer, 289

Prostatic hypertrophy, 123

Prostatitis, 123

Prosthesis, penile, 112

Protection, ineffective, 652–657

Protein, latex allergy reaction, 526

Prune juice, for constipation, 258

Pruritus, 123

Psoriasis, 123

Psychiatric conditions, chronic pain and, 602

Psychiatric disorder, parental
  ineffective adolescent eating dynamics and, 333
  ineffective child eating dynamics and, 335
  ineffective infant feeding dynamics and, 376

Psychological disorder, delayed surgical recovery and, 768

Psychological dyspnea-hyperventilation, 207–210

Psychological strengths, 288

Psychological therapies, for compromised family coping, 293

Psychoneurological factors, for adult falls, 351

Psychosis, 123–124

Psychosocial factors, for nausea, in pregnancy, 568

Psychosocial issues, during pregnancy, 232

Psychospiritual support, for impaired comfort, 238

Psychotherapy, for post-trauma syndrome, 626

Psychotic disorders
  self-mutilation and, 706
  self-neglect and, 709

PTCA. See Percutaneous transluminal coronary angioplasty

PTSD. See Posttraumatic stress disorder

Pulmonary disease, fatigue and, 372

Pulmonary edema, 124

Pulmonary embolism (PE), 124

Pulmonary stenosis, 124

Pulmonary tuberculosis (TB), 146

Pulmonary venous return, total anomalous, 149

Pulse
  absent or diminished peripheral, 125
  neurovascular assessment for, 620

Pulse deficit, 124
Pulse oximetry, 125
Pulse pressure
   increased, 125
   narrowed, 125
Puncture, lumbar, 86
Purpura, 125
   thrombocytopenic, 148
PVD. *See* Peripheral vascular disease
Pyelonephritis, 125
Pyloric stenosis, 125
Pyloromyotomy, 125
Pyridoxine, for nausea, in pregnancy,
   568

## Q

Qigong, for fear, 375
Questions, for urge presentation, 485

## R

RA. *See* Rheumatoid arthritis
Rabies, 125
Racial/ethnic differences, in defensive
   coping, 284
Radial nerve dysfunction, 125
Radiation
   client receiving, 581–583
   contamination and, 269
Radiation-induced diarrhea (RID),
   324
Radiation therapy, 125–126
Radical neck dissection, 126
Radiotherapy
   dry eyes and, 349, 351
   fatigue and, 369
   impaired oral mucous membrane
      integrity and, 579, 584
Rage, 126
Range of motion (ROM), for impaired
   comfort, 237
Rape-trauma syndrome, 126, 657–660
Rash, 126
Rationalization, 126
Rats, in home, 126
Raynaud's disease, 126
RDS. *See* Respiratory distress syndrome
Readiness
   for coping
      community, 281–283
      family, 297–298

Readiness *(Continued)*
   for decision-making, enhanced,
      299–300
   emancipated, 303–304
   for enhanced childbearing process,
      233–236
   for enhanced comfort, 239–241
   for enhanced communication, 241–242
   for enhanced exercise engagement,
      344–347
   for enhanced grieving, 415–418
   for enhanced health literacy, 527–528
   for enhanced health self-
      management, 425–426
   for enhanced home maintenance
      behaviors, 433–434
   for enhanced hope, 435–436
   for enhanced knowledge, 524–525
   for enhanced nutrition, 572–574
   for enhanced parenting, 612–614
   for enhanced power, 629–630
   for enhanced relationship, 662–663
   for enhanced religiosity, 665–667
   for enhanced resilience, 674–675
   for enhanced sleep, 731–733
   for family processes, 366–368
   for infant behavior, organized, 493
   for self-care, 684–686
   for self-concept, 696–698
   for spiritual well-being, 744–746
Receptacle, urinary, 476
Reconciliation, medication, 623
Recovery, delayed surgical, 767–770
Rectal bleeding, 127
Rectal fullness, 126–127
Rectal lump, 127
Rectal pain, 127
Rectal surgery, 127
Rectocele repair, 127
Reflex, sucking, 143
Reflex incontinence, 127
Refugees, PTSD in, 626
Regression, 127
Regretful, 127
Regulation, mood, impaired, 560–561
Regulatory problem, of disorganized
   infant behavior, 489
Regulatory-situational stimuli, auto-
   nomic dysreflexia and, 188
   risk for, 191

Rehabilitation, 127
Rehabilitative behavioral learning
    model, 632
Relapse prevention strategies
    for obesity, 586
    for overweight, 589
Relationship, 127
    in dysfunctional family processes,
        362
    enhanced, readiness for, 662–663
    ineffective, 660–662
        risk for, 663–664
Relationship-focused intervention, in
    enhanced relationship, 663
Relaxation techniques, 127–128
Religiosity, 128
    enhanced, readiness for, 665–667
    impaired, 664–665
        risk for, 667–668
Religious concerns, 128
Relocation stress syndrome, 128,
    668–672
    risk for, 672
Renal dysfunction, electrolyte imbal-
    ance and, 337
Renal failure, 128
    acute/chronic, child, 128
    nonoliguric, 128
Renal perfusion, in risk for shock, 719
Repair, shoulder, 136
Reproductive-urological stimuli, auto-
    nomic dysreflexia and, 188
    risk for, 191
Resection
    large bowel, 83
    small bowel, 138
Resilience
    enhanced, readiness for, 674–675
    impaired, 673–674
        risk for, 675–676
Resistance exercises, 345
    for impaired physical mobility, 551
Respirations, stertorous, 141
Respiratory acidosis, 128
Respiratory conditions, of neonate, 129
Respiratory disease, decreased activity
    tolerance due to, 161–164
Respiratory distress, 129
Respiratory distress syndrome (RDS),
    126, 129

Respiratory infections, acute childhood,
    129
Respiratory syncytial virus (RSV),
    129, 131
Restless leg syndrome, 129
Restraints, for acute confusion, 250
Retention, urinary, 153
Retinal detachment, 129
Retinopathy, diabetic, 129
Retinopathy of prematurity (ROP), 130
Rh factor incompatibility, 130
Rhabdomyolysis, 130
Rheumatic fever, 130
Rheumatoid arthritis (RA), 125, 130
    impaired physical mobility and, 553
Rhythm, in decreased cardiac output,
    210
Rib fracture, 130
Richmond Agitation Sedation Scale,
    250
Ridicule of others, 130
Ringworm
    of body, 130
    of nails, 130
    of scalp, 130
Risk
    for adult falls, 351–358
    for adult pressure injury, 640–641
    for allergic reaction, 172–175
    for aspiration, 180–185
    for autonomic dysreflexia, 191
    for bleeding, 192–194
    for child falls, 358–361
    for child pressure injury, 648
    for childbearing process, ineffec-
        tive, 236
    for chronic functional constipation,
        267–268
    for complicated immigration transi-
        tion, 470–472
    for compromised human dignity,
        439–440
    for confusion, acute, 255
    for constipation, 260–261
    for contamination, 273
    for decreased activity tolerance, 164
    for decreased cardiac output, 218
    for decreased cardiac tissue perfu-
        sion, 218–222
    for deficient fluid volume, 392

Risk *(Continued)*
for delayed child development, 316
for delayed infant motor development, 319–320
for disorganized infant behavior, 493–494
for disturbed family identity syndrome, 466–467
for disturbed personal identity, 469–470
for disuse syndrome, 326–330
for dry eye, 350–351
for dysfunctional gastrointestinal motility, 405
for electrolyte imbalance, 337–338
for elopement attempt, 339–340
for female genital mutilation, 378–380
for frail elderly syndrome, 394–395
for hypothermia, 458
perioperative, 461–464
for imbalanced fluid volume, 380–383
for impaired cardiovascular function, 222–223
for impaired emancipated decision-making, 305–306
for impaired liver function, 528–532
for impaired oral mucous membrane, 584
for impaired parenting, 614–615
for impaired religiosity, 667–668
for impaired resilience, 675–676
for ineffective activity planning, 166–167
for ineffective cerebral tissue perfusion, 228–230
for ineffective home maintenance behaviors, 434
for ineffective lymphedema self-management, 538
for ineffective relationship, 663–664
for infection, 494–498
for injury, 505–507
corneal, 508–510
thermal, 774–777
urinary tract, 516–519
for iodinated contrast media, adverse reaction to, 278–281
for latex allergy reaction, 525–527

Risk *(Continued)*
for loneliness, 532–534
for low self-esteem
chronic, 703
situational, 703–705
for neonatal hyperbilirubinemia, 444–445
for neonatal pressure injury, 652
for occupational injury, 510–514
for overweight, 591–595
for perioperative positioning injury, 615–619
for peripheral neurovascular dysfunction, 619–620
for peripheral tissue perfusion, ineffective, 797
for physical trauma, 802–804
for poisoning, 620–624
for post-trauma syndrome, 627–629
prone health behavior, 420–422
for relocation stress syndrome, 672
for self-mutilation, 708
for shock, 717–720
for sudden infant death, 758–759
for surgical site infection, 499–504
for unstable blood glucose level, 406–411
for unstable blood pressure, 194–197
for urge urinary incontinence, 488–489
Roaches, invasion of home with, 130
Rocking, in labor pain, 608
Rodents, in home, 126
Role
conflict, parental, 110–111, 676–678
in dysfunctional family processes, 362
performance
altered, 130
ineffective, 679–681
strain, caregiver, 223–227
Rolled sheet, for positioning, 617
ROP. *See* Retinopathy of prematurity
Rosenberg Self-Esteem Scale, 699, 702, 704
Rotation-oscillation power toothbrush, for impaired dentition, 309
Rotavirus vaccine, for diarrhea, 324
RSV. *See* Respiratory syncytial virus
Rubella, 131
childhood communicable diseases, 37

Rubeola, 91
Rubor, extremity, 131
Ruptured disk, 131

S

SAD. *See* Seasonal affective disorder
Sadness, 131
    frail elderly syndrome and, 393, 395
Safe environment, providing, 506
Safe sex, 131
    teaching, ineffective sexual pattern, 714
Safety
    childhood, 131
    medication, 505–506
    risks in, client with, 506
Salicylates, 655
Saliva substitutes, in dry mouth, 565
Salivary flow rate, in dry mouth, 564
Salivary glands, in dry mouth, 563
Salmonella, 131
Salpingectomy, 131–132
Sarcoidosis, 132
Sarcoma, Kaposi's, 79
Sarcopenia
    frail elderly syndrome and, 393, 395
    impaired sitting and, 720
    impaired standing and, 747
Sarcopenic obesity, frail elderly syn-
        drome and, 393, 395
SARS. *See* Severe acute respiratory
        syndrome
SBARR acronym, 765
SBE. *See* Self-breast examination
Scabies, 132
    childhood communicable diseases,
        37
SCAN. *See* Suspected child abuse and
        neglect
Scared, 132
Schizophrenia, 132–133
School-age
    enhanced religiosity in, 667
    nursing intervention in, for delayed
        child development, 315–316
Sciatica, 133
Scoliosis, 133
Screening questionnaire, self-reported,
        628
Screening Tool of Older People's
    Prescriptions (STOPP), 394

Screening Tool to Alert Right Treat-
    ment (START), 394
Seasonal affective disorder (SAD),
    131
Seatbelts, in impaired wheelchair
    mobility, 560
Sedatives, for delirium, 249
Sedentary lifestyle, 84, 133, 681–684
    at-risk population, 681–682
    client outcomes, 682
    defining characteristics, 681
    dysfunctional gastrointestinal motil-
        ity and, 400, 405
    frail elderly syndrome and, 393, 395
    nursing interventions, 682–684
    related factors, 681
Seizure
    disorders, adult, 133–134
    disorders, child, 134
    febrile, 134
Self, negative feelings about, 100
Self-breast examination (SBE), 132,
    134
Self-care
    assessment of, 685
    barriers to, 685
    deficit, 134
        bathing, 134, 686–689
        dressing, 134, 689–691
        feeding, 134, 691–694
        toileting, 134, 694–696
    enhanced, readiness for, 684–686
Self-catheterization, intermittent,
    479–480
Self-concept, 134
    readiness for enhanced, 696–698
Self-destructive behavior, 134
Self-directed violence, risk for,
    832–834
Self-esteem
    chronic low, 134, 698–700
        associated conditions, 698
        at-risk population, 698
        client outcomes, 698–699
        defining characteristics, 698
        low, risk for, 703
        nursing interventions, 699–700
        related factors, 698
        risk for, 703
    situational low, 134, 700–702

Self-esteem *(Continued)*
    associated conditions, 701
    at-risk population, 701
    client outcomes, 701
    defining characteristics, 701
    nursing interventions, 701–702
    related factors, 701
    risk for, 703–705
Self-harm, in risk for self mutilation, 706
Self-management
    health
        enhanced, readiness for, 425–426
        family, ineffective, 426–428
        ineffective, 422–424
    system of
        in nutrition, 572–573
        for obesity, 585
        for overweight, 589, 593
Self-mutilation, 134, 705–707, 766
    associated conditions, 706
    at-risk population, 706
    client outcomes, 706
    defining characteristics, 705
    nursing interventions, 706–707
    related factors, 705–706
    risk for, 708
Self-neglect, 708–710
    associated conditions, 709
    client outcomes, 709
    defining characteristics, 709
    nursing interventions, 710
    related factors, 709
Self-report
    able to provide
        for acute pain, 595–596
        for chronic pain, 601–602
    unable to provide
        for acute pain, 596
        for chronic pain, 602
Self-report pain tool, 596, 599–600, 602
Senile dementia, 134–135
Sensation disorders
    delayed child development and, 314, 316
    delayed infant motor development and, 317
    fear and, 374
    frail elderly syndrome and, 393, 395

Sensation disorders *(Continued)*
    impaired skin integrity and, 722
    ineffective home maintenance behaviors and, 431, 434
    risk for adult falls and, 352
    risk for child falls and, 359
    risk for delayed infant motor development and, 320
Sensitivity, oral temperature, impaired dentition and, 308
Sensory integration dysfunction, ineffective infant feeding dynamics and, 376
Separation anxiety, 135
Sepsis
    child, 135
    signs of, 654
Septic shock, 136
Septicemia, 135
Serum 25-hydroxyvitamin D concentration, decreased, frail elderly syndrome and, 393, 395
Serum creatinine, in contrast induced nephropathy, 279
Serum lactate levels, monitor, in risk for shock, 719
Service animal, 135
Severe acute respiratory syndrome (SARS), 135
Severe allergic reaction (anaphylaxis), 173–174
Sexual abuse, in sexual dysfunction, 712
Sexual assault nurse examiner, 658
Sexual assault response team, 658
Sexual behavior, in sexual dysfunction, 716
Sexual dysfunction, 135, 711–713
    associated conditions, 711
    at-risk population, 711
    client outcomes, 711
    defining characteristics, 711
    nursing interventions, 711–713
    related factors, 711
Sexual harassment victim, 135
Sexual history, dysfunction, 711
Sexuality
    adolescent, 135–136
    education, in ineffective sexuality pattern, 717
    pattern, ineffective, 136, 713–717

Sexually transmitted disease (STD), 136, 140
Sexually transmitted infections, in sexual dysfunction, 714
Shaken baby syndrome, 136
Shakiness, 136
Shame, 136
Shared decision-making, 677–678
Sheath system, 479–480
Shingles, 136
Shivering, 136
Shock
  cardiogenic, 136
  hypovolemic, 136
  risk for, 717–720
  septic, 136
Short-term insomnia, 520–522
Shoulder
  repair, 136
  replacement, total joint, 150
Sick sinus syndrome, risk for ineffective cerebral tissue perfusion, 228–229
SIDS. *See* Sudden infant death syndrome
Sitting
  impaired, 720–721
  problems, 137
Situational crisis, 137
Situational low self-esteem, 134, 700–702
  associated conditions, 701
  at-risk population, 701
  client outcomes, 701
  defining characteristics, 701
  nursing interventions, 701–702
  related factors, 701
  risk for, 703–705
Situational low self-esteem, risk for, adolescent maturational issues and, 90
Sjögren's syndrome, impaired oral mucous membrane integrity and, 579, 584
SJS. *See* Stevens-Johnson syndrome
Skin breakdown
  comprehensive plan for, 639
  pressure-related, 637, 645
Skin cancer, 137
Skin condition, in impaired physical mobility, 554

Skin disorders, 137
Skin integrity, impaired, 721–726
  associated conditions, 722
  at-risk population, 722
  client outcomes, 722
  defining characteristics, 721
  nursing interventions, 722–726
  related factors, 721–722
  risk for, 726–728
Skin turgor, change in elasticity in, 137
Skin-to-skin contact (SSC), for comfort of newborns, 240
Sleep, 137
  deprivation, 138, 729–731
    associated conditions, 729
    at-risk population, 729
    client outcomes, 729
    defining characteristics, 729
    nursing interventions, 729–731
    related factors, 729
  enhanced, readiness for, 731–733
  pattern, disturbed, 138, 733–734
  problems, 138
  quality and patterns, in impaired memory, 541
Sleep apnea, 138
  sleep deprivation and, 729
Sleep history
  in disturbed sleep pattern, 733
  in insomnia, 520
Sleep hygiene, 732
Sleep-related enuresis, sleep deprivation and, 729
Sleep-related painful erections, sleep deprivation and, 729
Sleep-wake cycle, acute confusion and, 249
Slide board transfer, in impaired transfer ability, 798
Slowed gastric motility, nursing interventions for, 401–405
Slurring, speech, 138
Small bowel resection, 138
Small for gestational age (SGA), newborn, 103
Smell, loss of ability to, 138
Smoking
  behavior, 138
  compromised host defenses and, 500
  delayed child development and, 315

Smoking *(Continued)*
  delayed infant motor development
      and, 318
  history, pregnancy and, 232
  status, of pregnant clients, 235
Social interaction, impaired, 138,
      735–737
  associated conditions, 735
  at-risk population, 735
  client outcomes, 735
  defining characteristics, 735
  nursing interventions, 735–737
  related factors, 735
Social isolation, 138, 737–739
  for additional interventions, 736
  associated conditions, 737
  at-risk population, 737
  client outcomes, 738
  defining characteristics, 737
  nursing interventions, 738–739
  related factors, 737
Social media, for metabolic imbalance
      syndrome, 545
Social support
  inadequate
      frail elderly syndrome and, 393,
          395
      maladaptive grieving and, 412,
          414
  for ineffective coping, 285
  through facilitation, 685
Social support systems
  for impaired parenting, 611
  for obesity, 586
  for overweight, 590, 593
Socioeconomic, risk for caregiver role
      strain and, 228
Socioeconomic status, of caregiver,
      224–225
Sociopathic personality, 138
Sodium, decreased/increased, 138
Soft-bristled toothbrush, for impaired
      dentition, 310–311
Soft drinks, stop intake of, in impaired
      oral mucous membrane, 581
Soft tissue injuries, chronic pain and,
      601
Soft toothbrush, in impaired oral
      mucous membrane, 582
Somatization disorder, 139

Sore nipples, breastfeeding and, 139
Sore throat, 139
Sorrow, 139
  chronic, 739–741
      associated conditions, 739
      at-risk population, 739
      client outcomes, 739–740
      defining characteristics, 739
      nursing interventions, 740–741
      related factors, 739
Spastic colon, 139
Specialized boots, for disuse syndrome,
      327
Specific phobia, 114
Speech, slurring of, 138
Speech disorders, 139
Speech-language pathologist (SLP), 773
  for impaired verbal communica-
      tion, 246
Spina bifida, 101–102, 139
Spinal cord injury, 139–140
  chronic pain and, 601
Spinal fusion, 140
Spinal injury, dysreflexia and, 479
Spiritual care, of readiness for self-care,
      685
Spiritual distress, 140, 741–743
  associated conditions, 742
  at-risk population, 742
  client outcomes, 742
  defining characteristics, 741
  nursing interventions, 742–743
  related factors, 741–742
  risk for, 743–744
Spiritual well-being, 140
  readiness for enhanced, 744–746
Spirituality
  in defensive coping, 284
  in enhancing coping, 288
Splenectomy, 140
Spontaneous ventilation, impaired,
      818–823
  associated conditions, 819
  client outcomes, 819
  defining characteristics, 819
  nursing interventions, 819–823
  related factors, 819
Sprains, 140
Squat transfer, in impaired transfer
      ability, 799

Stable blood pressure, risk for unstable, 140

Stage 1 pressure injury
  in impaired skin integrity, 723–724
  in impaired tissue integrity, 788

Stage 2 pressure injury
  in impaired skin integrity, 723
  in impaired tissue integrity, 788

Stage 3 pressure injury
  in impaired skin integrity, 723
  in impaired tissue integrity, 788

Stage 4 pressure injury
  in impaired skin integrity, 723
  in impaired tissue integrity, 788–789

STAMPEDAR acronym, 830

Standing
  impaired, 746–748
    associated conditions, 747
    client outcomes, 747
    defining characteristics, 747
    nursing interventions, 747–748
    related factors, 747
  pivot transfer, in impaired transfer ability, 799
  problems, 140

Stapedectomy, 140

"Start low and go slow" approach, for impaired physical mobility, 552

Stasis ulcer, 140, 152

State-organization system, of disorganized infant behavior, 489

STD. *See* Sexually transmitted disease

ST-elevation myocardial infarction (STEMI), 141

STEMI. *See* ST-elevation myocardial infarction

Stenosis
  mitral, 94
  pulmonary, 124
  pyloric, 125

Stent, coronary artery, 141

Sterilization surgery, 141

Stevens-Johnson syndrome (SJS), 137, 141

Stigma, in impaired memory, 542

Stillbirth, 141

Stimulus control techniques
  for enhanced nutrition, 573
  for obesity, 586
  for overweight, 590, 593

Stoma, 141

Stomatitis, 141
  treatment of, 582

Stool
  hard/dry, 141
  loose, 86

Strength training, in metabolic imbalance syndrome, 544

Strep throat, 141

Stress, 141
  overload, 748–749
  parenting, 613

Stress syndrome, relocation, 668–672
  risk for, 672

Stress urinary incontinence, 142, 480–484
  associated condition, 480
  client outcomes of, 481
  defining characteristics of, 480
  nursing interventions, 481–484
  related factors in, 480
  at risk population, 480

Stressors
  dysfunctional gastrointestinal motility and, 400, 405
  in ineffective community coping, 290
  in ineffective coping, 285
  ineffective protection and, 653

Stretching, for impaired physical mobility, 551

Stridor, 142

Stroke, 142
  fatigue and, 369
  heat, nursing interventions for, 446–448

Stroke volume, altered, risk for, decreased cardiac output, 218

Stuttering, 142

Subarachnoid hemorrhage, 142

Subarachnoid hemorrhagic stroke, 230

Subjective Global Nutrition Assessment (SGNA)
  for imbalanced nutrition, 577
  for ineffective child eating dynamics, 335

Substance
  misuse of, 142
    adolescent and, 143
    in pregnancy, 143
  withdrawal of, 143

Substance abuse
  pregnancy, 232
  in self-neglect, 710
Substance withdrawal syndrome, acute,
      749–752
  associated conditions, 750
  at-risk population, 750
  client outcomes, 750
  defining characteristics, 749
  nursing interventions, 750–752
  related factors, 750
  risk for, 752–754
Sucking reflex, 143
Suck-swallow response, ineffective
      infant, 755–758
Suction, nasogastric, 99
Sudden infant death syndrome (SIDS),
      137, 143
  risk for, 758–759
Suffocation, risk for, 143, 760–762
  associated factors, 760
  client outcomes, 760
  nursing interventions, 760–762
  risk factors, 760
Sugar-containing soft drinks, in
      impaired oral mucous membrane,
      581
Suicidal behavior, risk for, 762–767
  associated conditions, 763
  at-risk population, 763
  client outcomes, 763
  nursing interventions, 763–767
  related factors, 762–763
Suicidal ideation, 764
Suicide
  attempt, 143
  risk for, 701
  warning signs of, 764
Sun-blocking clothing, 775
Sunglasses, for ultraviolet light, 510
Sunscreen, 775
Support groups, in readiness for en-
      hanced family coping, 298
Support resources, for enhanced rela-
      tionship, 663
Support system, inadequate, 143
Supportive social networks, for defi-
      cient knowledge, 523
Suppressed inflammatory response, frail
      elderly syndrome and, 393, 395
Suppression, urge, 487–488

Surfing, urge, 473
Surgery
  corneal, nearsightedness, 99
  heart, keyhole, 80
  laser, 83
  Lasik eye, 83
  lung, 86
  nausea after, 569
  perioperative care, 144
  postoperative care, 144
  preoperative care, 144
  rectal, 127
  sterilization, 141
Surgical client
  general interventions for, 616–619
  nursing interventions for, in imbal-
      anced fluid volume, 381–383
Surgical recovery, delayed, 144, 767–770
  associated conditions, 768
  at-risk population, 768
  client outcomes, 768
  defining characteristics, 768
  nursing interventions, 768–770
  related factors, 768
  risk for, 770
Surgical site infection, 144
  risk for, 499–504
Surgical wound infection, delayed
      surgical recovery and, 768
Suspected child abuse and neglect
      (SCAN)
  child, 144–145
  parent, 145
Suspicion, 145
Swallowing
  difficulties, 145
  impaired, 771–774
Swaying, in labor pain, 608
Symptomatic urinary tract infection,
      479
Syncope, 145
Syndrome
  chronic pain, 606
  compartment, 620
  post-trauma, 624–627
    risk for, 119, 627–629
  rape-trauma, 126, 657–660
  relocation stress, 668–672
    risk for, 672
Syphilis, 145
Systemic lupus erythematosus, 145

# T

Tachycardia, 146
  in risk for shock, 718
Tachypnea, 146
Tai chi, for fear, 375
Tardive dyskinesia, 146
Targeted temperature hypothermia,
  nursing interventions for, 455–456
Taste abnormality, 146
TB. *See* Tuberculosis
TBI. *See* Traumatic brain injury
TD. *See* Traveler's diarrhea
Teachable moments, 525
Tear volume, reduced, dry eyes and,
  349, 351
Teeth, in impaired oral mucous mem-
  brane, 580
Temperature
  body, imbalance, risk for, 776
  core, 776
  decreased, 146
  high, 146
  hypothermia, targeted, nursing
    interventions for, 455–456
  regulation, impaired, 146
Temperature measurement
  in ineffective thermoregulation,
    778–780
  nursing interventions for
    hyperthermia in, 446–451
    hypothermia in, 452–458,
      461–464
TEN. *See* Toxic epidermal necrolysis
TENS. *See* Transcutaneous electrical
  nerve stimulation
Tension, 147
Terminal illness, as factor for ineffective
  coping, 294
Terminally ill
  adult, 147
  child
    adolescent, 147
    infant/toddler, 147
    preschool, 147
    school-age/preadolescent, 147
  death of child or parent, 147–148
Testicular self-examination (TSE),
  152
Tetralogy of Fallot, 148
Tetraplegia, 148

Text4Baby, in disturbed maternal-fetal
  dyad, 540
The Joint Commission National Patient Safety Goals, 193–194
Therapeutic beds, for impaired bed
  mobility, 546–547
Therapeutic communication techniques, for impaired verbal communication, 245
Therapeutic hypothermia, 455
Therapeutic isolation
  decreased diversional activity en-
    gagement and, 330
  impaired social interaction and, 735
Therapeutic mouthwashes, for impaired
  dentition, 310
Therapeutic relationship, in ineffective
  sexuality pattern, 714
Thermal injury
  cold, 776
  risk for, 774–777
    associated conditions, 775
    at-risk population, 775
    client outcomes, 775
    nursing interventions, 775–777
    risk factors, 774
Thermometer, calibrated, 776
Thermoregulation, ineffective, 148,
  777–780
  associated conditions, 777
  at-risk population, 777
  client outcomes, 777
  defining characteristics, 777
  nursing interventions, 778–780
  related factors, 777
  risk for, 781
Thoracentesis, 148
Thoracotomy, 148
Thought disorders, 148
Thought pattern, disturbed, 784–786
  associated conditions, 784
  at-risk population, 784
  client outcomes, 784–785
  defining characteristics, 784
  nursing interventions, 785–786
  related factors, 784
Thrombocytopenic purpura, 148
Thromboembolism prophylaxis, injury
  associated with, in impaired bed
  mobility, 548

Thrombophlebitis, 149
Thrush, oral, 106
Thyroidectomy, 149
TIA. *See* Transient ischemic attack
Tic disorder, 149
Timed toileting regimen, 476
Timed Up & Go Test, 354–355
Tinea
    capitis, 149
    corporis, 149
    cruris, 149
    pedis, 149
Tinea unguium, 149
Tinnitus, 149
Tissue damage, integumentary, 149
Tissue integrity, impaired, 786–791
    associated conditions, 787
    at-risk population, 787
    client outcomes, 787
    defining characteristics, 786
    nursing interventions, 787–791
    related factors, 786–787
    risk for, 791–792
Tissue oxygenation, decreased, impaired skin integrity and, 722
Tissue perfusion
    decreased, impaired skin integrity and, 722
    peripheral, 149
        ineffective, 792–796
Tobacco, use of, in disturbed maternal-fetal dyad, 540
Toddler, nursing intervention in, for delayed child development, 315–316
Toilet training, 149
Toileting
    problems, 149
    self-care deficit, 694–696
    timed, regimen, 476
Tonsillectomy, adenoidectomy and, 145–146, 149
Toothache, 149
Toothbrush
    for bleeding disorder, 582
    for impaired dentition, 309
    for impaired oral mucous membrane, 580
    for mucositis, 582
Toothette, 655

Topical local anesthetic treatment, for pediatric, 599
Total anomalous pulmonary venous return, 149
Total hip arthroplasty (THA), in ineffective sexuality pattern, 715
Total hip replacement, 150
Total joint replacement, 150
Total knee replacement, 150
Total parenteral nutrition (TPN), 150
Touch, in post-trauma syndrome, 626
Tourette's syndrome (TS), 150, 152
Towels, for positioning, 617
Toxemia, 150
Toxic epidermal necrolysis (TEN), 147, 150
TPN. *See* Total parenteral nutrition
Tracheal defect, impaired swallowing and, 771–772
Tracheoesophageal fistula, 150
Tracheostomy, 150
Traction
    casts and, 150–151
    orthopedic, 106–107
Training
    bladder
        for stress urinary incontinence, 487
        for urge urinary incontinence, 487
    pelvic floor, for urge urinary incontinence, 486–488
Transcutaneous electrical nerve stimulation (TENS)
    in labor pain, 608
    unit, 147
Transfer ability, 151
    impaired, 797–802
        associated conditions, 797
        client outcomes, 797–798
        defining characteristics, 797
        nursing interventions, 798–802
        related factors, 797
Transient ischemic attack (TIA), 149, 151
Translation-specific scoring instructions, for impaired memory, 542
Transplant
    kidney, 80
    liver, 85

Transurethral resection of the prostate (TURP), 151–152, 382
Trauma
    impaired swallowing and, 771–772
    physical, risk for, 151, 802–804
    in pregnancy, 151
Traumatic brain injury (TBI), 146, 151
    survivors of, 296
Traumatic event, 151
Travel history, 495
Traveler's diarrhea (TD), 146, 151
    acute, 324
Tricuspid atresia, 151
Trigeminal neuralgia, 151
Truncus arteriosus, 151
Trust
    enhancement of feelings of, 239
    for person and provider, 685
TS. See Tourette's syndrome
TSE. See Testicular self-examination
Tubal ligation, 152
Tube feeding, 152
Tuberculosis (TB), 146, 152
Tubular necrosis, kidney, acute, 99
Tumor, kidney, 81
TURP. See Transurethral resection of the prostate

U

Ulcer
    peptic, 112, 152
    stasis, 140, 152
Ulcerative colitis, 152
Umbilical cord, prolapsed, 123
Underpads, for toileting self-care deficit, 694
Unilateral lung disease, in impaired gas exchange, 397
Unilateral neglect, 100, 804–806
    client outcomes, 805
    compensatory strategies for, 557
    defining characteristics, 804–805
    nursing interventions, 805–806
    of one side of body, 152
Unintentional perioperative hypothermia, nursing interventions for, 462–463
Unsanitary food preparation, dysfunctional gastrointestinal motility and, 400, 405

Unsanitary living conditions, 152
Unstable blood glucose level, risk for, 406–411
Unstable blood pressure, risk for, 194–197
Unstageable pressure injury, 636, 644–645, 724
    in impaired tissue integrity, 789
Upper airway anomaly, impaired swallowing and, 771–772
Upper respiratory infection, 152
Urge suppression, 487–488
Urge surfing, 473
Urge urinary incontinence, 484–488
    risk for, 488–489
Urgency, to urinate, 152
Urinary catheter, 152–153
    indwelling
        in disability-associated urinary incontinence, 477
        in risk for urinary tract injury, 517
    proper placement, 518
Urinary diversion, 153
Urinary elimination
    impaired, 153
    monitoring, 517
Urinary incontinence, 153
    disability-associated, 473–477
        associated condition, 474
        client outcomes of, 474
        defining characteristics of, 474
        nursing interventions, 474–477
        related factors in, 474
        at risk population, 474
    mixed, 477–480
    stress, 480–484
    urge, 484–488
        risk for, 488–489
Urinary receptacle, 476
Urinary retention, 153, 810–814
    associated conditions, 810
    at-risk population, 810
    client outcomes, 810
    defining characteristics, 810
    nursing interventions, 810–814
    related factors, 810
    risk for, 815
Urinary tract infection (UTI), 153
    symptomatic, 479

Urinary tract injury, risk for, 516–519
  associated condition, 516–517
  client outcomes of, 517
  nursing interventions, 517–519
  risk factors, 516
  at risk population, 516
Urinate, urgency to, 152
Urine
  color of, in imbalanced nutrition, 577
  loss, factors of, 481
Urolithiasis, 153
US Alcohol Use Disorders Identifica-
    tion Test (USAUDIT), 363
US Dietary Guidelines, 572
Uterine atony
  in labor, 153
  in postpartum, 153
UTI. *See* Urinary tract infection

**V**

VAD. *See* Ventricular assist device
Vaginal changes, atrophic, 486
Vaginal hysterectomy, 153
Vaginitis, 153
Vagotomy, 153
Valsalva maneuver, 259
Value system conflict, 153
Varicose veins, 153
Vascular access device (VAD), damage
    to, 280–281
Vascular dementia, 153
Vascular disease
  ineffective home maintenance
      behaviors and, 431, 434
  perioperative positioning injury
      and, 615
  risk for adult falls and, 352
Vascular obstruction, peripheral neuro-
    vascular dysfunction and, 619
Vascular trauma, risk for, 815–818
  associated condition, 815
  client outcomes, 815
  monitoring infusion, 817–818
  nursing interventions, 816–818
  risk factors, 815
Vasectomy, 154
Vein
  damage, 280–281
  varicose, 153
Venereal disease, 154

Venous insufficiency, in ineffective
    peripheral tissue perfusion,
    794–795
Venous oxygen saturation, in impaired
    gas exchange, 396
Venous thromboembolism (VTE),
    154–155, 782
Ventilated client, mechanically,
    154
Ventilation-perfusion imbalance, im-
    paired gas exchange and, 395
Ventilator, client on, 582
Ventilator-associated events, 582
Ventilator-associated pneumonia,
    582
Ventilator support, impaired spontane-
    ous ventilation, 820–823
Ventricular assist device (VAD), 154
Ventricular fibrillation, 154
Verbal communication, impaired,
    242–246
  associated condition, 243
  defining characteristics of, 242–243
  related factors, 243
  at risk population, 243
Verbal relaxation therapy, for impaired
    comfort, 238
Verbal therapeutic communication, for
    labile emotional control, 343
Vertigo, 154
Veterans, 154
Veterans of Armed Services, in spiritual
    distress, 743
Vibrotactile stimulation, for neonatal
    abstinence syndrome, 571
Vigorous-intensity physical activity
  for obesity, 586
  for overweight, 589
Violence, 766
  other-directed, risk for, 701, 829–832
    associated condition, 829
    client outcomes, 829
    nursing interventions, 830–832
    risk factors, 829
Violent behavior, 154
Viral gastroenteritis, 154–155
Viral infections, fatigue and, 372
Virus
  respiratory syncytial, 129
  West Nile, 155

Vision impairment, 155
Vital signs, in risk for shock, 719
Vitamin D deficiency
    in impaired memory, 541
    in metabolic imbalance syndrome, 545
Vocal cord dysfunction, impaired swallowing and, 771–772
Volume, fluid
    deficient, 383–388
        risk for, 392
    excess, 388–392
    imbalance, risk for, 380–383
Vomiting, 155
    chronic, impaired dentition and, 308
    oral care for, 568
VTE. *See* Venous thromboembolism

## W

Waist circumference, elevated, in metabolic imbalance syndrome, 544
Walking, impaired, 155, 834–837
    associated condition, 834
    client outcomes/goals, 834
    defining characteristics, 834
    nursing interventions, 835–837
    related factors, 834
    special considerations, 836–837
Wandering, 155, 837–840
    client outcomes, 838
    defining characteristics, 837
    nursing interventions, 838–840
    related factors, 837
Warming measures, active, 776
Waste, contamination and, 269
Weakness, 155
Weight
    bearing, for impaired comfort, 237
    gain, 155
    loss, 155

Wellness-seeking behavior, 155
Wernicke-Korsakoff syndrome, 155
West Nile virus, 155
Wheelchair
    mobility, impaired, 555–560
        associated condition, 555
        client outcomes of, 556
        defining characteristics of, 555
        nursing interventions of, 556–560
        related factors, 555
        at risk population, 555
    use problems, 155
Wheezing, 155
White blood cell count, decreased in, 654
Whooping cough, 113–114
Wilms' tumor, 155
Withdrawal
    from alcohol, 155
    from drugs, 155
Wound care, postoperative interventions and, 502
Wounds
    compromised host defenses and, 500
    debridement of, 155
    dehiscence of, 156
    evisceration of, 156
    infection of, 156
    open, 156

## X

Xerostomia, 564
    in impaired oral mucous membrane, 581

## Y

Yoga, for fear, 375